Sarcoidosis

Sarcoidosis

Donald N Mitchell MD FRCP
Hon Consultant Physician
Royal Brompton and University College Hospitals
London, UK

David R Moller MD
Professor of Medicine and Director
Sarcoidosis Clinic and Research Program
Department of Medicine
The Johns Hopkins University School of Medicine
Baltimore, Maryland, USA

Stephen G Spiro BSc MD FRCP
Professor of Respiratory Medicine and Honorary Consultant Physician
University College London and The Royal Brompton Hospital
London, UK

Athol Wells MBChB MD FRACP FRCP FRCR
Professor of Respiratory Medicine and Head of Interstitial Lung Disease Unit
The Royal Brompton Hospital
London, UK

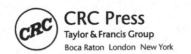

CRC Press
Taylor & Francis Group
Boca Raton London New York

CRC Press is an imprint of the
Taylor & Francis Group, an **informa** business

First published in 2012 by Hodder Arnold

Published in 2020 by CRC Press
Taylor & Francis Group
6000 Broken Sound Parkway NW, Suite 300
Boca Raton, FL 3487-2742

First issued in paperback 2020

ISBN-13: 978-0-367-57676-9 (pbk)
ISBN-13: 978-0-340-99211-1 (hbk)

Visit the Taylor & Francis Web site at
http://www.taylorandfrancis.com

and the CRC Press Web site a
http://www.crcpress.com

British Library Cataloguing in Publication Data
A catalogue record for this book is available from the British Library

Library of Congress Cataloging-in-Publication Data
A catalog record for this book is available from the Library of Congress

Cover Design: Helen Townson
Cover image © Scott Camazine/Science Photo Library
Typeset in 9.5/11.5 pt Minion by Datapage

Dedication for Donald Mitchell
To Dora; Ann and Robin; Ian and Susie and grandchildren Geir, James and Harriet

Dedication for Stephen Spiro
To Alison for 40 years of unfailing support and encouragement

Dedication for Athol Wells
To Pepi and her children, Athina and Maria

Dedication for David R. Moller
To Teresa, Stephanie and Christopher

AND to Donald for his inspirational dedication to a lifetime of relentless research and insight into the understanding of this mercurial condition. He is regarded with great affection and respect by all those who have known and worked with him. We are so pleased to have been part of this project.

Contents

Contributors

Penny Agent BSc (Hons) DMS
Deputy Director Rehabilitation and Therapies, Royal Brompton &
Harefield NHS Foundation Trust

Theingi Aung
Department of Endocrinology, Oxford Centre for Diabetes,
Endocrinology and Metabolism, Churchill Hospital, University of
Oxford, UK

Helen Booth
Consultant Thoracic Physician and Honorary Senior Lecturer,
University College London Hospitals, London, UK

James Boyer MD
Ensign Professor of Medicine, Emeritus Director, Yale Liver Center,
Digestive Disease Section, Department of Medicine, Yale University
School of Medicine, USA

Jeremy S Brown
Reader in Respiratory Infection/Honorary Consultant, University
College London and University College London Hospitals Trust,
London, UK

Andrew Bush MD FRCP FRCPCH
Professor of Paediatric Respirology, Imperial College;
Consultant Paediatric Chest Physician, Royal Brompton &
Harefield NHS Foundation Trust, London, UK

David R Cave MD PhD MRCP [UK]
Professor of Medicine, Department of Medicine, University of
Massachusetts, USA

Viquar Chamoun
Consultant Neurologist, Stoke Mandeville Hospital, Aylesbury,
Bucks

Bryan Corrin
Emeritus Professor of Pathology, London University, Honorary
Senior Clinical Research Fellow, National Heart and Lung Institute,
Imperial College, London; Honorary Consultant Pathologist,
Royal Brompton Hospital, London

Paul A Corris MB-BS FRCP
Transplant Institute, Institute of Cellular Medicine, Newcastle
University and Freeman Hospital, Newcastle Upon Tyne, UK

Tamera Corte BSc(Med) MBBS(Hons) FRACP PhD
Royal Brompton Hospital, London; Royal Prince Alfred Hospital,
Sydney, Australia; University of Sydney, Sydney, Australia

Derek Cramer MIScT CE Dip M.
Consultant Clinical Scientist, Head of Lung Function Unit, Royal
Brompton & Harefield NHS Foundation Trust, London, UK

Paul Cullinan
Occupational and Environmental Medicine, Royal Brompton
Hospital, London, UK

Ann Dewar
Electron Microscope Unit, Imperial College, Royal Brompton
Hospital, London, UK

Ameet Dhar BSc MRCP
Specialist Registrar and Honorary Clinical Research Fellow,
St. Mary's Hospital and Imperial College London, UK

Jacqueline Donovan MChem MSc DipRCPath
Principal Clinical Scientist, Department of Clinical Biochemistry,
Royal Brompton Hospital, London, UK

Roland M du Bois MA MD FRCP
National Jewish Health, Denver, Colorado, USA

Stephen R Durham BA Hons MB Bchir MA MRCP (UK) MD FRCP
Professor of Allergy & Respiratory Medicine,
Honorary Consultant Physician, Imperial College of Medicine,
National Heart and Lung Institute and Royal Brompton Hospital,
London, UK

Anthony J Edey MRCP FRCR
Clinical Fellow in Thoracic Imaging, The Royal Brompton &
Harefield NHS Foundation Trust, Department of Imaging,
London, UK

Gavin Giovannoni
Neuroscience & Trauma Centre, Blizard Institute, Barts and The
London School of Medicine and Dentistry, London, UK

Nicole Goh
Austin Hospital, Melbourne, Australia

Bernie Graneek BSc MB BS FRCP AFOM
Consultant Occupational Physician, Royal Marsden
NHS Foundation Trust, Honorary Senior Lecturer,
Department of Occupational & Environmental Medicine,
National Heart & Lung Institute, London, UK

David M Hansell FRCP FRCR MD
Professor of Thoracic Imaging, The Royal Brompton & Harefield
NHS Foundation Trust, Department of Imaging, London, UK

Patricia L Haslam PhD FRCPath
Emeritus Reader, National Heart & Lung Institute, Imperial College, London; Honorary Consultant, Royal Brompton Hospital, London, UK

Claire Hooper MBBS FRANZCO
Department of Ophthalmology, University of Sydney and Moorfields Eye Hospital, London, UK

James Hooper BSc MD FRCPath
Consultant Chemical Pathologist, Department of Clinical Biochemistry, Royal Brompton Hospital, London, UK

Michael B Hughes DM FRCP
Honorary Professorial Fellow, National Heart and Lung Institute, Imperial College London, Hammersmith Hospital Campus, London, UK

Niki Karavitaki
Department of Endocrinology, Oxford Centre for Diabetes, Endocrinology and Metabolism, Churchill Hospital, University of Oxford, UK

Peter Kelleher MRCP (Ire) PhD FRCPath
Immunology Section, Division of Infectious Diseases, Imperial College, London and Host Defence Unit, Royal Brompton Hospital, London, UK

Michael W Kemp MSc MCB FRCPath
Consultant Clinical Scientist, Department of Clinical Biochemistry, Royal Brompton Hospital, London, UK

Patrick TF Kennedy MB BCh BAO BMedSci MRCP MD
Senior Lecturer and Consultant Hepatologist, Barts and The London School of Medicine and Dentistry, London, UK

Ajit Lalvani MA DM FRCP FSB
Chair of Infectious Diseases Director, Tuberculosis Research Unit, National Heart and Lung Institute, Imperial College London, UK

Matthew Lane MB ChB MRCP
Transplant Institute, Institute of Cellular Medicine, Newcastle University and Freeman Hospital, Newcastle Upon Tyne, UK

Sue Lightman FRCP FRCOphth PhD FMedSci
UCL/Institute of Ophthalmology and Moorfields Eye Hospital, London, UK

Eric Lim MB ChB MD MSc FRCS(C-Th)
Consultant Thoracic Surgeon, Royal Brompton Hospital; Senior Lecturer, National Heart and Lung Institute, Imperial College, London, UK

J C Lyne
Cardiology Department, Royal Brompton Hospital, Royal Brompton & Harefield NHS Foundation Trust, Sydney Street, London, UK

Kate Maclaran MBchB BSc
Clinical Research Fellow, Imperial College London; Chelsea and Westminster Hospital London; Royal Brompton Hospital, Sydney Street, London, UK

Toby M Maher MB MSc PhD MRCP
Consultant Respiratory Physician, Interstitial Lung Disease Unit, Royal Brompton Hospital, Sydney Street, London, UK

Estella Matutes
Reader and Consultant Haematologist, Royal Marsden Hospital, London, UK

Robin J McAnulty PhD
Reader in Lung Pathobiology, Centre for Respiratory Research, University College London, London, WC1E 6JJ

Andrew Menzies-Gow
Royal Brompton & Harefield NHS Foundation Trust, London, UK

Robert F Miller MBBS FRCP CBiol FSB
Department of Infection and Population Health, University College London, UK

Donald N Mitchell MD FRCP
Honorary Consultant Physician, Royal Brompton Hospital, London, UK; Honorary Consultant Physician, UCLH NHS Foundation Trust, London; Honorary Consultant Physician, St. Mary's NHS Foundation Trust, London. Formerly: Senior Clinical Scientific Staff, Medical Research Council, London, UK

David R Moller MD
Professor of Medicine and Director, Sarcoidosis Clinic and Research Program, Department of Medicine, The Johns Hopkins University School of Medicine, Baltimore, Maryland, USA

Nilesh Morar MBChB FCDerm MMedDerm DPhil (Oxon)
Consultant Dermatologist, Chelsea and Westminster Hospital NHS Foundation Trust; Honorary Senior Lecturer, Imperial College London, London, UK

Neal Navani
Consultant in Thoracic Medicine and Honorary Senior Lecturer, University College London Hospital, London, UK

Andrew G Nicholson
Consultant Pathologist, Royal Brompton Hospital, London, Professor of Respiratory Pathology, National Heart and Lung Institute, Imperial College, London, UK

P J Oldershaw
Cardiology Department, Royal Brompton Hospital, Royal Brompton and Harefield NHS Foundation Trust, Sydney Street, London, UK

Helen Parfrey BM BCh MA PhD FRCP
University Lecturer and Honorary Consultant in Respiratory Medicine, University of Cambridge School of Clinical Medicine and Papworth Hospital *NHSFT* Cambridge, UK

Siddhartha Parker MD MA
Gastroenterology Fellow, Dartmouth-Hitchcock Medical Center, Lebanon, USA

Helen Parrott BSc (Hons)
Clinical Lead Physiotherapist, Royal Brompton and Harefield NHS Foundation Trust, London, UK

Nisha Patel BSc (Hons) MBBS MRCP (Lond)
Specialist Registrar in Gastroenterology, St Mary's Hospital, London, UK

Jeremy M Pfeffer FRCP FRCPsych
Consultant Psychiatrist and Honorary Senior Lecturer,
Royal Brompton Hospital and National Heart and Lung Institute,
London, UK

Paul E Pfeffer MA MRCP
Specialist Registrar in Respiratory Medicine,
Royal London Hospital, London, UK

Lucy Pigram
Clinical Nurse Specialist, Interstitial Lung Diseases Unit,
NIHR Respiratory Biomedical Research Unit,
Royal Brompton Hospital, London, UK

Michael I Polkey PhD FRCP
Professor of Respiratory Medicine, Royal Brompton Hospital/
National Heart and Lung Institute, London, UK

Joanna C Porter PhD FRCP
Senior Lecturer in Medicine, MRC Laboratory of Molecular Cell
Biology, University College London, London;
Honorary Consultant in Respiratory Medicine, University College
London Hospitals NHS Trust, London, UK

Elspeth Potton MA MRCP
Wellcome Trust Clinical Training Fellow, University College London
and University College London Hospitals Trust, London, UK

Priyajit Bobby Prasad MBBS FACP FRCPI
Consultant Gastroenterologist, Chelsea and Westminster Hospital,
London, UK

Anisur Rahman PhD FRCP
Professor of Rheumatology, Centre for Rheumatology Research,
University College London, London, UK

Elisabetta Renzoni
Royal Brompton & Harefield NHS Foundation Trust, London, UK

Hesham Saleh MBBCh FRCS FRCS (ORL–HNS)
Consultant Rhinologist/Facial Plastic Surgeon, Honorary Senior
Lecturer, Charing Cross and Royal Brompton Hospitals, Imperial
College, London, UK

Gurpreet Sandhu MBBS FRCS FRCS (ORL–HNS)
Consultant Otolaryngologist/Head & Neck Surgeon, Honorary
Senior Lecturer, Charing Cross and Royal National Throat, Nose
and Ear Hospital, University College, London, UK

H O Savage
Cardiology Department, Royal Brompton Hospital, Royal Brompton
& Harefield NHS Foundation Trust, Sydney Street, London, UK

John Scadding
Honorary Consultant Neurologist, National Hospital for Neurology
and Neurosurgery, Queen Square, London, UK

Pallav L Shah
Consultant Physician, Royal Brompton Hospital, Sydney Street,
London, UK

Om P Sharma MD FRCP Master FCCP FACP DTM&H
Professor of Medicine, Keck School of Medicine, Los Angeles, USA

Penny J Shaw MBBS MRCP DMRD FRCR
Department of Radiology, University College London Hospital,
London, UK

Farhana Shora
Royal Brompton & Harefield NHS Foundation Trust, London, UK

Anita K Simonds
Clinical and Academic Dept Sleep & Breathing,
Royal Brompton & Harefield NHS Foundation Trust,
London, UK

Dr Suveer Singh BSc PhD FRCP DICM EDIC FFICM
Consultant Respiratory Physician; Honorary Clinical Senior
Lecturer, Department of Respiratory Medicine, Chelsea and
Westminster Hospital, Imperial College London, UK

Paolo Spagnolo MD PhD
Department of Oncology, Haematology and Respiratory Diseases;
University of Modena and Reggio Emilia, Modena, Italy

Stephen G Spiro BSc MD FRCP
Professor of Respiratory Medicine; Honorary Consultant Physician,
University College Hospital and The Royal Brompton Hospital,
London, UK

Richard Staughton MA MB BChir FRCP
Emeritus Consultant Dermatologist, Daniel Turner Skin Clinic,
Chelsea and Westminster Hospital, London, UK

John C Stevenson, MB BS FRCP FESC MFSEM
Consultant Physician and Reader, National Heart & Lung Institute,
Royal Brompton Hospital, London, UK

Laura Tanner MRCP (UK) Resp
Transplant Institute, Institute of Cellular Medicine, Newcastle
University and Freeman Hospital, Newcastle Upon Tyne, UK

Anthony Newman Taylor FRCP FFOM FMedSci
Principal, Faculty of Medicine, Imperial College London,
London, UK

Magali N Taylor BSc MBBS FRCR
Department of Radiology, University College London Hospital,
London, UK

Muhunthan Thillai BA MBBS MRCP
Wellcome Trust Research Training Fellow, Specialist Registrar in
Respiratory Medicine, Tuberculosis Research Unit, National Heart
and Lung Institute, Imperial College London, UK

Edward Thompson
Emeritus Professor, Institute of Neurology, Queen Square,
London, UK

S Richard Underwood MD FRCP FRCR FESC FACC FASNC
Professor of Cardiac Imaging, National Heart and Lung Institute,
Imperial College London, Royal Brompton Hospital,
Sydney Street, London, UK

Violeta Vucinic–Mihailovic MD PhD
President of the Serbian Association of Sarcoidosis; Professor of
Internal Medicine and Pulmonology, Medical School, University of
Belgrade; Head of the Department of Sarcoidosis and other
granulomatous diseases at the Clinic of Pulmonary Diseases,
Clinical Centre Belgrade, Serbia

Simon Ward BSc Hons
Senior Chief Clinical Respiratory Physiologist, Head of Lung
Function Unit, Royal Brompton & Harefield NHS Foundation Trust,
London, UK

John A H Wass
Department of Endocrinology, Oxford Centre for Diabetes,
Endocrinology and Metabolism, Churchill Hospital,
University of Oxford, UK

Kshama Wechalekar MB BS DRM DNB (Nuclear Medicine)
Consultant in Nuclear Medicine, Royal Brompton Hospital,
Sydney Street, London, UK

Athol Wells MBChB MD FRACP FRCP FRCR
Professor of Respiratory Medicine and Head of Interstitial
Lung Disease Unit, The Royal Brompton Hospital, London, UK

Melissa Wickremasinghe
Tuberculosis Research Unit, National Heart and Lung Institute,
Imperial College, London, UK

Robert Wilson MD FRCP
Host Defence Unit, Royal Brompton Hospital,
London, UK

Stephen John Wort
Clinical Senior Lecturer and Honorary Consultant, Pulmonary
Hypertension and Critical Care Medicine, Royal Brompton Hospital,
London, UK

Foreword

Many teams of doctors and scientists throughout the world have made and continue to make huge contributions to solve the multifaceted problems and mysteries of sarcoidosis. We have certainly come a very long way from the many early descriptions of probable sarcoidosis as a separate entity, described in the earlier chapters.

The international conferences on sarcoidosis which have taken place regularly since 1958 reflect the world wide interest and the determination of the leaders in the field, to work globally together on this fascinating disorder. Whilst the contributors to this book are largely from the UK it is certainly not an isolationist endeavour and many of them have collaborated closely with their overseas colleagues. The great progress made in so many other parts of the world is fully acknowledged in the detailed references. The purpose of this book is to provide a timely overview of the current state of our knowledge on the Art and Science of sarcoidosis – to provide a stimulus to those trying to fill the many gaps in our understanding and at the same time to help clinicians provide optimal care for their patients.

It is the huge diversity in both the clinical and basic scientific aspects of sarcoidosis which make it such a challenge. This extreme diversity also makes it very difficult for hard pressed doctors to handle, and for scientists working in widely differing disciplines, to keep the whole spectrum of this condition in perspective. This book sets out to inform us where there are new facts, not least in the major advances in immunology and genetics. In addition it also importantly discusses the principles underlying individual patient management such as investigation, diagnosis, treatment and prognosis. The disorder ranges from an asymptomatic self limiting condition to a life threatening situation, resistant to all medication and retrievable in some case only, by lung transplantation. It explains the difficulties confounding clinical trials which have rightly led doctors to resist the temptation of premature indulgence in setting guidelines on best practice. This is so because in the face of such diversity, generalisations, as is implicit in guideline protocols, cannot be applied. Indeed they may do more harm than good.

Nevertheless the book does most usefully set out practical suggestions to enable physicians to handle the variables in a constructive and sophisticated way to individualise management of patients in the best possible way, within the present state of our knowledge.

On first sight it may seem odd that for a book which covers sarcoidosis in every organ of the body, there is no single chapter on the commonest site of all, namely that of the lung (i.e. pulmonary sarcoidosis). Naturally there is a straightforward explanation for this. So many of the chapters in every section of this book, in fact focus comprehensively on pulmonary involvement, so that to attempt to cover all aspects of pulmonary sarcoid in a single chapter would become repetitive, redundant or both.

The fascination of sarcoidosis where the cause(s) remain unclear is that on the one hand the clinical and pathological features are so characteristic that the identification of the condition in individual cases is not difficult. However, and on the other hand, the multiplicity and diversity of organ involvement, the variability of the time course and the rates and types of progression are so variable, that categorisation of cases into subgroups for rigorous clinical studies becomes exceedingly difficult. This unpredictability has led many physicians towards a nihilistic attitude towards medical intervention; sadly this attitude may have denied a large number of patients optimum care.

This book strongly supports a closely reasoned but more positive approach. The art is to explain to patients that this variability means that generalizations can be very misleading and that the imposition of rigid templates of management should be avoided. One needs to go further and impress upon them that by close and long term monitoring, this will reveal and identify the unique evolutionary pattern in individual patients, enabling the physician to plan a personalized management plan for each. In other words appropriate and timely introduction of intervention as well as appropriate reduction of therapies can be titrated against each individual patient's clinical course. This book also explores the more subtle concept of suppressing the tissue response (usually with corticosteroids) until the active driving force, whatever it is, has ceased. This approach is both rational and practical. This is also fundamental to good patient management and means that any attempt by NHS management to cut costs by fragmenting or reducing meticulous follow up by specialist services must be strongly resisted. sarcoidosis can be a long term condition requiring long term specialist care, often using specialized equipment and tests. The occasional chest X-ray with simple spirometry is not adequate.

One of the most extraordinary features of sarcoidosis is that, in a condition where identification is often so easy, it is the driving factors which still remain so elusive. This is so in spite of the fact that so many world class doctors and scientists have sought the cause(s) so diligently, and have been fully aware of the probability that the full explanation will eventually lie in a complex interaction between host responses, external agents and/or environmental factors.

There are very few medical conditions where we understand every aspect of their cause, pathogenesis, evolution and treatment. Until this utopia is reached it is right to stand back every now and then to review the current state of our knowledge. Not only does this approach reveal potential new lines to follow, but it also allows a collation of updated information to help practicing clinicians review and revise their current practices and explain things more clearly to their patients. This book does exactly that.

Professor Dame Margaret Turner Warwick
DBE DM PhD FRCP FAcad. Med. Sci
Emeritus Professor of Medicine London University.
Past Professor of Medicine, the Heart and Lung
Institute and Consultant Physician,
Royal Brompton Hospital

Preface

This book has its origins in the classic monograph written by Professor J. Guy Scadding and published in 1967 to worldwide acclaim. One of us (DNM) was privileged to collaborate with him in the preparation of a second edition, published in 1985.

Sadly, Professor Scadding died in 1999. In order to accommodate an update of the earlier editions and to include the expansion of our knowledge over the intervening years, we felt it appropriate to present 'Sarcoidosis' as a new book written on a multi-author basis with colleagues distinguished by their special interest and clinical practice within the multifactorial aspects of sarcoidosis.

We wish to express our thanks to Professor John Gibson, Dr Kenneth Citron and to our many other clinical and clinical research colleagues for their wisdom and advice. Accordingly, we hope that the text may go some little way toward a commemoration of Guy's outstanding contributions not only to sarcoidosis, but to medicine overall.

Finally, we owe a particular debt of gratitude to Philip Shaw, Sarah Penny, Mischa Barrett, Joanna Koster and Caroline Makepeace of Hodder Education for their advice and forbearance throughout the preparation of the manuscript, and to our secretaries, Donna Basire, Terri Cartwright and Sheila Campbell-Smith, whose commitment and dedication were indispensable.

Donald Mitchell
Athol Wells
Stephen Spiro
David Moller

PART I

HISTORICAL SURVEY, DEFINITION AND EPIDEMIOLOGY

Sarcoidosis in history

OM P SHARMA

Sarcoidosis, a commonplace inflammatory disease character-ized by the formation of non-caseating granulomas, occurs worldwide; no race, sex or age is out of its reach. Its chameleon-like multisystem presentation involving more than one organ in the body lets it easily cross the artificial boundaries of medical specialties. The innovative and indivi-dual approaches by international scientists of different dis-ciplines have contributed to an engrossing historical account of the disease (Scadding 1967; Scadding and Mitchell 1985).

THE BEGINNINGS

In 1869, Dmitri Mendeleev published the periodic table of elements; John Tyndall described the Tyndall effect, namely that a beam of light passing through colloidal solution can be observed from the side; Pere Armand David, a French missionary in China, described the giant panda; Paul Langerhans dissected the pancreas and discovered the islets of Langerhans; surgeon Johann Friedrich August von Esmarch demonstrated the use of a prepared first-aid bandage on the battlefield. The first issue of the scientific journal *Nature* appeared and the Suez Canal opened with an elaborate ceremony. The year 1869 welcomed Harvey Cushing, Mahatma Gandhi, André Gide, Henri Matisse, Mary Mallon (the 'Typhoid Mary'), and bade farewell to Hector Berlioz, Augustine Saint-Beuve, Mirza Ghalib (Indian poet) and Peter Roget (lexicographer).

Sarcoidosis specialists, however, remember 1869 for the contribution of Jonathan Hutchinson (1828–1913), one of the most extraordinary general practitioners of all time. A leading authority on syphilis, leprosy, neurological disorders, ocular inflammation, and diseases of the skin, he taught medicine in Polyclinic, one of the first postgraduate schools in London. He was on the teaching staff of various medical

and surgical societies, including the Medical Society of London and the Royal College of Surgeons, of which he was president in 1889. His personal museum in Haselmere became a miniature university where he regularly lectured. The vast collection of the drawings and sketches from his museum went to Johns Hopkins School of Medicine, Baltimore, USA (James 1968).

Hutchinson described a 58-year-old coal-wharf worker with purple, symmetrical skin plaques on the legs and hands that had gradually developed over the preceding two years. The lesions were neither tender nor painful. The patient had suffered also from gout and finally died of renal failure. Hunter, in an informative historical article, suggested that this case might have been of the same condition described subsequently as Mortimer's malady and most likely was the first recorded case of cutaneous sarcoidosis; however, no such claim was made at that time (Hutchinson 1877; Hunter 1936). Hutchinson's other patient, Mrs Mortimer, a 64-year-old woman, had raised, dusky red skin lesions on the face and forearms. There was no ulceration. Six months later the lesions had increased in size and extent. The lobule of the ear and the bridge of the nose swelled up and became red, and hard. Hutchinson opined that the disease was not tuberculosis and was unlike other types of lupus lesions. He presented the case to a meeting of the Dermatological Society of London where it was decided that a biopsy should be obtained. The patient, however, did not relish the prospect of having a piece of her skin removed and promptly disappeared, robbing Hutchinson of the priority in histological description of sarcoidosis granuloma. The disease, however, acquired the eponym of Mortimer's malady (Hutchinson 1898) (Fig. 1.1).

In 1869, Hutchinson and his wife Elizabeth traveled to Norway to meet Norwegian doctors interested in leprosy. Hutchinson met Dr Hansen of Bergen, a recognized leprosy

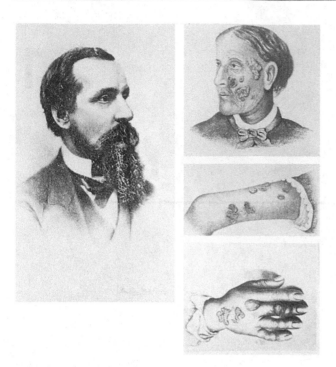

Figure 1.1   Jonathan Hutchinson (1828–1913) and Mrs Mortimer, courtesy of Dr D. G. James.

specialist. He also examined a collection of pathological drawings in the University Museum collection. Among these drawings there was one of a healthy Swedish sailor whose skin lesions were similar to those of Hutchinson's patient John W. The patient, however, did not have gout.

Caesar Boeck (1845–1917) coined the term 'sarkoid' because the lesion resembled sarcoma, and he published a study of 24 cases of 'benign miliary lupoids'; some of the cases showed involvement of the lungs, conjunctiva, bone, lymph nodes, spleen, and nasal mucous membrane. Thus the malady that started as a curious skin ailment in London became Boeck's multisystem sarcoidosis in Oslo (Boeck 1899).

Lupus pernio

In 1889, Ernest Besnier described a 34-year old patient with reddish-blue swellings of the nose, ears and upper extremities, for which he coined the terms 'lupus pernio' or 'lupus asphyxiation'. He referred to Hutchinson's chilblains but asserted that, based on the distribution of the lesion, the two conditions were distinct (Besnier 1889). In 1892, Tenneson reported another example of lupus pernio and described its essential histology of 'predominance of epithelioid cells and a variety of giant cells' in the skin lesions (Tenneson 1889). In the reports published by Besnier and Tenneson, wax models of the appearance of the patients were used to illustrate skin lesions. Lucien-Marie Pautrier (1876–1959), another Frenchman and Professor of Dermatology at Strasbourg and Lausanne, gets the credit for pointing out that the disease, because of its multisystem distribution, should be regarded as reticulo-endotheliosis (Pautrier 1937). Nevertheless, in France the disease became known as the malady of Besnier, Boeck and Schaumann (Turiaf 1971) (Fig. 1.2).

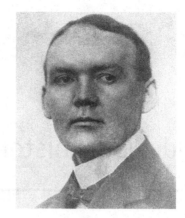

Figure 1.2   Jorge Schaumann (1879–1953), courtesy of Dr Yutaka Hosoda, Japan.

Bone lesions

Karl Kreibich (1869–1932) was born on 20 May 1869 in Prague and graduated in 1894 from the German Medical Faculty in Prague. In 1909 he succeeded Pick as Professor of Dermatology and later became Dean (1913) and Rector (1923) of the German University in Prague. Three of his 200 scientific papers were on lupus pernio. In one of his patients he noted lattice-like rarefactions of the terminal phalanges. It was the first description linking bone lesions (cysts) with lupus pernio (Kreibich 1904).

Jorgen Schaumann (1879–1953), a dermatologist at Saint Goran's Hospital and the Finsen Institute in Stockholm, Sweden, provided the common pathological basis for diverse clinical aspects of multisystem sarcoidosis. He called it 'lymphogranulomatosis benigna' and distinguished it from Hodgkin's malignant granuloma in a Zambaco prize-winning essay written in 1914, but published later (Schaumann 1936).

Erythema nodosum

Sven Löfgren (1910–1978) was born in Stockholm. During his medical training he came under the tutelage of Westergren and Schaumann. It was Löfgren who obtained tissue biopsies and linked erythema nodosum, the skin manifestation originally described by Robert Willan, and bilateral hilar adenopathy as a manifestation of acute sarcoidosis. The combination of erythema nodosum and hilar adenopathy is now known as Löfgren's syndrome (Fig. 1.3).

Löfgren argued that sarcoidosis was unlike and unrelated to tuberculosis and, thus, pulled sarcoidosis out of the shadows of tuberculosis and brought it into the limelight as a common disorder with good prognosis. He also described renal sarcoidosis and associated hypercalcemia (Löfgren 1953).

The Kveim test

Ansgar Kveim (1892–1966), a Norwegian dermatologist, made the important observation that sarcoid lymph node

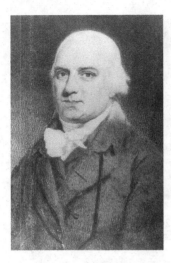

Figure 1.3   Robert Willan (1757–1812) first described erythema nodosum. Courtesy of Dr D. G. James.

tissue inoculated into the skin gave rise to a granulomatous papule in a sarcoidosis patient. Because the reaction did not occur in normal subjects or in one patient with lupus vulgaris, he contended that the papule was specific to sarcoidosis and advocated that the test might differentiate sarcoidosis from tuberculosis (Kveim 1941). In 1954, Siltzbach and Erlich conducted the first large-scale trial testing the Kveim antigen. Of the 200 subjects, with biopsy-proven sarcoidosis, 86 percent yielded a positive response; there were only 4 percent false-positive reactions (Siltzbach and Ehrlich 1954). Dr Geraint James proposed that the test be called the Kveim–Siltzbach test in honor of Louis Siltzbach's contribution in purifying the antigen and standardizing the test (James 1977).

Ocular manifestations

Schumacher and Berring, independently, first drew attention to iritis accompanying sarcoidosis. In addition they also noted the involvement of parotid and submaxillary glands in these patients (Schumacher 1909; Berring 1910) At the same time, Christian Heerfordt (1871–1953), a Danish ophthalmologist, drew attention to 'febris uveoparotidea subchronica', a combination of uveitis and enlargement of the parotid glands. He noted that the condition was chronic and frequently complicated by cranial nerve palsies, especially of the seventh nerve, and pleocytosis of the cerebrospinal fluid (Heerfordt 1909). Further observations by Bruins Slot, Longcope and Pierson, Pautrier, and Waldenstrom established uveoparotid fever as yet another manifestation of sarcoidosis (Bruins Slot 1938; Longcope and Pierson 1937; Pautrier 1937; Waldnestrom 1937).

Biochemical abnormalities

In 1935, Salvesen described four patients in Oslo with sarcoidosis, three of whom had considerable hyperglobulinemia of over 5 g/100 mL (Salveson 1935). Electrophoretic studies showed that the increase in globulin was principally in the gamma fraction and associated with low albumin levels. It was further demonstrated that, with acute onset of disease, serum levels of IgM and IgA were markedly elevated while IgG levels remained within normal range. On the other hand, patients with pulmonary infiltration had elevated levels of serum IgG, reflecting the chronic nature of the disease.

In 1939, Harrell and Fisher reported that hypercalcemia was present in six of their eleven patients at some time during the course of sarcoidosis (Harrell and Fisher 1939). In 1952, Longcope and Freiman reported that 11 of their 44 patients had high serum calcium (Longcope and Freiman 1952). Adams and associates showed that calcitriol, the most active metabolite of vitamin D, causes hypercalcemia in sarcoidosis and that macrophages from patients with active disease are the source of this hormone. Mason and associates identified a similar metabolite in sarcoid granuloma (Adams et al. 1983; Mason et al. 1984).

Serum angiotensin–converting enzyme

Jack Lieberman's original observation in 1974 of raised concentration of serum angiotensin-converting enzyme (SACE) in 15 out of 17 patients with sarcoidosis focused attention on the enzyme as a biological marker for sarcoidosis. Increased SACE activity is due to stimulation of activated macrophages and non-caseating granulomas (Lieberman 1975).

Immunological alterations

The lack of response to tuberculin was first described by Boeck in 1916. It was recognized that the depression of delayed hypersensitivity response was also seen with other antigens such as trichophytin, *Candida albicans*, histoplasmin, coccidioidin, tetanus toxoid, streptokinase–streptodoranase, measles, mumps and dinitrochlorobenzene.

Harold Israel helped to establish sarcoidosis as an illness with immunological aberration. He studied the response of sarcoidosis patients to BCG vaccination, the interrelationship between sarcoidosis and tuberculosis. Further in-vivo and in-vitro studies have now shown that sarcoidosis patients have depressed delayed-type sensitivity, hyperactivity of cellular and humoral immune systems, high levels of serum immune complexes, accumulation of T-cells at the site of activity, increased cytokine activity, and granuloma formation (Israel and Sones 1958; Moller 2002).

Bronchoalveolar lavage (BAL)

Although rigid bronchoscopy to remove secretions from the lungs and airways has been used for decades, the practice of obtaining biological specimens from the lungs for diagnostic and research purposes is relatively new. In the late 1960s many reports appeared recommending the use of fiberoptic bronchoscopy to retrieve specimens from the lungs of patients with sarcoidosis and other interstitial lung disease. These studies provided – and continue to provide – valuable insights into the granulomatous process, but so far have failed to reveal the etiology of sarcoidosis (Reynolds and Newball 1974).

Radiological classification

In 1942, Peter Kerley in Great Britain noted the radiological association of erythema nodosum and bilateral hilar adenopathy in sarcoidosis, and James, Thompson and Wilcox obtained, eventually, histological association in 1956 (Kerley 1942; James *et al.* 1956). In 1958, Professor Wurm developed the radiological staging of pulmonary sarcoidosis based on plain chest roentgenograms. The system was adopted and freely used by clinical investigators all over the world until the appearance of computerized tomography (CT) that mercilessly exposed the limitations of plain chest radiography. CT can detect mediastinal and hilar lymph nodes not seen on a plain chest X-ray film; high-resolution CT is helpful when pulmonary parenchymal disease is present. CT and magnetic imaging studies are of limited value in diagnosing sarcoidosis (Wurm *et al.* 1958).

Lung function

Nils Svanborg (1920–1997) was born in Umea. He published the first authoritative monograph describing pulmonary function abnormalities in sarcoidosis in great detail (Svanborg 1961) (Fig. 1.4).

MORE RECENT DEVELOPMENTS

The Royal Northern Hospital's Sarcoidosis Clinic, London

Spurred on by the studies of Boeck and Schaumann and many others on the European continent, many British physicians began to explore and study the disease from every angle. None was more influential and erudite than Professor John Guyet Scadding who was stimulated to take up sarcoidosis by Isidore Snapper (1889–1973), Professor of Clinical Medicine at the University of Amsterdam.

Scadding consolidated his vast personal experience of the disease, gathered at Hammersmith Hospital and Brompton Chest Hospital, now the Royal Brompton, in the widely acclaimed book *Sarcoidosis*, first published in 1967. At the Hammersmith Hospital in London, Scadding collaborated with Sheila Sherlock (later Dame Sheila, 1918–2001) on a study of aspiration liver biopsy in sarcoidosis. The test became the most valuable tool for diagnosing sarcoidosis and remained so for decades before being replaced by bronchoscopy (Scadding 1967).

The credit for making sarcoidosis a household word, however, goes to David Geraint James, a pupil of Scadding

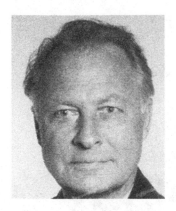

Figure 1.4   N. Svanborg (1920–1997) was the first physiologist to publish an exhaustive account of lung function changes in sarcoidosis.

and husband of Sheila Sherlock, who in 1953 started the renowned sarcoidosis clinic in a small north London hospital. The clinic in its heyday had attracted sarcoidosis specialists from all over the world. The Royal Northern Sarcoidosis Clinic, as it was called, became a sarcoidosis Mecca. Among many others, Harold Israel, Carol Johns, Guy Scadding, Sven Löfgren, Yutaka Hosoda, Louis Sitzbach, Ladislav Levinsky, Edwin Kendig, Jacques Chretien, Newton Bethlem, Takateru Izumi, William Jones Williams, Ronald Crystal, Gianfranco Rizzato, Samir Gupta, Donald Mitchell, Ulrich Costabel, Jan Costa Waldenstrom, Friedrich Wegener, Richard DeRemee, Sheila Sherlock, Margaret Turner-Warwick, Olof Selroos and Branislav Djuric participated in meetings and exchanged ideas at the Royal Northern Hospital. Neither the clinic nor the hospital exists now.

Sir William Osler and the Johns Hopkins Medical Center, Baltimore

In the earlier decades of the twentieth century sarcoidosis was not a significant illness in the USA; its evidence remains surrounded in the veil of tuberculosis. Sarcoidosis was not included in the 1907 edition of *Diseases of the Lungs* written by Dr Robert Babcock and published by D. Appleton and Co. of New York. It was not to be seen in any of the editions of William Osler's *Textbook of Medicine* or in the tomes by Austin Flint and George Pepper.

Nevertheless, the 14-year-old African-American admitted to the Johns Hopkins Medical Center, published in the *American Journal of Medical Sciences*, reported by Osler, most likely had sarcoidosis. The patient had bilateral parotid and lacrimal enlargement, lung disease and pleural involvement. At autopsy, no evidence of tuberculosis was found (Osler 1898).

There was a close relationship between Hutchinson and Osler, who often visited the former at Haselmere; Osler had descended from the American branch of the Hutchinsons of Lincolnshire. It is unclear how this family was related to Jonathan Hutchinson's family, but being Quakers bearing the same family names, and lived within close proximity, it was more than likely that the two families were close. Osler was instrumental in moving the valuable contents of Hutchinson's Haselmere museum to Johns Hopkins Medical School in Baltimore.

In 1937, the first significant publication about sarcoidosis in America appeared. It was a 75-page review from Johns Hopkins Hospital by Warfield Longcope. This event took place almost six decades after the first recorded case of sarcoidosis by Hutchinson (Longcope 1936).

International conferences

In June 1958, David Geraint James invited a group of international doctors to the Brompton Hospital in London for the first international meeting on sarcoidosis. Twenty-eight participants from eight countries came (Fig. 1.5). These doctors had researched and written about the disease. Before the conference they had only read each other's articles but had not met. The London conference was followed by the second conference, held in Washington in June 1960. Dr Martin Cummings, who for a brief period believed that sarcoidosis was caused by pine pollens, organized the meeting. The third conference was held in Stockholm in 1963 (Fig. 1.6).

Jude Turiaf (1904–1989), Professor of Medicine at Hospital Bichat, Paris, organized the fourth world conference on sarcoidosis in September 1966 (Fig. 1.7). The proceedings contain voluminous information crammed into 782 pages. Jacques Chretien (1923–2003), editor of the *French Thoracic Society Journal* and Honorary Fellow of the Royal College of

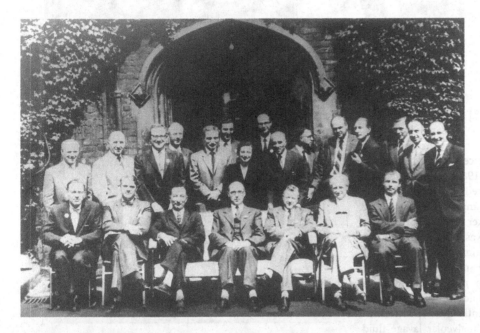

Figure 1.5 There were only 22 participants at the 1958 London conference including one woman, Dr. Ingrid Gilg. This photograph was taken in the grounds of the Brompton Hospital, London. Dr J. G. Scadding (sitting, centre) presided. Courtesy of Dr D. G. James.

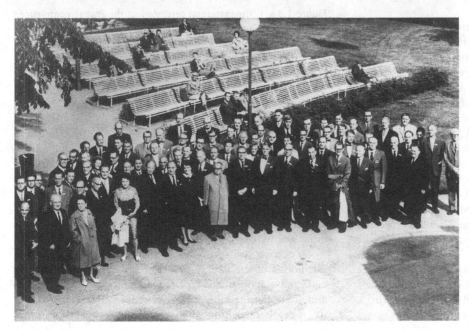

Figure 1.6 There was a large international participation in the Stockholm Conference organized by Dr Sven Lofgren in 1963. Courtesy of Dr D. G. James.

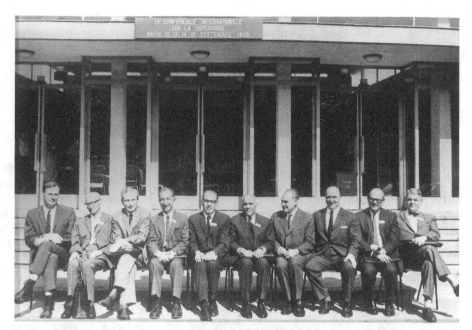

Figure 1.7   The International Committee on Sarcoidosis assembled for the Paris Conference in 1966 (from left to right): T. H. Hurley (Melbourne), E. A. Uehlinger (Zurich), J. S. Chapman (Dallas), H. Israel (Philadelphia), L. E. Siltzbach (New York), J. Turiaf (Paris), L. Levinsky (Prague), D. G. James (London), M. M. Cummings (Washington) and S. Lofgren (Stockholm). Courtesy of Dr D. G. James.

Physicians, London, organized the 1981 world conference in Paris where monoclonal antibodies in sarcoidosis first appeared.

The seventh international conference held in New York, organized by Louis Siltzbach (1906–1980), emphasized the immunological aberrations associated with sarcoidosis. Jack Lieberman recognized serum angiotensin-converting enzyme (SACE) as a biochemical marker of active sarcoidosis. Carol Johnson Johns (1923–2000) was the captain of the tenth international conference in Baltimore in 1984. Victor McKusick (1921–2008) delivered a memorable opening lecture, 'Sarcoidosis: a case study in nosology (McKusick 1986). The concept of *activity* of sarcoidosis was extensively discussed in the context of then recently developed techniques of gallium scanning and bronchoalveolar lavage fluid analysis.

Japan has hosted three world conferences on sarcoidosis and has an active Sarcoidosis Association (JAS). Dr Yutaka Hosoda organized the sixth world congress in 1972 in Tokyo with 300 delegates representing 22 countries; Dr Takateru Izumi, Professor of Medicine at Kyoto University, organized the 1991 conference in Kyoto jointly with the eleventh annual meeting of the Japan Society of Sarcoidosis; and Professor Masayuki Ando hosted the seventh WASOG conference in Kumamoto in 1999.

Geraint James encouraged Ladislav Levinsky to host participants from 37 countries at the 1969 world conference on sarcoidosis in Prague (Figs. 1.8 and 1.9). The conference resulted in an extensive 653-page book. Manuel Freitas e Costa, Professor of Respiratory Disease in the University Medical School, Lisbon, organized in 1989 a sarcoidosis conference that attracted 322 delegates; there were 76 oral presentations and 76 posters. In 1997, Professor Ulrich Costabel's conference in Essen paid tribute to German pioneers in the field including Alexander Bittorf, Erich Kuznitsky, Paul Langerhans, Theodore Langhans, Erwin Uehlinger, Friedrich Wegener,

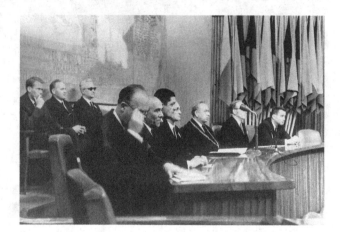

Figure 1.8   The inaugural ceremony at the Prague conference, 1969, in the venerable Aula Magna, the fourteenth-century assembly hall of Charles University. The platform party included Louis Siltzbach, Ladislav Levinksy, organizer, Jude Turiaf, and D. Geraint James. Courtesy of Dr D. G. James.

H. Eule, J. Meier-Sydow and Professor Carl Wurm. The latter in 1958 developed the radiological staging of pulmonary sarcoidosis that was adopted by clinical investigators all over the world.

On 22 February 2003, the Indian Association of Sarcoidosis and other Granulomatous Disorders (IASOG) was formed. It held its first annual meeting on 12 January 2004, organized by Dr Ashok Shah.

Stockholm was the venue of the first world congress on sarcoidosis of the twenty-first century. It was held in June 2002 and was organized by Drs Olof Selroos, Anders Eklund and Johan Grunewald. The conference is remembered for its in-depth exposition of the cytokine network leading to

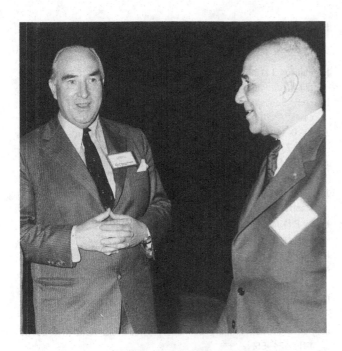

Figure 1.9 Two European giants of sarcoidosis: Dr D. Geraint James (UK) and Dr Jude Turiaf (France).

granuloma formation and discourses about genetic make-up predisposing to various phenotypes of sarcoidosis.

The ninth WASOG meeting, in association with BAL International Conference, was held in Athens, Greece, in June 2008. More than 250 international clinicians and scientists attended the conferences; they were 104 oral and poster presentations encompassing various clinical and basic science aspects of sarcoidosis and interstitial lung disease. At the time of writing, the next WASOG conference is scheduled to be held in Maastricht, Netherlands. Once again, there will be an intense scrutiny and research concentrated towards finding out the cause of sarcoidosis (Table 1.1).

WASOG, and the sarcoidosis journal

Professor Gianfranco Rizzato organized a world conference in Milan in 1987 and at the same time he took the opportunity to found the World Association of Sarcoidosis and Other Granulomatous Disorders (WASOG). This infrastructure enables specialists worldwide to exchange information and meet at regular intervals to keep the sarcoidosis spirit alive. In 1984, Dr Rizzato founded *Sarcoidosis*, a journal devoted to

Table 1.1 International sarcoidosis meetings, 1958–2009.

1958	First International Conference on Sarcoidosis (DG James, London)
1960	Second International Conference on Sarcoidosis (MM Cummings, Washington)
1963	Third International Conference on Sarcoidosis (S Löfgren, Stockholm)
1966	Fourth International Conference on Sarcoidosis (J Turiaf, Paris)
1969	Fifth International Conference on Sarcoidosis (L Lewinsky, Praha)
1971	First European Sarcoidosis Conference (E Martin, Genebra)
1972	Sixth International Conference on Sarcoidosis (KK Tamura, Y Hosada, Tokyo) (Fig. 1.10)
1975	Seventh International Conference on Sarcoidosis and Other Granulomatous Disorders (LE Siltzbach, New York)
1976	Second European Sarcoidosis Conference (H Eule, East Berlin)
1978	Eighth International Conference on Sarcoidosis and Other Granulomatous Disorders (W Jones Williams, Cardiff)
1980	Third European Sarcoidosis Conference (S Goldman, Novi-Sad)
1981	Ninth International Conference on Sarcoidosis and Other Granulomatous Disorders (J Chretian, Paris)
1983	Fourth European Sarcoidosis Conference (A Blasi, Sorrento)
1984	Tenth International Conference on Sarcoidosis and Other Granulomatous Disorders (Carol Johns, Baltimore)
1986	Fifth European Sarcoidosis Conference (H Klech, Vienna)
1987	Eleventh International Conference on Sarcoidosis and Other Granulomatous Disorders (G Rizzato, Milan)
1989	First WASOG meeting (MEE Costa, Lisbon)
1991	Second WASOG meeting (S Oshima, T Izumi, Kyoto)
1993	Third WASOG meeting (OP Sharma, Los Angeles)
1995	Fourth WASOG Meeting (R Dubois, DN Mitchell, London)
1997	Fifth WASOG Meeting (U Costabel, Essen)
1999	Sixth WASOG Meeting (M Ando, Kumamoto)
2001	First International WASOG Conference on Diffuse Lung Diseases (M Bocceri, Venice)
2002	Seventh WASOG Meeting (O. Selroos, A. Eklund, J. Gruenwald, Stockholm)
2003	Second International WASOG Conference on Diffuse Lung Diseases (P Rottoli, Siena)
2005	Eighth WASOG Meeting (LS Newman, RP Baughman, Denver)
2006	Third International WASOG Conference on Diffuse Lung Diseases (N Crimi, Catalina)
2007	Fourth International WASOG Conference on Diffuse Lung Diseases (Y Yoshizawa, Tokyo)
2008	Ninth WASOG Meeting and 11th BAL International Conference (ISH Constantopoulos, NM Siafakas, Athens)
2009	Fifth International WASOG Conference on Diffuse Lung Diseases (IM Judson, Charleston)

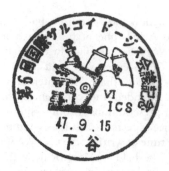

Figure 1.10   The Japanese Post Office issued a special stamp celebrating the VI International Conference on Sarcoidosis in 1972 in Tokyo, Japan. Courtesy of Dr Yutaka Hosoda.

sarcoidosis and other granulomatous disorders (Rizzato 2005). In 2008, Robert Baughman and Cesare Saltini took over the joint editorship of the journal, now called *Sarcoidosis Vasculitis and Diffuse Lung Diseases*. The journal is available online at www.sarcoidosis.it.

CONCLUSION

Sarcoidosis, a multisystem granulomatous disease, has a distinguished medical history that stretches over all the continents and covers the last 150 years. The last five decades have seen rapid progress in the understanding of clinical, radiological, physiological, biochemical and immunological aspects of the granulomatous process. Advances in the field of medical genomics and proteomics may hold the key to its etiology.

REFERENCES

Adams J, Sharma O, Gacad M, Singer F (1983). Metabolism of 25-hydroxyvitamin D3 by cultured pulmonary alveolar macrophages in sarcoidosis. *J Clin Invest* 72: 1856–60.

Berring P (1910). Zur Kentinis des Boeckschen Sarkoids. *Z Dermatol* 17: 404–12.

Boeck C (1899). Multiple benign sarcoid of the skin. *Norsk Mag Laegevid* 14: 1321–45.

Besnier E (1889). Lupus pernio de la face. *Ann Derm Syph (Paris)* 10: 33–6.

Bruins Slot W (1938). Ziekte van Besnier-Boeck – Febris uveoparotidea (Heerfordt). *Ned Tijdschr Genesk* 80: 2859–62.

Harrell GT, Fisher S (1939). Blood chemical studies in Boeck's sarcoid with particular reference to protein, calcium and phosphatase values. *J Clin Pathol* 18: 687–93.

Heerfordt CF (1909). Uber eine febris uveo-parotidea subchronica. *Graefes Arch Ophthalmol* 70: 254–8.

Hunter F (1936). Hutchinson–Boeck's disease (generalized sarcoidosis): historical note and report of a case with apparent cure. *New Engl J Med* 214: 246–52.

Hutchinson J (1877). Anomalous diseases of skin and fingers: case of livid papillary psoriasis? In: *Illustrations of Clinical Surgery*. J & A Churchill, London, pp. 42–3.

Hutchinson J (1898). Mortimer's malady: a form of lupus pernio. *Arch Surg (London)* 9: 307–15.

Israel H, Sones M (1958). Sarcoidosis: clinical observations in 160 cases. *Arch Intern Med* 102: 766–76.

James D (1968). Historical aspects of sarcoidosis. *Clio Medica* 3: 265–71.

James DG (1977). Sarcoidosis and respiratory disorders: Festschrift in honour of Louis Siltzbach. *Mt Sinai Med J* 44: 683–879.

James D, Thomson A, Wilcox A (1956). Erythema nodosum as a manifestation of sarcoidosis. *Lancet* 2: 218–21.

Kerley P (1942). The significance of the radiological manifestations of erythema nodosum. *Br J Radiol* 15: 155–65.

Kreibich K (1904). Uber lupus pernio. *Arch Derm Syph (Wien)* 71: 3–12.

Kveim A (1941). En ny og specifikk Kutan-reaksjon ved Boeck's sarcoid. *Nord Med* 9: 169–72.

Lieberman J (1975). Elevation of serum angiotensin converting enzyme (ACE) level in sarcoidosis. *Am J Med* 59: 365–72.

Löfgren S (1953). Primary pulmonary sarcoidosis. *Acta Med Scand* 145: 424–55.

Longcope W (1936). The generalized form of Boeck's sarcoid. *Trans Assoc Am Phys* 51: 94–102.

Longcope W, Frieman D (1952). A study of sarcoidosis. *Medicine (Baltimore)* 31: 1–132.

Longcope W, Pierson J (1937). Boeck's sarcoidosis (sarcoidosis). *Bull Johns Hopkins Hosp* 60: 223–96.

Mason R, Frankel T, Chan Y (1984). Vitamin-D conversion by sarcoid lymph node homogenate. *Ann Intern Med* 100: 59–61.

McKusick V (1986). Sarcoidosis: a case study in nosology. *J New York Acad Sci* 465: 1–2.

Moller D (2002). What causes sarcoidosis? *Curr Opin Pulm Med* 8: 429–34.

Osler W (1898). On chronic symmetrical enlargement of the salivary and lachrymal glands. *Am J Med Sci* 11: 1–4.

Pautrier L (1937). Syndrome de Heerfordt et maladie de Besnier–Boeck–Schaumann. *Bull Mem Soc Med Hop Paris* 53: 1608–20.

Reynolds H, Newball H (1974). Analysis of proteins and respiratory cells obtained from human lungs by bronchial lavage. *J Lab Clin Med* 84: 559–73.

Rizzato G (2005). History of WASOG and current activities. *Eur Respir Mon* 32: 335–6.

Salvesen HA (1935). The sarcoid of Boeck, a disease of importance to internal medicine. *Acta Med Scand* 86: 127–51.

Scadding JF (1967). *Sarcoidosis*. Eyre & Spottiswoode, London.

Scadding JG, Mitchell DN (1985). *Sarcoidosis*, 2nd edn. Chapman & Hall, London.

Schaumann J (1936). Lymphogranulomatosis benigna in the light of prolonged clinical observations and autopsy findings. *Br J Dermatol* 48: 399–46.

Schumacher H (1909). Iridocyclitis chronica. *Munch Med Wschr* 56: 2664–70.

Siltzbach L, Erlich J (1954). The Nickerson–Kveim reaction in sacoidosis. *Am J Med* 16: 790–803.

Svanborg N (1961). Studies on the cardiopulmonary function in sarcoidosis. *Acta Med Scand* 170(suppl.): 366.

Tenneson H (1889). Lupus pernio. *Ann Derm Syph (Paris)* **10**: 333–6.

Turiaf J (1971). Ernest Besnier (1831–1909) et Lucien-Marie Pautrier (1876–1959). In: Levinsky L, Macholda F (eds). *Fifth International Conference on Sarcoidosis*. Universita Karlova Press, Prague, pp. 57–62.

Waldenstrom J (1937). Some observations on uveoparotitis and allied conditions with special reference to the symptoms from the nervous system. *Acta Med Scand* **91**: 53.

Wurm K, Renidell H, Heilmeyer L (1958). *Der Lungeboeck in Rontgenbild*. Georg Thieme Verlag, Stuttgart.

Defining sarcoidosis

OM P SHARMA

More than a century ago, Jonathan Hutchinson, a British dermatologist, identified the first case of sarcoidosis at King's College Hospital, London. He considered the disease an unusual type of lupus, unrelated to tuberculosis and leprosy (Hutchinson 1877). In June 1881, Hutchinson delivered a lecture to the Royal College of Surgeons, London, and expanded on his observation and said that the new lupus-like lesion, consisting of symmetrical skin lesions involving the face and hands, was due to a constitutional peculiarity or diathesis (Hutchinson 1898). In the decades following the turn of the nineteenth century, several publications independently witnessed the blossoming of this dermatological curiosity into a multisystem clinical disorder.

Although clinical features of sarcoidosis became familiar, there was no simple and clear definition of the disease. It was then, as now, hard to provide a concise definition of a disease whose cause was not known (Hutchinson 1881).

When clinicians recognize a group of patients with symptoms and signs that do not conform to the pictures of previously described diseases, they define the new illness on the basis of clinical description. To be accepted as a case of the new disease, the patient must show the stated combination of clinical symptoms and signs (Scadding 1963). When knowledge has accumulated, to this initial workable definition may be added more objective anatomical, radiological, biochemical, immunological and other laboratory features (Riker and Clark 1949). This philosophical thinking led Scadding to recommend the following definition:

> Sarcoidosis is a disease characterized by the formation in all of several affected tissues of epithelioid-cell tubercles without caseation, though fibrinoid necrosis may be present at the centers of a few, proceeding either to resolution or to conversion into hyaline fibrous tissue.

This statement emphasized the histological features, and course, but did not include the multisystem clinical nature of the illness. Scadding, however, indicated that to his definition may be added the description of organs most frequently involved, including the lymph nodes, lungs, liver, spleen, skin, eyes, small bones of the hands and feet, and salivary glands.

As knowledge of sarcoidosis began to accumulate, practitioners of different disciplines added new information – particularly in biochemistry, radiology, immunology and genetics. This expanded the scope of sarcoidosis (Scadding 1967).

In June 1960, the international conference on sarcoidosis held in Washington, DC, revisited the issue and produced a comprehensive descriptive definition (Hardy 1961):

> Sarcoidosis is systemic granulomatous disease of undetermined etiology and pathogenesis. Mediastinal and peripheral lymph nodes, lungs, liver, spleen, skin, eyes, phalangeal bones, parotid glands are most often involved, but other tissues may be affected. The Kveim reaction is frequently positive, and tuberculin-type hypersensitivities are frequently depressed. Other important laboratory findings are hypercalciuria and increased serum immunoglobulins. The characteristic histologic appearance of epithelioid tubercles with little or no necrosis is not pathognomonic, and tuberculosis, fungal infections, beryllium disease, and local sarcoid reaction must be excluded. The diagnosis should be regarded as established for clinical purposes in patients who have consistent clinical features with biopsy evidence of epithelioid tubercles or a positive Kveim test.

Three decades elapsed before Yamamoto and colleagues, at the Kyoto world congress on sarcoidosis in 1991, provided a modified descriptive definition based on the prototype presented at the 1960 Washington conference (Yamamoto et al. 1993):

> Sarcoidosis is a multisystem disorder of unknown cause(s). It commonly affects young and middle-aged adults and frequently presents with bilateral hilar lymphadenopathy, pulmonary infiltration, ocular and

skin lesions. Liver, spleen, lymph nodes, salivary glands, heart, nervous system, muscles, bones, and other organs may also be involved. The diagnosis is established when clinico-radiological findings are supported by histological evidence of non-caseating epithelioid cell granulomas. Granulomas of known causes and local sarcoid reaction must be excluded. Frequently observed immunological features are depression of cutaneous delayed-type hypersensitivity and increased helper cell (CD4)/suppressor cell (CD8) ratio at the site of involvement. Circulating immune complexes along with signs of B-cell hyperactivity may also be detectable. Other markers of the disease include elevated levels of serum angiotensin-converting enzyme (ACE), increased uptake of radioactive gallium, abnormal calcium metabolism and abnormal fluorescein angiography. The Kveim–Siltzbach test, when appropriate cell suspension is available, may be of diagnostic help. The course and prognosis may correlate with the onset and extent of the disease. An acute onset with erythema nodosum or asymptomatic hilar adenopathy usually heralds a self-limiting course, whereas an insidious onset, especially with multiple extra-pulmonary lesions, may be followed by relentless fibrosis of the lungs and other organs. . . . Corticosteroids relieve symptoms, suppress the formation of granulomas and normalize the SACE levels and the gallium uptake.

In 1999, the ATS/ESR/WASOG expert panel refined and updated the definition (Joint Statement of ACT 1999; Fig. 2.1):

Sarcoidosis is a multisystem disorder of unknown cause. It commonly affects young and middle-aged adults and frequently presents with bilateral hilar adenopathy, pulmonary infiltration, ocular and skin lesions. The liver, spleen, lymph nodes, salivary glands, heart, nervous system, muscles, bones and other organs may also be involved. The diagnosis is established when clinico-radiographic findings are supported by histological evidence of non-caseating epithelioid cell granulomas. Granulomas of unknown causes and local sarcoid reactions must be excluded. Frequently observed immunological features are depression of cutaneous delayed type-hypersensitivity and a heightened Th1 immune response at sites of disease. Circulating immune complexes along with signs of B-cell hyperactivity may also be found. The course and prognosis may correlate with the mode of the onset, and the extent of the disease. An acute onset with erythema nodosum or asymptomatic bilateral hilar adenopathy usually heralds a self-limiting course, whereas an insidious onset, especially with multiple extra-pulmonary lesions, may be followed by relentless, progressively fibrosis of the lungs and other organs.

The disease occurs worldwide. Its frequency, pulmonary and extrapulmonary manifestations, response to treatment and prognosis are extraordinarily similar. Despite the resemblance, there are certain inexplicable distinctive features of the disease related to geography and race. African-Americans have a higher incidence of chronic skin lesions; Scandinavians have higher frequency of erythema nodosum; ocular and myocardial sarcoidosis manifestations are uniquely common in Japanese patients; Italians tend to have abnormal calcium metabolism; and Indians experience the highest occurrence of constitutional manifestations of fever, weight loss, joint pains and adenopathy.

Although genetics and racial background influence the presentation, course and prognosis of the disease, the epidemiological data from many countries suffer from fundamental problems in finding and diagnosing sarcoidosis, but the scientific enquiry into the cause of sarcoidosis has

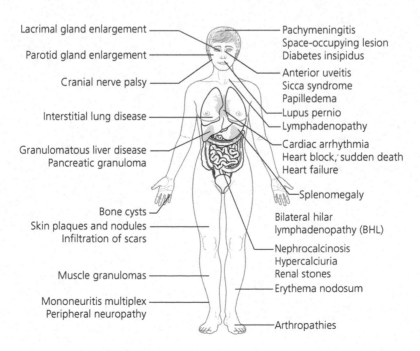

Figure 2.1   Multisystem manifestations of sarcoidosis.

gained a significant momentum (Baughman *et al.* 2001). Each advance in knowledge brings us closer to the enigma that continues to elude us, namely the etiology of sarcoidosis. As long as the cause or causes remain unknown, a succinct definition of sarcoidosis will remain a dream. Meanwhile, Scadding's original observation is a helpful, brief, practical and working definition:

> Sarcoidosis is a multisystem disease of unknown cause characterized by the formation in all or several affected tissues of epithelioid-cell tubercles without caseation, though fibrinoid necrosis may be present at the centers of a few. Based on the genetic makeup, the disease may proceed either to resolution or to conversion into hyaline fibrosis of the involved organs.

We are not yet ready for a more overarching definition.

REFERENCES

Baughman R, Teirstein A, Judson M *et al.* (2001). Clinical characteristics of patients in a case–control study of sarcoidosis. *Am J Respir Crit Care Med* **164**: 1485–89.

Hardy H (1961). Definition of sarcoidosis: Proceedings of the International Conference on Sarcoidosis, 1960. *Am Rev Tuberc* **84**(5, part 2): 2–4.

Hutchinson J (1877). Anomalous diseases of skin and fingers: case of livid papillary psoriasis? In: *Illustrations of Clinical Surgery*. J & A Churchill, London, pp. 42–3.

Hutchinson J (1881). *The Pedigree of Disease Being: Six Lectures on Temperament, Idiosyncrasy and Diathesis*. William Wood & Co, New York, pp. 73–88.

Hutchinson J (1898). Mortimer's malady: a form of lupus pernio. *Arch Surg* (London) **9**: 307–15.

Joint Statement of the American Thoracic Society (ATS), the European Respiratory Society (ERS) and the World Association of Sarcoidosis and other Granulomatous Disorders (WASOG) (1991). *Am J Respir Crit Care Med* **160**: 736–55.

Ricker W, Clark M (1949). Sarcoidosis: a clinico-pathologic review of 300 cases, including 22 autopsies. *Am J Clin Path* **19**: 725.

Scadding JG (1963). Principles of definition in Medicine. *Lancet* **1**: 323–5.

Scadding JG (1967). *Sarcoidosis*. Eyre & Spotttiswoode, London, pp. 38–44.

Yamamoto M, Sharma O, Hosoda Y (1993). The 1991 descriptive definition of sarcoidosis. In: *Proceedings of the Twelfth World Congress on Sarcoidosis, Kyoto, Japan*. Edizioni Bongraf, Sigilim Srl, Milan, pp. 33–6.

Epidemiology

PAUL CULLINAN

INTRODUCTION

Much of this book – and certainly the majority of its non-clinical chapters – is concerned with the considerable body of knowledge relating to the detailed pathophysiology of sarcoidosis. For most bioscientists, clinical or otherwise, this is a natural focus; their aim, even if it is at times oblique, is to reach an understanding of the mechanisms of the disease sufficient to permit its satisfactory treatment. In some contrast, the epidemiological approach is concerned primarily with etiology, an understanding of the cause(s) of the disease that will allow it ultimately to be prevented. The distinction is not absolute – considerations of cause and mechanism frequently accompany each other – but the approaches are sufficiently different that epidemiologists and basic scientists frequently misunderstand each other.

The epidemiological approach has as its basis the axiom that observation of the distribution of a disease among and between populations is a powerful tool, and that such observation leads to the generation of etiological hypotheses that might explain differences in such distributions. The subsequent testing of these hypotheses takes place in populations of affected people with appropriate comparison to unaffected people, sometimes through experiment but more commonly through 'observational' methods such as cohort or case–control analysis. In general the approach is iterative – very few if any epidemiological studies are definitive – and it is often painstaking. Nonetheless, if successful the gain is substantial; unfortunately, in the case of sarcoidosis, much remains to be done.

DIFFICULTIES

There are several features of sarcoidosis that make it intrinsically difficult for epidemiological study. These include the variability in its clinical presentation and the accompanying lack of a readily applied and indisputable case definition.

Expert consensus suggests that the diagnosis is established when clinical and/or radiographic features are present together with histological evidence of non-caseating, epithelioid granulomas (Joint Statement 1999), a definition that requires access to sophisticated diagnostic services. Such access probably has important social and other determinants (Rabin *et al.* 2004). Moreover, like many respiratory diseases, other conditions with similar presentations and perhaps more established etiologies must be 'excluded', a process that is inevitably variable and frequently subjective. Because the disease has a variable course – often brief and self-limiting but occasionally persistent or progressive – the distinction between prevalent and incident disease is not always easy.

A further difficulty arises from the observation that a high proportion of people with sarcoidosis are asymptomatic, their 'disease' being detected only by 'chance'. This finding is best established for pulmonary sarcoidosis where between a third and a half of patients report no symptoms but have their condition recognized usually through chest radiography undertaken for another purpose (Table 3.1). It seems probable that a similar situation pertains for sarcoid at other sites. Taken together, these difficulties result in a degree of 'misclassification' of disease and, in comparative studies, of non-disease – although given the low prevalence of sarcoidosis the latter is unlikely to be very important.

STUDY POPULATIONS

It is not easy to assemble sufficiently large, representative populations of patients with sarcoidosis for epidemiological

Table 3.1   Proportion of patients with pulmonary sarcoid whose condition was asymptomatic at presentation.

Reference	Country	Method of case ascertainment	Proportion of cases asymptomatic at presentation
(Sutherland et al. 1965)	UK	Radiographic screening	56%
BTTA (1969)	UK	Hospital clinics	31%
(Hillerdal et al. 1984)	Sweden	Population health screening	68%
(Hennessy et al. 1988)	USA	Hospital clinics	52%
Milman and Selroos (1990)	Scandinavia (various)	Radiographic screening + hospital clinics	35–58%

study; and in this context it is worth noting that mortality attributed to sarcoidosis is too rare to be of great use.

Perhaps the most widely used method, and one which is particularly suited to detailed study, is the 'case registry' of patients receiving hospital care. Such registries generally include patients with well-characterized disease, although misclassification is by no means avoided altogether. This apparent benefit is offset by difficulties in defining and enumerating a base population, making the estimation of disease rates very difficult; by the difficulty of separating incident from prevalent cases; and further by the variability in clinical features which means that patients may present to a number of different clinical specialties. In some settings, uncertainties over differential access to relevant hospital care may compound these difficulties (Gorham et al. 2004). Variations on the 'hospital series' include registries based on primary care populations such as insurance schemes in the United States or family practices in the United Kingdom. While they seldom include sufficient information for detailed study, such registries probably provide more valid information on disease rates and trends.

In the days when mass radiography was widely practiced it provided a valuable if limited tool for the epidemiological study of sarcoidosis. Thus population-based chest X-ray screening in several European countries and occupational screening, notably in the US military and in Japanese railway workers, have been used to derive and compare rates of prevalent and, in some cases, incident disease. These approaches have the advantages of size (often very large populations are included), of available information on denominators and of their capacity to detect incidental disease. On the other hand, they are limited to the detection of disease that includes pulmonary involvement, are dependent on the assiduousness with which suspected cases are investigated further, and – particularly for the study of causative factors – by the often narrow spectrum of the study population or information that is available. In any case the approach is seldom used now.

ONE DISEASE, ONE CAUSE?

While tempting, it is probably unrealistic to consider that sarcoidosis has a single 'cause'. Certainly, in the 130 years since the condition was first described, as a skin disorder (Hutchinson 1877), many have been considered but none – with

the exception of inhaled beryllium – has yet survived scrutiny (Box 3.1). There is good evidence to suggest that the granulomas that are characteristic of sarcoidosis develop as an immunological response to a persistent, poorly degradable antigenic stimulus; infectious agents and both inorganic and organic particulates can initiate the formation of pulmonary immune granulomas, particularly when they have low biodegradability and/or persistence within macrophages (Boros 1986a). The obvious analogy is with mycobacterial infection (Narayanan 1988), but schistosomal organisms appear to have a similar capacity (Boros 1986b). Several features of the distribution of sarcoidosis broadly favor an infective etiology, albeit one that might have a delayed onset of clinical presentation; the disease is roughly as common in men as in women, tends to present in youth (although rarely in childhood), and there is limited evidence of clustering in time and space. These issues are considered in more detail later. Whatever the environmental stimuli – and most would consider sarcoidosis to be the result of such – it is very probable that constitutional or genetic factors play an important role in both susceptibility and the mode of presentation.

Box 3.1 Selected agents considered in the etiology of sarcoidosis (none except beryllium is definitively established)

Infective agents
- mycobacterial (TB)
- mycobacterial (non-tuberculous)
- bacterial
- mycoplasma
- viral

Organic agents
- pine pollen
- bird antigens
- moulds

Mineral agents
- beryllium
- clay (pica)
- talc
- silica
- zirconium
- other metal dusts

DISTRIBUTIONS

How common is sarcoidosis?

Sarcoidosis is often short-lived and self-limiting, but it is in some cases a chronic disease that persists for many years, although it is seldom cited as a cause of death. Consequently the relationship between its incidence (the number of new cases over a defined time period) and its prevalence (the number of cases at a defined time point) may not be easy to determine.

Available measures of prevalence suggest that sarcoidosis is not a common condition. Mass radiographic surveys in Scandinavia in the 1950s and 60s suggested an overall prevalence of 28 per 100 000 (Milman and Selroos 1990); estimates from the UK in the same period were broadly similar, varying from 9 per 100 000 (McGregor 1961) to 36 per 100 000 (Anderson et al. 1963) of those screened. Similar studies from other parts of the world, however, reveal considerable variation.

Bauer and Löfgren (1964) compiled the findings of 29 such surveys from 24 countries, in ten instances nationwide. While the highest estimate of prevalence was in Sweden (64 per 100 000), far lower estimates (0.2 per 100 000) were made in Portugal and South America. Such variability may reflect differences in etiological exposures and susceptibility, but it probably reveals also differences in diagnostic practice and in the age, sex and morbid distributions of the screened populations.

Incidence rates derived from mass radiography campaigns also vary and probably for the same reasons. Annual estimates derived from nationwide screening programs in Scandinavia range from 14 per 100 000 (Riddervold 1964; Fog and Wilbek 1974) to 42 per 100 000 (Wallgren 1958). These are close to those measured in men working for the US Navy who were subjected to regular chest radiography; annual, age-adjusted incidence rates in that population varied from 7.6 per 100 000 in white men to 81.8 per 100 000 in African-American men (Sartwell and Edwards 1974). Reassuringly similar estimates were derived from a UK trial of BCG vaccination for tuberculosis in which regular chest radiography was used. There, Sutherland and colleagues (1965) reported annual incidence rates of sarcoidosis of between 8.0 and 12.7 per 100 000 among young men and women. Similarly, following a 'general health' screening program in Uppsala, Sweden, in which the take-up rate was 64 percent, the annual incidence was reported to be 24 per 100 000 of those screened (Hillerdal et al. 1984). In contrast, the incidence among Japanese railway workers undergoing annual chest radiography was much lower – just 1.5 per 100 000 (Hiraga et al. 1974).

For the reasons outlined above, one would expect estimates of disease incidence that are derived from case registries to be lower than those arising from mass surveys. Broadly speaking this is manifest, with the difference approximating to the proportion of (pulmonary) cases that are asymptomatic. Thus the overall incidence among patients registered with family practices in the UK was 5.0 per 100 000 (Gribbin et al. 2006), very close to the figure measured in insured populations and case registries in the USA (Henke et al. 1986; Rybicki et al. 1997) and again but earlier in the UK (BTTA 1969). That such

figures are likely to underestimate the true incidence was confirmed by a four-fold difference when 'special efforts' were made rather than a reliance only on a retrospective examination of case records in the Isle of Man (Parkes et al. 1985). The relatively low incidence in Japan – around 1 per 100 000 – seems to be confirmed using the case-register approach (Morimoto et al. 2003).

Considered together, this evidence indicates, with perhaps surprising consistency, that the overall annual incidence of sarcoidosis in western Europe and the USA is between 5 and 10 per 100 000. The point prevalence of disease is perhaps twice as high, reflecting its sometimes chronic nature. These figures suggest, cumulatively, a lifetime risk of disease of about 1 per cent (Rybicki et al. 1997). Evidence from other parts of the world is far more limited, but what is available suggests lower disease frequencies in Japanese and possibly South American populations.

Data on temporal trends in the incidence of sarcoidosis are not easily interpreted but except in certain instances suggest no important changes over the relatively brief time periods examined. Rates of new disease changed little in a large UK population over three time periods between 1991 and 2003 (Gribbin et al. 2006), and nor did they in Japan between 1960 and 1988 (Yamaguchi et al. 1989) or East Germany between 1970 and 1985 (Scharkoff 1987). In the USA, age-adjusted mortality rates increased but only marginally over a 12-year period between 1979 and 1991; from 1.3 to 1.6 per 100 000 and from 1.9 to 2.5 per 100 000 in men and women respectively (Gideon and Mannino 1996). In stark contrast, the incidence among naval personnel in the USA fell between 1975 and 2001 (Gorham et al. 2004) and especially in black men; it is not clear how far this decline was attributable to (differential) changes in ascertainment or diagnostic practice.

Age, sex and race

Sarcoidosis has been reported to present in childhood but this appears to be very unusual. No cases under the age of 15 years were reported from surveys in the Isle of Man (Parkes et al. 1985), mainland UK (BTTA 1969) or the USA (Henke et al. 1986). In a Japanese series of 2079 cases, half of whom were identified through mass radiography, just 29 (1.4 percent) were children aged under ten years (Hosoda et al. 1976). Similarly, the disease is very rarely recognized anew in the elderly (Gribbin et al. 2006).

Consistently, the peak age of incidence is reported to be in young adulthood (25–40 years) with perhaps a second crest in the sixth decade, more obviously in women. This broad pattern has been observed using different study methods in Scandinavian (Milman and Selroos 1990), North American (Sartwell and Edwards 1974; Henke et al. 1986; Baughman et al. 2001) and British (BTTA 1969; Gribben et al. 2006) populations. A slightly later average age of onset in women has been seen in the Isle of Man (Parkes et al. 1985) and in Sweden (Hillerdal et al. 1984); and there is some evidence of an upward shift over time in both men and women (Morimoto et al. 2003; Byg et al. 2003) – although, as above, this may reflect temporal variations in ascertainment and diagnostic practice.

A similarly consistent finding has been the observation that sarcoidosis is more frequent among women than men, although the difference seems to be less marked than many believe. Earlier studies, employing a variety of methods, indicated substantial sex differences. A survey of cases presenting to hospital clinics in the UK in the 1960s, for example, suggested that the incidence among women was 40 percent higher than among men (BTTA 1969), a pattern found elsewhere in the same country (Sutherland et al. 1965) and also in Sweden in the same era (Milman and Selmoos 1990). Studies of occupational groups tend, of course, to be less useful in this respect. More recent evidence, for example from the UK (Gribbin et al. 2006), suggests a far smaller sex difference. In any case, such variation does not necessarily reflect differences in exposure or susceptibility but may be the result of systematic bias in disease ascertainment arising, for example, from differential access to diagnostic services. Interestingly, the experience of the Uppsala screening program in Sweden suggests that, in that setting, women were less likely than men to have their disease detected by chance (Hillerdal et al. 1984).

As suggested above, there seem to be important 'racial' differences in rates of sarcoidosis. Any such observations need to be considered with care since they may in fact represent differences in exposure and/or disease ascertainment rather than any innate differences in susceptibility. Moreover they depend crucially on valid estimates of the appropriate denominators which are seldom available for studies of case registries. That susceptibility may be important, however, is suggested by the consistent finding of inter-racial differences in disease phenotype. Studies of both civilian and military men and women in the USA indicate that the disease has a higher incidence among black than white people (Sartwell et al. 1974; Gideon and Mannino 1996; Rybicki et al. 1997; McDonough and Gray 2000), the reported differences being between five- and ten-fold. Similar observations have been made in the UK (Edmondstone and Wilson 1985) and in South Africa (Benatar 1997).

There is good evidence, from both clinical and epidemiological experience, that different racial groups tend to present with different phenotypes of disease (Baughman et al. 2001). Thus erythema nodosum is more common in white European and North American populations than in black or Japanese populations (Pietinalho et al. 1996), whereas eye and skin presentations seem respectively to be more frequent in black or Puerto Rican groups. In general, extrathoracic – and thus 'widespread' – disease is reported more often in people of African origin than in white patients (Israel and Washburne 1980). While these patterns are usually attributed to complex interactions between innate susceptibility and environmental exposure(s) (Kreider et al. 2005), it is likely that, at least in some parts of the world, they reflect differential access to medical or screening services (Rabin et al. 2004).

Place

As with most aspects of the distribution of this complex disease, geographical comparisons of the frequency of sarcoi-

dosis depend critically on the quality of its ascertainment. For example, the apparent rarity of the disease in rural Africa almost certainly, but to an unknown degree, reflects under-recognition and the very real difficulty of distinguishing the disease from endemic tuberculosis. Even in countries with broadly equal access to necessarily sophisticated diagnostic services and with broadly similar views on what constitutes a case of the disease, reported geographical differences – as with those for age, sex and race – require careful deliberation.

What evidence there is from such settings suggests that the prevalence of sarcoidosis is higher at higher latitudes and roughly displays a north–south gradient. Explanations for this are uncertain at best, but it is noteworthy that other complex diseases (such as multiple sclerosis) whose causes are unknown but where infective etiologies have been postulated follow a similar geographical pattern. Intra-country comparisons, in which ascertainment and diagnosis are probably more uniform, have been less convincing. In a hospital case series from the UK (BTTA 1969), the highest incidence of disease was in the most southern of four study areas with a steady decrease northward, although the maximum distance between centers was just 600 miles. Estimates made in the USA and summarized by Bresnitz and Strom (1983) suggested, with reasonable consistency, that the disease was more frequent in those who currently resided in southern and eastern states; that this pattern was not solely attributable to race is indicated by the use of stratified analyses in several surveys suggesting that the risks for African-Americans living in these areas were consistently higher than for the white population.

Migrant studies have been used successfully for several diseases in which (early) infection may play a causal role; but not, it seems, for sarcoidosis. Interestingly, in their population-based case series from Rochester in the USA, Hennessy and colleagues (1988) reported that immigrants who had been resident in the community for fewer than five years were more likely than others to present with asymptomatic disease, probably as a result of routine medical screening including chest radiography. Thus, estimates of disease rates in this group are probably elevated artificially.

Clustering

Clustering of disease in place and/or time might indicate a shared environment (perhaps in relation to a transmissible agent) or a shared susceptibility (particularly for clustering among related persons) or, again, be a feature of selective ascertainment. There are several reports that the frequency of sarcoidosis among family members is higher than would be expected; their results reflect in part the care with which disease in non-index individuals was sought and identified. The highest frequency was found in an Irish population of 114 patients registered with a specialist clinic (Brennan et al. 1984). Eleven (9.6 percent) had one or more siblings with sarcoidosis (self-reported on questionnaire) suggesting a prevalence, in the sibling pool, of about 2.5 percent, a figure higher than that estimated for the general population. A similar proportion (10 percent) of African-American patients recruited in the USA were reported to have one or more affected siblings (Headings *et al.* 1976). A questionnaire survey of 406 patients attending a specialist clinic in the UK suggested that about 6 percent had one or more relatives with biopsy-proven sarcoidosis; the relative risk of disease in a sibling compared to the population prevalence was estimated to be between 36 and 73, indicative of significant familial clustering (McGrath *et al.* 2000). Findings from other studies using a variety of methods have reported much lower frequencies ranging between 0.8 and 4.6 percent (Sharma *et al.* 1976; Rybicki *et al.* 2001). The differences may relate to race; there is some evidence that familial aggregation is higher among white than black patients (Rybicki *et al.* 2001) and, perhaps unsurprisingly, among siblings than other relatives. Studies of affected families suggest a polygenic mode of inheritance with an important contribution from genes of the major histocompatibility complex (Schurmann *et al.* 2000).

Unarguably the most detailed study of disease clustering was that carried out among cases detected on the Isle of Man (Hills *et al.* 1987). In contrast to the above, the focus was on clustering in time and place. Using a method developed by Pike and Smith (1974) and with reference to a control group of patients selected at random from pathology and radiology records at the same hospital, there was a highly significant increase in links between cases whose places of residence, during an 'infective period' of five years before and two years after diagnosis, were separated by distances of less than 100 meters. No excess of residential links within 500 meters or of school or recreational links was found; a significant increase in workplace links may have reflected the fact that almost 10 per cent of cases were health workers in the (small) island's single hospital. An increase in case pairs diagnosed within one year of each other provided some evidence for temporal clustering within the same population.

This interesting approach merits further study in other settings. Unfortunately, other reports of 'clusters' depend only on small and uncontrolled case series of patients reported to have been 'in contact' with one another (Cummings *et al.* 1959; Terris and Chaves 1966; Stewart and Davidson 1982; Edmondstone and Wilson 1985), so their findings are difficult to interpret. Finally, Hosoda and colleagues (1976) failed to detect any evidence of time–space clustering in two areas of Japan.

Seasonal clustering of sarcoidosis, which would be suggestive of an infective etiology, has been examined in several settings. Studies of this sort are, of course, more straightforward for disease where the date of onset is readily established. This is not obviously the case for much sarcoidosis where the date of diagnosis may bear little relationship to the date of disease inception; but potentially useful information can be achieved by restricting analysis to cases of probable recent-onset disease. In Spain, among a population of patients with *erythema nodosum* and bilateral hilar lymphadenopathy, almost half had a diagnosis made between April and June (Bardinas *et al.* 1989). Similarly, Japanese patients with bilateral hilar lymphadenopathy, identified through a nation-wide case-finding exercise, were most frequently detected during the months June and July (Hosoda *et al.* 1976), a pattern that was recognized among both those identified by mass radiography and those presenting with symptomatic disease. In Greece, following mass radiography of almost 85 000 adults between 1980 and 1989, 70 percent of cases ($n = 40$) were identified between the months of March and May in each year; there were no diagnoses of asymptomatic stage I disease made between the months of July and November (Panayeas *et al.* 1991). In Norfolk, England, an 'outbreak' of eight cases of acute sarcoidosis, accompanied by arthropathy, was reported in May 1988 (Jawad *et al.* 1989); unfortunately, any family or other spatial contacts between the cases were not described.

ETIOLOGY

The fundamental purpose of the descriptive epidemiology of sarcoidosis, such as that outlined above, is the generaton of testable etiological hypotheses and, ultimately, the development of methods for primary disease prevention. Unhappily, few strong hypotheses have emerged and fewer still have proved robust enough to attract repeated analysis.

Perhaps the most valiant effort to explore etiology to date has been the ACCESS study, a large case–control analysis of hospital-ascertained patients and community controls in the USA (Rossman and Kreider 2007). Although ambitious in purpose and certainly fruitful in many respects – not least the demonstration that such work is possible – the study failed to provide any major advances in our understanding of causation. Indeed it might be argued that its (case–control) design was intrinsically unsuitable to the generation, rather than testing, of etiological hypotheses.

Infective agents

Probably the best candidate for an etiological hypothesis is infection. Several features of the distribution of sarcoidosis – its sex and age, and perhaps geographical, patterns and the (admittedly slim) evidence for spatial and seasonal clustering – suggest that the disease reflects an idiosyncratic response to an infective agent. The predilection for respiratory involvement favors, but does not confirm, an airborne transmission; the histological and immunological analogies with mycobacterial disease are well known, as is the observation that *erythema nodosum*, an established manifestation of 'acute' sarcoidosis, may be a consequence of infection with a variety of organisms.

Support for an infective – or at least a transmissible – etiology is lent by the passage experiments of Mitchell and colleagues (Mitchell and Rees 1969, 1970; Mitchell *et al.* 1976). In a murine model, these suggested that a granulomatous response could be produced by the inoculation of pooled, filtered homogenates or supernatants of mouse granulomatous tissue into other mice. Some other researchers have found it difficult to confirm these findings.

While most studies of potential causal organisms have focused on mycobacteria, it is worth reflecting that the reduction in the incidence of tuberculosis in many parts of the world has not apparently been followed by changes in the incidence of sarcoidosis; and while cardiac and salivary gland involvement are characteristic of sarcoidosis they are rare in established mycobacterial disease. Some studies have detected higher levels of mycobacterial antibodies in patients with sarcoidosis than in normal controls (Chapman and Speight 1964; Milman and Selroos 1990); and in the animal passage experiments described above, acid-fast organisms were found in some tissues, and mycobacteria with characteristics of *M. tuberculosis* were grown from some homogenates. The apparent inconsistency in this area may be explained by the technical difficulties in isolating cell-wall-deficient organisms; using an antibody raised against *M. tuberculosis* whole-cell antigen (HR37RV), Almenoff and colleagues (1996) identified cell-wall-deficient forms in patients with sarcoidosis.

The rapid development of molecular biology promises much in this field but has not yet provided consistent evidence. As with earlier methods, even new technologies have the limitations of imperfect sensitivity and specificity and failure to detect mycobacteria may reflect insensitive tools, whereas positive results may reflect contamination (Cosma *et al.* 2004). In a systematic review of 31 molecular studies, Gupta and associates (2007) reported that 26 percent of 874 patients had mycobacterial-positive findings, a prevalence between 10 and 20 times higher than in controls without sarcoidosis. There was considerable heterogeneity between the reports with detection rates varying from 0 to 100 percent (Rossman and Kreider 2007; Moller and Chen 2002; Brown *et al.* 2003).

It is difficult to judge such findings, and in any case the detection of an infectious relic does not necessarily imply cause since some infectious agents may traffic to established granulomas (Cosma *et al.* 2004). Conversely, at least some cases of sarcoidosis may be caused by a sustained immunological reaction to retained antigens of infective origin that are peculiarly difficult to detect. Through selective proteomic analysis of poorly soluble protein aggregates derived from affected tissues, Song and associates (2005) identified mycobacterial catalase–peroxidase (mKatG) – and circulating, specific IgG antibodies – in most sarcoidosis tissues but in none of the disease-free controls. Arguably, this might explain also the poverty of any therapeutic response to antimycobacterial treatment in most patients with sarcoidosis.

Attention has focused also on 'commensal' microorganisms of low virulence, notably *Propionibacter* species commonly implicated in acne. Abe and colleagues (1984) in Japan reported culture of *P. acnes* in 31 of 40 lymph nodes from 40 patients with sarcoidosis (and about 20 percent of patients with other diseases); this organism and others from the same species are capable of inducing granulomatous responses when injected into sensitized rabbits and rats (Yi *et al.* 1996; Ichiyasu *et al.* 1999). Subsequently Ishige, Eishi and their associates reported using PCR to look for propionibacterial DNA in lymph nodes of sarcoidosis patients, identifying evidence of the organisms in 80 and 98 of samples, respectively, both proportions higher than in referent patients without sarcoidosis (Ishige *et al.* 1999; Eishi *et al.* 2002). Furthermore, Ebe and associates (2000) reported that a recombinant protein from a *P. acnes* DNA expression library causes a proliferative response in peripheral blood mononuclear cells from some patients with sarcoidosis but not in healthy controls.

As with studies of mycobacterial infection, these promising findings have been somewhat dampened by evidence of

P. acnes in peripheral lung tissue and mediastinal lymph nodes of normal individuals, suggesting that *Propionibacter* species might be pulmonary commensals (Ishige *et al.* 2005). Nonetheless the implication that one or more widely prevalent organisms of relatively low pathogenicity may be important concurs with much of the epidemiology of sarcoidosis, and further studies such as these are probably warranted.

Occupational and 'environmental' exposures

The observation of 'Salem sarcoid' among women working in fluorescent light bulb factories in Massachusetts in the 1940s prompted both the recognition of inhaled beryllium as a cause of pulmonary granulomatous disease, and the search for other occupational causes of sarcoidosis. Perhaps unsurprisingly, given the approximately equal sex distribution of the disease, the findings have not been impressive. Some of this probably reflects the relatively primitive methods of identifying occupational exposures, many studies reliant on self-reports with no systematic attempts to collect objective information.

An exception was the ACCESS case–control study from which it was suggested that those with occupations in bird rearing, car manufacture, teaching, cotton manufacture and with exposure to radiation were at an increased risk; self-reported occupational exposures to insecticides, 'musty odours', air-conditioning and (non-occupationally) birds were isolated as particularly important (Newman *et al.* 2004). Many of these have been identified as causal in other granulomatous lung diseases and, as in other studies of occupational exposures, the question of disease misclassification deserves consideration. In contrast, no high-incidence occupational groups were identified in a series of cases identified through hospital clinics in Britain (BTTA 1969).

Cummings and associates (1959) reported an increased frequency of previous work in the lumber industry among US military patients with sarcoidosis, but this was not confirmed by subsequent study of patients identified through a specialist clinic (Buck and Sartwell 1961). Sarcoidosis developing in three firemen, all of whom had trained together, would point toward exposure to a common environmental antigen (Kern *et al.* 1993). Such findings and the (small) increase of sarcoidosis seen in some studies of firefighters (Prezant *et al.* 1999) and those living in rural areas (Kajdasz *et al.* 2001) have led to the hypothesis that the handling or burning of timber may lead to the development of sarcoidosis. More recently, it has been reported that the frequency of sarcoidosis among New York firefighters increased about four-fold following the World Trade Center incident in 2001 (Izbicki *et al.* 2007).

All such studies are hampered by the related issues of diagnostic ascertainment and the selection of a suitable referent population. An increased frequency of sarcoidosis in particular (often high-income) occupational groups was reported in Minnesota, USA (Hennessy *et al.* 1988) where 24 health professionals (14 physicians and 10 nurses) were included among the 129 identified cases, a proportion (19 percent of all cases) probably far higher than that in the general population. Similarly, Edmondstone (1988) observed that 15 percent of 156 cases identified through specialist hospital services were hospital workers, and 16 (10 percent) were nurses – although all of the latter group had 'substantial symptoms' and none had presented through employment screening services. Nonetheless, any study of occupation will need to dissociate the effects of differential access to diagnostic services.

Smoking

An intriguingly consistent findings has been the relatively low prevalence of cigarette smoking among patients with sarcoidosis; a selection of relevant studies is presented in Table 3.2. In some studies, decreasing risk estimates for those with heavier smoking habits have been observed (e.g. Bresnitz *et al.* 1986; Douglas *et al.* 1986).

A variety of biological explanations has been postulated. It is interesting that a similar inverse relationship has been reported in extrinsic allergic alveolitis (Arima *et al.* 1992), also a granulomatous pulmonary disease. Such relationships need, however, to be interpreted with care. In the study reported by Bresnitz and colleagues, for example, the association between smoking and sarcoidosis was not significant after statistical adjustment for socioeconomic status as measured by family income. Thus it is plausible that there may be an increase in ascertainment of sarcoidosis among high-income groups in whom cigarette smoking is less frequent.

CONCLUSION

Studying and interpreting the epidemiology of sarcoidosis is not easy. The disease is uncommon and, when suspected, requires relatively sophisticated techniques to distinguish it from other, more common diseases; much of it is asymptomatic. In such situations, particularly where diagnosis is difficult, determination and comparison of disease frequencies depends critically on access to diagnostic services. Bias in ascertainment, compounded by differences in diagnostic criteria and uncertainties about denominator populations, can easily lead to erroneous conclusions.

Nonetheless, several features of the disease's distribution across populations appear clear. Importantly it is primarily a disease of young adults with an approximately equal sex distribution, although perhaps a little more common in women. It is rare in childhood. Racial differences in incidence

are difficult to distinguish from confounding exposures, but it is probably a disease more common in black populations and there is good evidence of differences in disease presentation across races. Geographical differences exist and although difficult to interpret there may be an increasing frequency of disease with increasing latitude. Spatial clusters have been reported, but perhaps more interestingly has been their apparent rarity. What may be an 'acute' form of the disease appears to present more commonly in spring months. There has been no clear change in disease frequency, within populations, across time.

To date, analytic epidemiological studies, using observational techniques to test specific hypotheses arising from descriptive surveys, have been unconvincing; in large part because few such hypotheses have been developed. However it seems reasonable to suggest that sarcoidosis is an idiosyncratic response to one or more relatively common environmental agents. By analogy with berylliosis, some have suggested a role for (unidentified) inorganic, airborne dusts. Given the age distribution of the disease this seems intrinsically improbable; an occupationally encountered agent, furthermore, would be unlikely to manifest with an approximately equal sex distribution. Alternatively, and plausibly in the light of its pathological similarities with pulmonary tuberculosis, many have suggested that sarcoidosis is an unusual response to an environmental infectious agent or persistent antigen.

It is clear that novel approaches are required to explain many of the epidemiological features of the disease. Future studies will most probably continue to take advantage of the relative efficiency of the case–control design but will require more careful consideration of disease ascertainment and the selection of an appropriate referent group than has been typical to date. Further examination of the infective question might profitably employ newer techniques of molecular analysis of the polymorphic bacterial 16S-rRNA gene to characterize the composition of bacterial (and other microbiological) communities from the tissues of affected patients.

REFERENCES

Abe C, Iwai K, Mikami R, Hosoda Y (1984). Frequent isolation of *Propionibacterium acnes* from sarcoidosis lymph nodes. *Zentralbl Bakteriol Mikrobiol Hyg A* 256: 541–7.
Almenoff PL, Johnson A, Lesser M, Mattman LH (1996). Growth of acid-fast L forms from the blood of patients with sarcoidosis. *Thorax* 51: 530–3.

Table 3.2   Smoking in sarcoidosis: selected case-referent studies.

Reference	Country	Referent population	Number of patients (sarcoidosis)	Proportion ever smoking	Odds ratio
Terris and Chaves (1966)	USA	Hospital outpatients	240	53%	0.80
Douglas *et al.* (1986)	UK	General population	183	22%	0.36
Harf *et al.* (1986)	France	Healthy volunteers	101	25%	0.26
Bresnitz *et al.* (1986)	USA	Hospital outpatients	51	55%	0.70
Newman *et al.* (2004)	USA	General population	736	45%	0.62

Anderson R, Brett GZ, James DG, Siltzbach LE (1963). The prevalence of intrathoracic sarcoidosis. *Med Thorac* **20**: 152–62.

Arima K, Ando M, Ito K *et al.* (1992). Effect of cigarette smoking on prevalence of summer-type hypersensitivity pneumonitis caused by *Trichosporon cutaneum. Arch Environ Health* **47**: 274–8.

Bardinas F, Morera J, Fite E, Plasencia A (1989). Seasonal clustering of sarcoidosis. *Lancet* **2**(8660): 455–6.

Bauer HJ, Löfgren S (1964). International study of pulmonary sarcoidosis in mass chest radiography. *Acta Med Scand Suppl* **425**: 103–5.

Baughman RP, Teirstein AS, Judson MA *et al.* (2001). Clinical characteristics of patients in a case–control study of sarcoidosis. *Am J Respir Crit Care Med* **164**(10 Pt 1): 1885–9.

Benatar SR (1997). Sarcoidosis in South Africa: a comparative study in Whites, Blacks and Coloureds. *S Afr Med J* **52**: 602–6.

Boros DL (1986a). Immunoregulation of granuloma formation in murine schistosomiasis mansoni. *Ann NY Acad Sci* **465**: 313–23.

Boros DL (1986b). Experimental granulomatosis. *Clin Dermatol* **4**(4): 10–21.

Brennan NJ, Crean P, Long JP, Fitzgerald MX (1984). High prevalence of familial sarcoidosis in an Irish population. *Thorax* **39**: 14–18.

Bresnitz EA, Strom BL (1983). Epidemiology of sarcoidosis. *Epidemiol Rev* **5**: 124–56.

Bresnitz EA, Stolley PD, Israel HL, Soper K (1986). Possible risk factors for sarcoidosis: a case–control study. *Ann NY Acad Sci* **465**: 632–42.

Brown ST, Brett I, Almenoff PL *et al.* (2003). Recovery of cell wall-deficient organisms from blood does not distinguish between patients with sarcoidosis and control subjects. *Chest* **123**: 413–17.

BTTA (1969). Geographical variations in the incidence of sarcoidosis in Great Britain: a comparative study of four areas. A report to the Research Committee of the British Thoracic and Tuberculosis Association. *Tubercle* **50**: 211–32.

Buck AA, Sartwell PE (1961). Epidemiologic investigations of sarcoidosis. II: Skin sensitivity and environmental factors. *Am J Hyg* **74**: 152–73.

Byg KE, Milman N, Hansen S (2003). Sarcoidosis in Denmark, 1980–1994: a registry-based incidence study comprising 5536 patients. *Sarcoidosis Vasc Diffuse Lung Dis* **20**: 46–52.

Chapman JS, Speight M (1964). Further studies of mycobacterial antibodies in the sera of sarcoidosis patients. *Acta Med Scand Suppl* **425**: 61–7.

Cosma CL, Humbert O, Ramakrishnan L (2004). Superinfecting mycobacteria home to established tuberculous granulomas. *Nat Immunol* **5**: 828–35.

Cummings MM, Dunner E, Williams JH (1959). Epidemiologic and clinical observations in sarcoidosis. *Ann Intern Med* **50**: 879–90.

Douglas JG, Middleton WG, Gaddie J *et al.* (1986). Sarcoidosis: a disorder commoner in non-smokers? *Thorax* **41**: 787–91.

Ebe Y, Ikushima S, Yamaguchi T *et al.* (2000). Proliferative response of peripheral blood mononuclear cells and levels of antibody to recombinant protein from *Propionibacterium acnes* DNA expression library in Japanese patients with sarcoidosis. *Sarcoidosis Vasc Diffuse Lung Dis* **17**: 256–65.

Edmondstone WM (1988). Sarcoidosis in nurses: is there an association? *Thorax* **43**: 342–3.

Edmondstone WM, Wilson AG (1985). Sarcoidosis in Caucasians, Blacks and Asians in London. *Br J Dis Chest* **79**(1): 27–36.

Eishi Y, Suga M, Ishige I *et al.* (2002). Quantitative analysis of mycobacterial and propionibacterial DNA in lymph nodes of Japanese and European patients with sarcoidosis. *J Clin Microbiol* **40**: 198–204.

Fog J, Wilbek E (1974). [The epidemiology of sarcoidosis in Denmark]. *Ugeskr Laeger* **136**: 2183–91.

Gideon NM, Mannino DM (1996). Sarcoidosis mortality in the United States, 1979–1991: an analysis of multiple-cause mortality data. *Am J Med* **100**: 423–7.

Gorham ED, Garland CF, Garland FC *et al.* (2004). Trends and occupational associations in incidence of hospitalized pulmonary sarcoidosis and other lung diseases in Navy personnel: a 27-year historical prospective study, 1975–2001. *Chest* **126**: 1431–8.

Gribbin J, Hubbard RB, Le JI *et al.* (2006). Incidence and mortality of idiopathic pulmonary fibrosis and sarcoidosis in the UK. *Thorax* **61**: 980–5.

Gupta D, Agarwal R, Aggarwal AN, Jindal SK (2007). Molecular evidence for the role of mycobacteria in sarcoidosis: a meta-analysis. *Eur Respir J* **30**: 508–16.

Harf RA, Ethevenaux C, Gleize J *et al.* (1986). Reduced prevalence of smokers in sarcoidosis: results of a case–control study. *Ann NY Acad Sci* **465**: 625–31.

Headings VE, Weston D, Young RC, Hackney RL (1976). Familial sarcoidosis with multiple occurrences in eleven families: a possible mechanism of inheritance. *Ann NY Acad Sci* **278**: 377–85.

Henke CE, Henke G, Elveback LR *et al.* (1986). The epidemiology of sarcoidosis in Rochester, Minnesota: a population-based study of incidence and survival. *Am J Epidemiol* **123**: 840–5.

Hennessy TW, Ballard DJ, DeRemee RA *et al.* (1988). The influence of diagnostic access bias on the epidemiology of sarcoidosis: a population-based study in Rochester, Minnesota, 1935–1984. *J Clin Epidemiol* **41**: 565–70.

Hillerdal G, Nou E, Osterman K, Schmekel B (1984). Sarcoidosis: epidemiology and prognosis. A 15-year European study. *Am Rev Respir Dis* **130**: 29–32.

Hills SE, Parkes SA, Baker SB (1987). Epidemiology of sarcoidosis in the Isle of Man. 2: Evidence for space–time clustering. *Thorax* **42**: 427–30.

Hiraga Y, Hosoda Y, Odaka M (1974). Epidemiology of sarcoidosis in a Japanese working group: a ten-year study. In: Iwai K, Hosoda Y (eds). *Proceedings of the 6th International Conference on Sarcoidosis.* Tokyo, Japan, pp. 303–6.

Hosoda Y, Hiraga Y, Odaka M *et al.* (1976). A cooperative study of sarcoidosis in Asia and Africa: analytic epidemiology. *Ann NY Acad Sci* **278**: 355–67.

Hutchinson J (1877). Case of livid papillary psoriasis. In: *Illustrations of Clinical Surgery.* J&A Churchill, London, pp. 42–3.

Ichiyasu H, Suga M, Matsukawa A *et al.* (1999). Functional roles of MCP-1 in *Propionibacterium acnes*-induced, T cell-mediated pulmonary granulomatosis in rabbits. *J Leukoc Biol* **65**: 482–91.

Ishige I, Eishi Y, Takemura T *et al.* (2005). *Propionibacterium acnes* is the most common bacterium commensal in peripheral lung tissue and mediastinal lymph nodes from subjects without sarcoidosis. *Sarcoidosis Vasc Diffuse Lung Dis* **22**: 33–42.

Ishige I, Usui Y, Takemura T, Eishi Y (1999). Quantitative PCR of mycobacterial and propionibacterial DNA in lymph nodes of Japanese patients with sarcoidosis. *Lancet* **354**(9173): 120–3.

Israel HL, Washburne JD (1980). Characteristics of sarcoidosis in black and white patients. In: *Proceedings of the 8th International Conference on Sarcoidosis.* Alpha Omega, Cardiff, pp. 497–507.

Izbicki G, Chavko R, Banauch GI *et al.* (2007). World Trade Center 'sarcoid-like' granulomatous pulmonary disease in New York City Fire Department rescue workers. *Chest* **131**: 1414–23.

Jawad AS, Hamour AA, Wenley WG, Scott DG (1989). An outbreak of acute sarcoidosis with arthropathy in Norfolk. *Br J Rheumatol* **28**(2): 178.

Joint Statement of the American Thoracic Society (ATS), the European Respiratory Society (ERS) and the World Association of Sarcoidosis and Other Granulomatous Disorders (WASOG) (1999). *Am J Respir Crit Care Med* 160: 736–55.

Kajdasz DK, Lackland DT, Mohr LC, Judson MA (2001). A current assessment of rurally linked exposures as potential risk factors for sarcoidosis. *Ann Epidemiol* 11: 111–17.

Kern DG, Neill MA, Wrenn DS, Varone JC (1993). Investigation of a unique time–space cluster of sarcoidosis in firefighters. *Am Rev Respir Dis* 148(4 Pt 1): 974–80.

Kreider ME, Christie JD, Thompson B et al. (2005). Relationship of environmental exposures to the clinical phenotype of sarcoidosis. *Chest* 128: 207–15.

McDonough C, Gray GC (2000). Risk factors for sarcoidosis hospitalization among US Navy and Marine Corps personnel, 1981–1995. *Mil Med* 165: 630–2.

McGrath DS, Daniil Z, Foley P et al. (2000). Epidemiology of familial sarcoidosis in the UK. *Thorax* 55: 751–4.

McGregor I (1961). *The Two Year Mass Radiography Campaign in Scotland, 1957–1958* [abstract]. HMSO, Edinburgh.

Milman N, Selroos O (1990). Pulmonary sarcoidosis in the Nordic countries, 1950–1982: epidemiology and clinical picture. *Sarcoidosis* 7(1): 50–7.

Mitchell DN, Rees RJ (1969). A transmissible agent from sarcoid tissue. *Lancet* 2(7611): 81–4.

Mitchell DN, Rees RJ (1970). An attempt to demonstrate a transmissible agent from sarcoid material. *Postgrad Med J* 46: 510–14.

Mitchell DN, Rees RJ, Goswami KK (1976). Transmissible agents from human sarcoid and Crohn's disease tissues. *Lancet* 2(7989): 761–5.

Moller DR, Chen ES (2002). What causes sarcoidosis? *Curr Opin Pulm Med* 8: 429–34.

Morimoto Y, Kohyama S, Nakai K et al. (2003). Long-term effects of UV light on contractility of rat arteries *in vivo*. *Photochem Photobiol* 78: 372–6.

Narayanan RB (1988). Immunopathology of leprosy granulomas. Current status: a review. *Lepr Rev* 59(1): 75–82.

Newman LS, Rose CS, Bresnitz EA et al. (2004). A case–control etiologic study of sarcoidosis: environmental and occupational risk factors. *Am J Respir Crit Care Med* 170: 1324–30.

Panayeas S, Theodorakopoulos P, Bouras A, Constantopoulos S (1991). Seasonal occurrence of sarcoidosis in Greece. *Lancet* 338(8765): 510–11.

Parkes SA, Baker SB, Bourdillon RE et al. (1985). Incidence of sarcoidosis in the Isle of Man. *Thorax* 40: 284–7.

Pietinalho A, Ohmichi M, Hiraga Y et al. (1996). The mode of presentation of sarcoidosis in Finland and Hokkaido, Japan: a comparative analysis of 571 Finnish and 686 Japanese patients. *Sarcoidosis Vasc Diffuse Lung Dis* 13: 159–66.

Pike MC, Smith PG (1974). Case–control approach to examine diseases for evidence of contagion, including diseases with long latent periods. *Biometrics* 30: 263–79.

Prezant DJ, Dhala A, Goldstein A et al. (1999). The incidence, prevalence, and severity of sarcoidosis in New York City firefighters. *Chest* 116: 1183–93.

Rabin DL, Thompson B, Brown KM et al. (2004). Sarcoidosis: social predictors of severity at presentation. *Eur Respir J* 24: 601–8.

Riddervold L (1964). Sarcoidosis in Norway. *Acta Med Scand Suppl* 425: 111.

Rossman MD, Kreider ME (2007). Lesson learned from ACCESS (A Case Controlled Etiologic Study of Sarcoidosis). *Proc Am Thorac Soc* 4: 453–6.

Rybicki BA, Iannuzzi MC, Frederick MM et al. (2001). Familial aggregation of sarcoidosis: a case–control etiologic study of sarcoidosis (ACCESS). *Am J Respir Crit Care Med* 164: 2085–91.

Rybicki BA, Major M, Popovich J et al. (1997). Racial differences in sarcoidosis incidence: a 5-year study in a health maintenance organization. *Am J Epidemiol* 145: 234–41.

Sartwell PE, Edwards LB (1974). Epidemiology of sarcoidosis in the US Navy. *Am J Epidemiol* 99: 250–7.

Scharkoff T (1987). Apropos of the present level of epidemiologic knowledge on sarcoidosis. *Sarcoidosis* 4: 152–4.

Schurmann M, Lympany PA, Reichel P et al. (2000). Familial sarcoidosis is linked to the major histocompatibility complex region. *Am J Respir Crit Care Med* 162(3 Pt 1): 861–4.

Sharma OP, Neville E, Walker AN, James DG (1976). Familial sarcoidosis: a possible genetic influence. *Ann NY Acad Sci* 278: 386–400.

Song Z, Marzilli L, Greenlee BM et al. (2005). Mycobacterial catalase-peroxidase is a tissue antigen and target of the adaptive immune response in systemic sarcoidosis. *J Exp Med* 201: 755–67.

Stewart IC, Davidson NM (1982). Clustering of sarcoidosis. *Thorax* 37: 398–9.

Sutherland I, Mitchell DN, Hart PD (1965). Incidence of intrathoracic sarcoidosis among young adults participating in a trial of tuberculosis vaccines. *Br Med J* 2(5460): 497–503.

Terris M, Chaves AD (1966). An epidemiologic study of sarcoidosis. *Am Rev Respir Dis* 94(1): 50–5.

Wallgren S (1958). Pulmonary sarcoidosis detected by photofluorographic surveys in Sweden, 1950–1957. *Nord Med* 60: 1194–5.

Yamaguchi M, Hosoda Y, Sasaki R, Aoki K (1989). Epidemiological study on sarcoidosis in Japan: recent trends in incidence and prevalence rates and changes in epidemiological features. *Sarcoidosis* 6(2): 138–46.

Yi ES, Lee H, Suh YK et al. (1996). Experimental extrinsic allergic alveolitis and pulmonary angiitis induced by intratracheal or intravenous challenge with *Corynebacterium parvum* in sensitized rats. *Am J Pathol* 149: 1303–12.

Young RC, Hackney RL, Harden KA (1974). Epidemiology of sarcoidosis: ethnic and geographic considerations. *J Natl Med Assoc* 66: 386–8.

PART **II**

ETIOLOGY, PATHOLOGY, IMMUNOLOGY AND GENETICS

PART II

4

Etiology

MUHUNTHAN THILLAI, MELISSA WICKREMASINGHE, AJIT LALVANI, DAVID MOLLER AND DONALD MITCHELL

INTRODUCTION

There are a number of completely different hypotheses that relate to the etiology of sarcoidosis. Some of these are now of historic interest only and have been disproved to a certain extent. Others have been hinted at rather than explicitly stated in the literature, and some theories are ongoing with limited evidence for or against.

Among the suggestions that are of historic interest are those implied by the names proposed by Boeck and by Schaumann. Boeck postulated that the *multiple benign sarkoid* of the skin which he described in 1899 was a benign growth of connective tissue. Although he later recognized that the histology was similar to that of a tuberculoid granuloma, a variation of the name he suggested gradually crept into general use and is now used to describe the multisystem disease of which the skin eruption is one of several possible manifestations. In 1914, Schaumann altered the name to *lymphogranulomatosis benigna* for the generalized disease underlying sarcoid of the skin and lupus perino. In doing so he was suggesting that sarcoidosis might be regarded as a proliferative disease of lymphatic tissue, analogous in some respects to Hodgkin's disease. Like Boeck, he later came to the conclusion that the disease was probably related to tuberculosis. This is perhaps the theory which has persisted the most over the past century and there is some evidence to support it.

However, there are many arguments against a causal link between the two conditions and there are a number of other hypotheses with varying degrees of evidence. Evidence to support different hypotheses includes epidemiological observations, laboratory work with passage of granulomas through mice and clinical associations with other diseases. At present there is no widely accepted single cause of sarcoidosis.

TERRAIN SARCOIDIQUE

In the early twentieth century it was postulated that certain individuals may have an inherent tendency to react to a variety of different external stimuli by the production of non-caseating epitheliod-cell granulomas. This stereotypical inflammatory response at the site of inoculation, which is known as the sarcoid diathesis or *terrain sarcoidique* hypothesis, was first put forward as certain patients with the disease have a tendency for old scars to become infiltrated in the active stage of disease. However, aside from this infiltration, there is little other evidence that patients with sarcoidosis react with a sarcoid granuloma to non-specific stimuli.

An investigation into granulomatous reactions to a number of agents, including silica and phospholipids from hen's eggs and from human serum, showed that patients with sarcoidosis showed no evidence of abnormal reactivity to these substances (Refvem 1954). Intradermal tests in patients with sarcoidosis, those with zirconium granulomas and in healthy controls were performed with a number of stimuli including sodium stearate and a large number of metallic elements (Hurley and Shelley 1959). No difference was found in quality or intensity of reaction between the various groups apart from the disease-specific granulomatous response to zirconium. This suggests that the sarcoid granuloma is a single specific response to an inciting agent or possibly one of a number of agents.

EVIDENCE FOR A TRANSMISSIBLE AGENT

It may be that no external agent is needed to initiate and maintain the granulomatous changes found in sarcoidosis. This hypothesis raises the idea that the disease develops as a result of an intrinsic biochemical, genetic or cellular abnormality rather than by the stimulation of an external agent. This conjecture was advanced largely on the grounds that the sarcoid granuloma is biochemically different from other granulomas, principally in its synthesis of angiotensin-converting enzyme (Silverstein et al. 1976). However, these differences do not distinguish the sarcoid granuloma unequivocally from other granulomas as responses to known antigens may also show high levels of this enzyme (Farber et al. 1982).

The lack of evidence for a purely intrinsic cause has led many clinicians to believe that an external agent is involved in disease pathogenesis. If an external stimulus is involved, there are many questions that need to be answered. Is it a known pathogen? Is it unique to sarcoidosis? Is the presentation of disease merely a response in a person who is predisposed to an otherwise innocuous agent or agents?

Answers to these questions depend on the discovery and characterization of such agents. There has been much research into the identity of specific causal agents and, while there is as yet no conclusive proof for a specific cause, there is strong evidence pointing towards a transmissible factor that is involved in the pathogenesis of disease.

Transmission between individuals

A case–control study of residents on the Isle of Man (Parkes et al. 1985) found that 40 percent of 96 patients with sarcoidosis had prior contact with at least one person who had the disease, compared with fewer than 2 percent of controls. Of the sarcoidosis contact cases, 14 occurred within the same household and only nine of these were blood relatives. A total of 19 pairs of patients came into contact with one another at work, two were neighbours and 14 were friends. This study, along with further related work (Hills et al. 1987), suggests that some cases of sarcoidosis may be due to a communicable disease with direct transmission between susceptible individuals.

However, an alternative explanation for these findings is that the same data viewed from an occupational or environmental standpoint might be attributable to the sharing of a common environmental exposure which induces a hypersensitivity response in a large number of individuals. Retrospective analysis of the Isle of Man research showed that the studies only recorded a limited amount of occupational or household exposure data.

There are a number of case reports of transmission of sarcoidosis between individuals. A case series of four patients with recurrent pulmonary sarcoidosis has been described after lung transplant from donors with the disease (Klemen et al. 2000), while a number of cases of acquired sarcoidosis have been described in recipients of bone marrow from donors with active disease (Padilla et al. 2002). Conversely, sarcoidosis has been reported to have developed in non-sarcoid allografts after lung transplantation (Muller et al. 1996).

Animal studies

There are no naturally occurring in-vivo animal models for sarcoidosis. Animals such as cats and dogs have been identified as potentially having the disease, but such cases have been sparse in nature and poorly reported. Over the years a number of reports of attempts to transmit sarcoidosis to guinea pigs or hamsters by inoculation of granulomatous material from patients have been published (Santoianni and Ayala 1949). Work from the early part of the twentieth century was uncontrolled, usually based on single patients, and their results must be regarded as inconclusive but work from the latter part of the century has been more detailed. There is limited recent in-vivo animal work.

Detailed studies of Kveim injections into mice

A series of mouse experiments have been reported which were based on work carried out to investigate leprosy (Shepard 1960) in which homogenates of both human sarcoidosis tissue and normal tissue (as controls) were injected into the footpads of 12-week-old female CBA strain mice (Mitchell and Rees 1969, 1970a). Fresh sarcoidosis lymph nodes obtained from 26 patients and sarcoidosis spleens from two further patients served as the source of sarcoidosis material. As control tissues, lymph nodes were obtained from the para-aortic region in six otherwise healthy individuals, and from a routine varicose veins operation in one other person. Homogenates were prepared for all fresh tissues in 1 percent bovine albumin in saline solution to yield a 13.5 percent suspension.

Tissue homogenates were injected intraperitoneally, intravenously or into the hind footpads of the mice. Full-thickness biopsies, initially of the injected and later of the opposed footpad, were made 6–24 months after the injection. Mice that were sick were killed and their footpads and viscera were examined histologically. Assessments were made from coded sections that were examined routinely under polarized light to assist in the detection of foreign-body material.

Kveim tests were made in the ears with Lots 0025, 004 and 005 of CSL suspension (Hurley and Bartholomeusz 1968), between 9 and 17 weeks after inoculation of sarcoidosis or control-tissue homogenates. The Kveim tests were assessed microscopically after punch biopsy (4 mm) at intervals of 35–46 days after injection. Histological responses were categorized as positive, equivocal or negative. In a positive response the essential feature was the presence of one or more granulomas composed principally of epithelioid cells with occasional Langerhans-type giant cells. Negative responses included non-specific inflammatory changes, foreign-body reactions, scars with fibroblasts or fibrocytes and normal tissue. Of 193 footpads investigated from 114 mice injected with sarcoidosis homogenate, 57 showed positive responses and 46 equivocal responses after a mean interval of 15 months. Kveim tests were made in 111 of these mice; 21 showed a positive response and were associated with positive footpad histology. Of 173 footpads investigated from 78 mice inoculated with non-sarcoid homogenate, only one was positive and six equivocal after the same interval and Kveim tests in all 78 of these mice were negative (Fig. 4.1).

Mouse-to-mouse transmission was also found to occur with homogenates of granulomatous tissue of mice injected with sarcoidosis tissue homogenates being found capable of causing similar changes on injection into normal mice. At first passage, fresh homogenates from granulomatous footpads harvested at a mean interval of 15 months after injection of human sarcoidosis tissue homogenate were injected into the footpads of normal mice and led to changes interpreted as positive in 24 percent and equivocal in 48 percent. Comparable proportions were found in footpads injected with supernatant and filtrate of the supernatant, but autoclaved material produced no response. Up to six passages resulted in granulomatous changes in both the injected footpad and also in other footpads and in the lungs, liver, spleen and lymph nodes in a proportion of animals. Intravenous and intraperitoneal injections of granulomatous mouse-tissue homogenate were also found to produce changes in the organs of a proportion of mice.

Sarcoidosis-tissue homogenates retained in-vivo granuloma forming activity after storage for one week at +4 or −70°C but lost this activity after storage at −20°C and after irradiation with 2.5 mR. This inactivation with irradiation is in sharp contrast with the retention of selective activity by validated Kveim test suspensions after similar radiation (Mitchell et al. 1974).

Similar experiments with mice have found that granulomas after inoculation occurred after three months and persisted for at least one year without regression (Iwai and Takahashi 1976). In their experiments, they also found that irradiation of the sarcoidosis material resulted in a loss of in-vivo granuloma-forming activity. Some more recent studies have contradicted these findings. Notably, investigations of nude mice with a similar experimental setup found no ability to pass on a sarcoidosis granuloma to mice (Grizzanti and Rosenstreich 1988). One explanation for this may be the lack of T-cells in the mice which may be needed to form a granuloma in response to the injected antigens.

Crohn's disease has been investigated by a similar procedure using abnormal ileum and mesenteric lymph nodes from four patients who underwent bowel resection (Mitchell and Rees 1970b). Homogenates of these tissues were injected into mice footpads, intravenously and intraperitoneally 15–17 months later; granulomas were found in footpads in a substantial proportion of mice (40 percent positive, 30 percent equivocal) as well as in the mesenteric lymph nodes and bowels of some mice. No changes were found in other lymph nodes, the lungs or the spleen. Transmission of granulomatous changes from tissue originating from Crohn's disease was also found after

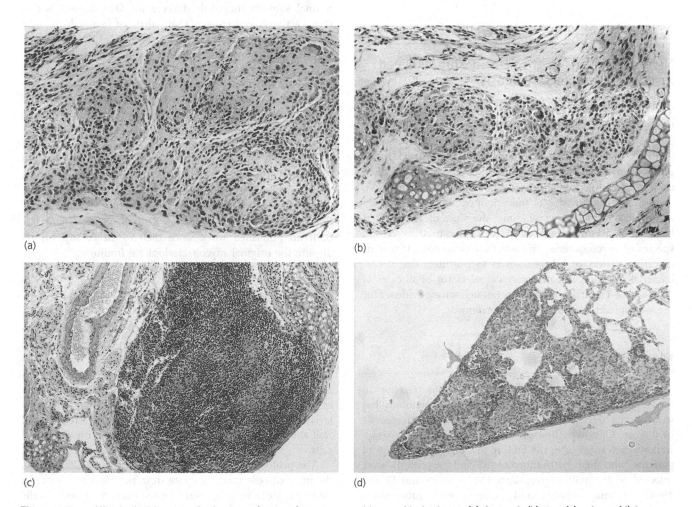

(a)   (b)   (c)   (d)

Figure 4.1   Histological images of mice granulomas after passage with sarcoidosis tissue: (a) footpad; (b) ear; (c) spleen; (d) lung.

successive passages. The effect of storage temperatures and irradiation was similar to that seen with sarcoidosis tissue homogenates.

These findings suggest that in sarcoidosis (and perhaps in Crohn's disease) there is a transmissible agent that can be passed repeatedly in mice, that is inactivated by autoclaving or by irradiation, and that can pass through a 0.2-micrometer filter.

The portfolio of mouse work in this area is not complete and still leaves open the question of the actual cause of activation of cells of the immune system which culminates in the formation of the sarcoidosis granuloma. Conflicting results from different studies may perhaps be explained by the different batches of Kveim reagent used in different studies, some of which were less stringently tested in humans than others. Notwithstanding, this work collectively suggests that, in at least some cases of human sarcoidosis, there is an agent present in the diseased tissue which is capable of producing anatomically dispersed granulomatous reactions in mice transmissible for at least five passages.

However, it does not answer the question as to the identity of that antigen or even whether it is an external one or rather something intrinsic to the host granulomatous response in sarcoidosis that can trigger the same response when inoculated into mice.

MYCOBACTERIA

Historical views on the relationship between mycobacteria and sarcoidosis

The similarity of the histological changes of sarcoidosis to those of mycobacterial disease, as well as the observed clinical associations between the conditions, led some early investigators to conclude that sarcoidosis was an unusual form of tuberculosis and could perhaps even be reclassified as non-caseating tuberculosis. When the term *tuberculosis* was first introduced, it was defined only in morbid anatomical terms. However, since the time of Koch it has been defined etiologically as the disease caused by certain species of mycobacteria. To state that sarcoidosis is a non-caseating variety of tuberculosis is to postulate that mycobacterial infection is a necessary causal factor of all cases of sarcoidosis. There is not currently enough strong evidence for the widespread acceptance of this statement.

Mycobacteriophages

The inability to consistently culture mycobacteria or to identify acid-fast bacilli from sarcoidosis granulomas has led some to suggest alternative methods for the pathogenesis of disease. One hypothesis relating sarcoidosis to mycobacteria was advanced after the finding that a high percentage of patients who had both tuberculosis and sarcoidosis were infected with mycobacteriophages (Mankiewicz and Beland 1964). Normal subjects and patients with tuberculosis produced phage-neutralizing antibodies while it was initially found that those with sarcoidosis showed no appreciable amount of these antibodies either to their own or to other mycobacteriophages. Mycobacteria resembling photochromagens emerged in cultures of virulent tubercle bacilli infected with mycobacteriophage.

It was suggested that sarcoidosis might develop in individuals infected with both tubercle bacilli and with mycobacteriophages but who were incapable of producing antibodies to mycobacteriophage. The tubercle bacilli under the influence of the phage may assume unrecognizable forms and be responsible for eliciting a non-caseating reaction.

In support of this view are reports that isolation of mycobacteria resembling *anonymous types* from sarcoidosis tissues was possible by serial culture in media enriched with phage-neutralizing rabbit sera. In guinea pigs infected with small doses of tubercle bacilli, infection with mycobacteriophage DSGA reduced the number of granulomas, made them more discrete, and diminished their survival time (Mankiewicz 1964). Further studies confirmed the isolation of mycobacteriophages from stools, tissue and sera of patients with tuberculosis and only occasionally from the stools of healthy subjects (Mankiewicz and Liivak 1967).

Later studies, however, disputed these findings and found no difference between the neutralizing activity of sera from patients with sarcoidosis and with tuberculosis against mycobacteriophages D29, Leo and R1. With sera from normal subjects they only differed for D29, against which their activity was lower than that of sarcoidosis and tuberculosis sera (Bowman and Daniel 1971). Further work reported on the failure of concurrent infection of guinea pigs with *M. tuberculosis* and with mycobacteriophage to produce sarcoid-like disease (Bowman et al. 1972).

A study into phage activity isolated five strains of bacteriophage with activity against mycobacteria from 17 patients whose sputum yielded tubercle bacilli. Most of the bacteriophages lysed human tubercle bacilli and one lysed *M. kanasasii*. No patients with sarcoidosis were studied (Redmond and Cater 1960). A more recent brief report does mention the isolation of mycobacteriophage from the stools of patients with sarcoidosis but does not elaborate earlier findings (Koz'min-Sokolov and Kostina 1971). There has been no published work since then to either support or dispute the original mycobacteriophage findings.

Cell-wall-deficient forms of mycobacteria

An alternative hypothesis to that of the mycobacteriophage involves the concept that an atypical form of mycobacteria is responsible for the pathogenesis of disease in sarcoidosis. These mycobacteria may be present within the granuloma in a form that it is not able to be cultured, such as a protoplast or L-form (otherwise known as cell-wall-deficient mycobacteria) which lacks the power to produce a characteristic cell wall and persists as an intracellular parasite of mesenchymal cells.

The protoplast may only rarely revert to a bacillary form, the infected cells might migrate to initiate foci of disease in other parts of the body, and in most cases the infected cells would be eliminated – though in some cases the intracellular infection may persist and give rise to progressive destructive changes. The affected individual may then show unusually efficient production of humoral antibody and abnormal cellular immune responses.

Such mycobacteria have been little studied and the difficulties associated with identification have led some to question their very existence. However, there are reports of findings of cell-wall-deficient mycobacteria after long culture of sarcoidosis granulomas (Cantwell 1981). Cell-wall-deficient forms of mycobacteria have been grown after prolonged culture of the blood of 19 out of 20 patients with sarcoidosis but were not found in a similar number of controls (Almenoff et al. 1996). Doubt has been cast on this remarkable finding by other groups who found no difference between sarcoidosis and controls in this respect (e.g. Brown et al. 2003).

Viral infections associated with mycobacteria

A related hypothesis to that of the mycobacteriophage is that, during the course of a mycobacterial infection, a low-grade virus might infect mesenchymal cells and so behave like a hypothetical protoblast form of tubercle bacillus (Hanngren et al. 1974). Viral infection would depress T-cell function and mycobacterial infection would stimulate B-cell function, but there is minimal evidence to support this hypothesis.

Arguments for and against the role of mycobacteria infection as a causal factor in sarcoidosis

Regardless of their exact role in the etiology of sarcoidosis, there are a number of studies to investigate the implications of mycobacteria as a causal agent. The evidence to support their role is summarized below.

HISTORICAL OBSERVATIONS OF THE CONCURRENCE OF BACTERIOLOGICALLY PROVEN MYCOBACTERIAL INFECTION IN PATIENTS WITH SARCOIDOSIS

Of all reported cases, the most difficult to explain as coincidental are those in which a clinical picture of mycobacterial tuberculosis merges imperceptibly into one of sarcoidosis and those cases of definite sarcoidosis in which mycobacteria are later isolated. Some patients present with atypical forms of mycobacterial lesions in the course of a disease which is otherwise characteristic of sarcoidosis. In others, the sudden and unexplained discovery of mycobacteria is accompanied by the disappearance of specific sarcoidosis features.

One such unusual case concerns a 17-year-old female patient in the United Kingdom who was initially investigated as a contact of her husband who had been diagnosed with pulmonary tuberculosis (Scadding 1960). Her chest radiograph at initial consultation was normal. A child born to her a year later was skin-tested as tuberculin-positive shortly after birth. Seven years after the patient was first seen, a small area of shadowing appeared on the radiograph of the upper zone of her right lung. She subsequently had a positive Mantoux test and tubercle bacilli were cultured from a gastric washing. Despite chemotherapy with appropriate anti-tuberculosis agents the chest shadowing slowly spread. Two years into treatment she was found to have a strongly positive Mantoux test and a liver biopsy revealed non-caseating granulomas.

The decision to add steroids to her treatment resulted in a dramatic improvement with rapid clearing of all lung shadows. The subsequent course of her disease was more constant with sarcoidosis with relapses on withdrawal of steroids. There are a number of equally unusual case reports in the literature but with the obvious associated difficulties of replication of results.

Non-caseating tubercles are occasionally the most prominent histological finding in otherwise definite mycobacterial disease. A study of 54 lymph nodes from cases of sarcoidosis and 49 diagnosed as chronic hyperplastic tuberculosis (due to the finding of acid fast bacilli in them) concluded that the two groups could be distinguished from each other histologically (Zettergren 1954). It is also recognized that non-caseating granulomas at the periphery of an obviously caseating focus of mycobacterial disease contain very few or no detectable acid-fast bacilli. The agent responsible for locally inciting granuloma formation at these sites is unidentified.

Failure to respond to anti-mycobacterial therapy does not in itself distinguish between sarcoidosis and tuberculosis. Occasional cases have been reported in which mycobacterial tuberculosis failed to respond to chemotherapy and where the infecting organism was shown to be sensitive in vitro. In other cases the diagnosis of chronic miliary tuberculosis with low tuberculin sensitivity seemed likely and was supported by the finding of acid-fast bacilli in lesions in a liver biopsy and in sputum although they did not grown on culture. However, anti-mycobacterial drugs were ineffective until corticosteroid treatment was added, bringing into doubt the original diagnosis. In fact, the differences, clinical and pathological, between sarcoidosis and indolent forms of tuberculosis are small. Indeed, there are even greater differences within the spectrum of tuberculosis from the healthy patient with remote latent infection as compared with the critically ill immunosuppressed patient with cavitating pulmonary disease. Therefore, the possibility that some cases of sarcoidosis are extreme examples of indolent granulomatous paucibacillary mycobacterial disease cannot currently be rejected outright.

MOLECULAR EVIDENCE OF MYCOBACTERIA FROM WITHIN SARCOID GRANULOMAS

A large point of contention regarding the link between mycobacteria and sarcoidosis rests with the ability by some to discover evidence of mycobacteria within sarcoid granulomas, a finding which has been disputed by others.

A number of studies have found evidence of mycobacterial DNA within histologically confirmed sarcoidosis tissue. DNA sequences coding for the mycobacterial 65 kDa antigen have been found in 11 out of 25 cases of sarcoidosis in patients from Austria where it was hypothesized that the mycobacteria detected were not due to M. tuberculosis as the insertion sequence 6110 of the *M. tuberculosis* complex (found in *M. tuberculosis*, *M. africanum*, *M. bovis* and BCG) was not detectable in any of the cases (Popper *et al.* 1997).

An investigation of sarcoidosis tissue samples using a nested polymerase chain reaction with primers corresponding to the insertion element IS6110 of *M. tuberculosis* complex found evidence of mycobacterial DNA in 9 out of 23 patients with sarcoidosis compared with only 1 out of 23 controls in patients from Spain (Fite *et al.* 2006). Mycobacterial RNA or rpo beta sequences have been found in 60 percent of sarcoidosis tissues but could not be detected in controls (Drake *et al.* 2002), and mycobacterial catalase–peroxidase has been identified in a subset of sarcoidosis tissues using a limited proteomics approach (Song *et al.* 2005). An analysis of five sarcoidosis spleens compared against control tissues identified mycobacterial RNA at a level 4.8 times higher in the controls (Mitchell *et al.* 1992).

A meta-analysis of 31 studies which all analyzed sarcoidosis tissues by PCR for nucleic acid amplification followed by identification of nucleic acid sequences specific for different types of mycobacteria concluded that 231 of 874 patients were positive for mycobacterial nucleic acids, and the odds of finding mycobacteria in sarcoidosis tissues versus controls was 9.67 (4.56–20.5), suggesting a potential link between mycobacteria and sarcoidosis in some cases (Gupta *et al.* 2007).

Animal studies have reported that, although human sarcoidosis samples may have been reported as being negative for mycobacteria, acid-fast bacilli had been seen in some granulomatous tissues of mice passaged from the sarcoid tissues of six patients (Mitchell and Rees 1983). These were found in the lungs of mice and also in the spleen between 5 and 17 months after the injection of the fresh homogenate or supernatant filtrate of mouse granulomatous tissue on the first to third passage from the original injection of sarcoidosis tissue 3–9 years previously. Mycobacteria having the characteristics of human *M. tuberculosis* were grown on Lowenstein–Jensen media from pooled homogenates of the lungs and spleens from mice in two of these serial passages. One of these originated in tissue from a patient with bilateral hilar lymphadenopathy who had a negative tuberculin test and a positive Kveim test.

Mouse lungs from the second passage and lungs and spleen from a third and fourth passage grew *M. tuberculosis*. Two of these passages resulted from supernatant passed through a 0.2-micrometer filter. The other originated from a patient with bilateral hilar lymphadenopathy, pulmonary infiltration and skin disease with positive Kveim and negative tuberculin tests. The findings that after several passages in mice acid-fast rods have appeared in some cases supports the suggestion that protoblast or an L-form of tubercle bacillus may act as an initiating agent of sarcoidosis.

EX-VIVO T-CELL RESPONSES TO MYCOBACTERIAL PROTEINS IN PATIENTS WITH SARCOIDOSIS

A role for mycobacterial organisms in the etiology of sarcoidosis is supported by recent studies that find mycobacterial proteins induce T- and B-cell responses in patients with sarcoidosis.

One of the authors and his colleagues employed a novel proteomic approach to detect potential pathogenic antigens in tissues from sarcoidosis patients (Song *et al.* 2005). This approach was based on the hypothesis that pathogenic tissue antigens would be poorly soluble with properties found in Kveim reagent (neutral-detergent insolubility, relative heat, acid and protease resistance) (Lyons *et al.* 1992). After biochemical extraction, sera from sarcoidosis patients were used to detect candidate tissue antigens. Mass spectrometry and protein immunoblotting led to the identification of the *M. tuberculosis* catalase–peroxidase protein (mKatG) as a tissue antigen. Using recombinant mKatG protein, we found circulating IgG directed to mKatG in about 50 percent of sarcoidosis patients (similar to PPD+ control patients), but in fewer than 5 percent of PPD− controls. Given that this approach was not predicated on any specific hypothesis regarding a microbial etiology of sarcoidosis, these findings provide unbiased support for a mycobacterial etiology in a subset of sarcoidosis.

Since the identification of mKatG as a candidate pathogenic antigen, several groups report that mycobacterial proteins induce T-cell responses in sarcoidosis. Using ELISpot technology, Drake and colleagues demonstrated INF-γ-expressing PBMC responses to ESAT-6 or an mKatG peptide in 15 of 26 sarcoidosis patients, 1 of 24 PPD− controls, and 7 of 8 PPD+ controls (Drake *et al.* 2007). This group also report that mycobacterial superoxide dismutase A (Allen *et al.* 2008) and antigen 85A (Hajizadeh *et al.* 2007) induce IFN-γ responses in PBMC of sarcoidosis patients, suggesting patients may have T-cell responses to multiple mycobacterial proteins. Dubaniewicz and colleagues report peripheral blood T-cell responses to mycobacterial heat-shock proteins in sarcoidosis (Dubaniewicz *et al.* 2007). A potential link of mycobacterial responses to MHC genes in sarcoidosis is suggested by the association of immune responses to ESAT-6 peptide NNALQNLARTISEAG and DRB1*1101 in African-Americans (Oswald-Richter *et al.* 2009).

Subsequent studies using recombinant mKatG protein found that patients with sarcoidosis mount Th1 responses to mKatG and other mycobacterial proteins found in PPD with greater frequency than control populations in both the USA and Sweden (Chen *et al.* 2008). We found over 80 percent of sarcoidosis patients demonstrated IFN-γ expressing CD4+ or CD8+ T cell responses to mKatG or PPD, suggesting a mycobacterial association in a majority of patients in the USA and northern Europe. Consistent with a pathogenic antigen, we found greater Th1 responses to mKatG in the lung than blood, with lower responses in patients undergoing treatment and absent responses in those with inactive sarcoidosis. Higher proportions of mKatG-reactive BAL cells were found in DRB1*0301+ Swedish patients compared to DRB1*0301− patients, suggesting a direct influence of MHC genotype on mKatG Th1 responses. Interestingly, patients with or without Löfgren syndrome had similar frequencies of mKatG specific IFN-γ-expressing blood T-cells, suggesting a mycobacterial link to both remitting and chronic sarcoidosis.

These studies add to the plethora of earlier studies linking mycobacterial organisms to sarcoidosis. Given this association, researchers need to explore specific pathogenic mechanisms responsible that lead to the pathobiological pathway of sarcoidosis instead of the more common recognized host response to mycobacterial organisms that leads to either an active infection or latency. One innate immune mechanism that could be involved in differentiating sarcoidosis from active infectious granulomatous diseases involves the acute-phase reactant, serum amyloid A, discussed in Chapter 6. Future pathogenetic insight will likely require a coordinated approach involving genetic, immunologic and innate host factors that may ultimately lead to disease-specific therapy or cure.

EPIDEMIOLOGICAL RELATIONSHIP BETWEEN TUBERCULOSIS AND SARCOIDOSIS

A number of epidemiological studies have shown that a high proportion of patients with sarcoidosis have been found to have a history of contact with tuberculosis. A description of two sibships details one which concerns eight cases of sarcoidosis and four of tuberculosis and the other which relates to four cases of sarcoidosis, three of tuberculosis and two having features of both diseases (Wurm et al. 1962). Comparisons of populations with highly distinguishable ethnic groups show that ethnicities with higher incidence of tuberculosis generally have a higher incidence of sarcoidosis. In the USA, black individuals are more liable to both tuberculosis and sarcoidosis than whites. In London, studies showing the changes in prevalence of abnormalities interpreted as due to tuberculosis and sarcoidosis were found from repeated mass radiographic surveys in an area with considerable proportions of peoples from Irish and West Indian backgrounds (Brett 1965). Among those born in the UK, the prevalence of both diseases diminished, and among West Indians both increased between the times of the two surveys. Thus, prevalence of sarcoidosis showed a change in the same direction as that of tuberculosis in each of three ethnic groups.

In stark contrast with the evidence put forward to propose a link between mycobacteria and the pathogenesis of sarcoidosis there are a number of arguments as to why such a causal relationship is less likely.

Actual incidence of mycobacterial isolation from sarcoidosis granulomas is low

The proportion of sarcoidosis cases from which tubercle bacilli are isolated is small. In some case series this has been reported as zero and in others it is no different from the incidence in the controls. In sharp contrast to earlier findings, several studies were either unable to detect mycobacterial DNA from the granulomatous lesions of patients with sarcoidosis or found that the incidence in sarcoidosis tissues was no different from that in controls (Bocart et al. 1992; Vokurka et al. 1997).

The variability of findings among these studies may be explained by the differences in case selection from a disorder presenting with a wide variety of clinical attributes, the fact that a number of different experimental methods have been used, and that patients have been studied from vastly different geographic regions.

An alternative explanation for this discordance may be that, due to the very definition of sarcoidosis, a mycobacterial infection has been excluded and should be taken into account when reading or analyzing such studies. The diagnosis of sarcoidosis has been rejected in a number of cases presenting otherwise characteristic features when intensive investigation has led to the isolation of M. tuberculosis (Kent et al. 1970).

Another explanation put forward is that the mycobacteria which cause sarcoidosis are no longer viable. This would explain why mycobacterial proteins have been detected within granulomas in some instances.

A final explanation may be that super-infecting mycobacteria migrate towards the site of sarcoid granulomas. This has been shown to be the case in some existing tuberculosis granulomas and may explain the variable findings in sarcoidosis (Cosma et al. 2004).

Lower tuberculin sensitivity in patients with sarcoidosis

Tuberculin sensitivity is lower in groups of patients with sarcoidosis than in unselected members of the population from which they are drawn, and this has been regarded as evidence against a mycobacterial etiology. This finding may be explained by the depressed skin immune response to specific antigens seen in sarcoidosis (Mathew et al. 2008); but when some groups of patients are investigated using an ex-vivo T-cell assay for diagnosis of tuberculosis, they are found to have responses no different from that of the normal population. An investigation into a Japanese cohort of patients found that only 3 of 90 tested with a commercially available interferon-γ assay used for diagnosis of tuberculosis had a positive response (Inui et al. 2008).

Difference in patterns of organ involvement between diseases

The common patterns of organ involvement in sarcoidosis differ significantly from those in tuberculosis. The uveal tract, the salivary and lacrimal glands, the heart and skeletal muscle and small bones of the hand and feet are often involved in sarcoidosis but are rarely seen in tuberculosis.

Conversely, the adrenal glands may be involved in caseating tuberculosis but almost never in sarcoidosis. One argument to explain this difference yet still support a mutual causality is due to the heterogeneity of the clinical spectrum of tuberculosis itself; different patterns of organ involvement are well recognized at different stages of disease. If sarcoidosis is also caused by mycobacteria, then it may simply display a different organ involvement to that of classical mycobacterial disease.

Strength of epidemiological evidence pointing towards a link

Despite some reports of similarities between the epidemiology of both diseases, a number of detailed epidemiological studies have shown differences between the geographical distributions of sarcoidosis and tuberculosis. There is evidence from the USA, Germany and Denmark that sarcoidosis is associated with residence in the countryside whereas tuberculosis is associated with living in urban areas.

Prevalence of sarcoidosis and tuberculosis in different parts of the same country shows no positive correlation. Despite some epidemiological evidence pointing towards a link between the two diseases in some countries, other studies dispute this. A combination of a nationwide sarcoidosis survey and the analysis of 460 000 people of working age in Japan concluded that there were large disparities between the prevalence of the two diseases, with tuberculosis prevalence being higher in the south of Japan while sarcoidosis was higher in the north (Hosoda et al. 2004).

DIFFERENCES IN TREATMENT STRATEGIES BETWEEN THE TWO DISEASES

The failure of antituberculosis chemotherapy to influence the course of sarcoidosis is difficult to reconcile with a direct etiological role for Mycobacterium tuberculosis. In addition, the mainstay of treatment of patients with sarcoidosis is with immunosuppressive drugs such as steroids. If mycobacteria were involved with the pathogenesis of sarcoidosis, it would be reasonable to expect that in at least a small percentage of cases the addition of such treatments would lead to the reactivation of tuberculosis. Such cases are extremely rare. Again, the argument that sarcoidosis is initiated by myco-bacteria which are no longer viable or active in disease pathogenesis goes some way towards explaining these issues.

NON–MYCOBACTERIAL MICROORGANISMS

Propionibacteria

Early studies first reported that Propionibacterium acnes could be frequently isolated from patients with sarcoidosis and hypothesized a possible link (Homma et al. 1978). Subsequent studies using PCR found evidence of P. acnes or P. granulosum rRNA in 15 out of 15 sarcoidosis lymph nodes compared with 2 out of 15 lymph nodes from patients with tuberculosis. Conversely, only three out of the sarcoidosis lymph nodes demonstrated evidence of mycobacteria (Ishige et al. 1999). A larger more recent study reported on 259 patients from five centers in Japan, Italy, Germany and the UK. Propionibacterial DNA was found in 106 of 108 sarcoidosis lymph node samples whereas mycobacterial DNA was only found in 0–9 percent of the lymph nodes (Eishi et al. 2002).

A study of formalin-fixed and paraffin-embedded biopsy samples of lymph nodes from nine patients from each of three groups (sarcoidosis, tuberculosis and non-specific lymphadenitis) used quantitative real-time PCR and in-situ hybridization for P. acnes (Yamada et al. 2002). A significant accumulation of P. acnes genomes was found in and around sarcoid granulomas, suggesting that the indigenous bacter-ium may be related to the cause of granulomatous inflam-mation in sarcoidosis.

An investigation into the presence of propionibacteria in the vitreous fluid of patients with sarcoid uveitis using PCR found P. acnes in 2 out of 6 samples and P. granulosum in 4 out of 6 samples (Yasuhara et al. 2005).

The majority of studies which describe the presence of propionibacteria in sarcoidosis tissue are from Japan and it may be that, in this region of the world, propionibacteria do have an etiological link with some cases of sarcoidosis. Studies investigating propionibacteria from Europe and North America have proven less convincing.

Viruses

An early investigation into viruses reported the isolation of a virus of the mumps–influenza–Newcastle disease group by serial inoculations into embryonated eggs of gastric material from four cases of sarcoidosis (Löfgren and Lundback 1950), but it was later concluded that the virus must have been a laboratory contaminant since the results could not be replicated in a laboratory that did not handle this virus. A culture of sarcoid lymph nodes and skin lesions by the plasma clot technique observed patchy degeneration of the outgrowing fibroblasts of a type they had not been observed in cultures of lymph nodes of other diseases (Lundbeck et al. 1959). Attempts to transfer a cytopathogenic effect to human embryonic lung cultures have been unsuccessful.

An investigation of 28 sarcoidosis lymph nodes, four lung biopsies, three Kveim test papules and three sarcoidosis spleen suspensions looked for evidence of viral infection by co-cultivation of lymphocytes from the sarcoidosis material with cultured human fibroblasts and of fibroblasts growing out of sarcoid tissues with human fibroblasts or with monkey Vero cells (Steplewski 1976). Some cytopathic effects were seen in the co-cultivation of lymphocytes from the sarcoidosis material with human fibroblasts, but transfer of the super-natant from these to fresh fibroblast cultures did not induce similar changes. All other tests for viral activity were negative and there was no electron microscopic evidence of viral agents. Isolation of an organism related to Mycoplasma orale type one has been shown from four of seven skin biopsy samples and two lymph nodes affected by sarcoidosis (Jansson et al. 1972). Patients with sarcoidosis had higher indirect hemagglutination titers against the isolated strain of Mycoplasma than did controls, but it seems possible that this was due to the generally enhanced humoral antibody response observed in sarcoidosis. However, M. orale type one is a common commensal and has been isolated from 25 percent of normal subjects and it has been argued there is no reason to suspect that it is pathogenic (Taylor-Robinson et al. 1964).

A number of other viruses have been investigated with respect to etiology of sarcoidosis and these include human herpesvirus 8, retroviruses, and Epstein–Barr virus. In each case there has been no definitive proof of a causal relation-ship, and instead it may be that in some studies the elevated virus antibody titer found in patients with sarcoidosis may be related to the ability of these patients to show enhanced humoral antibody responses to non-specific viral pathogens.

Nocardia-like organisms

An investigation into Nocardia reported the isolation of 17 organisms from 65 tissue samples from 36 patients with sarcoidosis using cultures in a variety of media incubated at various temperatures for periods of up to 3 months. Of these 17 organisms, four had the characteristics of *Nocardia*. The other 13 organisms were not described. This work has not been replicated.

Other candidate organisms

A number of other organic agents have been studied in depth but, as with mycobacteria and propionibacteria, there has been no conclusive evidence for their involvement in the pathogenesis of sarcoidosis.

One such study noted the high incidence of *Chlamydophila pneumoniae* infection associated with lung surgery and subsequently screened 39 patients with sarcoidosis, 26 with lung fibrosis (UIP) and 34 controls for the presence of *Chlamydophila*-specific antibodies in serum and bronchoalveolar lavage fluid (Gaede *et al.* 2002). They found that these antibodies were significantly higher in sarcoidosis patients compared to the controls. However, considering the high prevalence of such antibodies in the healthy population these findings might reflect *Chlamydophila* co-infection in the post-injured lungs of sarcoidosis patients.

An investigation into *Borrelia* looked for the presence of *Borrelia*-like organisms in cutaneous sarcoidosis by focus-floating microscopy (Derler *et al.* 2009). In a retrospective analysis of 38 cutaneous sarcoid tissues analyzed by immunohistochemistry with polyclonal anti-borrelia antibodies and assessment by focus floating microscopy, they found 34.2 percent of the sarcoidosis tissues had evidence of *Borrelia*-like organisms. PCR was performed in addition in 11 cases and was negative in all biopsies. Samples of erythema migrans served as positive controls. Thirty-six (92.3 percent) of 39 samples were positive by focus-floating microscopy, but only 46.6 percent gave positive results by PCR. Of 61 negative controls only one specimen was falsely positive.

Immunohistochemial evidence of *Rickettsia helvetica* has been found in 26 out of 30 tissue biopsy specimens from patients with sarcoidosis from one study from Sweden (Nilsson *et al.* 2002), a finding that has been not been replicated by others (Svendsen *et al.* 2009).

Borrelia burgdorferi has been intensively investigated and some groups have found evidence in some studies of the presence of *Borrelia*-like organisms within sarcoidosis granulomas. One study concluded that sarcoidosis may be a form of Lyme disease after finding that 27 of 33 patients with sarcoidosis had elevated levels of anti-borrelia antibody and that all patients' serum angiotensin-converting enzyme (ACE) levels decreased in conjunction with high doses of penicillin therapy (Hua *et al.* 1992). These findings have not been replicated in subsequent publications.

NON–ORGANIC CAUSAL AGENTS

A number of non-organic factors have been considered as possible causes or contributory causes of sarcoidosis. The high incidence of disease in the south-eastern area of the USA

coincided with the high content of beryllium in the soils of this region (Gentry *et al.* 1955), but the clinical differences between chronic beryllium disease and 'idiopathic' sarcoidosis, the clear relationship between known exposure to beryllium and the development of beryllium disease, and the absence of skin reactivity to beryllium in sarcoidosis, seems to rule out the possibility of a relationship between sarcoidosis and beryllium exposure.

A general correspondence of areas within the USA with the distribution of pine forests led to much investigation of the possibility that inhalation of pine pollen might be a causal factor in sarcoidosis (Cummings *et al.* 1956). Pine pollen has been shown to have acid-fast staining characteristics, contains an acid-fast lipid and an amino-acid resembling diamino-pimelic acid, and is capable of inducing epithelioid cell granulomas in tuberculin-sensitive guinea pigs, both at the site of intradermal injection and in the related lymph nodes (Cummings and Hudgins 1958). While pine pollen has components with granuloma-producing and immunogenic potentiality in the experimental animal, no evidence was obtained that any component caused or contributed to a progressive generalized granulomatosis; and epidemiological studies in other areas showed no relation between the distribution of pine forests and the incidence of sarcoidosis.

An investigation into a number of fire department rescue workers who were involved with the World Trade Center attacks in 2001 found that the incidence of sarcoidosis or sarcoid-like granulomatous pulmonary disease was significantly increased in this population (Izbicki *et al.* 2007).

A CASE–CONTROL ETIOLOGIC STUDY OF SARCOIDOSIS (ACCESS)

The ACCESS collaboration was a large multicenter study in North America which was initiated by the National Institutes of Health. It represents the largest case–controlled study to date to specifically investigate the etiological causes of sarcoidosis.

Seven hundred and six newly diagnosed patients with sarcoidosis and an equal number of age-, sex- and geographically placed matched controls were recruited for the study in the late 1990s. The major hypothesis of the investigation was that sarcoidosis occurs in genetically susceptible individuals through alteration of the immune response following exposure to environmental, occupational or infectious insults. The study investigated occupational and environmental factors using a detailed questionnaire. In addition, infectious agents in the blood were investigated by PCR of blood looking for a number of specific organisms and culture of blood for cell-wall-deficient mycobacteria. The study led to a number of publications but no single cause of sarcoidosis was identified.

The familial aggregation of sarcoidosis

This 2001 publication examined data on disease occurrence in 10 862 first-degree and 17 047 second-degree relatives of 706 age-, sex-, race- and geographically matched cases of sarcoidosis and controls who participated in the study from 1996 to 1999 (Rybicki et al. 2001). Siblings had the highest relative risk, followed by avuncular relationships, grand-parents and parents. White subsets had a higher risk when compared with African-Americans. A significantly elevated risk of sarcoidosis was observed among first- and second-degree relatives of sarcoidosis patients when compared with relatives of matched control subjects.

A case–control etiological study of sarcoidosis: environmental and occupational risk factors

This 2004 publication investigated the same patients with detailed questionnaires regarding suspected occupational and non-occupational exposures, and the data were assessed by univariable and multivariable analysis (Newman et al. 2004). A history of smoking cigarettes was less frequent among patients with sarcoidosis than controls. Positive associations between sarcoidosis and specific occupations were seen, such as agricultural employment, insecticide exposure or work in environments rich in mold or mildew. No single predomi-nant environmental cause of disease was identified.

Job and industry classifications associated with sarcoidosis in the ACCESS study

This 2005 publication further investigated the collated data with reference to Standard Industrial Classification (SIC) and Standard Occupational Classification (SOC) to assess occu-pational contributions to sarcoidosis risk (Barnard et al. 2005). A number of further detailed exposures were asso-ciated with sarcoidosis risk, including organic dust exposures, workers for suppliers of building materials, and those in hardware and gardening material work. Jobs associated with metal dust, metal fumes and work with childcare were negatively associated with the risk of sarcoidosis.

FURTHER ENVIRONMENTAL STUDIES

A number of other studies have looked more closely at non-organic stimuli in sarcoidosis. These include a study using a dataset similar to that used in the ACCESS studies which found that people who worked in occupations with potential metal exposures, in workplaces with high humidity, water drainage or musty odor (perhaps indicating a microbe-rich environment) may be at increased risk for sarcoidosis (Kucera et al. 2003), but concluded, however, that the complexity of occupational exposures makes it difficult to identify specific agents based on job title alone.

The follow-up of an earlier observation of geographic risk for sarcoidosis hospitalizations among African-Americans from South Carolina, USA, used univariable analysis and found that the use of wood stoves, fireplaces, non-public water supplies and living or working on a farm were all associated with increased risk of sarcoidosis (Kajdasz et al. 2001).

FURTHER EVIDENCE TO HELP ELUCIDATE THE ETIOLOGY

Cytokine-related therapies and the development of sarcoidosis

A rare paradoxical effect of anti-tumor necrosis factor alpha (anti-TNF-α) therapy is the emergence of sarcoid reactions. This is an intriguing property of these agents which are now widely used for rheumatological conditions but which have also paradoxically been used to treat refractory sarcoid (Baughman et al. 2005). Case reports described of sarcoidosis on anti-TNF therapy have presented predominantly in lung (Gonzalez-Lopez et al. 2006; Almodovar et al. 2007; Kudrin et al. 2007; Verschueren et al. 2007) and in skin, but there have also been reports in the bone marrow (Metyas et al. 2009) and as neurosarcoidosis (Sturfelt et al. 2007).

Recently a group of ten cases of sarcoid reactions were described on anti-TNF therapy for a variety of rheumatolo-gical conditions, with pulmonary and cutaneous involve-ment. From starting anti-TNF therapy the median time to onset of the reaction was 18 months (Daien et al. 2009). Clinical improvement occurred after discontinuation, with or without steroid treatment. Sarcoid reactions have also been described in the skin alone in the context of psoriatic and juvenile rheumatoid arthritis (Dhaille et al. 2010) and chronic plaque psoriaisis (Pink et al. 2010).

Although sarcoid reactions appear to occur independent of the indication for the anti-TNF therapy, most of the indications are rheumatological rather than for Crohn's disease. Interestingly there is a recognized association between rheumatoid arthritis and sarcoid even without anti-TNF therapy (Kucera 1989). The anti-TNF monoclonal antibodies and etanercept, a fusion protein containing the soluble TNF receptor, have each been implicated, suggesting a class effect. However, there is a suggestion that more cases have occurred with etanercept than with the monoclonal antibodies.

TNF-α is important for *Mycobacterium tuberculosis* con-tainment within granulomas and for mycobacterial granulo-ma development and maintenance (Kindler et al. 1989), and anti-TNF therapy is known to cause reactivation of tubercu-losis (Keane et al. 2001). However, granuloma formation can still occur during anti-TNF therapy both as sarcoid granu-lomas but also as tuberculous granuloma (Iliopoulos et al. 2006). The mechanisms of this paradoxical effect of anti-TNF are not clear (Sweiss and Baughman 2007) but may include increased T-cell production of interferon-γ promoting gran-uloma formation; rebound high levels of TNF-α occurring on anti-TNF therapy (Bhatia and Kast 2007); and increased frequency of infections with agents implicated in the etiology of sarcoid such as mycobacteria. Differentiating granulomas caused by active mycobacterial infection from sarcoid granulomas in this context is key, given the increased risk of tuberculosis on these agents.

Interferon-α, another cytokine therapy, is associated with sarcoidosis (Abdi et al. 1987; Goldberg et al. 2006); there is a reported incidence of sarcoidosis of 5 percent when used for the treatment of chronic hepatitis C infection (Hoffmann *et al.* 1998). A plausible explanation for interferon-α is stimulation of antigen presenting cells by promoting over-expression of MHC II antigens, release of pro-inflammatory cytokines and over-production of IFN-γ.

The biological therapies anti-TNF and IFN-α demonstrate the importance of cytokine disequilibrium in initiating granulomatous reactions and provide an interesting human model of emergent sarcoidosis.

Löfgren's syndrome

Löfgren's syndrome has a remission rate of 70–80 percent whereas patients with lupus pernio or fibrocystic pulmonary sarcoidosis rarely undergo remission. A study into the seasonality of sarcoidosis in 87 symptomatic recently diag-nosed patients with Löfgren's syndrome showed that, in these patients, the distribution of cumulative monthly presenta-tions peaked in spring and was lowest in autumn and winter (Sipahi Demirkok *et al.* 2006). This perhaps indicates that an environmental stimulus more abundant during these times may have a bearing on disease.

Several authors have written that predisposition to sarcoidosis is genetically determined and that genetics also appears to account for the variability in clinical phenotype and behavior (Spagnolo and du Bois 2007). In this context the association between Löfgren's syndrome and the extended HLA DRB1*0301/DQB1*0201 haplotype is probably the most extensively reproduced. Our current understanding of the biological evidence of variations in the human genome is far from complete, and the reported associations need to be verified in different ethnic populations.

Celiac disease

An investigation into the higher prevalence of celiac disease in one group's patients with sarcoidosis led to their advice for screening all sarcoidosis patients for celiac disease (Rutherford *et al.* 2004). A Cox proportional hazards ratio has been used to calculate the risk of subsequent sarcoidosis in 14349 indivi-duals found to have celiac disease between 1964 and 2003 (Ludvigsson *et al.* 2007). Conditional logistic regression was used to study the risk of celiac disease associated with prior sarcoidosis and celiac disease was found to be associated with a significantly increased risk of sarcoidosis (hazard ratio 4.03; CI 2.32–7.0). Prior sarcoidosis was significantly associated with an increased risk of celiac disease (odds ratio 3.58; CI 1.98–6.45). These findings suggest that celiac disease may be linked to an associated increased risk of sarcoidosis and that the etiology of both diseases may be linked.

Necrotizing sarcoid granulomatosis

This probable variant of sarcoidosis is characterized by large necrotizing granulomas which often involve the pulmonary arteries and veins (Popper *et al.* 2003). The clinical presenta-tion can be variable, with some patients presenting with cough, dyspnea, fever and chest pain while others can be relatively asymptomatic. Pleural involvement with pleuritis and/or pleural effusions is frequently present, as is pulmon-ary involvement with radiographs showing widespread nodular infiltrates and cavitation.

A report on the characteristics of 14 cases of necrotizing sarcoid granulomas showed that the mean age of onset was 37 years and the mean delay between onset of symptoms and diagnosis of disease was 12 months (Quaden *et al.* 2005). In 12 of the 14 patients, extrapulmonary symptoms were more common than respiratory symptoms which were only present in eight patients. Lung function was normal in 13 patients but TLCO diffusing capacity was slightly impaired in 8 of 11 patients tested. A CT scan showed a solitary nodule in four patients, bilateral nodules in three and pulmonary infiltrates in seven out of the 14 tested. One patient died from neurological complications despite treatment with cortico-steroids and immunosuppressive drugs. Two patients relapsed after initial treatment with corticosteroids and two relapsed after surgery. No relapse occurred in five untreated patients. During follow-up, lung cancer was detected in two patients after 26 months and eight years, respectively.

Orofacial granulomatosis

This uncommon syndrome presents with recurrent or pro-gressive orofacial swelling with lip and tongue enlargement with frequently salivary gland involvement and cranial neuro-pathies, particularly seventh nerve palsies (Mignogna *et al.* 2003). The histological findings usually show sarcoid-like non-caseating epitheliod cell granulomas. The cause is unknown but it may be a variant of either sarcoidosis or Crohn's disease. Intralesional or systemic corticosteroids may be helpful but it is often resistant to medical therapy. Surgery may be needed to treat the resulting disfigurement.

Orofacial graulomatosis is described as an uncommon clinicopathological entity occurring in patients who have oral lesions characterized by persistent or recurrent soft tissue enlargement, oral ulceration and a variety of other orofacial features which on biopsy show lymphedema and non-caseating granulomas (Hodgson *et al.* 2004) while a 20-year review of the condition describes orofacial granulomatosis as the presence of persistent enlargement of soft tissues of the oral and maxillary regions which are characterized by non-caseating granuloma-tous infiltration in the absence of otherwise proven sarcoidosis or Crohn's disease (Grave *et al.* 2009). The etiology of the oral lesions includes oral Crohn's disease (some patients go on to to develop full-blown Crohn's disease after a period of months to years), sarcoidosis and contact food allergies. The authors conclude that there is no single effective treatment but in many cases trials of therapy may not be necessary. A report of six cases of the disease concludes that there is a wide spectrum of presentation, even among a small cohort of patients (Poate *et al.* 2008).

Although a quarter of a century has passed since the condition was first identified in 1985, there is no consensus as to whether it is a distinct entity or as to whether it is merely a variant of sarcoidosis or Crohn's disease. The etiology of the disease is unknown but causes suggested include the same as those for sarcoidosis.

CONCLUSION

Despite much investigation over the past century there is still no widespread consensus as to what actually causes sarcoidosis. There is general acceptance that the disease is the result of an altered immune response in a genetically susceptible individual to a single or multiple exogenous antigenic stimuli. However, the exact nature of the inciting stimuli has yet to be pinned down.

The most likely candidates are mycobacteria, and there is evidence that mycobacteria are found within sarcoidosis tissue at a higher incidence than normal tissues. This may also be true for propionibacteria, particularly within a Japanese population. However, the actual role of these organisms in the etiology of disease is far from certain.

It may be that a large number of inciting agents are capable of causing disease in a susceptible host and this hypothesis is reflected by the range of presentations of sarcoidosis as well as the clinical variations that the course of the disease takes in different individuals. Alternatively, there may still be a single cause of disease, albeit it one that has yet to be fully elucidated.

REFERENCES

Abdi EA, Nguyen GK, Ludwig RN, Dickout WJ (1987). Pulmonary sarcoidosis following interferon therapy for advanced renal cell carcinoma. *Cancer* 59: 896–900.

Allen SS, Evans W, Carlisle J et al. (2008). Superoxide dismutase A antigens derived from molecular analysis of sarcoidosis granulomas elicit systemic Th-1 immune responses. *Respir Res* 9: 36.

Almenoff PL, Johnson A, Lesser M, Mattman LH (1996). Growth of acid-fast L forms from the blood of patients with sarcoidosis. *Thorax* 51: 530–3.

Almodovar R, Izquierdo M, Zarco P et al. (2007). Pulmonary sarcoidosis in a patient with ankylosing spondylitis treated with infliximab. *Clin Exp Rheumatol* 25: 99–101.

Barnard J, Rose C, Newman L et al. (2005). Job and industry classifications associated with sarcoidosis in A Case–Control Etiologic Study of Sarcoidosis (ACCESS). *J Occup Environ Med* 47: 226–34.

Baughman RP, Lower EE, Bradley DA et al. (2005). Etanercept for refractory ocular sarcoidosis: results of a double-blind randomized trial. *Chest* 128: 1062–47.

Bhatia A, Kast RE (2007). Tumor necrosis factor (TNF) can paradoxically increase on etanercept treatment, occasionally contributing to TNF-mediated disease. *J Rheumatol* 34: 447–9; author reply 449–50.

Bocart D, Lecossier D, De Lassence A et al. (1992). A search for mycobacterial DNA in granulomatous tissues from patients with sarcoidosis using the polymerase chain reaction. *Am Rev Respir Dis* 145: 1142–8.

Bowman BU, Daniel TM (1971). Further evidence against the concept of decreased phage neutralizing ability of serum of patients with sarcoidosis. *Am Rev Respir Dis* 104: 908–14.

Bowman BU, Amos WT, Geer JC (1972). Failure to produce experimental sarcoidosis in guinea pigs with *Mycobacterium tuberculosis* and mycobacteriophage DS6A. *Am Rev Respir Dis* 105: 85–94.

Brett GZ (1965). Epidemiological trends in tuberculosis and sarcoidosis in a district of London between 1958 and 1963. *Tubercle* 46: 413–16.

Brown ST, Brett I, Almenoff PL et al. (2003). Recovery of cell wall-deficient organisms from blood does not distinguish between patients with sarcoidosis and control subjects. *Chest* 123: 413–17.

Cantwell AR (1981). Variably acid-fast bacteria in a case of systemic sarcoidosis and hypodermitis sclerodermiformis. *Dermatologica* 163: 239–48.

Chen ES, Wahlstrom J, Song Z et al. (2008). T-cell responses to mycobacterial catalase–peroxidase profile a pathogenic antigen in systemic sarcoidosis. *J Immunol* 181: 8784–96.

Cosma CL, Humbert O, Ramakrishnan L (2004). Superinfecting mycobacteria home to established tuberculous granulomas. *Nat Immunol* 5: 828–35.

Cummings MM, Hudgins PC (1958). Chemical constituents of pine pollen and their possible relationship to sarcoidosis. *Am J Med Sci* 236: 311–17.

Cummings MM, Dunner E, Schmidt RH, Barnwell JB (1956). Concepts of epidemiology of sarcoidosis; preliminary report of 1194 cases reviewed with special reference to geographic ecology. *Postgrad Med* 19: 437–46.

Daien CI, Monnier A, Claudepierre P et al. (2009). Sarcoid-like granulomatosis in patients treated with tumor necrosis factor blockers: 10 cases. *Rheumatology* (Oxford) 48: 883–6.

Derler AM, Eisendle K, Baltaci M et al. (2009). High prevalence of 'Borrelia-like' organisms in skin biopsies of sarcoidosis patients from Western Austria. *J Cutan Pathol* 36: 1262–8.

Dhaille F, Viseux V, Caudron A et al. (2010). Cutaneous sarcoidosis occurring during anti-TNF-alpha treatment: report of two cases. *Dermatology* 220: 234–7.

Drake WP, Pei Z, Pride DT et al. (2002). Molecular analysis of sarcoidosis tissues for mycobacterium species DNA. *Emerg Infect Dis* 8: 1334–41.

Drake WP, Dhason MS, Nadaf M et al. (2007). Cellular recognition of *Mycobacterium tuberculosis* ESAT-6 and KatG peptides in systemic sarcoidosis. *Infect Immun* 75: 527–30.

Dubaniewicz A, Trzonkowski P, Dubaniewicz-Wybieralska M et al. (2007). Mycobacterial heat shock protein-induced blood T lymphocytes subsets and cytokine pattern: comparison of sarcoidosis with tuberculosis and healthy controls. *Respirology* 12: 346–54.

Eishi Y, Suga M, Ishige I et al. (2002). Quantitative analysis of mycobacterial and propionibacterial DNA in lymph nodes of Japanese and European patients with sarcoidosis. *J Clin Microbiol* 40: 198–204.

Farber HW, Fairman RP, Glauser FL (1982). Talc granulomatosis: laboratory findings similar to sarcoidosis. *Am Rev Respir Dis* 125: 258–61.

Fite E, Fernandez-Figueras MT, Prats R et al. (2006). High prevalence of *Mycobacterium tuberculosis* DNA in biopsies from sarcoidosis patients from Catalonia, Spain. *Respiration* 73: 20–6.

Gaede KI, Wilke G, Brade L et al. (2002). Anti-*Chlamydophila* immunoglobulin prevalence in sarcoidosis and usual interstitial pneumoniae. *Eur Respir J* 19: 267–74.

Gentry JT, Nitowsky HM, Michael M (1955). Studies on the epidemiology of sarcoidosis in the United States: the relationship to soil areas and to urban–rural residence. *J Clin Invest* 34: 1839–56.

Goldberg HJ, Fiedler D, Webb A et al. (2006). Sarcoidosis after treatment with interferon-alpha: a case series and review of the literature. *Respir Med* 100: 2063–8.

Gonzalez-Lopez MA, Blanco R, Gonzalez-Vela MC et al. (2006). Development of sarcoidosis during etanercept therapy. *Arthritis Rheum* 55: 817–20.

Grave B, McCullough M, Wiesenfeld D (2009). Orofacial granulomatosis: a 20-year review. *Oral Dis* 15: 46–51.

Grizzanti JN, Rosenstreich DL (1988). Effect of inoculation of sarcoid tissue into athymic (nude) mice. *Sarcoidosis* 5: 136–41.

Gupta D, Agarwal R, Aggarwal AN, Jindal SK (2007). Molecular evidence for the role of mycobacteria in sarcoidosis: a meta-analysis. *Eur Respir J* 30: 508–16.

Hajizadeh R, Sato H, Carlisle J et al. (2007). *Mycobacterium tuberculosis* antigen 85A induces Th-1 immune responses in systemic sarcoidosis. *J Clin Immunol* 27: 445–54.

Hanngren A, Biberfeldy E, Galands E, Redfem RJ et al. (1980). Is sarcoidosis due to an infectious interaction, between virus and mycobacterium? *Proceedings of the Sixth International Conference,* Tokyo. University of Tokyo Press, Tokyo: pp. 8–11.

Hills SE, Parkes SA, Baker SB (1987). Epidemiology of sarcoidosis in the Isle of Man. 2: Evidence for space–time clustering. *Thorax* 42: 427–30.

Hodgson TA, Buchanan JA, Porter SR (2004). Orofacial granulomatosis. *J Oral Pathol Med* 33: 252.

Hoffmann RM, Jung MC, Motz R et al. (1998). Sarcoidosis associated with interferon-alpha therapy for chronic hepatitis C. *J Hepatol* 28: 1058–63.

Homma JY, Abe C, Chosa H et al. (1978). Bacteriological investigation on biopsy specimens from patients with sarcoidosis. *Jpn J Exp Med* 48: 251–5.

Hosoda Y, Sasagawa S, Yamaguchi T (2004). Sarcoidosis and tuberculosis: epidemiological similarities and dissimilarities. A review of a series of studies in a Japanese work population (1941–1996) and the general population (1959–1984). *Sarcoidosis Vasc Diffuse Lung Dis* 21: 85–93.

Hua B, Li QD, Wang FM et al. (1992). *Borrelia burgdorferi* infection may be the cause of sarcoidosis. *Chin Med J* (English) 105: 560–3.

Hurley TH, Bartholomeusz CL (1968). The Kveim test in sarcoidosis. *Med J Aust* 2: 947–9.

Hurley HJ, Shelley WB (1959). Comparison of the granuloma producing capacity of normals and sarcoid granuloma patients: experimental analysis of the sarcoid diathesis theory. *Am J Med Sci* 237 685–92.

Iliopoulos A, Psathakis K, Aslanidis S et al. (2006). Tuberculosis and granuloma formation in patients receiving anti-TNF therapy. *Int J Tuberc Lung Dis* 10: 588–90.

Inui N, Suda T, Chida K (2008). Use of the QuantiFERON-TB Gold test in Japanese patients with sarcoidosis. *Respir Med* 102: 313–15.

Ishige I, Usui Y, Takemura T, Eishi Y (1999). Quantitative PCR of mycobacterial and propionibacterial DNA in lymph nodes of Japanese patients with sarcoidosis. *Lancet* 354: 120–3.

Iwai K, Takahashi S (1976). Transmissibility of sarcoid-specific granulomas in the footpads of mice. *Ann NY Acad Sci* 278: 249–59.

Izbicki G, Chavko R, Banauch GI et al. (2007). World Trade Center 'sarcoid-like' granulomatous pulmonary disease in New York City Fire Department rescue workers. *Chest* 131: 1414–23.

Jansson E, Hannuksela M, Eklund H et al. (1972). Isolation of a mycoplasma from sarcoid tissue. *J Clin Pathol* 25: 837–42.

Kajdasz DK, Lackland DT, Mohr LC, Judson MA (2001). A current assessment of rurally linked exposures as potential risk factors for sarcoidosis. *Ann Epidemiol* 11: 111–17.

Keane J, Gershon S, Wise RP et al. (2001). Tuberculosis associated with infliximab, a tumor necrosis factor alpha-neutralizing agent. *N Engl J Med* 345: 1098–104.

Kent DC, Houk VN, Elliott RC et al. (1970). The definitive evaluation of sarcoidosis. *Am Rev Respir Dis* 101: 721–7.

Kindler V, Sappino AP, Grau GE et al. (1989). The inducing role of tumor necrosis factor in the development of bactericidal granulomas during BCG infection. *Cell* 56: 731–40.

Klemen H, Husain AN, Cagle PT et al. (2000). Mycobacterial DNA in recurrent sarcoidosis in the transplanted lung: a PCR-based study on four cases. *Virchows Arch* 436: 365–9.

Koz'min-Sokolov BN, Kostina ZI (1971). [Detection of mycobacteriophages in tuberculosis and sarcoidosis patients]. *Probl Tuberk* 49: 74–5.

Kucera GP, Rybicki BA, Kirkey KL et al. (2003). Occupational risk factors for sarcoidosis in African-American siblings. *Chest* 123: 1527–35.

Kucera RF (1989). A possible association of rheumatoid arthritis and sarcoidosis. *Chest* 95: 604–6.

Kudrin A, Chilvers ER, Ginawi A et al. (2007). Sarcoid-like granulomatous disease following etanercept treatment for RA. *J Rheumatol* 34: 648–9.

Löfgren S, Lundback H (1950). Isolation of a virus from six cases of sarcoidosis, lymphogranulomatosis benigna Schaumann. *Acta Med Scand* 138: 71–5.

Ludvigsson JF, Wahlstrom J, Grunewald J et al. (2007). Coeliac disease and risk of sarcoidosis. *Sarcoidosis Vasc Diffuse Lung Dis* 24: 121–6.

Lundbeck H, Löfgren S, Nordenstam H (1959). Cultivation of sarcoidotic tissue from lymph nodes and skin. *Br J Exp Pathol* 40: 61–5.

Lyons DJ, Donald S, Mitchell DN, Asherson GL (1992). Chemical inactivation of the Kveim reagent. *Respiration* 59: 22–6.

Mankiewicz E (1964). The relationship of sarcoidosis to anonymous bacteria. *Acta Med Scand Suppl* 425: 68–73.

Mankiewicz E, Beland J (1964). The role of mycobacteriophages and of cortisone in experimental tuberculosis and sarcoidosis. *Am Rev Respir Dis* 89: 707–20.

Mankiewicz E, Liivak M (1967). Mycobacteriophages isolated from human sources. *Nature* 216: 485–6.

Mathew S, Bauer KL, Fischoeder A et al. (2008). The anergic state in sarcoidosis is associated with diminished dendritic cell function. *J Immunol* 181: 746–55.

Metyas SK, Tadros RM, Arkfeld DG (2009). Adalimumab-induced noncaseating granuloma in the bone marrow of a patient being treated for rheumatoid arthritis *Rheumatol Int.* Feb (4): 437–9.

Mignogna MD, Fedele S, Lo Russo L, Lo Muzio L (2003). The multiform and variable patterns of onset of orofacial granulomatosis. *J Oral Pathol Med* 32: 200–5.

Mitchell DN, Rees RJ (1969). A transmissible agent from sarcoid tissue. *Lancet* 2: 81–4.

Mitchell DN, Rees RJ (1970a). An attempt to demonstrate a transmissible agent from sarcoid material. *Postgrad Med J* 46: 510–14.

Mitchell DN, Rees RJ (1970b). Agent transmissible from Crohn's disease tissue. *Lancet* 2: 168–71.

Mitchell DN, Rees RJ (1983). Studies of transmissible agents in sarcoidosis. In: Proceedings of the 9th International Conference on Sarcoidosis, Paris. Pergaman Press, Oxford, pp. 132–41.

Mitchell DN, Bradstreet CM, Dighero MW et al. (1974). [Irradiated Kveim suspensions [letter]. *Lancet* 1: 734.

Mitchell IC, Turk JL, Mitchell DN (1992). Detection of mycobacterial rRNA in sarcoidosis with liquid-phase hybridisation. *Lancet* 339: 1015–17.

Muller C, Briegel J, Haller M et al. (1996). Sarcoidosis recurrence following lung transplantation. *Transplantation* 61: 1117–19.

Newman LS, Rose CS, Bresnitz EA et al. (2004). A case–control etiologic study of sarcoidosis: environmental and occupational risk factors. *Am J Respir Crit Care Med* 170: 1324–30.

Nilsson K, Pahlson C, Lukinius A et al. (2002). Presence of *Rickettsia helvetica* in granulomatous tissue from patients with sarcoidosis. *J Infect Dis* 185: 1128–38.

Oswald-Richter KA, Culver DA, Hawkins C *et al.* (2009). Cellular responses to mycobacterial antigens are present in bronchoalveolar lavage fluid used in the diagnosis of sarcoidosis. *Infect Immun* **77**: 3740–8.

Padilla ML, Schilero GJ, Teirstein AS (2002). Donor-acquired sarcoidosis. *Sarcoidosis Vasc Diffuse Lung Dis* **19**: 18–24.

Parkes SA (1985). Incudince of sarcoidosis in the Isle of Man. *Thorax* **40**(4): 284–7.

Pink AE Fonia A Smith CH Barker JN (2010). The development of sarcoidosis on antitumour necrosis factor therapy: a paradox, *Br J Dermatol.* **163** (3): 648–9.

Poate TW, Sharma R, Moutasim KA *et al.* (2008). Orofacial presentations of sarcoidosis: a case series and review of the literature. *Br Dent J* **205**: 437–42.

Popper HH, Klemen H, Colby TV, Churg A (2003). Necrotizing sarcoid granulomatosis: is it different from nodular sarcoidosis? *Pneumologie* **57**: 268–71.

Popper HH, Klemen H, Hoefler G, Winter E (1997). Presence of mycobacterial DNA in sarcoidosis. *Hum Pathol* **28**: 796–800.

Quaden C, Tillie-Leblond I, Delobbe A *et al.* (2005). Necrotising sarcoid granulomatosis: clinical, functional, endoscopical and radiographical evaluations. *Eur Respir J* **26**: 778–85.

Redmond WB, Cater JC (1960). A bacteriophage specific for *Mycobacterium tuberculosis*, varieties hominis and bovis. *Am Rev Respir Dis* **82**: 781–6.

Refvem O (1954). The pathogenesis of Boeck's disease (sarcoidosis): investigations on the significance of foreign bodies, phospholipides and hypersensitivity in the formation of sarcoid tissue. *Acta Med Scand Suppl* **294**: 1–146.

Rutherford RM, Brutsche MH, Kearns M *et al.* (2004). Prevalence of coeliac disease in patients with sarcoidosis. *Eur J Gastroenterol Hepatol* **16**: 911–15.

Rybicki BA, Iannuzzi MC, Frederick MM *et al.* (2001). Familial aggregation of sarcoidosis: a case–control etiologic study of sarcoidosis (ACCESS). *Am J Respir Crit Care Med* **164**: 2085–91.

Santoianni G, Ayala L (1949). [Title not available]. *Ann Ital Dermatol Sifilogr* **4**: 9–16.

Scadding JG (1960). *Mycobacterium tuberculosis* in the etiology of sarcoidosis. *Br Med J* **2**: 1617–23.

Shepard CC (1960). The experimental disease that follows the injection of human leprosy bacilli into foot-pads of mice. *J Exp Med* **112**: 445–54.

Silverstein E, Friedland J, Lyons HA, Gourin A (1976). Markedly elevated angiotensin converting enzyme in lymph nodes containing non-necrotizing granulomas in sarcoidosis. *Proc Natl Acad Sci USA* **73**: 2137–41.

Sipahi Demirkok S, Basaranoglu M, Dervis E *et al.* (2006). Analysis of 87 patients with Löfgren's syndrome and the pattern of seasonality of subacute sarcoidosis. *Respirology* **11**: 456–61.

Song Z, Marzilli L, Greenlee B *et al.* (2005). Mycobacterial catalase-peroxidase is a tissue antigen and target of the adaptive immune response in systemic sarcoidosis. *J Exp Med* **201**: 755–67.

Spagnolo P, Du Bois RM (2007). Genetics of sarcoidosis. *Clin Dermatol* **25**: 242–9.

Steplewski Z (1976). The serach for viruses in sarcoidosis. *Ann NY Acad Sci* **278**: 260–3.

Sturfelt G, Christensson B, Bynke G, Saxne T (2007). Neurosarcoidosis in a patient with rheumatoid arthritis during treatment with infliximab. *J Rheumatol* **34**: 2313–14.

Svendsen CB, Milman N, Nielsen HW *et al.* (2009). A prospective study evaluating the presence of Rickettsia in Danish patients with sarcoidosis. *Scand J Infect Dis* **41**: 745–52.

Sweiss NJ, Baughman RP (2007). Tumor necrosis factor inhibition in the treatment of refractory sarcoidosis: slaying the dragon? *J Rheumatol* **34**: 2129–31.

Taylor-Robinson D, Canchola J, Fox H, Chanock RM (1964). A newly identified oral mycoplasma (*M. orale*) and its relationship to other human mycoplasmas. *Am J Hyg* **80**: 135–48.

Verschueren K, Van Essche E, Verschueren P *et al.* (2007). Development of sarcoidosis in etanercept-treated rheumatoid arthritis patients. *Clin Rheumatol* **26**: 1969–71.

Vokurka M, LeCossier D, Du Bois RM *et al.* (1997). Absence of DNA from mycobacteria of the *M. tuberculosis* complex in sarcoidosis. *Am J Respir Crit Care Med* **156**: 1000–3.

Wurm K, Kehler E, Reichelt H (1962). [On the pathogenesis of sarcoidosis (Boeck's disease): multiple appearance of sarcoidosis in tuberculous families]. *Med Klin* **57**: 1760–4.

Yamada T, Eishi Y, Ikeda S *et al.* (2002). In-situ localization of *Propionibacterium acnes* DNA in lymph nodes from sarcoidosis patients by signal amplification with catalysed reporter deposition. *J Pathol* **198**: 541–7.

Yasuhara T, Tada R, Nakano Y *et al.* (2005). The presence of *Propionibacterium* spp. in the vitreous fluid of uveitis patients with sarcoidosis. *Acta Ophthalmol Scand* **83**: 364–9.

Zettergren L (1954). [Lymphogranulomatosis benigna; a clinical and histopathological study of its relation to tuberculosis]. *Acta Soc Med Ups Suppl* **59**: 1–180.

5

Pathology

BRYAN CORRIN, ANDREW G NICHOLSON AND ANN DEWAR

INTRODUCTION

Sarcoidosis is a multisystem granulomatous disease of unknown cause that is characterized by enhanced cellular hypersensitivity at sites of involvement. The lesions of sarcoidosis may be confined to one organ or disseminated widely. Autopsy studies show that asymptomatic sarcoidosis is much more common than is realized clinically (Hagerstrand and Linell 1964). Lymph nodes, the lungs, liver, spleen, skin and eyes are the organs most commonly affected, but virtually any part of the body may be involved. The distribution of the lesions is consistent with the lungs being the portal of entry of an unknown causative agent, the lymph nodes being affected by lymphatic spread from the lungs, and other organs being involved by a combination of lymphatic and blood spread, a situation entirely analogous with that in tuberculosis.

A diagnosis of sarcoidosis may be made in biopsy-negative patients if there are appropriate clinical features and other supportive investigations, but the minimal criteria for an established diagnosis of sarcoidosis include histological evidence of non-necrotizing epithelioid granulomas. The other criteria for an established diagnosis are consistent clinico-radiological features and the exclusion of agents known to cause granulomatous disease (Joint Statement 1999).

THE SARCOID GRANULOMA

The histological hallmark of sarcoidosis is the granuloma. This consists of a central collection of epithelioid cells and multinucleate giant cells of either Langhans or foreign-body type surrounded by a peripheral rim of lymphocytes (Plate 1).

Granulomas are, of course, found in a variety of conditions, notably tuberculosis, some fungal infections and chronic berylliosis. They may also be found in the vicinity of tumors. The granulomas of primary biliary cirrhosis resemble those of sarcoid and occasional patients have features of both these diseases (Fagan *et al.* 1983). Pulmonary granulomas have also been reported in HIV-infected patients receiving antiretroviral therapy (Naccache *et al.* 1999) and in leukemic patients being treated with interferon-α (Pietropaoli *et al.* 1999).

Sarcoid granulomas differ from those of tuberculosis in that they do not undergo caseation, although a little central necrosis is occasionally seen microscopically (Fig. 5.1). The giant cells often contain Schaumann and asteroid bodies (Plates 2 and 3) but these are not pathognomonic of sarcoidosis because they may be found in other forms of granulomatous inflammation. Schaumann bodies represent lysosomal residual bodies (Reid and Andersen 1988; Visscher *et al.* 1988), while asteroid bodies are aggregates of vimentin

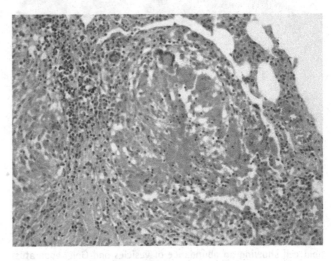

Figure 5.1 Although sarcoid granulomas are generally described as non-necrotizing, they often show a little central necrosis.

microfilaments and microtubules derived from the cytosphere, the radial arrangement of which determines the bodies' stellate form (Cain and Kraus 1983). Lymph nodes draining sarcoid tissue often contain small brown Hamazaki–Wesenberg bodies, which represent lysosomal ceroid pigment formed through the oxidation and polymerization of unsaturated fatty acids.

Epithelioid cells are derived from macrophages, but such is the transformation they undergo during this development that there are few ultrastructural similarities: gone are the phagosomes and lysosomes of a macrophage, replaced by cytoplasmic organelles more in keeping with a secretory cell. The immature epithelioid cell is rich in rough endoplasmic reticulum, as seen in cells synthesizing a proteinaceous secretion. Golgi apparatus and storage vesicles then appear, and in the mature epithelioid cell these organelles predominate (Fig. 5.2) (De Vos *et al.* 1990). Epithelioid cells secrete a variety of proinflammatory cytokines and fibrogenic cytokines, including transforming growth factor-β, tumor necrosis factor-α, RANTES and nitric oxide synthase (Mornex

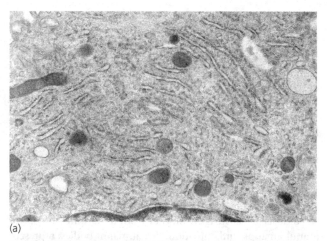
(a)

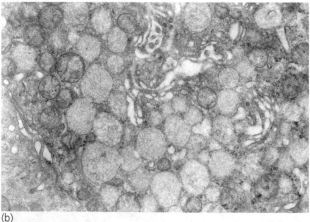
(b)

Figure 5.2   Electron micrographs of epithelioid cells in a pulmonary sarcoid granuloma. (a) An immature epithelioid cell showing abundant rough endoplasmic reticulum. The lysosomal dense bodies that characterize a macrophage are not evident. The electron-dense structures are mitochondria. (b) A mature epithelioid cell showing an abundance of vesicles and Golgi apparatus. Reproduced from Corrin B and Nicholson AG, *Pathology of the Lungs*, 3rd edn (2010), by permission of Churchill Livingstone.

et al. 1994; Myatt *et al.* 1994; Petrek *et al.* 1997; Shigehara *et al.* 1998; Tolnay *et al.* 1998; Facchetti *et al.* 1999). The enzyme dipeptidyl carboxypeptidase (EC3.4.15.1), which acts as a kininase but is best known by its trivial name angiotensin-converting enzyme, has been localized to the cytoplasm of the epithelioid cells (Pertschuk *et al.* 1981) which would therefore appear to be the source of the high serum levels of this enzyme that characterize granulomatous disease in general and sarcoidosis in particular. The granulomas are also responsible for the final hydroxylation and hence activation of vitamin D (Adams *et al.* 1983), thereby accounting for the hypercalcemia that is so frequently found in sarcoidosis (Papapoulos *et al.* 1979).

Closely associated with the centrally situated epithelioid cells are T-helper lymphocytes. T-suppressor lymphocytes are fewer in number and more peripherally situated (van den Oord *et al.* 1984; van Maarsseven *et al.* 1986). Antigen-presenting reticular cells are found at the periphery of the granulomas and B-lymphocytes between the granulomas (Fazel *et al.* 1992). Cytokine studies suggest that the T-helper lymphocytes are mainly of the Th1 phenotype, producing interleukin-2 and interferon-γ (Baumer *et al.* 1997; Minshall *et al.* 1997). Tissue gene-expression analyses have shown a gene network engaged in Th1-type responses to be significantly overexpressed in pulmonary sarcoidosis, with proteins MMP-12 and ADAMDEC1 emerging as likely mediators of lung damage and/or remodeling (Crouser *et al.* 2009). A switch to predominantly Th2 lymphocytes may underlie a change from healing by resolution to healing by fibrosis.

Spontaneous resolution is common, suggesting that the granulomas often resolve, but in other patients healing is by fibrosis (Plate 4). The latter process involves progressive hyalinization until Schaumann bodies are the only indication that extensive scarring is the result of granulomatous disease (Plate 3). However, active and healed granulomas are often seen together, suggesting that the unknown stimulus to the disease is a continuing one with new granulomas constantly replacing those that heal (Plate 4). Fibrosis may be evident histologically in new cases, indicating that the disease may be quite advanced before it causes symptoms.

HISTOPATHOLOGY

Involvement of the mediastinal lymph nodes is a prominent and probably early feature of sarcoidosis. The follicular architecture of the lymph nodes is often completely effaced by numerous non-necrotizing granulomas (Fig. 5.3). Similarly, in the lungs, many such granulomas may be seen. They are generally found scattered throughout otherwise unremarkable lung tissue (Plate 5), usually confined to the interstitium and only rarely involving air spaces. They may be so numerous that they become confluent, and rarely, large masses of sarcoid tissue are formed, the so-called nodular or conglomerate form of sarcoidosis (Plate 6) (Abramowicz *et al.* 1992; Malaisamy *et al.* 2009).

The pulmonary granulomas are preceded by a lymphocytic infiltrate (Rosen *et al.* 1978), but this is transient and is seldom evident by the time lung biopsy is undertaken.

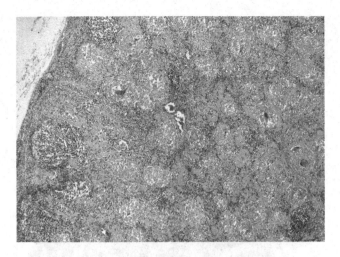

Figure 5.3   Lymph node containing prominent sarcoid granulomas.

Indeed, in contrast to extrinsic allergic alveolitis, which is also characterized by pulmonary granulomas, the histopathology of pulmonary sarcoidosis is generally notable in that it lacks a diffuse lymphocytic infiltrate (Plate 5). In the lungs the granulomas are most numerous along the lymphatics and are therefore particularly well seen in relation to the centriacinar bronchiolo-arterial bundles (Plate 7) and in the interlobular septa. They are very well developed in the main airways, including the mucosa, so this is a condition in which small fibreoptic bronchial biopsies frequently provide sufficient tissue for diagnostic purposes (Hsu *et al.* 1996). Also, because of their distribution along lymphatics, the granulomas come very close to arteries and veins and quite frequently involve all coats of these vessels in a granulomatous angiitis (Michaels *et al.* 1960; Rosen *et al.* 1979; Takemura *et al.* 1992) (Fig. 5.4). All sizes of vessel, from large elastic arteries to venules and lymphatics, may be affected, but veins are the vessels most commonly involved (Takemura *et al.* 1992). Indeed, sarcoidosis can sometimes cause veno-occlusive disease (Jones *et al.* 2009). Right heart strain has been attributed to this vascular involvement, although widespread pulmonary fibrosis is a more important cause (Battesi *et al.* 1978; Rodman *et al.* 1990). Rarely, sarcoidosis is combined with disseminated visceral giant cell angiitis (Gartside 1944; Lie 1991; Marcussen and Lund 1989; Shintaku *et al.* 1989). Such patients may have disseminated necrotizing granulomatosis, glomerulonephritis and systemic angiitis, as seen in Wegener's granulomatosis, combined with typical sarcoid granulomas. Vascular involvement is also prominent in what has been termed necrotizing sarcoid granulomatosis, which is considered more fully below.

DIFFERENTIAL DIAGNOSIS

When considering the differential diagnosis of sarcoidosis, infections such as tuberculosis always have to be considered. The only conclusive histological distinction is the identification of *Mycobacterium tuberculosis* by Ziehl–Neelsen staining, but features that favor sarcoidosis include granulomatous

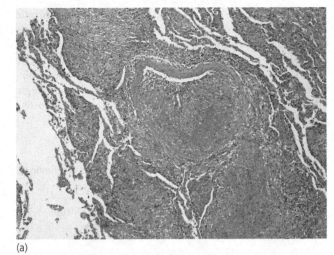

(a)

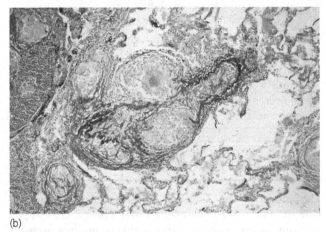

(b)

Figure 5.4   (a) Vascular involvement in pulmonary sarcoid (H&E). (b) Granulomas within and alongside a small vein, the lumen of which is occluded and the wall partly destroyed (Elastin–van Gieson stain). Reproduced from Corrin B and Nicholson AG, *Pathology of the Lungs*, 3rd edn (2010), by permission of Churchill Livingstone.

involvement of blood vessels and the presence of Schaumann bodies (Hsu *et al.* 1996).

Sarcoidosis also has to be distinguished from a giant cell reaction to foreign material, for which polarizing filters are indispensible (not forgetting that fragmented Schaumann bodies are usually birefringent). However, the onset of sarcoidosis is sometimes first evident in old scars containing foreign material. In general, sarcoid granulomas are more florid than the ordinary reaction to foreign material.

Sarcoid granulomas are also a well known phenomenon in lymph nodes draining tumors. They may also be seen close to a tumor in organs such as the lung and may even mask the tumor (Risbano *et al.* 2007). Overlooking lymphoma in a lymph node showing florid secondary granulomas is a notorious trap for the unwary pathologist. Reports of sarcoidosis being associated with lymphoma should be accepted only if the two diseases affect anatomically distinct sites and the appropriate clinical, radiographic and biochemical features of each disease are present (Karakantza *et al.* 1996).

Sarcoid-like granulomas characterize extrinsic allergic alveolitis but here they are generally more poorly formed, scanty, and seen on a background of diffuse chronic interstitial pneumonia, in contrast to pulmonary sarcoidosis in which well-formed granulomas are usually studded throughout otherwise normal alveolar tissue (Table 5.1). Even in very late sarcoidosis, lesions are generally recognizable as burnt-out granulomas, whereas in extrinsic allergic alveolitis the granulomas resolve without trace within a few months of last exposure to the responsible antigen.

Table 5.1   Comparison of the histological features of pulmonary sarcoidosis and extrinsic allergic alveolitis.

	Sarcoid	Extrinsic allergic alveolitis
Granulomas	Persistent, well formed	Evanescent, poorly formed
Interstitial pneumonitis	Inconspicuous	Prominent, peribronchiolar
Intraluminal fibrosis	Absent	Present
Lymph node involvement	Prominent	Absent

COURSE AND PROGNOSIS

The course of the disease is unpredictable. In about 60 percent of cases the lesions regress over a period of 2–5 years and the patient recovers. After spontaneous improvement relapse is unusual. Sometimes, however, the involved organs become progressively infiltrated and there is extensive fibrosis. In the lungs this results in upper-lobe volume loss and traction bronchiectasis. Based on the radiographic changes, four stages of thoracic sarcoidosis have been described:

1. bilateral hilar lymphadenopathy (Löfgren's syndrome);
2. bilateral hilar lymphadenopathy and lung involvement;
3. lung involvement without hilar lymphadenopathy;
4. irreversible pulmonary fibrosis.

However, except that stage 4 is obviously preceded by stages 2 or 3, these are modes of presentation rather than successive stages: lung involvement is not necessarily preceded by hilar lymphadenopathy.

An acute onset with erythema nodosum or asymptomatic bilateral hilar lymphadenopathy usually heralds a self-limiting course, whereas an insidious onset, especially with multiple extrapulmonary lesions, is more likely to be followed by relentless pulmonary fibrosis. Older patients and black people do less well than the young and whites. Advanced pulmonary sarcoidosis is often represented by upper-lobe honeycombing (Fig. 5.5 and Plate 8), which may be complicated by life-threatening saprophytic aspergillosis (Plate 9). An increased risk of pulmonary lymphoma and carcinoma has been identified in some studies (Askling *et al.* 1999; Bouros *et al.* 2002) but not in others (Seersholm *et al.* 1997).

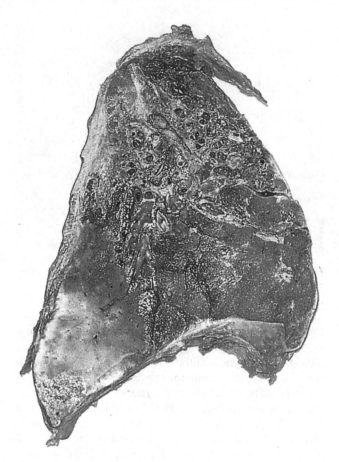

Figure 5.5   Late-stage pulmonary sarcoidosis: a whole lung slice showing fibrosis maximal in the upper lobe. Reproduced from Corrin B, Nicholson AG, *Pathology of the Lungs*, 3rd edn (2010), by permission of Churchill Livingstone and Dr N Gubbay, Cheltenham, UK.

The disease carries a mortality of about 5 percent, most of the deaths being attributable to either cardiac involvement or pulmonary fibrosis causing respiratory failure (Huang *et al.* 1981; Iwai *et al.* 1993; Perry and Vuitch 1995). Rare causes of death include chronic renal failure due to nephrosclerosis and the cerebral effects of meningovascular sarcoidosis. If lung transplantation is undertaken the disease may develop in the new lungs, and there is evidence that it derives from recipient immune cells (Johnson *et al.* 1993; Milman *et al.* 2005).

NECROTIZING SARCOID ANGIITIS AND GRANULOMATOSIS

Necrotizing sarcoid angiitis and granulomatosis combines the vasculitis and necrotizing granulomatosis seen in Wegener's granulomatosis with numerous non-necrotizing sarcoid granulomas (Liebow 1973). Women are affected more than men and the age range is wide with a mean of about 35 years (Saldana 1978; Churg *et al.* 1979; Koss *et al.* 1980; Churg 1983; Chittock *et al.* 1994; Quaden *et al.* 2005). Some patients are asymptomatic but most have non-specific respiratory symptoms accompanied by malaise (Quaden *et al.* 2005).

The condition is usually confined to the lungs. Chest radiographs show multiple nodules or masses measuring up to several centimeters in diameter, most numerous in the lower zones. Occasionally the lesions are unilateral or even single (Stephen *et al.* 1976; Saldana 1978). Cavitation is rare. Patients with diffuse infiltrates are occasionally encountered (Quaden *et al.* 2005).

Although evidence of extrapulmonary involvement is generally uncommon, hilar lymph node enlargement was a feature of more than half the patients in one series (Churg *et al.* 1979), and granulomas may be found in these nodes. Ocular and central nervous system involvement has also been reported (Churg *et al.* 1979; Beach *et al.* 1980; Dykhuizen *et al.* 1997; Strickland-Marmol *et al.* 2000; Quaden *et al.* 2005), and in some patients the disease has been associated with dacroadenitis and ulcerative colitis (Legall *et al.* 1996) or cutaneous involvement (Shirodaria *et al.* 2003). Generally, however, the disease is confined to the lungs and the prognosis is good, resolution occurring either spontaneously or following corticosteroid therapy (Chittock *et al.* 1994).

Pathologically, the lesions of necrotizing sarcoid granulomatosis form irregular areas of induration, which microscopically consist of confluent aggregates of epithelioid and giant cell granulomas with surrounding fibrosis and chronic inflammation (Fig. 5.6). The granulomas are identical to those seen in sarcoidosis and, as in sarcoidosis, they tend to follow lymphatic pathways in the bronchovascular bundles, the interlobular septa and the pleura, and may show a small central area of necrosis. However, there are also larger areas of coagulative necrosis, reminiscent of those seen in Wegener's disease (Fig. 5.7). Regression of the inflammation may leave the necrotic areas surrounded only by hyaline connective tissue. Various patterns of vasculitis may be seen, all involving both arteries or veins, and destroying the vessel wall to a varying extent. The vessels may show discrete granulomas, a more diffuse proliferation of giant cells and epithelioid macrophages, or merely lymphocyte and plasma cell infiltration (Figs 5.7 and 5.8). There may also be bronchial involvement, as in both sarcoidosis and Wegener's granulomatosis.

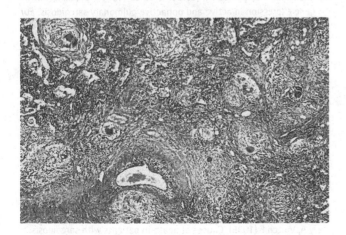

Figure 5.6 Necrotizing sarcoid granulomatosis. The lung contains numerous non-necrotizing epithelioid and giant cell granulomas and a necrotizing arteritis is also evident. Reproduced from Corrin B and Nicholson AG, *Pathology of the Lungs*, 3rd edn (2010), by permission of Churchill Livingstone.

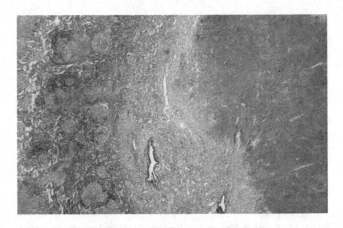

Figure 5.7 Necrotizing sarcoid granulomatosis. This low-power view shows non-necrotizing sarcoid-like granulomas (*left*) in conjunction with a large area of necrosis (*right*). Reproduced from Corrin B and Nicholson AG, *Pathology of the Lungs*, 3rd edn (2010), by permission of Churchill Livingstone.

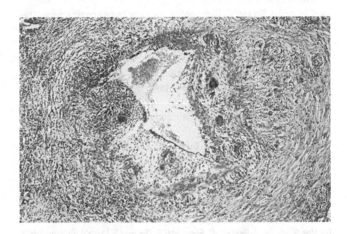

Figure 5.8 Necrotizing sarcoid granulomatosis. A pulmonary artery shows a granulomatous vasculitis. Reproduced from Corrin B and Nicholson AG, *Pathology of the Lungs*, 3rd edn (2010), by permission of Churchill Livingstone.

The differential diagnosis is chiefly from Wegener's granulomatosis and infection. The distinction from Wegener's is usually not difficult because well-formed non-necrotizing sarcoid granulomas are not a feature of Wegener's. Differentiation from infection may be more difficult and require negative special stains and culture. Whether the condition is to be distinguished from sarcoid is a moot point. It has been suggested that necrotizing sarcoid granulomatosis merely represents a variant of sarcoidosis in which mass lesions form, so-called nodular sarcoidosis (Plate 6) (Churg *et al.* 1979; Popper *et al.* 2003). This is supported by reports of raised levels of serum angiotensin-converting enzyme, selective migration of T-helper lymphocytes to the lung, and development of the disease in one of a family with a strong history of sarcoidosis (Spiteri *et al.* 1987; Lazzarini *et al.* 2008). Furthermore, as noted above, vascular involvement is frequently seen in sarcoidosis (Rosen *et al.* 1977). However, the broad areas of necrosis seen in necrotizing sarcoid granulomatosis are not a feature of classic sarcoidosis. In one case, onset coincided with *Chlamydia pneumoniae* infection (Tauber *et al.* 1999).

REFERENCES

Abramowicz MJ, Ninane V, Depierreux M et al. (1992). Tumour-like presentation of pulmonary sarcoidosis. Eur Respir J 5: 1286–7.

Adams JS, Sharma OP, Glacad MA, Singer FR (1983). Metabolism of 25-hydroxyvitamin D3 by cultured pulmonary alveolar macrophages in sarcoidosis. J Clin Invest 72: 1856–60.

Askling J, Grunewald J, Eklund A et al. (1999). Increased risk for cancer following sarcoidosis. Am J Respir Crit Care Med 160: 1668–72.

Battesi JP, Georges R, Basset F, Saumon G (1978). Chronic cor pulmonale in pulmonary sarcoidosis. Thorax 33: 76–84.

Baumer I, Zissel G, Schlaak M, MullerQuernheim J (1997). Th1/Th2 cell distribution in pulmonary sarcoidosis. Am J Respir Cell Molec Biol 16: 171–7.

Beach RC, Corrin B, Scopes JW, Graham E (1980). Necrotizing sarcoid granulomatosis with neurologic lesions in a child. J Pediatr 97: 950–3.

Bouros D, Hatzakis K, Labrakis H, Zeibecoglou K (2002). Association of malignancy with diseases causing interstitial pulmonary changes. Chest 121: 1278–89.

Cain H, Kraus B (1983). Immunofluorescence microscopic demonstration of vimentin filaments in asteroid bodies of sarcoidosis: comparison with electron microscopic findings. Virchows Arch B Cell Pathol 42: 213–26.

Chittock DR, Joseph MG, Paterson NAM, McFadden RG (1994). Necrotizing sarcoid granulomatosis with pleural involvement. Chest 106: 672–6.

Churg A (1983). Pulmonary angiitis and granulomatosis revisited. Hum Pathol 14: 868–83.

Churg A, Carrington CB, Gupta R (1979). Necrotizing sarcoid granulomatosis. Chest 76: 406–13.

Crouser ED, Culver DA, Knox KS et al. (2009). Gene expression profiling identifies MMP-12 and ADAMDEC1 as potential pathogenic mediators of pulmonary sarcoidosis. Am J Respir Crit Care Med 179: 929–38.

De Vos R, de Wolf-Peeters C, Facchetti F, Desmet V (1990). Plasmacytoid monocytes in epithelioid cell granulomas: ultrastructural and immunoelectron microscopic study. Ultrastruct Pathol 14: 291–302.

Dykhuizen RS, Smith CC, Kennedy MM et al. (1997). Necrotizing sarcoid granulomatosis with extrapulmonary involvement. Eur Respir J 10: 245–7.

Facchetti F, Vermi W, Fiorentini S et al. (1999). Expression of inducible nitric oxide synthase in human granulomas and histiocytic reactions. Am J Pathol 154: 145–52.

Fagan EA, Moore-Gillon JC, Turner-Warwick M (1983). Multiorgan granulomas and mitochondrial antibodies. New Engl J Med 308: 572–5.

Fazel SB, Howie SEM, Krajewski AS, Lamb D (1992). Lymphocyte-B accumulations in human pulmonary sarcoidosis. Thorax 47: 964–7.

Gartside IB (1944). Granulomatous arteritis in a lesion resembling sarcoidosis. J Pathol Bacteriol 56: 61–6.

Hagerstrand I, Linell F (1964). The prevalence of sarcoidosis in the autopsy material from a Swedish town. Acta Medica Scand Suppl 425: 171.

Hsu RM, Connors AF, Tomashefski JF (1996). Histologic, microbiologic, and clinical correlates of the diagnosis of sarcoidosis by transbronchial biopsy. Arch Pathol Lab Med 120: 364–8.

Huang CT, Heurich AE, Sutton AL, Lyons HA (1981). Mortality in sarcoidosis: a changing pattern of the causes of death. Eur J Respir Dis 62: 231–8.

Iwai K, Tachibana T, Takemura T et al. (1993). Pathological studies on sarcoidosis autopsy. I: Epidemiological features of 320 cases in Japan. Acta Pathol Jpn 43: 372–6.

Johnson BA, Duncan SR, Ohori NP et al. (1993). Recurrence of sarcoidosis in pulmonary allograft recipients. Am Rev Respir Dis 148: 1373–7.

Joint Statement of the American Thoracic Society (ATS), the European Respiratory Society (ERS) and the World Association of Sarcoidosis and Other Granulomatous Disorders (WASOG), adopted by the ATS Board of Directors and by the ERS Executive Committee (1999). Am J Respir Crit Care Med 160: 736–55.

Jones RM, Dawson A, Jenkins GH et al. (2009). Sarcoidosis-related pulmonary veno-occlusive disease presenting with recurrent haemoptysis. Eur Respir J 34: 517–20.

Karakantza M, Matutes E, Maclennan K et al. (1996). Association between sarcoidosis and lymphoma revisited. J Clin Pathol 49: 208–12.

Koss MN, Hochholzer L, Feigin DS et al. (1980). Necrotizing sarcoid-like granulomatosis: clinical, pathologic and immunopathologic findings. Hum Pathol 11(Suppl.): 510–19.

Lazzarini LC, de Fatima do Amparo Teixeira M et al. (2008). Necrotizing sarcoid granulomatosis in a family of patients with sarcoidosis reinforces the association between both entities. Respiration 76: 356–60.

Legall F, Loeuillet L, Delaval P et al. (1996). Necrotizing sarcoid granulomatosis with and without extrapulmonary involvement. Pathol Res Pract 192: 306–13.

Lie JT (1991). Combined sarcoidosis and disseminated visceral giant cell angiitis: a third opinion. Arch Pathol Lab Med 115: 210–11.

Liebow AA (1973). Pulmonary angiitis and granulomatosis. Am Rev Respir Dis 108: 1–18.

Malaisamy S, Dalal B, Bimenyuy C, Soubani A (2009). The clinical and radiologic features of nodular pulmonary sarcoidosis. Lung 187: 9–15.

Marcussen N, Lund C (1989). Combined sarcoidosis and disseminated visceral giant cell vasculitis. Pathol Res Pract 184: 325–30.

Michaels L, Brown NJ, Cory-Wright M (1960). Arterial changes in pulmonary sarcoidosis. Arch Pathol 69: 741–9.

Milman N, Andersen CB, Burton CM, Iversen M (2005). Recurrent sarcoid granulomas in a transplanted lung derive from recipient immune cells. Eur Respir J 26: 549–52.

Minshall EM, Tsicopoulos A, Yasruel Z et al. (1997). Cytokine mRNA gene expression in active and nonactive pulmonary sarcoidosis. Eur Resp J 10: 2034–9.

Mornex JF, Leroux C, Greenland T, Ecochard D (1994). From granuloma to fibrosis in interstitial lung diseases: molecular and cellular interactions. Eur Respir J 7: 779–85.

Myatt N, Coghill G, Morrison K et al. (1994). Detection of tumour necrosis factor alpha in sarcoidosis and tuberculosis granulomas using in-situ hybridization. J Clin Pathol 47: 423–6.

Naccache JM, Antoine M, Wislez M et al. (1999). Sarcoid-like pulmonary disorder in human immunodeficiency virus-infected patients receiving antiretroviral therapy. Am J Respir Crit Care Med 159: 2009–13.

Papapoulos SE, Frahjer LJ, Sandler LM et al. (1979). 1,25-dihydroxycholecalciferol in the pathogenesis of the hypercalcemia of sarcoidosis. Lancet ii: 627–30.

Perry A, Vuitch F (1995). Causes of death in patients with sarcoidosis: a morphologic study of 38 autopsies with clinicopathologic correlations. Arch Pathol Lab Med 119: 167–72.

Pertschuk LP, Silverstein E, Friedland J (1981). Immunohistologic diagnosis of sarcoidosis: detection of angiotensin-converting enzyme in sarcoid granulomas. *Am J Clin Pathol* **75**: 350–4.

Petrek M, Pantelidis P, Southcott AM *et al.* (1997). The source and role of RANTES in interstitial lung disease. *Eur Resp J* **10**: 1207–16.

Pietropaoli A, Modrak J, Utell M (1999). Interferon-alpha therapy associated with the development of sarcoidosis. *Chest* **116**: 569–72.

Popper HH, Klemen H, Colby TV, Churg A (2003). Necrotizing sarcoid granulomatosis: is it different from nodular sarcoidosis? *Pneumologie* **57**: 268–71.

Quaden C, Tillie-Leblond I, Delobbe A *et al.* (2005). Necrotising sarcoid granulomatosis: clinical, functional, endoscopical and radiographical evaluations. *Eur Respir J* **26**: 778–85.

Reid JD, Andersen ME (1988). Calcium oxalate in sarcoid granulomas: with particular reference to the small ovoid body and a note on the finding of dolomite. *Am J Clin Pathol* **90**: 545–58.

Risbano MG, Groshong SD, Schwarz MI (2007). Lung nodules in a woman with a history of breast cancer. *Chest* **132**: 1697–701.

Rodman DM, Lindenfeld JA (1990). Successful treatment of sarcoidosis-associated pulmonary hypertension with corticosteroids. *Chest* **97**: 500–2.

Rosen Y, Athanassiades TJ, Moon S, Lyons HA (1978). Nongranulomatous interstitial pneumonitis in sarcoidosis: relationship to development of epithelioid granulomas. *Chest* **74**: 122–5.

Rosen Y, Moon S, Huang C-T, Lyons HA (1977). Granulomatous pulmonary angiitis in sarcoidosis. *Arch Pathol Lab Med* **101**: 170–4.

Rosen Y, Vuletin JC, Pertschuk LP, Silverstein E (1979). Sarcoidosi: from the pathologist's vantage point. *Pathol Annu* **14**(Pt 1): 405–39.

Saldana MJ (1978). Necrotizing sarcoid granulomatosis: clinicopathologic observations in 24 patients [abstract]. *Lab Invest* **38**: 364.

Seersholm N, Vestbo J, Viskum K (1997). Risk of malignant neoplasms in patients with pulmonary sarcoidosis. *Thorax* **52**: 892–4.

Shigehara K, Shijubo N, Hirasawa M *et al.* (1998). Immunolocalization of extracellular matrix proteins and integrins in sarcoid lymph nodes. *Virchows Archiv* **433**: 55–61.

Shintaku M, Mase K, Ohtsuki H *et al.* (1989). Generalized sarcoid-like granulomas with systemic angiitis, crescentic glomerulonephritis, and pulmonary hemorrhage. *Arch Pathol Lab Med* **113**: 1295–8.

Shirodaria CC, Nicholson AG, Hansell DM *et al.* (2003). Lesson of the month: necrotizing sarcoid granulomatosis with skin involvement. *Histopathology* **43**: 91–3.

Spiteri MA, Gledhill A, Campbell D, Clarke SW (1987). Necrotizing sarcoid granulomatosis. *Br J Dis Chest* **81**: 70–5.

Stephen JG, Braimbridge MV, Corrin B *et al.* (1976). Necrotizing 'sarcoidal' angiitis and granulomatosis of the lung. *Thorax* **31**: 356–60.

Strickland-Marmol LB, Fessler RG, Rojiani AM (2000). Necrotizing sarcoid granulomatosis mimicking an intracranial neoplasm: clinicopathologic features and review of the literature. *Modern Pathol* **13**: 909–13.

Takemura T, Matsui Y, Saiki S, Mikami R (1992). Pulmonary vascular involvement in sarcoidosis: a report of 40 autopsy cases. *Hum Pathol* **23**: 1216–23.

Tauber E, Wojnarowski C, Horcher E *et al.* (1999). Necrotizing sarcoid granulomatosis in a 14-year-old female. *Eur Respir J* **13**: 703–5.

Tolnay E, Kuhnen C, Voss B *et al.* (1998). Expression and localization of vascular endothelial growth factor and its receptor flt in pulmonary sarcoidosis. *Virchows Archiv* **432**: 61–5.

van den Oord JJ, de Wolf-Peeters C, Fachetti F, Desmet VJ (1984). Cellular composition of hypersensitivity-type granulomas: immunohistochemical analysis of tuberculous and sarcoidal lymphadenitis. *Hum Pathol* **15**: 559–65.

van Maarsseven ACMT, Mullink H, Alons CL, Stam J (1986). Distribution of T-lymphocyte subsets in different portions of sarcoid granulomas: immunohistologic analysis with monoclonal antibodies. *Hum Pathol* **17**: 493–500.

Visscher D, Churg A, Katzenstein AL (1988). Significance of crystalline inclusions in lung granulomas. *Modern Pathol* **1**: 415–19.

6

Immunology

DAVID MOLLER, MUHUNTHAN THILLAI, AJIT LALVANI AND DONALD MITCHELL

INTRODUCTION

The pathologic hallmark of sarcoidosis is discrete, compact non-caseating granulomas. The granulomas comprise mainly epithelioid cells with CD4 lymphocytes, mature macrophages and multinucleated giant cells interspersed throughout the epithelioid core and CD8 lymphocytes in the periphery. The granulomatous inflammation leads to distortion of local architecture, tissue injury and fibrosis.

Granuloma formation is a form of host response to poorly soluble or insoluble foreign material that is evolutionarily conserved among both invertebrates and vertebrates. Current dogma contends that granulomas are designed to help protect (wall-off) harmful pathogens. This simplistic concept has recently undergone a reassessment from studies in zebrafish that suggest the granulomatous response to pathogenic mycobacteria is a pathogen-induced mechanism that facilitates their spread within the host (Davis and Ramakrishnan 2009). Unlike humans and mice, zebrafish lack an adaptive immune system. In humans and mice, both innate and adaptive immunity, orchestrated by key cytokines, chemokines and regulatory cells, lead to the development, maintenance and resolution of the granulomatous response (Kunkel *et al.* 1996).

The innate immune system is the first line of defense against foreign pathogens and is non-antigen-specific. Phagocytic cells, natural killer cells and dendritic cells express pattern-recognition receptors such as the Toll-like receptors (TLRs) that recognize molecular patterns on pathogens. Stimulation of these receptors triggers the release of cytokines such as TNF, IL-1 and IL-6, which leads to a generalized priming of the adaptive immune system.

Adaptive immunity involves T- and B-cell responses characterized by antigen specificity and memory. In granulomatous inflammation, pathogenic antigens are internalized by antigen-presenting cells (APCs) (dendritic cells, macrophages), processed to yield antigenic peptide fragments loaded onto MHC class I or II molecules for display on the surface of APCs. The MHC/peptide complex is interrogated by T-cells with antigen-specific receptors that, when accompanied by co-stimulation, results in the production of specific effector or regulatory cytokines. Naive T-cells develop into subsets of T-cells with specific transcriptional and cytokine profiles following exposure to cytokines and antigen (Swain 1994). T-helper (Th1) lymphocytes express the transcription factor Tbet and produce IFN-γ, IL-2 and lymphotoxin; Th2 lymphocytes express GATA-3 and produce IL-4, IL-5 and IL-13; Th17 cells express RORγt and produce IL-17 and IL-21. Regulatory T-cells express Foxp3 and produce IL-10 and/or TGF-β.

Granulomatous inflammation is typically polarized towards either a Th1, Th2 or Th17 cytokine profile depending on the nature of the inciting stimuli. For example, mycobacterial (PPD) antigens induce Th1-dominant granulomatous responses, schistosomal egg antigens (SEA) tend to elicit Th2 responses, and hypersensitivity pneumonitis may involve dominant Th17 responses (Scott *et al.* 1989; Chensue *et al.* 1994). These effector cytokines collaborate with pro-inflammatory cytokines such as TNF to enhance the innate immune response (phagocytosis, oxidative burst) which together orchestrate the granulomatous response (Chiu *et al.* 2003).

Despite the fact that granuloma-inducing agents in sarcoidosis first interact with cells of the innate immune system, relatively little is known about the relevant mechanisms. Our current concepts of sarcoidosis derive largely from studies of the adaptive immune system, so it is helpful from both an historical and pathobiologic perspective to review these studies first.

ADAPTIVE IMMUNITY

Research on the immunological basis of sarcoidosis was dramatically changed with the advent of bronchoalveolar lavage (BAL). Prior to this, studies were restricted to analysis of peripheral blood and serum. These early studies showed that patients with sarcoidosis were typified by circulating lymphopenia. This finding, along with the clinical observation that most sarcoidosis had cutaneous anergy, led to the concept that sarcoidosis is a disease of immunodeficiency. Use of BAL allowed researchers to sample the phenotype and function of inflammatory cells at sites of inflammation. With BAL, researchers documented the remarkable accumulation of activated CD4+ T-cells in the lungs of patients with pulmonary sarcoidosis (Hunninghake and Crystal 1981). This finding led to a paradigm shift to the concept that sarcoidosis is a disease of enhanced (not suppressed) T-cell immunity at sites of granulomatous inflammation. Shortly thereafter, the concept of sarcoidosis as a Th1 polarized disorder was established and is now recognized as a hallmark of the disease (Moller 1999; Zissel et al. 2007).

T-cells

One of the earliest analyses of the differential cell composition of BAL fluid demonstrated a remarkable accumulation of lymphocytes in sarcoidosis compared to other lung diseases (Yeager et al. 1977). Normally, lymphocytes comprise ~10 percent of BAL cells, alveolar macrophages ~90 per cent with <1–2 percent neutrophils or eosinophils. In sarcoidosis, the proportion of BAL lymphocytes averages 20–40 percent but may be as high as 80 percent. A seminal finding in sarcoidosis was that these lymphocytes were dominantly CD4+ T-cells (Hunninghake and Crystal 1981). Literally hundreds of studies have confirmed this, in general finding an average CD4:CD8 ratio of BAL lung T-cells of 3–5:1 compared to 2:1 in healthy individuals (Costabel 1997). In fewer than 10 percent of sarcoidosis patients are there greater numbers of CD8+ than CD4+ T-cells in BAL fluid.

Lung T-cells in pulmonary sarcoidosis express surface and cytosolic molecules consistent with recent activation. Approximately 5–10 percent of lung T-cells are IL-2R+, 30–50 percent are class II MHC DR+, >50 percent express the late activation marker VLA-1 (very late activation antigen-1, CD49a), and greater numbers of lung T-cells express the cell-cycle-related nuclear antigen Ki67 (Saltini et al. 1988). The surface density of the CD3:T-cell receptor complex on sarcoidosis BAL T-cells is reduced, consistent with activation through the T-cell antigen receptor (TCR) pathway (Du Bois et al. 1992). Sarcoidosis BAL lung T-cells have a phenotype of memory (CD45R0 + /RA −) T-cells (Dominique et al. 1990; Fazel et al. 1994).

Polarized Th1 disorder

A hallmark of sarcoidosis is that T-cells at sites of granulomatous inflammation express a highly polarized Th1 cytokine profile (Moller 1999). The Th1-defining cytokine IFN-γ enhances phagocytosis, antigen presentation and microbial killing, activating mononuclear phagocytes by up-regulation of oxidant pathways and synergizing with other pro-inflammatory cytokines such as TNF to facilitate and cellular trafficking through the induction of adhesion molecules and chemokines. The initial study of IFN-γ reported that BAL cells from sarcoidosis patients spontaneously produced significantly higher amounts of IFN-γ than BAL cells than from control subjects, a finding that predated the definition of Th1 and Th2 T-cell subsets (Robinson et al. 1985). Subsequently, investigators examined both Th1 and Th2 cytokines in parallel to establish the highly dominant Th1 polarization and lack of Th2 responses at sites of disease in sarcoidosis (Walker et al. 1994; Moller et al. 1996).

Earlier studies described the spontaneous expression of IL-2, a Th1-associated cytokine, in BAL cells from patients with sarcoidosis (Pinkston et al. 1983; Hunninghake et al. 1983). IL-2 enhances T-cell activation and proliferation, and has important anti-apoptotic effects on T-cells. The IL-2 receptor protein and mRNA was subsequently found to be up-regulated in mononuclear cells isolated from sites of active disease but not up-regulated in peripheral blood mononuclear cells (PBMCs), suggesting a compartmentalization of immune activation (Hancock et al. 1987; Konishi et al. 1988).

Consistent with a polarized Th1 response, critical Th1 immunoregulatory cytokines such as IL-12 and IL-18 are up-regulated at sites of granulomatous inflammation (Moller et al. 1996; Greene et al. 2000; Shigehara et al. 2000b). IL-12, probably the most potent Th1 promoting cytokine, is produced by activated mononuclear cells and dendritic cells, inducing Th1 differentiation in naive T-cells. Significant levels of spontaneous IL-12 protein and mRNA expression are observed in BAL cells from sarcoidosis patients, supporting the hypothesis that dysregulated expression of this cytokine may play a pivotal role in the pathogenesis of sarcoidosis (Moller et al. 1996). Spontaneous IL-12 mRNA and protein expression from alveolar macrophages correlate with disease activity, with higher levels observed in patients with active disease compared with either patients with inactive disease or healthy controls (Minshall et al. 1997; Kim et al. 2000; Shigehara et al. 2000a).

IL-18 is a second major immunoregulatory Th1 cytokine that is upregulated in sarcoidosis. IL-18 does not induce Th1 differentiation but is necessary for optimal induction of IFN-γ expression in T-cells and natural killer (NK) cells. IL-18 and IL-18 receptor expression is increased in the sarcoidosis lung, and is associated with increased expression of IFN-γ, IL-2 and local T-cell activation (Greene et al. 2000; Shigehara et al. 2000b). During active pulmonary sarcoidosis, locally enhanced levels of IL-18 and IL-12 may act synergistically to enhance local IFN-γ expression in the lung (Shigehara et al. 2001).

IL-15, a cytokine with functions similar to IL-2, may also play a role in sarcoidosis. IL-15 secretion from BAL cells and

PBMC is significantly higher in patients with active sarcoidosis compared with patients with inactive sarcoidosis or healthy controls (Zissel *et al.* 2000). Increased IL-15 expression in alveolar macrophages potentiates cytokine-primed (IL-2 or TNF) T-cell proliferation via up-regulation of the IL2 receptor complex, which also binds IL-15 (Agostini *et al.* 1996a). IL-27, a cytokine involved with T-cell activation and induction of IFN-γ, is also up-regulated in sarcoidosis (Larousserie *et al.* 2004).

The function of these Th1 cytokines depends on the expression of their receptors on local inflammatory cells. Increased mRNA expression of both IL-12 receptor subunits (β1 and β2 subunits) is significantly increased in BAL cells from patients with sarcoidosis compared with patients with tuberculosis, asthma or healthy controls (Taha *et al.* 1999). Surface expression of the IL-12Rβ2 subunit, necessary for a high-affinity IL-12β2 receptor and a marker of Th1 differentiation, is upregulated on BAL T-cells from patients with sarcoidosis (Rogge *et al.* 1999). Increased expression of the IL-18 receptor is also increased on CD4+ BAL T-cells compared to T-cells from the peripheral blood of patients with sarcoidosis (Katchar *et al.* 2003).

Th2 cytokines

Studies have consistently found a lack of up-regulation or decrease in the expression of Th2 cytokines in sarcoidosis (Walker *et al.* 1994; Hoshino *et al.* 1995; Moller *et al.* 1996; Minshall *et al.* 1997). For example, using in-situ hybridization, one study demonstrated preferential expression of IL-2, IFN-γ, IL-12 and IL-10, but not IL-3, IL-4 or IL-5 in BAL cells from patients with active and inactive sarcoidosis (Minshall *et al.* 1997). A possible exception involves the Th2 cytokine, IL-13. One study reports expression of IL-13 mRNA expression in BAL cells and PBMC from sarcoidosis patients (Hauber *et al.* 2003), but this finding has not been confirmed by other studies (Prasse *et al.* 2000; Miyazaki *et al.* 2002). Whether IL-13 is preferentially expressed in certain sarcoidosis phenotypes (e.g. chronic fibrotic sarcoidosis) remains uncertain.

Th17 cytokines

Recently, an alternate effector T-cell lineage (Th17) has been described (Harrington *et al.* 2005). Subsets of Th17+ cells express IL-17, IL-21 and IL-22, cytokines that stimulate pro-inflammatory cytokines such as TNF, IL-6, IL-1 and TGF-β. Th17+ T-cells develop in response to TGF-β, IL-6 or IL-21 and depend on IL-23 for maintenance of their phenotype. Th17+ T-cells have been described in tuberculosis, suggesting these subsets play a role in mycobacterial host defense (Khader and Cooper 2008). A role for Th17+ T-cells in hypersensitivity pneumonitis has also been described (Simonian *et al.* 2009). Conceptually Th17+ cells could enhance or replace Th1 responses that drive granulomatous inflammation in sarcoidosis, but the lack of reports to date suggests

that Th17+ T-cells are unlikely to undermine the concept of sarcoidosis as a dominant Th1 disorder.

Regulatory T-cells

Current concepts in immunology describe regulatory T-cells (Tregs) as master regulators of the immune response; both 'natural' constitutive and peripherally induced adaptive forms of Tregs have been described, usually constituting 5–10 percent of circulating T-cells in healthy individuals (Sakaguchi 2005). A subset of natural Tregs are characterized by high levels of expression of CD25 and the transcription factor forkhead box P3 (FoxP3), but many other subsets have been described. Tregs regulate T-cell responses through cytokines such as IL-10 (e.g. Tr1 cells), TGF-β (e.g. Th3 cells) and by contact-dependent suppression of antigen-presenting cells.

In sarcoidosis, Miyara and colleagues described an increased frequency of FoxP3+ T-cells in blood, lung and tissues consistent with an increase in natural Tregs in sarcoidosis (Miyara *et al.* 2006). They showed that isolated BAL CD25bright T-cells from sarcoidosis patients exhibit anti-proliferative activity, but do not completely inhibit TNF and IFN-γ production and were not effective in suppressing in-vitro granuloma formation (Miyara *et al.* 2006; Taflin *et al.* 2009). Swedish investigators observed that FoxP3 intensity (MFI) in the CD4+ FoxP3+ BALF T-cells of patients was decreased significantly compared to healthy controls, which may indicate lower suppressive Treg activity in sarcoidosis (Idali *et al.* 2008). These studies suggest that a deficiency in Treg function could be critical to the pathogenesis of sarcoidosis, though further studies are clearly needed to clarify their role in regulating Th1 responses.

PRO-INFLAMMATORY CYTOKINES

TNF family and receptors

TNF plays a critical role in granuloma formation, synergizing with IFN-γ or IL-4 in mediating macrophage activation and granuloma formation (Wynn *et al.* 1993; Chensue *et al.* 1994,1997). In active pulmonary sarcoidosis, BAL cells spontaneously release TNF from BAL cells in vitro (Bachwich *et al.* 1986; Baughman *et al.* 1990) with higher levels of TNF in patients with severe or progressive disease (Muller-Quernheim *et al.* 1992). Levels of the TNF soluble receptors, p55 and p75, that inhibit the bioactivity of TNF, are significantly elevated in the sera of sarcoidosis patients compared with healthy controls, suggesting a mechanism for limiting the pro-inflammatory effects of TNF (Armstrong *et al.* 1999). The central role of TNF in experimental granulomatous inflammation, and the therapeutic benefit of inhibiting this cytokine with anti-TNF therapies, allow a primary role for TNF in sarcoidosis pathogenesis.

Other members of the TNF family of proteins and receptors are also up-regulated at sites of granulomatous inflammation in sarcoidosis, though their contributions in sarcoidosis are less well established. LTα, LTβ and the TNF-related ligands CD70 and TNF-related receptors (TNFR1/p75, 4-1BB and LTβ-R) are expressed within the sarcoidosis lung (Agostini *et al.* 1996b; Boussaud *et al.* 1998; Katchar *et al.* 2001; Agyekum *et al.* 2003). The receptor Fas (CD95) which shares sequence homology with TNFR1/p55 and Fas ligand (FasL) is expressed in the tissue, serum and BAL of patients with sarcoidosis, suggesting a role for Fas-mediated apoptosis in the regulation of granulomatous inflammation (Dai *et al.* 1999; Shikuwa *et al.* 2002).

Other pro-inflammatory cytokines

Many other pro-inflammatory cytokines are up-regulated at sites of granulomatous inflammation in sarcoidosis. Macrophage migration inhibitory factor (MIF) was one of the first cytokines to be described in sarcoidosis in a study that showed elevated concentrations in the sera of patients with sarcoidosis compared to controls (Umbert *et al.* 1976). MIF is induced by IFN-γ with effects on macrophage trafficking and activation. Interleukin-1 (IL-1α and IL-1β), the IL-1 receptor and IL-1 receptor antagonist (IL-1ra) are expressed in sarcoidosis BAL fluid and cells and within sarcoidosis granulomas (Wewers *et al.* 1987; Yamaguchi *et al.* 1988; Chilosi *et al.* 1988). Some studies suggest the ratio of IL-1ra/IL-1β is higher in patients with sarcoidosis versus healthy controls (Kline *et al.* 1993) and correlates with clinical course (Mikuniya *et al.* 2000).

Osteopontin (OPN) is an acidic glycoprotein, inducible in macrophages by IFN-γ, that binds adhesion molecules to regulate neovascularization, wound healing and trafficking of T-cells to sites of inflammation (Li *et al.* 2003). A deficiency of OPN leads to impaired granuloma formation in some models of granulomatous inflammation (O'Regan *et al.* 2001). Studies document increased expression of OPN in sarcoidosis tissues as well as in infectious granulomatous disease, being most intensely expressed within epithelioid histiocytes and multinucleated giant T-cells (Carlson *et al.* 1997; O'Regan *et al.* 1999). Since OPN plays a role in the early induction of Th1 cytokine responses through a CD44-dependent induction of IL-12 expression in macrophages (Ashkar *et al.* 2000), OPN likely contributes to Th1 polarization in sarcoidosis.

GM-CSF, a pleomorphic cytokine induced by IL-18, can activate and induce the proliferation of alveolar macrophages (Trapnell and Whitsett 2002). GM-CSF mRNA is spontaneously produced by T-cells from patients with sarcoidosis and may track with disease progression or remission (Itoh *et al.* 1993).

Interleukin-6 (IL-6) has broad immunostimulatory effects, activating both B- and T-cells. IL-6 is found within cells in the periphery of sarcoidosis granulomas and is produced by alveolar macrophages (Steffen *et al.* 1993; Bost *et al.* 1994). Patients with active sarcoidosis have significantly higher levels of IL-6 in BAL compared with patients with inactive sarcoidosis and healthy controls (Homolka and Muller-Quernheim 1993; Girgis *et al.* 1995; Hoshino *et al.* 1995).

The effect of IL-6 on B-cells in sarcoidosis may contribute to the hypergammaglobulinemia that is characteristically observed in sarcoidosis.

Immunoregulatory cytokines

Transforming growth factor-beta (TGF-β) has potent immunosuppressive and anti-inflammatory effects as well as pro-fibrotic effects. TGF-β is expressed at sites of granulomatous inflammation by immunohistochemistry (Limper *et al.* 1994). Importantly, Zissel and co-workers found spontaneous TGF-β expression by BAL macrophages was lower in patients requiring therapy than in patients with active disease not requiring therapy (Zissel *et al.* 1996). These findings suggest a critical role for TGF-β in down-regulating the Th1 inflammation in sarcoidosis. A role for TGF-β in promoting fibrosis in chronic sarcoidosis is discussed below.

IL-10 has profound anti-inflammatory effects and is a key regulator of T-cell immunity, autoimmunity and infection. In experimental models of mycobacterial infection, IL-10 deficiency limits the extent of granulomatous inflammation and is associated with better control of disease (Florido *et al.* 2002). IL-10 mRNA and protein expression are described in patients with sarcoidosis though it is uncertain if the constitutive level of IL-10 expression differs from the healthy homeostatic lung environment (Hoshino *et al.* 1995; Moller *et al.* 1996; Zissel *et al.* 1996). Some studies suggest that IL-10 levels vary with disease activity or corticosteroid therapy (Minshall *et al.* 1997; Bingisser *et al.* 2000; Fuse *et al.* 2000). Given the critical role of IL-10 in regulating immune responses in general, it seems highly probable that IL-10 producing T-cells and mononuclear phagocytes play a critical role in determinating clinical course in sarcoidosis.

CHEMOKINES AND CHEMOKINE RECEPTORS

Chemokines are generally small peptides that signal through evolutionarily conserved G-protein coupled receptors and effect chemotaxis for specific leukocyte populations (Mackay 2001). Four chemokine families (CC, CXC, C, CX3C) are known. The differential expression of chemokines and their receptors determine which subsets of T-cells and monocytes traffic to sites of inflammation, thus regulating local immune responses. For example, CCR5 and CXCR3 have been associated with Th1 lymphocytes, and CCR4 and CCR8 have been associated with Th2 lymphocytes (Sallusto *et al.* 1998).

The chemokines and chemokine receptors that have been described to be up-regulated in sarcoidosis are those generally associated with Th1 immune responses. For example, the chemokine ligands macrophage inflammatory proteins 1α (CCL3) and 1β (CCL4) and RANTES (CCL5) are up-regulated in sarcoidosis BAL cells and may track with disease chronicity (Standiford *et al.* 1993; Iida *et al.* 1997; Ziegenhagen *et al.* 1998; Petrek *et al.* 2002). The receptor for these chemokines is CCR5, which is up-regulated on sarcoidosis BAL cells (Katchar *et al.* 2003). CXC chemokines induced by IFN-γ include MIG (CXCL9) and IP-10 (CXCL10), both of which are up-regulated in sarcoidosis. IP-10 protein and mRNA expression are increased in BAL fluid and cells in sarcoidosis, localized to epithelioid cells and macrophages (Agostini et al. 1998; Miotto et al. 2001). MIG mRNA expression is inducible in alveolar macrophages from sarcoidosis patients (Horton et al. 1997). These three IFN-γ-induced chemokines signal through CXCR3, which is highly expressed on activated Th1 cells isolated from sarcoidosis patients (Agostini et al. 1998; Katchar et al. 2003).

Other chemokines and chemokine receptors up-regulated in sarcoidosis include the monocyte chemoattractant proteins, MCP-1 (CCL2), MCP-3 (CCL7) and MCP-4 (CCL13) and their receptor CCR2, CXCL16, MIP-3α (CCL20) and fractalkine (CX3CL1) (Car et al. 1994; Hashimoto et al. 1998; Petrek et al. 2002). Interleukin-8 (IL-8) has broad pro-inflammatory effects and is classified as a CXC chemokine (CXCL8). Patients with sarcoidosis have elevated levels of IL-8 in BAL fluid which correlate with numbers of CD3 + BAL cells and disease severity (Car et al. 1994; Girgis et al. 1995). It is likely these chemokines and their receptors play key roles in the trafficking of CD4 + T-cells and monocytes to sites of granuloma formation, though their individual contributions remain uncertain.

In contrast to the up-regulation of Th1-associated chemokines and their receptors, studies show that Th2-associated chemokines and their receptors are down-regulated in sarcoidosis. For example, the Th2 chemokines CCL22, eotaxin (CCL11) and receptors CCR3, CCR4, CCR8 and CXCR4 show little expression in sarcoidosis cells or BAL fluid (Katoh et al. 2000; Panina-Bordignon et al. 2001; Katchar et al. 2003).

T-CELL RECEPTOR GENES

Although the accumulation of activated CD4 + T-cells indicates they are central to the pathogenesis of sarcoidosis, direct evidence that sarcoidosis is an antigen-driven disorder remained presumptive until studies of T-cell receptor (TCR) expression in this disease (Moller 1998). T-cell specificity results from the expression of the antigen-specific $\alpha\beta^+$ or $\gamma\delta^+$ T-cell receptor genes, each chain of which is the product of the genetic rearrangement of TCR variable (V), diversity (D)(α,β only), and joining (J) regions (Hedrick et al. 1988). A specific VDJ arrangement recognizes MHC–peptide complexes on antigen-presenting cells (MHC class II for CD4 + T-cells, MHC class I for CD8 + T-cells). T-cell activation requires both TCR stimulation by MHC-peptide (signal 1) plus co-stimulation by surface receptors (e.g. CD28, CD40L) that interact with antigen-presenting cells expressing counter receptors (e.g. B7, CD40) (signal 2) in the presence of differentiating cytokine signals (signal 3).

SARCOIDOSIS AS AN ANTIGEN–DRIVEN DISORDER

Studies of TCR expression in sarcoidosis demonstrated the selective expansion of oligoclonal populations of $\alpha\beta^+$ BAL

T-cells expressing specific V, D or J gene segments in the sarcoidosis lung (Moller et al. 1988; Forman et al. 1994; Forrester et al. 1994; Bellocq et al. 1994). Importantly, Grunewald and Eklund reported the striking expansion of Vα2.3+ (AV2S3) T-cells in the lungs of Swedish patients with an HLA-DR17 genetic background (HLA-DRB1*0301/ DRB3*0101) (Grunewald et al. 1992,2000; Planck et al. 2003). This was the first study to link biased TCR gene expression to a specific MHC genotype, thus defining two of the three components of the trimolecular complex that determines T-cell specificity (Moller and Chen 2002). Oligoclonal $\alpha\beta$ + T-cells with specific Vβ (BV) genes were shown to traffic to the site of newly formed granulomas in the skin (a Kveim reaction site), suggesting these T-cells accumulate in response to 'sarcoidosis antigens' (Klein et al. 1995). Selective expansion of oligoclonal populations of T-cells have also been documented in the blood, some with TCR hypervariable region amino acid similarities, suggesting circulation of antigen-expanded T-cells in sarcoidosis (Grunewald et al. 1995; Silver et al. 1996). These studies are consistent with the concept that sarcoidosis is associated with oligoclonal expansion of T-cells stimulated by conventional MHC-restricted antigen-driven responses. Direct assessment of the peptide specificities driving these TCR-specific T-cells has remained elusive, though recent progress has been made in defining candidate pathogenic antigens in sarcoidosis.

Some but not all studies find that $\gamma\delta^+$ T-cells, predominantly of the Vγ9 + Vδ2 + subset (normally < 10 percent of blood T-cells), circulate in greater proportions in the blood of patients with sarcoidosis compared to control subjects (Moller 1998). However, since $\gamma\delta^+$ T-cells are rarely found around granulomas in lymph nodes or skin, a role of this T-cell subset in the pathogenesis of sarcoidosis remains uncertain.

B–CELLS

There is evidence that B-cells are activated in sarcoidosis. Clinical studies document that sarcoidosis is often associated with broad-based, non-clonal hypergammaglobulinemia. The fact that IgG-1, -2 and -3 isotypes are most frequently increased in patients with sarcoidosis suggests an association with Th1 cytokine responses. IL-6, which has known B-cell stimulatory effects and is up-regulated in sarcoidosis, is frequently implicated in promoting the hypergammaglobulinemia. Elevated levels of immune complexes are also present in the serum, BAL and tissues of patients with sarcoidosis and associate with disease activity (Selroos et al. 1980). Whether the hypergammaglobulinemia and immune complexes reflect a disease-specific antibody response has not been determined. Microbial-specific antibodies have been noted in many patients with sarcoidosis, but almost all lack validation as disease-specific antigens. Possible exceptions include the recent description of circulating IgG to specific mycobacterial or propionibacterial antigens, observations supported by studies of corresponding antigen-specific T-cell responses to these microbial agents in sarcoidosis.

IDENTIFICATION OF PATHOGENIC SARCOIDOSIS ANTIGENS

A major goal in understanding the pathobiology of sarcoidosis is to identify pathogenic antigens that drive the local Th1 responses in sarcoidosis. In an attempt to detect pathogenic T-cell antigens in sarcoidosis tissues, one of the authors and his colleagues used a novel proteomic approach using matrix-associated laser desorption/ionization time-of-flight (MALDI-TOF) mass spectrometry. This approach led to the identification of *Mycobacterium tuberculosis* catalase–peroxidase (mKatG) as a tissue antigen and target of the adaptive immune response in sarcoidosis (Song *et al.* 2005). Notably, a follow-up study of sarcoidosis patients from the USA and Sweden found remarkable similarities in the T-cell responses to mKatG despite widely differing clinical, genetic and prognostic features between these cohorts (Chen *et al.* 2008). Over 70 percent of sarcoidosis patients from the USA and Sweden had Th1-specific responses to either mKatG or PPD in the lung or blood. In unpublished studies, we find mKatG reactive CD4+ Th1 cells in the lung have an effector memory phenotype, some with polyfunctional Th1 cytokine expression (IFN-γ and TNF). Immune responses to other mycobacterial antigens have also been reported (details in Chapter 4). These findings support the hypothesis that mKatG is a prototypic pathogenic antigen in sarcoidosis at least in the USA and Sweden, supporting a mycobacterial etiology of sarcoidosis in a subset of patients. In Japan, studies suggest antigens derived from propionibacterial organisms are pathogenic in sarcoidosis (Ebe *et al.* 2000).

Another approach to identify pathogenic antigens in sarcoidosis is to examine the sequence of peptides that bind to specific MHC genes known to be associated with sarcoidosis risk. This approach is based on the observation that distinct amino acid sequences or 'pockets' are present in MHC class I and II molecules which can be used to predict specific peptide binding sequences. One recent study provided data that the specific amino acids within pocket number four of DRβ and nine of DQβ were associated with risk of developing sarcoidosis, suggesting the possibility of predicting peptide antigens involved in sarcoidosis (Rossman *et al.* 2008). Swedish investigators capitalized on the observation that HLA-DRB1*0301 is highly associated with remitting sarcoidosis (Grunewald and Eklund 2009). These researchers eluted peptides from affinity-purified HLA-DR molecules from HLADRB1*0301 positive BAL cells, identifying 78 potential autoantigens (e.g. vimentin, ATP synthase) using mass spectrometry (Wahlstrom *et al.* 2007). However, direct evidence that any of these peptides stimulate AV2S3+ lung T-cells that are expanded in these patients remains unreported (Wahlstrom *et al.* 2009). The discovery of AV2S3 stimulating peptides could allow the identification of autoantigens or define the phenotype of T-cells associated with spontaneous disease remission.

INNATE IMMUNITY

Despite the fact that innate immunity is the first line of defense against infecting pathogens and is critical to the initiation, development and regulation of adaptive T- and B-cell responses, relatively few studies have been conducted regarding specific innate mechanisms involved in sarcoidosis pathogenesis. Mononuclear phagocytes form a major component of sarcoidosis granulomas and are critical innate immunoregulatory cells.

Macrophages

Macrophages express different phenotypes (classical, alternative, regulatory) depending on the cytokine milieu to which they are exposed. Classically activated macrophages are induced by INFγ and have enhanced antimicrobial function with up-regulated expression of pro-inflammatory cytokines, ox–redox molecules and proteases.

In sarcoidosis, alveolar (BAL) macrophages demonstrate a classically activated phenotype. Sarcoidosis BAL cells constitutively produce TNF-, IL-1-, IL-12-, IL-6- and Th1-associated chemokines (Muller-Quernheim 1998). These cells demonstrate enhanced function as antigen-presenting cells in part from the up-regulated expression of co-stimulatory molecules including MHC surface expression (Lem *et al.* 1985; Venet *et al.* 1985). Activated alveolar macrophages from patients with sarcoidosis express both B7-1(CD80) and B7-2 (CD86) isoforms that act as co-stimulatory molecules on T-cells (Nicod and Isler 1997; Agostini *et al.* 1999), though the B7-1 isoform may be preferentially expressed (Kaneko *et al.* 1999). This differential expression of B7-1 may favor the priming of naive T-cells to a Th1 phenotype on antigen presentation in sarcoidosis.

Consistent with a state of activation, expression of the pro-inflammatory nuclear transcription factor NFκB is up-regulated while anti-inflammatory PPARγ is decreased in sarcoidosis BAL cells compared to control cells (Greene *et al.* 2000; Culver *et al.* 2004). A recent study reported that gene networks involved in Th1 responses are up-regulated in sarcoidosis, including those expressed by alveolar macrophages (Crouser *et al.* 2009). For example, metalloproteinase MMP-12 and ADAMDEC1 transcripts are highly expressed (> 25-fold) in sarcoidosis lung tissues; protein expression is increased in BAL samples from patients with sarcoidosis, correlating with disease severity, suggesting these are mediators of lung damage and/or remodeling.

NK cells and NKT cells

NK cells play an important role in the initiation of inflammation, providing a source of pro-inflammatory cytokines such as IFN-γ (Brohee *et al.* 1987). NKT cells express an invariant TCR receptor (Vα24Jα18-Vβ11) and recognize CD1d-restricted antigens. One study found NKT cells were absent or greatly reduced in peripheral blood and lung from patients with both acute and resolved sarcoidosis, except in the subset with Löfgren's syndrome (Ho *et al.* 2005). NKT cells were not observed in mediastinal lymph nodes or granulomatous tissues. Since CD1d expression on antigen-presenting cells of patients was normal, the authors suggested the loss of immunoregulation by CD1d-restricted NKT cells could play a role in the persistent T-cell activity that characterizes sarcoidosis.

Dendritic cells

Dendritic cells (DCs) are central professional antigen-presenting cells that initiate and orchestrate immune responses, but few studies exist in sarcoidosis (Zaba et al. 2010). One study found that patients with sarcoidosis have low numbers of circulating immature dendritic cells but increased numbers of mature dendritic cells in biopsy samples, suggesting that dendritic cells may be preferentially recruited from the peripheral blood to granulomas (Ota et al. 2004). Another study suggests that the decreased cutaneous delayed-type hypersensitivity (DTH) responses to recall antigens in sarcoidosis is related to decreased function of circulating DCs (Mathew et al. 2008). Given their critical role in antigen presentation, further studies of DCs are necessary.

Toll-like receptors and related proteins

Toll-like receptors (TLR) and nucleotide-binding oligomerization domain (NOD)-like receptors have common structural components that bind to different conserved structural motifs on microorganisms. TLR and NOD-like receptor signaling pathways result in activation of transcription factors including NFκB that regulate cytokine expression. One study found TLR2 and TLR4 surface expression is higher in PMBC from sarcoidosis patients compared to controls (Wiken et al. 2009). In this study, synthetic TLR2 ligands, the TLR2 agonist S. aureus peptidoglycan and the NOD2 ligand MDP stimulated the production of TNF and IL-1. One of the authors and colleagues reported that BAL cells from sarcoidosis patients had greater surface expression of TLR2 and production of cytokines in response to synthetic TLR ligands compared to controls, most of whom had chronic obstructive lung disease (Chen et al. 2010). The fact that mycobacterial, propionibacterial and other microbial organisms contain TLR2-stimulating ligands suggests that exposure to these microbes could activate local inflammatory cells in sarcoidosis in a TLR2-dependent manner. We also report that an endogenous ligand of TLR2, serum amyloid A, is present within granulomas in sarcoidosis and stimulates BAL cells in sarcoidosis.

Serum amyloid A

We have reported data that serum amyloid A (SAA), an acute-phase reactant and amyloid precursor protein, accumulates in both soluble and aggregated forms within sarcoidosis granulomas (Chen et al. 2010). The intensity, focality and heterogeneity in the distribution of SAA was not seen in any other infectious or non-infectious granulomatous disease. The extent of SAA staining correlated with the number of CD3 + T-cells in the granuloma and not CD68 + macrophages, suggesting that the extent of expression of SAA

in sarcoidosis is pathogenically linked to local Th1 immune responses. In sarcoidosis patients, SAA regulates the expression of cytokines (TNF, IFN-γ, IL-10) involved in granuloma formation, mediated in part through TLR2. Serum amyloid A also stimulates sarcoidosis BAL cells through the receptor for advanced glycation end products (RAGE) to produce pro-inflammatory cytokines (unpublished data). RAGE is expressed within sarcoidosis granulomas, and may contribute to the genetic basis of clinical disease (Campo et al. 2007). Potentially, aggregates of SAA could serve as a 'seed' for further amyloid-like, non-Congophilic protein aggregation within granulomas, providing ongoing TLR2 stimulation that promotes progressive granulomatous inflammation in chronic sarcoidosis.

PRO-FIBROTIC MESENCHYMAL GROWTH FACTORS

The determinants of fibrosis in sarcoidosis are unknown. Histological studies indicate a preference for circumferential matrix deposition within the granulomas. Tissue injury from chronic inflammation can lead to fibrosis, but the underlying mechanisms and regulation are unclear.

Pro-fibrotic factors are present at sites of granulomatous inflammation in sarcoidosis. Fibronectin, a growth factor and chemoattractant for fibroblasts, is released by alveolar macrophages in pulmonary sarcoidosis (Bitterman et al. 1983; Suganuma et al. 1995). Other mesenchymal growth factors in the sarcoidosis lung include transforming growth factor (TGF-β1), platelet-derived growth factor, insulin-like growth factors, connective tissue growth factor, and fibroblast growth factors.

TGF-β1 is likely to play a central role in a fibrotic outcome in chronic sarcoidosis since this cytokine promotes fibrogenesis at many levels, including the induction of fibronectin and the α5β1 fibronectin receptor. Limper and colleagues showed that TGF-β1 localizes within the granuloma in sarcoidosis, particularly within epithelioid histiocytes (Limper et al. 1994). The TGF-β1 binding proteoglycan decorin, fibronectin and the fibronectin receptor localize in the fibrotic tissue surrounding granulomas. Higher levels of the profibrotic PDGF and insulin-like growth factor-1 (IGF-1) protein and mRNA expression are seen in BAL from patients with sarcoidosis but not in healthy controls (Homma et al. 1995; Bloor et al. 2001). Connective tissue growth factor, a member of the IGF superfamily, also is up-regulated in sarcoidosis (Allen et al. 1999).

How profibrotic factors collaborate with the ongoing T-cell-mediated inflammation to promote fibrosis is unclear. INF-γ has direct antifibrotic effects while Th2 cytokines such as IL-4 and IL-13 promote fibrogenesis. Thus, Th1-mediated granulomatous inflammation is far less fibrogenic than Th2-driven granulomatous inflammation (Chensue et al. 1994). Thus, many investigators have postulated that there is a transition from a Th1-dominant to a Th2-dominant cytokine responses in chronic, fibrotic sarcoidosis. There are no data to directly support this hypothesis. Given this lack of supporting evidence, it seems likely that fibrogenesis in sarcoidosis occurs dominantly within the milieu of an ongoing Th1 tissue response that, despite the presence of IFN-γ (or perhaps because of its associated tissue damage), results in organ fibrosis.

A PROPOSED MODEL OF SARCOIDOSIS

Immunological data can be used to develop the following hypothetical model of sarcoidosis (Fig. 6.1).

Specific microbial agents (e.g. mycobacterial or propionibacterial organisms) infect a genetically susceptible person. An over-exuberant innate immune reaction results in local aggregration of misfolded SAA and leaves remnant microbial antigens that also drive an exaggerated (hypersensitivity) adaptive Th1 response to disease-relevant pathogenic tissue antigens. Granulomatous inflammation develops around insoluble aggregated SAA and other host proteins. Serum amyloid A and binding matrix proteins trap microbial or autoantigens within granulomas, while soluble SAA, released from tissue granulomas, stimulates TLR2 and other innate receptors to promote production of TNF, Th1-promoting IL-12 and IL-18 and anti-inflammatory IL-10 (which limits severity and necrosis). If the innate/adaptive response is able to clear tissue antigens and aggregated SAA, remission of disease occurs – mediated by the immunosuppressive effects of TGF-β. Failure to clear pathogenic antigens and SAA aggregates results in a failure to down-regulate the Th1 responses, allowing TGF-β and other profibrotic factors to promote local fibrosis within the context of ongoing, low-grade tissue injury.

CONCLUSION

Remarkable progress has been made in our understanding of the immunopathogenesis of sarcoidosis. From an earlier concept of sarcoidosis as an immunodeficiency disorder, there is now consensus that sarcoidosis is a disease of enhanced, immunologic hypersensitivity to pathogenic tissue antigens (Box 6.1).

The concept of sarcoidosis as a highly polarized Th1 disorder remains a cornerstone, encompassing many immunological observations within a consistent model. Other more recent findings are provocative, but remain to be sufficiently validated to be elevated as a disease-defining hallmark.

Recent studies have also identified attractive candidate pathogenic antigens that drive the local immune responses associated with the granulomatous inflammation. Much work remains to be done, but it is clear that these candidate microbial antigens stimulate T- and B-cell immune responses consistent with promoting local immune responses consistent with the pathobiology of disease. Further studies are needed to define the roles of specific subsets of effector and regulatory T-cells with known antigenic specificity in the inflammatory process and how they determine clinical course. When combined with genetic and clinical phenotyping data, further immunological studies may lead to novel immunotherapeutic strategies designed to suppress or even prevent sarcoidosis.

Box 6.1 Immunological hallmarks

Validated
- CD4+ T-cell infiltration
- Polarized Th1 cytokine, chemokine and chemokine receptor expression
- Oligoclonal expansion of T-cell receptor αβ+ T-cells consistent with conventional antigen stimulation
- Classically activated macrophages in non-fibrotic disease

Candidates
- Regulatory T-cell deficiency
- Antigen-specific Th1 responses to microbial antigens
- Toll-like receptor activation

REFERENCES

Agostini C, Trentin L, Facco M et al. (1996a). Role of IL-15, IL-2, and their receptors in the development of T cell alveolitis in pulmonary sarcoidosis. *J Immunol* **157**: 910–18.

Agostini C, Zambello R, Sancetta R et al. (1996b). Expression of tumor necrosis factor-receptor superfamily members by lung T lymphocytes in interstitial lung disease. *Am J Respir Crit Care Med* **153**: 1359–67.

Agostini C, Cassatella M, Zambello R et al. (1998). Involvement of the IP-10 chemokine in sarcoid granulomatous reactions. *J Immunol* **161**: 6413–20.

Agostini C, Trentin L, Perin A et al. (1999). Regulation of alveolar macrophage–T-cell interactions during Th1-type sarcoid inflammatory process. *Am J Physiol* **277**: L240–50.

Agyekum S, Church A, Sohail M et al. (2003). Expression of lymphotoxin-beta (LT-beta) in chronic inflammatory conditions. *J Pathol* **199**: 115–21.

Allen JT, Knight RA, Bloor CA, Spiteri MA (1999). Enhanced insulin-like growth factor binding protein-related protein 2 (connective tissue

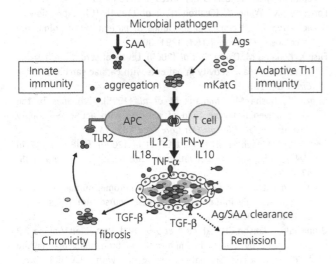

Figure 6.1   Hypothetical model of sarcoidosis, adapted from Chen *et al.* (2010).

growth factor) expression in patients with idiopathic pulmonary fibrosis and pulmonary sarcoidosis. *Am J Respir Cell Mol Biol* 21: 693–700.

Armstrong L, Foley NM, Millar AB (1999). Inter-relationship between tumour necrosis factor-alpha (TNF-α) and TNF soluble receptors in pulmonary sarcoidosis. *Thorax* 54: 524–30.

Ashkar S, Weber GF, Panoutsakopoulou V et al. (2000). Eta-1 (osteopontin): an early component of type-1 (cell-mediated) immunity. *Science* 287: 860–4.

Bachwich PR, Lynch JP, Larrick J et al. (1986). Tumor necrosis factor production by human sarcoid alveolar macrophages. *Am J Pathol* 125: 421–5.

Baughman RP, Strohofer SA, Buchsbaum J, Lower EE (1990). Release of tumor necrosis factor by alveolar macrophages of patients with sarcoidosis. *J Lab Clin Med* 115: 36–42.

Bellocq A, Lecossier D, Pierre-Audigier C et al. (1994). T cell receptor repertoire of T lymphocytes recovered from the lung and blood of patients with sarcoidosis. *Am J Respir Crit Care Med* 149: 646–54.

Bingisser R, Speich R, Zollinger A et al. (2000). Interleukin-10 secretion by alveolar macrophages and monocytes in sarcoidosis. *Respiration* 67: 280–6.

Bitterman PB, Rennard SI, Adelberg S, Crystal RG (1983). Role of fibronectin as a growth factor for fibroblasts. *J Cell Biol* 97: 1925–32.

Bloor CA, Knight RA, Kedia RK et al. (2001). Differential mRNA expression of insulin-like growth factor-1 splice variants in patients with idiopathic pulmonary fibrosis and pulmonary sarcoidosis. *Am J Respir Crit Care Med* 164: 265–72.

Bost TW, Riches DW, Schumacher B et al. (1994). Alveolar macrophages from patients with beryllium disease and sarcoidosis express increased levels of mRNA for tumor necrosis factor-alpha and interleukin-6 but not interleukin-1 beta. *Am J Respir Cell Mol Biol* 10: 506–13.

Boussaud V, Soler P, Moreau J et al. (1998). Expression of three members of the TNF-R family of receptors (4-1BB, lymphotoxin-beta receptor, and Fas) in human lung. *Eur Respir J* 12: 926–31.

Brohee D, Mertens G, Vanachter O et al. (1987). NK cells in sarcoidosis. *Chest* 92: 1127–8.

Campo I, Morbini P, Zorzetto M et al. (2007). Expression of receptor for advanced glycation end products in sarcoid granulomas. *Am J Respir Crit Care Med* 175: 498–506.

Car BD, Meloni F, Luisetti M et al. (1994). Elevated IL-8 and MCP-1 in the bronchoalveolar lavage fluid of patients with idiopathic pulmonary fibrosis and pulmonary sarcoidosis. *Am J Respir Crit Care Med* 149: 655–9.

Carlson I, Tognazzi K, Manseau EJ et al. (1997). Osteopontin is strongly expressed by histiocytes in granulomas of diverse etiology. *Lab Invest* 77: 103–8.

Chen ES, Wahlstrom J, Song Z et al. (2008). T cell responses to mycobacterial catalase–peroxidase profile a pathogenic antigen in systemic sarcoidosis. *J Immunol* 181: 8784–96.

Chen ES, Song Z, Willett MH et al. (2010). Serum amyloid A regulates granulomatous inflammation in sarcoidosis through Toll-like receptor-2. *Am J Respir Crit Care Med* 181: 360–73.

Chensue SW, Warmington K, Ruth J et al. (1994). Cytokine responses during mycobacterial and schistosomal antigen-induced pulmonary granuloma formation: production of Th1 and Th2 cytokines and relative contribution of tumor necrosis factor. *Am J Pathol* 145: 1105–13.

Chensue SW, Warmington K, Ruth JH et al. (1997). Mycobacterial and schistosomal antigen-elicited granuloma formation in IFN-gamma and IL-4 knockout mice: analysis of local and regional cytokine and chemokine networks. *J Immunol* 159: 3565–73.

Chilosi M, Menestrina F, Capelli P et al. (1988). Immunohisto-chemical analysis of sarcoid granulomas. Evaluation of Ki67+ and interleukin-1+ cells. *Am J Pathol* 131: 191–8.

Chiu BC, Freeman CM, Stolberg VR et al. (2003). Cytokine-chemokine networks in experimental mycobacterial and schistosomal pulmonary granuloma formation. *Am J Respir Cell Mol Biol* 29: 106–16.

Costabel U (1997). CD4/CD8 ratios in bronchoalveolar lavage fluid: of value for diagnosing sarcoidosis? *Eur Respir J* 10: 2699–700.

Crouser ED, Culver DA, Knox KS et al. (2009). Gene expression profiling identifies MMP-12 and ADAMDEC1 as potential pathogenic mediators of pulmonary sarcoidosis. *Am J Respir Crit Care Med* 179: 929–38.

Culver DA, Barna BP, Raychaudhuri B et al. (2004). Peroxisome proliferator-activated receptor gamma activity is deficient in alveolar macrophages in pulmonary sarcoidosis. *Am J Respir Cell Mol Biol* 30: 1–5.

Dai H, Guzman J, Costabel U (1999). Increased expression of apoptosis signalling receptors by alveolar macrophages in sarcoidosis. *Eur Respir J* 13: 1451–4.

Davis JM, Ramakrishnan L (2009). The role of the granuloma in expansion and dissemination of early tuberculous infection. *Cell* 136: 37–49.

Dominique S, Bouchonnet F, Smiejan JM, Hance AJ (1990). Expression of surface antigens distinguishing 'naïve' and previously activated lymphocytes in bronchoalveolar lavage fluid. *Thorax* 45: 391–6.

Du Bois RM, Kirby M, Balbi B et al. (1992). T-lymphocytes that accumulate in the lung in sarcoidosis have evidence of recent stimulation of the T-cell antigen receptor. *Am Rev Respir Dis* 145: 1205–11.

Ebe Y, Ikushima S, Yamaguchi T et al. (2000). Proliferative response of peripheral blood mononuclear cells and levels of antibody to recombinant protein from *Propionibacterium acnes* DNA expression library in Japanese patients with sarcoidosis. *Sarcoidosis Vasc Diffuse Lung Dis* 17: 256–65.

Fazel SB, Howie SE, Krajewski AS, Lamb D (1994). Increased CD45RO expression on T lymphocytes in mediastinal lymph node and pulmonary lesions of patients with pulmonary sarcoidosis. *Clin Exp Immunol* 95: 509–13.

Florido M, Cooper AM, Appelberg R (2002). Immunological basis of the development of necrotic lesions following *Mycobacterium avium* infection. *Immunology* 106: 590–601.

Forman JD, Klein JT, Silver RF et al. (1994). Selective activation and accumulation of oligoclonal V beta-specific T cells in active pulmonary sarcoidosis. *J Clin Invest* 94: 1533–42.

Forrester JM, Wang Y, Ricalton N et al. (1994). TCR expression of activated T cell clones in the lungs of patients with pulmonary sarcoidosis. *J Immunol* 153: 4291–302.

Fuse K, Kodama M, Okura Y et al. (2000). Levels of serum interleukin-10 reflect disease activity in patients with cardiac sarcoidosis. *Jpn Circ J* 64: 755–9.

Girgis RE, Basha MA, Maliarik M et al. (1995). Cytokines in the bronchoalveolar lavage fluid of patients with active pulmonary sarcoidosis. *Am J Respir Crit Care Med* 152: 71–5.

Greene CM, Meachery G, Taggart CC et al. (2000). Role of IL-18 in CD4+ T lymphocyte activation in sarcoidosis. *J Immunol* 165: 4718–24.

Grunewald J, Eklund A (2009). Lofgren's syndrome: human leukocyte antigen strongly influences the disease course. *Am J Respir Crit Care Med* 179: 307–12.

Grunewald J, Janson CH, Eklund A et al. (1992). Restricted V alpha 2.3 gene usage by CD4+ T lymphocytes in bronchoalveolar lavage fluid from sarcoidosis patients correlates with HLA-DR3. *Eur J Immunol* 22: 129–35.

Grunewald J, Hultman T, Bucht A et al. (1995). Restricted usage of T cell receptor V alpha/J alpha gene segments with different nucleotide but identical amino acid sequences in HLA-DR3+ sarcoidosis patients. Mol Med 1: 287–96.

Grunewald J, Berlin M, Olerup O, Eklund A (2000). Lung T-helper cells expressing T-cell receptor AV2S3 associate with clinical features of pulmonary sarcoidosis. Am J Respir Crit Care Med 161: 814–18.

Hancock WW, Muller WA, Cotran RS (1987). Interleukin 2 receptors are expressed by alveolar macrophages during pulmonary sarcoidosis and are inducible by lymphokine treatment of normal human lung macrophages, blood monocytes, and monocyte cell lines. J Immunol 138: 185–91.

Harrington LE, Hatton RD, Mangan PR et al. (2005). Interleukin 17-producing CD4+ effector T cells develop via a lineage distinct from the T helper type 1 and 2 lineages. Nat Immunol 6: 1123–32.

Hashimoto S, Nakayama T, Gon Y et al. (1998). Correlation of plasma monocyte chemoattractant protein-1 (MCP-1) and monocyte inflammatory protein-1alpha (MIP-1alpha) levels with disease activity and clinical course of sarcoidosis. Clin Exp Immunol 111: 604–10.

Hauber HP, Gholami D, Meyer A, Pforte A (2003). Increased interleukin-13 expression in patients with sarcoidosis. Thorax 58: 519–24.

Hedrick SM, Engel I, McElligott DL et al. (1988). Selection of amino acid sequences in the beta chain of the T cell antigen receptor. Science 239: 1541–4.

Ho LP, Urban BC, Thickett DR et al. (2005). Deficiency of a subset of T-cells with immunoregulatory properties in sarcoidosis. Lancet 365: 1062–72.

Homma S, Nagaoka I, Abe H et al. (1995). Localization of platelet-derived growth factor and insulin-like growth factor I in the fibrotic lung. Am J Respir Crit Care Med 152: 2084–9.

Homolka J, Muller-Quernheim J (1993). Increased interleukin 6 production by bronchoalveolar lavage cells in patients with active sarcoidosis. Lung 171: 173–83.

Horton MR, McKee CM, Farber JM, Al E (1997). Hyaluronan fragments synergize with IFN-g to induce the C-X-C chemokine MIG in mouse macrophages and alveolar macrophages from patients with sarcoidosis. Am J Resp Crit Care Med 155: A501.

Hoshino T, Itoh K, Gouhara R et al. (1995). Spontaneous production of various cytokines except IL-4 from CD4+ T cells in the affected organs of sarcoidosis patients. Clin Exp Immunol 102: 399–405.

Hunninghake GW, Crystal RG (1981). Pulmonary sarcoidosis: a disorder mediated by excess helper T-lymphocyte activity at sites of disease activity. New Engl J Med 305: 429–34.

Hunninghake GW, Bedell GN, Zavala DC et al. (1983). Role of interleukin-2 release by lung T-cells in active pulmonary sarcoidosis. Am Rev Respir Dis 128: 634–8.

Idali F, Wahlstrom J, Muller-Suur C et al. (2008). Analysis of regulatory T cell associated forkhead box P3 expression in the lungs of patients with sarcoidosis. Clin Exp Immunol 152: 127–37.

Iida K, Kadota J, Kawakami K et al. (1997). Analysis of T cell subsets and beta chemokines in patients with pulmonary sarcoidosis. Thorax 52: 431–7.

Itoh A, Yamaguchi E, Furuya K et al. (1993). Correlation of GM-CSF mRNA in bronchoalveolar fluid with indices of clinical activity in sarcoidosis. Thorax 48: 1230–4.

Kaneko Y, Kuwano K, Kunitake R et al. (1999). Immunohistochemical localization of B7 costimulating molecules and major histocompatibility complex class II antigen in pulmonary sarcoidosis. Respiration 66: 343–8.

Katchar K, Wahlstrom J, Eklund A, Grunewald J (2001). Highly activated T-cell receptor AV2S3(+) CD4(+) lung T-cell expansions in pulmonary sarcoidosis. Am J Respir Crit Care Med 163: 1540–5.

Katchar K, Eklund A, Grunewald J (2003). Expression of Th1 markers by lung accumulated T cells in pulmonary sarcoidosis. J Intern Med 254: 564–71.

Katoh S, Matsumoto N, Fukushima K et al. (2000). Elevated chemokine levels in bronchoalveolar lavage fluid of patients with eosinophilic pneumonia. J Allergy Clin Immunol 106: 730–6.

Khader SA, Cooper AM (2008). IL-23 and IL-17 in tuberculosis. Cytokine 41: 79–83.

Kim DS, Jeon YG, Shim TS et al. (2000). The value of interleukin-12 as an activity marker of pulmonary sarcoidosis. Sarcoidosis Vasc Diffuse Lung Dis 17: 271–6.

Klein JT, Horn TD, Forman JD et al. (1995). Selection of oligoclonal V beta-specific T cells in the intradermal response to Kveim–Siltzbach reagent in individuals with sarcoidosis. J Immunol 154: 1450–60.

Kline JN, Schwartz DA, Monick MM et al. (1993). Relative release of interleukin-1 beta and interleukin-1 receptor antagonist by alveolar macrophages: a study in asbestos-induced lung disease, sarcoidosis, and idiopathic pulmonary fibrosis. Chest 104: 47–53.

Konishi K, Moller DR, Saltini C et al. (1988). Spontaneous expression of the interleukin 2 receptor gene and presence of functional interleukin 2 receptors on T lymphocytes in the blood of individuals with active pulmonary sarcoidosis. J Clin Invest 82: 775–81.

Kunkel SL, Lukacs NW, Strieter RM, Chensue SW (1996). Th1 and Th2 responses regulate experimental lung granuloma development. Sarcoidosis Vasc Diffuse Lung Dis 13: 120–8.

Laroussserie F, Pflanz S, Coulomb-L'Hermine A et al. (2004). Expression of IL-27 in human Th1-associated granulomatous diseases. J Pathol 202: 164–71.

Lem VM, Lipscomb MF, Weissler JC et al. (1985). Bronchoalveolar cells from sarcoid patients demonstrate enhanced antigen presentation. J Immunol 135: 1766–71.

Li X, O'Regan AW, Berman JS (2003). IFN-gamma induction of osteopontin expression in human monocytoid cells. J Interferon Cytokine Res 23: 259–65.

Limper AH, Colby TV, Sanders MS et al. (1994). Immunohistochemical localization of transforming growth factor-beta 1 in the non-necrotizing granulomas of pulmonary sarcoidosis. Am J Respir Crit Care Med 149: 197–204.

Mackay CR (2001). Chemokines: immunology's high impact factors. Nat Immunol 2: 95–101.

Mathew S, Bauer KL, Fischoeder A et al. (2008). The anergic state in sarcoidosis is associated with diminished dendritic cell function. J Immunol 181: 746–55.

Mikuniya T, Nagai S, Takeuchi M et al. (2000). Significance of the interleukin-1 receptor antagonist/interleukin-1 beta ratio as a prognostic factor in patients with pulmonary sarcoidosis. Respiration 67: 389–96.

Minshall EM, Tsicopoulos A, Yasruel Z et al. (1997). Cytokine mRNA gene expression in active and nonactive pulmonary sarcoidosis. Eur Respir J 10: 2034–9.

Miotto D, Christodoulopoulos P, Olivenstein R et al. (2001). Expression of IFN-gamma-inducible protein; monocyte chemotactic proteins 1, 3, and 4; and eotaxin in TH1- and TH2-mediated lung diseases. J Allergy Clin Immunol 107: 664–70.

Miyara M, Amoura Z, Parizot C et al. (2006). The immune paradox of sarcoidosis and regulatory T cells. J Exp Med 203: 359–70.

Miyazaki E, Nureki S, Fukami T et al. (2002). Elevated levels of thymus- and activation-regulated chemokine in bronchoalveolar lavage fluid from patients with eosinophilic pneumonia. Am J Respir Crit Care Med 165: 1125–31.

Moller DR (1998). Involvement of T cells and alterations in T cell receptors in sarcoidosis. Semin Respir Infect 13: 174–83.

Moller DR (1999). Cells and cytokines involved in the pathogenesis of sarcoidosis. Sarcoidosis Vasc Diffuse Lung Dis 16: 24–31.

Moller DR, Chen ES (2002). Genetic basis of remitting sarcoidosis: triumph of the trimolecular complex? Am J Respir Cell Mol Biol 27: 391–5.

Moller DR, Konishi K, Kirby M et al. (1988). Bias toward use of a specific T cell receptor beta-chain variable region in a subgroup of individuals with sarcoidosis. J Clin Invest 82: 1183–91.

Moller DR, Forman JD, Liu MC et al. (1996). Enhanced expression of IL-12 associated with Th1 cytokine profiles in active pulmonary sarcoidosis. J Immunol 156: 4952–60.

Muller-Quernheim J (1998). Sarcoidosis: immunopathogenetic concepts and their clinical application. Eur Respir J 12: 716–38.

Muller-Quernheim J, Pfeifer S, Mannel D et al. (1992). Lung-restricted activation of the alveolar macrophage/monocyte system in pulmonary sarcoidosis. Am Rev Respir Dis 145: 187–92.

Nicod LP, Isler P (1997). Alveolar macrophages in sarcoidosis coexpress high levels of CD86 (B7.2), CD40, and CD30L. Am J Respir Cell Mol Biol 17: 91–6.

O'Regan AW, Chupp GL, Lowry JA et al. (1999). Osteopontin is associated with T cells in sarcoid granulomas and has T cell adhesive and cytokine-like properties in vitro. J Immunol 162: 1024–31.

O'Regan AW, Hayden JM, Body S et al. (2001). Abnormal pulmonary granuloma formation in osteopontin-deficient mice. Am J Respir Crit Care Med 164: 2243–7.

Ota M, Amakawa R, Uehira K et al. (2004). Involvement of dendritic cells in sarcoidosis. Thorax 59: 408–13.

Panina-Bordignon P, Papi A, Mariani M et al. (2001). The C-C chemokine receptors CCR4 and CCR8 identify airway T cells of allergen-challenged atopic asthmatics. J Clin Invest 107: 1357–64.

Petrek M, Kolek V, Szotkowska J, Du Bois RM (2002). CC and C chemokine expression in pulmonary sarcoidosis. Eur Respir J 20: 1206–12.

Pinkston P, Bitterman PB, Crystal RG (1983). Spontaneous release of interleukin-2 by lung T lymphocytes in active pulmonary sarcoidosis. New Engl J Med 308: 793–800.

Planck A, Eklund A, Grunewald J (2003). Markers of activity in clinically recovered human leukocyte antigen-DR17-positive sarcoidosis patients. Eur Respir J 21: 52–7.

Prasse A, Georges CG, Biller H et al. (2000). Th1 cytokine pattern in sarcoidosis is expressed by bronchoalveolar CD4+ and CD8+ T cells. Clin Exp Immunol 122: 241–8.

Robinson BW, McLemore TL, Crystal RG (1985). Gamma interferon is spontaneously released by alveolar macrophages and lung T lymphocytes in patients with pulmonary sarcoidosis. J Clin Invest 75: 1488–95.

Rogge L, Papi A, Presky DH et al. (1999). Antibodies to the IL-12 receptor beta 2 chain mark human Th1 but not Th2 cells in vitro and in vivo. J Immunol 162: 3926–32.

Rossman MD, Thompson B, Frederick M et al. (2008). HLA and environmental interactions in sarcoidosis. Sarcoidosis Vasc Diffuse Lung Dis 25: 125–32.

Sakaguchi S (2005). Naturally arising Foxp3-expressing CD25+CD4+ regulatory T cells in immunological tolerance to self and non-self. Nat Immunol 6: 345–52.

Sallusto F, Lenig D, Mackay CR, Lanzavecchia A (1998). Flexible programs of chemokine receptor expression on human polarized T helper 1 and 2 lymphocytes. J Exp Med 187: 875–83.

Saltini C, Hemler ME, Crystal RG (1988). T lymphocytes compartmentalized on the epithelial surface of the lower respiratory tract express the very late activation antigen complex VLA-1. Clin Immunol Immunopathol 46: 221–33.

Scott P, Pearce E, Cheever AW et al. (1989). Role of cytokines and CD4+ T-cell subsets in the regulation of parasite immunity and disease. Immunol Rev 112: 161–82.

Selroos O, Klockars M, Kekomaki R et al. (1980). Circulating immune complexes in sarcoidosis. J Clin Lab Immunol 3: 129–32.

Shigehara K, Shijubo N, Ohmichi M et al. (2000a). Enhanced mRNA expression of Th1 cytokines and IL-12 in active pulmonary sarcoidosis. Sarcoidosis Vasc Diffuse Lung Dis 17: 151–7.

Shigehara K, Shijubo N, Ohmichi M et al. (2000b). Increased levels of interleukin-18 in patients with pulmonary sarcoidosis. Am J Respir Crit Care Med 162: 1979–82.

Shigehara K, Shijubo N, Ohmichi M et al. (2001). IL-12 and IL-18 are increased and stimulate IFN-gamma production in sarcoid lungs. J Immunol 166: 642–9.

Shikuwa C, Kadota J, Mukae H et al. (2002). High concentrations of soluble Fas ligand in bronchoalveolar lavage fluid of patients with pulmonary sarcoidosis. Respiration 69: 242–6.

Silver RF, Crystal RG, Moller DR (1996). Limited heterogeneity of biased T-cell receptor V beta gene usage in lung but not blood T cells in active pulmonary sarcoidosis. Immunology 88: 516–23.

Simonian PL, Roark CL, Born WK et al. (2009). Gammadelta T cells and Th17 cytokines in hypersensitivity pneumonitis and lung fibrosis. Transl Res 154: 222–7.

Song Z, Marzilli L, Greenlee BM et al. (2005). Mycobacterial catalase-peroxidase is a tissue antigen and target of the adaptive immune response in systemic sarcoidosis. J Exp Med 201: 755–67.

Standiford TJ, Rolfe MW, Kunkel SL et al. (1993). Macrophage inflammatory protein-1 alpha expression in interstitial lung disease. J Immunol 151: 2852–63.

Steffen M, Petersen J, Oldigs M et al. (1993). Increased secretion of tumor necrosis factor-alpha, interleukin-1-beta, and interleukin-6 by alveolar macrophages from patients with sarcoidosis. J Allergy Clin Immunol 91: 939–49.

Suganuma H, Sato A, Tamura R, Chida K (1995). Enhanced migration of fibroblasts derived from lungs with fibrotic lesions. Thorax 50: 984–9.

Swain SL (1994). Generation and in vivo persistence of polarized Th1 and Th2 memory cells. Immunity 1: 543–52.

Taflin C, Miyara M, Nochy D et al. (2009). FoxP3+ regulatory T cells suppress early stages of granuloma formation but have little impact on sarcoidosis lesions. Am J Pathol 174: 497–508.

Taha RA, Minshall EM, Olivenstein R et al. (1999). Increased expression of IL-12 receptor mRNA in active pulmonary tuberculosis and sarcoidosis. Am J Respir Crit Care Med 160: 1119–23.

Trapnell BC, Whitsett JA (2002). Gm-CSF regulates pulmonary surfactant homeostasis and alveolar macrophage-mediated innate host defense. Annu Rev Physiol 64: 775–802.

Umbert P, Belcher RW, Winkelmann RK (1976). Lymphokines (MIF) in the serum of patients with sarcoidosis and cutaneous granuloma annulare. Br J Dermatol 95: 481–5.

Venet A, Hance AJ, Saltini C et al. (1985). Enhanced alveolar macrophage-mediated antigen-induced T-lymphocyte proliferation in sarcoidosis. J Clin Invest 75: 293–301.

Wahlstrom J, Dengjel J, Persson B *et al.* (2007). Identification of HLA-DR-bound peptides presented by human bronchoalveolar lavage cells in sarcoidosis. *J Clin Invest* **117**: 3576–82.

Wahlstrom J, Dengjel J, Winqvist O *et al.* (2009). Autoimmune T cell responses to antigenic peptides presented by bronchoalveolar lavage cell HLA-DR molecules in sarcoidosis. *Clin Immunol* **133**: 353–63.

Walker C, Bauer W, Braun RK *et al.* (1994). Activated T cells and cytokines in bronchoalveolar lavages from patients with various lung diseases associated with eosinophilia. *Am J Respir Crit Care Med* **150**: 1038–48.

Wewers MD, Saltini C, Sellers S *et al.* (1987). Evaluation of alveolar macrophages in normals and individuals with active pulmonary sarcoidosis for the spontaneous expression of the interleukin-1 beta gene. *Cell Immunol* **107**: 479–88.

Wiken M, Grunewald J, Eklund A, Wahlstrom J (2009). Higher monocyte expression of TLR2 and TLR4, and enhanced pro-inflammatory synergy of TLR2 with NOD2 stimulation in sarcoidosis. *J Clin Immunol* **29**: 78–89.

Wynn TA, Eltoum I, Cheever AW *et al.* (1993). Analysis of cytokine mRNA expression during primary granuloma formation induced by eggs of *Schistosoma mansoni*. *J Immunol* **151**: 1430–40.

Yamaguchi E, Okazaki N, Tsuneta Y *et al.* (1988). Interleukins in pulmonary sarcoidosis. Dissociative correlations of lung interleukins 1 and 2 with the intensity of alveolitis. *Am Rev Respir Dis* **138**: 645–51.

Yeager H, Williams MC, Beekman JF *et al.* (1977). Sarcoidosis: analysis of cells obtained by bronchial lavage. *Am Rev Respir Dis* **116**: 951–4.

Zaba LC, Smith GP, Sanchez M, Prystowsky SD (2010). Dendritic cells in the pathogenesis of sarcoidosis. *Am J Respir Cell Mol Biol* **42**: 32–9.

Ziegenhagen MW, Schrum S, Zissel G *et al.* (1998). Increased expression of pro-inflammatory chemokines in bronchoalveolar lavage cells of patients with progressing idiopathic pulmonary fibrosis and sarcoidosis. *J Investig Med* **46**: 223–31.

Zissel G, Homolka J, Schlaak J *et al.* (1996). Anti-inflammatory cytokine release by alveolar macrophages in pulmonary sarcoidosis. *Am J Respir Crit Care Med* **154**: 713–19.

Zissel G, Baumer I, Schlaak M, Muller-Quernheim J (2000). In-vitro release of interleukin-15 by broncho-alveolar lavage cells and peripheral blood mononuclear cells from patients with different lung diseases. *Eur Cytokine Netw* **11**: 105–12.

Zissel G, Prasse A, Muller-Quernheim J (2007). Sarcoidosis: immunopathogenetic concepts. *Semin Respir Crit Care Med* **28**: 3–14.

7

Genetics

PAOLO SPAGNOLO AND ROLAND M DU BOIS

INTRODUCTION

There is considerable epidemiological evidence to support the existence of a genetic predisposition to sarcoidosis (McGrath et al. 2001a; Grunewald 2008). For instance, the prevalence, incidence and severity of the disease vary widely between different races. However, sarcoidosis is not due to defects in a single major gene or chemical pathway but instead appears to be a complex/multifactorial disease likely to result from the interaction of environmental factors and multiple genes, some with a major disease effect but many with a relatively minor effect. Genetic factors are also likely to contribute to the wide variety of clinical presentations, progression as well as prognosis observed in sarcoidosis. Indeed, some believe that sarcoidosis may represent a 'family' of diseases, including Löfgren's syndrome, non-resolving/progressive lung disease, and granulomatous uveitis – each with potentially distinct genetic associations. In this respect, berylliosis could also be considered as a subset of the broad grouping 'sarcoidosis' and almost certainly was historically (Grutters et al. 2003a).

GENETIC STUDIES

Familial clustering of sarcoidosis has been reported in several populations. It was first described in two German sisters in 1923 (Martenstein 1923), and since then studies in various ethnicities have confirmed that family members of sarcoidosis patients have a several-fold increased risk of disease compared with the general population (Pietinalho et al. 1999; Rybicki et al. 2001; McGrath et al. 2000). While these findings could be attributed to a shared exposure to the putative sarcoidosis antigen(s), it seems more likely that they are a result of a shared genetic predisposition.

Few linkage studies have been performed in sarcoidosis, mainly owing to difficulties in recruiting large numbers of familial cases. Using a genome-wide approach, Schurmann and co-workers genotyped 122 affected siblings from 55 German families for seven DNA polymorphisms in the major histocompatibility complex (MHC) region on chromosome 6 and reported a genetic linkage of sarcoidosis to the class III region (Schurmann et al. 2000). In a follow-up study, the same team investigated an expanded cohort of 63 German families including affected siblings by using a larger number of genetic markers (225 microsatellites). Linkage was confirmed within the MHC region with the most prominent peak nearer the class II loci, but including the same marker identified in the first study (D6S1666). Six additional minor peaks on chromosomes 1, 3, 7, 9 and X were also identified (Schurmann et al. 2001a). However, given the wide spacing between the microsatellite markers used in this study, spurious positive and negative findings could not be excluded as a certain number of minor peaks would be expected by chance alone.

Further refinement of the MHC region map and a single nucleotide polymorphism (SNP) scan of a 16.4 Mb linkage peak centered at chromosome 6p21, identified a 15 kb disease-associated segment containing the butyrophilin-like 2 (BTNL2) gene in the MHC class II region (Valentonyte et al. 2005a). In a German cohort including familial and sporadic cases, Valentonyte and co-workers observed that the rs2076530 A allele was associated with sarcoidosis in both familial and case–control samples. The BTNL2 gene is a member of the immunoglobulin superfamily with likely co-stimulatory activities in T-cell activation based on its homology to B7-1 (Stammers et al. 2000). Further, Valentonyte and colleagues showed that the risk allele causes a functional change (the lack of the C-terminal IgC domain and transmembrane helix), which disrupts the membrane localization and hence function of the protein. The BTNL2 gene is in close proximity to the human leukocyte antigen (HLA)-DRB1 region. However, the authors reported that the BTNL2 variant associated with sarcoidosis represented a risk factor independent of HLA class II alleles, despite almost complete linkage disequilibrium (LD) with HLA-DRB1. Following this report, Rybicki and colleagues investigated the same BTNL2 polymorphism as well as a further nine variants in an African-American family cohort and in two case–control cohorts, one African-American and one white. They confirmed that the rs2076530 A allele is associated with an increased risk for sarcoidosis in their white population, while no association was observed in either African-American cohort (Rybicki et al. 2005). Although both of these studies came to the same conclusion regarding a BTNL2 allele predisposing to sarcoidosis, the issue of whether the BTNL2 associations are due to LD with HLA alleles is far from being satisfactorily resolved. Indeed, while our group's data on two large cohorts of sarcoidosis patients from the United Kingdom and the Netherlands showed odds ratios (ORs) for the putative rs2076530 A susceptibility allele comparable to previous studies, on regression analysis we found higher ORs for disease susceptibility associations with HLA-DRB1*12 and DRB1*14 (Spagnolo et al. 2007). Recently, Li and colleagues sequenced six coding exons within BTNL2, and identified a previously unknown one-base-pair deletion (c.450delC) in exon 3, which could cause a frameshift at amino acid position 150, thus introducing 96 additional amino acids (Li et al. 2009). However, the c.450delC genotype frequencies did not differ between patients ($n = 210$) and controls ($n = 201$). Of note, despite recent data suggesting a potential immunological role for BTNL2, its functional status in humans remains largely undetermined.

In the Sarcoidosis Genetic Analysis (SAGA) study in African-Americans, 380 markers were genotyped in 229 families with 519 pairs consisting of 338 affected sib pairs, 116 discordantly affected pairs (one sib had sarcoidosis and the other was healthy), and 15 unaffected sib pairs (Iannuzzi et al. 2005). A number of statistically significant peaks were identified, with the most prominent one at D5S2500 on chromosome 5q11 ($p = 0.0005$). Of note, agreement for linkage between the scans performed in the German and African-American populations were found only at chromosome 1p, 3p and 9q. Further, the lack of any positive linkage signal with the HLA region in the SAGA study highlights the complex (and probably race-specific) genetics underlying susceptibility to sarcoidosis.

In a follow-up fine-mapping study on African-Americans, additional microsatellite markers were used to refine regions with significant linkage. Sarcoidosis susceptibility alleles were identified on chromosome 5p15.2 and protective alleles on chromosome 5q11.2 (Gray-McGuire et al. 2006). Subsequent phenotypic analysis of these genome-wide scans showed the strongest linkage signals on chromosome 1p36 for radiographic resolution of sarcoidosis lesions and on chromosome 18q22 for the presence of cardiac or renal involvement (Rybicki et al. 2007). A limitation of linkage studies is confounding to admixture. This is particularly true for African-Americans who are known to be admixed with European-Americans and other populations to varying degrees (Parra et al. 1998). However,

Thompson and co-workers further analyzed the SAGA sample using linkage analysis stratified by genetically determined ancestry and confirmed the peaks on chromosome 5. In addition, they observed an additional susceptibility locus at 2q37 (Thompson et al. 2006).

Franke and co-workers recently performed a 100k genome-wide association study using 83,360 SNPs on 382 Crohn's disease (CD) patients, 398 sarcoidosis (SA) patients, and 394 healthy controls (Franke et al. 2008). Twenty-four SNPs most strongly associated with the combined CD/SA phenotype were selected for verification in an independent sample of 1317 patients (660 CD and 657 SA) and 1091 controls. The most significant association ($p = 0.036$) was observed on chromosome 10p12.2 (rs1398024 A allele) with an odds ratio for both diseases of 0.81. Finer mapping of the 10p12.2 locus pointed to yet unidentified variant/s in the C10ORF67 gene region as the most likely underlying risk factors.

More recently, a genome-wide association study (GWAS) looking at 440000 SNPs has been performed in 499 German individuals with sarcoidosis and 490 healthy controls. The strongest association signal mapped to the annexin A11 (ANXA11) gene on chromosome 10q22.3, and was validated in an independent cohort of 1649 cases, and 1832 controls. Finer mapping of the region identified a common non-synonymous SNP (rs1049550, R230C) as the variant most strongly associated with sarcoidosis (Hofmann et al. 2008). Annexin A11 appears to exert a number of regulatory functions in calcium signaling, cell division, vesicle trafficking and apoptosis (Moss and Morgan 2004), and has been implicated in the pathogenesis of several autoimmune disorders – including rheumatoid arthritis, systemic lupus erythematosus and Sjögren syndrome – by giving rise to autoantibodies (Jorgensen et al. 2000). In sarcoidosis, a dysfunction of annexin A11 could affect the apoptosis pathway, hence modifying the balance between apoptosis and survival of activated inflammatory cells. Nevertheless, the functional relevance of rs1049550, if any, in disease pathogenesis remains unknown.

MAJOR HISTOCOMPATIBILITY COMPLEX GENES

The major histocompatibility complex is located on chromosome 6p21 and is composed of three classes: MHC classes I, II and III. MHC class I mainly includes the HLA-A, HLA-B and HLA-C genes; MHC class II contains the HLA-DR, HLA-DQ and HLA-DP sub-classes. The MHC class III region is located between the class I and class II regions and contains tumor necrosis factors (TNF) alpha and beta, the complement proteins (C4A, C4B, C2, Bf), enzymes involved in steroid synthesis (CYP21A, CYP21B) and heat-shock proteins (HSPA1A, HSPA1B and HSPA1L) (Cooke and Hill 2001). Both CD4+ and CD8+ T-lymphocytes can only recognize antigens when they are presented with a self-MHC molecule. Specifically, HLA class I molecules bind peptides derived from endogenous antigen (endogenous pathway), while exogenous antigen is internalized by endocytosis and processed in the context of HLA class II molecules (endocytic pathway).

Peptide binding assays using natural and synthetic peptides show that natural polymorphisms of HLA molecules can influence both the specificity and affinity of peptide binding. Therefore, it is apparent that certain HLA molecules bind and present individual antigens in specific diseases and sarcoidosis is hypothesized to be one such disease (Hammer *et al.* 1994; Sturniolo *et al.* 1999).

Human leukocyte antigen class I

HLA association studies began over 30 years ago and concentrated on HLA class I alleles (HLA-A, -B and -C) using serological typing. Varying and often controversial results were obtained, depending on the cohort and the ethnicity studied; however, HLA-B7 and HLA-B8 have been most commonly linked to sarcoidosis. The role of HLA-B7 is unclear as this allele has been found in increased frequency in African-American patients (a population with a high disease prevalence) (McIntyre *et al.* 1977) but significantly decreased in Japanese patients (a population with a low prevalence of disease) (Ina *et al.* 1989), and unchanged in Moravian Czechs (Lenhart *et al.* 1990). Conversely, the HLA-B8 allele association is more robust. This allele has been associated with sarcoidosis of acute onset and short duration in a number of studies across racial boundaries (Smith *et al.* 1981; Olenchock *et al.* 1981; Hedfors and Lindstrom 1983; Guyatt *et al.* 1982; Gardner *et al.* 1984). Interestingly, as more studies of sarcoidosis and HLA-B8 were published, it was noted that HLA-B8/DR3 genes were inherited as a unique disease risk haplotype in Caucasians, suggesting that disease associations with class I genes may be simply due to LD with class II genes (Hedfors and Lindstrom *et al.* 1983; Gardner *et al.* 1984; Kremer 1986; Krause and Goebel 1987). Indeed, based on our current understanding of the immunopathogenesis of sarcoidosis, the class II genes are more likely to be involved in antigen presentation. Nevertheless, a study of Scandinavian patients by Grunewald and co-workers indicated that HLA-B7 and HLA-B8 increased the risk of sarcoidosis independently of class II genes (Grunewald *et al.* 2004), suggesting that HLA class I alleles may have more influence on disease susceptibility and prognosis than had been previously thought.

Human leukocyte antigen class II

HLA class II genes have been extensively studied because of the increased expression of these molecules on activated alveolar macrophages, and based on the hypothesis that sarcoidosis is triggered by exogenous antigen(s). To date several HLA class II associations with sarcoidosis have been reported, supporting the concept that a number of HLA genes acting either in concert or independently predispose to sarcoidosis. However, the high and variable LD within the MHC region makes it difficult to determine which specific genes apart from HLA-DRB1 confer sarcoidosis risk. For instance, Grunewald and co-workers showed in their Scandinavian population that the associations of HLA-DRB1*15 with chronic disease and HLA-DRB1*03 with mild disease were synonymous with the HLA-DQB1*0602–chronic disease and HLA-DQB1*0201–mild

disease associations (Grunewald *et al.* 2004). The latter results mirrored the HLA–DQB1 sarcoidosis outcome association reported by our group in two independent cohorts of Caucasian patients (Sato *et al.* 2002).

The associations of sarcoidosis with HLA class II genes vary by cohort, ethnicity and race. In Japanese patients, HLA-DR5, -DR6, -DR8 and -DR9 have been associated with disease (Ishihara *et al.* 1996a,b). In Germans, HLA-DR5 has been linked with chronic disease, but HLA-DR3 with disease of acute onset and short duration (Nowack and Goebel 1987; Swider *et al.* 1999). This pattern of differential linkage according to clinical phenotypes has been confirmed in Scandinavian patients; indeed, HLA-DR14 and HLA-DR15 have been associated with persistent disease, while DR17 (DR3) predisposed to an acute and self-limiting form of sarcoidosis (Berlin *et al.* 1997). Interestingly, HLA-DR9 has been associated with disease risk in Japanese patients, but with disease protection in Scandinavians (Berlin *et al.* 1997). The HLA-DR associations were more consistent across different populations when only the 'protective' alleles were considered. Both HLA-DR1 and HLA-DR4 have been found to be 'protective' in Scandinavians, Japanese, Italians, and in a study including UK, Polish and Czech patients (Foley *et al.* 2001). The latter study showed position 11 of the HLA-DRB1 sequence to be the most variable, with three susceptibility alleles all coding for small hydrophilic amino acids, and two protective alleles coding for amino acids with bulky, hydrophobic, aliphatic side-chains. Because the residue at position 11 is involved in the beta sheet that keeps the HLA-DR alpha and beta chain together, alteration in hydrophilicity/hydrophobicity may be important in HLA-DR heterodimer formation/conformation, thus modifying the HLA-DR protein-binding profile. This association would therefore suggest a specific interaction between the still unknown sarcoidosis trigger(s) and the host immune system (Foley *et al.* 1999).

Despite the limited number of reports to date, the HLA-DP locus is extremely interesting due to the finding that chronic beryllium disease (CBD), a systemic granulomatous disease often indistinguishable from sarcoidosis, is strongly associated with the presence of a glutamic acid residue at position 69 of the HLA-DPB1 beta chain (Richeldi *et al.* 1993). The immunopathological and clinical similarities between CBD and sarcoidosis suggest that these two disorders may also share a common genetic background. However, no association has been found with the Glu69+ allele in sarcoidosis patients (Maliarik *et al.* 1998a; Foley *et al.* 1999; Schurmann *et al.* 2000), whereas the HLA-DPB1 amino acids Val36+ and Asp55+ have been associated with sarcoidosis risk but only in African-American cases (Maliarik *et al.* 1998a).

In a study limited to African-Americans, 225 patients with family members as controls were genotyped for six microsatellite markers covering the MHC region (Rybicki *et al.* 2003). Interestingly, the authors observed that HLA-DQB1, and not HLA-DRB1, represented the strongest association with sarcoidosis in African-Americans. Subsequently, a follow-up study found that HLA-DQB1*0201 was transmitted to affected offspring only half as often as expected, whereas DQB1*0602 was transmitted to affected offspring ∼20 percent more than expected, and was associated with radiographic disease progression (Iannuzzi *et al.* 2003).

Recently, an association in Dutch patients between severe disease and the haplotype DRB1*150101/DQB1*0601 has been reported; however, due to the almost complete LD between these alleles among Caucasians, it was not possible to tease out the primary association (Voorter *et al.* 2005). Similar results had been previously shown by Sato and colleagues in a large study including patients from UK and the Netherlands. They found DQB1*0201 to be strongly associated with mild sarcoidosis, as assessed by chest radiographs, whereas a chronic course of disease was common among individuals carrying the DQB1*0602 allele (Sato *et al.* 2002). In the same study it was reported that carriage of the DQB1*0201 allele was significantly increased among both patients presenting with Löfgren's syndrome and patients with erythema nodosum (EN). In a follow-up study, Grutters and colleagues genotyped the DQB1*0201, DRB1*0301 as well as the variant at position −307 of the TNF-α gene (TNF2), which had been previously associated with Löfgren's syndrome (Swider *et al.* 1999), in an expanded cohort of patients. Although the strongest association was observed with DQB1*0201 (OR = 8.6 vs 6.7 and 6.8 for DRB1*03 and TNF2, respectively), the authors reported that the LD between DQB1*0201 and DRB1*03 was almost complete. The extended HLA haplotype including DQB1*0201, DRB1*0301 and TNF2 was present in 76 percent of Löfgren's patients (versus 24 percent of controls) and represented a clear risk factor for Dutch patients with Löfgren's syndrome (OR = 9.9) (Grutters *et al.* 2003b). More recently, Grunewald and Eklund characterized and HLA-DRB1 typed 301 patients with Löfgren's syndrome (Grunewald and Eklund 2009). Of note, while 95 percent of DRB1*03-positive patients had a resolving disease (defined as disease duration < 2 years), as many as 49 percent of DRB1*03-negative patients developed a non-resolving disease. These results suggest that carriage of DRB1*03 allele not only predisposes to Löfgren's syndrome but also influences its course. Löfgren's syndrome, a form of acute and usually self-limiting sarcoidosis presenting with fever, erythema nodosum, arthralgia and bilateral hilar lymphadenopathy (Löfgren and Lundback 1952), is almost exclusive to Caucasians, with the highest incidence reported amongst Scandinavians (Grunewald and Eklund 2001); conversely, this particular disease phenotype is limited to a small number of case reports among Japanese individuals. Of note, HLA-DRB1*03 is also extremely rare in Japan. On the other hand, cardiac sarcoidosis is more common than in Caucasians with cardiac involvement, being the most common cause of death from sarcoidosis in Japan. Cardiac sarcoidosis has been originally associated with the TNFA2 allele (Takashige *et al.* 1999). However, further studies showed that the strongest association was with the HLA-DQB1*0601 allele (Naruse *et al.* 2000). The TNFA2 allele was not in LD with the HLA-DQB1*0601 allele and may therefore represent an additional genetic risk factor for cardiac sarcoidosis.

NON-MHC GENES

The HLA-DRB1 associations predominate in the sarcoidosis genetic literature, and it is now commonly accepted that variation in the HLA-DRB1 genes influence sarcoidosis susceptibility and phenotypes. However, in roughly half of the patients the HLA genes do not seem to play any role, highlighting the importance of studying other genes, either MHC-associated or located in other chromosomal areas (Grutters *et al.* 2003a).

Infection susceptibility genes

MANNOSE-BINDING LECTIN (MBL)

MBL is a serum protein that binds oligosaccharides on the surface of pathogens, and triggers complement activation. Based on the hypothesis that the disease may be triggered by microbial agents, polymorphisms within MBL have been investigated in sarcoidosis. However one study of MBL gene promoter and exon 1 variants in British patients and controls found no associations with susceptibility to sarcoidosis, age of disease onset, or severity of disease (Foley *et al.* 2000).

HUMAN NATURAL-RESISTANCE-ASSOCIATED MACROPHAGE PROTEIN 1 (NRAMP1)

NRAMP1 has been associated with susceptibility to tuberculosis (Bellamy *et al.* 1998). The importance of the NRAMP1 gene in animal models of granulomatous disorders and its putative role in macrophage activation make it an attractive candidate gene in sarcoidosis. Maliarik and co-workers analyzed several NRAMP1 gene polymorphisms in a case–control study including individuals of African-American origin and found that a (CA)(n) repeat in the 5′ region of the gene was protective against sarcoidosis (Maliarik *et al.* 2000). However, the role of NRAMP1 in this disease needs to be clarified.

CASPASE RECRUITMENT DOMAIN 15 (CARD15)/ NUCLEOTIDE-BINDING OLIGOMERIZATION DOMAIN PROTEIN 2 (NOD2)

The caspase recruitment domain 15/nucleotide-binding oligomerization domain protein 2 (CARD15/NOD2) gene encodes a leukocyte receptor of the innate immune system. It recognizes intracellular bacterial lipopolysaccharides and activates nuclear factor-kappa B (NF-κB) (Girardin *et al.* 2003). CARD15 is also implicated in the pathogenesis of granulomatous diseases such as Blau syndrome and Crohn's disease (Miceli-Richard *et al.* 2001; Hugot *et al.* 2001). Polymorphisms within CARD15 have been also investigated in sarcoidosis with conflicting results. Schurmann and co-workers evaluated the four main CARD15 variants and found no association with sarcoidosis among German patients (Schurmann *et al.* 2003). Similarly, when the entire coding region was screened, the CARD15 polymorphism frequencies in UK sarcoidosis patients did not differ from those previously reported in control populations (Ho *et al.* 2005). No association between CARD15 variants and disease was found in Danish subjects (Milman *et al.* 2007). However, more recently, Sato and colleagues reported an association between the CARD15 functional polymorphism 2104T (702W) and severe pulmonary sarcoidosis, as assessed by radiographic stage of disease and pulmonary function test. Furthermore, and more interestingly, all patients carrying both CARD15 2104T and the CCR5 HHC haplotype – which had been previously associated with persistent parenchymal lung disease (Spagnolo et al. 2005) – had radiographic stage IV at presentation, suggesting that CARD15 and CCR5 may influence disease course and progression once sarcoidosis is established (Sato et al. 2010).

Antigen processing genes

TRANSPORTER ASSOCIATED WITH ANTIGEN PROCESSING (TAP)

Whole proteins require antigen processing before they can be immunologically recognized via the class I- or class II-restricted antigen presentation pathways. Variations within TAP genes may therefore theoretically modify the transport and presentation of antigenic peptide to CD4+ T-lymphocytes required to trigger the immunological cascade responsible for granuloma formation. TAP1 and TAP2 genes, located in the HLA class II region, encode subunits of a heterodimeric complex that functions in the endogenous antigen-processing pathway. In one study, significant differences between cases and controls were observed at the TAP2 locus in both UK and Polish populations although they are likely to be due to LD with the HLA-DR alleles (Foley et al. 1999,2001). However, Ishihara and co-workers did not reproduce the same findings in a cohort of Japanese patients (Ishihara et al. 1996c).

HLA-DMA AND HLA-DMB

The HLA-DMA and HLA-DMB genes map to an area between the HLA-DQ and HLA-DP loci of the MHC class II region (Kelly et al. 1991). HLA-DM functions in the class II antigen presentation pathway and is essential in preparing newly synthesized class II molecules for antigen binding (Fling et al. 1994). The low-molecular-weight proteins (LMP) genes, LMP2 and LMP7, encode two of the proteosome subunits involved in antigenic processing. However, studies of the HLA-DMA and HLA-DMB genes, and the LMP2 and LMP7 genes in Japanese sarcoidosis patients, did not reveal any association between variation at these loci and susceptibility to sarcoidosis (Ishihara et al. 1996c,d).

Cytokines and cytokine receptor genes

TUMOR NECROSIS FACTOR (TNF)

The TNF gene complex is located within the MHC region between the complement cluster region and the HLA-B locus and includes the TNF-α and lymphotoxin-α (previously known as TNF-β) genes. TNF-α is thought to be critical in mononuclear cell recruitment as well as in granuloma formation (Muller-Quernheim 1998); therefore, it is not surprising that the TNF gene complex has been extensively studied in the search for candidate susceptibility genes. An association between the rarer allele of a functional promoter polymorphism, which leads to increased TNF-α production (TNFA2), and Löfgren's syndrome has been reported (Seitzer et al. 1997; Swider et al. 1999). The same association has been confirmed in a large cohort of British and Dutch patients, suggesting that TNFA2 predicts a more favorable course of disease (Grutters et al. 2002). The latter study also showed that another rare allele of the TNF-α promoter, −857T, was associated with risk of sarcoidosis in both populations.

Nevertheless, the functional relevance of the reported TNF associations remains obscure and they may simply be in LD with the causative site(s) located elsewhere within the MHC region.

INTERLEUKIN 1 (IL-1)

The importance of IL-1 in granulomatous inflammation is well established. Hutyrova and colleagues investigated a number of polymorphisms within the IL-1α and IL-1β genes as well as an 86-bp variable number tandem repeat polymorphism in intron 2 of the interleukin-1 receptor antagonist (IL-1Ra) gene and found that the IL-1α -889 C/C genotype was significantly over-represented among sarcoidosis patients (n=95) compared with healthy controls (n=199), both from Czech Republic (Hutyrova et al. 2002). These results confirmed the association of an IL-1α marker and risk of sarcoidosis previously reported by Rybicki and co-workers (Rybicki et al. 1999). In a study among African-Americans of six markers closely linked to certain candidate cytokine genes, they identified two alleles associated with sarcoidosis. If both the IL-1α*137 and F13A*188 alleles were present, there was a 6-fold increased risk of disease, rising to a 15-fold increase in patients with a family history of sarcoidosis. The F13A marker is close to the gene for IRF-4 (a member of the interferon regulatory factor family – a transcription factor). However, a subsequent study including two large cohorts of patients and controls from two different European countries failed to reproduce this association in either population (Grutters et al. 2003c). Therefore, the previously reported associations may have been due to linkage disequilibrium within the IL-1 gene cluster between the IL-1α −889 C allele and an unidentified locus that confers the risk of sarcoidosis. Indeed, linkage disequilibrium does vary across different ethnicities and could account for the failure to reproduce similar findings in UK and Dutch populations.

INTERLEUKIN-7 RECEPTOR-ALPHA (IL7R-α)

This gene encodes a receptor highly expressed on both naive and memory T-cells. Recently, Heron and colleagues analyzed the frequency of six SNPs within IL7R in 475 sarcoidosis patients and 465 healthy controls (Heron et al. 2009). Replication of one significantly associated SNP was carried out in an independent cohort of patients and controls. Importantly, the SNP associated with sarcoidosis (rs10213865) was shown to be in complete linkage disequilibrium with a functional non-synonymous coding variant in exon 6 (rs6897932, T244I). Similar results were observed in the combined analysis of 663 individuals with sarcoidosis and 586 controls, thus suggesting that IL7R-α genetic polymorphisms may confer risk for sarcoidosis.

Chemokine receptor genes

The abnormal trafficking and accumulation of lymphocytes and macrophages represent a key step in sarcoidosis pathophysiology. This process results from the interaction between chemokines and specific G-protein-coupled receptors, which are both up-regulated at sites of granulomatous inflammation (Luster 1998; Agostini et al. 2002). Since the expression of chemokines and chemokine receptors is under genomic control, several studies have evaluated whether variations in these genes influence the susceptibility to sarcoidosis.

C–C CHEMOKINE RECEPTOR 2 (CCR2)

The CCR2 gene, which encodes for one of the main receptors for monocyte chemoattractant proteins (MCPs) (Charo and Ransohoff 2006), has been extensively studied with remarkable, although controversial, results. A SNP resulting in a conservative amino acid substitution (V64I) has been associated with a lower prevalence of sarcoidosis in a Japanese population, with a similar but not significant trend observed in a Czech population (Hizawa et al. 1999; Petrek et al. 2000). This polymorphism is also known to have a protective effect against progression of HIV infection to acquired immunodeficiency syndrome (AIDS) (Michael et al. 1997; Smith et al. 1997). Our group has investigated eight SNP (including V64I) across the CCR2 gene in 304 Dutch individuals (90 non-Löfgren's sarcoidosis, 47 Löfgren's syndrome, and 167 controls) and found that a particular haplotype (haplotype 2), which includes four unique SNPs, was strongly associated with Löfgren's syndrome as compared to both non-Löfgren's sarcoidosis patients and controls (Spagnolo et al. 2003). Of note, CCR2 haplotype 2 seemed to predispose to Löfgren's syndrome only in patients who also carried the HLA-DRB1*0301-DQB1*0201 allele. This association has subsequently been validated in an expanded cohort of Dutch patients and in two independent patient populations from Spain and Sweden (Spagnolo et al. 2008). However, these findings have not been replicated by Valentonyte and colleagues in a case–control and family-based study in individuals of German origin. Whether this is due to issues of case definition, subset ascertainment or true ethnic variation is unclear. However, the authors confirmed strong linkage disequilibrium across the genomic area where CCR2 lies (3p21) and showed positive linkage results ($p = 0.034$), thus suggesting that a susceptibility gene in the surrounding chromosomal region may exist (Valentonyte et al. 2005b).

C–C CHEMOKINE RECEPTOR 5 (CCR5)

CCR5 acts as a receptor for the chemokines 'macrophage inflammatory protein' (MIP)-1α (CCL3), MIP-1β (CCL4), and 'regulated upon activation, normally T-cell expressed and secreted' (RANTES/CCL5) (Alkhatib et al. 1996). Much of the information available on the functional consequences of CCR5 gene polymorphisms stems from studies of HIV-1-infected individuals as CCR5 is also the major co-receptor for the HIV type-1 virus. Individuals homozygous for a 32-base-pair deletion (Δ32/Δ32), resulting in a truncated protein that fails to reach the cell surface, are highly resistant to HIV infection (Samson et al. 1996). In addition to the Δ32 polymorphism, our group evaluated a further eight variations in 248 British subjects (106 patients and 142 controls) and in a second cohort of 281 Dutch individuals (112 patients and 169 controls). No differences in the genotype and allele frequencies of the CCR5 polymorphisms between patients and controls were observed in either the British or Dutch populations. However, one of the identified haplotypes (HHC) was strongly associated in both British and Dutch patients with the presence and persistence of parenchymal lung disease, as assessed by radiographic stage (II-III-IV vs stages 0-I) (Spagnolo et al. 2005). These findings could not be reproduced by a subsequent study by Fischer and co-workers (Fischer et al. 2008). On the other hand, these authors observed that two CCR5 promoter alleles – which are part of the HHC haplotype – were associated with Löfgren's syndrome, but only in female patients.

OTHER CANDIDATE GENES

CLARA-CELL 10 KD PROTEIN (CC10)

CC10 exhibits potent anti-inflammatory properties. In a case–control study in a Japanese population from Hokkaido (Ohchi et al. 2004), the A allele frequency of the G38A polymorphism was found to be significantly increased in sarcoidosis ($p = 0.0002$). In addition, the same A allele was associated with progressive disease ($p < 0.0001$). Furthermore, in the presence of IFN-γ, the 38A construct displayed significantly lower reporter activities, compared with the 38G construct ($p = 0.0177$). However, these associations have not been validated in a subsequent study including both Dutch and Kyoto Japanese sarcoidosis patients and healthy controls (Janssen et al. 2004). Of note, in the latter study the authors observed a significant difference between the Kyoto and Hokkaido control populations, but not between the two Japanese groups of patients. Significant differences were also observed in the A38G allele frequencies distribution between Dutch and Japanese subjects. These findings emphasize the need to study multiple ethnically and geographically distinct but homogeneous disease and control populations before drawing firm conclusions.

PROSTAGLANDIN–ENDOPEROXIDE SYNTHASE 2 (PTGS2)

PTGS2, also known as cyclooxygenase 2 (COX-2), is involved in the enzymatic conversion of arachidonic acid to prostanoids, which provide an essential homeostatic control in normal tissues and regulate inflammation. Hill and colleagues investigated the distribution of a G to C promoter polymorphism at position −765 in 198 patients and 166 healthy controls (Hill *et al.* 2006). Of note, the −765 variant appears to be functional, with the C allele having lower promoter activity. Carriage of the −765C allele was associated with both susceptibility to sarcoidosis and persistent pulmonary disease. The −765C association with sarcoidosis was also replicated in a smaller independent dataset. However, owing to the lack of clinical data, the association with poorer outcome could not be verified in this latter patient population.

FAS

Fas is a cell-surface receptor, which − once triggered by its cognate ligand (*Fas* ligand) − initiates a cascade of events within the cell culminating in cell apoptosis (Locksley *et al.* 2001). Available evidence suggests a critical role for apoptosis in persistence of granulomatous inflammation in sarcoidosis. Wasfi and colleagues investigated the frequency of three *Fas* promoter variants (−1377, −690, −670) and deduced haplotypes in White and African-American sarcoidosis patients and matched controls. Two associations were observed (haplotype −1377G/−690T/−670G with disease risk, and haplotype −1377G/−690C/−670A with disease protection), although only in African-Americans (Wasfi *et al.* 2008). While the race specificity of these findings is intriguing, the reported associations need to be validated in independent patient and control populations.

VASCULAR ENDOTHELIAL GROWTH FACTOR (VEGF)

Vascular endothelial growth factor − an endothelial cell-specific mitogen − is a potent mediator of vascular permeability, and promotes angiogenesis. Its biological activities are mediated through two high-affinity receptor tyrosine kinases: VEGF receptor 1 (VEGFR-1) and VEFG receptor 2 (VEGFR-2). VEGF is believed to play a major role in disease pathogenesis as suggested by an increased angiogenesis-inducing ability of activated alveolar macrophages in bronchoalveolar lavage (BAL) specimens from patients with pulmonary sarcoidosis (Meyer *et al.* 1989). In a study of 103 Japanese patients and 146 healthy controls, Morohashi and co-workers observed that the rs3025039 T-allele was significantly more common among controls, thus suggesting that carriage of this allele may protect from sarcoidosis (Morohashi *et al.* 2003). More recently, Pabst and colleagues suggested that polymorphisms within VEGF and its receptors may influence both disease predisposition and prognosis (Pabst *et al.* 2010). They studied 300 Caucasian patients and 381 matched controls and observed several genetic associations: between VEGFR-1 variants and sarcoidosis susceptibility, between VEGF variants and acute disease, and between different VEGFR-2 variants and both acute and chronic course of sarcoidosis.

While VEGF and its receptors appear plausible candidate genes in sarcoidosis predisposition and prognosis, the reported associations need to be validated in larger populations from different ethnic groups.

VITAMIN D RECEPTOR (VDR)

The active metabolite of vitamin D, 1,25-dihydroxyvitamin D3 (1,25(OH)$_2$D3), is produced at sites of sarcoidosis granulomas and plays a key role in multinucleated giant cell formation (Ohta *et al.* 1986; Sharma 1996). This hormone exerts its effects by interacting with the nuclear vitamin D receptor (VDR), encoded by a gene mapping to chromosome 12. A polymorphism in intron 8 leads to three genotypes, bb, bB and BB, with the common bb genotype being associated with reduced mRNA expression. An increased frequency of the rare B allele has been reported in Japanese sarcoidosis patients (Niimi *et al.* 1999); however, this finding has not been replicated either in a German Caucasian or in an African-American population (Guleva and Seitzer 2000; Rybicki *et al.* 2004).

ANGIOTENSIN-CONVERTING ENZYME (ACE)

Angiotensin-converting enzyme is secreted by the epithelioid cells at sites of sarcoidosis granulomatous inflammation, and serum ACE levels, commonly elevated in sarcoidosis, are thought to reflect the body granuloma load (Lieberman 1989). However, 28–47 percent of the phenotypic variation in serum ACE levels in both healthy individuals and patients is accounted for by the presence (I) or absence (D) of a 287 base-pair sequence in intron 16 of the ACE gene (Rigat *et al.* 1990; Furuya *et al.* 1996). This polymorphism has therefore been investigated extensively in sarcoidosis but association studies worldwide have produced inconsistent results. The D allele, which is associated with higher serum ACE levels, has been associated with increased sarcoidosis risk in African-Americans and in sarcoid-affected family members from a German population (Maliarik *et al.* 1998b; Schurmann *et al.* 2001b), whereas other studies in both Caucasians and Japanese have failed to reproduce the same finding (Arbustini *et al.* 1996; Tomita *et al.* 1997; McGrath *et al.* 2001b).

GENE EXPRESSION STUDIES

A recent study suggested that gene array expression profiling of transbronchial biopsies may detect a set of genes that differentiate patients with self-limiting ($n = 8$) from those with progressive-fibrotic ($n = 7$) pulmonary sarcoidosis (Lockstone *et al.* 2010). In particular, genes related to host immune activation, proliferation and defense were upregulated in the progressive-fibrotic group. Furthermore, the authors observed similarity in gene expression profiles between progressive-fibrotic pulmonary sarcoidosis and hypersensitivity pneumonitis but not idiopathic pulmonary fibrosis. The results of this study need to be confirmed in independent patient populations, and possibly expanded to other disease phenotypes. Nevertheless, gene signature profiles may help predict disease course in individual patients, thus offering impetus to refine the treatment of sarcoidosis.

CONCLUSION

The search for the sarcoidosis antigen continues, but irrespective of its nature, it seems inevitable that the development of the disease will be determined by exposure to that antigen in a genetically susceptible individual. In addition, genes that influence specific disease manifestations are likely to be largely separate from those underlying disease susceptibility. We are eventually beginning to unravel the complex mix of genes that determine that genetic susceptibility.

In sarcoidosis genetic literature, case–control association studies have often reported conflicting results due to sampling methodology (population stratification, small sample size, patient misclassification) and, probably, transethnic differences in disease mechanisms. If sarcoidosis genetics is to move forward, then new methodological approaches are needed. Analysis of homogeneous disease phenotypes, thus avoiding some of the inherent biases on *classical* case–control studies, will offer the most in this regard. Tighter phenotype definition, larger cohorts of patients as well as a familial and case–control approach are also essential in order to gain a clearer picture of the genetics of sarcoidosis in the future. Some of the genes that could potentially affect an individual's susceptibility to disease and the course of any established disease have been identified. Much work remains to be done, but a fuller understanding of the genetic basis of sarcoidosis is likely to open up new therapeutic avenues, for the treatment of both this disease and other granulomatous disorders.

REFERENCES

Agostini C, Meneghin A, Semenzato G (2002). T-lymphocytes and cytokines in sarcoidosis. *Curr Opin Pulm Med* 8: 435–40.

Alkhatib G, Combadiere C, Broder CC et al. (1996). CC CKR5: a RANTES, MIP-1alpha, MIP-1beta receptor as a fusion cofactor for macrophage-tropic HIV-1. *Science* 272: 1955–8.

Arbustini E, Grasso M, Leo G et al. (1996). Polymorphism of angiotensin-converting enzyme gene in sarcoidosis. *Am J Respir Crit Care Med* 153: 851–4.

Bellamy R, Ruwende C, Corrah T et al. (1998). Variations in the NRAMP1 gene and susceptibility to tuberculosis in West Africans. *New Engl J Med* 338: 640–4.

Berlin M, Fogdell-Hahn A, Olerup O et al. (1997). HLA-DR predicts the prognosis in Scandinavian patients with pulmonary sarcoidosis. *Am J Respir Crit Care Med* 156: 1601–5.

Charo IF, Ransohoff RM (2006). The many roles of chemokines and chemokine receptors in inflammation. *New Engl J Med* 354: 610–21.

Cooke GS, Hill AV (2001). Genetics of susceptibility to human infectious disease. *Nat Rev Genet* 2: 967–77.

Fischer A, Valentonyte R, Nebel A et al. (2008). Female-specific association of C-C chemokine receptor 5 gene polymorphisms with Löfgren's syndrome. *J Mol Med* 86: 553–61.

Fling SP, Arp B, Pious D (1994). HLA-DMA and -DMB genes are both required for MHC class II/peptide complex formation in antigen-presenting cells. *Nature* 368: 554–8.

Foley PJ, Lympany PA, Puscinska E et al. (1999). Analysis of MHC encoded antigen-processing genes TAP1 and TAP2 polymorphisms in sarcoidosis. *Am J Respir Crit Care Med* 160: 1009–14.

Foley PJ, Mullighan CG, McGrath DS et al. (2000). Mannose-binding lectin promoter and structural gene variants in sarcoidosis. *Eur J Clin Invest* 30: 549–52.

Foley PJ, McGrath DS, Puscinska E et al. (2001). Human leukocyte antigen-DRB1 position 11 residues are a common protective marker for sarcoidosis. *Am J Respir Cell Mol Biol* 25: 272–7.

Franke A, Fischer A, Nothnagel M et al. (2008). Genome-wide association analysis in sarcoidosis and Crohn's disease unravels a common susceptibility locus on 10p12.2. *Gastroenterology* 135: 12017–15.

Furuya K, Yamaguchi E, Itoh A et al. (1996). Deletion polymorphism in the angiotensin I converting enzyme (ACE) gene as a genetic risk factor for sarcoidosis. *Thorax* 51: 777–80.

Gardner J, Kennedy HG, Hamblin A, Jones E (1984). HLA associations in sarcoidosis: a study of two ethnic groups. *Thorax* 39: 19–22.

Girardin SE, Boneca IG, Viala J et al. (2003). Nod2 is a general sensor of peptidoglycan through muramyl dipeptide (MDP) detection. *J Biol Chem* 278: 8869–72.

Gray-McGuire C, Sinha R, Iyengar S et al. (2006). Genetic characterization and fine mapping of susceptibility loci for sarcoidosis in African Americans on chromosome 5. *Hum Genet* 120: 420–30.

Grunewald J (2008). Genetics of sarcoidosis. *Curr Opin Pulm Med* 14: 434–9.

Grunewald J, Eklund A (2001). Human leukocyte antigen genes may outweigh racial background when generating a specific immune response in sarcoidosis. *Eur Respir J* 17: 1046–8.

Grunewald J, Eklund A (2009). Löfgren's syndrome: human leukocyte antigen strongly influences the disease course. *Am J Respir Crit Care Med* 179: 307–12.

Grunewald J, Eklund A, Olerup O (2004). Human leukocyte antigen class I alleles and the disease course in sarcoidosis patients. *Am J Respir Crit Care Med* 169: 696–702.

Grutters JC, Sato H, Pantelidis P et al. (2002). Increased frequency of the uncommon tumor necrosis factor -857T allele in British and Dutch patients with sarcoidosis. *Am J Respir Crit Care Med* 165: 1119–24.

Grutters JC, Sato H, Welsh KI, du Bois RM (2003a). The importance of sarcoidosis genotype to lung phenotype. *Am J Respir Cell Mol Biol* 29: S59–62.

Grutters JC, Ruven HJT, Sato H et al. (2003b). MHC haplotype analysis in Dutch sarcoidosis patients presenting with Lofgren's syndrome. In: Grutters JC, (ed). *Genetic Polymorphisms and Phenotypes in Sarcoidosis*. Thesis, University Utrecht, pp. 85–96.

Grutters JC, Sato H, Pantelidis P et al. (2003c). Analysis of IL6 and IL1A gene polymorphisms in UK and Dutch patients with sarcoidosis. *Sarcoidosis Vasc Diff Lung Dis* 20: 20–7.

Guleva I, Seitzer U (2000). Vitamin D receptor gene polymorphism in patients with sarcoidosis. *Am J Respir Crit Care Med* 162: 760–1.

Guyatt GH, Bensen WG, Stolmon LP et al. (1982). HLA-B8 and erythema nodosum. *Can Med Assoc J* 127: 1005–6.

Hammer J, Bono E, Gallazzi F et al. (1994). Precise prediction of major histocompatibility complex class II-peptide interaction based on peptide side chain scanning. *J Exp. Med* 180: 2353–8.

Hedfors E, Lindstrom F (1983). HLA-B8/DR3 in sarcoidosis: correlation to acute onset disease with arthritis. *Tissue Antigens* 22: 200–3.

Heron M, Grutters JC, van Moorsel CH et al. (2009). Variation in IL7R predisposes to sarcoid inflammation. *Genes Immun* 10: 647–53.

Hill MR, Papafili A, Booth H et al. (2006). Functional prostaglandin-endoperoxide synthase 2 polymorphism predicts poor outcome in sarcoidosis. *Am J Respir Crit Care Med* 174: 915–22.

Hizawa N, Yamaguchi E, Furuya K et al. (1999). The role of the C-C chemokine receptor 2 gene polymorphism V64I (CCR2-64I) in sarcoidosis in a Japanese population. *Am J Respir Crit Care Med* **159**: 2021–3.

Ho LP, Merlin F, Gaber K *et al.* (2005). CARD 15 gene mutations in sarcoidosis. *Thorax* **60**: 354–5.

Hofmann S, Franke A, Fischer A *et al.* (2008). Genome-wide association study identifies ANXA11 as a new susceptibility locus for sarcoidosis. *Nat Genet*. **40**: 1103–6.

Hugot JP, Chamaillard M, Zouali H *et al.* (2001). Association of NOD2 leucine-rich repeat variants with susceptibility to Crohn's disease. *Nature* **411**: 599–603.

Hutyrova B, Pantelidis P, Drabek J *et al.* (2002). Interleukin-1 gene cluster polymorphisms in sarcoidosis and idiopathic pulmonary fibrosis. *Am J Respir Crit Care Med* **165**: 148–51.

Iannuzzi MC, Maliarik MJ, Poisson LM, Rybicki BA (2003). Sarcoidosis susceptibility and resistance HLA-DQB1 alleles in African Americans. *Am J Respir Crit Care Med* **167**: 1225–31.

Iannuzzi M C, Iyengar SK, Gray-McGuire C *et al.* (2005). Genome-wide search for sarcoidosis susceptibility genes in African Americans. *Genes Immun* **6**: 509–18.

Ina Y, Takada K, Yamamoto M *et al.* (1989). HLA and sarcoidosis in the Japanese. *Chest* **95**: 1257–61.

Ishihara M, Ishida T, Inoko H *et al.* (1996a). HLA serological and class II genotyping in sarcoidosis patients in Japan. *Jpn J Ophthalmol* **40**: 86–94.

Ishihara M, Inoko H, Suzuki K *et al.* (1996b). HLA class II genotyping of sarcoidosis patients in Hokkaido by PCR-RFLP. *Jpn J Ophthalmol* **40**: 540–3.

Ishihara M, Ohno S, Mizuki N *et al.* (1996c). Genetic polymorphisms of the major histocompatibility complex-encoded antigen-processing genes TAP and LMP in sarcoidosis. *Hum Immunol* **45**: 105–10.

Ishihara M, Naruse T, Ohno S *et al.* (1996d). Analysis of HLA-DM polymorphisms in sarcoidosis. *Hum Immunol* **49**: 144–6.

Janssen R, Sato H, Grutters JC *et al.* (2004). The Clara cell10 adenine38guanine polymorphism and sarcoidosis susceptibility in Dutch and Japanese subjects. *Am J Respir Crit Care Med* **170**: 1185–7.

Jorgensen CS, Levantino G, Houen G *et al.* (2000). Determination of autoantibodies to annexin XI in systemic autoimmune diseases. *Lupus* **9**: 515–20.

Kelly AP, Monaco JJ, Cho SG, Trowsdale J (1991). A new human HLA class II-related locus, DM. *Nature* **353**: 571–3.

Krause A, Goebel KM (1987). Class II MHC antigen (HLA-DR3) predisposes to sarcoid arthritis. *J Clin Lab Immunol* **24**: 25–7.

Kremer JM (1986). Histologic findings in siblings with acute sarcoid arthritis: association with the B8,DR3 phenotype. *J Rheumatol* **13**: 593–7.

Lenhart K, Kolek V, Bartova A (1990). HLA antigens associated with sarcoidosis. *Dis Markers* **8**: 23–9.

Li Y, Pabst S, Lokhande S *et al.* (2009). Extended genetic analysis of BTNL2 in sarcoidosis. *Tissue Antigens* **73**: 59–61.

Lieberman J (1989). Enzymes in sarcoidosis: angiotensin-converting enzyme (ACE). *Clin Lab Med* **9**: 745–55.

Locksley RM, Killeen N, Lenardo MJ (2001). The TNF and TNF receptor superfamilies: integrating mammalian biology. *Cell* **104**: 487–501.

Lockstone HE, Sanderson S, Kulakova N *et al.* (2010). Gene-set analysis of lung samples provides insight into pathogenesis of progressive, fibrotic pulmonary sarcoidosis, *Am J Respir Crit Care Med* [epub ahead of print].

Löfgren S, Lundback H (1952). The bilateral hilar lymphoma syndrome: a study of the relation to tuberculosis and sarcoidosis in 212 cases. *Acta Medica Scand* **142**: 265–73.

Luster AD (1998). Chemokines: chemotactic cytokines that mediate inflammation. *New Engl J Med* **338**: 436–45.

Maliarik MJ, Chen KM, Major ML *et al.* (1998a). Analysis of HLA-DPB1 polymorphisms in African-Americans with sarcoidosis. *Am J Respir Crit Care Med* **158**: 111–14.

Maliarik MJ, Rybicki BA, Malvitz E *et al.* (1998b). Angiotensin-converting enzyme gene polymorphism and risk of sarcoidosis. *Am J Respir Crit Care Med* **158**: 1566–70.

Maliarik MJ, Chen KM, Sheffer RG *et al.* (2000). The natural resistance-associated macrophage protein gene in African Americans with sarcoidosis. *Am J Respir Cell Mol Biol* **22**: 672–5.

Martenstein H (1923). Knochveranderungen bei lupus pernio. *Zentralbl Haut und Geschlechts-krankheiten sowie deren Grenzgebiete* **7**: 208.

McGrath DS, Daniil Z, Foley P *et al.* (2000). Epidemiology of familial sarcoidosis in the UK. *Thorax* **55**: 751–4.

McGrath DS, Goh N, Foley PJ, du Bois RM (2001a). Sarcoidosis: genes and microbes: soil or seed? *Sarcoidosis Vasc Diffuse Lung Dis* **18**: 149–64.

McGrath DS, Foley PJ, Petrek M *et al.* (2001b). Ace gene I/D polymorphism and sarcoidosis pulmonary disease severity. *Am J Respir Crit Care Med* **164**: 197–201.

McIntyre JA, McKee KT, Loadholt CB *et al.* (1997). Increased HLA-B7 antigen frequency in South Carolina blacks in association with sarcoidosis. *Transplant Proc* **9**: 173–6.

Meyer KC, Kaminski MJ, Calhoun WJ, Auerbach R (1989). Studies of bronchoalveolar lavage cells and fluids in pulmonary sarcoidosis: enhanced capacity of bronchoalveolar lavage cells from patients with pulmonary sarcoidosis to induce angiogenesis in vivo. *Am Rev Respir Dis* **140**: 1446–9.

Miceli-Richard C, Lesage S, Rybojad M *et al.* (2001). CARD15 mutations in Blau syndrome. *Nat Genet* **29**: 19–20.

Michael NL, Louie LG, Rohrbaugh AL *et al.* (1997). The role of CCR5 and CCR2 polymorphisms in HIV-1 transmission and disease progression. *Nat Med* **3**: 1160–2.

Milman N, Nielsen OH, Hviid TV, Fenger K (2007). CARD15 single nucleotide polymorphisms 8, 12 and 13 are not increased in ethnic Danes with sarcoidosis. *Respiration* **74**: 76–9.

Morohashi K, Takada T, Omori K *et al.* (2003). Vascular endothelial growth factor gene polymorphisms in Japanese patients with sarcoidosis. *Chest* **123**: 1520–6.

Moss S, Morgan R (2004). The annexins. *Genome Biol* **5**: 219.

Muller-Quernheim J (1998). Sarcoidosis: immunopathogenetic concepts and their clinical application. *Eur Respir J* **12**: 716–38.

Naruse TK, Matsuzawa Y, Ota M *et al.* (2000). HLA-DQB1*0601 is primarily associated with the susceptibility to cardiac sarcoidosis. *Tissue Antigens* **56**: 52–7.

Niimi T, Tomita H, Sato S *et al.* (1999). Vitamin D receptor gene polymorphism in patients with sarcoidosis. *Am J Respir Crit Care Med* **160**: 1107–9.

Nowack D, Goebel KM (1987). Genetic aspects of sarcoidosis: class II histocompatibility antigens and a family study. *Arch Intern Med* **147**: 481–3.

Ohchi T, Shijubo N, Kawabata I *et al.* (2004). Polymorphism of Clara cell 10-kD protein gene of sarcoidosis. *Am J Respir Crit Care Med* **169**: 180–6.

Ohta M, Okabe T, Ozawa K *et al.* (1986). In-vitro formation of macrophage-epithelioid cells and multinucleated giant cells by 1 alpha,25-dihydroxyvitamin D3 from human circulating monocytes. *Ann NY Acad Sci* **465**: 211–20.

Olenchock SA, Heise ER, Marx JJ *et al.* (1981). HLA-B8 in sarcoidosis. *Ann Allergy* **47**: 151–3.

Pabst S, Karpushova A, Diaz-Lacava A *et al.* (2010). VEGF gene haplotypes are associated with sarcoidosis. *Chest* **137**: 156–63.

Parra EJ, Marcini A, Akey J *et al.* (1998). Estimating African American admixture proportions by use of population-specific alleles. *Am J Hum Genet* **63**: 1839–51.

Petrek M, Drabek J, Kolek V *et al.* (2000). CC chemokine receptor gene polymorphisms in Czech patients with pulmonary sarcoidosis. *Am J Respir Crit Care Med* **162**: 1000–3.

Pietinalho A, Ohmichi M, Hirasawa M *et al.* (1999). Familial sarcoidosis in Finland and Hokkaido, Japan: a comparative study. *Respir Med* **93**: 408–12.

Richeldi L, Sorrentino R, Saltini C (1993). HLA-DPB1 glutamate 69: a genetic marker of beryllium disease. *Science* **262**: 242–4.

Rigat B, Hubert C, Alhenc-Gelas F *et al.* (1990). An insertion/deletion polymorphism in the angiotensin I-converting enzyme gene accounting for half the variance of serum enzyme levels. *J Clin Invest* **86**: 1343–6.

Rybicki BA, Maliarik MJ, Malvitz E *et al.* (1999). The influence of T cell receptor and cytokine genes on sarcoidosis susceptibility in African Americans. *Hum Immunol* **60**: 867–74.

Rybicki BA, Kirkey KL, Major M *et al.* (2001). Familial risk ratio of sarcoidosis in African-American sibs and parents. *Am J Epidemiol* **153**: 188–93.

Rybicki BA, Maliarik MJ, Poisson LM *et al.* (2003). The major histocompatibility complex gene region and sarcoidosis susceptibility in African Americans. *Am J Respir Crit Care Med* **167**: 444–9.

Rybicki BA, Maliarik MJ, Poisson LM, Iannuzzi MC (2004). Sarcoidosis and granuloma genes: a family-based study in African-Americans. *Eur Respir J* **24**: 251–7.

Rybicki BA, Walewski JL, Maliarik MJ *et al.* (2005). The BTNL2 gene and sarcoidosis susceptibility in African Americans and Whites. *Am J Hum Genet* **77**: 491–9.

Rybicki BA, Sinha R, Iyengar S *et al.* (2007). Genetic linkage analysis of sarcoidosis phenotypes: the Sarcoidosis Genetic Analysis (SAGA) study. *Genes Immun* **8**: 379–86.

Samson M, Libert F, Doranz BJ *et al.* (1996). Resistance to HIV-1 infection in caucasian individuals bearing mutant alleles of the CCR-5 chemokine receptor gene. *Nature* **382**: 722–5.

Sato H, Grutters JC, Pantelidis P *et al.* (2002). HLA-DQB1*0201: a marker for good prognosis in British and Dutch patients with sarcoidosis. *Am J Respir Cell Mol Biol* **27**: 406–12.

Sato H, Williams HR, Spagnolo P *et al.* (2010). CARD15/NOD2 polymorphisms are associated with severe pulmonary sarcoidosis. *Eur Respir J* **35**: 324–30.

Schurmann M, Lympany PA, Reichel P *et al.* (2000). Familial sarcoidosis is linked to the major histocompatibility complex region. *Am J Respir Crit Care Med* **162**: 861–4.

Schurmann M, Reichel P, Muller-Myhsok B *et al.* (2001a). Results from a genome-wide search for predisposing genes in sarcoidosis. *Am J Respir Crit Care Med* **164**: 840–6.

Schurmann M, Reichel P, Muller-Myhsok B *et al.* (2001b). Angiotensin-converting enzyme (ACE) gene polymorphisms and familial occurrence of sarcoidosis. *J Intern Med* **249**: 77–83.

Schurmann M, Valentonyte R, Hampe J *et al.* (2003). CARD15 gene mutations in sarcoidosis. *Eur Respir J* **22**: 748–54.

Seitzer U, Swider C, Stuber F *et al.* (1997). Tumour necrosis factor alpha promoter gene polymorphism in sarcoidosis. *Cytokine* **9**: 787–90.

Sharma OP (1996). Vitamin D, calcium, and sarcoidosis. *Chest* **109**: 535–9.

Smith MJ, Turton CW, Mitchell DN *et al.* (1981). Association of HLA B8 with spontaneous resolution in sarcoidosis. *Thorax* **36**: 296–8.

Smith MW, Carrington M, Winkler C *et al.* (1997). CCR2 chemokine receptor and AIDS progression. *Nat Med* **3**: 1052–3.

Spagnolo P, Renzoni EA, Wells AU *et al.* (2003). C-C chemokine receptor 2 and sarcoidosis: association with Lofgren's syndrome. *Am J Respir Crit Care Med* **168**: 1162–6.

Spagnolo P, Renzoni EA, Wells AU *et al.* (2005). C-C chemokine receptor 5 gene variants in relation to lung disease in sarcoidosis. *Am J Respir Crit Care Med* **172**: 721–8.

Spagnolo P, Sato H, Grutters JC *et al.* (2007). Analysis of BTNL2 genetic polymorphisms in British and Dutch patients with sarcoidosis. *Tissue Antigens* **70**: 219–27.

Spagnolo P, Sato H, Grunewald J *et al.* (2008). A common haplotype of the C-C chemokine receptor 2 gene and HLA-DRB1*0301 are independent genetic risk factors for Löfgren's syndrome. *J Intern Med* **264**: 433–41.

Stammers M, Rowen L, Rhodes D *et al.* (2000). BTL-II: a polymorphic locus with homology to the butyrophilin gene family, located at the border of the major histocompatibility complex class II and class III regions in human and mouse. *Immunogenetics* **51**: 373–82.

Sturniolo T, Bono E, Ding J *et al.* (1999). Generation of tissue-specific and promiscuous HLA ligand databases using DNA microarrays and virtual HLA class II matrices. *Nat Biotechnol* **17**: 555–61.

Swider C, Schnittger L, Bogunia-Kubik K *et al.* (1999). TNF-alpha and HLA-DR genotyping as potential prognostic markers in pulmonary sarcoidosis. *Eur Cytokine Netw* **10**: 143–6.

Takashige N, Naruse TK, Matsumori A *et al.* (1999). Genetic polymorphisms at the tumour necrosis factor loci (TNFA and TNFB) in cardiac sarcoidosis. *Tissue Antigens* **54**: 191–3.

Thompson CL, Rybicki BA, Iannuzzi MC *et al.* (2006). Reduction of sample heterogeneity through use of population substructure: an example from a population of African American families with sarcoidosis. *Am J Hum Genet* **79**: 606–13.

Tomita H, Ina Y, Sugiura Y *et al.* (1997). Polymorphism in the angiotensin-converting enzyme (ACE) gene and sarcoidosis. *Am J Respir Crit Care Med* **156**: 255–9.

Valentonyte R, Hampe J, Huse K *et al.* (2005a). Sarcoidosis is associated with a truncating splice site mutation in BTNL2. *Nat Genet* **37**: 357–64.

Valentonyte R, Hampe J, Croucher PJ *et al.* (2005b). Study of C-C chemokine receptor 2 alleles in sarcoidosis, with emphasis on family-based analysis. *Am J Respir Crit Care Med* **171**: 1136–41.

Voorter CE, Drent M, van den Berg-Loonen EM (2005). Severe pulmonary sarcoidosis is strongly associated with the haplotype HLA-DQB1*0602-DRB1*150101. *Hum Immunol* **66**: 826–35.

Wasfi YS, Silveira LJ, Jonth A *et al.* (2008). Fas promoter polymorphisms: genetic predisposition to sarcoidosis in African-Americans. *Tissue Antigens* **72**: 39–48.

PART **III**

INVESTIGATIONS

8

Radiology of the lungs and pleura

ANTHONY J EDEY AND DAVID M HANSELL

IMAGING TECHNIQUES

Chest radiography

The posterior–anterior chest radiograph remains central to the imaging and follow-up of patients with sarcoidosis. While conventional projection radiography is the oldest of all medical imaging tests, the technology for image acquisition has been transformed over the last two decades. Traditional film/screen systems for image acquisition provided images with very high spatial resolution but were limited by a narrow exposure range. A further problem with film as a means of image storage was that it was physically cumbersome and suffered from image degradation with time. The development of stimulable phosphor plate radiography and, more recently, flat-panel detector technology has overcome these problems. Despite a slight quantitative reduction in the spatial resolution of the images, these newer techniques have maintained or improved the diagnostic quality of images (Volk et al. 2004). In fact, the linear photoluminensce-dose response of these 'filmless' systems has led to a significant improvement in the visualization of previously hidden areas (e.g. behind the mediastinum on a frontal radiograph), as well as reducing the number of repeat radiographs required due to under- or over-exposure. Significantly, the ionizing radiation dose to the patient is substantially lower with flat-panel detector digital radiography: when compared with other techniques the effective dose is about 50 percent that of film/screen systems and 75 percent that of phosphor plate systems, resulting in minimal radiation exposure (Bacher et al. 2003). Finally, the development of patient archiving and communication systems (PACS) has meant that these digital images can be stored and reviewed from multiple locations within the hospital or remotely.

Computed tomography

Computed tomography (CT) of the thorax is a highly sensitive technique for elucidating subtle parenchymal abnormalities not visible on the chest radiograph, and is better able to detect otherwise hidden mediastinal lymph node enlargement (Leung et al. 1991; Grenier et al. 1994). Optimal parenchymal imaging is achieved with high-resolution reconstruction algorithms and narrow collimation (typically 1–1.5 mm slice thickness) (Leung et al. 1991; Lee et al. 1994).

High-resolution images may be acquired in one of two ways: either as part of a volumetric study or alternatively as interspaced images separated by 10–20 mm using a 'step-and-shoot' technique. Volumetric acquisition provides high-resolution images of the entire thorax and, with modern multidetector CT scanners, a complete set (up to 350 images) may be obtained in under a second. In the breathless patient, the speed of the examination is valuable as it minimizes respiratory motion artifacts.

A further advantage of volumetric datasets is that they are amenable to post-processing techniques such as maximum intensity projection (MIP) reformats, which increase the detection of small nodules and may increase confidence in interpretation (Remy-Jardin et al. 1996; Beigelman-Aubry et al. 2005). While interspaced images take longer to acquire, and are usually acquired over several breath holds, their major advantage is the significant reduction in ionizing radiation. A typical volumetric CT of the chest entails an effective dose of up to 8 mSv (Leswick *et al.* 2005) (compared to 3 mSv background radiation the average UK resident receives annually), whereas an interspaced HRCT produces a dose of around 1 mSv. Further reductions in dose can be achieved, without comprising diagnostic quality, by using lower than normal CT tube currents (Lee *et al.* 1994).

INDICATIONS FOR CT IMAGING

It is difficult to incorporate CT into a simple diagnostic algorithm that covers all eventualities. However, there are a number of situations in which CT undoubtedly plays an important role in the diagnosis of sarcoidosis (Mana *et al.* 1995).

First, in patients with atypical clinical or radiographic findings, CT often increases the diagnostic likelihood of sarcoidosis by detecting pathognomonic features not visible on the radiograph. Second, for patients with a normal chest radiograph but clinical features of the disease, the superior sensitivity of CT for the detection of parenchymal disease is useful for assessing thoracic involvement. Detection of occult thoracic involvement is particularly valuable when assessing patients with suspected sarcoidosis in another organ which may be difficult or high risk to biopsy (e.g. the central nervous system) as it helps to support the diagnosis without the need for biopsy.

Routine radiological follow-up of pulmonary sarcoidosis is almost invariably by chest radiography. Radiography allows monitoring of parenchymal and nodal disease, as well as the detection of supervening fibrosis with minimal exposure of the patient to radiation. After the diagnosis has been made, CT offers no particular advantage to radiographs in monitoring uncomplicated cases. However, unexpected or unexplained changes in symptomatology may prompt referral for CT to detect possible complications of sarcoidosis, including mycetoma formation, vascular involvement or bronchial stenosis.

CT is a routine part of the pre-transplant evaluation of a patient with end-stage pulmonary sarcoidosis and facilitates surgical planning. For example, demonstration of bronchiectasis is an indication for a double lung transplant because of the increased risk of microbial colonization which could put a single allograft at risk of cross- contamination from the native lung (Shah 2007). An additional advantage is the identification of mycetomas, which are associated with worsened post-transplant outcome (Hadjiliadis *et al.* 2002) and are therefore a relative contraindication to surgery (Shah 2007). However, data supporting the validity of pre-transplantation CT are lacking and pre-transplant imaging can be misleading with a significant (5 percent) false positive rate for the detection of early mycetomas (Marom *et al.* 1999). Despite this, CT is still undertaken in this group of patients.

MORPHOLOGICAL STAGES OF SARCOIDOSIS

While a number of radiographic staging systems for sarcoidosis have been reported, the most widely cited is that

developed by Scadding in 1961 and modified by DeRemee in 1983. This radiographic classification is simply a means of categorizing cases by appearance and applies to postero-anterior chest radiographs (and not CT findings). Stage 0 disease denotes a normal chest radiograph, stage I disease shows bilateral hilar lymphadenopathy with or without mediastinal nodal enlargement (Fig. 8.1), stage II disease describes bilateral hilar lymphadenopathy associated with parenchymal shadowing (Fig. 8.2), stage III disease is

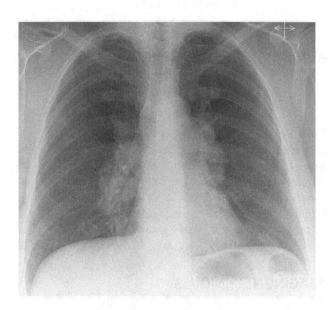

Figure 8.1   Stage I sarcoidosis: symmetrical bilateral hilar and bronchopulmonary lymphadenopathy causing well-defined lobulated contours of the hila.

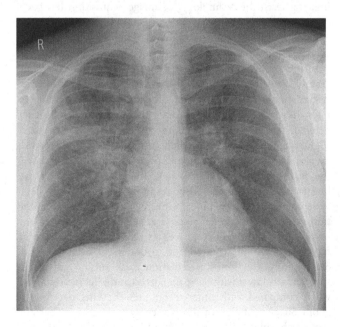

Figure 8.2   Stage II sarcoidosis: extensive perihilar parenchymal involvement with a conglomerate mass of nodules adjacent to the right hilum, with bihilar lymphadenopathy.

parenchymal involvement with no evidence of lymph node enlargement (Fig. 8.3), while stage IV disease is parenchymal infiltration with definite fibrosis (Fig. 8.4).

Stage at presentation varies widely according to geographic location and ethnicity (Siltzbach *et al.* 1974). However, an overall trend emerges from published data. Stage I is the most common at clinical presentation (about half of all cases), followed by stage II (about 25 percent), while stages 0, III and IV account for the remainder (about 10, 10 and 5 percent, respectively) (Siltzbach *et al.* 1974; Hillerdal *et al.* 1984). Older patients appear to be less likely to be stage I at diagnosis (Hillerdal *et al.* 1984).

These radiographic groups are referred to as stages, but it should be emphasized that they do not indicate a continuum

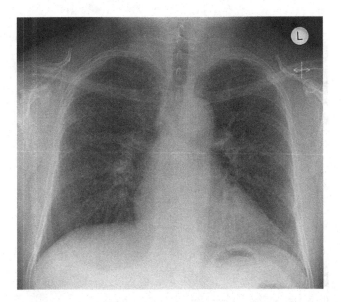

Figure 8.3   Stage III sarcoidosis: parenchymal involvement (in this case a miliary nodular pattern), with no obvious lymphadenopathy.

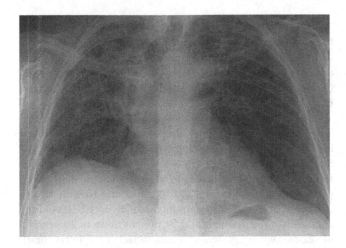

Figure 8.4   Stage IV sarcoidosis: architectural distortion and volume loss in the upper lobes with elevation of the hila and coarse reticulation indicative of fibrosis.

of disease inevitably progressing from one stage to the next but are descriptive categories. Imaging findings cannot be used in isolation as a guide to prognosis; the clinical presentation, age and ethnicity of the patient, among other factors, all have a bearing on long-term outcome (Nagai *et al.* 1999). For example, resolution of radiographic (and clinical) signs is most common in patients who present with acute symptoms such as erythema nodosum or polyarthropathy (Scadding 1961).

However, numerous observational trials have demonstrated a relationship between the radiographic staging of sarcoidosis and prognosis (Scadding 1961; Kirks *et al.* 1973; Siltzbach *et al.* 1974; Hillerdal *et al.* 1984; Joint Statement of ATS 1999). The likelihood of spontaneous remission reduces with increasing stage. Smellie and Hoyle analyzed the natural history of stage I disease in 66 patients (Smellie and Hoyle 1957): in two-thirds of patients presenting with stage I, bihilar lymphadenopathy either resolved spontaneously or remained unchanged over time. Where nodal disease resolved spontaneously, regression was typically rapid and occurred within 6 months of presentation. The remaining patients developed parenchymal opacities (i.e. progressed to stage II disease) (Smellie and Hoyle 1957).

Chronic lymph node enlargement can potentially cause errors of interpretation for patients who subsequently develop a malignancy and may mislead unwary observers to upstage disease. In this context, review of old images is crucial for establishing longstanding nodal enlargement. Patients presenting with stage II disease show spontaneous radiographic and clinical resolution in up to 70 percent of cases (Hillerdal *et al.* 1984). In those patients who do not show resolution, the majority develop fibrosis of varying extents; with approximately 10 percent evolving to stage III, and similar proportions remaining static or regressing to stage I (Scadding 1961). In contrast, patients with stage III disease at presentation show resolution in about 40 percent of cases (Hillerdal *et al.* 1984). In those patients with persistent radiographic changes the vast majority showed evidence of fibrosis (Scadding 1961).

In summary, radiographic staging of sarcoidosis reflects broad prognostic trends. Spontaneous remission occurs in 53–87 percent of patients with stage I disease; in 24–74 percent of patients with stage II disease; in 10–27 percent of patients with stage III disease; and in no patients with stage IV disease (Siltzbach *et al.* 1974).

IMAGING FEATURES OF SARCOIDOSIS

Lymph node enlargement

Thoracic lymph node enlargement is a common, but not invariable, feature of sarcoidosis and is evident on chest radiography at presentation in up to 90 percent of cases (Sider and Horton 1990). Two patterns of distribution are considered typical of sarcoidosis: symmetrical hilar lymphadenopathy and bilateral hilar lymphadenopathy with paratracheal nodal enlargement (the latter is eponymously named Garland's triad (Garland 1947)) (Figs 8.5 and 8.6).

The presence of hilar lymphadenopathy is indicated radiographically by an abnormal, well-demarcated, lobulated hilar contour. Typically, both the tracheobronchial and more distal bronchopulmonary lymph nodes are involved (Smellie and Hoyle 1957), and occasionally the nodal enlargement may be mistaken for dilatation of the pulmonary arteries. The degree of nodal enlargement in sarcoidosis ranges from minimal (just over 1 cm in diameter on CT) to massive. Regardless of size, it is rare for enlarged nodes to cause compression of the adjacent structures in early sarcoidosis as they have an essentially granulomatous and compliant content. However, as nodes become fibrotic or calcified they may occasionally result in local compressive effects. In the literature there are case reports of extrinsic compression of the major pulmonary arteries (Damuth *et al.* 1980), the superior vena cava (Brandstetter *et al.* 1981a) and the main airways (Talbot *et al.* 1959).

In sarcoidosis, hilar lymphadenopathy tends to be symmetrical; asymmetrical nodal enlargement broadens the differential diagnosis to include tuberculosis and lymphoma. However, asymmetrical hilar involvement is relatively common; in one CT series it was reported in just under 50 percent of biopsy-proven cases of sarcoidosis (Sider and Horton 1990). True unilateral involvement is less common and is probably present in 1–5 percent of cases (Rockoff and Rohatgi 1985). There is general consensus that, when asymmetry is present, the right-sided nodes tend to be larger than those on the left (Sider and Horton 1990; Gawne-Cain and Hansell 1996; Patil and Levin 1999). Asymmetrical, or

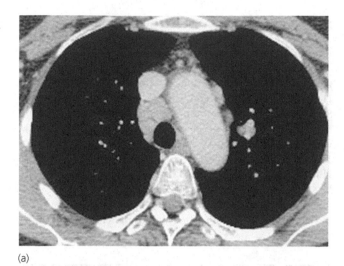

(a)

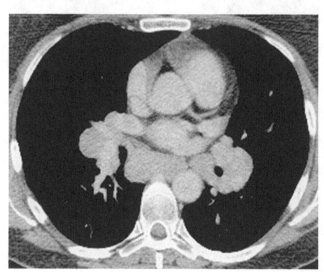

(b)

Figure 8.6   CT through the mediastinum, illustrating (a) non-calcified enlarged right paratracheal, and (b) subcarinal and symmetrical bihilar lymph node enlargement. Note that despite the large volume of the nodes there is no significant compression of the airways or other mediastinal structures.

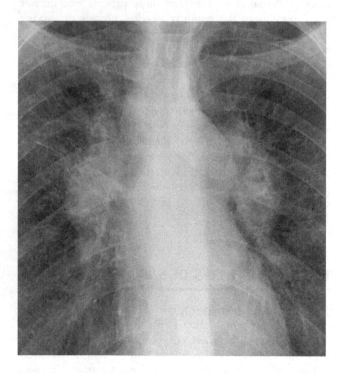

Figure 8.5   Garland's triad: right paratracheal and symmetrical bihilar lymphadenopathy, characteristic of sarcoidosis in the correct clinical context. In addition, gross subcarinal nodal enlargement (a relatively common site of nodal enlargement in sarcoidosis) is visible as increased retrocardiac opacification and obscuration of the superior aspect of the azygo-esophageal line.

truly unilateral, hilar lymphadenopathy appears to be more common at presentation in patients over the age of 50 years and may become symmetrical as the disease progresses (Rabinowitz *et al.* 1974; Rockoff and Rohatgi 1985; Conant *et al.* 1988).

While the combination of bihilar and paratracheal lymphadenopathy accounts for over 80 percent of cases identified on chest radiography, it is clear from CT studies that lymph node involvement is usually not confined to these regions. Additional involvement of the middle mediastinum, particularly the pretracheal region (Sider and Horton 1990), is almost universal. Anterior mediastinal nodal (including paracardiac) involvement may be present in up to 20 percent of cases, while posterior mediastinal (e.g. retrocrural) involvement is much less common. However, the benefit conferred by CT of enhanced detection of lymph nodes outside the classic distribution is debatable; in the absence of bihilar lymphadenopathy detection of mediastinal lymph node enlargement on either CT or chest radiography should raise doubts about the diagnosis of sarcoidosis. An advantage of CT scanning over radiography is the detection of peripheral lymph nodes (e.g. axillary and supraclavicular nodes) which are present in up to one-third of cases of sarcoidosis (Joint Statement of ATS 1999). Detection of peripheral lymphadenopathy may provide an alternative site to the mediastinum for diagnostic sampling. This is obviously advantageous, especially as it is reported to have equal diagnostic sensitivity to mediastinal nodal sampling (Yanardag *et al.* 2007).

Calcification of lymph nodes is detectable on CT in around 40 percent of sarcoidosis cases and the extent of calcification seems to be related to the duration of disease (Murdoch and Müller 1992; Gawne-Cain and Hansell 1996). However, calcification is also common in other granulomatous disease such as tuberculosis. Two features help to discriminate between sarcoidosis and tuberculous lymph nodes (Gawne-Cain and Hansell 1996). First, sarcoidosis tends to produce focal, central calcification which is delicate in appearance and has been likened to sprinkled icing-sugar (Fig. 8.7), as opposed to tuberculosis which more commonly produces diffuse calcification (Gawne-Cain and Hansell 1996; Müller and Silva 2008).

Second, predictably for a systemic disease, calcified nodes in sarcoidosis tend to be bilateral whereas in TB they are more often unilateral, following the path of lymphatic drainage. Finally, eggshell calcification has been reported to occur in sarcoidosis but is relatively uncommon (McLoud *et al.* 1974) (Plate 10).

In summary, symmetrical bihilar, paratracheal and subcarinal lymph node enlargement (readily seen on CT) which often shows central calcification is typical of stage I and II in sarcoidosis. Lymph node features which reduce the likelihood of sarcoidosis and increase likelihood of malignancy are marked nodal asymmetry, isolated mediastinal nodal enlargement (without hilar nodes), and recurrence of lymphadenopathy following complete radiological remission (Baughman 2007).

Parenchymal nodules

Nodules may be smooth or have an irregular contour and range in size from 1 to 20 mm in diameter. Micronodules (measuring less than 3 mm) are the most prevalent; nodules measuring more than 10 mm are described variously as airspace, large nodular, alveolar or pseudoalveolar (Brauner *et al.* 1989).

MICRONODULES

Parenchymal nodularity identified on chest radiography is often part of a mixed pattern of opacities. In a review of 150 radiographs (Kirks *et al.* 1973), most patients had more than one pattern of involvement; these comprised pure nodular, mixed reticulonodular densities, or pure reticulation. A reticulonodular pattern is the most common (Kirks *et al.* 1973; Müller *et al.* 1989b) and is likely to be the result of the superimposition of nodules on thickened interlobular septa or intralobular opacities (Müller and Silva 2008). Nodules tend to be small, ranging from 1 to 5 mm in diameter (Talbot *et al.* 1959), and are most profuse in the mid and upper zones (Müller *et al.* 1989b). Small nodular, parenchymal opacities are an almost universal finding on CT in patients with pulmonary sarcoidosis, and may be found at any radiographic stage of the disease. Nodules are identifiable in 80–100 percent of cases on HRCT (Brauner *et al.* 1989; Müller *et al.* 1989a; Grenier *et al.* 1994; Abehsera *et al.* 2000; Akira *et al.* 2005) but are least common in the presence of established fibrosis (Brauner *et al.* 1989). The relative scarcity of nodules in the context of established fibrosis is unsurprising as their histopathologic correlate is of aggregates of granulomas and as such they often represent reversible disease (Nishimura *et al.* 1995).

While it is not infrequent for nodules to be an isolated finding, they are most commonly seen in the context of other manifestations of sarcoidosis. Thus, in a review of 44 patients by Brauner, nodules were the only sign of disease in around 40 percent of cases but were identified in conjunction with other evidence of disease in 60 percent of cases (Brauner *et al.* 1989). Micronodules tend to lie in a perilymphatic distribution (Nishimura *et al.* 1995). Therefore, they are most prolific around the peribronchovascular bundles, the subpleural region (and by extension the fissures) and along the interlobular septa (Fig. 8.8). This distribution of nodules results in the characteristic signs visible on CT of 'beading' of the fissures and nodularity of the bronchovascular bundle (Brauner *et al.* 1989; Miller *et al.* 1995; Abehsera *et al.* 2000) (Fig. 8.9). Typically, this nodular infiltration of the lymphatics is symmetrical and has a predisposition for the mid and upper zones (Brauner *et al.* 1989). Notably, thickening of the bronchovascular bundles radiates peripherally from the hilar

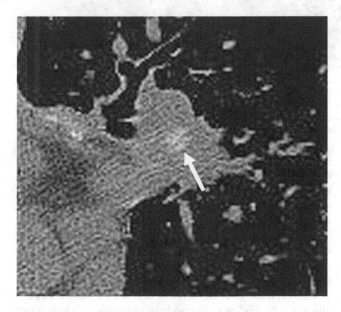

Figure 8.7   'Icing-sugar' calcification of hilar lymph nodes typical of sarcoidosis. This is a magnified prone CT section at the left hilum adjacent to the apical segmental bronchus of the left lower lobe.

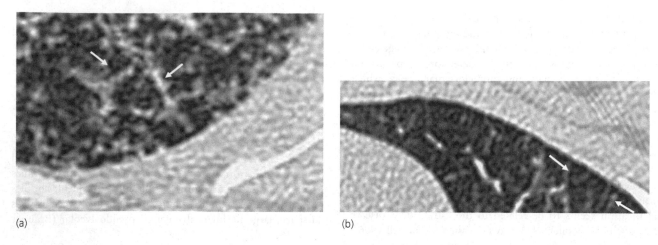

(a)   (b)

Figure 8.8   Interlobular septa are the lymphatic drainage pathway of the pulmonary lobules and are commonly thickened in sarcoidosis. Thickening may be (a) nodular or (b) smooth.

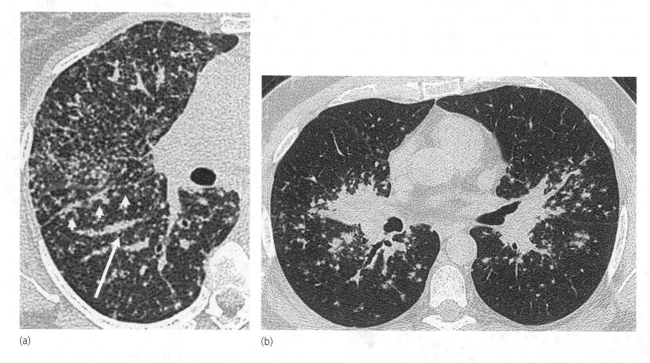

(a)   (b)

Figure 8.9   Micronodular sarcoidosis on HRCT. A perilymphatic distribution of granulomas typical of sarcoidosis, resulting in (a) 'beading' of the fissures (arrowheads), nodularity of the bronchovascular bundles (arrow), and (b) a predilection for the perihilar regions with, in this example, development of conglomerate hilar masses.

regions, a distribution that is often diagnostically useful (Nishino *et al.* 2009). Rows of micronodules on the visceral pleura of the lung may result in visible 'pseudoplaques' (Remy-Jardin *et al.* 1990; Bottaro *et al.* 2004; Hansell *et al.* 2008).

AIRSPACE OR LARGE NODULAR OPACITIES

Larger nodules measuring over 10 mm are a less common finding than micronodules. The terms nodular (Sharma *et al.* 1973), acinar (Kirks *et al.* 1973), alveolar (Rabinowitz *et al.* 1974) and pseudoalveolar sarcoidosis have been used inter-

changeably to describe these larger parenchymal nodules. On a chest radiograph, the nodule margins are usually poorly defined, hazy or fluffy and are commonly bilateral (Sharma *et al.* 1973). A nodular pattern of parenchymal involvement has been reported on CT in 15–27 percent of cases (Bergin *et al.* 1989; Nakatsu *et al.* 2002; Akira *et al.* 2005), but some reports suggest that the prevalence is higher in Afro-Caribbean patients (Malaisamy *et al.* 2009).

On CT, these opacities tend to have an irregular contour, obscure the visibility of the underlying vessels and may have visible air bronchograms (which may also be radiographically evident) – hence the term alveolar or pseudoalveolar opacities. The histopathological correlate of these large

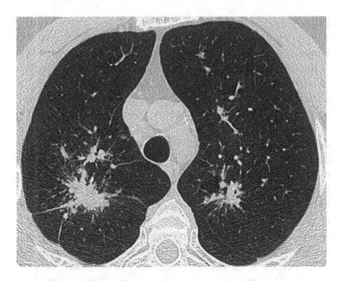

Figure 8.10 Air-space or large nodular sarcoidosis. Focal conglomerates of nodules result in an appearance of localized consolidation with an irregular border with micronodules in the immediate vicinity (the galaxy sign).

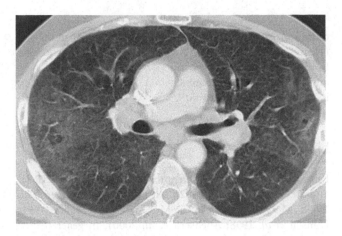

Figure 8.11 Ground-glass opacification as a feature of sarcoidosis is usually accompanied by other CT signs, including lymphadenopathy. In this case the ground glass has a subtle texture but no tractional airway dilatation to indicate fibrosis. Nevertheless, ground-glass opacification may be due to fine fibrosis or micronodular infiltration of the interstitium.

nodules is innumerable coalescent granulomatous foci which are more concentrated in the center of the lesion (Nishimura *et al.* 1993, 1995). Infiltration of the airspaces by a dense granulomatous infiltrate results in visible air bronchograms and histopathological analysis has demonstrated fibrosis and microscopic honeycombing surrounding these dilated airways (Nishimura *et al.* 1993). Careful inspection of these opacities on CT shows them to be composed of a conglomeration of much smaller nodules and, at their periphery, individual nodules can be resolved with distinct margins (Fig. 8.11). This CT appearance has been coined the 'sarcoid galaxy'. In a study by Nakatsu these features were identified in all patients (16 of 59) with nodules measuring over 10 mm (Nakatsu *et al.* 2002).

As with micronodules, large nodules tended to have a peribronchovascular distribution and favor the mid and upper zones. In a very small minority, large nodules may cavitate (Nakatsu *et al.* 2002). In the absence of infection, this rare feature is believed to be the result of ischemic necrosis of the granulomatous core (Rohatgi and Schwab 1980).

Ground-glass opacification

Ground-glass opacification describes areas of increased parenchymal density in which vessels and airways are visible on a non-contrast CT. It is a rare radiographic manifestation of sarcoidosis.

In a review of 1600 patients with sarcoidosis, only 10 patients (0.6 percent) were identified with diffuse ground-glass opacification and all of them had typical mediastinal and hilar lymph node enlargement (Tazi *et al.* 1994). Interestingly, this sign was most prevalent in Caucasian smokers. Rabinowitz and colleagues coined the phrase 'hilar haze' to describe the loss of clarity to the hilar regions due to regional ground-glass opacification (Rabinowitz *et al.* 1974). The hilar haze is most

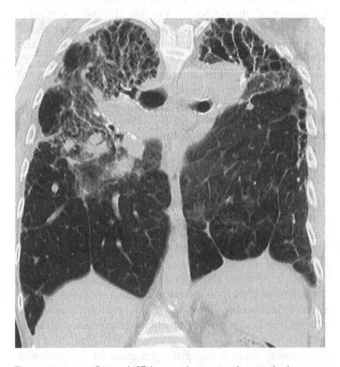

Figure 8.12 Coronal CT image demonstrating marked upper-lobe volume loss causing elevation of the hila and juxtaphrenic peaks. There is severe tractional dilatation of the upper-lobe airways indicating fibrosis.

evident when hilar nodes regress and may persist after the nodal enlargement has resolved (Rabinowitz *et al.* 1974).

CT is more sensitive for the detection of ground-glass opacification and has been reported in 16–83 percent of patients with sarcoidosis (Brauner *et al.* 1989; Murdoch and Müller 1992; Hansell *et al.* 1998; Abehsera *et al.* 2000; Lynch 2003). However, it is unusual for it to be the sole CT manifestation of sarcoidosis (Hansell *et al.* 2005). When present, ground-glass opacification tends to be multifocal (Hansell 2005) (Fig. 8.12).

The histopathological correlates of ground-glass opacification are microscopic granulomatous inflammation (Remy-Jardin *et al.* 1993; Nishimura *et al.* 1995) and fine fibrosis (Remy-Jardin *et al.* 1993), both of which displace air and, thus, increase the parenchymal density, in turn resulting in ground-glass opacification.

Linear opacities

Linear opacities may be a feature of sarcoidosis on HRCT and are identifiable in 24–82 percent of cases (Brauner *et al.* 1989; Müller *et al.* 1989a; Murdoch and Müller 1992; Hansell *et al.* 1998; Abehsera *et al.* 2000). In general, they are a less frequent finding than nodules (Lynch 2003). Reticular opacities may be due either to thickening of the interlobular septa (visible as thin linear structures conforming to the outline of the pulmonary lobule) (Remy-Jardin *et al.* 1994) or subpleural lines (thin curvilinear opacities 1 cm from the pleural surface and paralleling the pleura) (Abehsera *et al.* 2000). The term 'non-septal lines' is used to categorize other lines of variable thickness without a precise anatomical distribution and includes peripheral hilar lines and other translobular lines (Murdoch and Müller 1992; Remy-Jardin *et al.* 1994; Abehsera *et al.* 2000). Thickening of the interlobular septa is more frequent than thickening of non-septal lines (present in 89 percent and 72 percent of cases, respectively, in a cohort of 18 subjects – Murdoch and Müller (1992)) – and can be a useful sign as its presence may increase confidence in a diagnosis of sarcoidosis.

Small airways involvement

Air-trapping on expiratory CT, as a feature of sarcoidosis, was first reported by Gleeson *et al.* (1996), and is present in nearly all cases of sarcoidosis regardless of radiographic staging (Hansell *et al.* 1998; Davies *et al.* 2000; Magkanas *et al.* 2001; Terasaki *et al.* 2005). Air-trapping, as a manifestation of small airways dysfunction, is seen on CT as a mosaic attenuation pattern that becomes more apparent on expiration (Hansell 2001).

However, there is some disagreement, in the particular context of sarcoidosis, as to the functional significance of small airways disease (Gleeson *et al.* 1996; Hansell *et al.* 1998; Magkanas *et al.* 2001). For example, the extent of air-trapping does not correlate well with evidence of obstruction (Terasaki *et al.* 2005) (see section on stucture–function studies). Nevertheless, it is clear that bronchial walls are infiltrated by granulomas (and, thus, bronchial and transbronchial biopsies have a high diagnostic yield) and it seems plausible that this leads to small airways obstruction.

While the presence of air-trapping is a useful ancillary sign of sarcoidosis, in isolation its significance is harder to interpret as it may be present in apparently healthy subjects and involve up to 25 percent of the lung area on CT (Dalal and Hansell 2006).

Fibrosis

Fibrosis, reflecting irreversible damage to the lung, is the sequel to inflammatory sarcoidosis in 20–25 percent of cases (Abehsera *et al.* 2000) (Fig. 8.13). Radiographically, fibrosis is demonstrated by the presence of persistent linear opacities, typically in the mid and upper zones, associated with signs of upper lobe volume loss and architectural distortion (elevation of the hilar structures, the presence of phrenic peaks and distortion of the fissures) (Kirks *et al.* 1973). The extent of radiographically detectable changes ranges from limited linear scarring to conglomerate densities in the upper lobes, resembling progressive massive fibrosis at its extreme (Kirks *et al.* 1973). Fibrocystic disease is relatively common and results in upper zone emphysematous bullae or thick-walled cavities associated with upper-lobe volume loss and is often accompanied by increased transradiancy in the lower zones as a result of hyperinflation of the spared lung (Rabinowitz *et al.* 1974; Hansell 2005).

Architectural distortion is characteristic of fibrosis on CT and results in fissural distortion with loss of regularity and deformation of the interlobular septa. The bronchocentric nature of granulomatous infiltration in sarcoidosis means that the large airways may also be distorted, causing angulation or crossing of bronchi and deformation of the bronchial lumen, as well as tractional dilatation. The predilection for fibrosis to affect the upper zones results in striking retraction of the bronchi and main pulmonary arteries. Abehsera and co-workers reviewed the CT findings in 80 patients with stage IV sarcoidosis and noted three distinctive patterns of fibrosis: 47 percent had prominent bronchial distortion which was mainly central (Fig. 8.14); 29 percent had honeycombing which was predominantly peripheral and in the upper zones (Fig. 8.15); and 24 percent had a linear pattern (Abehsera *et al.* 2000). Interestingly, in the same study these patterns of fibrosis showed some correlation with the duration of the disease process with bronchial distortion seen after approximately 14 years of the disease, as

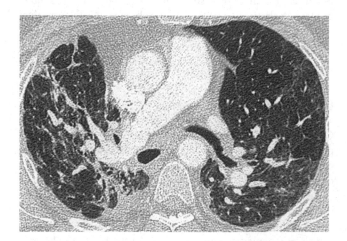

Figure 8.13   Contrast-enhanced axial CT image showing upper-zone fibrosis causing marked posterior retraction and distortion of the main pulmonary arteries and bronchi.

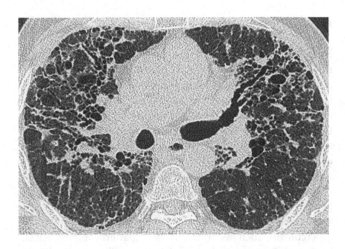

Figure 8.14   HRCT image through the upper lobes showing honeycombing. Honeycombing may be seen in fibrotic sarcoidosis in up to a third of cases.

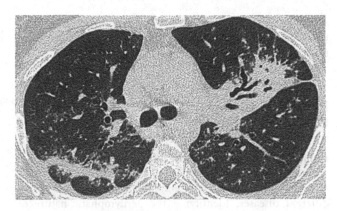

Figure 8.16   Conglomerate fibrotic opacities in a perihilar distribution may mimic progressive massive fibrosis (more usually seen in the setting of pneumoconiosis). In this image there is evidence of tractional airway dilatation in the left perihilar opacity. The accompanying micronodular opacities are typical of sarcoidosis.

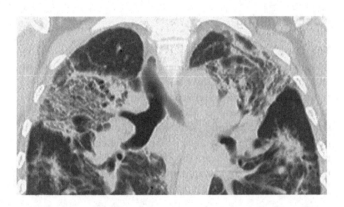

Figure 8.15   Detail from a coronal CT, showing fibrosis with reticular and linear opacities. Note the perihilar predilection of fibrosis and its tendency to 'stream' off the hila.

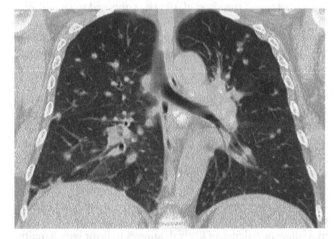

Figure 8.17   Sarcoidosis mimicking metastatic malignancy. Multifocal nodular opacities (between 5 and 10 mm) with some CT features similar to those described in air-space sarcoidosis.

opposed to honeycombing or linear opacities (10 and 9 years, respectively). In cases in which linear opacities predominate, the opacities tend to 'stream' off the hilar structures, resulting in a pathognomonic appearance; this presumably reflects a perilymphatic distribution of fibrosis (Fig. 8.16).

Finally, perihilar conglomerate masses (opacities greater than 3 cm in diameter that may envelope the bronchi and vessels) may be seen in fibrotic sarcoidosis. These conglomerate opacities are very similar to the appearance of progressive massive fibrosis (Abehsera *et al.* 2000; Chong *et al.* 2006) (Fig. 8.17).

Cavitary sarcoidosis

Pulmonary cavitary lesions are a very rare manifestation of sarcoidosis. Cavitary lesions are air-containing lesions of more than 1 cm diameter with a clearly defined wall and are

distinct from honeycombing, which tends to have cysts of more uniform size and no normal lung separating individual cysts (Hours *et al.* 2008).

In the largest series of cavitary sarcoidosis, 23 patients were identified from a large database ($n = 1060$) with atypical features of sarcoidosis (excluding those with aspergillomas) (Hours *et al.* 2008). In these patients, just over 50 percent had stage IV disease, but there was clinical evidence of ongoing disease activity in 75 percent of the cohort and nearly all had evidence of extrapulmonary involvement. Cavitary lesions were most commonly multiple (91 percent) and contained internal septations. Interestingly, pericavitary alveolar consolidation and ground-glass opacification were usually present, so it seems likely that the lesions represent ischemic evolution of conglomerate sarcoidosis granulomas – as noted in Nakatsu's report of the galaxy sign (Nakatsu *et al.* 2002). The natural history of cavitary lesions seems to be variable with about 50 percent improving with time, 25 percent progressing and 25 percent being stable (Hours *et al.* 2008).

PATTERNS OF SARCOIDOSIS MIMICKING OTHER DISEASES

Perilymphatic involvement

Micronodules are a radiographic feature of numerous different diseases. Identifying the perilymphatic nature of micronodules, typical of sarcoidosis, is key to reducing the differential diagnosis as it allows discrimination from diseases with randomly distributed micronodules – such as miliary tuberculosis, fungal infections and metastatic deposits (Webb *et al.* 2001; Webb 2006).

Perilymphatic diseases with nodules, most notably lymphangitis carcinomatosis, lymphoma and silicosis, may be more problematic. Lymphangitis is unilateral in about 35 percent of cases (Honda *et al.* 1999), as opposed to sarcoidosis, in which a truly unilateral distribution, as distinct from asymmetrical involvement, is very rare (Rockoff and Rohatgi 1985). Thus, in practice, while lymphangitis is often associated with a relevant clinical history of malignancy, unilateral perilymphatic disease should be regarded with suspicion, even in the absence of known malignancy, and should prompt further investigation.

Honda and co-workers evaluated the differences between sarcoidosis, lymphangitis and lymphoma on HRCT (Honda *et al.* 1999). In this study of 40 patients, the degree of subpleural involvement and interlobular septal thickening was found to be significantly greater in lymphangitis than in lymphoma or sarcoidosis. Therefore, interlobular septal thickening as a dominant feature of a perilymphatic disease may alter the balance of likely diagnoses to favor lymphangitis over sarcoidosis. Subpleural involvement with identification of pseudoplaques is relatively common in sarcoidosis (found in the upper lobes of 58 percent of cases with sarcoidosis; half of these pseudoplaques contain calcification (Remy-Jardin *et al.* 1990), but may also be found in coal-worker's pneumoconiosis, lymphangitis carcinomatosis and normal control patients (Remy-Jardin *et al.* 1990). As a consequence, pseudoplaques, as an isolated finding, may be difficult to interpret but in conjunction with other parenchymal signs may provide useful support for sarcoidosis.

Finally, silicosis may result in a similar appearance to sarcoidosis but a distinction can usually be made based on the history and the appearance of the nodules. Nodules in silicosis differ from those in sarcoidosis in three ways: they have a more uniform distribution and, unlike sarcoidosis, do not predominate in the perihilar regions; they are usually slightly larger; and they are slightly more dense (Chong *et al.* 2006). A further useful observation is that sarcoidosis micronodules are often associated with architectural distortion and this, in combination with the temporal and clinical course of the disease, may allow confident differentiation from other perilymphatic diseases (Nishino *et al.* 2009).

Airspace or large nodular sarcoidosis

Multifocal airspace sarcoidosis can mimic consolidating diseases such as organizing pneumonia or lymphoma (Nunes *et al.* 2007) and may prompt invasive diagnostic procedures (Fig. 8.18). Rarely, infection may mimic the CT appearances of alveolar sarcoidosis. Furthermore, while originally believed to be specific for sarcoidosis, the presence of micronodules surrounding a focus of consolidation (the galaxy sign) has also been reported in tuberculosis. Heo and co-workers reviewed 86 patients with active tuberculosis and detected clusters of small nodules (analagous to the galaxy sign) in 10 percent of cases (Heo *et al.* 2005). In a small number of cases with the galaxy sign, there were no ancillary features of tuberculosis, such as a tree-in-bud pattern. Nevertheless, large nodules around the peripheries are likely to be due to sarcoidosis unless there is evidence of a tree-in-bud infiltrate or ill-defined centrilobular nodules, both suggestive of tuberculosis.

Honeycombing

The cause of honeycombing as a manifestation of sarcoidosis has yet to be fully elucidated. Rarely it may be diffuse and occasionally the distribution of honeycombing will mimic that of usual interstitial pneumonia (UIP) (Padley *et al.* 1996; Abehsera *et al.* 2000) (Fig. 8.19). In this very small subset of patients with diffuse honeycombing, it is possible that there is co-existent UIP. Regardless of the radiological appearances, the diagnosis of sarcoidosis can usually be made on clinical and histopathological grounds (Abehsera *et al.* 2000).

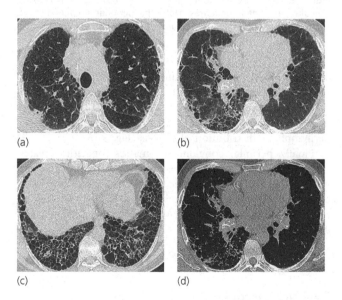

(a)   (b)

(c)   (d)

Figure 8.18   Example of histologically proven sarcoidosis mimicking usual interstitial pneumonia (UIP). HRCT images at the level of the aortic arch, the pulmonary trunk and the costophrenic recesses. There is fibrosis characterized by predominantly basal honeycombing. Note the calcified bihilar lymph nodes. This manifestation of pulmonary sarcoidosis is rare.

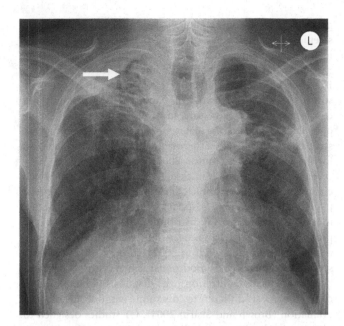

Figure 8.19   Chest radiograph showing fibrobullous destruction in both upper zones. On the right there is an intracavitary body (demarcated by an air-crescent) and marked thickening of the adjacent pleural surface, characteristic of mycetoma formation.

Fibrobullous destruction

Chronic, fibrotic (stage IV) sarcoid commonly results in cysts or thick-walled cavities, usually in the upper zones (Rabinowitz *et al.* 1974; Israel *et al.* 1982; Akira *et al.* 2005). The resulting fibrotic cavities can be difficult to distinguish from tuberculosis. However, ancillary signs such as bilateral (typical of sarcoidosis), rather than unilateral nodal calcification, may be useful for helping to distinguish between tuberculous and sarcoidosis-related fibrotic cavities. Occasionally, gross destruction of the upper-zone lung parenchyma, in the absence of fibrosis, can result in massive bullus formation; this very rare phenomenon may be a cause of so-called 'vanishing lung' disease (Miller 1981).

Cavitary sarcoidosis

It is very rare to find true cavitary sarcoidosis, in which the cavity wall is composed of non-caseating granulomas with minimal fibrosis (Rockoff and Rohatgi 1985; Nakatsu *et al.* 2002; Hours *et al.* 2008). Therefore, other more common cavitating lesions should be excluded before a confident diagnosis of sarcoidosis is made, specifically Wegener's granulomatosis and cavitating infections (particularly typical and atypical tuberculosis) (Nunes *et al.* 2007; Hours *et al.* 2008).

COMPLICATIONS OF FIBROSIS

Aspergillomas may form within fibrotic cavities associated with sarcoidosis and are typically found in late-stage disease

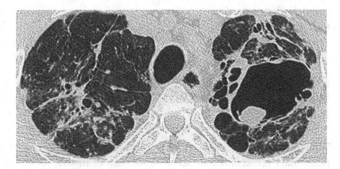

Figure 8.20   HRCT image through the lung apices. A mycetoma is seen within a region of fibrobullous destruction on the left. Note the background changes consistent with fibrotic sarcoidosis.

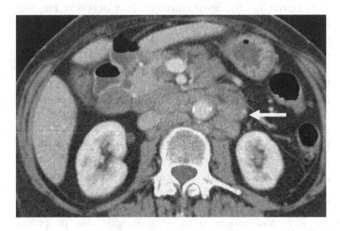

Figure 8.21   Abdominal lymph node enlargement is relatively common in sarcoidosis but may be difficult to distinguish from other causes (benign or malignant) on imaging grounds alone. In this example there is a mantle of enlarged para-aortic nodes.

(stage IV) (Israel *et al.* 1982; Tomlinson and Sahn 1987). In the developed world, sarcoidosis is probably the most common cause of mycetomas and is particularly common in Afro-Caribbeans (Israel *et al.* 1982). Radiographically, mycetomas are characterized by a mass of soft-tissue density within a lung cavity, separated from the cavity wall by an air crescent (Franquet *et al.* 2001). The earliest feature of fungal infection in the cavity, thickening of the pleural surface adjacent to the cavity, may be detected on a radiograph or CT (Sansom *et al.* 2000) (Figs 8.20 and 8.21). However, CT is more sensitive at detecting early mycetoma formation, which initially manifests as delicate soft tissue density fronds within the lumen of the cavity. Subsequent coalescence of the strands results in a visible fungal ball with a crescent of air interposed between it and the cavity wall (Roberts *et al.* 1987).

Identification of mycetoma formation is important for two reasons. First, erosion by the fungal ball into the hypervascular cavity wall results in hemoptysis in 74 percent of patients (Glimp and Bayer 1983), and in a small minority of patients – about 5 percent – hemorrhage may be life-threatening (Sansom *et al.* 2000). The second important point is that detection of a mycetoma is a relative contra-indication to transplantation (Hadjiliadis *et al.* 2002).

EXTRATHORACIC MANIFESTATIONS OF SARCOIDOSIS VISIBLE ON THORACIC IMAGING

Thoracic imaging incidentally incorporates a range of extra-pulmonary structures that show abnormalities in sarcoidosis. Autopsy series of patients with pulmonary sarcoidosis show hepatic and splenic involvement to be present in 40–60 percent (Lynch 2003). However, radiologically detectable hepatic disease is demonstrated in a smaller number of patients (4–38 percent) (Deutch *et al.* 1987; Britt *et al.* 1991; Warshauer *et al.* 1994; Folz *et al.* 1995), and CT may be normal even in patients with known hepatic involvement (Folz *et al.* 1995). Hepatic involvement most commonly causes organomegaly in about 40 percent of cases (Warshauer *et al.* 1994), but in a smaller number of cases (5 percent) coalescent granulomas may result in focal lesions that measure 2–10 mm in diameter and are of low density on contrast-enhanced CT (Warshauer *et al.* 1994). It is uncommon for hepatic involvement to be symptomatic (fewer than 5 percent of patients) (Joint Statement of ATS 1999; Lynch 2003). Splenic abnormalities are more frequent than hepatic abnormalities (25–60 percent) (Deutch *et al.* 1987; Britt *et al.* 1991; Folz *et al.* 1995; Warshauer *et al.* 1994) and, when present, are associated with other detectable abdominal abnormalities in about 50 percent of cases (Folz *et al.* 1995). The spectrum of splenic involvement is similar to that seen in the liver and ranges from organomegaly due to portal hypertension resulting from hepatic infiltration or direct splenic involvement (Warshauer *et al.* 1994), to nodular

granulomatous lesions. Nodular hepatic and, to a lesser extent, splenic infiltration poses potential diagnostic difficulties on imaging alone and has a broad differential diagnosis, including metastatic disease, lymphoma and infection (Britt *et al.* 1991). However, if a biopsy from an extrahepatic organ has demonstrated features of sarcoidosis and the CT features are consistent with hepatic sarcoidosis or the serum alkaline phosphatase is raised, the diagnosis is most likely to be hepatic sarcoidosis, provided that there is no other clinical explanation for the abnormalities (Judson 2002).

Sarcoidosis can result in extensive abdominal lymph node enlargement, seen on thoracic imaging in about 45 percent of patients (Folz *et al.* 1995). Nodal enlargement typically occurs in a para-aortic and caval distribution or in the region of the porta-hepatis and celiac axis, while retrocrural nodes are relatively uncommon (Judson 2002). In the context of widespread abdominal lymph node enlargement (with or without hepatic or splenic infiltration), the diagnosis of lymphoma is often the most difficult to discount without histological evaluation (Brown and Skarin 2004). CT studies designed to differentiate benign and malignant abdominal lymph node enlargement have shown variable outcomes. Thus, in a review of patients with sarcoidosis or non-Hodgkin's lymphoma, enlarged nodes in the retrocrural space were found to be significantly more prevalent in lymphoma – seen in 18 percent of sarcoidosis cases but 70 percent of lymphoma (Britt *et al.* 1991). Furthermore, in the same study, lymph nodes tended to be larger in lymphoma and to form a confluent mass of nodes more often than in sarcoidosis (Fig. 8.22). However, in an earlier case series, the CT appearances (including size, location, contour, density, relationship to the aorta and inferior vena cava and presence of mass effect) of lymph nodes were not significantly different for a range of benign and malignant diseases including sarcoidosis (Deutch *et al.* 1987). While the

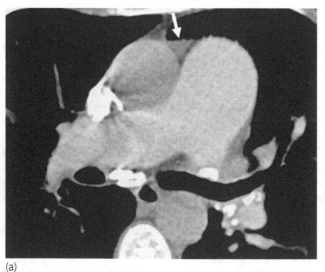

(a)

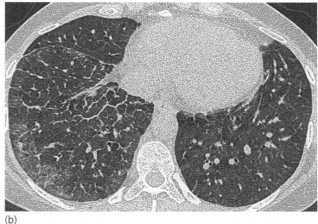

(b)

Figure 8.22   Histopathologically confirmed pulmonary veno-occlusive disease secondary to sarcoidosis. (a) Dilatation of the main pulmonary trunk relative to the ascending aorta (ratio > 1) is a relatively specific CT sign of pulmonary hypertension. An additional, less specific, finding ('the bikini sign') is fluid in the superior pericardial recess (arrow). (b) When signs of pulmonary hypertension are present, diffuse interlobular septal thickening should raise the possibility of pulmonary veno-occlusive disease (pleural effusions, an uncommon feature of sarcoidosis, may also be present).

findings in this study by Britt and associates differ from earlier series in which some of the points detailed were found to be useful discriminators, it seems that, on balance, a cautious approach to markedly enlarged abdominal lymph nodes is warranted.

Cardiac and osseous involvement is less common in sarcoidosis. Myocardial sarcoidosis is only clinically apparent in about 5 percent of patients (although autopsy studies suggest that subclinical involvement is more prevalent) (Joint Statement of ATS 1999). While granulomatous infiltration can affect any site in the heart, myocardial involvement is by far the most common site of disease (Doughan and Williams 2006). Identification of myocardial sarcoidosis is best achieved using gadolinium-enhanced cardiac MRI, and has a reported sensitivity and specificity of 100 percent and 78 percent, respectively (Smedema et al. 2005). By contrast, routine thoracic imaging using unenhanced HRCT is unable to detect direct myocardial involvement although it may demonstrate pericardial effusions (found in 3–19 percent of cases with cardiac involvement – Doughan and Williams (2006)). Finally, sarcoidosis of the bony thoracic cage and vertebral column can also be detected, but these lesions are rare and may be either lytic (most frequently) or sclerotic (Rockoff and Rohatgi 1985).

PLEURAL INVOLVEMENT

Schaumann first observed pleural involvement in sarcoidosis in 1933 but it is relatively uncommon, occurring in about 3 percent of cases (Soskel and Sharma 2000). In a comprehensive review of the literature, Soskel and Sharma noted that pleural involvement with sarcoidosis is most frequent in stage III disease, which accounts for 35 percent of cases. Pleural effusions are the most common manifestation, reported in 0.7–10 percent of cases (Chusid and Siltzbach 1974; Sharma and Gordonson 1975; Beekman et al. 1976; Soskel and Sharma 2000; Huggins et al. 2006). The effusions are usually lymphocytic and exudative (Huggins et al. 2006) but may occasionally be due to chyle (Cappell et al. 1993; Jarman et al. 1995). In a group of 181 patients, all with histopathological evidence of pulmonary sarcoidosis, ultrasonography (a highly sensitive technique for demonstrating fluid) detected effusions in only 5 patients (2.8 percent). The effusion was due to pleural involvement by sarcoidosis in just two cases, while parapneumonic collections and cardiac failure accounted for the pleural fluid in the remaining cases (Almoosa et al. 2006).

When present, effusions tend to be modest in size and unilateral (Soskel and Sharma 2000). Importantly, bilateral effusions are uncommon and their presence should raise doubts about the diagnosis or raise the possibility of complicating features, such as pulmonary veno-occlusive disease or cardiac dysfunction. Chylous effusions are very rare and are believed to result from obstruction of the thoracic duct by very large lymph nodes (Cappell et al. 1993; Jarman et al. 1995).

Other signs of pleural involvement include pneumothorax (Froudarakis et al. 1997), pleural thickening (Brauner et al.

1992; Murdoch and Müller 1992), or pleural nodules (Remy-Jardin et al. 1990; Bottaro et al. 2004). Pneumothoraces have been reported in up to 4 percent of patients with pulmonary sarcoidosis (Soskel and Sharma 2000). While some studies suggest that the frequency of pneumothoraces increases with the radiographic stage of disease (Sharma et al. 1987), the nature of the relationship between pneumothorax and sarcoidosis has been debated; some authors claim it to be a chance association whereas others have suggested that the association is due to rupture of subpleural blebs or necrosis of a subpleural granuloma (Kirks et al. 1973; Lake et al. 1978; Sharma et al. 1987; Akelsson et al. 1990; Flora et al. 1991).

Finally, pleural thickening visible on CT may be seen in longstanding cases. This is thought to represent inward retraction of extrathoracic soft tissue and extra-pleural fat rather than a true pleural abnormality (Brauner et al. 1992; Lynch 2003).

VASCULAR INVOLVEMENT

Pulmonary hypertension

Pulmonary hypertension complicates sarcoidosis in up to 5 percent of patients (Nunes et al. 2006). While chest radiography is relatively insensitive for the detection of pulmonary hypertension (Weitzman et al. 1974), signs, when present, include dilatation of the pulmonary trunk and main pulmonary arteries with peripheral 'pruning' (Matthay et al. 1981). CT signs of pulmonary hypertension are more sensitive and specific than radiography. A ratio of > 1, for the diameter of the pulmonary trunk to the ascending aorta, and dilatation of the segmental pulmonary arteries strongly correlate with the presence of pulmonary hypertension in patients both with and without fibrosis (Tan et al. 1998; Devaraj et al. 2008). In a study by Tan and associates, dilatation of the pulmonary artery alone had a sensitivity and specificity of 87 percent and 89 percent, respectively, while the combination of dilatation of the pulmonary trunk and the presence of dilated segmental pulmonary arteries was 100 percent specific for the presence of pulmonary artery hypertension (Tan et al. 1998).

In two studies of patients ($n = 60$) with sarcoidosis and pulmonary hypertension, there was an association with fibrosis (detected on chest radiography) in 66 percent of cases (Sulica et al. 2005; Nunes et al. 2006). However, the observation that pulmonary hypertension is also found in the absence of fibrosis implies that mechanisms other than lung destruction play a role its development. Histological evidence of vascular involvement is almost universal in sarcoidosis – 100 percent of cases in one post-mortem series (Takemura et al. 1992) – implying that an intrinsic vasculopathy is a likely additional cause for pulmonary hypertension (Hours et al. 2008).

It is also possible that the extent of venous infiltration may be a factor. In a study of 22 patients with pulmonary hypertension and sarcoidosis, CT features of veno-occlusive disease (ground-glass opacification and thickened interlobular septa) were also a frequent observation (Nunes et al. 2006). In the same study, this hypothesis was given credence by the histological demonstration of veno-occlusive disease in 4 out of 5 patients who underwent transplantation for sarcoidosis with pulmonary hypertension (Fig. 8.23). However, other causes of pulmonary hypertension have also been demonstrated, including direct compression of the proximal pulmonary arteries by mediastinal lymph node enlargement or fibrosing mediastinitis (Baughman 2007) (Fig. 8.24).

Necrotizing sarcoidosis granulomatosis

Necrotizing sarcoidosis granulomatosis is a rare disease, originally described by Liebow (1973). Histologically, it is characterized by the presence of numerous parenchymal sarcoid-like granulomas, non-caseating necrosis and granulomatous-, giant cell- or lymphocytic-type vasculitis involving both arteries and veins (Quaden et al. 2005).

There has been an ongoing debate since the original description as to whether the disease is a sarcoid reaction with an underlying necrotizing angiitis or sarcoidosis with necrosis of the granulomas and vessels. To date, there have been about 115 reported cases involving many sites in the body but, most commonly, the lungs (Strickland-Marmol et al. 2000). Hilar and/or mediastinal lymph node enlargement, present in around half of cases (Chittock et al. 1994; Quaden et al. 2005), in association with pulmonary nodules is the most common radiographic manifestation of necrotizing sarcoid granulomatosis (Chittock et al. 1994). CT findings include discrete airspace opacities (50 percent), multiple nodules (30 percent) or a solitary pulmonary nodule (20 percent) (Quaden et al. 2005). Although cavitation is more frequent (up to 15 percent) than in alveolar sarcoidosis,

the radiological signs of these two entities share many features; however, it appears that they are distinct phenomena (Nunes et al. 2007) (Fig. 8.25). A further potentially valuable indicator of the diagnosis is the presence of pleural thickening, an unusual feature of sarcoidosis. It was noted in 5 of 7 patients in one series (Chittock et al. 1994), but this may be an exaggeration of the association as in another study it was only detected in 1 of 14 patients (Quaden et al. 2005). Given its rarity, and particularly in cases with cavitation or a solitary pulmonary nodule, infection, malignancy or a granulomatous vasculitis should all be excluded before the diagnosis is reached and in most cases biopsy confirmation is needed (Quaden et al. 2005). Overall the prognosis of necrotizing sarcoidosis granulomatosis tends to be favorable.

MEDIASTINAL INVOLVEMENT

Fibrosing mediastinitis or sclerosing mediastinitis is a rare condition characterized by excessive fibrosis in the mediastinum. There are at least six reported cases in the literature of sarcoidosis-related fibrosing mediastinitis (Gordonson et al. 1973; Kinney et al. 1980; Radke et al. 1980; Devaraj et al. 2007; Hamilton-Craig et al. 2009). This condition is associated with significant morbidity and occasional mortality and may lead to dyspnea, or symptoms related to obstruction of the mediastinal vasculature, most commonly superior vena cava obstruction (Gordonson et al. 1973; Kinney et al. 1980; Radke et al. 1980; Devaraj et al. 2007; Hamilton-Craig et al. 2009). Widening of the mediastinum is the only radiographic indicator of fibrosing mediastinitis (Radke et al. 1980). On CT, a visible localized or diffuse

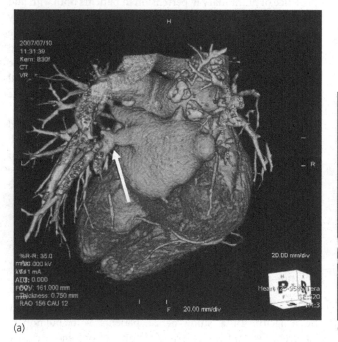

(a)

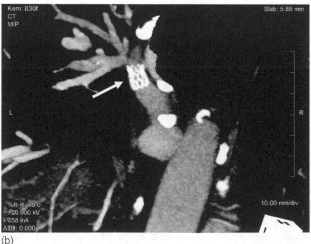

(b)

Figure 8.23   Pulmonary hypertension due to a stenosis of the right inferior pulmonary vein resulting from sarcoidosis. (a) Volume-rendered CT of the heart showing the pulmonary venous confluence. The right inferior pulmonary vein shows a clear stenosis (arrowed). (b) Maximum intensity projection (MIP) image of the right inferior pulmonary vein following endovascular stenting.

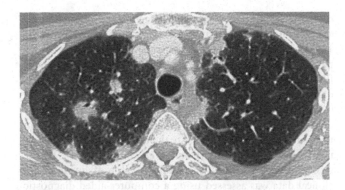

Figure 8.24   Necrotizing granulomatous sarcoidosis: a rare example of histologically proven necrotizing sarcoid granulomatosis. The nodular patten in this example is indistinguishable from alveolar sarcoidosis. Note the left-sided posterior pleural thickening which may be associated with this entity.

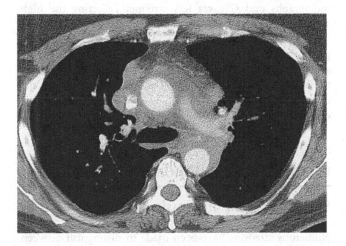

Figure 8.25   Biopsy-proven fibrosing mediastinitis secondary to sarcoidosis, with diffuse infiltration of the mediastinal fat by abnormal soft tissue. Mediastinal structures may be compressed and obstructed in some cases.

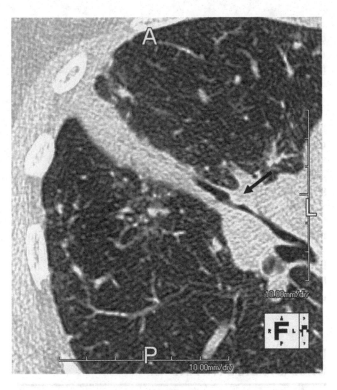

Figure 8.26   Endobronchial sarcoidosis. A smooth nodular endobronchial lesion (arrow) is shown with distal subsegmental atelectasis. Note the surrounding micronodular parenchymal changes.

soft-tissue mediastinal mass typically obliterates the adjacent fat planes and causes compression of adjacent structures (Devaraj *et al.* 2007) (Fig. 8.26).

LARGE AIRWAY INVOLVEMENT

Large airway involvement in sarcoidosis can occur anywhere from the epiglottis to the respiratory bronchioles (Miller *et al.* 1995). Tracheal involvement is rare but can result in stenosis (Brandstetter *et al.* 1981b; Henry and Cho 1983). Bronchial involvement is relatively frequent. Lenique and associates demonstrated smooth or nodular bronchial wall thickening in 39 of 60 patients with sarcoidosis (65 percent), with focal luminal narrowing present in 25 percent (Lenique *et al.* 1995). However, while bronchial abnormalities demonstrated on CT showed a significant correlation with endo-

scopic and transbronchial biopsy findings, CT is unable to differentiate mucosal thickening and secretions from granulomatous infiltration (Lenique *et al.* 1995). Bronchial stenoses may result from granulomatous inflammation of the bronchial wall, distortion resulting from fibrosis and, very rarely, from extrinsic compression from lymph nodes (Mendelson *et al.* 1983; Udwadia *et al.* 1990; Lynch 2003). Bronchiectasis distal to a stenotic lesions (unrelated to parenchymal fibrosis) is not uncommon (Udwadia *et al.* 1990) but rarely symptomatic (Lynch 2003).

MALIGNANT DISEASES WITH SARCOID-LIKE RESPONSE

The presence of non-caseating granulomas in patients with malignancy who do not fulfil the criteria for systemic sarcoidosis is referred to as a sarcoid-like reaction (Cohen and Kurzrock 2007). Sarcoid-like reactions have been reported in 4 percent of patients with carcinomas, including breast, renal, gastrointestinal and testicular (Cohen and Kurzrock 2007). However, they occur most commonly in hematological malignancies, affecting up to 14 percent and 7 percent of patients with Hodgkin's and non-Hodgkin's lymphoma, respectively (Brincker 1986).

Non-caseating granulomas are usually formed in lymph nodes draining the cancer, but may also occur in the stroma of the organ surrounding the primary neoplasm, and in distant lymph nodes, the spleen or the liver (Chowdhury et al. 2009). The majority of sarcoid-like reactions occur in patients undergoing follow-up for malignancy and develop long after the original disease (up to 17 years) (Hunsaker et al. 1996).

Thoracic sarcoid-like reactions have similar imaging findings to sarcoidosis, ranging from isolated bihilar lymph node enlargement to perilymphatic nodularity or even airspace opacities (Hunsaker et al. 1996; Chowdhury et al. 2009). This is important as the radiological manifestations of granulomatous infiltration may be misconstrued as metastatic nodal or pulmonary disease, rather than a benign (reactive) condition and, thus, substantially alter management (Hunsaker et al. 1996). At least two studies have found that the presence of sarcoid-like reactions in Hodgkin's lymphoma is associated with prolonged survival times and a lower incidence of herpes zoster in these patients (O'Connell et al. 1975; Sacks et al. 1978).

DIAGNOSTIC SENSITIVITY AND SPECIFICITY OF RADIOGRAPHY AND CT

The combination of characteristic clinical and chest radiographic findings may be sufficient to make the diagnosis of sarcoidosis without histological confirmation. The American Thoracic Society states that for patients with stage I or II disease the diagnosis can be made reliably in 98 and 89 percent of cases, respectively, but is less accurate for patients in stage III (52 percent) and stage 0 (23 percent) (Joint Statement of ATS 1999).

While bilateral hilar lymph node enlargement may be seen in a range of diseases, it is uncommon for it to be symmetrical in any disease other than sarcoidosis. Thus, in a large study, only 4 percent of patients with lymphoma had bilateral hilar lymphadenopathy, while fewer then 1 percent of patients with bronchogenic malignancy had this distinctive radiographic feature (Winterbauer et al. 1973). Furthermore, in the same study, the presence of bihilar lymph node enlargement combined with cutaneous, ocular or joint symptoms was specific for sarcoidosis in all cases and allowed confident differentiation from malignant processes. In the context of tuberculosis, the frequency of bihilar lymphadenopathy is also very low (about 0.05 percent) (Sakowitz and Sakowitz 1977). However, bilateral hilar lymphadenopathy in the presence of a pleural effusion, anterior mediastinal mass, anemia or hepatosplenomegaly is suspicious for malignancy (Winterbauer et al. 1973).

HRCT of the chest is more sensitive than other imaging modalities for the detection of parenchymal abnormalities associated with infiltrative lung diseases. While there is wide variation in the CT features of sarcoidosis, some features are near pathognomonic and in many centers such findings may obviate histological confirmation of the diagnosis (Wells 1998). Some have argued that, in cases with typical radiographic features of sarcoidosis (particularly stage I and II

disease), CT does not improve diagnostic confidence and exposes the patient to unnecessary radiation (Mana et al. 1995). However, for those patients with more extensive parenchymal involvement or established fibrosis, the plain-film differential diagnosis may be broad and CT can increase diagnostic specificity and confidence (Padley et al. 1991; Grenier et al. 1991, 1994; Wells 1998). Grenier's team clearly demonstrated the benefits of CT over plain radiography in two studies designed to evaluate the role of imaging in diffuse infiltrative lung disease (Grenier et al. 1991,1994). In the second of these studies, the additive value of imaging and clinical data was assessed using a computer-aided diagnostic algorithm by applying a Bayesian model to a large population with diffuse lung disease. Supplementing clinical data with the CT data increased diagnostic sensitivity by almost 10 percent, double the increase seen when compared with additional plain radiographic data. However, in patients in whom the correct diagnosis was made with a high degree of confidence on clinical grounds, the difference between plain radiographs and CT was less striking, reflecting the high specificity of the radiograph in patients with typical features, but understating the role of CT in patients with less typical presentations. A further important observation is that the additional value of HRCT is proportional to the experience of the observer (Grenier et al. 1991) and may be a factor in the decision as to whether histological sampling is necessary or not.

PROGNOSTIC EVALUATION WITH IMAGING

Signs indicating progressive fibrotic disease

Numerous attempts have been made to distinguish between inflammatory (potentially reversible) and fibrotic lesions, as judged by CT, in order to predict outcome and guide therapeutic intervention. Architectural distortion (manifested as fissural distortion, tractional airway dilatation, and volume loss), honeycombing (or cystic airspaces) and coarse linear opacities in the presence of architectural distortion are all irreversible and associated with a poorer prognosis (Brauner et al. 1992; Murdoch and Müller 1992; Remy-Jardin et al. 1994). In essence, these signs simply imply the presence of established fibrosis which is associated with a poor response to therapy.

The presence of ground-glass opacification in sarcoidosis is of variable significance. Once thought to be a sign of 'alveolitis', it has become clear that it may result from a number of processes, including active inflammation (alveolitis), granulomatous infiltration of airspaces, or microscopic fibrosis (Austin 1989; Brauner et al. 1992; Wells 1998). As such, its presence may be reversible or irreversible. In a study of the significance of ground-glass opacification (Remy-Jardin et al. 1993) in the broader context of diffuse lung disease, identification of tractional airway dilatation within areas of ground-glass opacification was found to be indicative of underlying fibrosis. In the same study, ground-glass opacification not associated with tractional dilatation was likely to be due to inflammation. However, these signs are not infallible, and in a small number of cases fibrosis may be present but not cause local architectural distortion (Remy-Jardin et al. 1993).

Signs of reversibility

In a retrospective study of 20 patients with biopsy-proven sarcoidosis in whom clinical symptoms had resolved, either as a result of steroid therapy or spontaneously, follow-up CT showed complete resolution of irregularly marginated nodules (10–20 mm diameter) and alveolar consolidation in all patients, while nodules measuring 3–10 mm showed at least partial resolution at follow-up (Brauner et al. 1992). In patients with disease of relatively recent onset, micronodules showed resolution on subsequent imaging. However, in a small number of subjects with a relatively long disease course (> 2 years), micronodular opacities were unchanged over time. Hence, nodules, micronodules and alveolar consolidation are all believed to represent active, inflammatory lesions.

The impression that these CT features are potentially reversible has been corroborated in other studies. Murdoch and Müller (1992) analyzed changes over time in patients who required repeated CT imaging for clinical indications. In this study, nodularity of the bronchovascular bundle was a universal finding at presentation ($n = 18$), and improved in 79 percent of cases, deteriorated in 14 percent and remained stable in 7 percent. Notably, their results indicated that the presence of nodules on the presenting scan was a prognostically favorable sign, while the presence of predominantly linear opacities tended to be predictive of disease progression.

A single discrepancy between the above two studies was that interlobular septal thickening generally improved in Murdoch's study, while in Brauner's analysis there was no improvement in any case, and a tendency for septal thickening to increase.

STRUCTURE–FUNCTION STUDIES

Studies correlating CT morphological appearances and lung function test abnormalities have produced mixed results (Müller et al. 1989b; Remy-Jardin et al. 1994; Hansell et al. 1998; Abehsera et al. 2000; Davies et al. 2000; Magkanas et al. 2001; Terasaki et al. 2005). One difficulty in interpreting these data is the variety of methodologies, descriptive terms and different pulmonary function parameters assessed. Nevertheless, one common point emerges from several studies of patients at all morphologic stages of sarcoidosis, namely that nodular opacities are rarely associated with significant pulmonary function deficits.

Depending on how it is defined, airflow obstruction is reported in 5 to 63 percent of patients with sarcoidosis

and appears to be more common than a restrictive defect (Lavergne et al. 1999). Airflow obstruction (defined as $FEV_1/FVC < 70$ percent) can occur in all radiographic stages, but its frequency increases from stage I to IV (Lavergne et al. 1999). Four different mechanisms of airway involvement account for airflow obstruction: (1) proximal bronchial distortion due to fibrosis and (2) intrinsic narrowing of the proximal bronchial lumen due to granulomatous infiltration are relatively frequent, while (3) extrinsic compression of the proximal airways by enlarged lymph nodes is rare (Naccache et al. 2008); finally, (4) small airways disease may cause airflow obstruction, but its frequency and functional significance are debatable (Naccache et al. 2008). In most patients, it is likely that a combination of these factors results in airflow obstruction. While these patterns may be recognized on HRCT, they are not, in themselves, predictive of airflow obstruction. Thus, in a recent study (Naccache et al. 2008), bronchial and peribronchial abnormalities were found in patients both with and without airflow obstruction. However, when present, the severity of the dominant pattern of bronchial abnormality was found to show a significant negative correlation with airway obstruction. Similarly, the functional significance of air-trapping (an indirect sign of small airways disease) on CT is doubtful, and Terasaki et al. (2005) have suggested that cigarette smoking may be a confounding factor in studies that show a relationship between airflow obstruction and extent of air-trapping (Davies et al. 2000; Magkanas et al. 2001; Terasaki et al. 2005).

Interestingly, there is good evidence that the extent of reticulation present on CT correlates with obstructive pulmonary function tests (Handa et al. 2006; Hansell et al. 1998; Naccache et al. 2008) and it has been suggested that cicatricial emphysema may be a further cause of airflow obstruction not directly related to the airways (Hansell et al. 1998).

These structure–function observations are of little day-to-day clinical importance, but they yield useful insights applicable to clinical trials. For example, HRCT signs may allow patients with airflow obstruction to be stratified into those with a potentially reversible cause of obstruction (e.g. granulomatous infiltration of the bronchial wall) or an irreversible cause (e.g. related to fibrosis), and thus predict response to therapy (de Jong et al. 2005).

CONCLUSION

Imaging continues to play an important role in the management and diagnosis of sarcoidosis. While sarcoidosis has a wide range of imaging manifestations, chest radiography remains useful in the diagnosis of stage I and II disease (with typical patterns of lymph node enlargement) and HRCT increases diagnostic confidence in stage III and IV sarcoidosis, as well as in those patients with atypical features. Further useful insights have been gained from HRCT into disease progression and its prediction, and from structure–function correlations.

REFERENCES

Abehsera M, Valeyre D, Grenier P et al. (2000). Sarcoidosis with pulmonary fibrosis: CT patterns and correlation with pulmonary function. Am J Roentgen 174: 1751–7.

Akelsson IG, Eklund A, Skold CM, Tornling G (1990). Bilateral spontaneous pneumothorax and sarcoidosis. Sarcoidosis 7: 136–8.

Akira M, Kozuka T, Inoue Y, Sakatani M (2005). Long-term follow-up CT scan evaluation in patients with pulmonary sarcoidosis. Chest 127: 185–91.

Almoosa KF, Ryu JH, Mendez J et al. (2006). Management of pneumothorax in lymphangioleiomyomatosis: effects on recurrence and lung transplantation complications. Chest 129: 1274–81.

Austin JH (1989). Pulmonary sarcoidosis: what are we learning from CT? Radiology 171: 603–4.

Bacher K, Smeets P, Bonnarens K et al. (2003). Dose reduction in patients undergoing chest imaging: digital amorphous silicon flat-panel detector radiography versus conventional film-screen radiography and phosphor-based computed radiography. Am J Roentgen 181: 923–9.

Baughman RP (2007). Pulmonary hypertension associated with sarcoidosis. Arthritis Res Ther Suppl 2: S8.

Beekman JF, Zimmet SM, Chun BK et al. (1976). Spectrum of pleural involvement in sarcoidosis. Arch Intern Med 136: 323–30.

Beigelman-Aubry C, Hill C, Guibal A et al. (2005). Multi-detector row CT and postprocessing techniques in the assessment of diffuse lung disease. Radiographics 25: 1639–52.

Bergin CJ, Bell DY, Coblentz CL et al. (1989). Sarcoidosis: correlation of pulmonary parenchymal pattern at CT with results of pulmonary function tests. Radiology 171: 619–24.

Bottaro L, Calderan L, Dibilio D et al. (2004). Pulmonary sarcoidosis: atypical HRTC features and differential diagnostic problems. Radiol Med 107: 273–85.

Brandstetter RD, Hansen DE, Jarowski CI et al. (1981a). Superior vena cava syndrome as the initial clinical manifestation of sarcoidosis. Heart Lung 10: 101–4.

Brandstetter RD, Messina MS, Sprince NL, Grillo HC (1981b). Tracheal stenosis due to sarcoidosis. Chest 80: 656.

Brauner MW, Grenier P, Mompoint D et al. (1989). Pulmonary sarcoidosis: evaluation with high-resolution CT. Radiology 172: 467–71.

Brauner MW, Lenoir S, Grenier P et al. (1992). Pulmonary sarcoidosis: CT assessment of lesion reversibility. Radiology 182: 349–54.

Brincker H (1986). Sarcoid reactions in malignant tumours. Cancer Treat Rev 13: 147–56.

Britt AR, Francis IR, Glazer GM, Ellis JH (1991). Sarcoidosis: abdominal manifestations at CT. Radiology 178: 91–4.

Brown JR, Skarin AT (2004). Clinical mimics of lymphoma. Oncologist 9: 406–16.

Cappell MS, Friedman D, Mikhail N (1993). Chyloperitoneum associated with chronic severe sarcoidosis. Am J Gastroenter 88: 99–101.

Chittock DR, Joseph MG, Paterson NA, McFadden RG (1994). Necrotizing sarcoid granulomatosis with pleural involvement: clinical and radiographic features. Chest 106: 672–6.

Chong S, Lee KS, Chung MJ et al. (2006). Pneumoconiosis: comparison of imaging and pathologic findings. Radiographics 26: 59–77.

Chowdhury FU, Sheerin F, Bradley KM, Gleeson FV (2009). Sarcoid-like reaction to malignancy on whole-body integrated (18)F-FDG PET/CT: prevalence and disease pattern. Clin Radiol 64: 675–81.

Chusid EL, Siltzbach LE (1974). Sarcoidosis of the pleura. Ann Intern Med 81: 190–4.

Cohen PR, Kurzrock R (2007). Sarcoidosis and malignancy. Clin Dermatol 25: 326–33.

Conant EF, Glickstein MF, Mahar P, Miller WT (1988). Pulmonary sarcoidosis in the older patient: conventional radiographic features. Radiology 169: 315–19.

Dalal PU, Hansell DM (2006). High-resolution computed tomography of the lungs: the borderlands of normality. Eur Radiol 16: 771–80.

Damuth TE, Bower JS, Cho K, Dantzker DR (1980). Major pulmonary artery stenosis causing pulmonary hypertension in sarcoidosis. Chest 78: 888–91.

Davies CW, Tasker AD, Padley SP et al. (2000). Air trapping in sarcoidosis on computed tomography: correlation with lung function. Clin Radiol 55: 217–21.

de Jong PA, Müller NL, Pare PD, Coxson HO (2005). Computed tomographic imaging of the airways: relationship to structure and function. Eur Respir J 26: 140–52.

DeRemee RA (1983). The roentgenographic staging of sarcoidosis: Historic and contemporary perspectives. Chest 83: 128–33.

Deutch SJ, Sandler MA, Alpern MB (1987). Abdominal lymphadenopathy in benign diseases: CT detection. Radiology 163: 335–8.

Devaraj A, Griffin N, Nicholson AG, Padley SP (2007). Computed tomography findings in fibrosing mediastinitis. Clin Radiol 62: 781–6.

Devaraj A, Wells AU, Meister MG et al. (2008). The effect of diffuse pulmonary fibrosis on the reliability of CT signs of pulmonary hypertension. Radiology 249: 1042–9.

Doughan AR, Williams BR (2006). Cardiac sarcoidosis. Heart 92: 282–8.

Flora G, Dostanic D, Jakovic R, Sharma OP (1991). Pneumothorax in sarcoidosis. Sarcoidosis 8: 75–9.

Folz SJ, Johnson CD, Swensen SJ (1995). Abdominal manifestations of sarcoidosis in CT studies. J Comput Assist Tomogr 19: 573–9.

Franquet T, Müller NL, Gimenez A et al. (2001). Spectrum of pulmonary aspergillosis: histologic, clinical, and radiologic findings. Radiographics 21: 825–37.

Froudarakis ME, Bouros D, Voloudaki A et al. (1997). Pneumothorax as a first manifestation of sarcoidosis. Chest 112: 278–80.

Garland LH (1947). Pulmonary sarcoidosis: the early roentgen findings. Radiology 48: 333–54.

Gawne-Cain ML, Hansell DM (1996). The pattern and distribution of calcified mediastinal lymph nodes in sarcoidosis and tuberculosis: a CT study. Clin Radiol 51: 263–7.

Gleeson FV, Traill ZC, Hansell DM (1996). Evidence of expiratory CT scans of small-airway obstruction in sarcoidosis. Am J Roentgen 166: 1052–4.

Glimp RA, Bayer AS (1983). Pulmonary aspergilloma: diagnostic and therapeutic considerations. Arch Intern Med 143: 303–8.

Gordonson J, Trachtenberg S, Sargent EN (1973). Superior vena cava obstruction due to sarcoidosis. Chest 63: 292–3.

Grenier P, Valeyre D, Cluzel P et al. (1991). Chronic diffuse interstitial lung disease: diagnostic value of chest radiography and high-resolution CT. Radiology 179: 123–32.

Grenier P, Chevret S, Beigelman C et al. (1994). Chronic diffuse infiltrative lung disease: determination of the diagnostic value of clinical data, chest radiography, and CT and Bayesian analysis. Radiology 191: 383–90.

Hadjiliadis D, Sporn TA, Perfect JR et al. (2002). Outcome of lung transplantation in patients with mycetomas. Chest 121: 128–34.

Hamilton-Craig CR, Slaughter R, McNeil K *et al.* (2009). Improvement after angioplasty and stenting of pulmonary arteries due to sarcoid mediastinal fibrosis. *Heart Lung Circ* **18**: 222–5.

Handa T, Nagai S, Fushimi Y *et al.* (2006). Clinical and radiographic indices associated with airflow limitation in patients with sarcoidosis. *Chest* **130**: 1851–6.

Hansell DM (2001). Small airways diseases: detection and insights with computed tomography. *Eur Respir J* **17**: 1294–313.

Hansell DM (2005). Miscellaneous diffuse lung diseases. In: Hansell DM, (ed.). *Imaging of Diseases of the Chest*, 4th edn. Elsevier Mosby, Philadelphia, pp. 631–53.

Hansell DM, Milne DG, Wilsher ML, Wells AU (1998). Pulmonary sarcoidosis: morphologic associations of airflow obstruction at thin-section CT. *Radiology* **209**: 697–704.

Hansell DM, Bankier AA, MacMahon H *et al.* (2008). Fleischner Society: glossary of terms for thoracic imaging. *Radiology* **246**: 697–722.

Henry DA, Cho SR (1983). Tracheal stenosis in sarcoidosis. *Southern Med J* **76**: 1323–4.

Heo JN, Choi YW, Jeon SC, Park CK (2005). Pulmonary tuberculosis: another disease showing clusters of small nodules. *Am J Roentgen* **184**: 639–42.

Hillerdal G, Nou E, Osterman K, Schmekel B (1984). Sarcoidosis: epidemiology and prognosis. A 15-year European study. *Am Rev Respir Dis* **130**: 29–32.

Honda O, Johkoh T, Ichikado K *et al.* (1999). Comparison of high resolution CT findings of sarcoidosis, lymphoma, and lymphangitic carcinoma: is there any difference of involved interstitium? *J Comput Assist Tomogr* **23**: 374–9.

Hours S, Nunes H, Kambouchner M *et al.* (2008). Pulmonary cavitary sarcoidosis: clinico-radiologic characteristics and natural history of a rare form of sarcoidosis. *Medicine* (Baltimore) **87**: 142–51.

Huggins JT, Doelken P, Sahn SA *et al.* (2006). Pleural effusions in a series of 181 outpatients with sarcoidosis. *Chest* **129**: 1599–604.

Hunsaker AR, Munden RF, Pugatch RD, Mentzer SJ (1996). Sarcoid-like reaction in patients with malignancy. *Radiology* **200**: 255–61.

Israel HL, Lenchner GS, Atkinson GW (1982). Sarcoidosis and aspergilloma: the role of surgery. *Chest* **82**: 430–2.

Jarman PR, Whyte MK, Sabroe I, Hughes JM (1995). Sarcoidosis presenting with chylothorax. *Thorax* **50**: 1324–5.

Joint Statement of the American Thoracic Society ATS (1999), the European Respiratory Society (ERS) and the World Association of Sarcoidosis and Other Granulomatous Disorders (WASOG), adopted by the ATS Board of Directors and by the ERS Executive Committee (1999). *Am J Respir Crit Care Med* **160**: 736–55.

Judson MA (2002). Hepatic, splenic, and gastrointestinal involvement with sarcoidosis. *Sem Respir Crit Care Med* **23**: 529–41.

Kinney EL, Murthy R, Ascunce G *et al.* (1980). Sarcoidosis: rare cause of superior vena caval obstruction. *Pennsylvania Med* **83**: 31.

Kirks DR, McCormick VD, Greenspan RH (1973). Pulmonary sarcoidosis: roentgenologic analysis of 150 patients. *Am J Roentgen Rad Ther Nucl Med* **117**: 777–86.

Lake KB, Sharma OP, Van Dyke JJ (1978). Pneumothorax in sarcoidosis. *Rev Interamer Radiol* **3**: 33–6.

Lavergne F, Clerici C, Sadoun D *et al.* (1999). Airway obstruction in bronchial sarcoidosis: outcome with treatment. *Chest* **116**: 1194–9.

Lee KS, Primack SL, Staples CA *et al.* (1994). Chronic infiltrative lung disease: comparison of diagnostic accuracies of radiography and low- and conventional-dose thin-section CT. *Radiology* **191**: 669–73.

Lenique F, Brauner MW, Grenier P *et al.* (1995). CT assessment of bronchi in sarcoidosis: endoscopic and pathologic correlations. *Radiology* **194**: 419–23.

Leswick DA, Webster ST, Wilcox BA, Fladeland DA (2005). Radiation cost of helical high-resolution chest CT. *Am J Roentgen* **184**: 742–5.

Leung AN, Staples CA, Müller NL (1991). Chronic diffuse infiltrative lung disease: comparison of diagnostic accuracy of high-resolution and conventional CT. *Am J Roentg* **157**: 693–6.

Liebow AA (1973). Pulmonary angiitis and granulomatosis. *Am Rev Respir Dis* **108**: 1–18.

Lynch JP (2003). Computed tomographic scanning in sarcoidosis. *Sem Respir Crit Care Med* **24**: 393–418.

Magkanas E, Voloudaki A, Bouros D *et al.* (2001). Pulmonary sarcoidosis: correlation of expiratory high-resolution CT findings with inspiratory patterns and pulmonary function tests. *Acta Radiol* **42**: 494–501.

Malaisamy S, Dalal B, Bimenyuy C, Soubani AO (2009). The clinical and radiologic features of nodular pulmonary sarcoidosis. *Lung* **187**: 9–15.

Mana J, Teirstein AS, Mendelson DS *et al.* (1995). Excessive thoracic computed tomography scanning in sarcoidosis. *Thorax* **50**: 1264–6.

Marom EM, McAdams HP, Palmer SM *et al.* (1999). Cystic fibrosis: usefulness of thoracic CT in the examination of patients before lung transplantation. *Radiology* **213**: 283–8.

Matthay RA, Schwarz MI, Ellis JH *et al.* (1981). Pulmonary artery hypertension in chronic obstructive pulmonary disease: determination by chest radiography. *Invest Radiol* **16**: 95–100.

McLoud TC, Putman CE, Pascual R (1974). Eggshell calcification with systemic sarcoidosis. *Chest* **66**: 515–17.

Mendelson DS, Norton K, Cohen BA *et al.* (1983). Bronchial compression: an unusual manifestation of sarcoidosis. *J Comp Assist Tomogr* **7**: 892–4.

Miller A (1981). The vanishing lung syndrome associated with pulmonary sarcoidosis. *Br J Dis Chest* **75**: 209–14.

Miller BH, Rosado-de-Christenson ML, McAdams HP, Fishback NF (1995). Thoracic sarcoidosis: radiologic–pathologic correlation. *Radiographics* **15**: 421–37.

Müller NL, Kullnig P, Miller RR (1989a). The CT findings of pulmonary sarcoidosis: analysis of 25 patients. *Am J Roentgen* **152**: 1179–82.

Müller NL, Mawson JB, Mathieson JR *et al.* (1989b). Sarcoidosis: correlation of extent of disease at CT with clinical, functional, and radiographic findings. *Radiology* **171**: 613–18.

Müller NL, Silva IS (2008). Sarcoidosis. In: Müller NL, Silva IS (eds). *Imaging of the Chest*. Saunders Elsevier, Philadelphia, pp. 668–89.

Murdoch J, Müller NL (1992). Pulmonary sarcoidosis: changes on follow-up CT examination. *Am J Roentgen* **159**: 473–7.

Naccache JM, Lavole A, Nunes H *et al.* (2008). High-resolution computed tomographic imaging of airways in sarcoidosis patients with airflow obstruction. *J Comput Assist Tomogr* **32**: 905–12.

Nagai S, Shigematsu M, Hamada K, Izumi T (1999). Clinical courses and prognoses of pulmonary sarcoidosis. *Curr Opin Pulmon Med* **5**: 293–8.

Nakatsu M, Hatabu H, Morikawa K *et al.* (2002). Large coalescent parenchymal nodules in pulmonary sarcoidosis: 'sarcoid galaxy' sign. *Am J Roentgen* **178**: 1389–93.

Nishimura K, Itoh H, Kitaichi M *et al.* (1993). Pulmonary sarcoidosis: correlation of CT and histopathologic findings. *Radiology* **189**: 105–9.

Nishimura K, Itoh H, Kitaichi M *et al.* (1995). CT and pathological correlation of pulmonary sarcoidosis. *Sem Ultra CT MR* **16**: 361–70.

Nishino M, Lee KS, Itoh H, Hatabu H (2009). The spectrum of pulmonary sarcoidosis: variations of high-resolution CT findings and clues for specific diagnosis. *Eur J Radiol* **73**: 66–73.

Nunes H, Humbert M, Capron F *et al.* (2006). Pulmonary hypertension associated with sarcoidosis: mechanisms, haemodynamics and prognosis. *Thorax* **61**: 68–74.

Nunes H, Brillet PY, Valeyre D *et al.* (2007). Imaging in sarcoidosis. *Sem Respir Crit Care Med* **28**: 102–20.

O'Connell MJ, Schimpff SC, Kirschner RH *et al.* (1975). Epithelioid granulomas in Hodgkin disease: a favorable prognostic sign? *J Am Med Assoc* **233**: 886–9.

Padley SP, Hansell DM, Flower CD, Jennings P (1991). Comparative accuracy of high resolution computed tomography and chest radiography in the diagnosis of chronic diffuse infiltrative lung disease. *Clin Radiol* **44**: 222–6.

Padley SP, Padhani AR, Nicholson A, Hansell DM (1996). Pulmonary sarcoidosis mimicking cryptogenic fibrosing alveolitis on CT. *Clin Radiol* **51**: 807–10.

Patil SN, Levin DL (1999). Distribution of thoracic lymphadenopathy in sarcoidosis using computed tomography. *J Thor Imag* **14**: 114–17.

Quaden C, Tillie-Leblond I, Delobbe A *et al.* (2005). Necrotising sarcoid granulomatosis: clinical, functional, endoscopical and radiographical evaluations. *Eur Respir J* **26**: 778–85.

Rabinowitz JG, Ulreich S, Soriano C (1974). The usual unusual manifestations of sarcoidosis and the 'hilar haze': a new diagnostic aid. *Am J Roentgen Rad Ther Nucl Med* **120**: 821–31.

Radke JR, Kaplan H, Conway WA (1980). The significance of superior vena cava syndrome developing in a patient with sarcoidosis. *Radiology* **134**: 311–12.

Remy-Jardin M, Beuscart R, Sault MC *et al.* (1990). Subpleural micronodules in diffuse infiltrative lung diseases: evaluation with thin-section CT scans. *Radiology* **177**: 133–9.

Remy-Jardin M, Giraud F, Remy J *et al.* (1993). Importance of ground-glass attenuation in chronic diffuse infiltrative lung disease: pathologic–CT correlation. *Radiology* **189**: 693–8.

Remy-Jardin M, Giraud F, Remy J *et al.* (1994). Pulmonary sarcoidosis: role of CT in the evaluation of disease activity and functional impairment and in prognosis assessment. *Radiology* **191**: 675–80.

Remy-Jardin M, Re *et al.* (1996). Diffuse infiltrative lung disease: clinical value of sliding-thin-slab maximum intensity projection CT scans in the detection of mild micronodular patterns. *Radiology* **200**: 333–9.

Roberts CM, Citron KM, Strickland B (1987). Intrathoracic aspergilloma: role of CT in diagnosis and treatment. *Radiology* **165**: 123–8.

Rockoff SD, Rohatgi PK (1985). Unusual manifestations of thoracic sarcoidosis. *Am J Roentgen* **144**: 513–28.

Rohatgi PK, Schwab LE (1980). Primary acute pulmonary cavitation in sarcoidosis. *Am J Roentgen* **134**: 1199–203.

Sacks EL, Donaldson SS, Gordon J, Dorfman RF (1978). Epithelioid granulomas associated with Hodgkin's disease: clinical correlations in 55 previously untreated patients. *Cancer* **41**: 562–7.

Sakowitz AJ, Sakowitz BH (1977). Bilateral hilar lymphadenopathy: an uncommon manifestation of adult tuberculosis. *Chest* **71**: 421–3.

Sansom HE, Baque-Juston M, Wells AU, Hansell DM (2000). Lateral cavity wall thickening as an early radiographic sign of mycetoma formation. *Eur Radiol* **10**: 387–90.

Scadding JG (1961). Prognosis of intrathoracic sarcoidosis in England: a review of 136 cases after five years' observation. *Br Med J* **2**: 1165–72.

Shah L (2007). Lung transplantation in sarcoidosis. *Sem Respir Crit Care Med* **28**: 134–40.

Sharma OP, Gordonson J (1975). Pleural effusion in sarcoidosis: a report of six cases. *Thorax* **30**: 95–101.

Sharma OP, Hewlett R, Gordonson J (1973). Nodular sarcoidosis: an unusual radiographic appearance. *Chest* **64**: 189–92.

Sharma SK, Pande JN, Mukhopadhay AK *et al.* (1987). Bilateral recurrent spontaneous pneumothoraces in sarcoidosis. *Jpn J. Med* **26**(1): 69–71.

Sider L, Horton ES (1990). Hilar and mediastinal adenopathy in sarcoidosis as detected by computed tomography: 3. *J Thorac Imag* **5**(2): 77–80.

Siltzbach LE, James DG, Neville E *et al.* (1974). Course and prognosis of sarcoidosis around the world. *Am J Med* **57**: 847–52.

Smedema JP, Snoep G, van Kroonenburgh MP *et al.* (2005). Evaluation of the accuracy of gadolinium-enhanced cardiovascular magnetic resonance in the diagnosis of cardiac sarcoidosis. *J Am Coll Cardiol* **45**: 1683–90.

Smellie H, Hoyle C (1957). The hilar lymph-nodes in sarcoidosis with special reference to prognosis. *Lancet* **273**: 66–70.

Soskel NT, Sharma OP (2000). Pleural involvement in sarcoidosis. *Curr Opin Pulmon Med* **6**: 455–68.

Strickland-Marmol LB, Fessler RG, Rojiani AM (2000). Necrotizing sarcoid granulomatosis mimicking an intracranial neoplasm: clinicopathologic features and review of the literature. *Mod Pathol* **13**: 909–13.

Sulica R, Teirstein AS, Kakarla S *et al.* (2005). Distinctive clinical, radiographic, and functional characteristics of patients with sarcoidosis-related pulmonary hypertension. *Chest* **128**: 1483–9.

Takemura T, Matsui Y, Saiki S, Mikami R (1992). Pulmonary vascular involvement in sarcoidosis: a report of 40 autopsy cases. *Hum Pathol* **23**: 1216–23.

Talbot FJ, Katz S, Matthews MJ (1959). Bronchopulmonary sarcoidosis; some unusual manifestations and the serious complications thereof. *Am J Med* **26**: 340–55.

Tan RT, Kuzo R, Goodman LR *et al.* (1998). Utility of CT scan evaluation for predicting pulmonary hypertension in patients with parenchymal lung disease. *Chest* **113**: 1250–6.

Tazi A, Sfemmes-Baleyte T, Soler P *et al.* (1994). Pulmonary sarcoidosis with a diffuse ground glass pattern on the chest radiograph. *Thorax* **49**: 793–7.

Terasaki H, Fujimoto K, Müller N *et al.* (2005). Pulmonary sarcoidosis: comparison of findings of inspiratory and expiratory high-resolution CT and pulmonary function tests between smokers and nonsmokers. *Am J Roentgen* **185**: 333–8.

Tomlinson JR., Sahn SA (1987). Aspergilloma in sarcoid and tuberculosis. *Chest* **92**: 505–8.

Udwadia ZF, Pilling JR, Jenkins PF, Harrison BD (1990). Bronchoscopic and bronchographic findings in 12 patients with sarcoidosis and severe or progressive airways obstruction. *Thorax* **45**: 272–5.

Volk M, Hamer OW, Feuerbach S, Strotzer M (2004). Dose reduction in skeletal and chest radiography using a large-area flat-panel detector based on amorphous silicon and thallium-doped cesium iodide: technical background, basic image quality parameters, and review of the literature. *Eur Radiol* **14**: 827–34.

Warshauer DM, Dumbleton SA, Molina PL *et al.* (1994). Abdominal CT findings in sarcoidosis: radiologic and clinical correlation. *Radiology* **192**: 93–8.

Webb WR (2006). Thin-section CT of the secondary pulmonary lobule: anatomy and the image. *Radiology* **239**: 322–38.

Webb WR, Müller NL, Naito H (2001). *High-resolution CT of the Lung*, 3rd edn. Lippincott Williams & Wilkins, Philadelphia.

Weitzman S, Pocock WA, Hawkins DM, Barlow JB (1974). Observer variation in radiological assessment of pulmonary vasculature. *Br Heart J* **36**: 280–90.

Wells A (1998). High-resolution computed tomography in sarcoidosis: a clinical perspective. *Sarcoid Vasc Diff Lung Dis* **15**: 140–6.

Winterbauer RH, Belic N, Moores KD (1973). Clinical interpretation of bilateral hilar adenopathy. *Ann Intern Med* **78**: 65–71.

Yanardag H, Caner M, Papila I *et al.* (2007). Diagnostic value of peripheral lymph node biopsy in sarcoidosis: a report of 67 cases. *Can Respir J* **14**: 209–11.

9

Radiologically guided interventional procedures

MAGALI N TAYLOR AND PENNY J SHAW

INTRODUCTION

This chapter covers radiologically guided tissue sampling in the diagnosis of sarcoidosis. The different techniques and equipment are described. Sarcoidosis offers a broad range of potential biopsy sites. Histologically, diagnosis is based on the identification of non-caseating epithelioid granulomas. Diagnosis by biopsy can usually be obtained (Teirstein *et al.* 2005), but may be insufficient to make a diagnosis as other conditions are associated with non-caseating granulomas. The diagnosis must be made from consideration of the clinical presentation, radiological manifestations together with laboratory tests.

Imaging with contrast-enhanced computed tomography (CT) will locate the site of disease, and its proximity to nearby structures. In most cases of suspected sarcoid, tissue is obtained via transbronchial lung biopsy at the time of bronchoscopy, or via an open lung biopsy through video-assisted thoracoscopy (VATS) or mini-thoracotomy. In a significant proportion of cases, sarcoid is included as a differential diagnosis, most commonly with TB, lymphoma and malignancy. In this situation the radiologist can identify the optimum site for tissue sampling, the mode of access, and choice of imaging modality. The location for sampling will be influenced not only by the site most likely to provide a diagnosis, but also the safest route.

METHODS OF TISSUE SAMPLING

Imaging technique

The imaging technique used to guide tissue sampling will depend on the anatomical site. In some cases of suspected sarcoid, tissue can be obtained using ultrasound (US) to sample superficial nodes (Fig. 9.1) or organs such as the liver. Ultrasound has the advantage of being readily available, fast and radiation-free, but visualization of the target lesion and surrounding structures is not always satisfactory; the deeper the lesion is to the skin, the poorer the resolution. Color Doppler is used to assess surrounding vascular structures as well as the vascularity of the lesion.

Tissue sampling of pulmonary and mediastinal lesions is usually performed using CT. Unlike ultrasound, CT will depict a lesion partially or completely surrounded by air, and allow better visualization of surrounding vascular structures (Fig. 9.2).

Positron emission tomography (PET) is playing an increasingly important role in the diagnosis and staging of many diseases. Tissue involved by sarcoid demonstrates increased fluorodeoxyglucose (FDG) uptake which can be assessed both visually and quantitatively. Involved lymph nodes may show increased uptake when not enlarged by CT criteria (in most anatomical locations this is a node

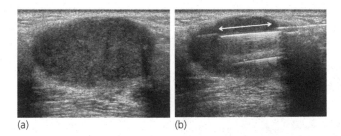

(a)   (b)

Figure 9.1   (a) Ultrasound depicting an abnormal lymph node that has become enlarged, more rounded and has lost its normal fatty hilum. (b) Ultrasound-guided lymph node biopsy was performed using a Temno 16G biopsy needle. The recess of the needle measures 2 cm (double-ended arrow) and the cutting cannula will be fired over this.

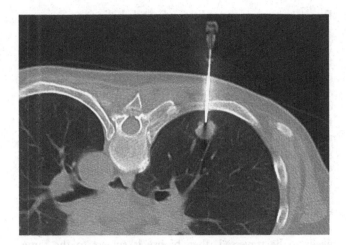

Figure 9.2 CT-guided biopsy of an intrapulmonary nodule using a Cook coaxial biopsy system (patient prone). The 16G outer needle is in position. Through this, an 18G biopsy needle will be introduced, and multiple cores taken.

measuring less than 1 cm in short axis diameter). Nodes and tissue demonstrating increased FDG activity can then be targeted for sampling (Fig. 9.3).

Magnetic resonance imaging (MRI) is reserved for guiding biopsies in patients with bone, soft tissue or articular lesions that are not well visualized by US or CT, providing a diagnostic yield of over 90 percent (Carrino *et al.* 2007).

Needles

Tissue may be obtained by using fine-needle aspiration (FNA) for cytology, or core biopsy for histology. Where possible, the latter is preferable as it has greater diagnostic yield in benign disease (Grief *et al.* 1999), with a sensitivity of 70 percent compared with 20–50 percent for FNA. This is in contrast to malignant disease where the yield is similar with a

sensitivity of 90–95 percent (Klein *et al.* 1996). Access to a cytologist during the procedure has been shown to increase the diagnostic yield of FNA.

The commonly used FNA and biopsy needles are pictured in Figure 9.4. The needles used for FNA are generally 20 to 23 gauge in size. FNA involves using a fine needle (which may be attached to a syringe under suction) and moving the needle gently in and out within the lesion to obtain cells. There are many types of needle available such as the Westcott, Chiba, Franseen and Rotex. The advantage of the Westcott is that it resembles a core biopsy needle, having a recess just proximal to the needle tip which allows small cores of tissue to be obtained in 50 percent of biopsies. The greater the gauge of the needle, the smaller its outer diameter, which not only is disadvantageous in terms of obtaining an adequate sample but the increased flexibility of the needle makes it more difficult to position. FNA, however, is more cost effective than a core biopsy and may be currently under-used (Tambouret *et al.* 2000).

The core biopsy needles are generally 14 to 18 gauge in size, the greater rigidity giving more torque and therefore improved ease of placement, especially for deeper lesions. They are available in a variety of lengths. They use a spring-loaded mechanism that fires an inner notched stylet and an outer cutting cannula when activated. Commonly used needles of this type include the Bard Biopty biopsy system, the handle portion of which is reusable, but rather heavy. Newer needles such as the Cook Quickcore and Bauer Temno biopsy devices have an inner stylet which is advanced prior to the firing of the cutting cannula, and they are disposable. The needles are designed with both a 1 cm and a 2 cm 'throw', the latter producing better cores. A coaxial system involves passing a cutting needle (usually 18 gauge), through a thin-walled introducer needle (usually 16 gauge). In this way, multiple cores can be obtained through a single pass, thereby reducing potential complications, and the duration of the procedure (Fig. 9.5).

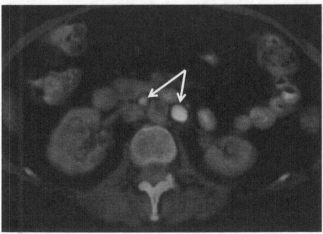

(a)

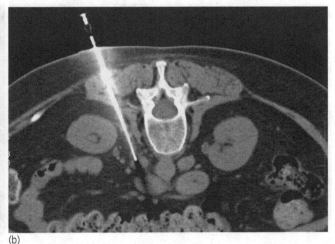

(b)

Figure 9.3 (a) Fused CT/PET scan at the level of the kidneys, showing increased FDG uptake in two para-aortic lymph nodes (arrows) (patient supine). (b) The left para-aortic node was targeted for biopsy using a Cook coaxial biopsy system (patient supine). The 16G outer needle is in position with its tip in the node. The biopsy needle will be introduced, to take samples 1 cm or 2 cm distal to the tip, depending on the node size.

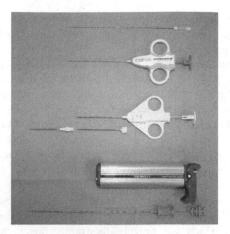

Figure 9.4   Photograph depicting the commonly used sampling needles: (a) 20G Westcott FNA needle; (b) 16G Temno biopsy system; (c) coaxial Cook 16G/18G biopsy system; d) Biopty biopsy system, with an 18G (pink) needle.

SITES FOR TISSUE SAMPLING

Sarcoidosis, being a multi-organ disease, presents a variety of sites for potential tissue diagnosis. Percutaneous sampling is performed by the radiologist, in the presence of accessible disease, when transbronchial lung or open lung biopsy is not feasible or is non-diagnostic, or where the presentation is atypical. The common sites for tissue sampling are illustrated in Figure 9.6. They include nodal and extranodal sites. A transbronchial approach using endoscopic US (EBUS) is preferable for central intrathoracic disease to sample suspected hilar or mediastinal nodes. This has largely superseded CT-guided biopsy for hilar node sampling (Fig. 9.7). Transesophageal sampling is useful for suspicious subcarinal or celiac axis lymph nodes. Mediastinoscopy or percutaneous biopsy may be indicated for mediastinal lymphadenopathy.

Percutaneous sampling of nodal disease

Sarcoid may be diagnosed histologically by obtaining tissue from abnormally appearing lymph nodes. Enlarged supraclavicular, cervical, axillary and inguinal nodes are most accessible under US guidance. Involved nodes are usually enlarged, appear rounded and lose their central fatty hilum – features that can be appreciated on both CT and US. Involved nodes may also demonstrate increased FDG activity, although generally not as high as nodes infiltrated with malignancy, and this helps identify nodes for sampling. Superficial nodes may be biopsied under US, whereas mediastinal nodes are sampled using CT guidance. When mediastinal nodal sampling is to be performed percutaneously, an approach avoiding lung parenchyma is preferable (Fig. 9.8). If lung needs to be traversed, then biopsy is subject to the same contraindications and potential complications as for a percutaneous lung biopsy (see below). Hilar nodes are usually not easily accessible percutaneously, due to their central (deep) location, and close proximity to major pulmonary vessels. Retroperitoneal nodes are ideally biopsied under CT guidance, with a coaxial system providing multiple cores for immunohistochemistry to allow differentiation from lymphoma (Fig. 9.9), whereas mesenteric nodes are biopsied under US.

Percutaneous transthoracic sampling of pulmonary lesions

Pulmonary lesions in sarcoid are not usually targeted for biopsy unless the diagnosis is uncertain and there is no suitable alternative. Pulmonary lesions are now sampled with a cutting needle rather than FNA. Use of a coaxial system increases the yield further, allowing multiple cores to be obtained through a single pleural pass, and thereby also

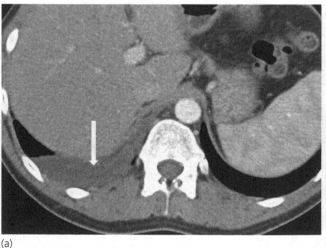

(a)

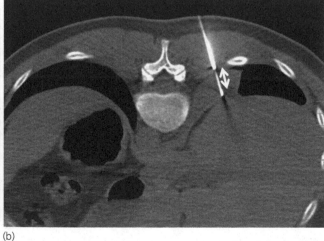

(b)

Figure 9.5   (a) Contrast-enhanced CT image of the lung bases showing a necrotic mass in the right lower lobe (arrow) (patient supine). (b) Biopsy of the lesion using a Cook coaxial system (patient prone). The inner 18G stylet has been advanced through the 16G outer needle. In this biopsy, the recess (double-ended arrow), where the core will be taken, measures 2 cm in length. The cutting cannula is about to be fired over the recess to obtain the biopsy.

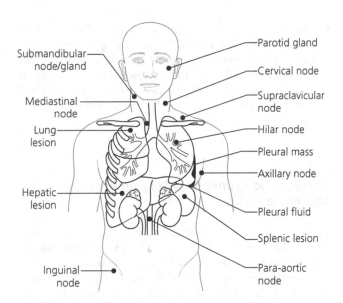

Figure 9.6   Common sites for percutaneous sampling.

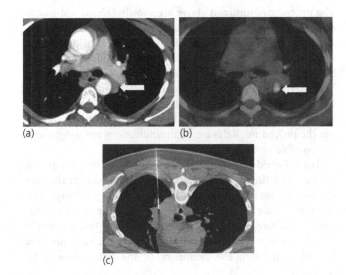

Figure 9.7   Contrast-enhanced CT image showing a left hilar node (arrow) interposed between the left main pulmonary artery and the descending aorta (patient supine). (b) Fused PET/CT image showing increased FDG uptake in the node (arrow). (c) The lymph node was targeted for CT-guided biopsy (patient prone).

reducing the pneumothorax rate. Because pulmonary and mediastinal lesions are either partially or completely surrounded by air, and because of their relation to major vascular structures, sampling is performed using CT guidance. Peripheral lesions are targeted as these require less lung parenchyma to be traversed, and pulmonary vessels at the periphery of the lung are smaller, thus reducing the risk of significant hemorrhage.

The procedure is limited with small lesions that can move in and out of the biopsy plane depending on the phase of respiration.

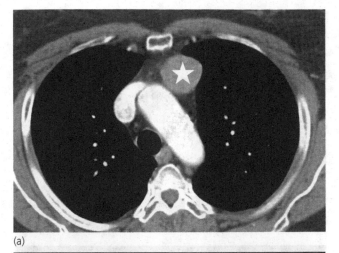

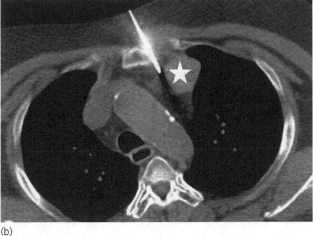

Figure 9.8   (a) Contrast-enhanced CT showing an enhancing nodal mass in the anterior mediastinum (star). (b) Biopsy of this mass was performed under CT using a coaxial Cook 16G/18G biopsy system.

Percutaneous sampling of extranodal, extrathoracic disease

The same methods described above can be used to sample extrathoracic disease.

- *Liver*. The liver is usually sampled with an 18G core biopsy needle using US guidance (Fig. 9.10). Normal liver parenchyma should be traversed en route to the lesion to reduce the risk of intraperitoneal hemorrhage, but should not be excessive which increases parenchymal hemorrhage.
- *Spleen*. FNA under US guidance is the method of choice with focal lesions, owing to the risk of bleeding with core biopsies. FNA was found to be a safe procedure being diagnostic in 83 percent of patients but in only 58 percent with benign lesions (Kang *et al.* 2007). As with liver biopsies, lesions which are peripheral but not directly subcapsular should be targeted to reduce the risk of bleeding. Some radiologists advocate performing sampling on arrested respiration to avoid lacerating the splenic capsule.

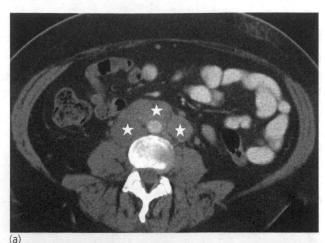

(a)

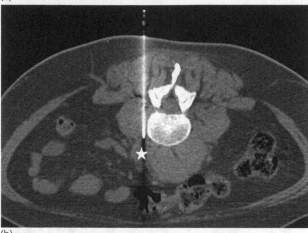

(b)

Figure 9.9 (a) Contrast-enhanced CT showing para-aortic lymphadenopathy (stars). (b) These nodes were biopsied under CT using a 16G/18G Cook coaxial system (patient prone).

- *Parotid and salivary glands.* US-guided core biopsy of focal lesions is accurate in differentiating benign from malignant disease and avoids surgery in a significant number of patients. It is superior to FNA (Buckland 1999; Kesse *et al.* 2002).

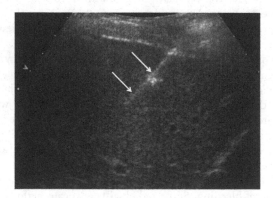

Figure 9.10 Ultrasound-guided biopsy of a liver lesion using an 18G Biopty biopsy system (arrows).

- *Pleura.* US-guided aspiration provides fluid for cytology and microbiology. Pleural biopsies using an 18G biopsy needle can be performed under US provided there is an accompanying effusion. Targeted pleural biopsies using an oblique approach without an effusion are performed under CT guidance (Fig. 9.11). Sarcoidosis can rarely present with a chylothorax.

Therapeutic bronchial artery angiography and embolization

Massive hemoptysis is defined as coughing up more than 600 mL of blood in 48 hours. Chronic cavitary sarcoid infected with an aspergilloma is an uncommon cause. Bronchial arteriography is initially required prior to embolization, as 95 percent of the hemoptysis comes from the bronchial arteries (Jackson 1996) (Fig. 9.12).

PROCEDURES

The procedures outlined above are mostly carried out in the outpatient setting, during allocated appointments or as day cases. A full blood count and coagulation screen is performed routinely before any biopsy. Aspirin and clopidogrel should be stopped 5 and 14 days respectively prior to the procedure. The international normalized ratio (INR) should be less than or equal to 1.4. The patient should be fasted. Written informed consent is obtained from the radiologist carrying out the procedure. Relevant contraindications are sought and the possible complications are discussed.

For CT-guided procedures, the position of needle entry is marked with the use of a surface grid positioned over the area of interest on the patient's skin prior to scanning. The procedures are carried out under local anesthetic, and sedation is rarely needed. Several samples are taken (usually 2 to 5 passes). Where the lesions appears partially necrotic (usually centrally), the periphery of the lesion should be sampled.

Samples are sent to both histology/cytology and microbiology. FNA samples are smeared on to slides, fixed with alcohol and sent to cytology. A saline wash of the needle is taken for microbiology. Core biopsies are placed in formalin for histopathology and immunochemistry and in saline for microbiology. The samples should reach the relevant departments without delay.

Following superficial lymph node FNA/biopsy, patients can go home straight away provided there are no immediate complications. For transpulmonary biopsies, patients are monitored in the programmed investigation unit in the radiology department for 5 hours after the procedure. A chest X-ray is taken at 1 hour and 4 hours post biopsy to check for a pneumothorax and to identify if it is increasing in size. A pneumothorax is usually apparent at the time of the procedure and high-flow oxygen should be administered as this increases the rate of pneumothorax reabsorption. The patient should be biopsy-side down where possible to reduce

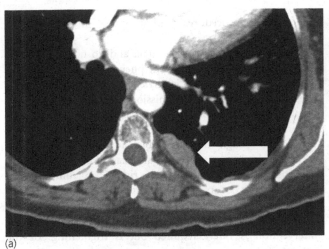
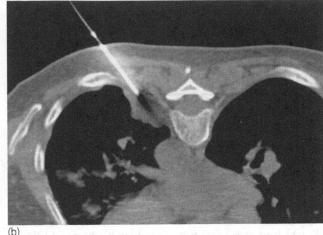

(a)   (b)

Figure 9.11   (a) Contrast-enhanced CT showing a left posterior, pleurally based mass (arrow) (patient supine). b) The mass was biopsied under CT using a coaxial Cook 16G/18G system (patient prone).

the risk of pneumothorax, and heart rate, blood pressure, respiratory rate and pulse oximetry should be monitored regularly. Prior to patient discharge, the symptoms of delayed or expanding pneumothorax are explained. For deep node/mass biopsies that do not require a transpulmonary approach, the patient should be similarly monitored but chest radiography is not necessary.

Following liver and splenic FNA/biopsy, the patient should be placed biopsy-side down to reduce the risk of

bleeding. Following a period of observation in the unit, patients are sent home the same day provided there are no complications evident. There is a significant risk of delayed bleeding (>24 hours), and patients should be made aware of symptoms relating to this prior to discharge, and have a reliable person present overnight.

CONTRAINDICATIONS

The contraindications to needle biopsy are summarized in Box 9.1. Where there is a need to traverse lung, relative contraindications include pulmonary fibrosis and emphysema, as a pneumothorax in these circumstances could be life-threatening. Biopsy may be possible if the lesion is peripheral and lung parenchyma is not traversed. It is important that the patient is cooperative and able to lie still in the supine or prone position for up to 40 minutes. Each patient is

Figure 9.12   Bronchial angiogram showing hypertrophied left bronchial artery. The inferior left bronchial artery has been catheterized via the aorta (arrow). Courtesy of Dr Duncan Brennand, University College London Hospital.

Box 9.1 Relative contraindications to needle biopsy

General
- Bleeding disorders, thrombocytopenia, anticoagulant therapy
- Uncooperative patient/inability to lie still

Specific to lung
- Poor lung function (FEV$_1$ <40% or multiple bullae)
- Pulmonary fibrosis
- Pneumonectomy
- Pulmonary hypertension
- Small nodules <5 mm diameter

Specific to liver
- Ascites
- Biliary obstruction

FEV$_1$, forced expiratory volume in 1 second.

considered individually, following discussion at the relevant multidisciplinary meeting.

COMPLICATIONS

The complications of needle biopsy are summarized in Box 9.2. Risk–benefit must always be considered.

The main complications of lung biopsies or biopsies passing through the lung are pneumothorax and hemorrhage (which may produce hemoptysis) (Fig. 9.13). Contrary to popular belief, the complication rate does not increase by using a larger cutting needle as opposed to a fine needle. In keeping with other studies, a 2002 survey performed in the UK, which reviewed data from 5444 lung biopsies and FNAs, found no difference in the complication rates between the two methods (Richardson *et al.* 2002). The pneumothorax

rate for both procedures is in the range of 3–42 percent (Lacasse *et al.* 1999).

Most pneumothoraces are small and do not require any intervention. When a significant pneumothorax does occur, aspiration via a 3-way tap is carried out, and only rarely is a chest drain and overnight admission necessary. Patients with emphysema or pulmonary fibrosis are at increased risk of a pneumothorax, as are those with small central lesions, and those who cough uncontrollably during the procedure. Where multiple pleural passes are made, or where fissures are crossed, this also increases the risk of a pneumothorax.

Hemoptysis occurs in 4–5 percent of biopsies (Richardson *et al.* 2002), being more common in those patients with pulmonary hypertension. It usually resolves quickly and intervention is rarely required but is frightening for the patient.

A systemic arterial embolism (SAAE) is a potentially fatal complication of interventional lung procedures. Its incidence may not be as rare as previously thought, and its sequelae can be subclinical (Hiraki *et al.* 2007). It occurs as a result of air being introduced into the pulmonary venous circulation and subsequently occluding the cerebral or coronary arteries via the left atrium and ventricle, either from a pulmonary vein communicating with atmospheric air though the needle, or a pulmonary vein communicating with an airway through the needle tract. The former is more likely to occur if the patient takes a breath in (thereby causing a negative pressure gradient) while the stylet/cutting needle is being removed post-sampling or reintroduced pre-sampling. To minimize this risk, the hub of the introducer needle which remains in the lesion is occluded with the operator's thumb in the interim period; arrested respiration at this time may also prevent this scenario. The latter situation usually occurs when the patient coughs during the procedure. Prompt recognition of air embolism and treatment is important. A CT scan of the head and neck should be performed to confirm the diagnosis. The patient should be placed in the right lateral decubitus position (left side up), until definitive treatment with hyperbaric oxygen therapy can be instigated. Some centers

---

Box 9.2 Complications of needle biopsy

General
- Vascular: bleeding/hematoma/pseudoaneurysm
- Infection (rare)
- Damage to local structures
- Non-diagnostic/need for repeat procedure

Specific to lung
- Pneumothorax
- Hemorrhage along the tract
- Hemoptysis
- Air embolism (rare)
- Empyema

Specific to liver
- Pneumothorax
- Bile leak
- Pseudoaneurysm

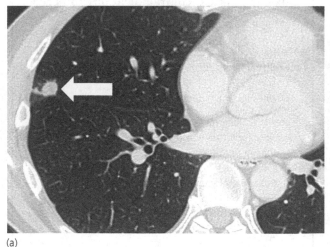

(a)

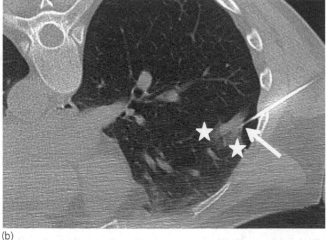

(b)

Figure 9.13   (a) CT scan demonstrating a small pulmonary nodule (arrow). (b) Biopsy of the nodule resulted in a small pneumothorax (arrow) and peri-lesional ground-glass change in keeping with hemorrhage (stars).

advocate routinely scanning the entire chest after the procedure to look for complications, including air within the left cardiac chambers, so that treatment can be instigated even with subclinical SAAEs. Death from needle biopsy of the lung occurs in 0.07–0.15 percent (Richardson *et al.* 2002; Tomiyama *et al.* 2006).

The main complication of hepatic and splenic FNA or biopsy is bleeding, which may be delayed (>24 hours). Bleeding is most commonly subcapsular or parenchymal (seen on 23 percent of ultrasound images obtained after liver biopsy), and less commonly into the biliary tree (hemobilia) in the case of liver biopsies, or into the peritoneal cavity (Reddy and Schiff 1996). There is also a small risk of pneumothorax for lesions close to the hemi-diaphragms.

PITFALLS

If FNA or biopsy is non-diagnostic it should be repeated or an alternative method of sampling considered. Sarcoid-like granulomas are commonly found in Hodgkin's lymphoma and less commonly in association with non-Hodgkin's lymphoma. In some cases, this sarcoid granulomatous process may be so extensive as to mask the underlying malignancy (Dunphy *et al.* 2000). Granulomatous sarcoid-like reactions may also occur in lymph nodes that drain seminomas, carcinomas, and less commonly sarcomas. It is important to be aware of this when sampling mediastinal or hilar nodes in the presence of a lung nodule/mass, or with extensive retroperitoneal lymphadenopathy.

REFERENCES

Buckland JR, Manjaly G, Violaris N, Howlett DC (199). Ultrasound-guided cutting-needle biopsy of the parotid gland. *J Laryngol Otol* 113: 988–92.

Carrino JA, Khurana B, Ready JE *et al.* (2007). Magnetic resonance imaging-guided percutaneous biopsy of musculoskeletal lesions. *J Bone Joint Surg Am* 89: 2179–87.

Dunphy CH, Panella MJ, Grosso LE (2000). Low-grade B-cell lymphoma and concomitant extensive sarcoidlike granulomas. *Arch Pathol Lab Med* 124: 152–6.

Greif J, Marmor S, Schwarz Y *et al.* (1999). Percutaneous core needle biopsy versus fine needle aspiration in diagnosing benign lung lesions. *Acta Cytol* 43: 756–60.

Hare SS, Gupta A, Goncalves ATC *et al.* (2011). Systemic arterial air embolism after percutaneous lung biopsy. *Clin Radiol* 66: 589–96.

Hiraki T, Fujiwara H, Sakurai J *et al.* (2007). Nonfatal systemic air embolism complicating percutaneous CT-guided transthoracic needle biopsy: four cases from a single institution. *Chest* 132: 684–90.

Jackson J (1996). Interventional radiology within the thorax. In: Watkinson A, Adam A (eds). *Interventional Radiology: A Practical Guide*. Radcliffe Medical Press, Oxford, pp. 147–72.

Kang M, Kalra N, Gulati M *et al.* (2007). Image-guided percutaneous splenic interventions. *Eur J Radiol* 64: 140–6.

Kesse KW, Manjaly G, Violaris N, Howlett DC (2002). Ultrasound-guided biopsy in the evaluation of focal lesions and diffuse swelling of the parotid gland. *Br J Oral Maxillofac Surg* 40: 384–8.

Klein JS, Salomon G, Stewart EA (1996). Transthoracic needle biopsy with a coaxially placed 20-gauge automated cutting needle: results in 122 patients. *Radiology* 198: 715–20.

Lacasse Y, Wong E, Guyatt G, Cook D (1999). Transthoracic needle aspiration biopsy for the diagnosis of localised pulmonary lesions: a meta-analysis. *Thorax* 54: 884–93.

Reddy KR, Schiff ER (1996). Complications of liver biopsy. In: Taylor MB, (ed.). *Gastrointestinal Emergencies*, 2nd edn. Williams & Wilkins, Baltimore.

Richardson CM, Pointon KS, Manhire AR, Macfarlane JT (2002). Percutaneous lung biopsies: a survey of UK practice based on 5444 biopsies. *Br J Radiol* 75: 731–5.

Tambouret R, Geisinger KR, Powers CN *et al.* (2000). The clinical application and cost analysis of fine-needle aspiration biopsy in the diagnosis of mass lesions in sarcoidosis. *Chest* 117: 1004–11.

Teirstein AS, Judson MA, Baughman RP *et al.* (2005). The spectrum of biopsy sites for the diagnosis of sarcoidosis. *Sarcoid Vasc Diffuse Lung Dis* 22: 139–46.

Tomiyama N, Yasuhara Y, Nakajima Y *et al.* (2006). CT-guided needle biopsy of lung lesions: a survey of severe complication based on 9783 biopsies in Japan. *Eur J Radiol* 59: 60–4.

10

Staging and monitoring pulmonary sarcoidosis: pulmonary function tests and other variables

ATHOL WELLS, HELEN PARFREY, SIMON WARD AND DEREK CRAMER

INTRODUCTION

Although chest radiographic abnormalities are present in 85–95 percent of patients with sarcoidosis, many are asymptomatic whereas other patients experience progressive respiratory compromise or disabling systemic symptoms. The Scadding chest radiographic staging system, although providing broad prognostic distinctions between patient cohorts, does not reliably distinguish between reversible, stable and progressive lung disease in individual patients. These uncertainties cause major management difficulties for clinicians, especially in distinguishing between strategies of observation without immediate treatment, therapeutic intervention to reverse disease and treatment of irreversible disease to minimize further damage and symptomatic deterioration.

As the majority of deaths from sarcoidosis result from respiratory failure, the precise staging of pulmonary disease severity and the reliable detection of disease progression are both central to accurate management. However, there is no universally agreed definition of 'active' pulmonary disease (Turner-Warwick *et al.* 1986). Systemic symptoms correlate poorly with the extent of pulmonary involvement. Respiratory symptoms, including cough, exertional dyspnea and chest discomfort, are often minor until the pulmonary reserve is seriously compromised, but may be prominent in other cases in which there is mild underlying lung disease. Physical findings in the lungs tend to be minimal in mild to moderate pulmonary sarcoidosis: even when radiographic infiltrates are extensive, crackles are present in fewer than 20 percent of cases. The reliable identification of clinically significant changes in pulmonary disease has also proved problematic. Many tests used to assess baseline disease severity are not well suited to monitoring progression and other tests have not been validated for the identification of change. In routine practice, most clinical algorithms for serial monitoring make use of chest radiography and spirometric volumes, based on the ready availability of these tests.

In this chapter, we discuss difficulties in the staging and monitoring of pulmonary disease severity in sarcoidosis. The limitations of other tests used historically for these purposes are summarized, to highlight the central role of pulmonary function tests, which are discussed in detail. Quality assurance in pulmonary function estimation and the determination of fitness to fly in the pulmonary function laboratory are also reviewed.

QUANTIFICATION OF PULMONARY DISEASE SEVERITY

Historically, the severity of pulmonary sarcoidosis has been quantified by the degree of exercise tolerance, chest radiographic abnormalities and pulmonary function tests. However, it has long been recognized that, in diffuse lung disease, the level of pulmonary function impairment is a more accurate indicator of the histological severity of pulmonary disease than the severity of respiratory symptoms or findings on chest radiography (Keogh and Crystal 1980). This truism applies especially to pulmonary sarcoidosis.

As a measure of disease severity, exertional dyspnea is both insensitive and non-specific. In health, there is considerable pulmonary reserve: pulmonary disease may be moderately advanced before there is significant limitation in day-to-day life. Not infrequently, DLco levels of 50–60 percent of predicted normal are associated with little or no reduction in exercise tolerance, and this is especially the case when disease progression has been insidious, allowing adaptation to loss of pulmonary function. By contrast, in more rapidly progressive disease, in which the slow process of adaptation has not occurred, lesser reductions in DLco and lung volumes may cause significant limitation. The non-specific nature of dyspnea is an even more important constraint. Cardiac involvement, pulmonary vascular disease, anemia, proximal myopathy due to corticosteroid therapy and, especially, the musculoskeletal complications of sarcoidosis (resulting in increased respiratory work during locomotion) may all contribute to limiting dyspnea in sarcoidosis, even when pulmonary function tests are normal or near to normal. Distressing cough due to airway inflammation is sometimes triggered by exertion and this may make it difficult to assess whether exercise intolerance is primarily due to pulmonary parenchymal disease.

The severity of chest radiographic findings is also an imprecise guide to underlying disease severity, except in the minority of patients with overt extensive fibrotic abnormalities. Abnormalities are present on chest radiography in 85–95 percent of patients with sarcoidosis, but a significant minority is entirely asymptomatic. As discussed elsewhere in more detail, bilateral hilar adenopathy is the most frequent chest radiographic abnormality, occurring in up to 80 percent of cases. Among the 20–50 percent of patients with radiographic pulmonary parenchymal involvement, most do not have gross scarring or major distortion of the lung parenchyma: lesser abnormalities range from very minor limited linear change to more extensive reticulonodular infiltration, ground-glass opacification, alveolar opacities and large nodules.

The most common pattern is one of reticulonodular opacities, seen in 85–90 percent. Importantly, these changes are generally most prominent in the middle and upper zones, and this can lead to an over-estimation of disease severity. Upper-zone changes tend to be more readily visualized on chest radiography and often overstate overall disease severity, owing to the two-dimensional nature of the chest radiograph. It is not uncommon to find that, on high-resolution computed tomography (HRCT), abnormalities that are apparently prominent on chest radiography are relatively limited and associated with normal HRCT findings in a large part of the total lung volume. More importantly, the upper zones of the lung contribute little to pulmonary function and, thus, regionally severe disease confined to the upper lobes may be associated with normal exercise tolerance and little reduction in pulmonary function indices.

By contrast, in an important minority of patients, fibrotic contraction may lead to upward displacement of the hila with distortion of accompanying blood vessels and fissures. In these cases, a large proportion of the lung may contract down into a relatively small fibrotic volume, with the result that radiographic appearances may seriously understate disease severity.

Thus, the level of symptoms is a notoriously unreliable guide and the chest radiograph may seriously overstate or understate disease severity. Experienced chest physicians have come to understand that, in patients with apparently alarming upper-zone radiographic abnormalities, it is correct to question whether disease is truly clinically significant and, in some cases, to defer therapeutic intervention if the level of pulmonary function impairment is relatively mild. In essence, decisions on treatment should not be based on the chest radiograph in isolation.

In principle, it might be supposed that HRCT should play a useful ancillary role in the staging of pulmonary sarcoidosis, in allowing a more accurate estimation of the global morphologic extent of disease. However, the role of HRCT in this regard remains contentious. Based on accumulated experience in one leading center (Costabel and Guzman 2001), it was argued that thoracic HRCT was warranted in approximately 30 percent of patients with sarcoidosis in order to clarify chest radiographic findings, with the added advantage that HRCT patterns 'pathognomonic' of sarcoidosis are useful in atypical cases when the diagnosis of sarcoidosis is elusive. Moreover, as discussed elsewhere in detail, HRCT may provide prognostic information in some cases, as certain patterns (nodules, septal lines, consolidation) generally regress with therapy whereas others (irregular coarse lines, cysts, honeycombing, traction bronchiectasis, architectural distortion) are reliably irreversible (Remy-Jardin et al. 1994; Hansell et al. 2005).

However, although it can be argued that HRCT should be performed at presentation in most patients with chest radiographic abnormalities, in order to provide more reliable information on disease severity, this view has yet to be validated. Correlations between HRCT findings and pulmonary function tests have been explored in several studies. In the largest of these, the accuracy of HRCT was evaluated in the assessment of functional impairment in 95 patients with confirmed pulmonary sarcoidosis (Remy-Jardin et al. 1994). The extent of each abnormal pattern was quantified for upper, mid and lower zones as a percentage 'score' by means of visual estimation. The scores for each type of abnormality were summed to provide an overall HRCT severity score (range 0–84). However, correlations between individual HRCT patterns and pulmonary function indices were weak. From this study, it can be concluded that the extent of disease on HRCT is not a good predictor of functional impairment in any individual patients.

These findings highlight the dilemma faced by clinicians in the use of HRCT in staging pulmonary disease. HRCT provides a great deal of morphological information and it might be supposed that it should provide important clinical information when integrated with pulmonary function tests. However, no easily used HRCT scoring system has been validated for this purpose. An attempt has been made to reduce the complexity of HRCT scoring (Drent et al. 2003), adapted from a more complex system (Oberstein et al. 1997). This approach consisted of the semi-quantitative scoring of the extent of thickening or irregularity of the bronchovascular bundle, intra-parenchymal nodules, septal and non-septal lines, parenchymal consolidation, focal pleural thickening and enlargement of lymph nodes, graded using a four-point scale (0: no lesions found; 1: up to 33 percent; 2: up to 66 percent, and 3: more than 66 percent), with sub-scores summed to provide an overall HRCT score of disease extent. However, although moderate correlations were seen with pulmonary function variables (including FEV_1, FVC and DLco), with Spearman's rank correlation coefficient range of -0.43 to -0.71, this system has yet to be integrated into clinical practice. A readily applicable HRCT scoring system needs to be rapid, easy to learn and reproducible. No HRCT system that satisfies these criteria has been shown to provide useful information in routine clinical practice.

Thus, the staging of disease severity using symptomatic severity and the morphological extent of disease on chest radiography and HRCT is fraught with difficulty. In this context, pulmonary function estimation plays a crucial role.

PULMONARY FUNCTION TESTS IN THE STAGING OF DISEASE SEVERITY

Before pulmonary function tests (PFTs) are considered in detail, their most important limitation in the staging of pulmonary sarcoidosis needs to be highlighted.

Normal pulmonary function values have been defined in a number of populations and are expressed as a normal range, which is computed from patient age, gender and height, with significant ethnic variation. Normality in values for FEV_1, FVC and DLco ranges from 80 to 120 percent of the value predicted for these variables. Herein lies an important problem. The clinician has no knowledge of pulmonary function values in an individual patient before the onset of disease. In a patient presenting with apparently minor reduction in spirometric volumes to, for example, 75 percent of predicted normal, the clinician has no means of knowing whether these values represent a very minor fall from premorbid values of 80 percent of predicted, a very major fall from premorbid values of 120 percent of predicted, or a reduction that lies somewhere in between.

This problem is common to the use of PFTs in all forms of diffuse lung disease. However, in many other diseases, such as idiopathic pulmonary fibrosis and the other idiopathic interstitial pneumonias, pulmonary function impairment tends to be more severe, on average, than in pulmonary sarcoidosis, and the confounding effect of variation in the normal range tends to be less important. Similarly, in the minority of sarcoidosis patients with severe pulmonary disease, major reductions in pulmonary function indices can be interpreted with confidence. By contrast, in the majority of patients with pulmonary sarcoidosis, lung function impairment is relatively mild, or values lie within the normal range. In this context, pulmonary function values are equally influenced by disease severity and by variation in normal premorbid values. As discussed later, this difficulty can only be addressed by integrating pulmonary function data with clinical and radiographic findings in a 'gestalt' assessment of disease severity.

Pulmonary function tests in sarcoidosis are abnormal in approximately 20 percent of patients with radiographic stage I disease, and in 20–80 percent of patients with stage II to IV chest radiographic appearances. Although pulmonary sarcoidosis is widely viewed as an interstitial lung disease, based on the presence of non-caseating granulomas in the alveolar walls, small lymphatics, perivascular and peribronchiolar regions, histological abnormalities frequently involve the larger airways and, less commonly, the respiratory muscles. Moreover, cardiac involvement and pulmonary vascular disease (which is increasingly diagnosed in sarcoidosis) also have a variable, and sometimes major, impact on pulmonary function variables, especially on measures of gas transfer and arterial gases. Thus, lung function abnormalities in sarcoidosis may arise from any pulmonary compartment. As a result, the wide spectrum of patterns of functional impairment in sarcoidosis includes airflow obstruction, lung restriction, a mixed obstructive/restrictive ventilatory effect, and disproportionate reduction in gas transfer (suggestive of a pulmonary vasculopathy).

In many sarcoidosis patients with severe parenchymal lung disease, there is prominent lung restriction and this is most commonly associated with chest radiographic stages III and IV (Romer 1982; Neville et al. 1983; Alhamad et al. 2001). However, lung restriction is not confined to this subgroup of patients but can be associated with any chest radiographic stage. A restrictive ventilatory defect, with reductions in FVC of 15–25 percent, in combination with reductions in DLco of 25–50 percent, has occurred in patients with radiological stage 0 disease (Harrison et al. 1991; Alhamad et al. 2001). Reductions in the diffusing capacity for carbon monoxide (DLco) have been reported in up to 50 percent of patients with sarcoidosis, but this is usually less severe than in patients with idiopathic pulmonary fibrosis (Lynch et al. 1997).

Airflow obstruction has been more prevalent than lung restriction in a number of sarcoidosis cohorts and has been found in up to 60 percent of cases. It has been argued that airflow obstruction is an early feature of sarcoidosis, corresponding to granulomatous bronchiolitis and preceding the development of fibrotic disease. However, in one longitudinal study, airflow obstruction occurred at all radiographic stages of disease and was the most common pulmonary physiologic abnormality, increasing in prevalence with increasing chest radiographic stage (Harrison et al. 1991). In HRCT studies of sarcoidosis patients with established disease, the predominant morphological findings associated with airflow obstruction have been fibrotic reticular abnormalities, peribronchial thickening and mosaic attenuation (Gleeson et al. 1996; Hansell et al. 1998). These associations are likely to correspond to the historical chest radiographic observation that airflow obstruction may accompany distortion due to surrounding parenchymal fibrosis (Levinson et al. 1977), corresponding to the histological observation of peribronchiolar fibrosis (Carrington 1976) and explaining why airflow obstruction does not respond to treatment in most cases. Endoluminal fibrotic stenoses of large airways, as a sequel to endobronchial granulomatous lesions, may occasionally result in severe airflow obstruction (Chambellan et al. 2005), but this mechanism of airflow obstruction appears to be much less prevalent than peribronchial fibrosis in fibrotic interstitial disease. Very rarely, airflow obstruction may be due to airway compression by enlarged lymph nodes.

In spite of the presence of major airflow obstruction in an important subgroup of patients, FVC and DLco levels have been regarded historically as the most accurate pulmonary function measures of pulmonary involvement in sarcoidosis. However, it will be obvious from the discussion above that 'average' statements of this type fail to take into account the heterogeneous spectrum of patterns of pulmonary function impairment encountered. Indeed, FEV_1 levels were more tightly linked to global morphological abnormalities on HRCT than FVC or DLco levels, in one study (Hansell et al. 1998), in keeping with the fact that FEV_1 levels are reduced in both obstructive and restrictive disorders, whereas FVC levels are less impaired in mild to moderate airflow obstruction. However, spirometric volumes do not reflect disease severity in a third subset of patients with disproportionate reduction in DLco. Thus, it must be concluded that no single pulmonary function test is equal to the accurate staging of pulmonary disease in all cases.

A more logical approach is to evaluate the pattern of pulmonary function impairment in individual patients and to select as the cardinal measure of severity the most impaired variable among FEV_1, FVC, DLco and, in end-stage disease, po_2 levels. For the purpose, minimum baseline staging should include the measurement of spirometric volumes and measures of gas transfer at initial evaluation. Only by this means can the pattern of pulmonary function impairment be fully understood in individual patients. Ideally, plethysmographic volumes should also be evaluated at baseline, to refine the assessment of airflow obstruction and lung restriction, and because this allows subsequent monitoring of TLC levels as a substitute for FVC in patients who develop contraindications to spirometry – such as chest wall pain and glaucoma.

It should be acknowledged that no studies exist that establish, either in sarcoidosis or in diffuse lung disease in general, that FVC is intrinsically more accurate in staging and monitoring disease than other measures of volume including TLC, VA and slow VC (which may be less variable than FVC). Similarly, alternatives measures of airflow obstruction include RV, TLC, airflow at low lung volumes, evaluation of the expiratory flow volume curve and the RV/TLC ratio, which may be particularly useful in the identification of obstruction in the presence of restriction: none of these variables has been formally compared to FEV_1 levels and the FEV_1/FVC ratio. Spirometric variables have a primary role in sarcoidosis in the evaluation of patterns of ventilatory impairment for historical reasons, including cost and ease of measurement in the outpatient clinic. However, mixed ventilatory patterns are common in sarcoidosis. Thus, the integration of spirometric and plethysmographic variables, in order to deconstruct obstructive and restrictive components, adds usefully to pulmonary function evaluation.

The accuracy of pulmonary function tests in initial staging can be evaluated by examining the linkage between individual variables and mortality, an approach that has provided invaluable insights in idiopathic pulmonary fibrosis and other forms of progressive fibrotic lung disease. However, when examined across the whole range of disease severity, baseline pulmonary function tests values have not consistently been predictive of long-term mortality in sarcoidosis. Thus, in this regard, sarcoidosis differs strikingly from idiopathic pulmonary fibrosis, a disease in which mortality has been consistently linked to the severity of impairment of a number of pulmonary function variables at presentation. This difference is likely to reflect the major variability in responsiveness to treatment in sarcoidosis. In idiopathic pulmonary fibrosis, disease invariably progresses sooner or later despite treatment. By contrast, some sarcoidosis patients with severe pulmonary impairment have striking regression of disease with treatment and, in other cases, therapeutic intervention results in the prevention or slowing of progression of irreversible disease.

Even in advanced disease, pulmonary function variables do not reliably predict outcome in pulmonary sarcoidosis. In one retrospective cohort study, a variety of demographic and clinical variables, including selected pulmonary function variables, were examined against mortality in patients with advanced sarcoidosis awaiting lung transplantation (Shorr et al. 2003). Data from 405 patients listed on the United Organ Sharing Network (UNOS) between 1995 and 2000 were evaluated. African-American ethnicity, the use of supplemental oxygen and elevated mean pulmonary artery pressure predicted mortality at two years. However, FVC levels did not differ significantly between survivors and non-survivors (41.3 ± 13.5 percent vs 43.1 ± 13.1 percent). Importantly, given the malignant prognostic significance of pulmonary hypertension, measures of gas transfer (DLco and Kco levels) were not collected in this study.

In the most recent guidelines for the assessment and management of pulmonary sarcoidosis, minimum recommended pulmonary function staging consisted of the measurement of spirometric volumes (Joint Statement 1999). It is likely that this recommendation will be expanded when revised guidelines are eventually issued. The frequency of disproportionate reduction in DLco levels in pulmonary sarcoidosis is increasingly recognized, even when there is no other overt evidence of pulmonary vascular disease, and, thus, gas transfer should routinely be measured at baseline. However, the importance of DLco estimation in not confined to the evaluation of interstitial lung disease. Pulmonary hypertension has traditionally been viewed as a rare complication of sarcoidosis, a view that was endorsed by echocardiographic findings in a large series of Japanese patients with sarcoidosis. However, in chronic pulmonary sarcoidosis, pulmonary arterial hypertension has a significant prevalence – approaching 50 percent in one report (Baughman et al. 2006) – in sarcoidosis patients with chronic exercise intolerance.

In diffuse lung disease at large, and in idiopathic pulmonary fibrosis in particular, the degree of reduction in spirometric and plethysmographic volumes is not reliably predictive of the presence of pulmonary hypertension. In sarcoidosis, the identification of pulmonary hypertension is complicated by the multiplicity of mechanisms of pulmonary vasculopathy, other than changes secondary to severe interstitial disease, discussed in detail elsewhere in this book. Thus, the measurement of DLco at baseline provides a means of identifying patients more likely to have severe pulmonary vascular disease as well as those at higher risk of developing pulmonary hypertension later in the course of disease. However, the difficulty of detecting pulmonary vascular disease in the presence of interstitial lung disease must be emphasized. The cardinal pulmonary function profile, a reduction in DLco levels which is disproportionate to lung volumes, should prompt further investigation for pulmonary hypertension (Burke et al. 1987). This pattern of pulmonary function impairment does not distinguish between a primary pulmonary vasculopathy and secondary pulmonary hypertension.

Traditionally, reductions in Kco levels (the DLco/VA ratio) have been used to quantify disproportionate reductions in DLco. In more recent reports, a high FVC/DLco ratio has indicated a higher likelihood of pulmonary hypertension (Steen et al. 1992; Nathan et al. 2007). It is likely that the two ratios provide approximately equivalent information but this view needs to be confirmed in future studies. In principle, it might be expected that the FVC/DLco ratio should be less reproducible as it is subject to the variability of both spirometric and gas transfer measurement, whereas Kco is measured with a single maneuver. Importantly, disproportionate reduction in DLco is only an approximate guide as to the likelihood of pulmonary hypertension. No single value of either ratio has been identified as an optimal diagnostic threshold. In part this reflects the considerable reserve in the pulmonary circulation, such that considerable ablation of the pulmonary vasculature may occur before pulmonary hypertension supervenes. Thus, measurements of Kco levels or the FVC/DLco ratio are useful in triggering investigations to confirm or exclude pulmonary hypertension but are not diagnostic in isolation. The likelihood of underlying pulmonary hypertension is further increased when a disproportionate reduction in gas transfer is associated with severe resting hypoxia or major arterial oxygen desaturation with minor exertion.

Arterial gases at rest are of relatively little value in the baseline evaluation of pulmonary sarcoidosis, unless disease is advanced or there is prominent exercise limitation and pulmonary hypertension is suspected. In common with other fibrotic diffuse lung diseases, hypoxia in pulmonary sarcoidosis is usually associated with pco_2 levels that are slightly reduced or at the lower limit of normal, except in end-stage disease. In the absence of pulmonary hypertension, severe hypoxia is a late feature, due to the protective effect of alveolar hyperventilation which allows preservation of po_2 levels in association with significant widening of the alveolar–arterial oxygen gradient.

The role of exercise testing in the staging of pulmonary sarcoidosis is uncertain. As in idiopathic pulmonary fibrosis, maximal exercise testing has no role in routine evaluation. However, in selected cases, maximal exercise testing may be useful in the evaluation of unexplained troublesome dyspnea, which is not explained by resting pulmonary and cardiac investigations. Exercise testing is used to reproduce the limitation described by the patient. If exercise is limited by severe desaturation, it can be concluded that investigations at rest have understated the degree of cardiopulmonary limitation. In other patients with undue exercise limitation, there is little or no desaturation or widening of the alveolar–arterial oxygen gradient at the end of maximal exercise and it is possible to conclude that limitation is due to chest discomfort, loss of fitness or musculoskeletal factors. Thus, maximal exercise testing is more often useful in demonstrating the absence of significant cardiopulmonary limitation than in quantifying the exact impact of pulmonary disease.

The six-minute walk test is now widely performed in the routine evaluation of diffuse lung disease, but at present there are no compelling data to support a similar utility in pulmonary sarcoidosis. More than in most other forms of idiopathic diffuse lung disease, the six-minute walk test needs to be interpreted with caution in pulmonary sarcoidosis as its performance is heavily influenced by musculoskeletal factors, pulmonary vasculopathy and separate cardiac involvement, as well as by deconditioning and the beneficial effects of rehabilitation. However, although not currently recommended in routine staging, the six-minute walk test may be useful for a number of reasons. Significant reduction in the six-minute walk distance may provide a useful 'gestalt' statement of the overall impact of pulmonary and extrapulmonary sarcoidosis on exercise tolerance. The test, which better reflects normal daily activity than maximal exercise testing, sometimes demonstrates much better exercise tolerance than described by the patient. In advanced disease, the test may be useful in the appraisal of the need for ambulatory oxygen. Finally, striking exercise desaturation may alert the clinician to the possibility of underlying pulmonary hypertension.

ASSESSMENT OF 'PULMONARY DISEASE ACTIVITY'

Up to this point, the evaluation of pulmonary disease severity has been discussed in detail. An additional clinical goal has been the assessment of pulmonary *disease activity*, which can loosely be defined as the presence of clinically significant inflammatory disease.

From time to time, the equation of active disease with reversible disease has led to confusion. While regression of disease with treatment is reliably indicative of major inflammation, many patients with irreversible disease continue to deteriorate. In these cases, ongoing inflammation, although a minority component, with little or no impact on chest radiographic or pulmonary function findings, continues to drive disease progression. Thus, 'disease activity' and disease severity are not synonymous and baseline symptoms, pulmonary function impairment and chest radiographic abnormalities do not reliably identify a higher risk of subsequent decline in individual patients.

The limitations of HRCT in this regard are summarized above. A number of other tests explored in the identification of 'active disease' are reviewed briefly here and are discussed in greater detail elsewhere in this book.

Gallium-67, taken up by activated macrophages and T-lymphocytes, was once widely used to assess sarcoid activity. Gallium uptake localizes in many inflammatory and neoplastic processes and is not specific for sarcoidosis. The sensitivity of gallium uptake has been as high as 94 percent in the detection of active pulmonary disease (as judged by deteriorating pulmonary function indices), although specificity was low at 67 percent (Kohn et al. 1982). In this series, in 20 patients with clinical remission of disease, there was a reduction or complete regression of abnormal gallium uptake in all cases. However, in this and other series, the utility of gallium scanning has been limited by its low specificity: abnormal uptake is often present in patients with stable disease. Additional limitations include the lack of a readily applicable threshold for the amount of abnormal gallium uptake that constitutes pulmonary 'disease activity', the absence of a simple reproducible method of quantifying change in signal, and the radiation burden associated with the test. Thus, gallium scanning is no longer routinely used as a means of assessing pulmonary disease.

FDG PET scanning shows some promise, although its role in the assessment and monitoring of pulmonary sarcoidosis is not yet clearly defined. In one small study, PET scanning was more sensitive than gallium scanning in detecting active pulmonary disease (100 vs 81 percent), and was much more sensitive in identifying extrapulmonary involvement (90 vs 48 percent) (Nishiyama et al. 2006). The added clinical value of PET scanning, over baseline pulmonary function tests and chest radiography, has yet to be evaluated in the routine staging of pulmonary disease severity. However, PET scanning may eventually have a role in rationalizing long-term treatment to prevent disease progression in selected patients with irreversible disease. A reduction in abnormal pulmonary signal has been observed following steroid therapy (Teirstein et al. 2007; Braun et al. 2008) and after administration of infliximab (Keijsers et al. 2008). However, until these changes have been shown to predict the longer term stabilization of disease, the marginal availability and expense of the test dictates that this use of serial PET scanning will be largely confined to pharmaceutical studies.

A bronchoalveolar lavage (BAL) lymphocytosis is seen in over 85 percent of patients with pulmonary sarcoidosis, with an increase the CD4/CD8 ratio in 50–60 percent; but neither finding has reliably denoted clinically significant pulmonary 'disease activity', as judged by subsequent disease progression. A BAL neutrophilia has been associated with more progressive disease in one report (Ziegenhagen et al. 2003), and in a second study the absence of a BAL neutrophilia was predictive of spontaneous disease regression in newly diagnosed steroid-naive patients with sarcoidosis (Drent et al. 1999). However, these observations have not led to the widespread use of BAL to evaluate 'disease activity': BAL is performed routinely in some units but is not performed at all in other centers. Moreover, repeat BAL in order to assess responsiveness to therapy has not been validated. It should be stressed that these reservations do not detract from the larger utility of BAL in diagnosis, discussed elsewhere. However, it appears that despite statistically significant trends in patient cohorts, there are too many exceptions in individual cases to justify a central role for the BAL evaluation of 'disease activity' in routine prognostic evaluation.

Serum biomarkers have been similarly unsatisfactory in the identification of active pulmonary disease. Although elevated in 30–80 percent of patients with sarcoidosis, serum ACE levels may be normal in active disease and do not correlate with chest radiographic stage (Shorr et al. 1997). Similarly, the correlation between the extent of nodular change and consolidation on HRCT and the serum ACE level is weak (Leung et al. 1998). Improvements in the sensitivity of serum ACE, with the discovery of the insertion/deletion polymorphism of the ACE gene in the 1990s and the use of genotype-specific reference ranges, have been counterbalanced by a reduction in an already low specificity (Stokes et al. 1999). In the recent British Thoracic Society Guidelines for the diagnosis and management of interstitial lung disease

(BTS 2008), it was concluded that serum ACE levels do not add usefully to the pulmonary function tests and imaging in the staging and monitoring of pulmonary disease.

Among a number of other studied serum biomarkers, the most attention has been given to soluble interleukin-2 receptors (sIL-2r), which are released by activated T-cells, reflect granulomatous inflammation and are found in the BAL fluid and serum of patients with sarcoidosis. The possible role of sIL-2r as a marker of sarcoid activity and disease progression has been explored in several studies (Keicho et al. 1990; Muller-Quernheim et al. 1991; Ziegenhagen et al. 1997; Grutters et al. 2003). However, although sIL-2r levels correlated with the percentage and absolute BAL lymphocyte counts in the most positive clinical report, they were not linked to subsequent need for treatment, radiographic evolution or pulmonary function outcome (Grutters et al. 2003). Moreover, the correlation between sIL-2 levels and BAL lymphocyte levels was not seen in another study (Muller-Quernheim et al. 1991).

In conclusion, the pursuit of a separate measure of pulmonary 'disease activity', over and above the evaluation of disease severity, has not enhanced routine clinical evaluation, despite attempts to amalgamate a number of variables in disease activity indices. In the end, conclusions on the likely activity of disease must be based on clinical commonsense. Overtly severe disease has a track-record of repeated disease progression and is more likely to progress in future. The duration of disease is a further important consideration: in disease of short duration, moderately severe pulmonary disease is indicative of a high likelihood of a progressive course. As discussed above, although symptoms and chest radiographic findings should be taken into account, pulmonary function tests provide the most accurate severity information for management purposes. However, in many cases with pulmonary disease of mild to moderate severity, accurate treatment decisions cannot be made from baseline severity in isolation but must be based on observed changes in disease severity with time.

DETECTION OF CHANGE IN PULMONARY DISEASE SEVERITY

Pulmonary function tests in the monitoring of change

In routine practice, serial PFTs and chest radiography are the cornerstone of monitoring. However, in pulmonary sarcoidosis there is a paucity of studies in which serial data are 'validated' against long-term outcome in the detection of change. This contrasts with idiopathic pulmonary fibrosis, in which lung function trends have been examined against mortality, leading to current recommendations that FVC and DLco levels should be monitored at 3- to 6-month intervals. This disparity may reflect the lack of a gold standard for change in sarcoidosis and the relative absence of a mortality 'anchor' against which to validate pulmonary function trends. However, the established principles of monitoring change in idiopathic pulmonary fibrosis apply also to pulmonary sarcoidosis.

The estimation of FVC has the important advantages of simplicity and reproducibility. Changes in pulmonary function tests are expressed as percentage change from absolute baseline values. Changes in pulmonary function tests are calculated using absolute values rather than percentages of predicted levels, which are influenced by the timing of patient birthdays within the monitored time-period. The widespread use of threshold values for 'significant change' is based on the known reproducibility of individual variables to two standard deviations of change. A 10 percent change in FVC values is viewed as 'significant' (e.g. a fall from 2 L to 1.8 L) because FVC values differ by less than 10 percent in 95 percent of normal subjects, when repeated in the short term. It should not be forgotten that, based on these data, a spurious change in FVC values of 10 percent or more will occur on repeat testing in 5 percent of normal subjects and sarcoidosis patients alike, due to measurement variation.

It should also be acknowledged that no comparison has been made between percentage change from baseline, absolute change and percentage change in predicted normal values in the monitoring of interstitial lung disease. In principle, one or another approach might offer minor advantages but the weight of accumulated experience has dictated the current approach to pulmonary function monitoring. Similarly, the use of FVC, rather than other lung volumes, has been determined by the ready availability of simple spirometry and the perception that, for monitoring purposes, FVC and other volumes are essentially synonymous measures, unlike DLco. The perceived advantage of FVC over DLco in detecting change largely reflects the variability of DLco estimation, with a 15 percent change needed to reduce confounding by measurement variation. As discussed later, variability in DLco estimation can be significantly reduced by the daily calibration of lung function equipment against normal biological controls, but this is seldom practicable.

However, despite the primary role of serial FVC trends in pulmonary function monitoring, the value of combining trends in different pulmonary function variables must be emphasized. Measurement variation in any single variable may result equally in an over-statement or an *under-statement* of the degree of change. The integration of variables measured using separate techniques (i.e. spirometry and estimation of gas transfer) allows the clinician to reach the conclusion that there is an overall trend, even when 'significant change' is not apparent in all variables. The importance of this approach is best understood when Bayesian principles are applied to the detection of change. In sarcoidosis, changes in severity are less prevalent than in idiopathic pulmonary fibrosis, and measurement variation is thus a relatively more frequent confounder. For example, if the pre-test probability of a 10 percent change in FVC approximates 15 percent and the probability that this threshold will be reached due to measurement variation approximates 5 percent (as discussed above), the likelihood that a 10 percent alteration in FVC represents change will be only 75 percent (a likelihood ratio of 15 percent to 5 percent, or 3:1). A concurrent change in DLco increases the likelihood that there is truly a change in disease severity. The use of standardized thresholds for change

across all interstitial lung diseases, irrespective of their progressiveness, is an over-simplification which needs to be addressed in future guidelines.

The heterogeneity of patterns of pulmonary function impairment in pulmonary sarcoidosis is a further important consideration. It can be argued that the pulmonary function variables that are most important for routine monitoring in individual patients are those that are most impaired at baseline. In a patient with severe airflow obstruction, disease progression or regression will tend to manifest as a change in FEV_1. It is logical to focus on change in DLco when the baseline profile is one of a disproportionate reduction in DLco. Thus, no single PFT can be viewed as the primary arbiter of a change in disease severity in all sarcoidosis patients. The need to integrate pulmonary function trends creates obvious difficulties in pharmaceutical studies, in which a single primary end-point is required. However, it can only be concluded that, in routine practice, pulmonary function monitoring is more accurate when FEV_1, FVC and DLco trends are considered in combination and reconciled with the pulmonary function profile at baseline.

Chest radiography and HRCT in the monitoring of change

Although serial chest radiography is widely used in the detection of change, the evaluation of simple global changes in chest radiographic extent has been little studied. In published reports, more attention has been paid to detailed chest radiographic scoring systems, which are less user-friendly in routine practice.

The International Labor Office pneumoconiosis system (ILO 1980), developed to identify radiographic changes provoked by industrial dusts, requires the scoring of the profusion of interstitial opacities in three zones in each lung. Considerable radiological expertise is required. In one study (Judson *et al.* 2008), changes in ILO profusion scores were examined in exacerbations of sarcoidosis. Although profusion scores increased significantly during exacerbations in patients with a decline in spirometric volumes, agreement between observers was only moderate, leading the authors to conclude that this scoring technique should not be used in clinical practice. The limitations of the ILO scoring system were acknowledged in the British Thoracic Society sarcoidosis study (Gibson *et al.* 1996). A modified scoring system was developed in which radiographic abnormalities were classified into reticulonodular, masses, confluent shadows, and fibrotic change, each assigned a score based on extent and profusion (Muers *et al.* 1997). However, despite good inter-observer agreement, only changes in the reticulonodular (R) score and fibrosis (F) score correlated with trends in pulmonary function variables and dyspnea scores and the correlation coefficients were low. Thus, detailed scoring systems provide a small amount of additional information but are difficult to apply in daily clinical practice, owing to complexity and significant disagreement between observers.

Recently, the rapid assessment of chest radiographic change was evaluated in a cohort of patients enrolled in a double-blind randomized trial of infliximab in chronic pulmonary sarcoidosis (Baughman *et al.* 2009). Serial radiographic change was compared using the system described above (Muers *et al.* 1997) and, separately, a five-point scale for global change (markedly worsened, worsened, unchanged, improved, markedly improved). Inter-observer agreement between two expert readers was good for both systems. However, changes in FVC levels correlated more strongly with simple changes in global scores than with changes identified using the more complex system. Thus, chest radiographic change is best quantified in routine practice using a simple user-friendly global assessment of disease extent, without recourse to the evaluation of individual radiographic patterns. Essentially, more detailed chest radiographic scoring makes too many demands of a blunt instrument.

In pulmonary sarcoidosis, no validated serial HRCT scoring system has been developed. In some patients, it appears that HRCT is too sensitive, as minor regional change often has little or no correlation with pulmonary function trends. In other cases, significant pulmonary function trends are not associated with major HRCT change. At present, serial HRCT cannot be recommended, either in routine monitoring or as a primary end-point in pharmaceutical studies. Serial HRCT has an occasional role when other serial data are conflicting and need to be reconciled.

Staging pulmonary disease and monitoring change: which test?

In conclusion, no single test stands alone as an arbiter of either the baseline staging of pulmonary disease or the evaluation of change in disease severity. For both purposes, accurate evaluation requires the integration of symptoms, chest radiography and pulmonary function tests. Among these measures, it is clear that pulmonary function tests consistently provide the most reliable data, but only if their limitations are taken into account. In the baseline quantification of the severity of disease, the confounding effect of the wide range of normal values is a major constraint and the heterogeneity in patterns of pulmonary function impairment in sarcoidosis necessitates a flexible approach. The most frequent source of inaccuracy in the monitoring of disease is measurement variation, especially in patients in whom a low pre-test likelihood of true change is low: in this context, change in individual pulmonary function variables is often spurious.

Furthermore, no single chest radiographic variable or pulmonary function test is sufficiently robust to stand alone as the cardinal means of assessing severity and serial change in all patients. In the staging of disease severity, an integrated approach is required with the amalgamation of symptoms, pulmonary function variables and imaging data, in order to inform key management decisions. A multidisciplinary approach is even more important in the detection of change, again because trends in any single PFT may be confounded by measurement variation when the pre-test likelihood of change is low. In pharmaceutical studies, serial FVC estimation is an appropriate primary end-point, based on data in other interstitial lung diseases. However, in routine practice,

symptomatic change, trends in global radiographic appearances and pulmonary function trends in spirometric volumes and measures of gas transfer must be reconciled, although no clear guidance on this process exists in current guidelines (Joint Statement 1999). This precept applies equally to treatment responses and to changes in disease severity in other contexts. In conclusion, the multidisciplinary evaluation of pulmonary sarcoidosis, rather than an undue focus on any single test, is as important in the detection of change as it is in diagnosis and the staging of disease at a single point in time.

Among other tests, gallium scanning is largely discredited and PET scanning has yet to be validated, despite promising preliminary results. Proposed markers of disease activity, including serm ACE levels, BAL lymphocyte counts and serum IL-2 levels, have not been shown to provide useful staging information in clinical practice and have no defined role in the serial monitoring of pulmonary disease. Although sometimes highly useful in diagnosis, HRCT has not provided staging information that is demonstrably more accurate than the level of pulmonary function impairment and it has been frustratingly difficult to adapt HRCT to routine monitoring. Among these ancillary tests, PET scanning may have the greatest future promise, both for staging and for monitoring, based on pilot data. However, for the moment, pulmonary function tests and chest radiography remain central to both staging and monitoring of pulmonary disease.

QUALITY ASSURANCE: THE ACCURACY AND REPRODUCIBILITY OF PFTs

As PFT threshold values are used to signify 'significant' change, thorough quality control and quality assurance procedures are essential in lung function laboratories to ensure technical accuracy and to minimize measurement variability. Best practice includes the documentation and rigorous checking of quality control and quality assurance procedures to ensure that they meet recognized standards (Brusasco *et al.* 2005a,b). Details and guidelines pertaining to quality control and quality assurance relevant to routine lung function tests are specified by the American Thoracic Society / European Respiratory Society standards, which include information relating to calibration and verification of equipment.

The acquisition of biological control data is an essential part of this process (ARTP 2006; Cotes *et al.* 2006). Trend analyses of biological control data should be carried out frequently; generally, these data are produced by the performance of pulmonary function tests by staff members who do not have respiratory disease. In some pulmonary function laboratories, including the laboratory in the authors' institution, pulmonary function data are reacquired by staff members at the start of every day, in order to recalibrate equipment as necessary. Our experience leaves us in no doubt that daily recalibration is worthwhile, especially with regard to measures of gas transfer, which are notoriously less reproducible than lung volumes. In part, this reflects the greater technical complexity inherent in the measurement of gas transfer. We acknowledge that the demands of routine practice do not always permit so meticulous an approach. However, at the very least, we believe that biological control data should be acquired at weekly intervals, even though this is a more stringent recommendation than made in some guideline statements. For example, some protocols for the performance of PFTs in pharmaceutical trials in idiopathic pulmonary fibrosis recommend the monthly acquisition of biological control data. However, this is insufficiently rigorous, especially with regard to variables such as FVC and DLco, generally chosen as primary or co-primary endpoints. The identification of equipment malfunction may be particularly difficult as it is often undetected by routine calibration maneuvers but it will generally be disclosed by trend analyses.

Cotes and associates state that, for individual pulmonary function variables, a coefficient of variation (standard deviation/mean, $\times$ 100) of 4–8 percent should be expected in pulmonary function laboratories with 'high standards' (Cotes et al. 2006). However, coefficients of variation of 2–4 percent for routine tests (spirometric volumes, total lung capacity, measures of gas transfer) can be achieved for daily biological control data, with the stringent monitoring of performance, and careful quality assurance and quality control. In our own institution, the acquisition of daily biological control data during the last two decades has been associated with a root-mean-square coefficient of variation (RMSCV) of less than 4 percent for all routine lung function parameters. This may account for the observation that, in fibrotic idiopathic interstitial pneumonia (idiopathic pulmonary fibrosis, fibrotic non-specific interstitial pneumonia), serial trends in DLco have a greater prognostic significance against mortality in our population (Latsi et al. 2003) than in other cohorts, in which serial FVC trends have been more closely associated with long-term outcome. FVC estimation carries less intrinsic variability but rigorous quality assurance remains essential, given the recent observation that, in patients with idiopathic pulmonary fibrosis, relative declines in FVC of 5–10 percent from baseline values are predictive of increased mortality. In pulmonary sarcoidosis, the minimization of technical variability in the estimation of spirometric volumes is especially important as, in some patients, bronchial hyper-reactivity may cause fluctuations from day to day that are not generally seen in other diffuse lung diseases. If there is also a failure to institute rigorous quality assurance and quality control, the clinical significance of serial pulmonary function trends may be very difficult to interpret.

The reproducibility of MEF_{25} and RV is significantly lower than that of the other variables discussed above, even with the application of rigorous quality assurance. Relative measurement 'noise' and the attendant coefficient of variation for the measurement of MEF_{25} are relatively high because MEF values are usually very low ($<$ 2 L/s). The RV is calculated from two measured variables (functional residual capacity and expiratory reserve volume) and the coefficient of variation is increased, due to the summation of the intrinsic variability of two measured parameters. Thus, neither RV nor MEF_{25} is suited to the detection of significant functional change in clinical practice.

Inter-laboratory variability also requires consideration, especially at referral centers, as PFTs must be reconciled with those performed previously at local laboratories. Inter-laboratory variability will be minimized by rigorous quality assurance at both laboratories, which result in only minor discrepancies in FVC values as there is minimal variation in measurement techniques across laboratories. By contrast, DLco values are notoriously inconsistent between laboratories, even if rigorous quality assurance measures are in place. This reflects the many variations between laboratories in measurement technique that occur in gas transfer estimation. Thus, apparently significant gas transfer trends disclosed by measurements at separate laboratories should be viewed with skepticism, especially when spirometric values are stable.

The acquisition of biological control data is also an essential addition to other quality control procedures in the performance of maximal cardiopulmonary exercise tests. In our institution, it has proved possible for staff members to produce exercise data on a weekly basis (Roca et al. 1997). From published data, coefficients of variation should be less than 7 percent for maximal oxygen uptake (Roca et al. 1997), less than 5 percent for maximal carbon dioxide production, and less than 7 percent for maximal ventilation (Reville and Morgan 2000).

FITNESS-TO-FLY TESTS

A hypoxic inhalation test (i.e. a fitness-to-fly test) should be performed in patients with minor hypoxemia who wish to travel by air. The level of hypobaric hypoxemia reflects the level of hypoxemia during air travel as there is an inverse relationship between oxygen partial pressure and altitude. An altitude effect occurs during travel in a pressurized cabin as ambient pressure is decreased during ascent. Because commercial aircraft typically cruise at 12 000 meters and engineering and financial constraints preclude sea-level pressurization, aircraft cabins are pressurized to a maximum altitude of approximately 2500 meters. At this altitude, there is an oxygen partial pressure corresponding to breathing 15 percent oxygen at sea level (Seccombe et al. 2004). In individuals without respiratory disease, reductions in the partial pressure of arterial blood (Pao_2) at this altitude will generally fall to between 8.0 and 10.0 kPa (Spo_2 90–94 percent), depending in part on age and minute ventilation (Cramer et al. 1996). However, other factors causing the wide individual variation in response to a hypobaric environment are not well understood (Ernstring et al. 2000). For this reason, the British Thoracic Society recommends pre-flight assessments in patients with respiratory disease, even if hypoxemia is minimal (BTS 2002, 2004). Furthermore, pre-flight assessment is warranted in patients with severe lung function impairment and significant exercise intolerance, even in the absence of minor hypoxemia, as significant hypoxemia is seen in some patients with a normal Pao_2 at sea level, on breathing 15 percent oxygen.

The gold-standard means of pre-flight assessment, hypobaric chambers, are cumbersome to use and not widely available because of their expense. Substitute methods include hypoxic inhalation tests and predictive equations. Formal assessment using the hypoxic inhalation test is preferable as the level of hypoxemia, on breathing 15 percent oxygen, is highly variable for a given level of pulmonary function impairment. Predictive equations need to take this variability into account and, thus, often considerably overestimate the need for in-flight oxygen (Martin *et al.* 2007). During the hypoxic inhalation test, cabin altitude is simulated at sea level by the inhalation of a gas mixture containing 15 percent oxygen in nitrogen. The hypoxic gas mixture is inhaled from a Douglas bag for 20 minutes, with the measurement of arterial gases at the beginning and end of the test, and monitoring of oxygen saturation (Spo_2) and ECG throughout. From these measurements, the required flow rate of supplemental oxygen is ascertained. It is generally accepted that in-flight oxygen is needed (usually at 2 L/min via nasal prongs) if the Pao_2 is less than 6.6 kPa (83 percent Spo_2). However, it is important to recognize that short-term hyperventilation (as judged by $Paco_2$ levels) is common during the test and may mask hypoxemia. This should be taken into account, especially for long-haul flights.

An alternative technique is to seat the patient in the body plethysmograph and to reduce oxygen concentration within the body box to 15 percent ($Fio_2 = 0.15$) (Cramer *et al.* 1996). This allows oxygen requirements to be titrated accurately using nasal prongs.

REFERENCES

Alhamad EH, Lynch JP, Martinez FJ (2001). Pulmonary function tests in interstitial lung disease: what role do they have? *Clin Chest Med* 22: 715–50.

ARTP (2006). Working Groups on Standards of Care and Recommendations for Lung Function Departments: *Quality assurance for lung function laboratories*. Available at www.ARTP.org.uk.

Baughman RP, Engel PJ, Meyer CA et al. (2006). Pulmonary hypertension in sarcoidosis. *Sarcoid Vasc Diffuse Lung Dis* 23: 108–16.

Baughman RP, Desai S, Drent M et al. (2009). Changes in chest roentgenogram of sarcoidosis patients during a clinical trial of infliximab therapy: comparison of different methods of evaluation. *Chest* 136: 526–35.

Braun JJ, Kessler R, Constantinesco A, Imperiale A (2008). 18 F-FDG PET/CT in sarcoidosis management: review and report of 20 cases. *Eur J Nucl Med Mol Imaging* 35: 1537–43.

Brusasco V, Crapo R, Viegi G (2005a). ATS/ERS task force on standardisation of lung function testing: General considerations for lung function. *Eur Respir J* 26: 153–61.

Brusasco V, Crapo R, Viegi G (2005b). ATS/ERS task force on standardisation of lung function testing: Standardisation of the single breath determination of carbon monoxide uptake in the lung. *Eur Respir J* 26: 720–35.

BTS (2002). British Thoracic Society recommendations: Managing passengers with respiratory disease planning air travel. *Thorax* 57: 289–304.

BTS (2004). British Thoracic Society recommendations: Managing passengers with respiratory disease planning air travel – summary for primary care. Available at www.brit-thoracic.org.uk/.

BTS (2008). British Thoracic Society in collaboration with the Thoracic Society of Australia and New Zealand and the Irish Thoracic Society: Interstitial lung disease guideline. *Thorax* 63(Suppl. V): v1–58.

Burke CM, Glanville AR, Morris AJR et al. (1987). Pulmonary function in advanced pulmonary hypertension. *Thorax* 42: 151–5.

Carrington CB (1976). Structure and function in sarcoidosis. *Ann NY Acad Sci* 278: 265–83.

Chambellan A, Turbie P, Nunes H et al. (2005). Endoluminal stenosis of proximal bronchi in sarcoidosis: bronchoscopy, function and evolution. *Chest* 127: 472–81.

Costabel U, Guzman M (2001). Bronchoalveolar lavage in interstitial lung disease. *Curr Opin Pulm Med* 7: 255–61.

Cotes JE, Chinn DJ, Miller MR (2006). *Lung Function*, 6th edn. Blackwell, Oxford, p. 79.

Cramer D, Ward S, Geddes D (1996). Assessment of oxygen supplementation during air travel. *Thorax* 51: 202–3.

Drent M, Jacobs J, de Vries J et al. (1999). Does the cellular bronchoalveolar lavage fluid profile reflect the severity of sarcoidosis? *Eur Respir J* 13: 1338–44.

Drent M, De Vries J, Lenters M et al. (2003). Sarcoidosis: assessment of disease severity using HRCT. *Eur Radiol* 13: 2462–71.

Ernsting J, Nicholson AN, Rainford DJ (eds). (2000). *Aviation Medicine*, 3rd edn. Butterworth-Heinemann, Oxford.

Gibson GJ, Prescott RJ, Muers MF, Mitchell DN (1996). British Thoracic Society sarcoidosis study: Effects of long-term corticosteroid treatment. *Thorax* 51: 238–47.

Gleeson FV, Traill ZC, Hansell DM (1996). Evidence of expiratory CT scans of small-airway obstruction in sarcoidosis. *Am J Roentgen* 166: 1052–4.

Grutters JC, Fellrath JM, Mulder L et al. (2003). Serum soluble interleukin-2 receptor measurement in patients with sarcoidosis: a clinical evaluation. *Chest* 124: 186–95.

Hansell DM, Milne DG, Wilsher ML, Wells AU (1998). Pulmonary sarcoidosis: morphologic associations of airflow obstruction on thin section computed tomography. *Radiology* 209: 697–704.

Hansell DM, Armstrong P, Lynch DA, McAdams HP (eds). (2005). *Imaging of Diseases of the Chest*, 4th edn. Elsevier Mosby, St Louis, pp. 635–6.

Harrison BD, Shaylor JM, Stokes TC, Wilkes AR (1991). Airflow limitation in sarcoidosis: a study of pulmonary function in 107 patients with newly diagnosed disease. *Resp Med* 85: 59–64.

ILO (1980). *Guidelines for the Use of ILO International Classification of Radiographs of Pneumoconioses* [Occupational Safety Series 22]. International Labor Office, Geneva.

Joint Statement of the American Thoracic Society, European Respiratory Society and World Association of Sarcoidosis And Other Granulomatous Disorders (1999). *Am J Respir Crit Care Med* 160: 736–54.

Judson MA, Gilbert GE, Rodgers JK et al. (2008). The utility of the chest radiograph in diagnosing exacerbations of pulmonary sarcoidosis. *Respirology* 13: 97–102.

Keicho N, Kitamura K, Takaku F, Yotsumoto H (1990). Serum concentration of soluble interleukin-2 receptor as a sensitive parameter of disease activity in sarcoidosis. *Chest* 98: 1125–9.

Keijsers RGM, Verzijlbergen JF, van Diepen DM et al. (2008). 18 F-FDG PET in sarcoidosis: an observational study in 12 patients treated with Infliximab. *Sarcoid Vasc Diff Lung Dis* 25: 143–50.

Keogh BA, Crystal RG (1980). Pulmonary function testing in interstitial pulmonary disease. What does it tell us? *Chest* 78: 856–64.

Kohn H, Klech H, Mostbeck A, Kummer F (1982). 67-Ga scanning for assessment of disease activity and therapy decisions in pulmonary sarcoidosis in comparison to chest radiography, serum ACE and blood T-lymphocytes. *Eur J Nucl Med* 7: 413–16.

Latsi PI, du Bois RM, Nicholson AG et al. (2003). Fibrotic idiopathic interstitial pneumonia: the prognostic value of longitudinal functional trends. *Am J Respir Crit Care Med* 168: 531–7.

Leung AN, Brauner MW, Caillat-Vigneron N *et al.* (1998). Sarcoidosis activity: correlation of HRCT findings with those of 67Ga scanning, bronchoalveolar lavage, and serum angiotensin-converting enzyme assay. *J Comput Assist Tomogr* 22: 229–34.

Levinson RS, Metzger LF, Stanley NN *et al.* (1977). Airway function in sarcoidosis. *Am J Med* 62: 51–9.

Lynch JP, Kazerooni EA, Gaye SE (1997). Pulmonary sarcoidosis. *Clin Chest Med* 18: 755–85.

Martin SE, Bradley JM *et al.* (2007). Flight assessment in patients with respiratory disease: hypoxic challenge testing vs. predictive equations. *Q J Med* 100: 361–7.

Muller-Quernheim J, Pfeifer S, Strausz J, Ferlinz R (1991). Correlation of clinical and immunologic parameters of the inflammatory activity of pulmonary sarcoidosis. *Am Rev Respir Dis* 144: 1322–9.

Muers MF, Middleton WG, Gibson GJ *et al.* (1997). A simple radiographic scoring method for monitoring pulmonary sarcoidosis: relations between radiographic scores, dyspnea grade and respiratory function in the British Thoracic Society Study of Long-Term Corticosteroid Treatment. *Sarcoid Vasc Diff Lung Dis* 14: 46–56.

Nathan SD, Shlobin OA, Ahmad S *et al.* (2007). Pulmonary hypertension and pulmonary function testing in idiopathic pulmonary fibrosis. *Chest* 131: 657–63.

Neville E, Walker A, James DG (1983). Prognostic factors predicting outcome of sarcoidosis: an analysis of 818 patients. *Q J Med* 2: 525–33.

Nishiyama Y, Yamamoto Y, Fukunaga K *et al.* (2006). Comparative evaluation of 18F-FDG PET and 67-Ga scintigraphy in patients with sarcoidosis. *J Nucl Med* 47: 1571–6.

Oberstein A, Zitzewitz H von, Schweden F, Muller-Quernheim J (1997). Non-invasive evaluation of the inflammatory activity in sarcoidosis with high-resolution computed tomography. *Sarcoid Vasc Diff Lung Dis* 14: 65–72.

Remy-Jardin M, Giraud F, Remy J *et al.* (1994). Pulmonary sarcoidosis: role of CT in the evaluation of disease activity and functional impairment and in prognosis assessment. *Radiology* 191: 675–80.

Reville SM, Morgan M (2000). Biological quality control for exercise testing. *Thorax* 55: 63–6.

Roca J, Whipp BJ *et al.* (1997). ERS task force on standardization of clinical exercise testing: Clinical exercise testing with reference to lung diseases – indications, standardization and interpretation strategies. *Eur Respir J* 10: 2662–89.

Romer FK (1982). Presentation of sarcoidosis and outcome of pulmonary changes. *Dan Med Bull* 29: 27–32.

Seccombe LM, Kelly PT, Wong CK *et al.* (2004). Effect of simulated commercial flight on oxygenation in patients with interstitial lung disease and chronic obstructive pulmonary disease. *Thorax* 59: 966–70.

Shorr AF, Torrington KG, Parker JM (1997). Serum angiotensin converting enzyme does not correlate with radiographic stage at initial diagnosis of sarcoidosis. *Respir Med* 91: 399–401.

Shorr AF, Davies DB, Nathan ST (2003). Predicting mortality in patients with sarcoidosis awaiting lung transplantation. *Chest* 124: 922–8.

Steen VD, Graham G, Conte C *et al.* (1992). Isolated diffusing capacity reduction in systemic sclerosis. *Arthritis Rheum* 35: 765–70.

Stokes GS, Monaghan JC, Schrader AP *et al.* (1999). Influence of angiotensin converting enzyme (ACE) genotype on interpretation of diagnostic tests for serum ACE activity. *Aust NZ J Med* 29: 315–18.

Teirstein AS, Machac J, Almeida O *et al.* (2007). Results of 188 whole-body fluorodeoxyglucose positron emission tomography scans in 137 patients with sarcoidosis. *Chest* 132: 1949–53.

Turner-Warwick M, McAllister W, Lawrence R (1986). Corticosteroid treatment in pulmonary sarcoidosis: do serial lavage lymphocyte counts, serum angiotensin converting enzyme measurements, and gallium-67 scans help management? *Thorax* 41: 9903–13.

Ziegenhagen MW, Benner UK, Zissel G *et al.* (1997). Sarcoidosis: TNF-alpha release from alveolar macrophages and serum level of sIL-2R are prognostic markers. *Am J Respir Crit Care Med* 156: 1586–92.

Ziegenhagen MW, Rothe ME, Schlaak M, Muller-Quernheim J (2003). Bronchoalveolar and serological parameters reflecting the severity of sarcoidosis. *Eur Respir J* 21: 407–13.

11

Endoscopic techniques in diagnosis

NEAL NAVANI AND PALLAV L SHAH

INTRODUCTION

Flexible bronchoscopy is an important tool for the diagnosis of patients with sarcoidosis. It allows inspection and sampling of the major airways and biopsy of the lung as well as intrathoracic lymph nodes. Demonstration of non-caseating granulomas is central to the diagnosis of sarcoid along with consistent radiological and clinical features. A clinical diagnosis without biopsy may only be made in patients with classical Löfgren's syndrome (Iannuzzi *et al.* 2007). Prior to the introduction of flexible bronchoscopy by Ikeda and colleagues in 1968, patients with pulmonary sarcoidosis were required to undergo mediastinoscopy, rigid bronchoscopy or open lung biopsy to establish a diagnosis. Flexible bronchoscopy now allows endobronchial biopsy, bronchoalveolar lavage, transbronchial lung biopsy and transbronchial needle aspiration. Development of newer endoscopes also allows endobronchial and endoscopic ultrasound-guided sampling of mediastinal lymph nodes which have an increasing role in the pathological evaluation of intrathoracic lymph nodes in stage I and II sarcoidosis. Evolution of technology has allowed further advances in the bronchoscopy suite, including electromagnetic navigation and confocal microscopy. These techniques are all discussed in detail below.

FLEXIBLE BRONCHOSCOPY

Flexible bronchoscopy is a commonly performed initial investigation for the diagnosis of pulmonary sarcoidosis. The procedure is carried out in the ambulatory care setting with or without intravenous sedation. In those patients with reversible airway obstruction, a nebulized bronchodilator prior to the procedure may be of benefit. The videobroncho-scope (Fig. 11.1) is advanced via the nose or mouth until the true vocal cords are visible and topical lignocaine is instilled in order to achieve local anesthesia. Rarely, macroscopic abnormalities suggestive of sarcoidosis may be evident at the larynx or arytenoids (Mariotta *et al.* 1994). Passing the bronchoscope through the anesthetised true vocal cords allows visualization of the trachea. The endobronchial tree can then be easily examined down to the sub-segmental level.

Macroscopic granulomas may occur anywhere along the respiratory tract, and it is not uncommon for mucosal abnormalities to be evident in the endobronchial tree. The typical appearance varies from cobblestoning with whitish plaques to small isolated pale nodules (Plate 11). One study of 74 patients has reported that half of patients with stage I or stage II disease had endobronchial abnormalities while the prevalence of endobronchial abnormalities was higher at 83 percent in those with stage III disease (Bilaceroglu *et al.* 1999). In this setting, endobronchial biopsy (EBB) of these lesions has a high diagnostic yield particularly when the visible endobronchial nodules are biopsied.

EBB is performed by inserting specifically designated biopsy forceps into the working channel of the flexible

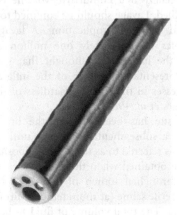

Figure 11.1   Distal tip of videobronchoscope.

bronchoscope. The forceps are advanced out of the distal end of the bronchoscope and then manipulated to the endobronchial abnormality under direct vision. The forceps are opened, then apposed to the target area and then closed. The forceps are then retracted and the biopsy samples obtained are placed in formalin for histological processing. Four to six biopsies are recommended.

EBB retains an important role in the patient with suspected sarcoidosis even when no macroscopic endobronchial abnormalities are present. Non-caseating granulomas may be observed from endobronchial biopsies in 30 percent of patients with normal endobronchial appearances (Shorr et al. 2001). Therefore it has been recommended that EBB via flexible bronchoscopy should be routinely performed in patients with suspected sarcoidosis. In order to maximize yield in patients without apparent endobronchial disease, it is suggested that six specimens in total may be obtained from the main carina and bilateral secondary carinae (Chapman and Mehta 2003).

Bronchoalveolar lavage

Bronchoalveolar lavage (BAL), performed during flexible bronchoscopy, has gained widespread acceptance as a minimally invasive method that provides important information about immunological, inflammatory and infectious processes taking place at the alveolar level. Studies have shown that cell types and their levels of function are comparable whether obtained from BAL or open lung biopsy.

The procedure should be carried out before other bronchoscopic investigations in order to avoid iatrogenic contamination of the lavage fluid, particularly with blood. There are no absolute contraindications to the performance of BAL beyond those commonly associated with bronchoscopy. Occasionally, the process is complicated by transient hypoxemia due to residual fluid in the alveoli. In patients with localized disease, lavage of the involved segment is more likely to provide the best results. However, in patients with a diffuse distribution of disease as commonly seen in sarcoidosis, the right middle lobe or lingula is lavaged most commonly because the anatomy allows maximal recovery of fluid and cells from these areas. Lavage in one site is usually adequate, especially if a cumulative volume of 100 mL or greater is instilled. Lavage should be confined to one lung, in order to avoid hypoxic complications. A lavage volume of 100 mL samples approximately one million alveoli (1.5–3 percent of the lung). It is thought that such a sample provides a representative picture of the inflammatory and immune processes in the alveoli regardless of the site of the lavage (Helmers et al. 1989).

Once the site has been chosen, the bronchoscope is advanced into a subsegmental bronchus until the lumen is occluded; this is referred to as the 'wedged' position. Optimal results may be obtained when the bronchoscope completely occludes the bronchial lumen of a 3rd or 4th bronchial subsegment. Sterile saline (at room temperature) is utilized as the lavage fluid. The total volume of fluid to be instilled has not been standardized. BAL typically involves the delivery of a total of 100–180 mL of fluid in 50–60 mL aliquots; larger volumes are occasionally used for research purposes.

Several methods are available for the recovery of the lavage fluid. Some centers use the same syringe to retrieve the sample by gentle continuous hand suction on the syringe. Suction should be gentle enough that visible airway collapse does not occur. A 250 mL or greater container is ideal, otherwise the liquid is rapidly suctioned all the way into the waste pump. Some centers employ tubing and several containers attached in series connected to a suction pump to recover the lavage fluid. With the latter method there is also the theoretical disadvantage that cellular components (and in particular macrophages) may become damaged or inactivated by the connection tubing, although this has not been substantiated. A further consideration is that a silicon container should be used in order to minimize adhesion to the wall of the container. Either low-pressure wall suction or a low pressure mechanical pump is used. However, it is difficult to control the suction pressure applied and in some patients there is significant airway collapse, which limits the fluid volume recovered. The total duration of lavage after wedging the bronchoscope is approximately five minutes. The first aliquot commonly returns the least volume and may contain a higher proportion of bronchial contaminant, so many operators choose to discard this sample as it may not accurately reflect alveolar constituents. The lavage fluid is then transferred to the microbiological and cytology laboratories for analysis.

Transbronchial lung biopsy

Transbronchial lung biopsy is a key investigation in the patient with suspected pulmonary sarcoidosis and its utility in the diagnosis of sarcoidosis was first documented in 1975 (Koerner et al. 1975). Subsequent cohort studies have demonstrated diagnostic yields of between 40 and 70 percent, with higher diagnostic rates seen in more advanced radiographic stages. Recently it has been shown that TBLB is more likely to be positive in those with a greater extent of parenchymal disease on high-resolution computed tomography (HRCT) scan (de Boer et al. 2009). However, TBLB may still obtain non-caseating granulomas in patients with radiographic stage I disease and even in patients with no obvious parenchymal disease on HRCT. Many patients with stage IV disease exhibit established pulmonary fibrosis with honeycombing, and TBLB may be associated with an increased risk of pneumothorax in this subgroup.

TBLB is carried out via flexible bronchoscopy whereby the biopsy forceps are inserted as far as possible into the distal airway, such that the tip of the forceps is no longer visible but assumed to be located within the lung parenchyma. The forceps is then withdrawn by 1 cm in order to reduce the likelihood of biopsy of the pleura. In inspiration the biopsy forces are opened and during expiration the forceps are advanced and closed, trapping lung parenchyma.

The main complications are bleeding and pneumothorax. One report summarizing five years of experience in a university teaching hospital (4273 bronchoscopies with 173 transbronchial biopsy procedures) described a 4 percent frequency of pneumothorax and 2.8 percent occurrence of significant bleeding (greater than 50 mL) (Pue and Pacht 1995). Real-time fluoroscopy allows the position of the forceps to be visualized during the procedure but does not appear to improve diagnostic yield nor reduce the incidence of complications in patients with sarcoidosis. Whether the specimen floats is an unreliable sign of alveolar content (Curley et al. 1998).

Several factors appear to influence the diagnostic yield from TBLB in patients with sarcoidosis. The number of biopsies taken has been evaluated and at least five to six biopsies should be taken to maximize the chance of a positive diagnosis (Descombes et al. 1997). This may be important since approximately a third of transbronchial biopsy attempts consist of bronchial mucosa rather than lung parenchyma. Larger forceps secure bigger specimens that have a higher diagnostic yield, but do not lead to increased risk of bleeding or pneumothorax (Loube et al. 1993). Operator experience may also significantly influence yield from TBLB.

Transbronchial cryobiopsy

This is a new technique devised to obtain better quality transbronchial lung biopsy specimens (Babiak et al. 2009). Patients who undergo the procedure require intubation in order to provide a secure airway and to facilitate repeated insertion and removal of the bronchoscope. It also ensures any complications can be managed efficiently. The cryoprobe is inserted through the instrument channel of the broncho-scope into a specified bronchial segment. The procedure is performed with either fluoroscopic guidance or electromagnetic navigation with the Superdimension procedure (see page 119). The probe is activated for 2–3 seconds and the freezing effect causes some of the adjacent lung to become adherent to the probe. The probe and bronchoscope are gently tugged and the whole sample is removed as a single unit. The piece of lung adherent to the probe is allowed to thaw and placed in formalin.

This technique provides much larger transbronchial lung biopsies (almost three times larger than conventional forceps biopsy) without any crush artifact. The main theoretical risks are a greater incidence of hemorrhage and pneumothoraces than conventional transbronchial lung biopsies. Although in one case series there were a few more cases of hemorrhage they did not require any additional intervention. The risks are minimized by correct placement of the probe to ensure that it is in the outer quarter of the lung zone where the blood vessels are smaller, but imaging is required to ensure that the probe is not in contact with the pleura.

Transbronchial needle aspiration

Transbronchial needle aspiration biopsy (TBNA) is an important procedure for the pathological confirmation of mediastinal lymphadenopathy. Since Wang first described the procedure via flexible bronchoscopy in 1978 in a patient with lung cancer, several reports have highlighted its utility in patients with suspected sarcoidosis.

During flexible bronchoscopy a dedicated TBNA needle is introduced into the working channel. While inserting the needle, the flexible bronchoscope should be kept as straight as possible, with its distal tip in the neutral position in order to prevent damage to the bronchoscope. The beveled end of the needle should be kept within the metal hub during its passage through the working channel in order to prevent damage to the working channel by the needle. Several methods have been described for performing TBNA. The jabbing technique involves the needle being opposed to the airway wall at the desired site and then the needle is inserted perpendicular to the airway wall by a jabbing movement. With this technique, the bronchoscope position is fixed, and the needle is pushed perpendicularly through the inter-cartilaginous space and into the lymph node. The piggy-back method is an alternative and requires that the bronchoscope with the extended needle is advanced as a unit, allowing the needle to penetrate the airway wall. Once the needle has entered the lymph node, it is then moved in and out within the lymph node while suction with a syringe is applied. Complications of significant bleeding or pneumothorax are rare.

Several needles for TBNA are commercially available. A 22-gauge needle provides cytological specimens while a 19-gauge needle allows histological cores to be obtained. It is a current area of debate as to whether a confident diagnosis of sarcoidosis may be made on cytology alone. Whether dealing with cytology or histology, however, pathologists are able to diagnose non-caseating granulomas only. Granulomas due to sarcoidosis have no specific pathological features to distinguish them from other granulomas, not even at histological examination. The pathology must always, therefore, be taken in the context of clinical and radiological findings.

A further area of concern of the use of cytology for the pathological diagnosis of sarcoidosis is that granulomas in mediastinal nodes have been described as a reaction to malignancy and anthracotic pigment. Histological specimens therefore may be preferred to exclude these other diagnoses, particularly lymphoma. Conversely, one study of TBNA of mediastinal nodes in patients with previous cancer reliably diagnosed granulomatous inflammation with no evidence of disease recurrence on clinical follow-up (Kennedy et al. 2008). The cytological criteria for the diagnosis of sarcoidosis are discussed further in Chapter 12.

All lymph nodes stations that lie adjacent to the airways are available to sampling by TBNA. The upper and lower paratracheal regions, subcarinal and hilar areas are accessible by conventional TBNA. Most operators elect to sample enlarged lymph nodes in the right paratracheal and subcarinal lymph node stations, which are both commonly involved in patients with stage I and II sarcoidosis. TBNA has a high sensitivity for the diagnosis of sarcoidosis in patients with enlarged mediastinal lymph nodes. In one study of 53 patients, non-necrotizing epithelioid granulomas were observed in 42 of 53 patients (79 percent), with similar results for stage I disease (27/33, 82 percent) and stage II disease (15/20, 75 percent) disease (Trisolini et al. 2008). Sensitivity of TBNA for the diagnosis of sarcoidosis ranges from 46 to 90 percent in the published literature to date (Bilaceroglu et al. 2004).

Several factors may affect the diagnostic yield of TBNA in patients with sarcoidosis. Aspirating more than one lymph node station and performing at least four to five aspirates (and up to seven) per lymph node may maximize yield (Chin *et al.* 2002). More experienced operators and those with specific training in TBNA may also obtain higher sensitivities. On-site evaluation of samples may reduce the number of inadequate specimens and also reduce the number of passes required in patients with suspected malignant lymphadenopathy, and results are also likely to be applicable to those with intrathoracic lymphadenopathy due to sarcoidosis.

A major advantage of TBNA is that it may be combined with the other bronchoscopic procedures to maximize diagnostic yield in patients with sarcoidosis. In one small study of 13 patients, non-caseating granulomata (with stain and culture negative for tuberculosis and fungi) were found in 7 of the 13 patients by TBLB, and in 6 of the 13 patients by TBNA (of which 4 patients had negative TBLB). The sensitivity of the combined procedure was 85 percent and higher than TBLB or TBNA in isolation (Leonard *et al.* 1997). TBNA may also prevent the need for mediastinoscopy in patients with enlarged intrathoracic lymphadenopathy due to sarcoidosis, and it offers the advantage of not requiring general anesthesia nor the morbidity and cost associated with an operation.

Limitations of TBNA in the diagnosis of sarcoidosis must also be recognized. A negative sample (inadequate or lymphocytes only) does not exclude the diagnosis and the negative predictive value of conventional TBNA in patients with suspected sarcoidosis is yet to be adequately established. Sampling of lymph nodes of less than 1 cm in short axis is not usually performed by conventional TBNA. Therefore the utility of the procedure in patients with stage III and IV sarcoidosis has not been investigated.

Despite the scientific evidence supporting the use of TBNA in sarcoidosis and its excellent safety profile, the procedure is under-utilized, for reasons that are not clear. A variable learning curve for the procedure and disappointing results may have led many operators to abandon the practice. However, TBNA remains an important technique for the pathological confirmation of sarcoidosis, either alone or when combined with other bronchoscopic methods.

node sampling, the US catheter must be withdrawn and replaced with a conventional TBNA needle and lymph node puncture is performed as described above. No data on the specific use of radial EBUS for the diagnosis of sarcoidosis are currently available.

In 2003, an integrated linear-array convex probe (BF-UC160FOL5, Olympus, Tokyo) was introduced that allows real-time aspiration of mediastinal and hilar nodes under direct vision (Krasnik *et al.* 2003). This uses an electronic scanning mechanism which scans a 90-degree window parallel to the insertion direction of the bronchoscope (Fig. 11.2). The frequency ranges from 5 to 12 kHz and the EBUS scope has a 30-degree offset viewing chip. Acoustic contact may be obtained by simply applying the transducer to the airway wall and may be enhanced by the use of a water-filled balloon covering the transducer.

The procedure is performed under conscious sedation, with the patient lying supine, through the oral route. The lymph nodes are systematically evaluated from the paratracheal to the hilar lymph nodes. Once the target lymph node is identified, a dedicated 22-gauge needle, contained in a sheath, is inserted into the working channel of the EBUS scope. It is important to verify that the sheath is seen to extend beyond the tip of the scope (visible as a small crescent) on the bronchoscopic image, in order to avoid inadvertent damage to the scope by the needle. The airway wall is penetrated with the needle and can be seen to enter the lymph node on the US image (Fig. 11.3). Suction is applied to the needle via a syringe and then, under direct vision, the needle is moved to and fro within the lymph node. Cytological specimens are obtained and smeared directly on to slides or injected into saline or a liquid fixative. Occasionally core biopsies are obtained and are placed into formalin.

EBUS-TBNA routinely allows access to upper and lower paratracheal lymph nodes, the subcarinal station as well as hilar nodes and some proximal intrapulmonary lymph nodes.

Recent data have confirmed that EBUS-guided TBNA has a superior yield to conventional TBNA for the diagnosis of sarcoidosis (Tremblay *et al.* 2009). Tremblay and colleagues

ENDOBRONCHIAL US-GUIDED TRANSBRONCHIAL NEEDLE ASPIRATION

Endobronchial ultrasound-guided transbronchial needle aspiration (EBUS-TBNA) is an important technique that is likely to develop into a key diagnostic tool for sarcoidosis with enlarged intrathoracic lymph nodes.

Initially a radial EBUS probe (miniprobe, UM-BS20-26R, Olympus Medical, Tokyo) was developed. This is an adapted vascular probe and comprises a radial ultrasound probe mounted on the tip of a flexible catheter. The miniprobe is a mechanical scanning ultrasound transducer and measures 2.6 mm in diameter with a frequency range of 20–30 kHz. The probe is covered with a balloon which is inflated with water in the airway in order to provide acoustic contact with the airways and allows per-bronchial structures and lymph nodes to be visualized. However, in order to allow lymph

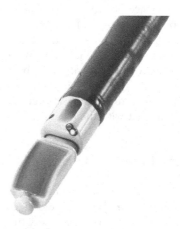

Figure 11.2   Note that the instrument channel and optical CCD chip are offset in the endobronchial ultrasound scope but end-on with the videobronchoscope.

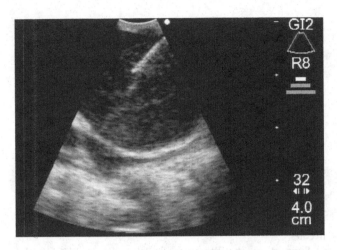

Figure 11.3   Endobronchial ultrasound image of 22-gauge needle within mediastinal lymph node due to sarcoidosis.

randomly allocated 50 patients with suspected stage I and II sarcoidosis to undergo either EBUS-TBNA or conventional TBNA using a 19-gauge needle. The diagnostic yield of EBUS-TBNA was 83.3 percent compared to 53.8 percent with conventional TBNA ($p < 0.05$). Other cohort studies have illustrated the value of EBUS-TBNA in pathologically confirming a diagnosis of sarcoid with sensitivities between 24 and 93 percent (Table 11.1). However, these studies generally had a high prevalence of sarcoid and it is unclear whether the results can be extrapolated to a general population of patients with undiagnosed mediastinal lymphadenopathy, particularly in tuberculosis endemic areas.

The available data suggest that EBUS-TBNA has a higher diagnostic yield than conventional bronchoscopic procedures, such as transbronchial biopsy, in cohorts of patients with high disease prevalence. It remains to be seen whether conventional bronchoscopy with endobronchial and transbronchial biopsies

can provide additional yield to EBUS-TBNA. Routine bronchoscopy following EBUS-TBNA at the same sitting is feasible and safe. However, the addition of routine bronchoscopy may be necessary only in those centers where rapid on-site evaluation of samples is not available.

A limitation of EBUS-TBNA for the diagnosis of sarcoidosis is that a negative sample does not exclude the disease, even if an adequate sample has been obtained. This is in part due to the sampling error of a 22-gauge needle.

One study has tested the feasibility of using biopsy forceps (Olympus FB-56D-1) to sample mediastinal lymph nodes via EBUS (Herth *et al.* 2008). The biopsy forceps are compatible with the 2 mm working channel of a linear EBUS scope and are equipped with rat-tooth forceps at the distal end. Seventy-five patients were selected with subcarinal lymph nodes greater than 25 mm in short axis. Under general anesthesia and via a rigid bronchoscope, the patients initially underwent standard EBUS-TBNA with a 22-gauge needle. This was then replaced with a flexible bronchoscope and a blind TBNA with a 19-gauge needle was performed at the site of the EBUS-guided TBNA puncture. Finally, the video-bronchoscope was replaced with an EBUS scope and the miniforceps positioned in the working channel. The forceps were advanced towards the visible puncture site made by the 19-gauge TBNA needle. The blunt tip of the forceps was then forced through the puncture site of the bronchial wall. Under direct US vision the miniforceps were opened and closed within the node obtaining biopsy specimens. Samples were placed in formalin. Of the 75 patients included in the study, 25 had sarcoidosis. The sensitivity of miniforceps biopsy (88 percent) was significantly higher when compared with using a 22-gauge needle (24 percent) or 19 gauge needle (36 percent). Although the study population was not selected on the clinical probability of having sarcoidosis (resulting in low disease prevalence), it is unclear why the sensitivity of EBUS-TBNA with a 22-gauge needle was lower than previously reported. One other multicenter study with a low prevalence

Table 11.1   Published studies (up to August 2009) of endobronchial US-guided transbronchial needle aspiration for the diagnosis of sarcoidosis stages I or II.

Reference	Study design	EBUS needle	No. of patients	ROSE	Sarcoidosis prevalence (% of study population)	Sensitivity of EBUS for the diagnosis of sarcoidosis
Herth *et al.* 2006	Prospective cohort	22G	502	No	1%	33%
Oki *et al.* 2007	Prospective cohort	22G	15	No	93%	93%
Wong *et al.* 2007	Cohort	22G	65	Yes	94%	92%
Garwood *et al.* 2007	Retrospective cohort	22G	49	Yes	98%	85%
Herth *et al.* 2008	Prospective cohort	Miniforceps 22G	75	No	33%	88% 24%
Tremblay *et al.* 2009	Randomized controlled trial	22G	50	No	94%	83%
Nakajima *et al.* 2009	Retrospective cohort	22G	38	Yes	92%	91%

ROSE, rapid on-site cytological evaluation.

of sarcoidosis has reported a similar sensitivity for EBUS-TBNA of 33 percent. In that study of 502 patients, 6 were found to have sarcoidosis. Two patients were diagnosed by EBUS-TBNA. Further studies are required on the utility of EBUS-TBNA with the standard 22-gauge needle and mini-forceps for the diagnosis of sarcoidosis. However, it is likely that EBUS-TBNA will become an important first-line, minimally invasive approach in patients with suspected sarcoidosis and enlarged mediastinal or hilar lymph nodes.

ENDOSCOPIC US–GUIDED MEDIASTINAL SAMPLING

Endoscopic ultrasound was first developed for evaluation of the pancreas but was soon adapted as an effective tool for sampling the posterior mediastinum; it has an important role in the diagnosis of lymph nodes due to sarcoidosis. The echoendoscope (Fig. 11.4) has a flexible tip with an ultrasound transducer engineered into the distal end.

In common with flexible bronchoscopy and EBUS-TBNA, the procedure is carried out in the ambulatory care setting with intravenous sedation. The echoendoscope is 13 mm in diameter and two types are in clinical use, radial and linear. The radial echoendoscope allows 360-degree ultrasound imaging of structures adjacent to the esophagus, but needle sampling is not possible. The linear version (EUS) provides a view parallel to the direction of the scope and is analogous to the linear EBUS. Under direct vision provided by the linear EUS, the left paratracheal, subcarinal and lower paraesophageal glands can be sampled. It is occasionally possible also to visualize lymph nodes in the aortopulmonary window. Owing to the anatomical location of the esophagus, left-sided lymph nodes are generally easier to sample. The right paratracheal lymph node and hilar lymph nodes cannot be sampled with this procedure.

The ultrasound appearance of lymph nodes in patients with sarcoidosis has been studied and found to be unreliable, particularly when tissue sampling is feasible. Several needles are available for use with linear EUS. Samples obtained by EUS-FNA with a 22-gauge needle are suitable for cytopathological analysis. Occasionally, core samples obtained by EUS-FNA can be sent for histopathological investigation; however, core tissue

samples are more reliably obtained using a 19-gauge Tru-Cut needle (Alliance Corp., McGaw Park, IL). This needle is specifically designed for compatibility with linear EUS. This method, however, requires that the mediastinal lymph node be at least 2 cm in diameter in the direction of the biopsy. Adding Tru-Cut biopsy to FNA may improve the diagnostic accuracy and the adequacy of sampling for a diagnosis of granulomatous disorders. Conflicting evidence exists on the importance of on-site evaluation of biopsy samples in EUS-guided fine-needle aspiration, but diagnostic yield appears to be maximized by performing three to five passes. The key advantages of EUS over EBUS are the improved ultrasound images produced by the larger EUS transducer and also potentially better samples obtained with the larger gauge and Tru-Cut needles.

Support in the literature for the use of EUS in the diagnosis of sarcoid is emerging. In an initial report from Hamburg in 2000, EUS-FNA diagnosed non-caseating granulomas in all 19 patients with enlarged lymph nodes and sarcoidosis (Fritscher-Ravens et al. 2000). In one retrospective cohort study of 127 patients who had mediastinal lymphadenopathy of unknown cause, EUS-FNA identified sarcoidosis with a sensitivity and specificity of 89 and 96 percent, respectively (Wildi et al. 2004). In another prospective cohort study, 50 patients with sarcoidosis underwent EUS-FNA (Annema et al. 2005). Sarcoidosis was confirmed in 41 patients (82 percent). Among the patients who had granulomas detected by EUS-FNA, 71 percent had a prior non-diagnostic bronchoscopy. Aspirated lymph nodes were in the paratracheal, aortopulmonary window, and paraesophageal regions.

Like EBUS-TBNA, EUS-guided mediastinal lymph node sampling has clear advantages over mediastinoscopy for the diagnosis of sarcoidosis from mediastinal lymph nodes. The procedure is performed on an outpatient, without general anesthesia, is painless and has a similar diagnostic sensitivity to mediastinoscopy. It is increasingly recognized that EUS may be combined in the same sitting with bronchoscopy and EBUS-TBNA so that endobronchial, bronchial and even transbronchial biopsies and lavage may also be performed. Recently, the endobronchial US probe has been placed in the esophagus for more convenient access to the posterior and left-sided lymph nodes, although this approach for the diagnosis of sarcoidosis has yet to be evaluated.

As with other techniques involving aspirates for cytology, a false-negative rate is appreciable (approximately 20 percent) and negative or inadequate samples should not be regarded as definitive.

FUTURE DIRECTIONS

Advances in technology are translating into new possibilities for the endoscopy suite. Among these are confocal laser fluorescent microscopy (CLFM) and electromagnetic navigation (EMN). These new techniques have exciting potential for improving the diagnosis of sarcoidosis and providing further insights into its pathophysiology.

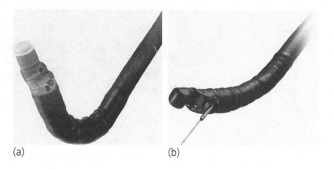

(a)   (b)

Figure 11.4   Endoscopic ultrasound scopes: (a) radial array; (b) linear array.

Confocal laser fluorescence microscopy for the lungs, also called alveoloscopy, is one such technique and allows for microscopic views of tissue *in vivo* (Thiberville *et al.* 2007). A 1.4 mm probe (BronchoFlex, Mauna Kea Technologies) is inserted into the working channel of the bronchoscope and advanced as distally as possible. The probe produces images of the mucosa with which it is in contact. It detects and produces a blue light to induce fluorescence similar to autofluorescence bronchoscopy. The probe is able to produce magnified images with a resolution of 5 μm, with a field of view of 600 μm, such that alveolar structures and macrophages can be visualized. This allows for evaluation at the microscopic level *in vivo*, a feat not possible in the past. No exogenous flourophore is required. This technology is still experimental and findings in patients with sarcoidosis await definition.

Advances have also been seen in electromagnetic navigation (EMN) for the sampling of mediastinal lymph nodes and peripheral lung parenchyma (Gildea *et al.* 2006). This new technology (Superdimension) particularly allows access to peripheral lung, not traditionally within reach of standard bronchoscopy. Data from the CT scan of the chest are merged with data obtained at endobronchial examination by the use of specific computer software. The patient is placed on a magnetic-field generator plate within the endoscopy suite. Specific landmarks such as the main carina, right upper-lobe carina, right middle-lobe carina, and the secondary carina on the left side are marked. These positions are identified at bronchoscopy and marked with the magnetic tracker, allowing co-registration of the patient data at bronchoscopy with the CT data. The system can then be used like a GPS system to navigate to specific target sites on the CT scan. The magnetic locatable guide in conjunction with a steerable catheter allows navigation to specific sites in the peripheral lung or for targeting mediastinal and hilar lymph nodes. Once in position, the sensor is withdrawn (leaving the catheter in place) and a biopsy of peripheral lung or mediastinal lymph node is performed. This EMN technique may be most beneficial in patients with discrete lesions in the peripheral lung parenchyma but can also be used to direct biopsy of areas of lung parenchyma that are thought to give highest yield on the basis of CT scan. Data are awaited on the utility of EMN in the diagnosis of sarcoidosis.

CONCLUSION

Endoscopic techniques are important initial investigations for patients who require pathological diagnosis of sarcoidosis. Bronchoscopy allows bronchoalveolar lavage, endobronchial and transbronchial biopsies which provide tissue for pathological and microbiological analysis. This may confirm the presence of non-caseating granulomas but also provide samples for microbiological exclusion of tuberculosis. The emerging techniques of endobronchial and endoscopic ultrasound have high diagnostic yields in patients with stages I and II sarcoidosis. They are likely to gain increasing importance in selected patients with enlarged intrathoracic lymph nodes due to sarcoidosis and may reduce the necessity for mediastinoscopy in the majority of cases.

REFERENCES

Annema JT, Veselic M, Rabe KF (2005). Endoscopic ultrasound-guided fine-needle aspiration for the diagnosis of sarcoidosis. *Eur Respir J* 25: 405–9.

Babiak A, Hetzel J, Krishna G, Fritz P *et al.* (2009). Transbronchial cryobiopsy: a new tool for lung biopsies. *Respiration* 78: 203–8.

Bilaceroglu S, Gunel O, Eris N *et al.* (2004). Transbronchial needle aspiration in diagnosing intrathoracic tuberculous lymphadenitis. *Chest* 126: 259–67.

Bilaceroglu S, Perim K, Gunel O *et al.* (1999). Combining transbronchial aspiration with endobronchial and transbronchial biopsy in sarcoidosis. *Monaldi Arch Chest Dis* 54: 217–23.

Chapman JT, Mehta AC (2003). Bronchoscopy in sarcoidosis: diagnostic and therapeutic interventions. *Curr Opin Pulm Med* 9: 402–7.

Chin R, McCain TW, Lucia MA *et al.* (2002). Transbronchial needle aspiration in diagnosing and staging lung cancer: how many aspirates are needed? *Am J Respir Crit Care Med* 166: 377–81.

Curley FJ, Johal JS, Burke ME, Fraire AE (1998). Transbronchial lung biopsy: can specimen quality be predicted at the time of biopsy? *Chest* 113: 1037–41.

de Boer S, Milne DG, Zeng I, Wilsher ML (2009). Does CT scanning predict the likelihood of a positive transbronchial biopsy in sarcoidosis? *Thorax* 64: 436–9.

Descombes E, Gardiol D, Leuenberger P (1997). Transbronchial lung biopsy: an analysis of 530 cases with reference to the number of samples. *Monaldi Arch Chest Dis* 52: 324–9.

Fritscher-Ravens A, Sriram PV, Bobrowski C *et al.* (2000). Mediastinal lymphadenopathy in patients with or without previous malignancy: EUS-FNA-based differential cytodiagnosis in 153 patients. *Am J Gastroenterol* 95: 2278–84.

Garwood S, Judson MA, Silvestri G *et al.* (2007). Endobronchial ultrasound for the diagnosis of pulmonary sarcoidosis. *Chest* 132: 1298–304.

Gildea TR, Mazzone PJ, Karnak D *et al.* (2006). Electromagnetic navigation diagnostic bronchoscopy: a prospective study. *Am J Respir Crit Care Med* 174: 982–9.

Helmers RA, Dayton CS, Floerchinger C, Hunninghake GW (1989). Bronchoalveolar lavage in interstitial lung disease: effect of volume of fluid infused. *J Appl Physiol* 67: 1443–6.

Herth FJ, Eberhardt R, Vilmann P *et al.* (2006). Real-time endobronchial ultrasound guided transbronchial needle aspiration for sampling mediastinal lymph nodes. *Thorax* 61: 795–8.

Herth FJ, Morgan RK, Eberhardt R, Ernst A (2008). Endobronchial ultrasound-guided miniforceps biopsy in the biopsy of subcarinal masses in patients with low likelihood of non-small cell lung cancer. *Ann Thorac Surg* 85: 1874–8.

Iannuzzi MC, Rybicki BA, Teirstein AS (2007). Sarcoidosis. *New Engl J Med* 357: 2153–65.

Kennedy MP, Jimenez CA, Mhatre AD *et al.* (2008). Clinical implications of granulomatous inflammation detected by endobronchial ultrasound transbronchial needle aspiration in patients with suspected cancer recurrence in the mediastinum. *J Cardiothorac Surg* 3: 8.

Koerner SK, Sakowitz AJ, Appelman RI *et al.* (1975). Transbronchinal lung biopsy for the diagnosis of sarcoidosis. *New Engl J Med* 293: 268–70.

Krasnik M, Vilmann P, Larsen SS, Jacobsen GK (2003). Preliminary experience with a new method of endoscopic transbronchial real time ultrasound guided biopsy for diagnosis of mediastinal and hilar lesions. *Thorax* **58**: 1083–6.

Leonard C, Tormey VJ, O'Keane C, Burke CM (1997). Bronchoscopic diagnosis of sarcoidosis. *Eur Respir J* **10**: 2722–4.

Loube DI, Johnson JE, Wiener D *et al.* (1993). The effect of forceps size on the adequacy of specimens obtained by transbronchial biopsy. *Am Rev Respir Dis* **148**: 1411–13.

Mariotta S, Valeri B, Guidi L, Bisetti A (1994). Endoscopic findings in arytenoid sarcoidosis. *Sarcoidosis* **11**: 40–41.

Nakajima T, Yasufuku K, Kurosu K *et al.* (2009). The role of EBUS-TBNA for the diagnosis of sarcoidosis: comparisons with other bronchoscopic diagnostic modalities. *Respir Med* **103**: 1796–800.

Oki M, Saka H, Kitagawa C *et al.* (2007). Real-time endobronchial ultrasound-guided transbronchial needle aspiration is useful for diagnosing sarcoidosis. *Respirology* **12**: 863–8.

Pue CA, Pacht ER (1995). Complications of fiberoptic bronchoscopy at a university hospital. *Chest* **107**: 430–2.

Shorr AF, Torrington KG, Hnatiuk OW (2001). Endobronchial involvement and airway hyperreactivity in patients with sarcoidosis. *Chest* **120**: 881–6.

Thiberville L, Moreno-Swirc S, Vercauteren T *et al.* (2007). In-vivo imaging of the bronchial wall microstructure using fibered confocal fluorescence microscopy. *Am J Respir Crit Care Med* **175**: 22–31.

Tremblay A, Stather DR, Maceachern P *et al.* (2009). A randomized controlled trial of standard vs endobronchial ultrasonography-guided transbronchial needle aspiration in patients with suspected sarcoidosis. *Chest* **136**: 340–6.

Trisolini R, Tinelli C, Cancellieri A *et al.* (2008). Transbronchial needle aspiration in sarcoidosis: yield and predictors of a positive aspirate. *J Thorac Cardiovasc Surg* **135**: 837–42.

Wildi SM, Judson MA, Fraig M *et al.* (2004). Is endosonography-guided fine-needle aspiration (EUS-FNA) for sarcoidosis as good as we think? *Thorax* **59**: 794–9.

Wong M, Yasufuku K, Nakajima T *et al.* (2007). Endobronchial ultrasound: new insight for the diagnosis of sarcoidosis. *Eur Respir J* **29**: 1182–6.

12

Bronchoalveolar lavage

PATRICIA L HASLAM

INTRODUCTION

Bronchoalveolar lavage (BAL) is a safe investigatory procedure that involves lavaging a selected subsegment of the lungs with sterile physiological saline via a fiberoptic bronchoscope to sample lung lining fluid containing free cells and other intrinsic or extrinsic inhaled components from the peripheral airways.

Following publication by Reynolds and Newball (1974) of their seminal report showing the potential of BAL in humans, research using BAL has provided a wealth of information about pathogenetic mechanisms in pulmonary sarcoidosis and many other diffuse lung diseases. During the first three decades, research was mainly devoted to elucidating the types of immune and inflammatory cells that accumulate in the peripheral airways in health and disease, and studying their subpopulations, phenotypes, products and functions (Klech and Pohl 1989; Klech and Hutter 1990; Klech et al. 1992). Extracellular components in BAL fluid were also investigated including cytokines, chemokines, growth factors, soluble adhesion molecules, immunoglobulins, complement components, coagulation products, specific products from granulocytes, enzymes and their inhibitors, oxidation products and antioxidants, lipid mediators, markers and mediators of fibrosis, extracellular matrix components, surfactant components, mediators and regulators of apoptosis, markers of cell damage or death, and many other components including infections or other inhaled environmental or occupational agents (Haslam and Baughman 1999a, b).

In the last decade, research has expanded to include also investigations of genetic susceptibility, gene expression profiles in BAL cells, antigen presentation, T-cell receptor analysis, regulatory T-cells, polymorphisms of cytokines such as TNF-α and of cell receptors such as Toll-like receptors, and proteomic profiling of BAL fluids.

In sarcoidosis, such studies have made a major contribution to understanding the key role played by T-lymphocyte subpopulations, macrophages, dendritic cells and their products in pulmonary inflammation and mechanisms of granuloma formation (Wahlstrom et al. 2001; Grünewald et al. 2002; Pabst et al. 2006; Grünewald and Eklund 2007; Sharma et al. 2008; Grutters et al. 2009; Zaba et al. 2010). They have also helped in the continuing search to identify potential etiologic agents (Hiramatsu et al. 2003; Oswald-Richter et al. 2010), and to clarify gene expression profiles and genetic susceptibility (Thonhofer et al. 2002; Rybicki et al. 2005; Chen and Moller 2007; Iannuzzi and Rybicki 2007; Grünewald et al. 2010).

It is outside the scope of this chapter to give further details on the research applications of BAL in sarcoidosis as these are included in other chapters of this book. The main aim of the present chapter is to describe the procedure of BAL and the important role it also plays in routine clinical investigation to assist in the diagnostic work-up of pulmonary sarcoidosis and many other diffuse lung diseases. BAL findings are rarely specifically diagnostic except in some lower respiratory tract infections, thoracic malignancies and some rare lung diseases. BAL cannot identify pathognomonic features in sarcoidosis; however, it can increase confidence in the diagnosis or help to exclude other diseases that must be considered in the differential diagnosis.

Numerous publications confirm that BAL differential cell counts, other cytological features or microbiological findings, when interpreted together with clinical, functional and HRCT findings, can increase confidence in the diagnosis of many lung diseases including sarcoidosis, hypersensitivity pneumonitis (HP), chronic berylliosis, pulmonary eosinophilias, and some of the idiopathic interstitial pneumonias (IIPs) (Klech and Pohl 1989; Klech and Hutter 1990; Klech et al. 1992). In certain other lung diseases, BAL can identify specific features that may establish the diagnosis and avoid the need for biopsy including infections, malignancies, alveolar lipoproteinosis (ALP), pulmonary hemosiderosis, pulmonary Langerhans cell histiocytosis (LCH), amioderone pneumonitis, and giant cell intersitial pneumonia in hard-metal lung disease (GIP) (Haslam 1984; Klech and Hutter 1990; Klech et al. 1992). Detection of inorganic dust fibers or particles in BAL can also be useful to confirm an occupational or environmental exposure or to demonstrate an unrecognized exposure in patients who report no occupational history (Johnson et al. 1986).

Throughout the 1970s, 80s and 90s it was common clinical practice to routinely include BAL in the pre-treatment diagnostic work-up of all patients with diffuse interstitial lung diseases (ILDs) who were well enough to undergo bronchoscopy. However, in recent years high-resolution computerized tomography (HRCT) has become an increasingly important diagnostic tool, and specialists now consider that in some situations HRCT appearances, in the appropriate clinical context, are sufficiently characteristic to confirm a suspected diagnosis without the need for BAL or lung biopsy (Costabel 2007; Wells et al. 2008). In 2002, an ATS/ERS International Committee published a new consensus terminology for the IIPs (Travis et al. 2002). This has also led to considerable changes in the way specialists approach the diagnosis and management of these and other ILDs (Wells et al. 2008).

Despite the above changes, some of which remain controversial, most experts still consider that, in patients with no contraindications to bronchoscopy, BAL remains a valuable investigatory tool that is still indicated whenever the preliminary clinical investigations plus HRCT fail to completely establish a confident diagnosis, or where there is a need for additional information to confirm, strengthen or to exclude a diagnosis (Costabel 2007; Wells et al. 2008; Ohshimo et al. 2009).

BRONCHOALVEOLAR LAVAGE PROCEDURE

The clinical applications of BAL have been hindered because for many years the procedure was not precisely standardized. In addition, BAL quantitative concentrations do not accurately reflect in-vivo levels of the components sampled by BAL because there is still no satisfactory method of determining the dilution factor during lavage. However, during the 1990s

the European Respiratory Society (ERS) made major efforts to improve standardization and published a series of guidelines and recommendations for the conduct and applications of BAL covering technical aspects (Klech and Pohl 1989), clinical applications (Klech and Hutter 1990; Klech et al. 1992), measurement of acellular components and standardization of the procedure (Haslam and Baughman 1999a,b). The main recommendations for a standard procedure in adults have recently been summarized in the ERS *Handbook Respiratory Medicine* (Haslam 2010) and are as follows.

BAL is preferably performed under local anesthesia using fiberoptic bronchoscopy. The first steps are essentially the same as for routine fiberoptic bronchoscopy – premedication with a sedating compound; local anesthesia with lidocaine, removing any excess prior to lavage; and generally semi-supine patient positioning. The additional steps for lavage involve:

- gently wedging the tip of the bronchoscope into an appropriate subsegmental bronchus – the right middle lobe (RML) is the recommended standard site in diffuse lung diseases and healthy controls, but the area of greatest radiographic abnormality in localized lung diseases;
- infusing standard aliquots of sterile physiological saline pre-warmed to body temperature through the application tube of the bronchoscope (four 60 mL aliquots to a maximum 240 mL is recommended);
- sequentially collecting the washings from each aliquot (keeping dwell time to the minimum) by gentle aspiration (very low suction pressure of 3.33–13.3 kPa / 25–100 mmHg to avoid airway collapse) into a container to which cells are poorly adherent (e.g. siliconized glass or a non-cell-adherent plastic such as polyethylene designed for suspension tissue cultures).

Additional procedures such as brushings, bronchial biopsy or transbronchial biopsy should not be performed before lavage as these can result in contamination of lavage samples with blood or bronchial components.

The side-effects of BAL are low and comparable to those of fiberoptic bronchoscopy alone except for a slightly increased risk of transient, minor post-lavage pyrexia. This risk is associated with large lavage introduction volumes and can be avoided by keeping total introduction volumes lower than 300 mL (Dhillon et al. 1986). However, total introduction volumes should not be less than 100 mL in order to sample a greater alveolar area relative to the bronchiolar area (Haslam and Baughman 1999b; Baughman and Rennard 1999). The smaller the introduction volumes the greater the risk of producing a predominantly 'bronchiolar' rather than 'bronchoalveolar' lavage.

In the past, a few workers proposed that the first 20 mL aliquot of lavage fluid recovered should be discarded as this was shown to contain a higher proportion of bronchial components than subsequent aliquots recovered. However, the ERS BAL task force does not favor discarding any aliquots as components that have diagnostic value may be selectively lost. Instead, the task force recommends using a larger lavage introduction volume (total 240 mL in four aliquots) and mixing together all the aspirates recovered, which dilutes and minimizes the effect of bronchial contamination (Haslam and Baughman 1999b; Baughman and Rennard 1999).

For routine clinical diagnostic purposes, it is preferable to use BAL prior to treatment. Therapy can result in changes in BAL cell counts and this may impede the diagnostic value. Smoking also causes significant alterations in levels and functions of BAL cells and other components. For this reason it is important to accurately record whether at the time of lavage the patient is a current, ex- or non-smoker and whether he or she is taking anti-inflammatory or other drugs. A record should also be made of the suspected diagnosis, any associated diseases, the lavage site, the total volume of instilled fluid, number of aliquots, and the total volume of fluid recovered.

PROCESSING OF BAL SAMPLES

The lavage step of the bronchoscopy procedure takes only a few minutes and, because cells deteriorate rapidly in saline, BAL samples should be delivered immediately to the laboratory for processing, which should commence within one hour to transfer the BAL cells into tissue culture medium in order to delay their further deterioration. All laboratory procedures must be conducted using non-cell-adherent containers and pipettes to avoid selective loss of adherent cell types.

- First, the total volume of the recovered BAL sample should be accurately measured.
- The gross appearance of the sample should be noted to record any abnormality such as 'milky appearance' (which is highly suggestive of ALP), excessive 'bloody appearance' (suggestive of acute hemorrhagic conditions) or other unusual coloration (such as blue coloration that can occur after exposure to printing inks).
- The sample should now be mixed to ensure even suspension, then divided into measured aliquots for delivery to different departments if a range of different laboratory investigations is required. This might be 20 mL or more for BAL cytology (and immunocytochemistry and flow cytometry, if required), 10 mL for microbiology, 20 mL for electron microscopy (if required) and 10 mL for biochemistry (if required).
- The aliquot of fluid for BAL cytological investigation should be well mixed and a viability test (e.g. trypan blue) used to check cell viability. The total number of cells per milliliter should then be counted using a hemocytometer (e.g. improved Neubauer Counting chamber) and a white-cell counting stain (e.g. Kimura stain). Frequently there are not enough cells per mL in the very dilute original BAL sample to obtain an accurate cell count. For this reason, many workers prefer to perform the cell count after the next step in the procedure.
- Centrifuge the neat BAL sample by low-speed centrifugation (300 g at 4°C for 10 min) to separate the cells and other insoluble components from the BAL supernatant

fluid. After removing the supernatant fluid and aliquoting it for storage at −70°C, the BAL cell pellet is then washed into serum-free tissue culture medium (Minimum Essential Medium containing 25 mM HEPES buffer) to maintain the pH at 7 in an open system. This preserves cell viability much better than saline (pH = 5).

- The cells are resuspended in a small volume of medium (1–2 mL) to achieve a more concentrated suspension than in the neat fluid. A cell count is performed as above to determine the number of cells per milliliter and calculate the absolute total cells and number per mL in the original fluid.
- Finally, the volume of the cell suspension is adjusted to achieve a suitable concentration (e.g. 1.5×10^6 cells/mL) to prepare cytocentrifuge slide preparations: 100 μL aliquots of the suspension containing 1.5×10^5 cells are suitable to prepare each cytocentrifuge slide preparation (spinning at 450 rpm for 4 min). Glass slides should be degreased and flamed before use to better promote cell adherence to the slide.

At least six slides should be prepared for each patient. After air-drying, two should be fixed in methanol (not formalin which can impair the staining of mast cells) and stained with an appropriate differential counting stain (May–Grünwald–Giemsa is most commonly used). The others should be used for any additional special stains that may be indicated. For example, it is of value to also routinely include a Gomori–Grocott silver stain to assist in demonstrating fungi and *Pneumocystis carinii*, and to include a Perl stain for ferric iron inclusions within macrophages which can indicate pulmonary hemosiderosis.

BAL samples are occasionally so heavily contaminated with mucus as to cause serious technical problems preventing processing. The presence of such excessive mucus from the airways indicates that these samples should be considered inadequate for accurate indication of alveolar events. Mucus can be removed by filtering the lavage sample through cotton gauze or nylon mesh, but this has the disadvantage that it can cause loss of some adherent cell types or other components such as inorganic dust fibers or *P. carinii*. Filtration is, therefore, not advisable when using lavage for routine diagnostic purposes. The majority of BAL samples from patients with diffuse lung diseases and from normal controls do not contain large amounts of mucus and can usually be processed without filtration. In occasional cases where heavy mucus does interfere with processing, a better alternative to filtration to avoid loss of components is to remove mucus from the separated BAL cells and other components *after* centrifugation, by treating the pellet with the mucolytic agent dithiothreitol.

Some workers consider that processing of BAL samples can be delayed for 24 hours. This is not advisable because, even in tissue culture medium, some cells – particularly granulocytes – are short-lived with apoptotic changes starting by 9 hours. Therefore, BAL cells and other insoluble components should ideally be separated and transferred into MEM + HEPES within 1 hour and slide preparations made ready for air-drying within 1–4 hours. Staining can be delayed if necessary.

DIFFERENTIAL BAL CELL COUNTING AND OTHER CYTOLOGICAL APPEARANCES

The routine standard approach to BAL cell counting is to perform a differential count of all the cells present and then express the count of each individual cell type as a percentage of the total BAL cells. This proportionate approach is used because it is not influenced by the unknown BAL dilution factor.

Although quantitative measurements of BAL cells per milliliter (and absolute total numbers) are inaccurate due to the unknown amount of dilution during BAL, these should be recorded because they can indicate gross increases or decreases compared with control ranges. This can assist in interpretation of changes in differential percentage BAL cell counts. For example, reduced percentages of lymphocytes relative to macrophage percentages in healthy smokers compared to non-smokers have been shown to be due to a significant increase in absolute numbers of macrophages and numbers/mL in the smokers, not to reduction in numbers of lymphocytes (Reynolds and Newball 1974).

BAL differential percentage cell counting is most commonly performed using May–Grünwald–Giemsa stained cytocentifuge slide preparations. The slides are examined by light microscopy initially at low power ($\times 10$ and $\times 25$ objectives) to scan and grade (0–5) the amount of mucus and erythrocytes present and to look for evidence of any unusual cytological features (such as inorganic dust particles or fibers, globules of lipoprotein, giant cells, malignant cells, or microorganisms) that may be present in addition to inflammatory cells. Ciliated bronchial or squamous epithelial cells may also occur, indicating the presence of contaminants from the upper airways.

A differential count should then be made of all the different types of cell present using a higher power magnification ($\times 40$ or $\times 60$ objectives) employing random field counting starting at the top left (avoiding the edges of the preparation which can be non-representative) and moving in a zig-zag pattern across the preparation counting all the cells until a total of at least 400 has been reached. The result for each cell type is then expressed as a percentage of the total cells counted (i.e. the differential percentage BAL cell count).

When using BAL as a diagnostic aid, it is important that all cell types present (not just inflammatory cell types) be included in the initial differential count to ensure that valuable information on percentages of other cell types (e.g. malignant cells, giant cells, epithelial cells) is not omitted. If more than 5 percent of epithelial cells are present, this indicates an abnormally high level of contamination of the sample with material from the upper airways and such samples should be considered inadequate as an accurate indicator of alveolar events (Klech and Pohl 1989; Haslam and Baughman 1999b). For research purposes on inflammatory cell types, differential counts can be recalculated if required to exclude other cell types.

It is also important to record abnormal cell appearances. In particular, this includes recording the percentages of foamy macrophages, multinucleate macrophages, giant cells, and the percentages of macrophages containing smoking-related particles, or refractile or birefringent particles indicative of inorganic dusts. Rarely, most of the macrophages may appear densely laden with particles similar to those in smokers but with an orange–brown appearance. This raises the suspicion of pulmonary hemosiderosis, and a Perl stain to test for hemosiderin-laden macrophages should be conducted.

In addition, in samples with very high counts of neutrophils, it is important to check whether there is any evidence of intracellular bacteria. This can indicate active bacterial pneumonia.

Fungal spores or hyphae should also be routinely screened for using a Gomori–Grocott silver stain, which can also detect *Pneumocystis carinii*. These microorganisms may also be seen in the routine May–Grünwald–Giemsa stained preparations.

NORMAL RANGES AND THE EFFECT OF SMOKING

In healthy non-smoking volunteers, the majority of the cells in BAL samples are macrophages and a few lymphocytes, but proportions of other cell types are very low. Smoking causes significant increases in the number of macrophages in BAL samples, which can be at least 4-fold higher (absolute and per mL) in healthy smokers compared with non-smokers, and there are also slight but significant increases in neutrophils (Reynolds and Newball 1974). Thus, it is essential to take smoking into account when defining normal ranges and interpreting the results of any BAL studies.

Owing to the historical absence of a standard BAL procedure, most centers established their own normal ranges using small numbers of volunteers. Published ranges show some variability especially when cell counts are expressed per milliliter or absolute numbers. However, results are very similar when cell counts are expressed as differential percentage counts (consistent with these not being influenced by dilution) (Klech and Pohl 1989; BAL Co-operative Group Steering Committee 1990). For practical purposes, the following normal ranges can be employed for differential percentage BAL cell counts:

- macrophages: ≥ 80 percent in non-smokers and ≥ 90 percent in smokers;
- lymphocytes: ≤ 20 percent in non-smokers and ≤ 10 percent in smokers;
- neutrophils: ≤ 3 percent in non-smokers and ≤ 4 percent in smokers (very occasionally higher);
- eosinophils: ≤ 0.5 percent in non-smokers and ≤ 3 percent in smokers;
- mast cells: ≤ 0.5 percent in non-smokers and smokers;
- plasma cells: 0 percent;
- ciliated or squamous epithelial cells: ≤ 5 percent.

Smoking-related inclusions are frequently present in macrophages from the smokers.

BAL CYTOLOGICAL FEATURES IN RARE LUNG DISEASES

Several rare orphan lung diseases must be considered in the differential diagnosis of diffuse ILDs. The HRCT pattern in these rare diseases may be sufficiently diagnostic in some cases, but others can remain unclear. A number of unusual BAL cytological features can assist in establishing the diagnosis of some of these diseases (Haslam 1984; Danel et al. 1992).

Alveolar lipoproteinosis (ALP)

One of the earliest and best known applications of BAL is to assist in diagnosis of ALP, which is characterized by abnormal accumulation of surfactant phospholipids and proteins in the peripheral airspaces. In primary idiopathic ALP, the accumulations can become so large that therapeutic whole-lung lavage may also be needed. In these classic cases, the gross appearance of the original BAL fluid is characteristically 'milky', suggesting this diagnosis. Confirmatory appearances are found in the BAL cytocentrifuge preparations, where there are characteristic acellular basophilic globules dispersed among granular acellular debris (Danel et al. 1992). Electron microscopy shows that the globules are large aggregates of lipoprotein (Gilmour et al. 1988). Staining an additional cytocentrifuge preparation with Periodic-acid–Schiff (PAS) combined with alcian blue can confirm the presence of PAS-positive phospholipidic material (pink staining) and distinguish it from mucins (blue staining). The BAL cells are of no diagnostic value. They are mainly macrophages, although the cytoplasm is often 'vacuolated' due to uptake of lipid. HRCT in classic cases with major accumulation shows a characteristic 'crazy paving' pattern. However, this may be less clear in patients with minor accumulation as can occur in early disease or in secondary ALP that can occur in association with long-term immunosuppressive therapy, silicosis, or very occasionally in patients with HP. BAL cytology shows the characteristic lipoprotein globules, but the other features seen in classic idiopathic ALP may be less evident (dense acellular debris and gross milky fluid) (Haslam et al. 1988). When ALP is detected, it is essential to establish whether this is primary idiopathic ALP or secondary ALP to select appropriate therapy. Therapeutic lung lavage may be needed only in idiopathic ALP.

Pulmonary hemosiderosis (PH)

The value of BAL as an adjunct to diagnosis of the pulmonary hemorrhagic disorders is well recognized (Haslam 1984; Danel et al. 1992; Klech et al. 1992). Acute hemorrhagic conditions should be considered if the original BAL fluid is very heavily contaminated with blood and the BAL cytocentrifuge preparations show very numerous erythrocytes (highest grade 5). This is invariably the BAL appearance in patients with bleomycin fibrosis, and to a lesser extent in occasional patients with collagen–vascular diseases. However,

the greatest value of BAL cytology in the hemorrhagic conditions is to assist in the diagnosis of chronic hemorrhage within the lungs (often 'occult') that can result in the development of PH. There are various possible causes including idiopathic pulmonary hemosiderosis, lung involvement in Goodpasture's syndrome, or development of PH secondary to persistent lower respiratory tract infections, lung transplantation, or even smoking. It may be asymptomatic or symptomatic. Clinically relevant PH is indicated when all or most of the BAL macrophages are heavily laden with hemosiderin. The BAL cells are mainly macrophages as in normal controls (which is very unusual in most diffuse interstitial lung diseases apart from LCH and RB-ILD, see below). However, the macrophages contain cytoplasmic inclusions resembling those in heavy smokers except that they have a distinctive orange–brown appearance suggestive of hemosiderin. A special stain for ferric iron, such as Perl stain, can confirm this.

Although BAL is a specific indicator of PH, it cannot differentiate between the various diseases that can give rise to this syndrome and it cannot accurately distinguish between asymptomatic and symptomatic stages. However, it is only in clinically relevant active PH that almost every macrophage is hemosiderin-laden; and a 'Golde scoring' approach can be used to distinguish such cases. Nevertheless, the clinician must take further steps to distinguish primary idiopathic PH or Goodpasture's syndrome from known causes of secondary PH to establish the final diagnosis.

Pulmonary Langerhans cell histiocytosis (LCH)

Another rare disease in which specific BAL findings can aid diagnosis is pulmonary LCH (Haslam 1984; Danel et al. 1992; Klech et al. 1992). This possible diagnosis is suspected when patients present with evidence of ILD, but with an apparently 'normal' BAL cell profile by light microscopy showing mainly macrophages containing dense smoking-related inclusions as in normal heavy smokers. LCH is a multisystemic, smoking-related disease, and the increases in Langerhans cells which characterize this disorder cannot be distinguished from macrophages in the conventional May–Grünwald–Giemsa stained BAL cytocentrifuge preparations. Special additional laboratory investigations must be undertaken. If electron microscopy (EM) is available, the most specific and definitive additional test is to examine samples of the BAL cells by EM. The presence of Langerhans cells containing characteristic intracytoplasmic X-bodies (granules of typical pentalaminar structure with a 'tennis racquet' shape at one end) can be specifically identified by ultrastructure. Small increases in Langerhans cells can also occur in BAL in smokers with and without other lung diseases, but in these situations counts do not exceed 5 percent of the total BAL cells. Counts higher than 5 percent are a strong diagnostic indicator of pulmonary LCH. Many centers do not have access to EM, and as an alternative they can use immunocytochemistry or flow cytometry to identify Langerhans cells by employing monoclonal antibodies to detect surface markers (CD1a and S-100 protein) expressed on these cells. Although less definitive than EM, CD1a is a highly specific marker for Langerhans cells and when expressed on more than 5 percent of the BAL cells this also strongly supports the diagnosis of LCH. However, counts of Langerhans cells can fluctuate at different stages of disease thus a negative BAL finding cannot exclude this diagnosis.

BAL IN SARCOIDOSIS AND OTHER NON-INFECTIOUS GRANULOMATOUS LUNG DISEASES

In contrast to the above rare lung diseases, malignancies, and respiratory infections (including *M. tuberculosis*), where highly specific BAL features can help to establish the diagnosis, there are no specific BAL features in the majority of other diffuse lung diseases including pulmonary sarcoidosis and other granulomatous lung diseases such as hypersensitivity pneumonitis (HP) and chronic beryllium disease. However, BAL cell counts often show typical profiles of increase in different types of immune and inflammatory cells, which may allow a diagnosis to be made with greater confidence.

The typical BAL cellular profile that supports the diagnosis of granulomatous lung diseases is the finding of predominant increases in percentages of lymphocytes (nearly all T-lymphocytes) together with decreased percentages of macrophages, but without or with only minor increases in other inflammatory cell types. Differences in percentages of lymphocytes, in profiles of other cell types, and in T-lymphocyte sub-populations (CD4/CD8 ratios) can help to differentiate between different granulomatous diseases, For example, striking increases in lymphocytes ≥50 percent are highly suggestive of hypersensitivity pneumonitis, while moderate increases ≥40 percent are more common in sarcoidosis and chronic beryllium disease. More details are given below.

Sarcoidosis

Nearly all patients with pulmonary sarcoidosis have increases in BAL lymphocyte percentages at the time of diagnosis (Haslam 1984; Klech *et al.* 1992; Costabel *et al.* 2005). Although BAL lymphocyte increases occur in other diseases, the BAL cellular profile most typical of sarcoidosis is the finding of decreases in macrophages together with moderate increases in lymphocytes (≤40 percent), and occasionally also minor increases in neutrophils. The macrophages usually resemble those in normal non-smokers and there is no increase in 'foamy' macrophages (unlike HP). The lymphocytes are mainly normal in appearance with no evidence of increased 'blast' forms. There have been numerous investigations of the clinical value of BAL cell counts in sarcoidosis, but the utility has been compromised by differences between study groups in the stage of disease (often not well defined) and by inaccurate use of the term 'activity' (often muddled with staging or erroneously equated with prognosis). Although in the 1970s there were reports that patients with

higher counts of lymphocytes ≥28 percent had more active disease and a poorer prognosis, subsequent studies have not confirmed this. It now appears that patients who progress unfavorably to develop chronic widespread parenchymal involvement (radiographic stages II and III) have significantly lower levels of BAL lymphocytes than patients at an earlier stage (stage I) (Lin *et al.* 1985). Indeed, patients with highly active acute onset disease (Löfgren's syndrome) have been reported to have the highest BAL lymphocyte counts even though they have the best prognosis (Ward *et al.* 1989). T-lymphocyte sub-population analysis shows that CD4/CD8 ratios are also very frequently increased in patients with Löfgren's syndrome (Drent *et al.* 1993a). Increased CD4/CD8 ratios also occur in around half of all patients with sarcoidosis; but normal or low ratios are also common, so this is not a sensitive marker for sarcoidosis. However, it has been reported that ratios ≥3.5 are highly specific for sarcoidosis and can be of value in diagnosis of that subgroup of patients (Drent *et al.* 2001; Welker *et al.* 2004). The use of ratios is still a controversial issue because very variable ratios including increased ratios occur in many other diffuse lung diseases.

While increases in BAL lymphocytes can support the diagnosis of sarcoidosis, they cannot guide decisions on when to commence corticosteroid treatment. Paradoxically, lower lymphocyte counts are found in patients who have progressed to parenchymal disease and fibrosis. Increases in BAL neutrophils have also been shown in these patients (Lin *et al.* 1985). Evidence of a relationship between increased BAL neutrophils and progressive deterioration has also been reported (Drent *et al.* 1999; Ziegenhagen *et al.* 2003). These reports support the view that BAL neutrophilia may be a useful marker of chronic progression in sarcoidosis indicating need for treatment. Unfortunately, BAL findings have not yet identified any reliable markers in sarcoidosis that can accurately monitor disease activity, guide the choice of drugs or doses or duration, or predict resolution.

Hypersensitivity pneumonitis (extrinsic allergic alveolitis)

BAL findings of striking increases in lymphocyte percentage counts ≥50 percent together with decreased percentages of macrophages in the presence or absence of various additional features as described below, can be of especial value in increasing confidence in the diagnosis of HP and reducing the likelihood of sarcoidosis or other ILDs (Haslam 1984; Klech *et al.* 1992; Selman 2003).

HP is triggered in susceptible individuals by immune hypersensitivity reactions to antigens in many inhaled organic dusts. For example, fungal and/or bacterial antigens in moldy hay can trigger 'farmer's lung disease', microbial antigens in contaminated air-conditioners can give rise to 'humidifier lung disease', and avian proteins in bird droppings can give rise to 'bird-breeders lung diseases'. Patients with repeated high-dose exposure (as in farmer's lung and pigeon breeder's lung) usually have a characteristic episodic course with repeated acute episodes. By contrast, patients with chronic low-dose exposure (as often occurs in budgerigar fancier's lung) can have an insidious subacute progressive course. In the longer term, the disease can progress to chronic irreversible fibrosis.

Nearly all patients with acute or subacute HP have very high BAL lymphocyte percentages usually ≥ 50 percent. As in sarcoidosis, most of the lymphocytes are T-lymphocytes but unlike sarcoidosis CD4+/CD8+ ratios are more frequently decreased (<2 in non-smokers, <1 in smokers) than increased (>3 in non-smokers, >2 in smokers). However, these ratios are too variable and non-disease specific to be of any reliable diagnostic value.

In addition to high BAL lymphocyte percentages, certain other BAL cytological appearances can further increase confidence in the diagnosis of HP. Unlike sarcoidosis where most BAL lymphocytes have the morphological appearance of normal small lymphocytes, in HP it is common to find 'blast forms' of lymphocytes among the BAL cells (Haslam et al. 1987). Occasional plasma cells have also been reported. An increased proportion of BAL macrophages may also have a characteristic 'foamy' appearance (Haslam 1994). In patients during acute episodes or in those with subacute disease for up to 3 months after antigen exposure, there are minor to moderate increases in neutrophils and mast cells in addition to the lymphocyte increases in BAL (Haslam et al. 1987; Drent et al. 1993b).

While none of these BAL markers by itself is a specific diagnostic marker, the full BAL profile of a striking increase in lymphocytes combined with minor to moderate increases in neutrophils and/or mast cells is a strong diagnostic indicator of HP with recent antigen exposure. In patients with other evidence suggestive of this diagnosis, such additional BAL findings can strengthen diagnostic confidence sufficiently to avoid the need for biopsy. Furthermore, the finding of this BAL profile in an ILD patient with an unclear diagnosis strongly indicates probable HP. Removal of patients from exposure can then be urgently implemented.

It is important to be aware that striking increases in BAL lymphocytes also occur in healthy workers exposed to these organic antigens without evidence of lung disease (who also have evidence of circulating specific antibodies to these antigens as in patients with HP). Thus, these changes in BAL appear to be a response to exposure rather than disease-specific. It has been suggested that asymptomatic individuals may have an unknown protective response. It is also of interest that most patients with HP are non-smokers and it has been speculated that smoking may have a suppressive effect on the immune hypersensitivity reactions associated with this disease (Hughes and Haslam 1990). These and many other questions remain under research investigation.

Chronic beryllium disease and other occupational granulomatous lung diseases caused by mineral dusts

Chronic beryllium disease (CBD) is a granulomatous occupational lung disease that results from inhalation of fumes or dusts from beryllium metal or its salts. It is clinically and histologically very similar to pulmonary sarcoidosis. The BAL differential cell count profile is also similar to that in sarcoidosis, showing macrophages together with moderate to marked increases in lymphocytes (which can exceed 50 percent). As in sarcoidosis, phenotypic analysis shows that the lymphocytes are T-lymphocytes. Also resembling sarcoidosis, CD4+/CD8+ ratios are significantly increased, but this appears to be a less variable finding than in sarcoidosis with increased ratios >3 in nearly all CBD patients (Newman et al. 1989).

An additional diagnostic test has been developed to specifically confirm beryllium sensitization in suspected CBD. This tests the ability of blood and BAL lymphocytes from the patient to proliferate in vitro when challenged with beryllium salts. Most of the proliferating cells are CD4+ T-cells (Saltini et al. 1989). The diagnostic specificity of this test has been reported to be 100 percent and the sensitivity is much higher using BAL than blood lymphocytes (Rossman et al. 1988).

Beryllium salts are soluble, so BAL cytology cannot provide any morphological evidence of beryllium exposure. However, a number of other inorganic dusts, such as aluminum, can also give rise to granulomatous occupational lung diseases often associated with moderate increases in BAL lymphocytes (Newman 1998). These diseases can also be indicated by the presence of insoluble refractile and/or birefringent inorganic dust particles within the cytoplasm of BAL macrophages. More information on BAL in occupational dust diseases is given below.

BAL IN OTHER OCCUPATIONAL LUNG DISEASES DUE TO MINERAL DUSTS

The initial clinical assessment of all patients with suspected ILD must include a detailed occupational history to establish whether there has been exposure to any of the other agents, in addition to beryllium, that can cause occupational ILDs. Exposures related to hobbies or the environment should also be recorded.

BAL has been widely applied as a research tool to study interstitial fibrosing lung diseases caused by exposure to fibrous mineral dusts such as asbestos, talc and glass fiber, and non-fibrous mineral dusts such as silica, coal, hard metal, antimony and iron (Costabel et al. 1992). The greatest clinical value of BAL in these diseases is to show that dust is present in the lungs confirming that exposure has taken place. This is not disease-specific because dust is also present in BAL from exposed workers without disease. However, BAL is useful:

- to provide direct evidence of specific dust exposure when this is required for medico-legal reasons;
- to identify potentially relevant inhaled dust in ILD patients who have no known exposure history;
- to identify inhaled dust in patients with a history of uncertain exposure;
- to identify the predominant types of dust/s in the lungs of patients with a history of mixed dust exposures;
- to help to exclude the coexistence of an ILD of another cause in a patient who may also have dust exposure.

BAL differential cell counts demonstrate typical patterns of inflammatory cells in the different mineral dust ILDs, but these are not disease-specific and are generally not of diagnostic value. One exception is hard-metal-associated GIP, where the presence of increased numbers of bizarre foreign-body type giant cells containing refractile particles of hard-metal can provide a highly specific indicator of this diagnosis.

More details of BAL findings in these occupational diseases are as follows.

Asbestosis and other ILDs caused by exposure to fibrous mineral dusts

When inhaled asbestos or other fibrous dusts are deposited in the peripheral airways, the fibers can become coated with iron-containing protein deposits to form 'dumb-bell' shaped ferruginous bodies. Ferruginous bodies can be detected and counted by light microscopy in routine May–Grünwald–Giemsa stained BAL cytocentifuge preparations. It is important not to pre-filter BAL samples or fibers and ferruginous bodies may be lost.

Classic asbestos bodies are regularly segmented and have a fine central fiber core, which is transparent (Haslam 1984; Costabel et al. 1992). Other fibrous dusts form ferruginous bodies which may be thicker and irregular in shape, such as the flat plate-like talc bodies (Haslam 1984). There is usually no need to conduct mineralogical analysis to identify the inhaled dust, because in most cases the exposure history is known. When there is no clear exposure history or there have been mixed exposures, mineralogical analysis can be performed. The most common method is energy dispersive X-ray microanalysis using BAL samples prepared for either transmission or scanning EM (Johnson et al. 1986). Uncoated fibers too small to form bodies can also be detected by EM and analyzed.

Many research studies have investigated whether quantifying the number of asbestos fibers in BAL samples can differentiate between exposed workers with and without asbestos-related diseases, but this has not yet proved of clinical value (Johnson et al. 1986; De Vuyst et al. 1998).

BAL differential cell counts in the asbestos-related diseases usually show only minor increases in inflammatory cells, and these are not of diagnostic value. The patterns are similar to those in the IIPs but the counts tend to be lower. Some workers exposed to asbestos but without evidence of disease have been reported to have increases in BAL lymphocytes, but it is unknown whether this has clinical prognostic relevance (Wallace et al. 1989). Levels of lymphocytes have also been reported to be higher in patients with pleural disease than in those without (Wallace et al. 1989). By contrast, in asbestosis findings are more variable but some reports have indicated that increases in lymphocyte percentages are associated with less severe impairment of lung function while increases in neutrophil and eosinophil percentages are associated with more severe impairment and with a longer duration of disease (Gellert et al. 1985).

In conclusion, BAL is useful to confirm or indicate dust exposure, but BAL cell counts are not of diagnostic value in ILDs caused by fibrous mineral dusts.

Hard-metal lung disease and other ILDs caused by exposure to non-fibrous mineral dusts

Non-fibrous crystalline or metallic dusts do not form ferruginous bodies. However, particles associated with these exposures can be detected by light microscopy within BAL macrophages. These particles are usually highly refractile or birefringent and are distinct from smoking-related particles. They can indicate exposure to dusts such as hard metal, crystalline silica, aluminum or chromium–cobalt–molybdenum alloys used in dentistry. Coal-dust exposure can also give rise to distinctive particles in macrophages, but these are not refractile unless crystalline silica is also present as in coal pneumoconiosis associated with progressive massive fibrosis (PMF). If there is no known exposure history, mineral dust particles within macrophages can also be identified by energy dispersive X-ray microanalysis using preparations fixed for scanning or scanning transmission EM (Johnson et al. 1986).

BAL differential cell count profiles in individuals exposed to crystalline silica or coal dust with or without disease are too non-specific and variable to be of diagnostic value. In silica exposure or disease, moderate increases in percentages of BAL lymphocytes and sometimes also in neutrophils can occur, but total BAL cell counts are usually normal or only slightly increased (Christman et al. 1985; Costabel et al. 1992). By contrast, in patients with simple coal pneumoconiosis, marked increases in total BAL cell counts have been reported (mainly due to increases in macrophages as occur in smokers), and also mild increases in neutrophil percentages (Rom et al. 1987). More marked increases in neutrophil percentages have been reported in PMF associated with coal pneumoconiosis (Wallaert et al. 1990).

Patients with mineral dust exposures that cause granulomatous lung diseases often have increases in BAL lymphocyte percentages as previously described.

BAL cytology is also valuable to detect rare cases of GIP in hard-metal lung disease. Bizarre giant cells can be detected among the BAL cells giving a specific indication of this diagnosis (Davison et al. 1983). The giant cells are distinct from the usual multinucleate macrophages that are commonly seen, for example in smokers. They are of the foreign-body type, often have more than 10 nuclei, and small refractile particles consistent with hard-metal exposure can often be detected in their cytoplasm and in other BAL macrophages. Energy dispersive X-ray microanalysis indicates the predominant component is tungsten (Davison et al. 1983; Johnson et al. 1986). Other components in alloys of hard metal include titanium, tantalum, nickel, chromium, niobium and vanadium. Cobalt is also added as a binding agent, but it is rarely found in the lungs of patients because it is soluble and rapidly cleared. It is thought to play an important role in pathogenesis because diamond polishers exposed to cobalt alone can develop cobalt lung which shows very similar features to hard-metal lung disease (Demedts et al. 1984).

Other inflammatory cells in BAL in hard-metal lung disease are variable and not of diagnostic value. Some workers have reported mild increases in lymphocytes with reduced CD4/CD8 ratios, while others have reported mild to moderate increases in neutrophils and sometimes also eosinophils (Davison et al. 1983; Massaglia et al. 1988). Giant cell counts have been observed to fall with progression from GIP to UIP during follow-up after removal from exposure (Davison et al. 1983). Thus, the absence of giant cells does not exclude the diagnosis of hard-metal lung disease. Demonstration of typical refractile particles within macrophages also indicates that this diagnosis should be considered.

BAL IN DRUG-INDUCED OR OTHER IATROGENIC LUNG DISEASES

A large number of drugs have the potential to cause pneumotoxic effects and it is essential to obtain a detailed history of all current and previous drug therapy in patients who present for investigation of suspected ILD. The drug-induced ILDs have a wide range of pathologies and their presentation may be acute or chronic. Early diagnosis is important to prevent irreversible lung damage. The varying pathologies associated with different drugs may include alveolar hemorrhage, diffuse alveolar damage, pulmonary edema, eosinophilic pneumonia, secondary alveolar lipoproteinosis, drug-induced interstitial pulmonary fibrosis, drug-induced hypersensitivity pneumonitis, and pulmonary thesaurismosis with hyperlymphocytosis.

BAL differential cell counts show different patterns of increased inflammatory cell types associated with different types of drugs (Israel-Biet et al. 1992). BAL lymphocytosis is a feature of HP induced by many drugs, including methotrexate, nitrofurantoin, BCG therapy and many others. Increases in eosinophils and less frequently in neutrophils may also occur, while occasionally some drugs (including tetracyclines and sulfasalazine) can induce eosinophilic pneumonia indicated by very striking and predominant increases in BAL eosinophils ≥ 40 percent. BAL is a valuable diagnostic aid in such cases, which often respond well to steroids. BAL is also a sensitive indicator of acute alveolar hemorrhage which is a notable feature of some drug-induced toxicities, including those induced by d-penicillamine and bleomycin.

Other iatrogenic diseases where BAL cytological features can be valuable diagnostic indicators include lipoid pneumonia induced by mineral oil such as in nose drops, where BAL macrophages contain large vacuoles of lipid, which stain strongly with Oil-Red-O. In addition, the drug amiodarone can induce the accumulation of numerous large lamellar inclusions of phospholipid within alveolar macrophages and other cells (thesaurismosis). This feature is a general effect of amiodarone treatment, but when it occurs in association with BAL lymphocytosis this is a strong indicator of amiodarone-induced pneumonitis (Danel et al. 1988; Israel-Biet et al. 1992). Radiation pneumonitis is another iatrogenic disease that is associated with increases in BAL lymphocytes, although BAL is more useful in these cases to exclude infections or spread of malignancy.

BAL IN OTHER PULMONARY EOSINOPHILIC DISEASES

In addition to drug-induced eosinophilic pneumonia, eosinophilic infiltrates in the lungs indicated by increases in BAL eosinophils can occur in many other lung diseases. Mild to moderate increases in BAL eosinophil percentages are frequently found in patients with idiopathic pulmonary fibrosis (IPF) and also occur in some patients with connective tissue diseases affecting the lungs. However, in all these cases the eosinophil increases are combined with increases in neutrophils, which are usually predominant. Minor increases in BAL eosinophils accompanied by more prominent increases in other inflammatory cell types have also been reported in very occasional patients with other more common diffuse lung diseases, including sarcoidosis, hypersensitivity pneumonitis and tuberculosis. However, the greatest value of BAL as an aid to the diagnosis of the eosinophilic lung diseases is to identify those disorders associated with especially striking and predominant increases in eosinophils in BAL. These include not only drug-induced eosinophilic pneumonia but also acute or chronic idiopathic eosinophilic pneumonia (Danel et al. 1992). These frequently result in life-threatening acute respiratory failure and BAL is a valuable diagnostic tool in critical care to distinguish these rare cases of eosinophilic pneumonia from other causes of acute lung injury, which is important so that treatment with steroids can commence as soon as possible (Dejaegher and Demedts 1984).

Other diseases where eosinophilia can be the predominant BAL finding − sometimes also with mild to moderate increases in lymphocytes but usually only with normal or slight increases in neutrophils − are allergic diseases, including asthma, Churg−Strauss syndrome and bronchopulmonary aspergillosis, and parasitic infections such as schistosomiasis.

In the appropriate clinical setting, BAL can be of great value to increase confidence in the diagnosis of eosinophilic lung diseases and especially of the eosinophilic pneumonias.

BAL IN PATIENTS WITH ACUTE RESPIRATORY FAILURE

In the critical care setting, BAL has been of considerable value to study pathogenic mechanisms in acute respiratory distress syndrome (ARDS), which is etiologically associated with a wide range of risk factors including sepsis, trauma, aspiration, smoke inhalation, near drowning and many others. A large body of BAL information is available on inflammatory cells and mediators, proteolytic enzymes and inhibitors, oxidants and antioxidants, and pulmonary surfactant composition (Baker et al. 1999; Aggarwal et al. 2000). The clinical utility of most of this information is not yet clear. However, it is long-established that BAL is of considerable value to assist in distinguishing bacterial and viral pneumonias or other infections from the many other possible causes of acute respiratory failure. BAL differential cell counts can also help to increase confidence in the diagnosis of ARDS, where patients classically show increases only in BAL neutrophils with exceptionally high percentage counts, usually above 60 percent and often above 80 percent during, the first week after presentation (Aggarwal *et al.* 2000). Sometimes, bacteria may be observed within the cytoplasm of the neutrophils and this is a useful indicator of an active bacterial infection. Rarely, patients may be encountered who have a very different BAL cell profile that is inconsistent with the diagnosis of ARDS. This can be very useful to distinguish other diseases that can result in respiratory failure. For example, striking increases in eosinophils can indicate eosinophilic pneumonia; or a profile of mainly macrophages containing large lamellar bodies of phospholipid can indicate amiodarone pneumonitis. Acute interstitial pneumonia with the histopathological feature of diffuse alveolar damage is another rare disease that may very occasionally be encountered, but no definitive BAL features have so far been reported in this very rare condition (see IIP section below).

BAL IN PATIENTS WITH LOWER RESPIRATORY TRACT INFECTIONS

A variety of bronchoscopic sampling techniques, including BAL, have long been used to assist the diagnosis of lower respiratory tract infections (LRTIs). However, contamination of the bronchoscope with irrelevant bacteria and other organisms from the oropharynx when it traverses the upper airways can present a major problem in distinguishing between such contaminants and meaningful infections. For this reason, very precise methodology is recommended by specialists in the field of respiratory infections to minimize contamination (Dombret and Chastre 1998). The two methods now considered to be of particular value are:

- the protected specimen brush (PSB) technique, which makes use of a double-lumen catheter with a PSB to collect uncontaminated samples directly from the lower respiratory tract;
- BAL using a fiberoptic bronchoscope following recommended precautions to reduce contamination, or alternatively using a protected transbronchoscopic balloon-tipped catheter.

Both PSB and BAL are very safe procedures, but the risk of minor bleeding is less with BAL so this is the preferred method for use in ventilated patients to diagnose pneumonias or in immunocompromised patients to diagnose opportunistic lung infections. BAL also has the advantage that it samples a larger alveolar area.

There are very strict requirements not only for the BAL procedure but also for handling of BAL specimens to obtain optimal microbiological results. These include aseptic procedure, lavaging the site of maximal involvement, rapid delivery to the laboratory within 30 minutes, and precautions to avoid any contamination of the BAL fluid with lidocaine. The techniques used for detetection of microorganisms (bacteria, viruses, fungi, protozoa, etc.) include using appropriately stained smears or cytocentrifuge preparations, quantitative culture techniques, immunocytochemical techniques and modern rapid diagnostic DNA/RNA techniques.

LRTIs in immunocompetent patients

Many studies have demonstrated that there is good agreement between positive quantitative BAL culture results (generally $>10^4$ CFU/mL) and PSB culture results for the diagnosis of the agents causing community-acquired pneumonia or nosocomial pneumonia in mechanically ventilated patients, and that both approaches have a similar high sensitivity and specificity (Chastre *et al.* 1995; Jourdain *et al.* 1997). Giemsa or Gram staining of BAL cytocentrifuge preparations or smears is also useful to rapidly identify BAL cells containing intracellular bacteria, which are present in most patients with active pneumonia but not in those without pneumonia (Chastre *et al.* 1995). It is important for optimal results that these diagnostic techniques be employed as soon as possible before commencement of antibiotic therapy. Precise identification of the infectious agent, often in >80 percent of patients with pneumonia using BAL or PSB, is valuable to select the optimal antibiotic for the individual patient. This helps to avoid empirical use of broad-spectrum antibiotics in patients without true infection, which can risk emergence of antibiotic-resistant strains. Microorganisms that commonly cause community-acquired or noocomial pneumonias include *Streptococcus pneumoniae*, *Haemophilus influenzae*, *Staphylococcus aureus*, *Moraxella catarrhalis*, *Mycoplasma pneumoniae*, *Legionella* species, *Chlamydia* species, Gram-negative enteric bacilli and *Pseudomonas aeruginosa*. Guidelines providing detailed advice on the diagnosis and management of these LRTIs are available (Torres *et al.* 2001; Woodhead *et al.* 2005).

LRTIs in immunocompromised patients

BAL is the preferred method to sample the lungs of patients with immunodeficiency when pulmonary infiltrates develop, raising suspicion of opportunistic infections. Although the diagnostic yield of BAL for opportunistic infections has been reported to be lower than with lung biopsies (transbronchial, VATS or open), the risk of complications using biopsy is higher in immunocompromised patients, so BAL is preferred initially because this can often provide a definitive diagnosis of an opportunistic infection (Bjermer *et al.* 1992). In particular, BAL is of proven value in acquired immunodeficiency syndrome (AIDS) to diagnose pulmonary opportunistic infections including *Pneumocystis carinii* pneumonia, invasive aspergillosis, mycobacterial infections, *Cryptococcus neoformans*, or *Pseudomonas aeruginosa* pneumonia. It is also of value in organ transplant recipients to assist in identifying *Pneumocystis carinii* pneumonia, cytomegalovirus pneumonitis, and other opportunists. Patients with malignant diseases frequently develop impaired immunity due to drug-induced immunosuppression, and patients with leukaemia or lymphoma have impaired cell-mediated immunity making them especially susceptible to *Cryptococcus*, tuberculosis, toxoplasmosis and *Nocardia*. Fungal infections, due to for example *Candida*, *Aspergillus*, *Histoplasma*, coccidiomycosis, *Cryptococcus* and blastomycosis, can also be a serious problem in immunocompromised patients. Other bacterial infections also occur, including *Legionella*. Virus infections that are also common in immunosuppressed patients include not only cytomegalovirus but also adenovirus, herpes simplex, varicella-zoster and respiratory syncytial viruses.

BAL IN THORACIC MALIGNANCIES

Early diagnosis of lung cancers is of crucial importance if there is to be any chance of successful treatment. Broncho-scopic techniques have long played a major role in the diagnosis and early detection. About 50–60 percent of all lung cancers develop in the central airways and may be detected bronchoscopically before they are radiologically evident. In recent years, the sensitivity and specificity for detecting and locating early malignant lesions have been much improved by the introduction of endobronchial ultrasound and/or fluorescence bronchoscopy using autofluorescence or photodynamic diagnosis to visualize malignant tissue. Bronchoscopic biopsies (bronchial or transbronchial), aspiration biopsies, bronchial brushings or bronchial washings can then be obtained from the affected sites for histological or cytological examination. BAL (as distinct from small-volume bronchial washings) has not been much used in routine thoracic oncology. This is probably because it was traditionally used by pulmonologists to investigate non-malignant lung diseases. However, during routine screening of BAL samples from a wide range of patients with suspected ILDs, malignant cells are occasionally demonstrated by BAL cytology when this diagnosis is not initially suspected. Several workers have also published studies of large groups of patients with primary lung cancer showing that BAL cytology has a similar diagnostic yield to bronchial washings and the yield can be higher than that for biopsies when tumor is not visible by bronchoscopy (Rennard *et al.* 1992). In particular, BAL can be of value in the diagnosis of peripheral lung tumors, including early peripheral nodules or diffuse peripheral lesions associated with adenocarcinoma or bronchoalveolar cell carcinoma. BAL cytology can also be of diagnostic value in malignancies other than primary lung cancers, for example hematological malignancies in the lung including B-cell lymphomas and Hodgkin's lymphoma (Rennard *et al.* 1992). Metastatic lesions and lymphangitic spread to the lungs from non-pulmonary tumors (e.g. breast cancer) has also been reported. Malignant cells can usually be easily detected in routine May–Grünwald–Giemsa stained BAL preparations. However, these preparations do not show the nuclear detail preferred for cytological confirmation of malignant cells. Therefore, additional Papanicolaou-stained slides can be prepared. When B-cell lymphomas are suspected, additional immunocytochemical or flow cytometric tests can be conducted using specific monoclonal antibodies to test for monoclonality of immunoglobulin class.

When malignant cells are detected during routine BAL screening of patients for ILDs, confirmatory tests should always be conducted with the assistance of a specialist pathologist or cytopathologist with experience of malignant cell cytology.

BAL IN IDIOPATHIC INTERSTITIAL PNEUMONIAS (IIPs)

A high proportion of patients presenting for investigation of diffuse lung disease are likely to have one of the IIPs or one of the systemic collagen–vascular diseases (CVDs) that can affect the lungs. BAL cannot establish the diagnosis of any of the IIPs or CVDs. However, if clinical observations and HRCT suggest one of these diseases but are inconclusive, certain characteristic BAL cell profiles can be supportive or suggest that an alternative needs to be considered (Wells *et al.* 2008).

The terminology of IIP was redefined in 2002 and this syndrome has now been split into a number of separate 'diseases' on the basis of defined histopathological, clinical and HRCT features, although etiologic agents have still not been identified (Travis *et al.* 2002). Before 2002, the syndrome IIP was termed 'idiopathic pulmonary fibrosis' in the USA and 'cryptogenic fibrosing alveolitis' in the UK and some other countries; and it was recognized that the syndrome probably contained a variable group of disorders. Using these previous terms, the main BAL findings for the syndrome (i.e. all the IIPs grouped together) during the 1970s, 80s and 90s were that nearly all patients had increases in BAL inflammatory cells, the most common profile being macrophages combined with moderate increases in neutrophils and sometimes also mild to moderate increases in eosinophils. Up to about 20 percent of patients also had mild to moderate increases in lymphocytes combined with increases in neutrophils and very occasionally also eosinophils. These earlier studies also provided evidence that higher counts of granulocytes – and in particular increases in eosinophils – were associated with more rapid progression and a poorer prognosis (Haslam *et al.* 1992). In addition, increases in lymphocytes were associated with a better prognosis and a better chance of improvement on corticosteroids (Haslam *et al.* 1992). These earlier findings have now been reconsidered following the reclassification of the syndrome into a number of separate diseases in 2002 (Travis *et al.* 2002). In particular, it now appears that BAL profiles that include increases in lymphocytes as well as granulocytes relate to different diseases usually with a better prognosis than those that include only increases in granulocytes, as described below.

1. The term *idiopathic pulmonary fibrosis* (IPF) is now reserved only for patients who have the histopathological feature of usual interstitial pneumonia (UIP) on surgical lung biopsies, an HRCT pattern consistent with UIP, and no increase in lymphocytes in BAL. These patients characteristically have a BAL profile of macrophages combined with moderate increases in neutrophils and sometimes also mild to moderate increases in eosinophils. Prognosis is poor and more effective treatments are urgently needed.

2. The term *non-specific interstitial pneumonitis* (NSIP) recognizes a new form of IIP that can be distinguished histopathologically from IPF/UIP by having the more cellular and homogeneous histological pattern of NSIP on surgical lung biopsies. Patients with NSIP generally have a more favorable prognosis than those with IPF/UIP. However, controversy exists about whether this may be a mixed group of disorders rather than a single disease entity, because several clinico-radiological-histopathological variants can be distinguished including cases with predominantly cellular NSIP, predominantly fibrotic NSIP, and a mixture of cellular and fibrotic patterns. The NSIP pattern is also commonly found in other ILDs, including HP and cryptogenic organizing pneumonia (COP). Therefore work is still in progress to further improve the classification of NSIP. Consistent with the more favorable prognosis compared to IPF, BAL cell profiles in cellular NSIP generally show a minor to moderate increase in lymphocytes in addition to increases in neutrophils and sometimes also eosinophils. However, patients with fibrotic NSIP often have BAL cell profiles similar to those in IPF/UIP with increases only in granulocytes. BAL cell counts are therefore not helpful in discriminating between fibrotic NSIP and IPF. The BAL cell profile in fibrotic NSIP is also similar to that in NSIP associated with collagen vascular diseases. Thus, BAL is of no value in differentiating between these ILDs.

3. The term *cryptogenic organizing pneumonia* (COP) is now used for the organizing pneumonia of unknown cause that was previously known as idiopathic bronchiolitis obliterans with organizing pneumonia (BOOP). BAL is of value to help to exclude other ILDs and other known causes of organizing pneumonia (e.g. viral pneumonias, drug toxicity). BAL cell profiles frequently show increases in lymphocytes in addition to granulocytes, but these occur in many other ILDs so their diagnostic value is very limited without supporting clinico-radiological-histopathological features.

4. The term *lymphoid interstitial pneumonia* (LIP) remains unchanged in the new classification. It is a very rare IIP, which is characterized by diffuse pulmonary lymphoid hyperplasia with predominantly interstitial changes. Studies of immunoglobulin gene rearrangement indicate that LIP is not neoplastic. BAL cell profiles have been reported to show increases in total and percentage counts of lymphocytes which can increase confidence in this disease if clinical features and HRCT are also supportive.

5. The term *respiratory bronchiolitis associated interstitial lung disease* (RB-ILD) denotes a smoking-related ILD characterized by accumulation of pigmented macrophages and mild inflammatory changes centering on respiratory bronchioles and neighboring alveoli, with mild alveolar septal thickening and fibrosis. Clinical features and HRCT appearances can also be suggestive. BAL cytology shows mainly macrophages heavily laden with smoking-related inclusions, sometimes accompanied by minor increases in neutrophils. These BAL findings can increase confidence in this diagnosis when clinical and HRCT findings are also consistent.

6. The term *desquamative interstitial pneumonia* (DIP) has unfortunately been retained in the new classification even though it is well known that the intra-alveolar accumulations of large mononuclear cells are alveolar macrophages, not desquamated alveolar epithelial cells as first thought. DIP is a rare smoking-related ILD, characterized histologically by accumulations of numerous pigmented macrophages in the alveolar spaces and mild alveolar septal thickening with or without fibrosis, but without the prominent bronchiolar inflammation seen in RB-ILD. BAL findings in DIP indicate that the cell profile typically shows many heavily pigmented macrophages as in RB-ILD, but usually combined with moderate increases in neutrophils, eosinophils and sometimes also lymphocytes. Thus, because of the similarity to other IIPs, BAL is of limited value in the diagnosis of DIP.

7. The term *acute interstitial pneumonia* (AIP) is now used to denote the acute-onset, very rapidly progressive cases of interstitial pulmonary fibrosis that were first described by Hamman and Rich (1935). This is now considered to be a separate IIP which is distinct from IPF. It is characterized by the finding of the histopathological feature of diffuse alveolar damage (DAD) in addition to a fibrosing pneumonitis. This disorder is so rare that there are few reports of BAL findings, but marked increases in neutrophils have been reported. However, striking increases in neutrophils are also the characteristic BAL finding in ARDS and pneumonia. Therefore, histology may be needed to diagnose AIP.

In conclusion, with regard to BAL in the IIPs it can be concluded that BAL findings are not of specific diagnostic value, but they can be of some value to increase diagnostic confidence or to exclude other ILDs that must be considered in the differential diagnosis.

BAL IN SYSTEMIC CONNECTIVE TISSUE DISEASES INVOLVING THE LUNGS

Patients with rheumatological connective tissue diseases may also develop associated interstitial lung disease. The clinical features and histopathological and HRCT patterns are variable and show many similarities to those in the IIPs. The diagnosis of the rheumatological disease often precedes the development of ILD, but in some cases ILD may be the preceding symptom. Subclinical alveolitis has also been demonstrated by BAL in patients with connective tissue diseases when chest radiographs and HRCT are normal (Wallaert *et al.* 1986; Wells *et al.* 2008). However, there are limited data on BAL findings in patients with ILD associated with connective tissue diseases and much of the information relates to systemic sclerosis (SS).

The most common BAL cell profile in the ILD associated with SS is macrophages combined with moderate increases in neutrophils either alone or sometimes together with eosinophils or lymphocytes. A significant correlation between increasing levels of BAL neutrophils and increasing extent of disease on HRCT and severity of lung functional impairment indicates that levels of BAL neutrophils may reflect severity of disease (Wells *et al.* 1994). BAL eosinophil increases, however, also occur early in the disease (Wells et al. 1998) and it has been reported that BAL eosinophilia is associated with a higher mortality, despite treatment, in SS patients with biopsy-proven NSIP (Bouros et al. 2002). Thus, BAL eosinophilia may be a potentially useful marker of disease progressiveness in the ILD of SS as has previously been suggested in IPF. BAL lymphocyte increases are less frequent than increases in neutrophils and eosinophils in SS and have been reported to occur especially in patients with a cellular HRCT pattern (Bouros et al. 2002).

BAL is therefore only of limited value to increase diagnostic confidence in ILD associated with SS, but the possibility that BAL eosinophilia may be a useful marker of disease progression needs to be followed up.

There are insufficient data on BAL in other connective tissue diseases with associated ILD to draw any clear conclusions about its clinical value. The few reports available indicate that increases in BAL neutrophils and/or lymphocytes (but not eosinophils) are the most common finding in the ILDs Sjögren's syndrome, polymyositis and dermatomyositis (Wallaert et al. 1992). As in SS and IPF, there is some evidence that higher levels of BAL neutrophils reflect more severe disease.

Further studies are needed to better clarify the clinical and research utility of BAL in the connective-tissue diseases involving the lungs.

BAL IN PEDIATRIC RESPIRATORY DISEASES

BAL is a valuable investigatory technique in pediatric respiratory medicine. However, there are important modifications of BAL procedure for use in infants and children. Readers who wish to obtain further details should refer to detailed published guidelines (see DeBlic et al. 2000).

BAL IN AIRWAYS DISEASES

BAL was initially developed to study patients with parenchymal lung diseases, so the procedure was designed to maximize sampling from the bronchoalveolar spaces rather than the upper airways. Alternative modifications of procedure to obtain 'bronchial' lavages are available (Gravelyn et al. 1988). However, numerous research studies have been conducted using conventional BAL in airways diseases including asthma and COPD. Nevertheless, there are no routine clinical applications of BAL in these airways diseases.

CONCLUSION

The routine clinical application of BAL is mainly confined to BAL cytology. It cannot identify specific diagnostic markers in sarcoidosis. However, BAL cell counts can increase confidence in the diagnosis if moderate increases in lymphocytes are present together with other clinico-radiological-histopathological features consistent with this diagnosis. BAL is also useful to assist in *excluding* a wide range of other diffuse lung diseases that need to be considered in the differential diagnosis. In addition, BAL continues to be a research tool of considerable value not only in sarcoidosis, but also in many other diffuse lung diseases.

Acknowledgment

Dr Haslam's emeritus work is part supported by the Royal Brompton and Harefield Charitable Fund no. B0437.

REFERENCES

Aggarwal A, Baker CS, Evans TW, Haslam PL (2000). G-GSF and IL-8 but not GM-CSF correlate with severity of pulmonary neutrophilia in acute respiratory distress syndrome. Eur Respir J 15: 895–901.

Baker CS, Evans TW, Randle BJ, Haslam PL (1999). Damage to surfactant-specific protein in acute respiratory distress syndrome. Lancet 353: 1232–7.

BAL Co-operative Group Steering Committee BAL (1990). Bronchoalveolar lavage constituents in healthy individuals, idiopathic pulmonary fibrosis, and selected comparison groups. Am Rev Respir Dis 141(Suppl. 5): S169–202.

Baughman RP, Rennard SI (1999). Bronchoalveolar lavage sampling and general approaches to correction for variability of dilution and lung permeability. Eur Respir Rev 9(66): 28–31.

Bjermer L, Rust M, Heurlin N et al. (1992). The clinical use of bronchoalveolar lavage in patients with pulmonary infections. Eur Respir Rev 2(8): 106–13.

Bouros D, Wells AU, Nicholson AG et al. (2002). Histopathologic subsets of fibrosing alveolitis in patients with systemic sclerosis and their relationship to outcome. Am J Respir Crit Care Med 165: 1581–6.

Chastre J, Fagon JY, Bornet-Lesco M et al. (1995). Evaluation of bronchoscopic techniques for the diagnosis of nosocomial pneumonia. Am J Respir Crit Care Med 152: 231–40.

Chen ES, Moller DR (2007). Expression profiling in granulomatous lung disease. Proc Am Thorac Soc 4: 101–7.

Christman JW, Emerson RJ, Graham WGB et al. (1985). Mineral dust and cell recovery from the bronchoalveolar lavage of healthy Vermont granite workers. Am Rev Respir Dis 132: 393–9.

Costabel U (2007). Ask the Expert: Diffuse interstitial lung disease. Breathe 4: 165–72.

Costabel U, Donner CF, Haslam PL et al. (1992). Clinical role of BAL in occupational lung diseases due to mineral dust exposure. Eur Respir Rev 2(8): 89–96.

Costabel U, Guzman J, Drent M (2005). Diagnostic approach to sarcoidosis. Eur Respir Mon 32: 259–64.

Danel C, Israel-Biet D, Venet A et al. (1988). Ultrastructural comparison of bronchoalveolar lavage (BAL) in patients under amiodarone with or without pulmonary symptoms. Eur Respir J 1(Suppl. 2): 254s.

Danel C, Israel-Biet D, Costabel U et al. (1992). The clinical role of BAL in rare pulmonary diseases. Eur Respir Rev 2(8): 83–8.

Davison AG, Haslam PL, Corrin B et al. (1983). Interstitial lung disease and asthma in hard metal workers: bronchoalveolar lavage, ultrastructural and analytical findings, and bronchial provocation tests. Thorax 38: 119–28.

DeBlic J, Midulla F, Barbato A et al. (2000). Bronchoalveolar lavage in children: report of ERS Task Force. Eur Respir J 15: 217–31.

Dejaegher P, Demedts M (1984). Bronchoalveolar lavage in eosinophilic pneumonia before and during corticosteroid therapy. *Am Rev Respir Dis* **129**: 629–32.

Demedts M, Gheysens B, Nagels J *et al.* (1984). Cobalt lung in diamond polishers. *Am Rev Respir Dis* **130**: 130–5.

De Vuyst P, Karjalainen A, Dumartier P *et al.* (1998). ERS Task Force Report: Guidelines for mineral fibre analysis in biological samples: report of the ERS Working Group. *Eur Respir J* **11**: 1416–26.

Dhillon DP, Haslam PL, Townsend PJ *et al.* (1986). Bronchoalveolar lavage in patients with interstitial lung diseases: side effects and factors affecting fluid recovery. *Eur J Respir Dis* **68**: 342–50.

Dombret MC, Chastre J (1998). The role of fibreoptic bronchoscopy in the diagnosis of bacterial infections. *Eur Respir Mon* **9**: 153–70.

Drent M, van Velzen-Blad H, Diamant M *et al.* (1993a). Relationship between presentation of sarcoidosis and T-lymphocyte profile: a study of bronchoalveolar lavage fluid. *Chest* **104**: 795–800.

Drent M, Velzen-Blad H, Diamant M *et al.* (1993b). Bronchoalveolar lavage in extrinsic allergic alveolitis: effect of time elapsed since antigen exposure. *Eur Respir J* **6**: 1276–81.

Drent M, Jacobs JA, De Vries J *et al.* (1999). Does the cellular bronchoalveolar lavage fluid profile reflect the severity of sarcoidosis? *Eur Respir J* **13**: 1338–44.

Drent M, Jacobs JA, Cobben NA *et al.* (2001). Computer program supporting the diagnostic accuracy of cellular BALF analysis: a new release. *Respir Med* **95**: 781–6.

Gellert AR, Langford JA, Winter RJD *et al.* (1985). Asbestosis: assessment by bronchoalveolar lavage and measurement of pulmonary epithelial permeability. *Thorax* **40**: 508–14.

Gilmour L, Talley F, Hook G (1988). Classification and morphometric quantification of insoluble material from the lung of patients with alveolar proteinosis. *Am J Pathol* **133**: 252–64.

Gravelyn TR, Pan PM, Eschenbacher WL (1988). Mediator release in an isolated airway segment in subjects with asthma. *Am Rev Respir Dis* **137**: 641–6.

Grunewald J, Brynedal B, Darlington P *et al.* (2010). Different HLA-DRB1 allele distributions in distinct clinical subgroups of sarcoidosis patients. *Respir Res* **11**(1): 11–25.

Grunewald J, Eklund A (2007). Role of CD4+ T-Cells in sarcoidosis. *Proc Am Thorac Soc* **4**: 461–4.

Grunewald J, Wahlstrom J, Berlin M *et al.* (2002). Lung restricted T-cell receptor AV2S3+ CD4+ T-cell expansions in sarcoidosis patients with a shared HLA-DRbeta chain conformation. *Thorax* **57**: 348–52.

Grutters JC, Drent M, van den Bosch JMM (2009). Sarcoidosis. In: duBois RM, Richeldi L (eds). *Intersitial Lung Diseases* [European Respiratory Monograph 46], pp. 126–54.

Hamman L, Rich AR (1935). Fulminating diffuse interstitial fibrosis of the lungs. *Trans Am Clin Climat Assoc* **51**: 154–63.

Haslam PL (1984). Bronchoalveolar lavage. *Semin Respir Med* **6**: 55–70.

Haslam PL (1994). Foamy macrophages in granulomatous lung diseases. *Sarcoidosis* **11**: 114–18.

Haslam PL (2010). Bronchoalveolar lavage. In: Palange P, Simonds A (eds). *ERS Handbook Respiratory Medicine*, European Respiratory Society publications, pp? 103–9.

Haslam PL, Bauer W, de Rose V *et al.* (1992). The clinical role of BAL in idiopathic pulmonary fibrosis. *Eur Respir Rev* **2**(8): 58–63.

Haslam PL, Baughman RP (eds) (1999a). Report of European Respiratory Society (ERS) Task Force: guidelines for measurement of acellular components and recommendations for standardization of bronchoalveolar lavage (BAL). *Eur Respir Rev* **9**(66): 25–157.

Haslam PL, Baughman RP (1999b). Editorial: Report of ERS Task Force: guidelines for measurement of acellular components and standardization of BAL. *Eur Respir J* **14**: 245–8.

Haslam PL, Dewar A, Butchers P *et al.* (1987). Mast cells, atypical lymphocytes and neutrophils in bronchoalveolar lavage in extrinsic allergic alveolitis: comparison with other interstitial lung diseases. *Am Rev Respir Dis* **135**: 35–47.

Haslam PL, Hughes DA, Dewar A, Pantin CFA (1988). Lipoprotein macroaggregates in bronchoalveolar lavage from patients with diffuse interstitial lung diseases: comparison with idiopathic alveolar lipoproteinosis. *Thorax* **43**: 140–6.

Hiramatsu J, Kataoka M, Nakata Y *et al.* (2003). *Propionibacterium acnes* DNA detected in bronchoalveolar lavage cells from patients with sarcoidosis. *Sarcoid Vasc Diff Lung Dis* **20**: 197–203.

Hughes DA, Haslam PL (1990). Effect of smoking on the lipid composition of lung lining fluid and relationship between immunostimulatory lipids, inflammatory cells and foamy macrophages in extrinsic allergic alveolitis. *Eur Respir J* **3**: 1128–39.

Iannuzzi MC, Rybicki BA (2007). Genetics of sarcoidosis: candidate genes and genome scans. *Proc Am Thorac Soc* **4**: 108–16.

Israel-Biet D, Danel C, Costabel U *et al.* (1992). The clinical role of BAL in drug-induced pneumonitis. *Eur Respir Rev* **2**(8): 97–9.

Johnson NF, Haslam PL, Dewar A *et al.* (1986). Identification of inorganic dust particles in bronchoalveolar lavage macrophages by energy dispersive X-ray microanalysis. *Arch Envir Health* **41**: 133–44.

Jourdain B, Joly-Guillou ML, Dombret MC *et al.* (1997). Usefulness of quantitative cultures of bronchoalveolar lavage fluid for diagnosing nosocomial pneumonia in ventilated patients. *Chest* **111**: 411–18.

Klech H, Hutter C (eds) (1990). Clinical guidelines and indications for bronchoalveolar lavage (BAL): report of the European Society of Pneumology Task Group on BAL. *Eur Respir J* **3**: 937–74.

Klech H, Pohl W (eds) (1989). Technical recommendations and guidelines for bronchoalveolar lavage (BAL): report of the European Respiratory Society of Pneumology Task Group on BAL. *Eur Respir J* **2**: 561–85.

Klech H, Hutter C, Costabel U (eds) (1992). Clinical guidelines and indications for bronchoalveolar lavage (BAL): report of the European Society of Pneumology Task Group on BAL. *Eur Respir Rev* **2**(8): 47–127.

Lin YH, Haslam PL, Turner-Warwick M (1985). Chronic pulmonary sarcoidosis: relationship between lung lavage cell counts, chest radiograph, and results of standard lung function tests. *Thorax* **40**: 501–7.

Massaglia GM, Avolio G, Barberis S *et al.* (1988). Pneumoconiosis caused by hard metals: a case series. In: Grassi C, Rizzato G, Pozzi E (eds). *Sarcoidosis and Other Granulomatous Disorders*, Elsevier Science, Amsterdam, pp. 709–10.

Newman LS (1998). Metals that cause sarcoidosis. *Semin Respir Infect* **13**(3): 212–20.

Newman LS, Kreiss K, King TE *et al.* (1989). Pathologic and immunologic alterations in early stages of beryllium disease. *Am Rev Respir Dis* **139**: 1479–86.

Ohshimo S, Bonella F, Cui A *et al.* (2009). Significance of bronchoalveolar lavage for the diagnosis of idiopathic pulmonary fibrosis. *Am J Respir Crit Care Med* **179**: 1043–7.

Oswald-Richter K, Sato H, Hajizadeh R *et al.* (2010). Mycobacterial ESAT-6 and katG are recognized by sarcoidosis CD4+ T-cells when presented by the American sarcoidosis susceptibility allele, DRB1*1101. *J Clin Immunol* **30**: 157–66.

Pabst S, Baumgarten G, Stremmel A *et al.* (2006). Toll-like receptor (TLR) 4 polymorphisms are associated with a chronic course of sarcoidosis. *Clin Exp Immunol* **143**: 420–6.

Rennard SI *et al.* (1992). Assessment of the clinical value of bronchoalveolar lavage in the diagnosis of cancer in the lung. *Eur Respir Rev* **2**(8): 100–5.

Reynolds HY, Newball HH (1974). Analysis of proteins and respiratory cells obtained from human lungs by bronchial lavage. *J Lab Clin Med* **84**: 559–73.

Rom WN, Bitterman PB, Rennard SI *et al.* (1987). Characterization of the lower respiratory tract inflammation of nonsmoking individuals with interstitial lung disease associated with chronic inhalation of inorganic dusts. *Am Rev Respir Dis* **136**: 1429–34.

Rossman MD, Kern JA, Elias JA *et al.* (1988). Proliferative response of bronchoalveolar lymphocytes to beryllium. *Ann Intern Med* **108**: 687–93.

Rybicki BA, Walewski JL, Maliarik MJ *et al.* (2005). The *BTNL2* gene and sarcoidosis susceptibility in African Americans and whites. *Am J Hum Genet* **77**: 491–9.

Saltini C, Winestock K, Kirby M *et al.* (1989). Maintenance of alveolitis in patients with chronic beryllium disease by beryllium-specific helper T cells. *New Engl J Med* **320**: 1103–9.

Selman M 2003. Hypersensitivity pneumonitis. In: Schwarz M, King T (eds). *Interstitial Lung Disease*, 4th edn. BC Decker, Hamilton Ontario, pp. 452–84.

Sharma S, Ghosh B, Sharma SK (2008). Association of *TNF* polymorphisms with sarcoidosis, its prognosis and tumour necrosis factor (TNF)-α levels in Asian Indians. *Clin Exp Immunol* **151**: 251–9.

Thonhofer R, Maercker C, Popper HH (2002). Expression of sarcoidosis related genes in lung lavage cells. *Sarcoid Vasc Diff Lung Dis* **19**: 59–65.

Torres A, Carlet J *et al.* (2001). Ventilator-associated pneumonia: report of ERS Task Force. *Eur Respir J* **17**: 1034–45.

Travis WD, King TE, Bateman ED *et al.* (2002). American Thoracic Society/European Respiratory Society international multidisciplinary consensus classification of idiopathic interstitial pneumonias. General principles and recommendations. *Am J Respir Crit Care Med* **165**: 277–304.

Wahlstrom J, Katchar K, Wigzell H *et al.* (2001). Analysis of intracellular cytokines in CD4+ and CD8+ lung and blood T cells in sarcoidosis. *Am J Respir Crit Care Med* **163**: 115–21.

Wallace JM, Oishi JS, Barbers RG *et al.* (1989). Bronchoalveolar lavage cell and lymphocyte profiles in healthy asbestos-exposed shipyard workers. *Am Rev Respir Dis* **139**: 33–8.

Wallaert B, Hatron PY, Grosbois JM *et al.* (1986). Subclinical pulmonary involvement in collagen–vascular diseases assessed by bronchoalveolar lavage: relationship between alveolitis and subsequent changes in lung function. *Am Rev Respir Dis* **133**: 574–80.

Wallaert B, Hoorelbeke A, Sibille Y *et al.* (1992). The clinical role of bronchoalveolar lavage in collagen–vascular diseases. *Eur Respir Rev* **2**(8): 64–8.

Wallaert B, Lassalle Ph, Fortin F *et al.* (1990). Superoxide anion generation by alveolar inflammatory cells in simple pneumoconiosis and progressive massive fibrosis of non-smoking coal workers. *Am Rev Respir Dis* **141**: 129–33.

Ward K, O'Connor C, Odlum C, Fitzgerald MX (1989). Prognostic value of bronchoalveolar lavage in sarcoidosis: the critical influence of disease presentation. *Thorax* **44**: 6–12.

Welker L, Jörres RA, Costabel U, Magnussen H (2004). Predictive value of BAL cell differentials in the diagnosis of interstitial lung diseases. *Eur Respir J* **24**: 1000–6.

Wells AU, Hansell DM, Rubens MB *et al.* (1994). Fibrosing alveolitis in systemic sclerosis: bronchoalveolar lavage findings in relation to computed tomographic appearance. *Am J Respir Crit Care Med* **150**: 462–8.

Wells AU, Hansell DM, Haslam PL *et al.* (1998). Bronchoalveolar lavage cellularity: lone cryptogenic fibrosing alveolitis compared with the fibrosing alveolitis of systemic sclerosis. *Am J Respir Crit Care Med* **157**: 1474–82.

Wells AU, Hirani N *et al.* (2008). Interstitial lung disease guideline: the British Thoracic Society in collaboration with the Thoracic Society of Australia and New Zealand and the Irish Thoracic Society. *Thorax* **63**(Suppl. 5): 1–58.

Woodhead M, Blasi F, Ewig S *et al.* (2005). Guidelines for the management of adult lower respiratory tract infections: report of ERS Task Force in collaboration with ESCMID. *Eur Respir J* **26**: 1138–80.

Zaba LC, Smith GP, Sanchez M, Prystowsky SD (2010). Dendritic cells in the pathogenesis of sarcoidosis. *Am J Respir Cell Mol Biol* **42**: 32–9.

Ziegenhagen MW, Rothe ME, Schlack M, Müller-Quernheim J (2003). Bronchoalveolar and serological parameters reflecting the severity of sarcoidosis. *Eur Respir J* **21**: 407–13.

13

Role of bone density measurement in the management of sarcoidosis

KATE MACLARAN AND JOHN C STEVENSON

INTRODUCTION

Osteoporosis, or a reduction in bone mass such that fracture may occur on minimal trauma, is an important worldwide cause of morbidity and mortality currently affecting more than 75 million people in the USA, Europe and Japan (World Health Organization 1994). The main clinical manifestations of osteoporosis are fractures of the proximal femur, vertebrae and distal forearm. It is estimated that around 50 percent of women and 20 percent of men will sustain an osteoporotic fracture during their lifetime (Van Staa *et al.* 2001).

In the UK it has been estimated that osteoporotic fractures cost the health service around £1.7 billion per year (Holroyd *et al.* 2008), and as a result of increasing longevity the prevalence of osteoporosis, and subsequent economic impact, is set to rise. Worldwide, hip fractures due to osteoporosis are expected to rise 3-fold by 2050 to a predicted 6.3 million fractures per year. In the USA, in 2005 osteoporosis-related fractures were estimated to cost $19 billion dollars per year and this has been predicted to rise to $25.3 billion by 2025 (National Osteoporosis Foundation 2009).

The National Institute of Health definition of osteoporosis as 'a skeletal disorder characterized by compromised bone *strength* predisposing to increased risk of fracture' (NIH 2001) reflects the contribution of both bone density and quality towards overall bone strength. Bone density is measured in grams of mineral per unit volume or area and is determined by peak bone mass, usually achieved by late teens, combined with the rate of loss later in life. Bone mass in men undergoes a gradual decline, from its peak, of approximately 0.5 percent per year. In women, however, there is a period of accelerated loss commencing around the time of the menopause, which results in the increased risk of osteoporosis associated with the female gender. Bone quality refers to micro-architecture, bone turnover, damage accumulation and mineralization and is being increasingly recognized as an important contributor towards fracture risk.

Bone involvement in sarcoidosis was recognized over a century ago by Kreibich (1904) although it was many years before a link between sarcoidosis and osteoporosis was recognized. In 1970 it was suggested that generalized osteoporosis was one of the earliest radiologically detectable signs of bone involvement in patients with sarcoidosis (Pygott 1970). However, it was not until computerized tomography (CT) scanning became more widely used that studies investigating bone density in sarcoidosis began. These studies have shown that the link between sarcoidosis and osteoporosis is far from straightforward and a direct causative effect has yet to be established. Here we will consider in greater detail the relationship between sarcoidosis and bone density and its implications for clinical practice. The other manifestations of sarcoidosis-associated bone disease are described in other chapters.

PATHOGENESIS

The etiology of osteoporosis is multifactorial and many individual risk factors have been identified (Box 13.1). In patients with sarcoidosis there are also several more disease-specific risk factors for reduced bone density. Each patient therefore needs to be considered individually to assess personal risk.

Individual risk factors of particular relevance to patients with sarcoidosis include immobility and corticosteroid treatment. Many patients with sarcoidosis will have limited exercise capacity and subsequently have decreased physical activity. Reduced physical activity is a well-recognized risk factor for osteoporosis and the effects of immobility on bone density have been demonstrated (del Puente *et al.* 1996).

Box 13.1 Risk factors for osteoporosis

Genetic
- Increasing age
- Female gender
- Family history of osteoporosis or fracture
- Caucasian or Asian

Constitutional
- Previous fragility fracture
- Low BMI ($< 19\,kg/m^2$)
- Early menopause (< 45 years)

Lifestyle
- Cigarette smoking
- Alcohol abuse
- Poor dietary calcium intake
- Immobility

Drugs
- Glucocorticoids (>7.5mg prednisolone/day)
- Heparin

Co-morbidities
- Rheumatoid arthritis
- Chronic liver disease
- Chronic kidney disease
- Hyperparathyroidism
- Hyperthyroidism
- Hypogonadism
- Malabsorption
- Anorexia nervosa
- Neuromuscular disease

Corticosteroids remain the mainstay of treatment for patients with sarcoidosis and are often required for prolonged periods. The relationship between corticosteroid treatment and bone loss has long been recognized, with the risk of corticosteroid-induced osteoporosis increasing with dose and duration of use. Corticosteroids can result in rapid bone loss and impairment of bone quality via increased bone resorption and reduced bone formation. The risk of fracture in the hip, wrist or spine increases significantly with oral corticosteroid use and falls rapidly after cessation (Van Staa et al. 2000). These acknowledged effects led to the development of guidelines for managing patients with any condition on long-term steroid treatment (Royal College of Physicians 2002).

In addition to individual risk factors, several disease-related hypotheses exist, suggesting metabolic mechanisms by which sarcoidosis may directly increase the risk of osteoporosis.

First, it has been shown that suffering from a chronic inflammatory condition such as rheumatoid arthritis (Gough et al. 1994) or inflammatory bowel disease (Bernstein et al. 2000) increases the risk of bone loss and fracture. This is thought to be due to the presence of pro-inflammatory cytokines that may stimulate osteoclastogenesis and subsequent osteoclast-mediated bone resorption. As sarcoidosis is an inflammatory T-cell-mediated disease, this is a potential mechanism for a direct effect on bone density. Furthermore, inflammatory conditions are often associated with poor nutritional status and reduced lean body mass, creating an environment unfavorable for bone formation.

Second, sarcoidosis is associated with hypercalcemia, hypercalciuria and elevated 1,25-dihydroxyvitamin D, and it has been suggested that these could act as risk factors for osteoporosis. Conclusive evidence as to whether these metabolic changes and their management (i.e. reducing calcium intake) reduce bone mass is lacking. Overproduction of 1,25-dihydroxyvitamin D within sarcoid granulomas may cause increased calcium absorption, and stimulate osteoclast-mediated bone resorption and bone turnover (Rizatto 1998; Conron et al. 2000). Increased bone turnover can reduce bone quality by increasing the proportion of immature bone. Elevated serum levels of 1,25-dihydroxyvitamin D have been associated with increased bone turnover and reduced BMD in women with sarcoidosis (Hamada et al. 1999). However, elevated 1,25-dihydroxyvitamin D was observed in sarcoid patients with normal bone density and in those with osteopenia (Meyrier et al. 1986), suggesting that other factors are contributing to alterations in bone density.

A more detailed description of calcium metabolism and its wider effects is found in other chapters.

It has also been hypothesized that granulomas could potentially induce a local osteoclastic reaction via mechanisms unrelated to overproduction of activated vitamin D (Fallon et al. 1981). Local production of osteoclast activating factor has been suggested as a mechanism which may lead to increased resorption (Meyrier et al. 1986). Activity such as this has been observed in multiple myeloma where cytokines acting as osteoclast activating factors are released and act as powerful stimulants of bone resorption. Further evidence for a local cause comes from a study of an osteopenic patient with skeletal sarcoidosis. From analysis of a bone biopsy the authors found that the granulomas were associated with histological features of bone remodeling and they concluded that this may cause increased bone turnover and subsequent diffuse osteopenia (Fallon et al. 1981). However, not all patients with osteopenia suffer from sarcoid bone lesions and therefore other mechanisms must also exist.

BONE DENSITY MEASUREMENT

Bone mineral densitometry is currently the best available non-invasive tool for assessing bone mass in clinical practice. The WHO has created diagnostic criteria for osteoporosis based on T scores generated from BMD measurements (Table 13.1). These values represent standard deviations

Table 13.1   WHO diagnostic criteria for osteoporosis (1994).

T score	Diagnosis
> -1.0	Normal bone density
-1.0 to -2.5	Osteopenia
< -2.5	Osteoporosis
< -2.5 with fragility fracture	Severe osteoporosis

from the peak bone mass of young adults. Limitations of this definition are that it was designed for use in postmenopausal Caucasian women and therefore may not be fully applicable to men, younger populations or other ethnicities. In these populations it is more appropriate to use z-scores which represent standard deviations from age, sex and ethnicity matched controls.

Measurement of bone density can be carried out in several different ways. Dual-energy X-ray absorptiometry (DXA) is the most commonly used and best established method in current clinical practice. This measures bone density by determining the absorption of two beams of photons at two different energies and is classically performed to assess bone density at the hip and lumbar spine (Figs 13.1 and 13.2). DXA has variable performance in predicting fracture risk depending on the site assessed. Owing to kyphosis, scoliosis and aortic calcification, which may produce falsely elevated vertebral BMD values, the hip/proximal femur is regarded as the preferred site for measuring BMD in older patients. The risk of fracture increases 1.5-fold overall for every standard deviation below the mean BMD. However, the gradient of risk increases to 2.6/SD for femoral neck BMD. DXA carries a low radiation dose (1 mrem for each site) and takes around 5 minutes at each site to perform.

Other techniques such as quantitative computed tomography (QCT) and ultrasonography can be used to assess BMD, although they have not yet taken on widespread clinical use. QCT can distinguish between cortical and trabecular bone, but it is costly and confers an increased

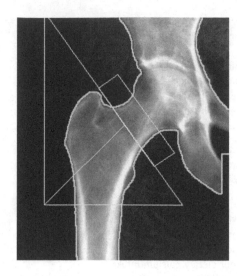

Figure 13.2   DXA image of femoral neck bone density in an unaffected woman.

radiation dose. Ultrasonography, which has the advantage of being cheap and portable, is often used to assess BMD at peripheral sites. It may have a role in risk assessment in areas with limited resources, but it has not been fully validated as a predictor of future fracture risk.

Biochemical markers of bone turnover exist, although these have yet to be used in general clinical practice. There may be a role in the future for their use in monitoring response to treatment, as they would be expected to pick up changes in bone turnover earlier than changes in bone density could be detected by DXA.

Bone density alone is not the best predictor of fracture risk as it has a low sensitivity and therefore the majority of fractures will occur in patients with bone density above −2.5. As previously discussed, bone fragility is not only due to BMD but can also be due to changes in the microarchitecture of bone and in matrix composition. In addition, risk factors such as age can be as important predictors of fracture risk as BMD, and several risk factors have been identified which act independently to BMD (Kanis *et al.* 2002).

These limitations of using BMD alone to assess fracture risk have led the WHO to create algorithms to predict individual risk more accurately. These tools undertake a more global evaluation of validated risk factors, alone or in combination with BMD measurements, to highlight when intervention may be appropriate.

The FRAX® algorithm (www.shef.ac.uk/FRAX) calculates 10-year probability of hip fracture or major osteoporotic fracture (clinical vertebral, hip, forearm or humerus fracture) based on clinical risk factors and femoral neck BMD. Figures have been calibrated for country-specific fracture and mortality data for ten countries worldwide. Thresholds for treatment have been suggested and also thresholds between which BMD would influence decision to treat. The algorithm does, however, have certain limitations. It has been designed for use in postmenopausal women and men over the age of 50 years and applies only to untreated patients. Additionally, it is unable to take into account the cumulative severity of

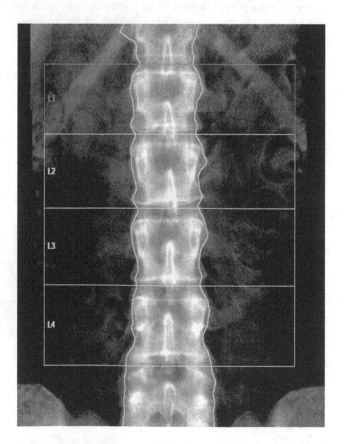

Figure 13.1   DXA image of lumbar spine bone density in an unaffected woman.

each risk factor, such as corticosteroid dose and duration. The algorithm can therefore be used as a guide for when treatment may be recommended but ultimately the clinician must make a judgment based in the individual case.

BONE DENSITY IN SARCOIDOSIS

Relatively few studies examining bone density in patients with sarcoidosis exist, and despite the many mechanisms potentially reducing bone density, studies frequently show conflicting results.

Untreated patients

It was initially suggested by Tervonen et al. (1974) that untreated patients with sarcoidosis may have an acute phase with abnormally high BMD but that BMD then went on to decline with time.

Subsequent studies in untreated patients have shown conflicting results. Several studies have shown a mild reduction in bone density in chronic sarcoid (Montemurro et al. 1991a; Rizzato et al. 1992; Rottoli et al. 1993) and postmenopausal women (Sipahi et al. 2004). In a group of patients with chronic untreated sarcoidosis the frequency of osteopenia was shown to be over 50 percent (Rizzato et al. 1992). These patients included males, premenopausal and postmenopausal females, with an average disease duration of 20 months. This study also made a comparison between early and longstanding untreated sarcoidosis and demonstrated deteriorating BMD z-scores with disease duration (z-score -1.19 ± 0.24 vs 0.32 ± 0.39, $p < 0.001$). BMD of 43 untreated patients in a trial investigating the prevention of corticosteroid-induced osteoporosis with alendronate showed reduced mean BMD within the osteopenic range at their initial measurement (Gonnelli et al. 1997). A more recent study demonstrated increased BMD in the trochanter but normal BMD elsewhere, despite increased biochemical markers of bone turnover (Heijckmann et al. 2007). It was suggested that sarcoidosis may therefore provide some form of protective effect on the bones.

Treated patients

Loss of bone density in corticosteroid-treated sarcoidosis patients has been observed (Rizzato et al. 1988), with over 70 percent of treated patients found to have reduced BMD compared to controls or untreated sarcoidosis patients. The rate of decline of BMD while on corticosteroid treatment was found to be especially rapid in postmenopausal women (Montemurro et al. 1990). However, treated premenopausal women have also been shown to have significantly lower spinal BMD compared to untreated and control groups (Sipahi et al. 2004). Alder et al. (2003) found that 80 percent of a group of both corticosteroid-treated and untreated patients had at least osteopenia. However, 50 percent of their patients had been referred for assessment of possible osteoporosis and therefore these figures may not apply to the general sarcoid population. In addition, they could not find any predictors for bone density from measurements of blood or urine calcium levels, markers of bone turnover, hormone levels or activity scores. Weight, age and corticosteroid use were the only factors showing an association with hip BMD. There may be some protection from intermittent corticosteroid use, but no trials have directly compared risks and benefits of different corticosteroid regimens with bone density as a primary outcome.

Comparisons between different corticosteroids have shown that they may be equally effective at treating sarcoidosis but have varying effects on bone density. For example, deflazacort appeared as effective as prednisolone in the long-term treatment of chronic sarcoidosis, but it may have less impact on bone density (Rizatto et al. 1997). Further investigation comparing different regimens is needed.

Fracture risk

The clinical impact of bone density in sarcoidosis in terms of fracture risk is even less well established. One study found that 20 percent of participants had vertebral deformities suggestive of fracture (Hiejkmann et al. 2007). This was despite an average bone density within normal limits, which led them to hypothesize that the increased fracture risk may be due to changes in bone structure not evident by bone densitometry, such as changes in matrix composition and micro-architecture. A 4-year follow-up study demonstrated that the rate of vertebral deformities had increased to 32 percent despite unchanged BMD (Heijkmann et al. 2008).

Certain limitations exist in studies investigating BMD in sarcoidosis, as disease activity and progression may introduce an inherent bias. Untreated groups are more likely to have less active disease and effect on bone is likely to be related to disease activity. Effects on bone density would be expected to differ in relation to the natural course of the disease, although no long-term follow-up studies have been performed on patients with chronic progressive disease.

MANAGEMENT

Individual assessment of fracture risk is vital. Age and BMD are the strongest independent risk factors for future fracture, so measurement of BMD by DEXA should be considered in all patients with sarcoidosis, especially when considering treatment with corticosteroids or if other risk factors are present. Patients with sarcoidosis are often young and may require lengthy or repeated courses of corticosteroids, making effective and safe bone protection essential.

Management of patients with established osteopenia or osteoporosis or prevention of corticosteroid-induced osteoporosis is more difficult in patients with sarcoidosis as some treatments may exacerbate hypercalcemia. While general guidelines for prevention and management of osteoporosis (Compston et al. 2009) provide valuable information, they may need to be adapted for use in the younger populations and to take into account the disturbances in calcium metabolism that can occur in sarcoidosis.

Lifestyle measures should be recommended to all patients, examples being regular weight-bearing exercise, cessation of smoking and reduction of alcohol. Calcium and vitamin D supplementation are often the first-line preventative measures for those at risk of osteoporosis, although these are not widely recommended in sarcoidosis owing to the risk of hypercalcemia and hypercalciuria. Some clinicians consider their use if serum and urine calcium parameters are within normal ranges and with regular monitoring (Conron *et al.* 2000).

Bisphosphonates have been shown to reduce corticosteroid-induced bone loss in sarcoidosis patients and could be considered in patients at high risk of osteoporosis. Alendronate has been demonstrated to prevent corticosteroid-induced bone loss in a randomized controlled trial of 43 sarcoidosis patients, with an increase in BMD of 0.8 percent in the group receiving alendronate compared to a loss of 4.5 percent in the placebo-treated group ($p < 0.01$) (Gonnelli *et al.* 1997). Limitations of bisphosphonates include their gastrointestinal side-effects, and their use is not generally recommended in women of reproductive age as their effects on fetal development are unknown. Of more concern is the long skeletal retention time of the more potent bisphosphonates, particularly when unpredicted adverse effects are emerging with long-term treatment. Although these are rare events, atrial fibrillation (Heckbert *et al.* 2008), osteonecrosis of the jaw (Seghizadeh *et al.* 2009) and inflammatory eye disease (Sharma *et al.* 2008) have been reported with bisphosphonate use. Furthermore, there are increasing reports of sub-trochanteric femoral fragility fractures (Goh *et al.* 2007; Lenart *et al.* 2008; Kwek *et al.* 2008; Neviaser *et al.* 2008; Leung *et al.* 2009) which may be due to over-suppression of bone remodeling leading to accumulation of fatigue damage. The more potent bisphosphonates, particularly those administered intravenously, may be more likely to cause such unwanted effects (Durie *et al.* 2005; Reid *et al.* 2009). While this may not be a problem in elderly osteoporotics with limited life-expectancy, considerable caution should be taken in young patients. In the authors' opinion, these drugs should not be given to patients under age 60 years unless there are compelling reasons, such as severe osteoporosis unresponsive to other agents.

Latest British Thoracic Society guidance (Bradley *et al.* 2008) recommends empirical use of a bisphosphonate in all corticosteroid-treated patients to reduce the effects on bone density. These recommendations are based on grade D evidence (i.e. non-analytical studies or expert opinion) and no large-scale studies have examined the clinical and economic efficacy of this strategy in sarcoidosis. Other strategies include treating only high-risk groups (those with prior fracture or aged over 65 years in which cases BMD assessment is not necessary), and in lower risk individuals using BMD assessment and giving treatment if their T score is −1.5 or below (RCP 2002).

In postmenopausal women, hormone replacement therapy with estrogen/progestogen, or estrogen alone if hysterectomized, should be considered, especially in those who are also seeking treatment for vasomotor menopausal symptoms. Estrogen has been shown to be effective in reducing the risk of both hip and vertebral fractures. The increased rates of bone loss observed in corticosteroid-treated postmenopausal women suggest some synergistic effect between these two conditions and emphasizes the need for adequate bone protection and regular monitoring of BMD in this population.

Evidence also exists for the use of calcitonin in sarcoidosis (Montemurro *et al.* 1991b), although this is not usually recommended unless there is a contraindication to bisphosphonate use. There are several other agents licensed for management of osteoporosis, such as strontium ranelate and parathyroid hormone. None of these agents has been specifically studied in sarcoidosis patients.

No specific recommendations exist for the monitoring of bone density in patients with sarcoidosis. Each patient should be assessed individually for risk factors and a DXA scan considered, especially prior to corticosteroid treatment. We suggest two-yearly monitoring of bone density while undergoing corticosteroid treatment. In patients with inactive disease not currently receiving corticosteroid therapy, routine assessment of bone density is not usually required. Again, individual risk factors should be taken into account and acted on if necessary.

REFERENCES

Alder RA, Funkhouser HL, Petkov VI, Berger MM (2003). Glucocorticoid-induced osteoporosis in patients with sarcoidosis. *Am J Med Sci* **325**: 1–6.

Bradley B, Branley HM, Egan JJ *et al.* (2008). Interstitial lung disease guideline: the British Thoracic Society in collaboration with the Thoracic Society of Australia and New Zealand and the Irish Thoracic Society. *Thorax* **63**(Suppl. 5): 1–58.

Bernstein CN, Blanchard JF, Leslie W *et al.* (2000). The incidence of fracture among patients with inflammatory bowel disease: a population-based cohort study. *Ann Intern Med* **133**: 795–9.

Compston J, Cooper A, Cooper C *et al.* (2009). National Osteoporosis Guideline Group (NOGG): Guidelines for the diagnosis and management of osteoporosis in postmenopausal women and men from the age of 50 years in the UK. *Maturitas* **62**: 105–8.

Conron M, Young C, Beynon HLC (2000). Calcium metabolism in sarcoidosis and its clinical implications. *Rheumatology* **39**: 707–13.

del Puente A, Pappone N, Mandes MG *et al.* (1996). Determinants of bone mineral density in immobilization: a study on hemiplegic patients. *Osteopor Int* **6**: 50–4.

Durie BGM, Katz M, Crowley J (2005). Osteonecrosis of the jaw and bisphosphonates. *New Engl J Med* **353**: 99–102.

Fallon MD, Perry HM, Teitelbaum SL (1981). Skeletal sarcoidosis with osteopenia. *Metab Bone Dis Rel Res* **3**: 171–4.

Goh S-K, Yang KY, Koh JSB *et al.* (2007). Subtrochanteric insufficiency fractures in patients on alendronate therapy: a caution. *J Bone J Surg (Br)* **89-B**: 349–53.

Gonnelli S, Rottoli P, Cepollaro C *et al.* (1997). Prevention of corticosteroid-induced osteoporosis with alendronate in sarcoid patients. *Calcif Tissue Int* **61**: 382–5.

Gough AK, Lilley J, Eyre S *et al.* (1994). Generalised bone loss in patients with early rheumatoid arthritis. *Lancet* **344**: 23–7.

Hamada K, Nagai S, Tsutsumi T, Izumi T (1999). Bone mineral density and vitamin D in patients with sarcoidosis. *Sarcoid Vasc Diff Lung Dis* 16: 219–23.

Heckbert SR, Li G, Cummings SR *et al.* (2008). Use of alendronate and risk of incident atrial fibrillation in women. *Arch Intern Med* 168: 826–31.

Heijckmann AC, Huijberts MS, De Vries J *et al.* (2007). Bone turnover and hip bone mineral density in patients with sarcoidosis. *Sarcoid Vasc Diff Lung Dis* 24: 51–8.

Heijckmann AC, Drent M, Dumitrescu B *et al.* (2008). Progressive vertebral deformities despite unchanged bone mineral density in patients with sarcoidosis: a 4-year follow-up study. *Osteopor Int* 19: 839–47.

Holroyd C, Cooper C, Dennison E (2008). Epidemiology of osteoporosis. *Best Pract Res Clin Endocrin Metab* 22: 671–85.

Kanis JA, Black D, Cooper C *et al.* (2002). International Osteoporosis Foundation; National Osteoporosis Foundation: A new approach to the development of assessment guidelines for osteoporosis. *Osteopor Int* 13: 527–36.

Kreibich K (1904). Uber lupus pernio. *Arch Dermatol Syphilol* 71: 3–16.

Kwek EBK, Koh JSB, Howe TS (2008). More on atypical fractures of the femoral diaphysis. *New Engl J Med* 359: 316–18.

Lenart BA, Lorich DG, Lane JM (2008). Atypical fractures of the femoral diaphysis in postmenopausal women taking alendronate. *New Engl J Med* 358: 1304–6.

Leung F, Lau T-W, To M *et al.* (2009). Atypical femoral diaphyseal and subtrochanteric fractures and their association with bisphosphonates. *Br Med J Case Reports* doi:10.1136/bcr.10.2008.1073.

Meyrier A, Valeyre D, Bouillon R *et al.* (1986). Different mechanism of hypercalciuria in Sarcoidosis. *Ann NY Acad Sci* 465: 575–86.

Montemurro L, Fraioli P, Riboldi A *et al.* (1990). Bone loss in prednisolone-treated sarcoidosis: a two-year follow-up. *Ann Ital Med Interna* (Rome) 5: 164–8.

Montemurro L, Fraioli P, Rizzato G (1991a). Bone loss in untreated longstanding sarcoidosis. *Sarcoidosis* 8: 29–34.

Montemurro L, Schiraldi G, Fraioli P *et al.* (1991b). Prevention of corticosteroid-induced osteoporosis with salmon calcitonin in sarcoid patients. *Calcif Tissue Int* 49: 71–6.

National Osteoporosis Foundation (2009). Disease statistics. Available at www.nof.org/osteoporosis/diseasefacts.htm.

Neviaser AS, Lane JM, Lenart BA *et al.* (2008). Low-energy femoral shaft fractures associated with alendronate use. *J Orthopaed Trauma* 22: 346–50.

NIH Consensus Development Panel on Osteoporosis Prevention, Diagnosis and Therapy (2001). Osteoporosis prevention, diagnosis and therapy. *J Am Med Assoc* 285: 320–3.

Pygott F (1970). Sarcoidosis in bone. *Postgrad Med J* 46: 505–6.

Reid DM, Devogelaer J-P, Saag K *et al.* (2009). Zoledronic acid and risedronate in the prevention and treatment of glucocorticoid-induced osteoporosis: a multicentre, double-blind, double-dummy, randomised controlled trial. *Lancet* 373: 1253–63.

Rizzatto G (1998). Clinical impact of bone and calcium metabolism changes in sarcoidosis. *Thorax* 53: 425–9.

Rizzato G, Tosi G, Mella C, Montemurro L *et al.* (1988). Prednisolone-induced bone loss in sarcoidosis: a risk especially frequent in postmenopausal women. *Sarcoidosis* 5: 93–8.

Rizzato G, Montemurro L, Fraioli P (1992). Bone mineral content in sarcoidosis. *Sem Respir Med* 13: 411–23.

Rizzato G, Riboldi A, Imbimbo B *et al.* (1997). The long-term efficacy and safety of two different corticosteroids in chronic sarcoidosis. *Respir Med* 91: 449–60.

Rottoli P, Gonnelli S, Silitro S *et al.* (1993). Alterations in calcium metabolism and bone mineral density in relation to the activity of sarcoidosis. *Sarcoidosis* 10: 161–2.

Royal College of Physicians (2002). Bone and Tooth Society of Great Britain, National Osteoporosis Society and Royal College of Physicians: Glucocorticoid-induced osteoporosis – guidelines on prevention and treatment. Royal College of Physicians, London.

Sedghizadeh PP, Stanley K, Caligiuri M *et al.* (2009). Oral bisphosphonate use and the prevalence of osteonecrosis of the jaw: an institutional inquiry. *J Am Dent Assoc* 140: 61–6.

Sharma NS, Ooi J-L, Masselos K *et al.* (2008). Zoledronic acid infusion and orbital inflammatory disease. *New Engl J Med* 359: 1410–11.

Sipahi S, Tuzun S, Ozaras R *et al.* (2004). Bone mineral density in women with sarcoidosis. *J Bone Mineral Metab* 22: 48–52.

Tervonen S, Karjalainen P, Valta R (1974). Bone mineral in sarcoidosis. *Acta Med Scand* 196: 497–503.

Van Staa T, Leufkens HGM, Abenhaim L *et al.* (2000). Use of oral corticosteroids and risk of fractures. *J Bone Mineral Res* 15: 993–1000.

Van Staa TP, Dennison EM, Leufkens HGM, Cooper C (2001). Epidemiology of fractures in England and Wales. *Bone* 29: 517–22.

World Health Organization (1994). Assessment of fracture risk and its application to screening for postmenopausal osteoporosis [report of a WHO study group]. *World Health Organization Technical Report Series* 843: 1–129.

14

Nuclear imaging in pulmonary sarcoidosis

KSHAMA WECHALEKAR, S RICHARD UNDERWOOD AND MICHAEL B HUGHES

INTRODUCTION

Sarcoidosis can affect any organ, most commonly the lungs (Lynch *et al.* 1997). One of its most recognizable manifestations is erythema nodosum, which has an excellent prognosis. Other presentations include extrathoracic lymphadenopathy, eye involvement and abnormal liver function. Kidney, central nervous system (CNS), heart and musculoskeletal involvement are seen in a minority. Management often needs a multidisciplinary approach.

The clinical picture is variable and can take an acute or a chronic course. Symptoms are often non-specific and can occur in other conditions. Up to a half of patients present with non-productive cough, dyspnea and chest pain and may predominantly have endobronchial or lung parenchymal involvement (Bechtel *et al.* 1981). Fatigue and impaired quality of life are more common in sarcoidosis than in healthy controls, but physical features such as clubbing or crackles are less common despite extensive pulmonary infiltrates on radiography (Lynch *et al.* 1997; Wirnsberger *et al.* 1998; De Vries *et al.* 2004). Almost two-thirds of patients run a benign course with spontaneous remission, but 10–30 percent of patients run a more chronic course (Judson *et al.* 2003). Chronic progressive pulmonary sarcoidosis can result in severe respiratory failure (Baughman *et al.* 1997).

There is no single diagnostic test for sarcoidosis and both structural imaging techniques such as X-ray computed tomography (CT) and magnetic resonance imaging (MRI) are used as well as functional imaging using radionuclides. The diagnosis is based on three criteria:

- a compatible clinical and/or imaging picture;
- histological evidence of non-caseating granulomas;
- exclusion of other diseases that might produce similar clinical or histology features.

History, examination, chest radiography and bronchoalveolar lavage (BAL) or biopsy are commonly the first steps. A variety of biochemical and hematology tests, eye examination, ECG and lung function tests are used to assess organ involvement. Radiology and radionuclide imaging are helpful for assessing the activity and extent of the disease.

SINGLE-PHOTON RADIONUCLIDE IMAGING

Gallium-67

Gallium is a non-specific marker of infection and inflammation, but it is also used to image malignant processes such as lymphoma. Normal distribution is to the liver, spleen, bone marrow, bone and the growth plates, with less intense uptake in the lacrimal and salivary glands and in the nasal mucosa, and low-grade uptake in the breast. Excretion is through the gut. Because this distribution is related to transferrin receptors, the normal distribution is altered by iron injection, radiotherapy, chemotherapy and congenital absence of the receptors.

After intravenous injection, gallium is mainly bound to transferrin, an iron transport protein, but in serum it also combines with hydroxyl ions to form gallate $[Ga(OH)^{4-}]$ (Weiner 1996). Infective, inflammatory or neoplastic processes have increased vascularity and a higher concentration of transferrin receptors, leading to higher uptake of gallium into macrophages and the neoplastic cells themselves. The gallium–transferrin complex is relatively large with slow cellular uptake, so imaging is performed 24–72 hours (typically 48 hours) after injection. Traditionally, planar whole-body or spot views are acquired, but emission tomographic imaging (SPECT) is becoming more common.

The combination of SPECT and X-ray CT imaging helps with localization of abnormalities, and this can be from either separate or combined SPECT and CT systems.

GALLIUM-67 IMAGING

The most common site of abnormal gallium uptake in patients with sarcoidosis is intrathoracic with the typical appearance of bilateral hilar and paratracheal uptake at the site of adenopathy and/or lung parenchymal uptake. Other common sites of abnormal uptake are the salivary and lacrimal glands, particularly the parotid glands and the bones. If a biopsy site for histological confirmation is not apparent clinically, gallium imaging can direct attention to clinically silent but involved organs. Small cutaneous or subcutaneous sarcoid infiltrations, including lupus pernio, are difficult to visualize because of physiological or pathological uptake in surrounding tissues such as the nose and sinuses. The sensitivity for detecting pulmonary sarcoidosis is 60–90 percent, but the specificity is low as gallium uptake is also seen in most interstitial lung diseases.

Typical patterns of uptake have been described as 'panda' and 'lambda' signs (Fig. 14.1), although these are not totally specific (Sulavik et al. 1993). The lambda pattern is formed from bilateral hilar and right paratracheal nodes and is seen in 72 percent of patients with sarcoidosis. The panda sign arises from lacrimal and parotid uptake and is seen in 79 percent of patients. Both patterns together are seen in 62 percent of patients. Other causes of the panda sign are HIV infection, Sjögren's syndrome, graft-versus-host disease, rheumatoid arthritis, and systemic lupus erythematosus and after head and neck irradiation for treatment of malignancies such as lymphoma.

Gallium scan shows extent of disease involvement on whole-body imaging as shown in Fig. 14.2. The prognostic role of abnormal gallium uptake has been studied by several groups. In an early study reduced or normalized gallium uptake during treatment was associated with maintained lung function and a good prognosis (Niden et al. 1986), but later studies have not confirmed this.

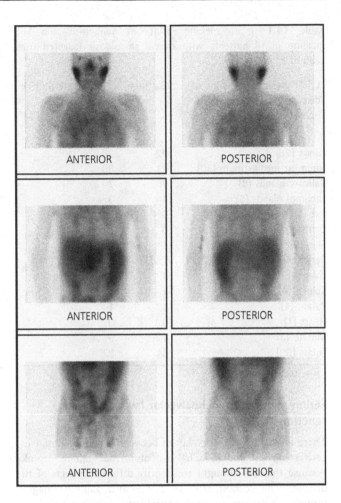

Figure 14.2   Planar gallium images in a patient with disseminated sarcoidosis, showing the panda sign (lacrimal, nasal and parotid uptake) with patchy lung uptake, splenomegaly and inguinal lymph nodal uptake.

COMPARISON BETWEEN GALLIUM SCINTIGRAPHY AND OTHER INVESTIGATIONS

Radiology

Various studies have compared gallium scintigraphy with radiology such as the chest X-ray and CT, but the former provides physiological information and the latter anatomy, and the techniques need not always agree. Functional abnormalities often precede structural changes and so, depending on the time of imaging with respect to the natural history of disease, one or other or both may be affected.

In a European multicenter study of over 600 patients with suspected intrathoracic disease, gallium scintigraphy was abnormal in 43 percent when the chest X-ray was normal (Rizzato and Blasi 1986). Conversely, 23 percent of patients with intrathoracic involvement on chest X-ray did not show gallium uptake (Table 14.1). There was no correlation between the X-ray staging of the disease and abnormal gallium uptake, but gallium was more sensitive in detecting changes such as improvement or relapse of disease.

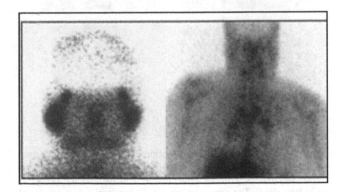

Figure 14.1   Gallium-67 scans showing (left) panda and (right) lambda patterns in sarcoidosis.

Table 14.1   Site-specific results of gallium-68 and SRS imaging in 18 patients with known sarcoidosis (adapted from Lebtahi *et al.* 2001).

Clinically involved sites of disease (no. of known involved sites)	Gallium	^{111}In-pentetreotide (SRS)
Lungs (26)	22	26
Hilum or mediastinum (30)	21	30
Salivary glands (8)	7	7
Lacrimal glands (5)	4	3
Eye (1)	0	0
Central nervous system (5)	0	3
Skin (8)	1	2
Peripheral lymph nodes (2)	1	2
Liver (5)	4	4
Spleen (4)	2	4
Palate (1)	1	1
Heart (1)	0	0
Muscle (3)	1	0
Totals (99)	64	82*

* $p < 0.001$

Serum markers, bronchoalveolar lavage and lung function

There is only a weak correlation between serum angiotensin-converting enzyme (SACE) and abnormal gallium uptake because they are thought to identify different aspects of the disease. The combination of SACE and gallium imaging improves both sensitivity and specificity such that if both are normal sarcoidosis is highly improbable (Nosal *et al.* 1979).

When bronchoalveolar lavage (BAL) was compared with gallium uptake in patients with pulmonary sarcoidosis, some authors (Crystal *et al.* 1981; Line *et al.* 1981) have reported strong correlation while others (Beaumont *et al.* 1982) have reported no correlation. These discrepant results may be due to different cellular responses in different stages of disease, such as T-lymphocytic alveolitis in early phase in BAL fluid and activated macrophages (weak gallium uptake) and granulomas in the later phase (strong gallium uptake) (Maña and van Kroonenburgh 2005).

Pulmonary function tests bear a weak correlation with gallium scan and BAL (Line *et al.* 1981), since lung function testing can be normal in the presence of mild to moderate alveolitis. Some studies found that even low-grade gallium uptake by the pulmonary parenchyma was associated with some degree of lung restriction, and others showed a close correlation between the degree of gallium uptake before treatment and the subsequent increase in vital capacity after corticosteroid therapy (Baughman *et al.* 1984).

CURRENT PRACTICE IN GALLIUM IMAGING

Gallium scintigraphy is most valuable in selected clinical settings as opposed to being required routinely for primary diagnosis or the assessment of prognosis or treatment response. It is valuable in cases of diagnostic difficulty and

particularly to define the extent and distribution of disease when SPECT and CT are combined (Plate 12).

In patients with a normal CXR but clinical features of extrathoracic disease such as the eye, the central nervous system or other single organ involvement gallium scintigraphy can assist with the diagnosis by detecting clinically silent disease and potentially identifying sites for biopsy. It can also be particularly helpful in distinguishing between fibrotic changes in the lungs from inactive disease and relapse of disease after discontinuing steroid therapy.

Somatostatin receptor imaging

Somatostatin receptor scintigraphy is a newer alternative to gallium. Somatostatin analogs such as octreotide and pentetreotide are labeled with indium-111, and the technique is most commonly used for imaging neuro-endocrine tumors. Somatostatin receptors are expressed by normal and activated lymphocytes and macrophages, but they are also expressed in granulomatous diseases including sarcoidosis (Fig. 14.3). Uptake is not specific for sarcoidosis and imaging cannot differentiate sarcoidosis from tumor.

Target-to-background ratio with SRS is significantly higher than with gallium scintigraphy, especially for lung and mediastinal involvement. This is because of the absence of physiological uptake of ^{111}In-pentetreotide in bone marrow or lungs and the energy of ^{111}In photons, which is better suited for the gamma camera.

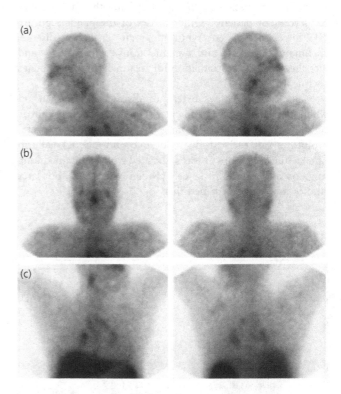

Figure 14.3   Planar ^{111}In-octreotide images showing abnormal uptake in the salivary glands and hilar nodes in a patient with known sarcoidosis (anterior projection left in (b) and (c), posterior projection right). The abnormal uptake in the lacrimal and salivary glands, hilar and mediastinal nodes is similar to the appearance with gallium, but note the better lesion-to-background ratio in the chest.

In one of the larger studies, 46 patients with known sarcoidosis were imaged 24 hours after injection of ^{111}In-pentetreotide using planar but not SPECT imaging (Kwekkeboom et al. 1998). With the exception of fine nodular parenchymal disease noticed on CT in one patient, known mediastinal, hilar and/or interstitial disease was recognized in all 37 patients with somatostatin receptor imaging, and abnormal uptake was seen in 7 patients with known disease but normal chest X-ray. Additional abnormalities were seen in the parotid glands and supraclavicular lymph nodes, the former correlating well with SACE. In 13 patients, extrapulmonary disease that was not previously identified was demonstrated, predominantly in the salivary glands, supraclavicular lymph nodes, nose, eyes and skin granulomas. However, 28 percent of the known sites of disease involvement such as in the skin, eyes, liver and central nervous system were not identified, and neither the degree nor the pattern of tracer uptake correlated with disease severity or clinical course. Follow-up imaging in 13 patients after corticosteroid therapy showed improved chest X-ray appearance in 6 patients, and 5 of these also showed improvements in the abnormal ^{111}In-pentetreotide uptake.

Lebtahi and associates compared gallium imaging to pentetreotide imaging in 18 patients with sarcoidosis (Lebtahi et al. 2001). Abnormal gallium uptake was seen in two-thirds of the clinically involved sites, but abnormal pentetreotide uptake was seen in 83 percent and the difference was greatest in patients receiving corticosteroid therapy. Gallium scintigraphy failed to detect bilateral thoracic involvement and a pseudotumoral lesion in the left temporal lobe (see Table 14.1). SRS detected central nervous system involvement in three of four patients and also confirmed three sites of clinically suspected bone involvement but missed seven extrathoracic sites. Among the treated patients (9/18), SRS detected significantly more sites than gallium scintigraphy ($p < 0.001$), especially for thoracic and CNS involvement, and appeared more accurate for evaluation of disease activity.

Depreotide is a newer somatostatin analog, which can be labeled and imaged with technetium-99m. Shorr et al. (2004) imaged 22 patients with biopsy-proven sarcoidosis using planar and SPECT imaging. All patients with abnormal chest X-rays had abnormal depreotide uptake, and there was a strong correlation between sarcoidosis activity, an abnormal scan, stage on X-ray and pulmonary function tests. Four patients with extrapulmonary disease (2 cardiac, 1 CNS, 1 skin) had abnormal uptake in the involved organ. Despite these encouraging results for sensitivity, the specificity of depreotide imaging for sarcoidosis is likely to be lower since abnormal uptake is also seen in malignancy. Unfortunately, there have been no substantial trials of depreotide imaging for sarcoidosis in recent years.

POSITRON-EMITTING RADIONUCLIDE IMAGING

[18]F-2-fluoro-2-deoxyglucose

[18]F-2-fluoro-2-deoxyglucose (FDG) is an analog of glucose that is transported, phosphorylated and metabolically trapped as FDG-6-phosphate in cells that metabolize glucose. It is the most widely used tracer that is used with positron emission tomography (PET) for the detection and staging of malignancies. However, it is not cancer-specific and abnormal uptake is seen in other tissues with increased glucose metabolism, including infection and inflammation.

In sarcoidosis, FDG uptake is seen in inflammatory cells such as neutrophils, activated macrophages and lymphocytes, and the amount of uptake is proportional to disease activity. FDG uptake can be measured as the standardized uptake value (SUV) and, provided that variables such as the state of fasting and injection to scan time are constant, the SUV can be used to assess response to treatment:

$$SUV = \frac{\text{uptake in MBq/mL in tissue (decay corrected)}}{\text{total MBq injected per body weight in grams}}.$$

Several cases have been reported of the incidental finding of sarcoidosis in patients imaged with FDG-PET for malignancy (Takanami et al. 2008; Ataergin et al. 2009). Abnormalities have been described in the brain, spinal cord, nerves, joints, bones, bone marrow, lymph nodes, eyes, heart, pleura, lung, muscles, larynx and elsewhere. Radiology and histology have confirmed sarcoidosis in most cases, and abnormal FDG uptake has resolved with corticosteroid treatment; but it can be difficult to distinguish the patterns of FDG uptake in sarcoidosis and disseminated malignancy.

In one of the largest retrospective studies, Teirstein et al. (2007) reviewed 188 FDG PET scans performed in 137 patients with proven sarcoidosis. The most common sites of abnormal FDG uptake were mediastinal (54 scans) and extrathoracic lymph nodes (30 scans) and the lung (24 scans). Twenty sites of occult disease were also identified. Abnormal lung uptake was seen in two-thirds of patients with radiographic stage II and III sarcoidosis, and absent lung uptake was common in patients with stage 0 and I disease and in burnt-out fibrotic stage IV disease. The authors concluded that FDG PET is valuable for identifying occult and reversible granulomas in patients with sarcoidosis.

Comparison of FDG PET and bronchoalveolar lavage

More recently, Keijsers et al. (2010) studied the relationship between FDG uptake and sarcoid activity by bronchoalveolar lavage (BAL) in a retrospective study of 77 consecutive patients with newly diagnosed and histologically proven pulmonary sarcoidosis. Patients were classified according to the conventional radiographic stages. The FDG uptake is thought to reflect disease activity and it identified more lesions in the mediastinum, hila and lung parenchyma by PET than conventional radiography. Combining the so-called inactive (0) and end stages (IV), FDG showed uptake in mediastinum/hila in all patients and parenchymal activity in 57 percent of patients. In stage I disease, defined as BHL without parenchymal involvement, 52 percent of patients demonstrated increased metabolic activity in the parenchyma. This shows increased sensitivity of FDG to detect active disease and inadequacy of conventional radiographic classification for staging sarcoidosis. This may have major impact on starting or discontinuation of immunosuppressive therapy.

Lymphocytosis in BAL fluid represents alveolitis and an increased CD4/CD8 ratio is highly specific for sarcoidosis. Increased BAL neutrophils are related to future pulmonary deterioration in terms of fibrosis and are known to be higher in stage IV disease. Severe parenchymal impairment on radiographic stage correlates positively with the SUV_{max} (FDG) of the lung parenchyma but inversely with the SUV_{max} of the mediastinum/hila. The extent of metabolic activity (SUV_{max}) in the mediastinum/hila correlates with the CD4/CD8 ratio in BAL (both diminish from stage I to stage IV), while the increase in metabolic activity in the lung parenchyma in stage IV correlates with an increase in the number of neutrophils. This study suggests that FDG uptake might replace the invasive procedure but more studies are needed to establish a firmer correlation between uptake pattern and cellular morphology (see Fig. 14.4).

Sarcoidosis or malignancy?

Disseminated malignancy, tuberculosis and lymphoma in particular have patterns of FDG uptake similar to sarcoidosis and it is important to exclude these conditions before diagnosing sarcoidosis from an abnormal FDG PET scan.

Alavi *et al.* (2002) studied 31 patients with known and suspected sarcoidosis and they identified three patterns of uptake (Table 14.2). In 71 percent of patients there was bilateral hilar uptake of FDG extending into the mediastinum and the lung, as in the typical pattern of gallium scintigraphy. In these patients the sarcoid lesions were also seen on CT and most patients had a diagnosis of sarcoidosis before PET imaging. In 19 percent of patients a discrepant pattern was seen with multiple foci of intense FDG uptake within and outside the chest and commonly also splenic uptake, but not necessarily corresponding with CT abnormalities. This pattern is indistinguishable from malignant disease and is a considerable diagnostic challenge for PET imaging alone,

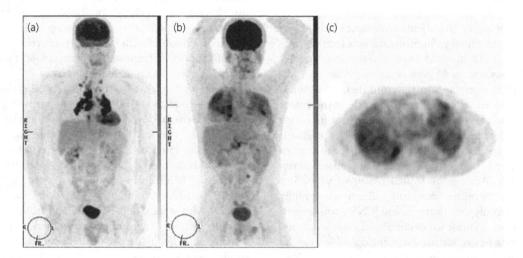

Figure 14.4   (a) FDG PET of a patient with abnormal activity in the mediastinum and hila without parenchymal or extrapulmonary activity. (b) FDG PET of a patient with abnormal activity in the mediastinum, hila, lungs and abdominal lymph nodes. BAL showed 7.8 percent lymphocytes, normal CD4/CD8 ratio and 1.1 percent neutrophils. (c) Transverse image in the same patient as (b), showing the affected lung parenchyma. Reproduced with permission from Springer Science + Business Media.

Table 14.2   Imaging patterns in sarcoidosis and malignancy (Alavi *et al.* 2002).

Patterns	CT	FDG	Conclusion
Typical (71%)	BHL and lung changes	BHL and lung uptake	Typical pattern of sarcoidosis; little overlap with malignancy
Discrepant (19%)	Solitary nodule	Intra- and extrathoracic abnormalities, splenic uptake	Difficult to differentiate between sarcoidosis and malignancy
Suspected metastases from unknown primary (10%)	Multiple small lung lesions but undetected primary	Matching uptake of FDG but undetected primary	Supports an inflammatory disorder such as sarcoidosis

BHL, bilateral hilar lymphadenopathy

although the discrepancy is less likely in lymphomas when CT normally shows large masses. The inflammatory uptake tends to change quickly with fewer lesions on CT but numerous lesions on PET, and this pattern should raise the suspicion of sarcoidosis. Ten percent of patients showed a third pattern with multiple small FDG avid lesions in the lung, suggesting metastases from an unknown primary tumor, but this pattern is also compatible with an inflammatory disorder like sarcoidosis. It should be noted that some primary tumors, such as bronchoalveolar carcinoma, do not have avid FDG uptake and that absence of a primary on FDG imaging does not necessarily exclude malignancy.

Comparison of FDG PET and gallium scintigraphy

Braun and associates compared FDG PET–CT and gallium SPECT in 12 patients with biopsy-proven sarcoidosis in several sites (Braun *et al.* 2008). The sensitivity of FDG and gallium was 86 and 67 percent, respectively. The falsely negative sites were in the pharynx, larynx, facial skin, stomach and liver for both techniques. However, both forms of imaging identified new sites that were not previously apparent, including abdominal, pelvic and peripheral lymph nodes, bone, muscle, pharynx, larynx and salivary glands.

Prager and associates compared FDG PET and gallium scintigraphy in the initial assessment of 24 patients with histologically proven sarcoidosis (Prager *et al.* 2008). Sixty-four lesions were detected by gallium and 85 by FDG, and the conclusion was that FDG was more suitable for imaging the mediastinum, the hila, the posterior lungs and extrathoracic lesions.

In a similar study, Nishiyama and associates compared FDG PET and gallium SPECT in 18 patients with sarcoidosis (Nishiyama *et al.* 2006). Gallium detected 17 of 21 (81 percent) pulmonary and 15 of 31 (48 percent) extrapulmonary sites, whereas FDG detected all 21 pulmonary sites and 28 of 31 (90 percent) extrapulmonary sites.

FDG in assessing response to treatment

Braun *et al.* (2008) used FDG PET to study the response to corticosteroid therapy in five patients. Incomplete regression was seen in two patients who were on tapering doses of steroids. Two patients in whom the steroids had been withdrawn because of clinical improvement showed complete remission. Persistent abnormal FDG uptake was seen in one patient with poor compliance to therapy. In all patients, FDG uptake correlated well with clinical evaluation and radiology (see Fig. 14.5).

Keijsers *et al.* (2008) reported FDG PET in 12 patients with refractory sarcoidosis treated with infliximab. Symptoms improved in 11 patients while chest X-ray staging did not change. FDG PET showed either improvement or normalization in the responding patients, and in the other a decrease in SUV of the lung parenchyma was associated with an improvement of vital capacity. The authors concluded that FDG uptake represented disease activity (Plate 13).

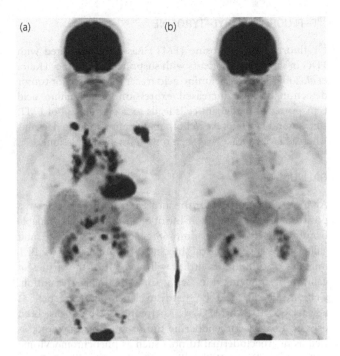

Figure 14.5   FDG PET maximum intensity projections in a 66-year-old woman with multisystem biopsy-proven sarcoidosis at primary staging (a) before and (b) after corticosteroid treatment. Initially there is abnormal uptake in the right supraclavicular, left axillary, mediastinal, bilateral hilar, para-aortic and inguinal lymph nodes with complete regression after treatment (only normal activity in brain, kidneys and bladder remains). With permission from Springer Science + Business Media.

Radiolabeled amino acids

CARBON-11 METHIONINE

Yamada *et al.* (1998) compared FDG and ^{11}C-methionine uptake in 31 patients with sarcoidosis. Methionine uptake represents *cell proliferation* as opposed to FDG which images *glucose utilization* (occurs as a result of inflammation). In this study, the authors examined whether PET could predict the clinical course of sarcoidosis by evaluating the different propensities of FDG and methionine accumulation in mediastinal and bilateral hilar lymphadinopathy. FDG and methionine uptake values showed no correlation among the total group of patients. In the patients with a high FDG uptake rate, the methionine uptake was relatively low, and vice versa. So the patients were divided according to the dominance of uptake.

The FDG-dominant group had a higher rate of remission (78 percent) and a lower rate of appearance of pulmonary involvement, while the methionine dominant group had a lower rate of remission (33 percent) and a higher rate of appearance of pulmonary involvement on follow-up imaging. The results suggest that methionine dominant group may develop progressive pulmonary involvement.

Patients with an abnormal chest X-ray and a high SACE but a normal PET scan may remain well without treatment, suggesting that FDG PET can be used to assess the need for suppressive therapy.

¹⁸F–FLUORO–METHYL–TYROSINE

¹⁸F-fluoro-methyl tyrosine (FMT) has been compared with FDG in sarcoidosis patients with suspected malignancy (Kaira et al. 2007). FMT is an amino acid tracer that is used for tumor detection because increased expression of an amino acid transporter in malignant cells leads to accumulation of FMT. They found FDG uptake in both malignant and sarcoid lesions whereas FMT uptake was seen only in malignant lesions.

GALLIUM-68

An intriguing prospect for the future is gallium–68, which is a positron emitter with a half-life of 68 minutes and is available from a long-lived germanium-68 generator. Gallium-67 and gallium-68 have identical biochemical properties, so PET imaging of gallium-68 citrate will have all of the virtues of gallium-67 imaging but with superior image resolution. Gallium-68 can also be used to label peptides such as 68Ga-DOTA(0)-Phe(1)-Tyr(3)-octreotide, which has been used to image neuroendocrine tumors such as carcinoid, as well as neuroectodermal tumors such as pheochromocytoma and paraganglioma. Will gallium-68 supplant gallium-67 and FDG PET in the nuclear imaging of sarcoidosis? It is possible, but time will tell.

CURRENT PRACTICE AND FUTURE PROSPECTS

The gallium scan has been the mainstay of nuclear imaging of sarcoidosis for several decades but new techniques such as SPECT–CT and PET–CT have provided additional value. The diagnosis of sarcoidosis rightly relies on histology, but in early disease with borderline hilar lymphadenopathy and in Löfgren's syndrome the gallium scan can support the diagnosis without invasive investigation. The advantage of gallium imaging is its ability to survey the whole body and to find extrapulmonary sites of disease, especially in patients with only single-organ involvement clinically. It shows sites of active inflammation and can help to differentiate fibrosis from active inflammation. It is able to detect relapses after treatment and can assess disease activity before lung transplantation.

Somatostatin analogs have better sensitivity than gallium except in extrapulmonary disease, but they are not specific and they cannot differentiate between benign and malignant uptake. Thus, they have not supplanted the gallium scan.

FDG PET gives a better three-dimensional map of inflammation in sarcoidosis than the gallium scan, especially when combined with CT. It is superior to gallium for assessing the extent of disease, potential biopsy sites and assessment of response to treatment of relapse, but it is not always so readily available.

CONCLUSION

Gallium-67, although not entirely specific for sarcoidosis, remains the inexpensive way of imaging active inflammation in thoracic and extrathoracic sarcoidosis and it has the advantage of whole-body imaging. Gallium-67 SPECT with near simultaneous CT for anatomical localization gives better definition of inflamed tissue than planar imaging

Somatostatin receptor scintigraphy is superior for imaging intrathoracic sites and CNS involvement in comparison with gallium imaging. FDG PET–CT is, at the moment, the best technique for imaging active sarcoidosis – if it is available.

New PET tracers such as gallium-68 are on the horizon and may change the imaging of sarcoidosis.

REFERENCES

Alavi A, Gupta N, Alberini JL et al. (2002). Positron emission tomography imaging in nonmalignant thoracic disorders. Semin Nucl Med 32: 293–321.

Ataergin S, Arslan N, Ozet A, Ozguven MA (2009). Abnormal 18F-FDG uptake detected with positron emission tomography in a patient with breast cancer: a case of sarcoidosis and review of the literature. Case Report Med 2009: 785047.

Baughman RP, Winget DB, Bowen EH, Lower EE (1997). Predicting respiratory failure in sarcoidosis patients. Sarcoid Vasc Diff Lung Dis 14: 154–8.

Baughman RP, Fernandez M, Bosken CH et al. (1984). Comparison of gallium-67 scanning, bronchoalveolar lavage, and serum angiotensin-converting enzyme levels in pulmonary sarcoidosis: predicting response to therapy. Am Rev Respir Dis 129: 676–81.

Beaumont D, Herry JY, Sapene M et al. (1982). Gallium-67 in the evaluation of sarcoidosis: correlations with serum angiotensin-converting enzyme and bronchoalveolar lavage. Thorax 37: 11–18.

Bechtel JJ, Starr T, Dantzker DR, Bower JS (1981). Airway hyperreactivity in patients with sarcoidosis. Am Rev Respir Dis 124: 759–61.

Bergin CJ, Bell DY, Coblentz CL, Chiles C et al. (1989). Sarcoidosis: correlation of pulmonary parenchymal pattern at CT with results of pulmonary function tests. Radiology 171: 619–24.

Braun JJ, Kessler R, Constantinesco A, Imperiale A (2008). 18F-FDG PET/CT in sarcoidosis management: review and report of 20 cases. Eur J Nucl Med Mol Imaging 35: 1537–43.

Crystal RG, Roberts WC, Hunninghake GW et al. (1981). Pulmonary sarcoidosis: a disease characterized and perpetuated by activated lung T-lymphocytes. Ann Intern Med 94: 73–94.

De Vries J, Rothkrantz-Kos S, van Dieijen-Visser MP, Drent M (2004). The relationship between fatigue and clinical parameters in pulmonary sarcoidosis. Sarcoids Vasc Diff Lung Dis 21: 127–36.

Judson MA, Thompson BW, Rabin DL et al. (2003). ACCESS Research Group: The diagnostic pathway to sarcoidosis. Chest 123: 406–12.

Kaira K, Oriuchi N, Otani Y et al. (2007). Diagnostic usefulness of fluorine-18-alpha-methyltyrosine positron emission tomography in combination with 18F-fluorodeoxyglucose in sarcoidosis patients. Chest 131: 1019–27.

Keijsers RG, Verzijlbergen JF, van Diepen DM et al. (2008). 18F-FDG PET in sarcoidosis: an observational study in 12 patients treated with infliximab. Vasc Diff Lung Dis 25(2): 143–9.

Keijsers RG, Grutters JC, van Velzen-Blad H et al. (2010). (18)F-FDG PET patterns and BAL cell profiles in pulmonary sarcoidosis. Eur J Nucl Med Mol Imaging 37: 1181–8.

Kwekkeboom DJ, Krenning EP, Kho GS et al. (1998). Somatostatin receptor imaging in patients with sarcoidosis. Eur J Nucl Med 25: 1284–92.

Lebtahi R, Crestani B, Belmatoug N et al. (2001). Somatostatin receptor scintigraphy and gallium scintigraphy in patients with sarcoidosis. J Nucl Med 42: 21–6.

Leung AN, Brauner MW, Caillat-Vigneron N et al. (1998). Sarcoidosis activity: correlation of HRCT findings with those of gallium scanning, bronchoalveolar lavage, and serum angiotensin-converting enzyme assay. J Comput Assist Tomogr 22: 229–34.

Line BR, Hunninghake GW, Keogh BA et al. (1981). Gallium-67 scanning to stage the alveolitis of sarcoidosis: correlation with clinical studies, pulmonary function studies, and bronchoalveolar lavage. Am Rev Respir Dis 123: 440–6.

Lynch JP, Kazerooni EA, Gay SE (1997). Pulmonary sarcoidosis. Clin Chest Med 18: 755–85.

Mäkinen TJ, Lankinen P, Pöyhönen T et al. (2005). Comparison of 18F-FDG and 68Ga PET imaging in the assessment of experimental osteomyelitis due to Staphylococcus aureus. Eur J Nucl Med Mol Imaging 32: 1259–68.

Maña J, van Kroonenburgh M (2005). Clinical usefulness of nuclear imaging techniques in sarcoidosis. Eur Respir Mon 32: 284–300.

Niden AH, Mishkin FS, Salem F et al. (1986). Prognostic significance of gallium lung scans in sarcoidosis. Ann NY Acad Sci 465: 435–43.

Nishiyama Y, Yamamoto Y, Fukunaga K et al. (2006). Comparative evaluation of 18F-FDG PET and gallium scintigraphy in patients with sarcoidosis. J Nucl Med 47: 1571–6.

Nosal A, Schleissner LA, Mishkin FS, Lieberman J (1979). Angiotensin-I-converting enzyme and gallium scan in noninvasive evaluation of sarcoidosis. Ann Intern Med 90: 328–31.

Prager E, Wehrschuetz M, Bisail B et al. (2008). Comparison of 18F-FDG and gallium citrate in sarcoidosis imaging. Nuklearmedizin 47(1): 18–23.

Rizzato G, Blasi A (1986). A European survey on the usefulness of gallium lung scans in assessing sarcoidosis: experience in 14 research centers in seven different countries. Ann NY Acad Sci 465: 463–78.

Shorr AF, Helman DL, Lettieri CJ et al. (2004). Depreotide scanning in sarcoidosis: a pilot study. Chest 126: 1337–43.

Sulavik SB, Spencer RP, Palestro CJ et al. (1993). Specificity and sensitivity of distinctive chest radiographic and/or gallium images in the noninvasive diagnosis of sarcoidosis. Chest 103: 403–9.

Takanami K, Kaneta T, Yamada T et al. (2008). FDG PET for esophageal cancer complicated by sarcoidosis mimicking mediastinal and hilar lymph node metastases: two case reports. Clin Nucl Med 33: 258–61.

Teirstein AS, Machac J, Almeida O et al. (2007). Results of 188 whole-body fluorodeoxyglucose positron emission tomography scans in 137 patients with sarcoidosis. Chest 132: 1949–53.

Weiner RE (1996). The mechanism of gallium localization in malignant disease. Nucl Med Biol 23: 745–51.

Wirnsberger RM, de Vries J, Breteler MH et al. (1998). Evaluation of quality of life in sarcoidosis patients. Respir Med 92: 750–6.

Yamada Y, Uchida Y, Tatsumi K et al. (1998). Fluorine-18-fluorodeoxy-glucose and carbon-11-methionine evaluation of lymphadenopathy in sarcoidosis. J Nucl Med 39: 1160–6.

15

IGRAs and sarcoidosis

MUHUNTHAN THILLAI AND AJIT LALVANI

INTRODUCTION

Swift and accurate diagnosis of sarcoidosis is paramount as conditions with similar clinical pictures such as tuberculosis or lymphoma require radically different yet equally prompt treatment. Current methods of diagnosis rely on a suggestive clinical and radiological picture supported by compatible histology from tissue samples obtained by invasive biopsy of affected organs. Obtaining a biopsy involves risks to the patient which may be significant in terms of morbidity as well as healthcare costs. For example, an iatrogenic pneumothorax after a transbronchial lung biopsy will require a prolonged inpatient stay with intercostal chest drainage. In addition, the histology of disease is non-specific and can be made only after excluding other differential diagnoses. There is no available test that can predict disease progression or response to treatment.

A greater understanding of the immune mechanisms and potential antigenic targets involved in sarcoidosis disease pathogenesis will help to develop more accurate diagnostic methods with potentially major and immediate advances for clinical practice. To this end, interferon-γ release assays (IGRAs) have been investigated in sarcoidosis for ex-vivo responses to specific antigens. The implied association between sarcoidosis and tuberculosis has resulted in much recent research focusing on T-cell responses to mycobacterial antigens in patients with proven sarcoidosis, but results of studies to date remain far from conclusive.

INTEFERON-GAMMA RELEASE ASSAYS IN THE DIAGNOSIS OF *MYCOBACTERIUM TUBERCULOSIS* INFECTION

The pathway from exposure to *M. tuberculosis* to disease is a multistep process that depends partly on the body's own immune defences. Bacilli may cause immediate disease or may lie dormant for decades. Approximately 5–10 percent of people infected with *M. tuberculosis* go on to develop active disease. The immune mechanisms that underly these different clinical outcomes are not fully understood.

The current strategy for diagnosis and treatment of latent tuberculosis infection (LTBI) in the developed world is based on 'targeted testing' – the identification of those at highest risk of progression from LTBI to active disease. Such individuals will stand to benefit most from preventative treatment, and this population includes people infected recently (within the last 2–3 years) and those with suppressed or immature immune systems regardless of when they acquired infection.

Diagnosis of LTBI was historically defined as a positive tuberculin skin test (TST) in an otherwise asymptomatic person exposed to TB with no clinical or radiographic signs of active disease. LTBI induces a strong cell-mediated immune response that is effectively exploited by the TST, which measures the delayed-type hypersensitivity response to intradermal inoculation of purified protein derivative (PPD) of tuberculin – a crude mixture of more than 200 proteins from *M. tuberculosis*.

The TST does have several drawbacks, the most important of which is its poor specificity in patients vaccinated with bacille Calmette–Guérin (BCG) due to cross-reactivity of the many antigens in PPD with BCG and *M. tuberculosis*. Further disadvantages include poor sensitivity in people with suppressed or immature cellular immunity (e.g. individuals infected with HIV), those with iatrogenic immunosuppression, and very young children. There are also logistical difficulties as the test requires a trained healthcare professional to perform the test, as well as a repeat visit by the patient for reading of the result.

Given these problems with the TST, much research in recent years has been focused on finding alternative superior methods of diagnosing LTBI. The extremely low bacterial burden in LTBI makes it almost impossible to detect the organism directly, and the weak humoral response makes serological testing unreliable. However, infection is found to evoke a strong T-cell response which is dominated by T-helper 1 (Th1) type CD4 T-cells that secrete interferon-gamma (IFN-γ).

Major advances in mycobacterial genomics in the 1990s resulted in the identification of a genomic segment – region of difference 1, or RD1 – which is deleted from all strains of BCG vaccine and most environmental mycobacteria (Behr *et al.* 1999). Of the nine open reading frames in this region, Rv3875 (early secretory antigenic target-6, ESAT-6) and Rv3874 (culture filtrate protein-10, CFP-10) were the first to be studied and it was found that both gene products are very strong targets of Th1 cells in infection with *M. tuberculosis*.

It was therefore postulated that a T-cell response to these antigens could serve as a specific marker of infection with *M. tuberculosis*, which would bypass the problem of false-positive TST results in individuals previously vaccinated with BCG. Antigen-specific T-cell assays traditionally had historically been confined to research laboratories as they required specialized equipment, radioisotopes, and suitable technical expertise. However, two assay platforms for rapid measurement of antigen-specific IFN-γ-secreting T-cell responses suitable for use in routine diagnostic service laboratories across the world were developed; these are now collectively known as IFN-γ release assays (IGRAs). Both assays exploit the fact that T-cells from people infected with *M. tuberculosis* become sensitized to ESAT-6 or CFP-10 *in vivo*, and release IFN-γ when they re-encounter the antigens *ex vivo*.

The rapid ex-vivo enzyme-linked immunospot (ELISpot) assay counts individual antigen-specific T-cells based on the principle that a highly sensitive T-cell assay that uses highly specific antigens from *M. tuberculosis* should result in a diagnostic test with high sensitivity and specificity. The assay directly enumerates antigen-specific T-cells that secrete IFN-γ, which appear as dark spots, where each spot is the 'footprint' of an individual T-cell specific for *M. tuberculosis*. Spots are counted using a magnifying lens or automated reader.

The alternate method is a whole-blood IFN-γ enzyme-linked immunoassay (ELISA) which measures the concentration of IFN-γ in the supernatant of a sample of diluted whole blood after incubation with the same antigens for 24 hours. Whole-blood IFN-γ ELISA was developed originally as an assay for detecting TB in cattle in the 1980s; it was adapted for use in humans in the 1990s using PPD, which was subsequently replaced by ESAT-6 and CFP-10. These antigens subsequently were complemented by a third antigen (TB7.7 from region of difference 11) and the format modified so that these antigens were coated onto the inner aspect of tubes for collecting blood.

Both assays are available commercially as quality-controlled, regulatory-approved diagnostic test kits. The two IGRAs have some similarities (e.g. both need to be processed within eight hours of taking a blood sample), as well as several key differences (e.g. ELISpot requires separation of white cells, which ensures a fixed number of white blood cells in the assay but is technically more complex to process).

Figure 15.1 is a diagrammatic representation of the TST, ELISpot and ELISA for diagnosing *M. tuberculosis* infection.

Both assays have sensitivity of 80–85 percent and a specificity approaching 100 percent for diagnosis of LTBI. ELISpot performs well in patients co-infected with HIV in young children, and published data in these patient populations is more extensive than with ELISA (Lalvani and Millington 2007). In LTBI, ELISpot probably has higher sensitivity than the TST, while ELISA seems to have similar sensitivity to the TST. In young children, ELISpot appears to have higher sensitivity than the TST, while ELISA may have similar sensitivity to the TST.

Unlike the TST, both tests seem to be relatively robust to co-infection with HIV in people with relatively low CD4 counts. For screening of iatrogenically immunosuppressed patients with rheumatic disorders before initiating anti-TNF therapy, IGRAs seem to be more sensitive than TST, and data with ELISA are currently more extensive than with ELISpot. Indeterminate results are more common with ELISA and are associated strongly with immunosuppression, young age, and old age, while indeterminate results with ELISpot are rare in all risk groups studied to date (Menzies *et al.* 2007).

Both assays are in routine use throughout much of the developed world and have been incorporated into national guidelines for the targeted testing of individuals with suspected LTBI. There are no universally agreed guidelines for the use of IGRAs in diagnosis of active TB, although an early diagnostic result may help guide management of patients with suspected active TB prior to the availability of further investigations (Fig. 15.2).

IGRAs can be used to rule out sarcoidosis when it is suspected in the differential diagnosis. The poor speed and sensitivity of existing diagnostic tools for both sarcoidosis and active tuberculosis causes delays in diagnosis. As infection with *M. tuberculosis* is a prerequisite for active TB, reliable determination of infection status could accelerate diagnostic assessment of a patient with suspected sarcoidosis by enabling rapid exclusion of TB.

Conversely, positive results with both TST and IGRA may help guide decisions about early initiation of presumptive treatment for tuberculosis while the results of cultures from patients with severe disease are awaited, and in patients with extrapulmonary disease, for whom culture is frequently negative. However, it is important to note that the use of

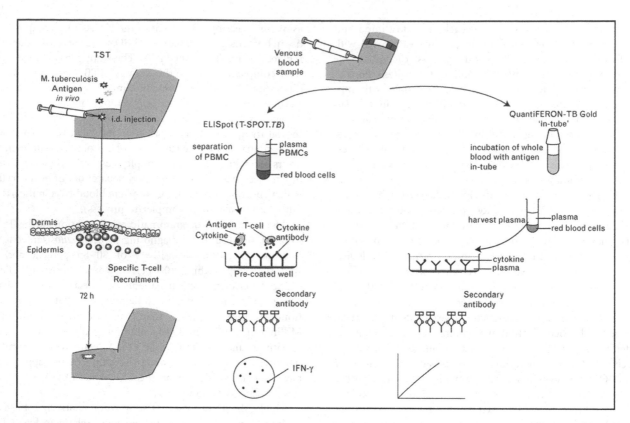

Figure 15.1   The TST (*left*) is performed when purified protein derivative is intradermally injected into the volar surface of the forearm. The delayed-type hypersensitivity response (induration) is measured 72 h later. ELISpot (*center*) uses peripheral blood mononuclear cells (including T-cells) which are separated from the blood sample by density centrifugation, and are washed, counted and then incubated with ESAT-6 and CFP-10 in a standard 96-well microtiter plate for 16–20 h. If the patient is infected with *M. tuberculosis*, T-cells will recognize the antigens and secrete IFN-γ. This cytokine is captured in the immediate vicinity of the cytokine-secreting T-cell by antibodies specific for IFN-γ coated on the bottom of each well. The cytokine-bound antibodies are subsequently detected with another antibody conjugated to an enzyme that catalyzes a colorimetric reaction resulting in visible spots, where each spot represents the footprint of one T-cell that responded to the antigens. These spots are counted and the frequency of *M. tuberculosis*-specific T-cells quantified. ELISA (*right*) uses whole blood from the patient. It is incubated with ESAT-6, CFP-10 and TB7.7 in the blood collection tube for 16–24 h. If the patient is infected with *M. tuberculosis*, T-cells will recognize the antigens and secrete IFN-γ. The tube is centrifuged and the plasma transferred to a 96-well microtiter plate. IFN-γ in the plasma is captured by antibodies specific for IFN-γ coated on the bottom of each well. The cytokine-bound antibodies are subsequently detected with another antibody conjugated to an enzyme that catalyzes a colorimetric reaction. The optical density of each well is measured and the concentration of IFN-γ determined using a standard curve. Reprinted with permission from Lalvani A, Thillai M (2008). 100-year update on the diagnosis of latent tuberculosis infection. *Horizons in Medicine* 20: 69–84.

IGRAs to rule out active tuberculosis in patients with suspected sarcoidosis is not validated or approved by any regulatory authorities.

RATIONALE FOR CAUSAL RELATIONSHIP OF MYCOBACTERIA WITH SARCOIDOSIS

The similarities between the histological changes and the clinical presentation of sarcoidosis with tuberculosis have led a number of investigators to postulate a role for mycobacteria in the etiology of sarcoidosis. Theories include that of direct disease causality, disease due to mycobacteriophages (Mankiewicz and Beland 1964), or viruses after mycobacterial infection (Nikoskelainen *et al.* 1974) and the implications of cell-wall-deficient mycobacteria found in the blood of patients with sarcoidosis (Almenoff *et al.* 1996).

Evidence put forward for such involvement includes historical observations of the concurrence of bacteriologically proven mycobacterial infection in patients with sarcoidosis, in which a number of cases of patients with proven tuberculosis go on to develop sarcoidosis (Scadding 1960). There is also some suggestion of a shared epidemiology between the two diseases in certain parts of the world (Brett 1965).

Proteomic techniques and nucleic acid amplification tests have all been used to show evidence of the presence of mycobacteria within sarcoidosis tissue. A meta-analysis of 31 studies, all of which analyzed sarcoidosis tissues by polymerase chain reaction (PCR) for nucleic acid amplification followed by identification of nucleic acid sequences specific for different types of mycobacteria, concluded that 231 of 874 patients were positive for mycobacterial nucleic acids and the odds of finding mycobacteria in sarcoidosis tissues versus controls was 9.67 (4.56–20.5), suggesting a potential link between mycobacteria and sarcoidosis in some cases (Gupta *et al.* 2007).

However, despite some evidence for the presence of mycobacterial involvement in the etiology of disease, other evidence points away from a causal relationship. This includes the lack of conclusive country-specific epidemiological

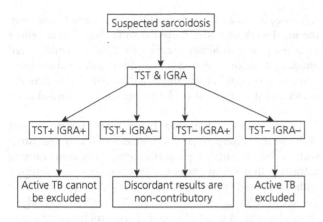

Figure 15.2   Suggested pathway for incorporation of T-cell-based interferon-γ release assays into the diagnostic algorithm for the *ruling out* of active tuberculosis in a patient with suspected sarcoidosis. This pathway should be placed in the context of a contemporary evidence base. Positive results for the tuberculin skin test (TST) and IGRA may help guide decisions about early initiation of presumptive treatment of tuberculosis while the results of culture tests from patients with severe disease are awaited and in those with extrapulmonary disease, for whom culture frequently is negative. Discordant results do not contribute to the diagnostic work-up of active TB or sarcoidosis. Negative results for TST and IGRA can be used as a 'rule-out test' to reliably exclude active TB with a high negative predictive value and may help guide the diagnosis towards sarcoidosis in a patient in whom the disease is suspected. In patients with very high pretest probability, however, active tuberculosis cannot be ruled out with as much certainty.

evidence for such a relationship, the differences in organ involvement between the two diseases, and the differences in treatment strategies. The fact that immunosuppressive therapies for sarcoidosis do not cause reactivation of any latent mycobacteria seems to point away from viable organisms being present within diseased granulomatous tissue. However, this does not discount the theory that immune responses to non-viable remnants of mycobacteria are responsible for some cases of sarcoidosis.

RATIONALE FOR ANTIGEN-SPECIFIC T-CELL RESPONSES

Kveim reagent is sarcoidosis material that has been prepared to certain exacting specifications. It is often derived from sarcoidosis spleen or lymph node tissue but can be prepared using most diseased tissue specimens. The reagent was historically used to diagnose disease in a method analogous to use of the TST in patients with tuberculosis. Intradermal inoculation of Kveim reagent caused a pathognomonic granuloma within 4–6 weeks at the site of injection (Siltzbach 1961) with high sensitivity (up to 80 percent) and specificity (>98 percent).

The immune mechanisms of this reaction are poorly understood and the antigenic targets of the granuloma-associated CD4+ T-cells that predate the immunopathology of disease are unknown. However, previous work has implicated an oligoclonal CD4+ T-cell infiltrate which precedes formation of the diagnostic local epitheliod intra-dermal granulomas. Analysis of the TCR V beta repertoire from Kveim reaction sites using a PCR technique demon-strated this oligoclonal pattern of V beta gene expression with limited junctional variability in the hypervariable section of the TCR (Klein *et al*. 1995). This implicates a small number of Kveim reagent derived targets with invoke host T-cell responses.

Work by a number of groups to remove non-protein-aceous material from Kveim has shown that these targets are likely to be proteins, as the resulting suspension after these treatments still has the ability to cause a Kveim reaction (Lyons *et al*. 1992).

INVESTIGATION OF T-CELL RESPONSES TO MULTIPLE MYCOBACTERIAL ANTIGENS

Based on the hypothesis that there exists a limited number of antigens within both Kveim reagent and sarcoid granulomas targeted by granuloma-associated T-cells, and that these antigens may be mycobacterial in origin, a number of research groups have investigated the use of the commercial TB interferon-γ release assays in patients with sarcoidosis. The majority have found no increase in response in this patient group. An investigation into a Japanese cohort of patients at low risk of LTBI found that only 3 of 90 tested with the IFN-γ ELISA assay used for diagnosis of tuberculosis had a positive response (Inui *et al*. 2008), and smaller unpublished studies from Europe have made similar findings.

However, mycobacterial antigens other than those found in RD1 have been investigated further with the belief that the antigens involved are not necessarily from viable mycobacter-ial organisms; rather, that they are responsible for initiating sarcoidosis in some patients through a mechanism that may be different from that from a standard tuberculosis infection.

Mycobacterium tuberculosis mycolyl transferase (Antigen 85A) is one of three secreted subunit proteins in *M. tuberculosis* that together form the Antigen 85 complex. IFN-γ ELISpot assays have been used to assess for recognition of this antigen by PBMCs from patients with sarcoidosis and controls. Reactivity to Ag85A whole protein was observed in 15 of 25 sarcoidosis subjects compared to 2 of 22 PPD-negative subjects ($p = 0.0006$) and to 14 of 16 PPD-positive subjects. Peptide-mapping studies identified four immunogenic Ag85A pep-tides, which induced Th1 immune responses in individual subjects, suggesting that multiple epitopes from this protein may have a role in antigen-specific T-cell recognition in some patients with sarcoidosis (Hajizadeh *et al*. 2007).

Early secreted antigenic target (ESAT-6) is one of the components of the IGRAs for diagnosis of TB infection but has also been investigated alone in patients with sarcoidosis. One study showed a significant difference among the sarcoidosis subjects (with 12 of 30 patients responding to the antigen) and PPD-negative control subjects who had only 1 of 26 responding positively ($p = 0.0014$). The same study further investigated bronchoalveolar lavage (BAL) fluid and found that one patient who had no recognition of ESAT-6 by

PBMC demonstrated strong BAL cell Th1 immune responses to ESAT-6 (Drake *et al.* 2007).

A further more detailed study by the same research group found that, when combined with the mycobacterial antigen mKatG, BAL T-cells from 32 out of 44 sarcoidosis patients displayed antigen-specific recognition to either of the whole proteins compared with 1 of 27 controls with other lung diseases ($p < 0.0001$). The primary cells responding to the antigens were shown to be CD4+ T-cells, although CD8+ T-cell responses were observed in the BAL of some of the sarcoidosis patients. Blocking of Toll-like receptor 2 reduced the strength of the observed immune response (Oswald-Richter *et al.* 2009).

Superoxide dismutase A (SodA) is a mycobacterial secreted virulence factor responsible for generating host cellular immune responses in infected hosts. The protein sequence has been identified from sarcoidosis tissue using PCR (Drake *et al.* 2002), and in one study SodA amplicons were detected in 12 of 17 sarcoidosis specimens, compared to 2 of 16 controls ($p = 0.001$) and in 3 of 3 tuberculosis specimens, and the sequences were shown to be identical to that found in *M. tuberculosis*. ELISpot analysis found that 6 of 12 sarcoidosis subjects recognized the SodA peptides, compared to 1 of 26 PPD-negative controls ($p = 0.002$) and 6 out of 11 PPD-positive subjects (Allen *et al.* 2008).

A follow-up to this work has been the development of a mouse model of pulmonary sarcoidosis. Mice were sensitized by subcutaneous injection of SodA and then challenged with intravenous injection of SodA or control. Subsequent histological analysis revealed hilar lymphadenopathy and non-caseating granulomas in the lungs of SodA-treated mice. BAL cells from these mice demonstrated CD4+ T-cell responses against SodA peptide, and this was present in the SodA-sensitized mice only (Swaisgood *et al.* 2010).

A study to investigate T-cell responses to non-mycobacterial proteins involved the sequencing of peptides eluted from HLA-DR molecules of bronchoalveolar lavage fluid to identify self-antigens in disease. It was based on a study showing that sarcoidosis patients expressing the HLA-DR allele DRB1*0301 are characterized by large accumulations in the lungs of CD4+ T-cells expressing the TCR AV2S3 gene segment (Wahlstrom *et al.* 2009).

Analysis of these antigenic peptides by reversed-phase HPLC and liquid chromatography plus mass spectrometry resulted in the identification of 78 amino acid sequences from self-proteins including vimentin and ATP synthase. Characterization of blood and lung T-cell autoimmune responses to these self-antigens may help in our understanding of the persistent pulmonary inflammation seen in sarcoidosis.

MYCOBACTERIAL CATALASE–PEROXIDASE (mKatG)

Although T-cell responses to a number of mycobacterial antigens have been investigated in sarcoidosis, the majority of these have been chosen for study based on their potential for responses in patients infected with mycobacteria. Aside from the intial work on SodA, there has so far been limited effort to investigate sarcoidosis material itself for potential T-cell antigens. A major exception is that of mycobacterial catalase–peroxidase (mKatG), a mycobacterial protein that is clinically relevant as it is involved in the conversion of isoniazid from the prodrug to the active form.

In one study, sarcoidosis tissue extracts were treated with neutral detergent and proteases, which is consistent with the known physical properties of the granuloma causing extracts within Kveim reagent. Tissue antigens were detected with immunoglobulin (Ig)G or F(ab')(2) fragments from pooled sarcoidosis sera in 9 of 12 (75 percent) sarcoidosis tissues but only 3 of 22 (14 percent) control tissues (Song *et al.* 2005).

One of these sarcoidosis tissue antigens was subsequently identified as mKatG using matrix-assisted laser desorption/ionization time-of-flight (MALDI-TOF) mass spectrometry. The identity of mKatG as a tissue antigen was further confirmed in a number of sarcoidosis tissues with immuno-blotting using anti-mKatG monoclonal antibodies. IgG antibodies to recombinant mKatG were also detected in a number of sera from patients with sarcoidosis.

T-cell responses to mKatG have subsequently been investigated and higher frequencies of mKatG-reactive, IFN-γ-expressing T-cells have been found in the peripheral blood of sarcoidosis patients compared with healthy controls in phenotypically diverse patient groups from North America and Sweden. Sarcoidosis patients who displayed T-cell responses to mKatG showed preferential accumulation of mKatG-reactive CD4+ Th1 cells in the lung, indicating a compartmentalized response (Chen *et al.* 2008). In addition, circulating mKatG-reactive T-cells were found in patients with active sarcoidosis only. The absence of these cells in patients with inactive disease may indicate that they play a role in causality of acute disease only.

Aims to identify the cells responsible for immune responses to mkatG peptides have indicated that CD4+ T-cells may be the cell type primarily responsible for these systemic responses. Recognition of mkatG is inhibited using monoclonal antibody against HLA-DR and HLA-DQ, but not HLA-DP and katG presented by antigen-presenting cells expressing DRB1*1101-induced Th1 responses from sarcoidosis T-cells. This demonstrates the likely immunological relevance of the association of HLA DRB1*1101 with sarcoidosis (Oswald-Richter *et al.* 2010).

Work investigating multiple cytokine production from subsets of T-cells has shown that CD4+ T-cells from the bronchoalveolar lavage fluid of patients with pulmonary sarcoidosis respond to mKatG by production of IFN-γ, TNF-α, and IL-2. CD8+ T-cells responded with IFN-γ only. Examination of a further subset of T-cells showed that AV2S3+ T-cells responded with IFN-γ secretion to mKatG to a significantly higher extent than AV2S3 T-cells. CD4+ T-cells from peripheral blood responded with both IFN-γ and TNF-α production after stimulation with mKatG (Wiken *et al.* 2010).

To date, mKatG is the only antigen identified using an immunologically based proteomic approach. Analysis of sarcoidosis spleen and lymph node tissue using more diverse techniques may yield still further proteins of interest.

LTBI AS A CONFOUNDING FACTOR IN PATIENTS WITH SARCOIDOSIS

The hypothesis that mycobacteria have a causal role in disease pathogenesis is not thought of as being universally applicable to all cases of sarcoidosis. IGRAs used for diagnosis of LTBI have been investigated in patients with sarcoidosis and it has been generally found that there is no increased response above the expected in this group. One point of contention with papers investigating T-cell responses to individual specific mycobacterial antigens is the somewhat unexplored possibility of patients being incidentally co-infected with latent tuberculosis infection which is unrelated to their sarcoidosis. Such a possibility would lead to false-positive responses in these individuals.

The difficulty lies in the stringent choice of study groups. The selection of a PPD-negative (assessed by a negative skin TST) control group may bias towards an increased incidence of LTBI in the sarcoidosis group. Some of the published studies are from regions of high incidence of background LTBI and where the sarcoidosis patients did not have TST results. Indeed, when studies have examined IGRAs in patients with sarcoidosis in areas of low levels of LTBI, the findings are generally negative (Inui et al. 2008).

An ideal study would involve sarcoidosis patients who are shown to have no evidence of latent TB infection. It could be hypothesized that any resulting T-cell responses to mycobacterial antigens other than those seen in RD1 would be due to sarcoidosis, rather than any latent TB infection. The inherent difficulty with this scenario is that, by removing all patients with LTBI from the sarcoidosis study group, the investigators may be selecting out cases of sarcoidosis that are actually caused in some way by mycobacteria, leaving only a cohort of patients with disease caused by other stimuli. This 'catch 22' is hard to resolve and will remain until an actual molecular mechanism for disease pathogenesis by mycobacterial proteins can be proven at least in some cases of sarcoidosis.

FUTURE WORK

The difficulty in investigating T-cell responses in peripheral blood and BAL fluid to mycobacterial antigens lies with our limited understanding of the T-cell infiltrate associated with the Kveim reagent. Well-validated Kveim reagent has almost total specificity; i.e. it does not produce a reaction in patients with other disorders including those with tuberculosis. However, if the active component within Kveim is a mycobacterial protein, it would be expected to cause a skin response in most patients with tuberculosis – which is not the case.

One explanation for this apparent disparity is that the antigens that have been investigated (including mKatG) may be more antigenic in patients with sarcoidosis than in those

with tuberculosis, and there is some evidence to support this theory. An alternative explanation is that, if sarcoidosis is caused by a number of different etiological factors, a subset of patients may have increased responses to mycobacterial antigens compared to controls. The difficulty here lies again with ensuring that the sarcoidosis patients chosen for the study do not have latent TB instead as a separate entity causing false-positive T-cell responses.

A number of areas of interest need to be further explored, including T-cell responses to self-antigens such as the HLA-bound peptides which are presented *in vivo* during pulmonary inflammation, as well as investigation of T-cell responses to other antigens in select cohorts (e.g. responses to propionibacteria in patients from Japan). A thorough analysis of these responses in large patient cohorts is needed before we can make any solid conclusions about T-cell responses to specific etiological agents.

REFERENCES

Allen SS, Evans W, Carlisle J et al. (2008). Superoxide dismutase A antigens derived from molecular analysis of sarcoidosis granulomas elicit systemic Th-1 immune responses. *Respir Res* 9: 36.

Almenoff PL, Johnson A, Lesser M, Mattman LH (1996). Growth of acid-fast L forms from the blood of patients with sarcoidosis. *Thorax* 51: 530–3.

Behr MA, Wilson MA, Gill WP et al. (1999). Comparative genomics of BCG vaccines by whole-genome DNA microarray. *Science* 284: 1520–3.

Brett GZ (1965). Epidemiological trends in tuberculosis and sarcoidosis in a district of London between 1958 and 1963. *Tubercle* 46: 413–16.

Chen ES, Wahlstrom J, Song Z et al. (2008). T-cell responses to mycobacterial catalase–peroxidase profile a pathogenic antigen in systemic sarcoidosis. *J Immunol* 181: 8784–96.

Drake WP, Pei Z, Pride DT et al. (2002). Molecular analysis of sarcoidosis tissues for mycobacterium species DNA. *Emerg Infect Dis* 8: 1334–41.

Drake WP, Dhason MS, Nadaf M et al. (2007). Cellular recognition of *Mycobacterium tuberculosis* ESAT-6 and KatG peptides in systemic sarcoidosis. *Infect Immun* 75: 527–30.

Gupta D, Agarwal R, Aggarwal AN, Jindal SK (2007). Molecular evidence for the role of mycobacteria in sarcoidosis: a meta-analysis. *Eur Respir J* 30: 508–16.

Hajizadeh R, Sato H, Carlisle J et al. (2007). *Mycobacterium tuberculosis* antigen 85A induces Th-1 immune responses in systemic sarcoidosis. *J Clin Immunol* 27: 445–54.

Inui N, Suda T, Chida K (2008). Use of the QuantiFERON-TB Gold test in Japanese patients with sarcoidosis. *Respir Med* 102: 313–15.

Klein JT, Horn TD, Forman JD et al. (1995). Selection of oligoclonal V beta-specific T-cells in the intradermal response to Kveim–Siltzbach reagent in individuals with sarcoidosis. *J Immunol* 154: 1450–60.

Lalvani A, Millington KA (2007). T- cell-based diagnosis of childhood tuberculosis infection. *Curr Opin Infect Dis* 20: 264–71.

Lyons DJ, Donald S, Mitchell DN, Asherson GL (1992). Chemical inactivation of the Kveim reagent. *Respiration* 59: 22–6.

Mankiewicz E, Beland J (1964). The role of mycobacteriophages and of cortisone in experimental tuberculosis and sarcoidosis. *Am Rev Respir Dis* 89: 707–20.

Menzies D, Pai M, Comstock G (2007). Meta-analysis: new tests for the diagnosis of latent tuberculosis infection: areas of uncertainty and recommendations for research. *Ann Intern Med* **146**: 340–54.

Nikoskelainen J, Hannuksela M, Palva T (1974). Antibodies to Epstein–Barr virus and some other herpesviruses in patients with sarcoidosis, pulmonary tuberculosis and erythema nodosum. *Scand J Infect Dis* **6**: 209–16.

Oswald-Richter K, Sato H, Hajizadeh R *et al.* (2010). Mycobacterial ESAT-6 and katG are recognized by sarcoidosis CD4+ T-cells when presented by the American sarcoidosis susceptibility allele, DRB1*1101. *J Clin Immunol* **30**: 157–66.

Oswald-Richter KA, Culver DA, Hawkins C *et al.* (2009). Cellular responses to mycobacterial antigens are present in bronchoalveolar lavage fluid used in the diagnosis of sarcoidosis. *Infect Immun* **77**: 3740–8.

Scadding JG (1960). Mycobacterium tuberculosis in the aetiology of sarcoidosis. *Br Med J* **2**: 1617–23.

Siltzbach LE (1961). The Kveim test in sarcoidosis: a study of 750 patients. *J Am Med Assoc* **178**: 476–82.

Song Z, Marzilli L, Greenlee BM *et al.* (2005). Mycobacterial catalase-peroxidase is a tissue antigen and target of the adaptive immune response in systemic sarcoidosis. *J Exp Med* **201**: 755–67.

Swaisgood CM, Oswald-Richter K, Moeller SD *et al.* (2010). Development of a sarcoidosis murine lung granuloma model using *Mycobacterium* superoxide dismutase A peptide. *Am J Respir Cell Mol Biol* **44**: 166–74.

Wahlstrom J, Dengjel J, Winqvist O *et al.* (2009). Autoimmune T-cell responses to antigenic peptides presented by bronchoalveolar lavage cell HLA-DR molecules in sarcoidosis. *Clin Immunol* **133**: 353–63.

Wiken M, Idali F, Al Hayjama A, Grunewald J, Eklund A, Wahlstrom J (2010). No evidence of altered alvedar macrophage polarization, but reduced expression of TLR2, in bronchoalvedar lavage calls in sarcoidosis. *Respir Res* **11**: 121.

16

The Kveim reaction

MUHUNTHAN THILLAI, DONALD MITCHELL AND AJIT LALVANI

INTRODUCTION

The diagnostic granuloma that forms after the intradermal injection of sarcoidosis tissue is named after the Norweigen pathologist Ansgar Kveim who first formally reported in 1941 that the injection of a heated suspension of sarcoid lymph node tissue caused a nodule to develop at the site of injection in 12 out of 13 patients with sarcoidosis (Kveim 1948). The reaction occurred between nine days and four weeks after injection and subsequent biopsy of the nodule revealed histological changes consistent with sarcoidosis. The reaction was not seen in an equivalent number of control patients without the disease.

Further validation of the reaction led to preparation of specific Kveim *reagents* for diagnostic use in sarcoidosis worldwide. The reagent cannot be currently used owing to the lack of availability of standardized bioactive in-vivo diagnostic material as well as the potential for the suspension to transmit prion diseases such as new-variant Cruetzfeldt–Jackob disease.

The Kveim reaction has been investigated intensively. It was found that a number of different sarcoid tissue specimens could be used for preparation, including spleen, lymph node and tonsil, but that individual reagents vary greatly in their ability to produce the diagnostic reaction (Danbolt 1951a). Immunological analysis has indicated that the delayed reaction occurs as a consequence of a select number of antigen-specific T-cells infiltrating the site of injection, but detailed histological and immunological investigations of the reaction have provided few answers (Klein *et al.* 1995).

PREPARATION OF KVEIM REAGENT AND ATTEMPTS TO ISOLATE THE ACTIVE COMPONENT

The majority of historical Kveim reagent was derived from spleen (owing to the large amount of tissue available) and lymph nodes – which were thought to have had a higher potential for the reaction despite the smaller amount of available material. A number of studies have shown that only a small proportion (about 1 in 5) of sarcoid spleens are suitable for use as an in-vivo diagnostic test, because of problems with weak reactivity or low specificity of the other batches (Mitchell *et al.* 1976).

The original method of preparation described by Kveim, among others, consisted of cutting the tissue into narrow pieces and rinsing it free of blood with cold sterile normal saline (Danbolt 1948). Batches of 30–35 g of tissue were ground up in a mortar with a sterile physiological saline solution to make a suspension of known strength, usually one part by weight of wet tissue to ten of the final suspension. The larger particles were allowed to separate by sedimentation and were then discarded. The supernatant particulate suspension was then used as the test material after adjustment of the pH to 7.2–7.4, sterilization by heating to 56–60°C for one hour on two successive days, and the addition of a preservative, usually 0.25% phenol. Reagents may also have been treated with 2.5 megarad of radiation in an attempt to inactivate any living organisms that may have been present. This basic method has been modified in a number of subtle ways, but the underlying principle was that Kveim reagent remained a relatively crude suspension of human sarcoid tissues.

After initial evaluations, a number of techniques were used to try to both increase the potency of Kveim reagent and identify the active component. The conclusions of this work are varied, but in general it was felt that the biologically active material within Kveim was particulate and was not water-soluble. It did not pass a Berkefeld or Seitz filter (Danbolt 1951b) and, while the opalescent supernatant after centrifugation at 2500 rpm retained activity, the clear supernatant after ultra-centrifugation at 30 000 rpm became inactive (Rogers and Haserick 1954). Work has shown that the particles sedimenting from spleen suspension in 15 minutes of centrifugation at 5500 g appeared to have the highest activity (Chase 1961). Particles sedimenting on further centrifugation at 10000 g showed only one-ninth of the activity, weight for weight, of the larger particles.

Removal of lipids by extraction in the cold with ether or with chloroform–methanol did not reduce activity, and ether extraction was actually thought to have increased activity. Repeated extraction with a series of hot organic solvents destroyed activity, and this was suspected of being due to the disruption of lipoprotein linkages. Boiling in aqueous suspension seemed to reduce but did not destroy potency. Much of this original work was carried out by Chase and Siltzbach who removed nucleoprotein by 2 M sodium chloride, apparently without reducing potency, and they found that the discarded nucleoprotein fraction was not active.

Exposure to sodium hydroxide at low concentrations appeared to reduce activity somewhat. Proteolytic enzymes, nucleases, hyaluronidase and neuraminidase appeared to have little effect in diminishing the granuloma-causing capacity of the reagent. Electron microscopy and acid phosphatases have been used to argue that the active component may be located in the cell membrane.

A final attempt by Chase and Siltzbach to concentrate the active component of Kveim reagent resulted in a validated suspension that was extracted with alcohol, ether and water, dispersed by sonication, and digested with pepsin, the remaining solid particles, amounting to about 90 percent of the initial dry weight, being suspended in phenolized buffer. This new suspension, designated type III, was found to produce granulomatous reactions in parallel tests with the original type I suspension in reactive sarcoidosis patients. Based on the much smaller weight of tissue needed to cause a reaction, the active component within this type III appeared to have been concentrated 9-fold (Siltzbach 1967).

Kveim reagents are known to retain activity after prolonged storage, even several years at temperatures around 4°C (Siltzbach and Ehrlich 1954). Although some reagents have retained their activity after storage for more than a decade, other batches of Kveim reagent have lost activity after just a few weeks of storage in similar conditions (Nelson and Schwimmer 1957).

The granuloma-producing potency of a sarcoid tissue correlated poorly with the clinical features of the patient who provided it, and tissue from patients who have no discernible reaction to Kveim reagent were themselves used to prepare Kveim of high diagnostic quality. When using lymph nodes as a source of material, some studies have indicated that the activity of the Kveim reagent increased as the nodes diminished in size. A study of tested suspensions from lymph nodes of 16 sarcoidosis patients found that the most potent were obtained from patients who responded weakly to a Kveim test (Putkonen 1964). In addition, a suspension prepared from a granulomatous papule at a previous test site was shown to produce a similar, though smaller, reaction.

Reactions to simultaneous tests with suspensions prepared from sarcoid spleen and from mediastinal lymph nodes indicated that reactions to the spleen suspension may have been weaker than those to lymph-node suspension. It was also felt that the active component was perhaps present in greater quantity in chronic compared to recent active lesions.

Suspensions made in a similar manner from normal tissues have usually resulted in negative reactions, but a minority of non-sarcoidosis tissues have been shown to produce Kveim-like reactions after injection into patients with sarcoidosis (Nelson 1949). The mechanisms for this, as with for the Kveim reaction itself, are not fully understood.

HISTOLOGY OF THE KVEIM REACTION

See Figs 16.1–16.3.

A typical diagnostic reaction in a patient with sarcoidosis consists of well-formed tuberculoid collections of epithelioid cells with or without giant cells and with limited lymphocytic infiltration which develops within 14 days. This initial appearance is not fully characteristic of the final result.

Rogers and Haserick (1954) described the evolution of the reaction in serial biopsies of reacting and non-reacting subjects. In the non-reactors, the test sites showed only slight perivascular infiltration with lymphocytes in the early stage. At 14 days there was a small collection of lymphocytes with a few small multinucleated cells, and there was virtually normal skin at 42 days.

In those who reacted to the Kveim, one patient developed an intense reaction with some central necrosis. The early changes at 3 days were similar to those in the non-reactors. However, by 6 days, there was a dense perivascular infiltration containing large pale-staining histiocytes, small deeply staining mononuclear cells, and some atypical pleomorphic cells. After 10 days, some central collagen degeneration with a few foci of necrosis was seen, the affected area being infiltrated with polymorphonuclear leukocytes, and surrounded by mononuclear leukocytes and histiocytes and pleomorphic cells.

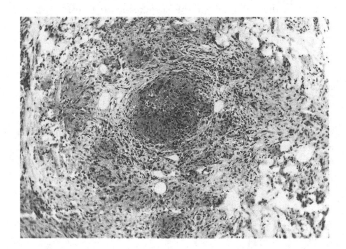

Figure 16.1   Histology of a Kveim test site (90 × magnification), 5 weeks after an intracutaneous injection of a test suspension.

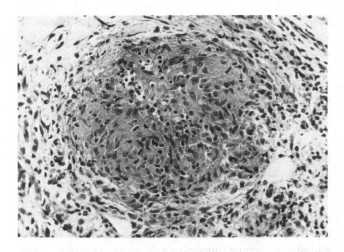

Figure 16.2   Histology of a Kveim test site (120 × magnification), 5 weeks after an intracutaneous injection of a test suspension.

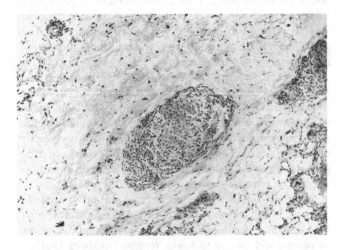

Figure 16.3   Biopsy site of Kveim reaction (90 × magnification), showing a single granuloma with minimal acceptability for a positive Kveim reaction.

At 13 days in patients who reacted to Kveim, the atypical cells had diminished and lymphocytes increased in number. Small collections of epithelioid cells, surrounded by lymphocytes, were recognizable near vessels, together with a few giant cells of Langerhans type. At 16 days, epithelioid cell tubercles were more evident, and lymphocytes less numerous. These changes had progressed at 25 days to large aggregations of epithelioid cells with scanty peripheral lymphocytes, and at 42 days to almost confluent epithelioid cell tubercles. By this time, the central necrotic area was well-defined and acellular.

Siltzbach studied the histology of developing Kveim reactions by serial injections at intervals of 1–4 weeks (Siltzbach 1961). At one week, the reaction consisted of mononuclear cells with small numbers of neutrophils, eosinophils and plasma cells. During subsequent weeks, the neutrophils, eosinophils and plasma cells diminished in numbers and epithelioid cells appeared. Electron microscopy of granulomatous Kveim test sites showed an ultrastructure generally similar to that of sarcoid granulomas.

IMMUNOLOGY OF THE KVEIM REACTION

The immunology of the Kveim reaction is somewhat similar to that of a sarcoid granuloma which shows a predominantly CD4+ T-cell infiltrate throughout with a scattering of CD 8+ T-cells at the periphery.

Studies have implicated a CD4+ T-cell infiltrate which characterizes the diagnostic local epitheliod intradermal granulomas as being oligoclonal. Polymerase chhain reaction (PCR) analysis of the T-cell receptor (TCR) V beta repertoire from Kveim reaction sites demonstrates this oligoclonal pattern of V beta gene expression with limited junctional variability in the hypervariable section of the TCR (Klein et al. 1995). This suggests that the Kveim reaction occurs as a direct result of T-cell infiltration into the site of injection in response to a small number of antigens within the material.

In direct in-vitro tests, a number of groups found that Kveim test suspensions inhibited migration of leukocytes from patients with sarcoidosis (Brostoff and Walker 1971), a finding that has since been questioned by others (e.g. Becker et al. 1972). Tests for production of leukocyte migration inhibition factor by cells stimulated with Kveim reagent have given similarly variable results. Kveim test suspensions have also been shown to inhibit leukocyte migration in a proportion of patients with Crohn's disease (Brostoff and Walker 1971).

Attempts to demonstrate antibodies against a component or components of Kveim have been reported in the literature. A study investigating the sera of 75 patients with biopsy-confirmed sarcoidosis and of 90 control subjects showed that, by using the passive hemagglutination method, the sarcoidosis subjects had a higher range of total antibody titers than the controls (Favez and Leuenberger 1972). A method to induce antibodies in rabbits by repeatedly injecting Kveim reagent intravenously resulted in sera from the infected animals showing up to three bands of protein precipitation against Kveim reagent, the identities of which were not confirmed (Bergmann et al. 1979).

There has so far been limited further effort to investigate Kveim reagent for these antigens with the notable exception of mycobacterial catalase–peroxidase (mKatG), a mycobacterial protein that has been identified from sarcoidosis tissue extracts treated in a manner similar to the preparation of Kveim reagent (Song et al. 2005). Tissue antigens were detected with immunoglobulin (Ig)G or F(ab′) 2 fragments from sarcoidosis sera in 9 of 12 sarcoidosis tissues but in only 3 of 22 control tissues; and matrix-assisted laser desorption/ionization time-of-flight mass spectrometry was used to identify mKatG as one of these antigens. Immunoblotting with anti-mKatG monoclonal antibodies and the detection of IgG antibodies to recombinant mKatG were used to confirm the presence mKatG in a number of sarcoidosis serum specimens.

Higher frequencies of mKatG-reactive, IFN-γ-expressing T-cells have been found in the peripheral blood of sarcoidosis patients compared with healthy controls in phenotypically diverse patient groups from North America and Sweden (Chen et al. 2008). Those sarcoidosis patients who displayed T-cell responses to mKatG showed preferential accumulation of mKatG-reactive CD4+ Th1 cells in the lung, indicating a compartmentalized response. This work indicates that mycobacterial antigens may have a role to play in some cases of sarcoidosis, but there has been limited further work to identify other antigens within Kveim reagent.

USE OF THE KVEIM REAGENT AS A DIAGNOSTIC TOOL

Although it is now not used in the diagnosis of sarcoidosis, the Kveim test enjoyed wisdespread use up until the 1980s when the concerns about transmission of prion diseases led to its gradual withdrawal. During several decades of use a number of clinical research studies helped to carefully define its use in patients with sarcoidosis. The generally accepted figures are that properly validated Kveim showed up to 80 percent sensitivity and almost 100 percent specificity when used in the diagnosis of sarcoidosis.

Historically, 1 mL disposable syringes with short-shank needles were used to allow passage of the Kveim reagent into the skin. The injection was usually made intracutaneously into the ulnar side of the upper part of the forearm, so that any residual scar remained inconspicuous. The result was a raised papule with a *peau d'orange* appearance. The epidermis at the test site was then marked with a tattoo using Gunter–Wagner Pelikan ink to allow ease of serial inspection and subsequent biopsy.

An area of induration about 3–4 mm in diameter with some surrounding erythema usually developed in the day or two after the injection and was thought non-specific and attributable to inflammatory response to trauma and to a particulate suspension. In Kveim reactive subjects, this erythema was slowly replaced, usually during the second week, by an area of palpable induration which developed into a dusky red papule and attained a diameter of up to 5 mm by 14 days. Thereafter, it persisted and often increased in size for a time up to 8 weeks. It was usually excised for biopsy at 4–6 weeks for histological confirmation of a sarcoid-like granuloma. Occasionally, a visible and palpable reaction persisted as long as the sarcoidosis remained active.

Rarely, the appearance of a papule at the test site was delayed. Records show a number of cases of the development of reaction papules at the site of injection several years after a Kveim test, these late reactions usually developing during a resurgence of activity of sarcoidosis. Ulceration of the site was relatively rare, although papules showed crusting, and a few underwent central softening. The size of reaction papules has been investigated for possible relationships with histology and to duration of sarcoidosis, but with no conclusive results.

The effect of systemic as well as intralesional corticosteroids on the response to Kveim reagent has also been much studied. The injection of 5 mg hydrocortisone together with the test suspension was found to inhibit the Kveim reaction in some cases (Rogers and Haserick 1954). Patients with active sarcoidosis on treatment with corticosteroids but showing a poor treatment response were shown to still develop granulomatous responses to Kveim tests. However, larger studies on patients at various stages of disease found that daily doses of regular oral prednisolone had an inhibitory effect on the reaction (Siltzbach and Waraich 1969).

Although early clinicians took the delayed appearance of a reaction papule as indicating a positive test, later observers concluded that the frequency of unspecific reactions necessitated a biopsy confirmation. Biopsy was usually performed 4–6 weeks after the injection in order to allow sufficient time for even the most delayed reactions to take place. A small amount (0.15 mL) of 1% procaine with adrenaline was injected to minimize capillary oozing, and a 3–4 mm diameter skin biopsy was taken from the center of the reaction.

Interpretation of the test required analysis of representative serial sections by an experienced observer who was usually kept blind to the clinical features. Microscopically, the essential feature of a response supporting a diagnosis of sarcoidosis was the presence of one or more granulomas composed principally of epithelioid cells, but a fairly wide range of histological patterns was acceptable as positive reactions in the interpretation of the Kveim result. In fact, all decisions on response were subject to a certain amount of observer variation. Further staining occurred to examine by polarized light for birefringent foreign-body material in such reactions and to rule out the presence of any active infectious agent.

In general, the majority of patients reacted within two years of the onset of sarcoidosis with the proportion falling with increasing duration of disease. Correspondingly, up to 90 percent of those with radiographic evidence of hilar lymph node enlargement reacted; while of those with pulmonary infiltration only, fewer than half reacted. The details of 2532 patients with pulmonary sarcodiosis and 805 with extrathoracic lesions only are shown in Tables 16.1 and 16.2.

When patients were retested, after periods up to one year, 84 percent still reacted; after 1–3 years, 68 percent; after 3–5 years, 50 percent; and after longer periods up to l5 years, 38 percent still reacted to Kveim reagent (Siltzbach 1961).

Table 16.1   Results of Kveim reactivity in patients with pulmonary sarcoidosis.

Radiological form of disease	Total tested	Positive	Equivocal	Negative
BHL with EN or arthropathy (Löfgren's)	461	395 (86%)	17 (4%)	49 (10%)
BHL only (stage 1)	957	691 (72%)	51 (5%)	215 (22%)
BHL with pulmonary infiltrates (stage 2)	450	329 (73%)	16 (4%)	105 (23%)
Pulmonary infiltrates (stage 3)	664	225 (34%)	46 (7%)	391 (59%)
Totals	2532	1640 (65%)	132 (5%)	760 (30%)

Table 16.2 Results of Kveim reactivity in patients with extrathoracic sarcoidosis only.

Organ involvement	Total tested	Positive	Equivocal	Negative
Uveitis	127	25 (20%)	7 (6%)	95 (74%)
EN	300	65 (22%)	14 (5%)	221 (73%)
Liver or spleen	41	17 (41%)	4 (10%)	20 (49%)
Lymph node	88	36 (41%)	7 (8%)	45 (51%)
Skin (excluding EN)	130	54 (42%)	5 (4%)	71 (54%)
Nerve	33	11 (33%)	1 (3%)	21 (64%)
Cardiac	16	3 (19%)	1 (6%)	12 (75%)
Other	70	12 (17%)	4 (6%)	54 (77%)
Totals	805	223 (28%)	43 (5%)	539 (67%)

MYCOBACTERIAL INFECTION AND BCG VACCINATION

Although Kveim suspensions that have been validated for their selectivity for sarcoidosis caused few reactions in patients with tuberculosis, some of the rejected Kveim suspensions were reported to cause granulomatous reactions in a higher proportion of tuberculosis patients than of other subjects. A study specifically looking at this phenomenon reported a significant difference in this respect between two suspensions prepared at different times from the cervical lymph nodes of the same patient with sarcoidosis (Israel et al. 1958). The first suspension of Kveim reagent produced granulomatous nodules in 12 of 57 tests in 28 patients with sarcoidosis and in 14 of 27 tests in 33 patients with tuberculosis. Two years later, a second suspension prepared from cervical nodes from the same patient gave well-defined granulomatous reactions in 13 of 46 patients with sarcoidosis but in none of 29 with tuberculosis. Such variable responses have been confirmed by other research groups, but examples of Kveim reagent that produced a response in patients with TB infection were discarded during validation and hence not used for clinical diagnosis.

A number of studies have investigated the effect of prior BCG vaccination on Kveim responses. The largest study to date involved 13 598 individuals who had been vaccinated with BCG as part of a large UK Medical Research Council-funded study into the protective effects of vaccination against tuberculosis (Hart et al. 1964). Fifty-eight of the individuals remained persistently tuberculin-negative during 8–10 years of close observation. Of these, 19 were available for further study, and were revaccinated; 7 converted and 12 failed to convert. Of the final group of 12 who still remained persistently negative, all were given Kveim injections using spleen J (a well-validated form of reagent) and 10 were found to have clinical evidence of a Kveim reaction, 7 of whom were categorized as positive by histology after analysis by a blinded pathologist. None of these 12 non-convertors to BCG had any medical history or clinical evidence suggesting previous sarcoidosis.

Explanations of this effect include the hypothesis that serial BCG vaccinations are responsible for priming the adaptive immune system to respond to Kveim reagent with the possibility that there is a cross-reactive antigen present in both BCG and Kveim. The argument against this theory is that individuals with two BCG vaccinations are not shown to have a higher incidence of Kveim reactivity than those vaccinated only once.

The 12 individuals in the study also showed a decreased response to an intradermal injection of *Candida* antigen, so an alternative explanation may be that the non-conversion to tuberculin after BCG vaccination was due to an underlying abnormality in the immune system associated with an increased reactivity to Kveim reagent. Smaller studies investigating this phenomonen have proved inconclusive.

THE KVEIM REACTION IN OTHER DISEASES

Apart from responses in patients with mycobacterial disease, the Kveim reagent has been investigated in a number of other diseases. The Mitsuda lepromin test in leprosy is analogous to the Kveim test in that both involve intradermal injection of diseased tissue. However, the Mitsuda test for leprosy does not reliably distinguish between diseased and healthy individuals as well as the Kveim reagent does for sarcoidosis.

Despite some studies showing significantly positive Kveim reactions in subgroups of patients with leprosy from China and Japan, the majority of investigations do not show that patients with leprosy are more likely to have a granulomatous reaction to Kveim reagent (Pearson et al. 1969). The weakly positive reactions in these two ethnic groups remain unexplained. There is little information about the reactivity of patients with sarcoidosis to lepromatin.

A number of investigations of Kveim reagent have been carried out in patients with Crohn's disease with the attempt to find a causal link with the two granulomatous diseases. One study showed that Kveim reactions reported as histologically positive were present in 38 of 74 patients (51 percent) with diagnosed Crohn's disease (Mitchell et al. 1970). However, this phenomenon appears restricted to certain preparations of Kveim material.

Patients with chronic brucellosis have an increased appearance of granulomas, particularly in the liver. A study of Kveim injections into 32 patients with chronic brucellosis showed a positive reactivity in 7; and in 11 who had serological evidence of brucellosis, 1 had a positive Kveim test and 4 had an equivocal result (Williams 1974). None of the patients had any clinical or radiological evidence of sarcoidosis.

CONCLUSION

The Kveim reaction is likely to be due to a limited number of protein (or perhaps lipoprotein) antigenic targets that induce an influx of CD4+ T-cells at the site of injection in sarcoidosis patients and the subsequent formation of the pathognomonic granulomas seen in disease. The delay in the reaction, which may occur after several weeks, may be related to the general systemic anergy seen in sarcoidosis, which in turn may be due to a disorder in the antigen processing pathway. However, unlike an allergic response or the immune response to other injections such as tuberculin in patients with tuberculosis, Kveim reactivity tends to diminish over time as the activity of sarcoidosis decreases.

Despite once being a sensitive and highly specific test for disease, the Kveim reagent is no longer used for diagnosis of disease. The clinical knowledge that has been built up over time remains inconclusive, and the lack of ability for in-vivo testing is a barrier to further such studies. However, recent advances in molecular biology, immunology and comparative proteomics allow us to further investigate the pathogenesis of disease using in-vitro models of sarcodiosis. Although the test itself may seem outdated, a better understanding of the immunopathology of the Kveim reaction may help our understanding of the disease itself and point towards newer immunology-based approaches for diagnosis of sarcoidosis.

REFERENCES

Becker FW, Krull P, Deicher H, Kalden JR (1972). Leucocyte-migration test in sarcoidosis. *Lancet* 1: 120–3.

Bergmann KC, Kirschnick AM, Djuric B (1979). Demonstration of an antigenic component in Kveim antigen. *Allergol Immunopathol* (Madr) 7: 249–52.

Brostoff J, Walker JG (1971). Leucocyte migration inhibition with Kveim antigen in Crohn's disease. *Clin Exp Immunol* 9: 707–11.

Chase MW (1961). The preparation and standardization of Kveim testing antigen. *Am Rev Respir Dis* 84(5 Pt 2): 86–8.

Chen ES, Wahlstrom J, Song Z et al. (2008). T-cell responses to mycobacterial catalase–peroxidase profile a pathogenic antigen in systemic sarcoidosis. *J Immunol* 181: 8784–96.

Danbolt N (1948). On the antigenic properties of tissue suspensions prepared from Boeck's sarcoid. *Acta Derm Venereol* 28: 151–7.

Danbolt N (1951a). On the skin test with sarcoid tissue suspension (Kveim's reaction). *Acta Derm Venereol* 31: 184–93.

Danbolt N (1951b). Progressive papule caused by injection of sarcoid tissue suspension (Kveim's test) in a patient with Boeck's sarcoid. *Acta Derm Venereol* 31: 446–8.

Favez G, Leuenberger P (1972). [Circulating antibodies directed against a constituent of lymphatic origin demonstrated during active sarcoidosis]. *Schweiz Med Wochenschr* 102: 129–31.

Hart PD, Mitchell DN, Sutherland I (1964). Associations between Kveim test results, previous BCG vaccination, and tuberculin sensitivity in healthy young adults. *Br Med J* 1: 795–804.

Israel HL, Sones M, Beerman H, Pastras T (1958). A further study of the Kveim reaction in sarcoidosis and tuberculosis. *New Engl J Med* 259: 365–9.

Klein JT, Horn TD, Forman JD et al. (1995). Selection of oligoclonal V beta-specific T-cells in the intradermal response to Kveim–Siltzbach reagent in individuals with sarcoidosis. *J Immunol* 154: 1450–60.

Kveim A (1948). Some remarks on the aetiology of Boeck's sarcoid. *Acta Derm Venereol* 28: 169.

Mitchell DN, Dyer NC, Cannon P et al. (1970). The Kveim test in Crohn's disease. *Postgrad Med J* 46: 491–4.

Mitchell DN, Sutherland I, Bradstreet CM, Dighero MW (1976). Validation and standardization of Kveim test suspensions prepared from two human sarcoid spleens. *J Clin Pathol* 29: 203–10.

Nelson CT (1949). Kveim reaction in sarcoidosis. *Arch Derm Syphilol* 60: 377–89.

Nelson CT, Schwimmer B (1957). The specificity of the Kveim reaction. *J Invest Dermatol* 28: 55–60; discussion, 60–1.

Pearson JM, Pettit JH, Siltzbach LE et al. (1969). The Kveim test in lepromatous and tuberculoid leprosy. *Int J Lepr Other Mycobact Dis* 37: 372–81.

Putkonen T (1964). Source of potent Kveim antigen. *Acta Med Scand Suppl* 425: 83–5.

Rogers FJ, Haserick JR (1954). Sarcoidosis and the Kveim reaction. *J Invest Dermatol* 23: 389–406.

Siltzbach LE (1961). The Kveim test in sarcoidosis: a study of 750 patients. *J Am Med Assoc* 178: 476–82.

Siltzbach LE (1967). [Clinical and experimental aspects of the Kveim test in sarcoidosis]. *Poumon Coeur* 23: 499–527.

Siltzbach LE, Ehrlich JC (1954). The Nickerson–Kveim reaction in sarcoidosis. *Am J Med* 16: 790–803.

Siltzbach LE, Waraich BA (1969). Effects of corticosteroid therapy on Kveim reactivity in sarcoidosis. *Am Rev Respir Dis* 99: 614–16.

Song Z, Marzilli L, Greenlee BM et al. (2005). Mycobacterial catalase–peroxidase is a tissue antigen and target of the adaptive immune response in systemic sarcoidosis. *J Exp Med* 201: 755–67.

Williams E (1974). Chronic brucellosis [letter]. *Br Med J* 2: 274.

17

Biochemical investigations

MICHAEL W KEMP, JACQUELINE DONOVAN AND JAMES HOOPER

INTRODUCTION

Critical evaluation of a biochemical investigation into a disease process requires answers to four questions:

- Do patients with the condition have different test results compared with normal controls?
- Do patients with specified test results have a higher probability of the condition compared with patients with other results for the test?
- Among patients having the same pre-test probability (i.e. the same clinical presentation), does the test distinguish those who have the condition from those who do not?
- Do patients who have the test performed have better outcomes compared with those who do not?

The answers to these questions provide information about the diagnostic sensitivity, specificity, positive and negative predictive values, and prognosis or risk stratification (Christenson 2007).

The ATS statement on sarcoidosis (1999), and the recent guideline from the British Thoracic Society on the diagnosis and treatment of interstitial lung disease (Wells and Hirani 2008), have indicated a role for biochemical investigations in the initial assessment and investigation of patients with sarcoidosis, but not in making the diagnosis. A suitably sensitive and specific biochemical marker for use in diagnosis is still to be identified.

SERUM ANGIOTENSIN-CONVERTING ENZYME (ACE)

Angiotensin-converting enzyme is a membrane-bound glycoprotein, expressed by the epithelial cells of many tissues, but is most abundant on the luminal surface of the vascular endothelium (Shen *et al.* 2008). Pulmonary epithelium has a higher ACE activity than that of other organs (Bader and Ganten 2008). In patients with sarcoidosis, the enzyme is also produced by epithelioid cells of the sarcoid granuloma, alveolar macrophages, and monocytes from peripheral blood. ACE activity in sarcoid lymph nodes is much higher than in lymph nodes from normal individuals (Allen *et al.* 1986). The enzyme is a zinc-dependent dipeptidyl carboxypeptidase, and requires the presence of chloride ions for activity.

The classical physiological role for ACE is to cleave a C-terminal histidyl-leucine dipeptide from the decapeptide angiotensin I to form the octapeptide angiotensin II, which is a potent vasopressor agent. However, ACE does not exhibit substrate specificity for angiotensin I alone, and will remove C-terminal dipeptides from a variety of peptides, including chemotactic peptide (a tripeptide), bradykinin (a nonapeptide), and neurotensin (a tridecapeptide). Large or folded molecules are not cleaved by ACE. The variety of substrates, and ubiquitous tissue distribution, suggest that ACE may play a role in physiological and pathological processes, apart from control of blood pressure and maintenance of electrolyte balance (Shen *et al.* 2008). ACE is found in many species, vertebrates and invertebrates, often as close sequence homologs to the human enzyme, and with very similar biochemical properties, which implies that ACE is highly evolutionarily conserved. Many organisms with the enzyme lack an identifiable renin–angiotensin system, supporting the existence of a range of other biological functions for ACE (Coates 2003).

Serum ACE in diagnosis

The first report of a relatively high activity of ACE in the blood of patients with active sarcoidosis was a chance observation in a study of the incidence of hypotension in patients with chronic lung disease. Serum ACE activity was elevated, when compared to controls, in 15 of a group of 17 patients with active sarcoidosis, diagnosed by chest X-ray, and tissue biopsy showing the presence of non-caseating granulomas, in the absence of tuberculosis, fungal infection or cancer (Liebermann 1975).

The initial optimism that serum ACE could be used as a diagnostic marker has not been realized; in many published series fewer than 50 percent of patients with sarcoidosis actually have elevated serum ACE activity (Studdy *et al.* 1980). Other studies have shown that elevations in ACE activity are not specific for sarcoidosis. Unfortunately elevated serum ACE activity has been reported in diseases that need to be excluded when making a diagnosis of sarcoidosis, such as tuberculosis, atypical mycobacterial infections and lymphoma (Studdy and Bird 1989). Other conditions in which elevations of serum ACE activity have been reported in some patients include alcoholic liver disease, hyperthyroidism, berylliosis, asbestosis and silicosis.

The poor specificity means that serum ACE is of limited use as a diagnostic tool. If there is good clinical or radiographic evidence for a diagnosis of sarcoidosis, then a raised serum ACE provides good supporting evidence, but a normal serum ACE does not exclude a diagnosis of sarcoidosis.

Serum ACE and disease monitoring

Initial evidence suggested that serum ACE could be used to monitor disease progression and steroid therapy. Initiation of prednisone therapy was shown to lead to a fall in serum ACE activity within 2 weeks (Liebermann 1975). In patients with an elevated serum ACE activity at diagnosis, disease remission, either spontaneously or as a result of steroid therapy, is mirrored by a fall in serum enzyme activity. Conversely, relapse is characterized by increasing serum ACE activity (Studdy and Bird 1989). The highest serum ACE activities are found in patients with widespread chronic active disease.

Early studies showed a good correlation between serum ACE activity and serial chest X-ray monitoring, with a weak correlation with radioisotope gallium lung scanning, and bronchiolar lavage cellular profiles. Other groups have not found any correlation between serum ACE activity and radiographic stage at initial diagnosis in patients with histologically confirmed sarcoidosis (Shorr *et al.* 1997). Current guidelines do not support the use of these methods of monitoring disease progression (high-resolution computed tomography and pulmonary function testing are now the methods of choice), and serum ACE is not considered to be of value in disease monitoring (Wells and Hirani 2008).

Measurement of serum ACE activity

Early assays for serum ACE relied on the use of the natural enzyme substrate, angiotensin I. These procedures were technically demanding, so synthetic substrates, such as hippuryl histidyl leucine, were developed (Friedland and Silverstein 1976). Hippuryl histidyl leucine is hydrolyzed to hippurate and the dipeptide histidyl leucine in a reaction catalyzed by ACE. Histidyl leucine then reacts with o-phthaldialdehyde to form a product that can be measured spectrofluorimetrically. This method was relatively simple and rapid to perform, but not easy to automate.

Current methods are almost exclusively based on the hydrolysis of furylacryloylphenylalanylglycylglycine to glycylglycine and furylacryloylphenylalanine (Holmquist *et al.* 1979). The reaction is catalyzed by ACE, and can be monitored spectrophotometrically. Commercially available kits have been developed and adapted for use on many automated analyzers. However, assessment of assay quality between laboratories in the United Kingdom has shown poor analytical performance, with many different reference ranges, leading to widely disparate clinical classification of external quality assessment samples, despite the use of the same assay substrate by most laboratories (Muller 2002).

Cerebrospinal fluid ACE in neurosarcoidosis

ACE activity can be detected in cerebrospinal fluid (CSF) from patients with neurosarcoidosis and from control subjects. Consistently elevated CSF ACE activity from neurosarcoid patients is yet to be demonstrated. There is little evidence that CSF ACE is derived from granulomas in the central nervous system in patients with neurosarcoid; indeed the likely sources of higher ACE activity in these patients are macrophages and lymphocytes in the CSF. The consensus opinion now is that measurement of CSF ACE is of little diagnostic use in the investigation of patients with neurosarcoidosis (Kellinghaus *et al.* 2004).

The ACE gene

The human ACE gene maps to chromosome 17q23, and is composed of 21 kilobases. Two isoforms of ACE exist in humans, one expressed in somatic tissues and one in germinal cells of the testes. Somatic ACE (sACE) is composed of 1306 amino acid residues with two active sites, and germinal ACE (gACE) has 732 residues, and one active site (Coates 2003).

The only well-documented allelic variant of ACE is the insertion/deletion (I/D) polymorphism in intron 16 of the ACE gene. Alleles can be either I or D, resulting in three possible genotypes, II, DD or ID. The frequency of the genotypes shows considerable variation among racial groups. The genotype also influences serum ACE activity, with DD individuals having almost twice the activity of II individuals, and ID individuals showing values somewhere between the other two genotypes (Sharma *et al.* 1997). The genetic balance of the reference group used to derive a reference range will obviously affect the values obtained, which may go some way towards explaining variations in reference ranges between laboratories. The use of genotype-specific reference ranges might well improve the poor sensitivity of serum ACE assays. However, this would require all patients to be genotyped as a matter of routine, which would be beyond the budget and

SERUM PROTEINS

Since a continuing hyperimmune response to an unknown agent at sites of disease activity is characteristic of sarcoidosis, it was thought that inflammatory markers might be of value in the monitoring of disease activity. Activation of monocyte–macrophages leads to the release of cytokines, such as tumor necrosis factor and interleukins 1 and 6, which stimulate hepatic synthesis and release of acute-phase proteins such as C-reactive protein (CRP) and serum amyloid A (SAA). However, a number of studies have shown that measurement of these proteins is of no value in the diagnosis of sarcoidosis, or in monitoring disease progression (Rothkrantz-Kos et al. 2003).

Electrophoresis of serum proteins shows a polyclonal gammopathy in about 50 percent of patients with untreated sarcoidosis (Nunes et al. 2007), and about 80 percent have an increase in the serum concentration of at least one individual immunoglobulin. Immunoglobulin G was reported to be elevated in 56 percent of white British patients, followed by IgA in 27 percent, and IgM in 13 percent. No correlation could be demonstrated between the stage of sarcoidosis, or the organs affected, and the immunoglobulin pattern or concentrations (Studdy et al. 1980).

Patients with sarcoidosis have an increased risk for the development of lymphoproliferative disorders, most commonly Hodgkin's disease or non-Hodgkin's lymphoma. This may be due to the tissue inflammatory response causing an increased chance of lymphocytes undergoing mutation and malignant transformation (Brincker 1995). The extended life of B-lymphocytes and plasma cells in patients with sarcoidosis may also increase the chance of malignant transformation. A rare but significant association between sarcoidosis and multiple myeloma has been described (Sen et al. 2002), and care must be taken to exclude the presence of a monoclonal gammopathy when increased concentrations of serum immunoglobulins are detected.

Rarely, hypogammaglobulinemia may be found in patients with sarcoidosis. Sarcoidosis in association with common variable immunodeficiency (CVID) has been demonstrated in a small number of patients, usually presenting with moderate pulmonary involvement, lymphadenopathy and hepatosplenomegaly. Sarcoid-like non-caseating granulomas appear frequently in patients with CVID, and may be found in lymphoid tissues, solid organs and skin. The diagnosis of sarcoidosis has been confirmed in only a few of these patients. Any patient with sarcoidosis presenting with hypogammaglobulinemia should be investigated further (Sutor and Fabel 2000).

LIVER FUNCTION TESTS

Liver function tests (LFTs) should be undertaken as part of the initial assessment of patients with sarcoidosis. Granulomas may be found in up to 80 percent of liver biopsy samples from patients with sarcoidosis, and mild abnormalities of LFTs are common, usually in the form of elevations of serum aminotransferase and alkaline phosphatase activities, and may not require any intervention (American Thoracic Society 1999). Granulomas are usually small, and found in the portal spaces. Rarely, significant hepatic complications may occur, including portal hypertension, cholestasis, or hepatic failure (Malnick et al. 2008).

SERUM AND URINE CALCIUM

Calcium metabolism

The maintenance of calcium homeostasis depends on the balance between absorption from the gut, bone turnover, urinary excretion, and protein binding. Hormonal regulation of these procedures is controlled by the secretion of vitamin D and parathyroid hormone, and influenced by thyroid and sex hormones. Vitamin D is hydroxylated initially in the liver to form 25-hydroxycholecalciferol, which is used by the body as a storage form of the vitamin. Further hydroxylation in the kidney, under the influence of the enzyme 1-α-hydroxylase, leads to the formation of 1,25-dihydroxycholecalciferol (calcitriol), which is biologically active. The rising concentration of calcitriol in renal tubular cells causes down-regulation of 1-α-hydroxylase, and up-regulation of 25-hydroxycholecalciferol 24-hydroxylase, leading to the formation of 24,25-hydroxycholecalciferol, which is biologically inactive. The sarcoid alveolar macrophage also possesses 1-α-hydroxylase activity, but the feedback mechanisms are not present (Conron et al. 2000).

The disordered calcium homeostasis seen in sarcoidosis is similar to that seen in vitamin D intoxication (Sharma 1996). Calcitriol has immunoregulatory activity, and has been shown to down-regulate the activation and proliferation of lymphocytes, probably by inhibiting interleukin-2 and interferon-γ activity, which are necessary to produce a granulomatous response. It is possible that the production of calcitriol by the sarcoid alveolar macrophage is an adaptive response to down-regulate T-cell activity at the sites of sarcoid granuloma formation (Conron et al. 2000).

Measurement of serum calcium: ionized or corrected?

Approximately 45 percent of the total calcium in plasma exists as free calcium ions, 5 percent is complexed with ions such as citrate or phosphate, and the remaining 50 percent of the total is bound to albumin. The three forms are in equilibrium, but only ionized calcium is biologically active.

Measurement of ionized calcium is technically difficult, and stringent precautions must be observed when collecting and processing samples to minimize pre-analytical errors (Boink et al. 1991). Most clinical laboratories report a serum calcium value corrected for the serum albumin concentration, using an equation derived by determining the linear regression relationship of calcium on albumin concentration in normal individuals. A typical equation is as follows:

corrected [Ca] (mmol/L)

$$= \text{total [Ca] (mmol/L)} + 0.02 \, (40 - [\text{albumin}] \, (\text{g/L}).$$

Equations such as this have entered into common use and are still being used, despite having been produced in excess of 20 years ago.

The relationship between serum calcium and albumin may be influenced by the analytical methods used to measure the two parameters. It would be good practice for each laboratory to derive its own linear regression equation for calcium on albumin, and not use published data (James *et al.* 2008).

Hypercalcemia

Hypercalcemia is present in approximately 11 percent of patients with sarcoidosis (Sharma 2000). There is no evidence that race, sex, age, occupation or season influence its development. Hypercalcemia is also transient in occurrence, may fluctuate, and may need to be monitored over a long period to get a true picture of its severity.

Although there are no nationally or internationally agreed guidelines for the treatment of hypercalcemia in sarcoidosis, a patient with a serum calcium concentration greater than 3.00 mmol/L, or renal complications in the presence of a lesser degree of hypercalcemia, requires treatment (Conron *et al.* 2000). If the serum calcium is in excess of 3.50 mmol/L, then emergency treatment may be required, by rehydration, administration of a loop diuretic to encourage urinary calcium excretion, and initiation of corticosteroid therapy.

Hypercalciuria

The mechanism of hypercalciuria in sarcoidosis is not fully understood, but is probably primarily due to increased calcium absorption from the gut, together with some bone resorption. The renal tubular maximum reabsorptive rate for calcium is not increased (Sharma 2000).

The prevalence of hypercalciuria in untreated patients with sarcoidosis is 40–60 percent, depending on the published series. Approximately 10 percent of patients may develop renal calculi. Patients may also develop nephrocalcinosis if either hypercalcemia or hypercalciuria is longstanding; nephrocalcinosis probably accounts for about half of the cases of renal impairment in patients with sarcoidosis (Conron *et al.* 2000). Patients with hypercalcemia usually have hypercalciuria; however not all patients with hypercalciuria have hypercalcemia (Studdy *et al.* 1980).

Management of hypercalciuria requires the risk of urinary stone formation to be kept to a minimum, by encouraging the patient to drink sufficient fluids to maintain a high urine output (Conron *et al.* 2000). Limiting dietary calcium intake, and minimizing exposure to sunlight, may also be useful. Corticosteroid therapy also reduces hypercalciuria, by inhibiting calcitriol synthesis. If the patient develops severe side-effects of corticosteroid therapy, then chloroquine or hydroxychloroquine can be used, both of which inhibit 1-α-hydroxylation in the kidney, thereby lowering the plasma calcitriol and calcium concentrations, and reducing urinary calcium excretion (Sharma 2000). The antifungal agent ketoconazole, which inhibits the cytochrome P450-linked enzyme systems involved in steroid synthesis, also inhibits 1-α-hydroxylase, and lowers plasma calcitriol and calcium concentrations, and can be used to treat hypercalcemia and hypercalciuria (Conron *et al.* 2000).

POTENTIAL SEROLOGICAL MARKERS FOR SARCOIDOSIS

It is impossible to predict the likely clinical course for patients with sarcoidosis, prompting research into biomarkers that may be of value in predicting outcome.

Serum enzymes are frequently of value in the diagnosis and management of disease, with ACE being of limited value in sarcoidosis. Lysozyme was reported to be of value, but has been shown to lack specificity and sensitivity (Turton *et al.* 1979). Chitotriosidase activity, produced by activated macrophages, has been reported to be elevated in patients with sarcoidosis, and initial studies have shown correlation with ACE activity in serum, radiological staging, and quantitative high-resonance CT score (Bargagli *et al.* 2008).

The inflammatory process seen in patients with sarcoidosis leads to the production of a number of cytokines, such as interleukin-2 (IL-2). Production of IL-2 causes T-cell activation; activated T-cells release a soluble form of the IL-2 receptor (sIL-2r) into the bloodstream. Assays for sIL-2r are available commercially, and may be useful in predicting disease severity (Rothkrantz-Kos *et al.* 2003). Other cytokines or soluble cytokine receptors that may be of value in the diagnosis or management of sarcoidosis include IL-18, IL-12 p40, and soluble tumor necrosis factor receptor II (Costabel *et al.* 2008).

Several proteins have been investigated as suitable disease markers. Lung epithelium-specific proteins (pneumoproteins), such as Clara Cell 16 (CC16), KL-6, and surfactant protein-D have been studied for their value in diagnosis and management. All showed a lack of specificity for sarcoidosis, so are of no value in diagnosis; CC16 and KL-6 may be of value in disease monitoring, and further studies should be performed (Janssen *et al.* 2003). Serum YKL-40, secreted by macrophages, has been shown to correlate positively with serum ACE activity, and inversely with lung carbon monoxide diffusion capacity (Johansen *et al.* 2005).

Proteomics analysis has been employed in the search for suitable biomarkers for human diseases, for example for markers of ovarian and lung cancer. The production of a sarcoidosis protein profile, using surface-enhanced laser desorption ionization time-of-flight mass spectrometry (SELDI-TOF-MS) may well be of value in the discovery of suitable biomarkers for sarcoidosis. It is likely that a combination of markers will be required because of the multifactorial nature of the disease. Preliminary results are encouraging, and large studies will be required to validate suitable markers (Bons *et al.* 2007).

REFERENCES

Allen RKA, Chai SY, Dunbar MS, Mendelsohn FAO (1986). In-vitro autoradiographic localization of angiotensin-converting enzyme in sarcoid lymph nodes. *Chest* **90**: 315–20.

American Thoracic Society (1999). Statement on sarcoidosis. *Am J Respir Crit Care Med* **160**: 736–55.

Bader M, Ganten D (2008). Update on tissue renin–angiotensin systems. *J Mol Med* **86**: 615–21.

Bargagli E, Maggiorelli C, Rottoli P (200). Human chitotriosidase: a potential new marker of sarcoidosis severity. *Respiration* **76**: 234–8.

Boink ABTJ, Buckley BM, Christiansen TF et al. (1991). IFCC recommendations on sampling, transport and storage for the determination of ionized calcium in whole blood, plasma and serum. *J Aut Chem* **13**: 235–9.

Bons JA, Drent M, Bouwman FG et al. (2007). Potential biomarkers for diagnosis of sarcoidosis using proteomics in serum. *Respir Med* **101**: 1687–95.

Brincker H (1995). Sarcoidosis and malignancy. *Chest* **108**: 1472–4.

Christenson RH (2007). Evidence-based laboratory medicine: a guide for critical evaluation of in-vitro laboratory testing. *Ann Clin Biochem* **44**: 111–30.

Coates D (2003). The angiotensin converting enzyme. *Int J Biochem Cell Biol* **35**: 769–73.

Conron M, Young C, Beynon HLC (2000). Calcium metabolism in sarcoidosis and its clinical implications. *Rheumatology* **39**: 707–13.

Costabel U, Ohshimo S, Guzman J (2008). Diagnosis of sarcoidosis. *Curr Opin Pulm Med* **14**: 455–61.

Friedland J, Silverstein E (1976). A sensitive fluorimetric assay for serum angiotensin-converting enzyme. *Am J Clin Path* **66**: 416–24.

Holmquist B, Bunning P, Riordan JF (1979). A continuous spectrophotometric assay for angiotensin converting enzyme. *Anal Biochem* **95**: 540–8.

James MT, Zhang J, Lyon AW, Hemmelgarn BR (2008). Derivation and internal validation of an equation for albumin-adjusted calcium. *BMC Clin Pathol* **8**: 12.

Janssen R, Sato H, Grutters JC et al. (2003). Study of Clara Cell 16, KL-6, and surfactant protein-D in serum as disease markers in pulmonary sarcoidosis. *Chest* **124**: 2119–25.

Johansen JS, Milman N, Hansen M et al. (2005). Increased serum YKL-40 in patients with pulmonary sarcoidosis: a potential marker of disease activity? *Resp Med* **99**: 396–402.

Kellinghaus C, Schilling M, Ludemann P (2004). Neurosarcoidosis: clinical experience and diagnostic pitfalls. *Eur Neurol* **51**: 84–8.

Liebermann J (1975). Elevation of serum angiotensin-converting enzyme (ACE) level in sarcoidosis. *Am J Med* **59**: 365–72.

Malnick S, Melzer E, Sokolowski N, Basevitz A (2008). The involvement of the liver in systemic diseases. *J Clin Gastroenterol* **42**: 69–80.

Muller BR (2002). Analysis of serum angiotensin-converting enzyme. *Ann Clin Biochem* **39**: 436–43.

Nunes H, Bouvry D, Soler P, Valeyre D (2007). Sarcoidosis. *Orphanet J Rare Dis* **2**: 46–53.

Rothkrantz-Kos S, van Dieijen-Visser MP, Mulder PGH, Drent M (2003). Potential usefulness of inflammatory markers to monitor respiratory functional impairment in sarcoidosis. *Clin Chem* **49**: 1510–17.

Sen F, Mann K, Madeiros J (2002). Multiple myeloma in association with sarcoidosis. *Arch Pathol Lab Med* **126**: 365–8.

Sharma OP (1996). Vitamin D, calcium, and sarcoidosis. *Chest* **109**: 535–9.

Sharma OP (2000). Hypercalcaemia in granulomatous disorders: a clinical review. *Curr Opin Pulm Med* **6**: 442–7.

Sharma P, Smith I, Maguire G et al. (1997). Clinical value of ACE genotyping in diagnosis of sarcoidosis. *Lancet* **349**: 1602–3.

Shen XZ, Xiao HD, Li P et al. (2008). New insights into the role of angiotensin-converting enzyme obtained from the analysis of genetically modified mice. *J Mol Med* **86**: 679–84.

Shorr AF, Torrington KG, Parker JM (1997). Serum angiotensin converting enzyme does not correlate with radiographic stage at initial diagnosis of sarcoidosis. *Respir Med* **91**: 399–401.

Studdy PR, Bird R (1989). Serum angiotensin converting enzyme in sarcoidosis: its value in present clinical practice. *Ann Clin Biochem* **26**: 13–18.

Studdy PR, Bird R, Neville E, James DG (1980). Biochemical findings in sarcoidosis. *J Clin Pathol* **33**: 528–33.

Sutor G, Fabel H (2000). Sarcoidosis and common variable immuno-deficiency. *Respiration* **67**: 204–8.

Turton CWG, Grundy E, Firth G et al. (1979). Value of measuring serum angiotensin 1 converting enzyme and serum lysozyme in the management of sarcoidosis. *Thorax* **34**: 57–62.

Wells AU, Hirani N (2008). Interstitial lung disease guideline: the British Thoracic Society in collaboration with the Thoracic Society of Australia and New Zealand and the Irish Thoracic Society. *Thorax* **63**: v1–58.

18

Sleep studies

ANITA K SIMONDS

SLEEP-DISORDERED BREATHING

Sleep-disordered breathing is a generic term covering obstructive sleep apnea, central sleep apnea with periodic breathing, and nocturnal hypoventilation.

Obstructive sleep apnea (OSA) is characterized by recurrent episodes of upper airway collapse during sleep, usually associated with sleep fragmentation, with fluctuations in blood pressure, heart rate and cardiac output. Partial episodes are called hypopneas. By contrast, in central sleep apnea the respiratory irregularity is most commonly associated with chronic heart failure or cerebral insult, such as neurosarcoid, and caused by unstable ventilatory drive. Nocturnal hypoventilation oocurs in individuals with ventilatory insufficiency and if unaddressed may lead to daytime ventilatory failure. It occurs in those with severe restrictive ventilatory defects, such as secondary to respiratory muscle weakness, morbid obesity or reduced ventilatory drive.

To characterize the nature and severity of sleep-disordered breathing, monitoring of respiration during sleep – a sleep study – is almost always required because effective management is hindered without a clear diagnosis. The extent of sleep apnea is expressed as the apnea/hypopnea index (AHI), the total of apneas and hyponeas per hour of sleep overnight.

SARCOID AND SLEEP-DISORDERED BREATHING

There have been few studies of the prevalence of sleep-related breathing disorders in patients with sarcoid. Mughal and associates assessed 70 consecutive patients (42 females) with biopsy-proven sarcoid using the Sleep Apnea / Sleep Disorders Questionnaire (SA/SDQ) which has a reported 81 percent specificity for the diagnosis of sleep apnea in the general population (Mughal *et al.* 2005). The Epworth sleepiness score, which is a measure of sleepiness, was also applied. The patient group had a mean age of 48 years, mean duration of diagnosis was 78 months, two-thirds were on steroid therapy (mean prednisolone dose 7 mg/day) or other immunosuppression, and 60 percent had two or more organs involved. Thirty-nine patients scored positively on the SA/SDQ and 14 had an elevated Epworth sleepiness score (normal score <10). This would suggest a prevalence of obstructive sleep apnea of 39 percent of the sarcoid patients, which is significantly higher than the prevalence in the general middle-aged population where obstructive sleep apnea occurs in 4 percent of men and 2 percent of women.

Turner and associates performed sleep studies on 83 patients with sarcoid and compared results with a control group of 91 patients seen in general pulmonary clinics (Turner *et al.* 1997). Seventeen percent of sarcoid patients were found to have sleep apnea compared to 3 percent of the control group. Prevalence was higher in males with sarcoid, and in those with lupus pernio.

INTRINSIC HYPERSOMNOLENCE AND FATIGUE

Hypersomnolence can be a feature of neurosarcoid (Rubinstein *et al.* 1988). Clearly in this situation the presence of sleep apnea should be excluded, and a label of instrinsic sleep disorder applied only if polysomnography has excluded other possible causes. As well as OSA, this could also include restless leg syndrome which becomes more prevalent with increasing age and is also seen in patients with polyneuropathy, cardiac failure, renal insufficiency and iron deficiency. Excessive sleepiness should be distinguished from fatigue which is well recognized in sarcoid (Lower *et al.* 2008). Fatigue, too, is a diagnostic label of exclusion and a sleep study is helpful to exclude other contributory conditions.

ETIOLOGICAL MECHANISMS AND PATHOPHYSIOLOGY OF SLEEP APNEA

Factors predisposing to upper airway collapse and obstructive sleep apnea include obesity (which may be exacerbated by steroid therapy) and upper airway lesions. There are case reports of laryngeal sarcoid mainly affecting the supraglottic larynx causing obstructive sleep apnea, and sarcoid lesions in the tongue and epiglottis also causing OSA (Fuso *et al.* 2001). Indeed, OSA was the presenting feature of the disease in one case and resolved after 2 months' treatment with steroid therapy. It should not be forgotten that OSA is a common condition, so OSA and sarcoid may coexist; however, weight gain (e.g. related to steroid therapy) may cause an individual with simple snoring to progress to significant obstructive sleep apnea.

Sarcoid lesions in the medullary, pontine and hypothalamic regions are most likely to be associated with central sleep apnea, but this is a rare finding. Granulomatous change in the hypothalamus may be seen at postmortem and either damage to this region or inhibition of brainstem projections to higher regions may be responsible. Speculatively, activated sarcoid macrophages may release interleukin-1 which is a sleep-promoting factor (Rubinstein *et al.* 1988).

WHEN TO SUSPECT A SLEEP DISORDER

Individuals with obstructive sleep apnea present with a constellation of daytime sleepiness, poor sleep quality, troublesome snoring and choking, and their bed partners often report erratic breathing (witnessed apneas) and restlessness. The Epworth sleepiness score can be used to quantitate sleepiness (Johns 1991).

Morning headaches or anorexia for breakfast may be seen in patients with nocturnal hypoventilation. Those with excessive sleepiness, or snoring and one other feature above such as choking and morning headaches, should have a sleep study. In addition, both central and obstructive sleep apnea is more common in those with heart failure, nocturnal hypoventilation is seen in those with significant respiratory muscle weakness, or marked restrictive ventilatory defect, and central sleep apnea more is prevalent in those with neurosarcoid; so there should be a low threshold to carry out sleep studies in these clinical situations.

A sleep study should also be considered in patients with disproportionate daytime hypoxemia compared to lung function results, and in those with pulmonary hypertension that is not easily explained on lung function results alone as nocturnal hypoxemia due to any sleep-related breathing disorder could be driving the progression of these complications.

WHAT TYPE OF SLEEP STUDY?

Investigations of breathing during sleep vary from simple overnight oximetry to respiratory polygraphy (monitoring of oronasal airflow/pressure, chest and abdominal movement, snoring, oximetry and position), and full polysomnography where, in addition to respiratory variables, electroencephalogram, electrooculogram and electromyogram signals are obtained so that sleep stages and their duration can be ascertained. Sleep studies can be carried out in the sleep laboratory or at home.

Oximetry can be useful in screening but is not specific or sensitive enough to give a clear diagnosis in all cases. The accuracy of diagnosis will depend on symptoms and pre-test probability. For example, in overweight sarcoid patients with snoring, witnessed apneas and daytime somnolence, a respiratory polygraphy study at hospital or home carried out and interpreted by an experienced team is usually satisfactory and will confirm or refute the diagnosis of OSA; see Figure 18.1. In those with neurosarcoid or sleepiness in whom a respiratory polygraphy study is negative, full polysomnography will be required. For the diagnosis of nocturnal hypoventilation, the addition of CO_2 measurement (e.g. transcutaneous CO_2 or end-tidal CO_2) to respiratory polygraphy will usually confirm the diagnosis.

Daytime somnolence can be quantified and differentiated from fatigue by a multiple sleep latency test, or Osler wake test. Web links to the National Institute of Clinical Excellence (NICE) and Scottish Intercollegiate guideline network (SIGN) recommendations for investigation and management of sleep-disordered breathing are listed later.

TREATMENT AND OUTCOME

Individuals with OSA should be advised about sensible strategies, such as weight loss and positional modification (e.g. sleeping with head of bed elevated). The standard treatment for moderate or severe obstructive sleep apnea syndrome is nasal continuous positive airway pressure therapy (CPAP) (Jenkinson *et al.* 1999; Stradling 2007). This rapidly reverses somnolence and corrects hypoxemia and cardiovascular consequences of the apnea events. Obvious upper airway lesions should be treated or resected if feasible. The mandibular advancement splint which fits over upper and lower teeth and lifts forward the mandible may be successful in patients who snore or who have mild OSA.

Nocturnal hypoventilation resulting in symptomatic nocturnal hypercapnia is best addressed by nocturnal noninvasive ventilation. Central sleep apnea is more difficult to address. For those with neurosarcoid, management with steroid therapy or cerebral irradiation may be successful. If the problem is occurring as a result of heart failure, then oxygen therapy or adaptive servo-ventilation may be effective (Philippe *et al.* 2006; Hastings *et al.* 2010), although the latter is still the subject of a large randomized trial.

Intrinsic somnolence (sleepiness in the absence of sleep-disordered breathing) may respond to dexmethylphenidate (Lower *et al.* 2008). In other conditions causing somnolence (e.g. narcolepsy), modafinil has now superseded methylphenidate and dexamphetamine as it has fewer side-effects. Modafinil has also been used to treat fatigue. However the European Medicine Agency's Committee for Medicinal Products for Human Use ruled in 2010 that modafinil

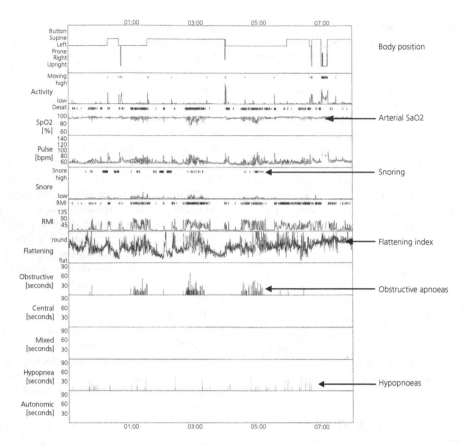

Figure 18.1   A respiratory polygraphy sleep study showing obstructive sleep apnoea in a patient with renal sarcoid who gained 20 kg in weight on therapy. Flattening index is a measure of airflow obstruction. Apnoeas/hypopnoea index is 19/hour. Epworth sleepiness score was 15/20 and the patient responded well to CPAP therapy.

should only be used for the treatment of narcolepsy and not in the management of intrinsic somnolence or fatigue.

CONCLUSION

Every major form of sleep-disordered breathing can be found in patients with sarcoidosis, and the prevalence of these sleep disorders is likely to be higher than in the general population. As a consequence, there should be a low threshold for considering sleep studies particularly in those with classic symptoms of obstructive sleep apnea and daytime somnolenece. There is also considerable overlap in symptoms of sleep apnea and sarcoid – fatigue, tiredness, night sweats – and so care should be taken not to automatically ascribe these symptoms to sarcoid.

Resolution of sleep-disordered breathing may occur with successful treatment of sarcoid; but if not, or if time is required for complete resolution, standard measures such as CPAP for OSA can prove very effective.

FURTHER READING

Guidelines for diagnosis and management of obstructive sleep apnea/hypopnea syndrome

SIGN guideline on management of obstructive sleep apnea/hypopnea syndrome in adults. Available at www.sign.ac.uk/pdf/sign73.pdf.
NICE guidance on CPAP therapy for obstructive sleep apnea/hypopnea syndrome (2008). Available at http://guidance.nice.org.uk/TA139.

REFERENCES

Fuso F, Maiolo C, Tramaglino LM *et al.* (2001). Orolaryngeal sarcoidosis presenting as obstructive sleep apnoea. *Sarcoid Vasc Diff Lung Dis* 18: 85–90.

Hastings PC, Vazir A, Meadows GE *et al.* (2010). Adaptive servo-ventilation in heart failure patients with sleep apnea: a real world study. *Int J Cardiol* 139: 17–24.

Jenkinson C, Davies RJO, Mullins R, Stradling JR (1999). Comparison of therapeutic and subtherapeutic nasal continuous positive pressure airway pressure for obstructive sleep apnoea: a randomised prospective parallel trial. *Lancet* 353: 2100–5.

Johns MW (1991). A new method for measuring daytime sleepiness: the Epworth sleepiness scale. *Sleep* 14: 540–5.

Lower EE, Harman S, Baughman RP (2008). Double-blind, randomized trial of dexmethlyphenidate for the treatment of sarcoidosis-associated fatigue. *Chest* 133: 1189–95.

Mughal MM, Golish J, Kavuri M *et al.* (2005). Sleep apnea in sarcoidosis. *Chest* 128: 230S.

Philippe C, Stoica-Herman M, Druout X *et al.* (2006). Compliance with and effectiveness of adaptive servoventilation versus continuous positive airway pressure in the treatment of Cheyne–Stokes respiration in heart failure over a six month period. *Heart* 92: 337–42.

Rubinstein I, Gray TA, Moldofsky H, Hoffstein V (1988). Neurosarcoidosis associated with hypersomnolence treated with corticosteroids and brain irradiation. *Chest* 94: 205–6.

Stradling J (2007). Obstructive sleep apnoea. *Br Med J* 335: 313–14.

Turner GA, Lower EE, Corser BC *et al.* (1997). Sleep apnea in sarcoidosis. *Sarcoid Vasc Diff Lung Dis* 14: 61–4.

PART **IV**

THE HEART, PULMONARY HYPERTENSION, THE UPPER RESPIRATORY TRACT, THE AIRWAYS, AND PULMONARY FIBROSIS

19

The heart

J C LYNE, H O SAVAGE AND P J OLDERSHAW

PREVALENCE

The first described case of cardiac sarcoid was published by Bernstein and associates in 1929. While cardiac sarcoidosis is more common than previously recognized, the true prevalence of this condition is unknown owing to the paucity of symptoms during life. Clinically significant cardiac involvement in truly unselected patients with sarcoidosis is probably impossible to ascertain, and most published studies have been carried out postmortem (Roberts et al. 1977; Fleming 1994).

Clinical evidence of myocardial involvement is present in approximately 5 percent of patients with sarcoidosis, although postmortem studies have documented subclinical cardiac involvement in 20–30 percent of cases (Iwai et al. 1994; Thomsen and Eriksson 1999; Chapelon-Abric et al. 2004). A number of autopsy studies carried out on patients with sarcoidosis in the USA quote cardiac involvement in 18–75 percent (Sharma et al. 1993; Perry and Vuitch 1995). In the UK, Fleming and co-workers retrospectively studied 50 patients and found 14 with cardiac sarcoidosis at necropsy (Fleming 1973). In 1967, Scadding studied a cohort of 267 patients with myocardial involvement of sarcoid and found only two patients with suggestive clinical features (Scadding 1967). In 1972, Ghosh and co-workers described six cases of myocardial sarcoidosis identified at autopsy (Ghosh et al. 1972). More recently, a 50-year experience at the Johns Hopkins Hospital was published; cardiac involvement was found in 7 percent of the 188 patients with sarcoid from their registry (Johns and Michele 1999). All published reports thus quote a variable prevalence of cardiac sarcoidosis, although those of Afro-Caribbean descent are thought to be three times more likely to develop cardiac sarcoid.

There are no large randomized trial data on cardiac sarcoidosis, but the literature suggests that making the diagnosis is clinically important. Unlike the situation in isolated pulmonary disease, cardiac involvement implies a particularly poor prognosis. Sudden cardiac death is well documented and may be the first presentation of this condition (Mikhail et al. 1974; Fleming 1988).

PATHOGENESIS

Myocardial pathology results from the presence of non-caseating granulomas, which can be seen on endomyocardial biopsy. Clinical manifestations usually depend on the location and extent of granulomatous inflammation. Non-caseating granulomas infiltrate the myocardium and heal to eventually become fibrotic scars (Sharma et al. 1993), resulting in contractile dysfunction from restrictive myocardium which, in severe disease, may lead to heart failure (Roberts et al. 1977; Silverman et al. 1978; Fleming 1994).

In terms of pathology, any part of the heart can be affected, from the endocardium through myocardium to the pericardium. In the myocardium, granulomas may involve any region of the heart, although the most common sites are the left ventricular free wall (96 percent), septum (73 percent), right ventricle (46 percent), right atrium (11 percent) and left atrium (7 percent) (Bargout and Kelly 2004). Transmural involvement is common and large portions of the ventricular wall may be replaced by fibrous tissue, potentially leading to progressive thinning and aneurysm formation, particularly of the right ventricular free wall. Chest pain has been described in up to 28 percent of patients and, since about half of these will have abnormal thallium perfusion scans, despite angiographically normal coronary arteries, this is thought to be secondary to microvascular spasm. Granulomas entangle small coronary arteries in a web of fibrosis, while leaving larger coronary arteries unaffected (Matsui et al. 1976; Roberts et al. 1977). Valve involvement is uncommon; however, dysfunction may result from infiltration of papillary muscles which leads to functional valvular impairment (Hapelon-Abric et al. 2004).

Involvement of the pericardium may be observed as effusions or pericarditis. The presence of significant pulmonary involvement with resultant raised pulmonary pressures may lead to right ventricular hypertrophy and, consequently, cor pulmonale. The conducting system of the heart is also particularly vulnerable to damage: tachyarrhythmia and conduction defects are not uncommon.

CLINICAL PRESENTATION

The diagnosis of cardiac sarcoidosis, based on a combination of clinical features and investigations, is often difficult owing to the non-specific nature of clinical manifestations. When cardiac dysfunction is the sole manifestation, the diagnosis is not usually entertained: a high index of suspicion is required in such instances to make a diagnosis, with early recourse to a combination of radiological and nuclear imaging.

Cardiac manifestations are largely dependent on the location and extent of granulomatous inflammation. The degree of infiltration may range from a few scattered lesions to extensive diffuse involvement. Owing to the potentially diffuse nature of the disease, cardiac involvement has a wide spectrum of clinical manifestations, frequently presenting with non-specific symptoms, but should be considered in any patient with symptoms of arrhythmia (palpitation, presyncope, syncope), exertional breathlessness or congestive heart failure. Systemic symptoms, including fatigue, malaise, fever and weight loss, may also occur.

Cardiac manifestations may precede, follow or occur concurrently with involvement of the lungs or other organs. However, myocardial involvement is common in patients with sarcoidosis who have cardiac symptoms and unusual in those without such symptoms. This was illustrated in a report of 101 patients with biopsy-proven pulmonary sarcoidosis, 19 of whom presented with cardiac symptoms (Smedema et al. 2005). An ECG was performed in all patients and most underwent further cardiac evaluation with echocardiography, radionuclide myocardial perfusion imaging, cardiac magnetic resonance imaging and, in a few cases, coronary angiography and/or endomyocardial biopsy. Cardiac sarcoidosis was diagnosed much more frequently in symptomatic patients (84 vs 4 percent).

It is noteworthy that isolated cardiac sarcoidosis is by no means a rare entity and the absence of pulmonary manifestations does not exclude the diagnosis. Therefore, in patients without a diagnosis, the following represent a spectrum of cardiac abnormalities that should raise suspicion:

- a conduction abnormality in a young patient, a patient with dilated cardiomyopathy and ventricular regional wall-motion abnormality, possibly with an inducible perfusion defect, particularly of the anteroseptal or apical segments;
- a sustained re-entrant ventricular tachycardia and a non-specific resting ECG abnormality;
- a restrictive cardiomyopathy of unknown etiology;
- presumed arrhythmogenic right ventricular cardiomyopathy/dysplasia and AV block in association with evidence of unexplained respiratory disease;

- patients with dyspnea which is out of proportion to pulmonary disease (either in definite sarcoidosis or in interstitial lung disease at large, with sarcoidosis in the differential diagnosis), particularly in the presence of congestive heart failure.

Sudden cardiac death related to unrecognized cardiac sarcoidosis is well documented, so any patient with diagnosed sarcoidosis should be screened with a 12-lead electrocardiogram, echocardiogram and Holter monitoring.

INVESTIGATIONS

There is no singular diagnostic test for cardiac sarcoidosis, so confirmation of definite cardiac involvement in sarcoidosis is a desirable but not an absolute prerequisite for the initiation of empirical treatment. As discussed earlier, the non-specificity of symptoms can create an overlap with other known conditions and, hence, affect the selection of appropriate tests to facilitate a diagnosis. Therefore it is not uncommon to find patients started on treatment based on a high clinical index of suspicion, without histological confirmation of the diagnosis, either from the heart or from elsewhere in the body.

Electrocardiography and ambulatory monitoring

The need to reconcile clinical features and the level of diagnostic confidence of cardiac sarcoidosis makes it a frustrating disease to diagnose. The ECG findings may be normal; however, repolarization abnormalities with non-specific ST-T wave changes (Roberts et al. 1977; Ahmad et al. 1992; Grief et al. 2008), arrhythmias and conduction disturbances are found in approximately 70 percent of patients who have systemic sarcoidosis (Chapelon-Abric et al. 2004), including 50 percent of those with no definitive clinical evidence of cardiac involvement (Grief et al. 2008). All degrees of conduction defects, including complete heart block, left and right bundle branch block, have been documented (Fleming 1988). First-degree heart block due to disease of the atrioventricular node or bundle of His, and various types of intraventricular conduction defects, are common among patients with cardiac sarcoidosis (Chapelon-Abric et al. 2004). These lesions may initially be silent, but can progress to complete heart block and cause syncope (Yoshida et al. 1997). Fibrosis in the cephalad portion on the interventricular septum is a constant finding in patients with abnormalities of the conduction system. Involvement of the ventricular septum and conduction system can lead to a variety of arrhythmias, including complete heart block and sudden cardiac death. Complete heart block is the most common finding in patients with clinically evident cardiac sarcoidosis, and occurs at a younger age in patients with sarcoidosis than in individuals with complete heart block due to other etiologies (Fleming 1994).

Supraventricular arrhythmias are infrequent in cardiac sarcoidosis. Arrhythmias that have been described include ectopic atrial activity, paroxysmal atrial tachycardia, atrial flutter, atrial fibrillation, and sinus arrest secondary to granulomatous involvement of the sinus node (Ahmad et al. 1992; Iwai et al. 1994). Holter monitoring can document and define subclinical rhythm disturbances missed on ECG (Suzuki et al. 1994). In one study, 38 consecutive patients with biopsy-proven sarcoidosis received 24 h Holter monitoring (Reuhl et al. 1997). More than 10 supraventricular ectopic beats occurred in 8 of 12 patients (66.7 percent) with clinical cardiac sarcoidosis, in 7 of 26 patients (26.9 percent) with no clinical evidence of cardiac sarcoidosis, and in 3 of 58 healthy control subjects (5 percent).

Most recently Mehta and associates interviewed ambulatory patients with sarcoidosis, evaluated with ECG, Holter monitoring, and transthoracic echocardiography (TTE). Those with symptoms or abnormal results were further studied with cardiac MRI (CMRI) or positron emission tomography (PET) scanning. The diagnosis of cardiac sarcoid was based on abnormalities detected by these imaging studies. Among the 62 patients evaluated, the prevalence of cardiac sarcoid was 39 percent. Patients with cardiac sarcoid had more cardiac symptoms than those without disease (46 vs 5 percent, respectively; $p < 0.001$), and were more likely to have abnormal Holter monitoring findings (50 vs 3 percent, respectively; $p < 0.001$) and TTE findings (25 vs 5 percent, respectively; $p < 0.02$) (Yazaki et al. 2001). The degree of pulmonary impairment did not predict cardiac sarcoid. This structured algorithm revealed that an abnormality found on any of the four baseline testing variables (i.e. symptoms, ECG, Holter monitoring, or TTE) was more sensitive for the diagnosis of cardiac sarcoid than the modified Japanese Ministry of Health and Welfare (JMHW) criteria for diagnosing sarcoid (Fleming 1994; Box 19.1).

The prevalence of ECG abnormalities has been correlated with the severity of cardiac involvement. Silverman and co-workers studied 84 patients and found 15 percent of patients without detectable cardiac involvement had ECG abnormalities. This was in contrast to 42 percent of patients with microscopically evident granulomas and up to 75 percent of patients with gross evidence of cardiac granulomas or infiltration, at autopsy, who had arrhythmia or conduction disturbances (Silverman et al. 1978).

Heart rate variability (HRV) analysis obtained during Holter monitoring provides a useful method to measure autonomic activity. It has been shown that HRV is decreased in patients with systemic sarcoidosis but the decrease is more apparent in patients with cardiac sarcoidosis. The clinical significance of this observation may be uncertain (Uslu et al. 2006), but the development of chronotropic incompetence may be a useful marker of cardiac infiltration.

Ventricular arrhythmia

Some patients with known systemic sarcoidosis develop symptomatic or electrocardiographically evident arrhythmias or conduction abnormalities prior to sarcoid-related sudden death; however sudden death can occur in the absence of a

---

Box 19.1 Guidelines for diagnosing cardiac sarcoidosis (Japan Society of Sarcoidosis and Other Granulomatous Disorders; adapted from Hiraga et al. (1993))

Histological diagnosis
Confirmed when myocardial biopsy specimens demonstrate non-caseating epithelioid cell granuloma with histological or clinical diagnosis of extracardiac sarcoidosis

Clinical diagnosis
Although myocardial biopsy specimens do not demonstrate non-caseating epithelioid cell granuloma, extracardiac sarcoidosis is diagnosed histologically or clinically and satisfies the following conditions and more than one of six basic diagnostic criteria
- more than two **major** criteria are satisfied;
- one **major** criterion and more than two **minor** criteria are satisfied

Major criteria:
- advanced AV block
- basal thinning of the interventricular septum
- positive cardiac gallium-67 uptake
- depressed ejection fraction of the left ventricle (LVEF <50%)

Minor criteria:
- abnormal ECG findings: ventricular arrhythmias (VT, multifocal or frequent PVCs), CRBBB, axis deviation or abnormal Q-wave
- abnormal echocardiography: regional abnormal wall motion or morphological abnormality (ventricular aneurysm, wall thickening)
- nuclear medicine: perfusion defect detected by ^{201}Tl myocardial scintigraphy or ^{99}Tc myocardial scintigraphy
- Gd-enhanced MRI: delayed enhancement of myocardium
- endomyocardial biopsy: interstitial fibrosis or monocyte infiltration over moderate grade

---

previous cardiac event (Reuhl et al. 1997). Among patients with cardiac sarcoidosis, sudden death due to ventricular tachyarrhythmia or conduction block accounts for 25–65 percent of deaths (Reuhl et al. 1997; Yazaki et al. 2001).

Sustained or unsustained ventricular tachycardia and ventricular premature beats are the second most common presentation of cardiac sarcoidosis. Electrocardiography identifies ventricular arrhythmia in as many as 22 percent of patients with sarcoidosis (Sekiguchi et al. 1980). Sarcoid granulomas in the ventricular myocardium can become the foci of abnormal automaticity, or may disrupt ventricular activation, conduction and recovery, leading to the creation of an arrhythmogenic substrate (Grief et al. 2008). Re-entrant substrate is formed, not only in association with the healing of cardiac granulomas in the inactive phase of cardiac sarcoidosis, but also in the active phase. Ventricular arrhythmia may also be the result of an ischemic event; involvement of the smaller coronary branches is well documented in sarcoidosis. As noted previously the larger conductance vessels are uninvolved.

Arrhythmias are often refractory to antiarrhythmic drugs, including amiodarone (Winters et al. 1991; Syed and Myers 2004). Therefore, although steroids may halt progression of left ventricular dysfunction, arrhythmias may warrant device implantation. There is limited experience with implantable cardioverter defibrillators (ICDs) in patients with cardiac sarcoidosis (Bajaj et al. 1988; Winters et al. 1991; Paz et al. 1994; Butany et al. 2006). Therefore, the main indications are thought to be similar to those in patients with other forms of cardiomyopathy: secondary prevention in survivors of sudden death or patients with refractory ventricular tachyarrhythmias who are at an increased risk of sudden cardiac death. In addition, some recommend an ICD as primary therapy of ventricular tachycardia owing to the relative lack of efficacy with antiarrhythmic drugs (Winters et al. 1991), and for primary prevention in selected patients with mild to moderate symptoms of heart failure and a left ventricular ejection fraction ≤35 percent (Butany et al. 2006).

For risk stratification, ventricular stimulation protocols have included stimulation of the right ventricle from two sites with drive-cycle lengths of 600 and 450 ms and up to three premature extra beats to prematurity of 240, 200 and 200 ms, burst pacing from 300 to 200 ms and repeating of the protocol with IV infusion of isoproterenol. The electrophysiological study (EPS) findings were considered positive if sustained (i.e. >30 s) ventricular tachycardia was provoked. While inducible ventricular arrhythmias predict spontaneous ventricular tachycardia and adverse outcomes in patients with ventricular dysfunction (Aizer et al. 2005), the value of an EPS only (without ablation) may be controversial in patients with cardiac sarcoidosis and preserved left ventricular function.

In addition, there is a high rate of recurrence of ventricular tachycardia or sudden death with antiarrhythmia drug therapy, even when guided by EPS (Winters et al. 1991). The role of EPS was further evaluated in a series of 32 patients with cardiac sarcoidosis at a single center who were referred for EPS for evaluation of symptoms (palpitations, syncope, pre-syncope or sudden death) and/or any ventricular arrhythmia including ventricular premature beats, unsustained or sustained ventricular tachycardia (VT), or ventricular fibrillation (VF) (Aizer et al. 2005). Six patients had experienced spontaneous VT or VF, while 10 patients had inducible sustained ventricular arrhythmias: 4 of 6 with spontaneous VT/VF and 6 of 26 without spontaneous ventricular arrhythmias. All of the 12 patients with spontaneous or inducible ventricular arrhythmias received an implantable cardiac defibrillator. The following findings were noted at a mean follow-up of 32 months:

- Nine of the 12 patients received appropriate ICD therapy during follow-up. In comparison, only 2 of 20 patients with neither spontaneous nor induced ventricular arrhythmias experienced SCD or sustained ventricular arrhythmias.
- Among patients with inducible or spontaneous ventricular arrhythmias, survival free of appropriate ICD therapy

at 5 years was 20 percent, while survival free of death or transplant was 90 percent.

Thus, EPS successfully identified patients with cardiac sarcoidosis who were likely to experience ventricular arrhythmias or sudden cardiac death. However, the role of EPS in risk stratification remains uncertain, since 80 percent of patients with inducible ventricular arrhythmias also had heart failure, with an average left ventricular ejection fraction of only 33 percent. As a result, most would probably have been considered for ICD placement regardless of the EPS results. Electrophysiological testing may prove to be of use early in symptomatic patients who do not have heart failure, and ICD therapy may be warranted in such patients who have a positive test. These observations constitute the rationale for the use of a pacemaker and the consideration of an implantable cardioverter defibrillator.

Ablation of ventricular arrhythmia can be helpful in some patients and may have a role in the treatment of cardiac sarcoidosis. In a series of eight patients, electrophysiology studies revealed evidence of scar-related re-entry with multiple monomorphic VTs induced (4 ± 2 VTs per patient) with both right bundle branch block and left bundle branch block QRS configurations (Koplan et al. 2006). Areas of low-voltage scar were present in the right ventricle in all eight patients, in the left ventricle in five (63 percent), and in the epicardium in two patients undergoing epicardial mapping. Ablation abolished one or more VTs in six patients (75 percent), but other VTs remained inducible in all but one patient. Post-ablation, some form of sustained VT recurred in six patients within 6 months. However, at longer follow-up (6 months to 7 years), four patients were free of VT with antiarrhythmia drugs and immune suppression. Cardiac transplantation was eventually required in five patients because of either recurrent VT (4) or heart failure (1). However incomplete ablation of the pulmotricuspid isthmus may be proarrhythmic, and cases of recurrent ventricular arrhythmia have been described (Reuhl et al. 1997).

Endomyocardial biopsy

This is a semi-invasive way to make a diagnosis of cardiac sarcoid. It is, however, the test that confirms myocardial involvement most reliably as it provides a histological diagnosis of non-caseating granulomas (Hagemann and Wurm 1980; Scadding and Mitchell 1985). Other histopathologic findings – such as myocardial interstitial fibrosis, heart muscle disarrangement and fragmentation, and inflammatory mononuclear cell infiltrates – support the diagnosis. Because of the diffuse nature of the disease, biopsy specimens may be positive in a minority of patients, so a negative myocardial biopsy by no means excludes the diagnosis. The yield from transvenous RV sampling remains notoriously poor because of the patchy nature of granulomatous distribution in the heart, and the fact that the sample area is usually the RV apex and apical septum, whereas granulomas are mostly found in the LV free wall and basal septum. The yield is usually not greater than 22 percent in most published series, but this may increase to 37 percent in patients with dilated cardiomyopathy. Hagemann and Wurm, in a review of 702 patients, reported that while 5 percent of their patients had clinical evidence of cardiac sarcoidosis, only 15 percent had cardiac lesions at necropsy (Hagemann and Wurm 1980). Scadding and Mitchell reported a far lower percentage with only 4 of the 500 patients reviewed having such evidence (Scadding and Mitchell 1985). It is, however, important to note that microscopic granulomas may also be present but, if not diffuse, are often missed. Therefore, the invasive nature of the test, problem of sampling error and limited descriptions in the literature of non-granulomatous changes that may be seen in cardiac sarcoidosis limit endomyocardial biopsy as a viable mode of investigating cardiac sarcoidosis.

TREATMENT

The treatment of cardiac sarcoidosis starts when a physician, who has a high index of suspicion, recognizes subtle signs that may be indicative of the presence of disease. This condition can be fatal if left untreated, so expert assistance should always be sought.

Corticosteroids have been the mainstay of treatment for over two decades. It is important to note, however, that there have been no randomized controlled trials looking at the use of corticosteroids in cardiac sarcoid, a situation that differs from treatment in pulmonary sarcoidosis (Pietnalho et al. 2002). Thus, a steroid-based approach to treatment remains mainly anecdotal, supported by reports in small case series (Shammas and Movahed 1994). Current practice is that, for patients with ECG changes or cardiac symptoms, systemic corticosteroids should be started. The aim of treatment is to control inflammation and fibrosis, in order to maintain cardiac structure and function.

Some studies involving patients with cardiac sarcoidosis suggest better survival rates among those treated with corticosteroids than those not treated (Ishikawa et al. 1984). In individual cases and small series, steroid use has also been shown to reverse mechanical and electrical abnormalities: however, prolonged use has also been reported to lead to increased risks of ventricular aneurysms (Ishikawa et al. 1984; Shammas and Movahed 1994). Higher success rates were demonstrated in patients who had treatment initiated before the onset of LV systolic dysfunction.

After an initial intravenous loading period, oral steroids such as prednisolone are administered daily with the aim to switch to steroid-sparing agents later in management. These agents, including azathioprine, hydroxychloroquine, ciclosporin and methotrexate, may also be started earlier in patients who do not respond to corticosteroids or who develop side-effects (Agbogu et al. 1995; Muller-Quernheim et al. 1999). Even though these agents have been studied extensively in pulmonary sarcoidosis and neurosarcoidosis, specific efficacy data are lacking in cardiac sarcoidosis and again their use is anecdotal (Lower et al. 1997). Demeter reports one case of myocardial sarcoidosis which was unresponsive to corticosteroids but treated successfully with cyclophosphamide (Demeter 1988).

Conventional treatment for heart failure is initiated when necessary and ACE inhibitors, beta-blockers and diuretics all have a role to play, provided there are no contraindications. Antiarrythmic agents are employed to treat lethal arrhythmias but the risk of heart block increases with their use. A permanent pacemaker is indicated when there is evidence of complete AV block or other high-grade conduction system disease is present. Glucocorticoids or other forms of anti-inflammatory therapy should be continued on an individual basis (as tolerated and as needed clinically) in a patient who has a pacemaker.

As discussed earlier, cardiac electrophysiology studies, mapping and ablation of these lethal arrhythmias, particularly VT, have been shown to be helpful in some patients. The general consensus is that prophylactic implantation of a cardiac defibrillator (ICD) should be offered to a patient with life-threatening or refractory arrhythmias as prognosis might be improved (Winters et al. 1991). Some patients may require consideration of heart transplantation where extensive myocardial involvement may be unresponsive to the aforementioned therapies. These patients often do well with a low recurrence of disease in the allograft (Valantine et al. 1987). In fact, patients with sarcoid cardiomyopathy undergoing orthotropic heart transplant had better short- and intermediate-term survival than seen in the majority of heart transplant recipients. The diagnosis of sarcoidosis should, therefore, not disqualify potential transplant candidates (Zaidi et al. 2007).

PROGNOSIS

Mortality in cardiac sarcoidosis is usually as a result of fatal arrhythmias or conduction defects leading to sudden cardiac death. A smaller percentage will develop rapidly progressive congestive cardiac failure secondary to extensive myocardial damage or a consequence of cor pulmonale. Some patients will, however, remain subclinical through life and mortality will be as a result of non-cardiac causes.

Variable survival rates in cardiac sarcoid have therefore been quoted. Many studies suggest that the 5-year mortality may exceed 50 percent (Yazaki et al. 2001). Other conservative reports suggest between 2 and 40 percent at 5 years (Fleming 1973; Roberts et al. 1977).

Yazaki and co-workers published their series of 95 Japanese patients with cardiac sarcoidosis between 1984 and 1996 (Yazaki et al. 2001). They observed overall survival rates of 85 percent at one year, 72 percent at three years, 60 percent at five years, and 44 percent at ten years. In the mean period of follow-up of 68 months, 29 patients (30 percent) died of congestive heart failure and 11 (12 percent) experienced sudden death. Predictors of mortality were analyzed among 75 of these patients treated with corticosteroids. Kaplan–Meier survival curves showed 5-year survival rates of 75 percent in steroid-treated patients and 89 percent in patients with LVEF ≥50 percent. Multivariate analysis identified New York Heart Association functional class, LV end-diastolic diameter, and sustained ventricular tachycardia as independent predictors of mortality.

CONCLUSION

Sarcoid involvement of the heart remains difficult to diagnose and a high index of suspicion is usually necessary. Early and expert assessment is needed to reach a diagnosis, and prompt initiation of treatment might be life-saving.

REFERENCES

Agbogu BN, Stern BJ, Sewell C et al. (1995). Therapeutic considerations in patients with refractory neurosarcoidosis. Arch Neurol 52: 875–9.

Ahmad K, Kim YH, Spitzer AR et al. (1992). Total nodal radiation in progressive sarcoidosis: case report. Am J Clin Oncol 15: 311–13.

Aizer A, Stern EH, Gomes JA et al. (2005). Usefulness of programmed ventricular stimulation in predicting future arrhythmic events in patients with cardiac sarcoidosis. Am J Cardiol 96: 276–82.

Bajaj AK, Kopelman HA, Echt DS (1988). Cardiac sarcoidosis with sudden death: treatment with the automatic implantable cardioverter defibrillator. Am Heart J 116: 557–60.

Bargout R, Kelly RF (2004). Sarcoid heart disease: clinical course and treatment. Int J Cardiol 97: 173–82.

Bernstein M, Konzelman FW, Sidlick DM (1929). Boeck's sarcoid: report of a case with visceral involvement. Arch Intern Med 4: 721–34.

Butany J, Bahl NE, Morales K et al. (2006). The intricacies of cardiac sarcoidosis: a case report involving the coronary arteries and a review of the literature. Cardiovasc Pathol 15: 222–7.

Chapelon-Abric C, de Zuttere D, Duhaut P et al. (2004). Cardiac sarcoidosis: a retrospective study of 41 cases. Medicine (Baltimore) 83: 315–34.

Demeter SL (1988). Myocardial sarcoidosis unresponsive to steroids: treatment with cyclophosphamide. Chest 94: 202–3.

Fleming HA (1973). Sarcoid heart disease. Br Med J 1: 174–5.

Fleming H (1994). Cardiac sarcoidosis. In: James D (ed.). Sarcoidosis and Other Granulomatous Disorders. Marcel Dekker, New York, pp. 323–34.

Fleming HA (1988). Death from sarcoid heart disease. United Kingdom series 1971–1986, 300 cases with 138 deaths. In: Grassi C, Rizzato G, Pozzi E (eds). Sarcoidosis and Other Granulomatous Disorders [11th world congress]. Elsevier, Amsterdam, p. 19.

Ghosh P, Fleming HA, Gresham GA et al. (1972). Myocardial sarcoidosis. Br Heart J 34: 769–73.

Grief M, Petrakopoulou P, Weiss M et al. (2008). Cardiac sarcoidosis concealed by arrhythmogenic right ventricular dysplasia/cardiomyopathy. Nat Clin Pract Cardiovasc Med 5: 231–6.

Hagemann GJ, Wurm K (1980). The clinical, electrocardiographic and pathological features of cardiac sarcoidosis. In: Jones Williams W, Davies BH (eds). Sarcoidosis and Other Granulomatous Diseases [8th international conference]. Alpha Omega, Cardiff, p. 601.

Hapelon-Abric C, de Zuttere D, DuHaut P et al. (2004). Cardiac sarcoidosis: a retrospective study of 41 cases. Medicine (Baltimore) 83: 315–34.

Hiraga H, Hiroe M, Iwai K et al. (1993). Guideline for Diagnosis of Cardiac Sarcoidosis [study report on diffuse pulmonary diseases]. Japanese Ministry of Health and Welfare, Tokyo, pp. 23–4

Ishikawa T, Kondoh H, Nakagawa S et al. (1984). Steroid therapy in cardiac sarcoidosis: increased left ventricular contractility concomitant with electrocardiographic improvement after prednisolone. Chest 85: 445–7.

Iwai K, Sekiguti M, Hosoda Y et al. (1994). Racial difference in cardiac sarcoidosis incidence observed at autopsy. Sarcoidosis 11: 26–31.

Johns CJ, Michele TM (1999). The clinical management of sarcoidosis: a 50-year experience at the Johns Hopkins Hospital. Medicine 78: 65–111.

Koplan BA, Soejima K, Baughman K et al. (2006). Refractory ventricular tachycardia secondary to cardiac sarcoid: electrophysiologic characteristics, mapping, and ablation. Heart Rhythm 3: 924–9.

Lower EE, Broderick JP, Brott TG et al. (1997). Diagnosis and management of neurological sarcoidosis. Arch Intern Med 157: 1864–8.

Matsui Y, Iwai K, Tachibana T et al. (1976). Clinicopathological study on fatal myocardial sarcoidosis. Ann NY Acad Sci 278: 455–69.

Mikhail JR, Mitchell DN, Bull KP (1974). Abnormal electrocardiographic findings in sarcoidosis. In: Kiwai, Hosoda Y (eds). Proceedings of 6th International Conference on Sarcoidosis. University of Tokyo Press, Tokyo, pp. 365–72.

Muller-Quernheim J, Kienast K, Held M et al. (1999). Treatment of chronic sarcoidosis with an azathioprine/prednisolone regimen. Eur Respir J 14: 1117–22.

Paz HL, McCormick DJ, Kutalek SP et al. (1994). The automated implantable cardiac defibrillator: prophylaxis in cardiac sarcoidosis. Chest 106: 1603–7.

Perry A, Vuitch F (1995). Causes of death in patients with sarcoidosis: a morphologic study of 38 autopsies with clinicopathologic correlations. Arch Pathol Lab Med 119: 167–72.

Pietinalho A, Tukiainen P, Haahtela T et al. (2002). Finnish Pulmonary Sarcoidosis Study Group: Early treatment of stage II sarcoidosis improves 5-year pulmonary function. Chest 121: 24–31.

Reuhl J, Schneider M, Sievert H et al. (1997). Myocardial sarcoidosis as a rare cause of sudden cardiac death. Forensic Sci Int 89: 145–53.

Roberts WC, McAllister HA, Ferrans VJ (1977). Sarcoidosis of the heart: a clinicopathologic study of 35 necropsy patients (group 1) and review of 78 previously described necropsy patients (group 11). Am J Med 63: 86–108.

Scadding JG (1967). Sarcoidosis. Eyre & Spottiswoode, London, p. 291.

Scadding JG, Mitchell DN (1985). The heart. In: .Sarcoidosis, 2nd edn. Chapman & Hall, London, pp. 329–48.

Sekiguchi M, Numao Y, Imai M et al. (1980). Clinical and histopathological profile of sarcoidosis of the heart and acute idiopathic myocarditis: concepts through a study employing endomyocardial biopsy. I: Sarcoidosis. Jpn Circ J 44: 249–63.

Sharma OP, Maheshwari A, Thaker K (1993). Myocardial sarcoidosis. Chest 103: 253–8.

Shammas RL, Movahed A (1994). Successful treatment of myocardial sarcoidosis with steroids. Sarcoidosis 11: 37–9.

Silverman KJ, Hutchins GM, Bulkley BH (1978). Cardiac sarcoid: a clinicopathologic study of 84 unselected patients with systemic sarcoidosis. Circulation 58: 1204–11.

Smedema JP, Snoep G, van Kroonenburgh MP et al. (2005). Cardiac involvement in patients with pulmonary sarcoidosis assessed at two university medical centers in the Netherlands. Chest 128: 30–5.

Suzuki T, Kanda T, Kubota S et al. (1994). Holter monitoring as a noninvasive indicator of cardiac involvement in sarcoidosis. Chest 106: 1021–4.

Syed J, Myers R (2004). Sarcoid heart disease. Can J Cardiol 20: 89–93.

Thomsen TK, Eriksson T (1999). Myocardial sarcoidosis in forensic medicine. *Am J Forensic Med Pathol* **20**: 52–6.

Uslu N, Akyol A, Gorgulu S *et al.* (2006). Heart rate variability in patients with systemic sarcoidosis. *Ann Noninvasive Electrocardiol* **11**: 38–42.

Valantine HA, Tazelaar HD, Macoviak J *et al.* (1987). Cardiac sarcoidosis: response to steroids and transplantation. *J Heart Transplant* **6**: 244–50.

Winters SL, Cohen M, Greenberg S *et al.* (1991). Sustained ventricular tachycardia associated with sarcoidosis: assessment of the underlying cardiac anatomy and the prospective utility of programmed ventricular stimulation, drug therapy and an implantable antitachycardia device. *J Am Coll Cardiol* **18**: 937–43.

Yazaki Y, Isobe M, Hiroe M *et al.* (2001). Prognostic determinants of long-term survival in Japanese patients with cardiac sarcoidosis treated with prednisone. *Am J Cardiol* **88**: 1006–10.

Yoshida Y, Morimoto S, Hiramitsu S *et al.* (1997). Incidence of cardiac sarcoidosis in Japanese patients with high-degree atrioventricular block. *Am Heart J* **134**: 382–6.

Zaidi AR, Zaidi A, Vaitkus PT (2007). Outcome of heart transplantation in patients with sarcoid cardiomyopathy. *J Heart Lung Transplant* **26**: 714–17.

Radionuclide imaging in cardiac sarcoidosis

KSHAMA WECHALEKAR, S RICHARD UNDERWOOD AND MICHAEL HUGHES

INTRODUCTION

Cardiac sarcoidosis can present with arrhythmia, heart failure or sudden death at any age. It is more frequent in younger patients and can even present in adolescence. The heart can be the sole site of involvement, and sudden death is common as a result of cardiac involvement that can be unrecognized in life.

Non-caseating granulomas can involve all cardiac structures such as the conduction system, papillary muscles, myocardium and pericardium. Myocardial involvement can present as hypertrophy or as abnormal regional function. Later on, myocardial scarring can replace the granulomas, leading to ventricular dilatation and remodeling, regional abnormalities or aneurysm. More diffuse involvement can lead to globally impaired function and left ventricular failure. Arrhythmias such as heart block can arise from involvement of conducting tissue, but tachyarrhythmias are also seen. Involvement of the pericardium can present with effusion.

Because early diagnosis and treatment can reduce morbidity and mortality it is important to investigate patients with possible cardiac involvement. The diagnosis of myocardial sarcoidosis can be either histological or clinical (Box 19b.1). Clinical diagnosis is difficult. The electrocardiogram, two-dimensional echocardiography, magnetic resonance imaging and radionuclide imaging using positron and single-photon emitters have been used, but no single test is dominant. Endomyocardial biopsy is insensitive because of the patchy nature of disease.

SINGLE-PHOTON IMAGING

Gallium-67

Gallium-67 has predominant gamma emissions at 93, 185 and 300 keV and a physical half-life of 78 hours. Injected

---

Box 19b.1 Criteria for the diagnosis of cardiac sarcoidosis

Histological diagnosis
Cardiac sarcoidosis is present when the histology of operative or endomyocardial biopsy specimens demonstrates epithelioid granuloma without caseation

Clinical diagnosis
In patients with histologically diagnosed extracardiac sarcoidosis and no other reason for myocardial abnormality, cardiac involvement is diagnosed when one component of item (a) and one or more of items (b–e) are present:

(a) complete right bundle branch block, left-axis deviation, atrioventricular block, ventricular tachycardia, premature ventricular contraction (>grade 2 in Lown's classification), or abnormal Q or ST–T changes on resting or Holter electrocardiography
(b) abnormal myocardial motion, regional myocardial thinning or thickening or dilatation of the LV
(c) abnormal myocardial perfusion scintigraphy in the absence of an ischemic cause or abnormal accumulation of gallium or technetium-99m pyrophosphate
(d) abnormal intracardiac pressure, low cardiac output or ejection fraction
(e) interstitial fibrosis or cellular infiltration of more than moderate grade in endomyocardial biopsies, even if the findings are non-specific.

Adapted from Japanese Ministry of Health and Welfare Guidelines (JMHWG) intravenously as gallium citrate, it is a non-specific marker of inflammation, infection and rapid cell division such as neoplasia. Normal biodistribution is to the liver, spleen, bone marrow, bone and the growth plates. Less intense uptake is seen in lachrymal and salivary glands and in the nasal mucosa. Low-grade uptake is seen in the breast tissue. Physiological uptake of gallium-67 is associated with conditions stimulating prolactin production or related to estrogenic hormone administration (Kim *et al.* 1977). It is excreted by the gut.

The mechanism of uptake of gallium into inflamed and neoplastic tissue is complex and may not be fully understood. After intravenous injection of gallium citrate, the gallium (as Ga^{3+}) is partly bound with high affinity to transferrin, an iron transport protein, and partly complexed with hydroxyl ions forming gallate ($Ga(OH)_4$) (Weiner 1996; Eguchi *et al.* 2000). The gallium–transferrin complex enters cells that express the transferrin receptor, such as macrophages and neoplastic cells, by endocytosis. Once inside the cell, both gallium moieties complex with the iron storage protein ferritin. The process of uptake can be slow and gallium scintigraphy is usually performed at 48 or 72 hours.

Scintigraphic localization of gallium into areas inflamed by sarcoid granulomas is helpful for the diagnosis and characterization of the disease as well as response to treatment, but uptake is also seen in other clinical conditions (Box 19b.2).

An advantage of gallium scintigraphy is the ability to image the whole body by either planar or tomographic imaging and to combine scintigraphy with X-ray computed tomography (CT) to aid localization (see Plate 15).

In patients with newly presenting arrhythmia, it is important to consider sarcoidosis in the differential diagnosis (Radulescu *et al.* 2010; Nomura *et al.* 2011). A study of patients with known cardiac sarcoidosis showed more frequent cardiac uptake in patients with ventricular tachycardia (VT) than in those without (71.4 vs 14.3 percent; $p < 0.05$) (Futamatsu *et al.* 2006). After steroid therapy, six of

the seven patients with VT who underwent repeat imaging showed reduced gallium uptake and there was no recurrence of VT.

Myocardial perfusion scintigraphy

Myocardial perfusion scintigraphy (MPS) has been used in patients with suspected myocardial sarcoidosis for many years. The longest established tracer is thallium-201, which has a main X-ray emission at 80 keV and a physical half-life of 72 hours. Injected as thallous chloride. it is a combined tracer of myocardial viability and perfusion and areas of reduced uptake after a resting injection indicate loss of viable myocardium. This is most commonly seen in ischaemic heart disease, but it can suggest myocardial replacement by fibrosis or granulomatous tissue if ischaemic heart disease is unlikely. Differentiation between ischaemic and inflammatory scarring is difficult, but the former commonly has profound defects corresponding with coronary territories and stress-induced defects caused by coronary obstruction. Even in the absence of ischaemic heart disease, thallium defects are not specific for sarcoidosis and they may be the result of other infiltrative disorders, inflammation or cardiomyopathy, as shown in Box 19b.2.

Related tracers of viability and perfusion are technetium-99m MIBI (methoxy isobutyl isonitrile) and tetrofosmin. These have some disadvantages for imaging viability and perfusion compared with thallium, but they have some physical advantages arising from the higher energy (140 keV) gamma photon and the shorter half-life (6 hours) of technetium-99m. Eguchi *et al.* (2000) studied 16 patients with sarcoidosis using MIBI or tetrofosmin MPS. Out of these, 6 patients were known to have cardiac involvement in the form of ventricular tachycardia, atrioventricular block or congestive heart failure. Twenty-five control subjects were also studied with the same technique. The total number of abnormal segments were highest in cardiac sarcoidosis (60 vs 32 percent in non-cardiac sarcoidosis, and 7 percent in controls; $p = 0.0001$). More frequent abnormalities were found in both ventricles compared with controls (LV 31 percent, RV 88 percent vs LV 0 percent, RV 32 percent; $p = 0.0001$). Left ventricular involvement was associated with heart block and congestive heart failure, and right ventricular involvement with right ventricular tachyarrhythmia.

The combination of MPS and gallium imaging can be helpful. In a study of 25 patients with sarcoidosis and no known ischaemic heart disease, six patients had resting thallium defects (Okayama *et al.* 1995). Four of these underwent gallium imaging and two had myocardial uptake of gallium. After steroid treatment there was clinical and scintigraphic improvement in two patients, with gallium uptake but no improvement in the other two.

In another study of 14 patients using gallium and MIBI perfusion, myocardial gallium uptake was seen in nine patients (Nakazawa *et al.* 2004). In seven of these, the site of gallium uptake corresponded with a MIBI defect and the gallium uptake was supressed by steroid therapy in all. Of the five patients without myocardial gallium uptake, two had MIBI defects and both had already received steroids.

Box 19b.2 Causes of gallium uptake in the heart

Endocardium
- Bacterial endocarditis, neoplasm

Myocardium
- Myocardial infarction, myocarditis, sarcoidosis, amyloidosis, Kawasaki's disease, secondary syphilis, myocardial abscess, histiocytic lymphoma

Epicardium
- Histiocytic lymphoma

Pericardium
- Neoplastic: melanoma, histiocytic lymphoma
- Infectious pericarditis: bacterial, viral, tuberculosis, histoplasmosis
- Non-infectious: inflammatory pericarditis, post pericardiotomy syndrome

Adapted from Skye and Rao (1983)

Imaging sympathetic innervation

Small fiber neuropathy occurs frequently in sarcoidosis and autonomic dysfunction can be a consequence. Iodine-123 meta-iodo-benzyl guanidine (mIBG) concentrates in presynaptic sympathetic nerve terminals following uptake by the uptake-1 mechanism normally used to replenish neuronal norepinephrine stores (Tobes *et al.* 1985). The tracer is commonly used to detect phaeochromocytoma and it can also be used to assess prognosis in patients with heart failure (Jacobson *et al.* 2010). It is normally imaged 15 minutes and 4 hours after intravenous injection, and both planar and emission tomographic imaging are relatively simple.

Meta-IBG imaging has been combined with MPS in patients with myocardial sarcoidosis. The defects of innervation were found to be larger than those of viability but the locations generally corresponded, suggesting that sympathetic innervation imaging may be more sensitive than myocardial scarring imaging (Misumi *et al.* 1996). In 32 of 45 consecutive patients with sarcoidosis who had abnormal thermal threshold testing indicating small fiber neuropathy, there was mild to moderate heterogeneity of sympathetic innervation but only a minority of these had abnormal autonomic function by tilt testing (Hoitsma *et al.* 2005). A case with improved sympathetic innervation after carvedilol in a patient with sarcoidosis, small fiber neuropathy and autonomic dysfunction has been described (Smulders *et al.* 2008).

These studies confirm that abnormal sympathetic innervation can be imaged in sarcoidosis, but prospective studies are required to establish whether mIBG can have a routine role in investigation.

POSITRON EMISSION TOMOGRAPHY

Positron emission tomography (PET) is a nuclear imaging technique using radiopharmaceuticals that emit positrons. The positron annihilates with an electron to produce 511 keV gamma photons emitted in opposite directions, and this allows localization of the events when the photons are detected simultaneously by opposing detectors. PET images have higher spatial resolution than SPECT and they also have the potential for quantification. It does, however, have the disadvantage of greater complexity, cost and the need for an on-site cyclotron for the very short-lived tracers.

The most commonly used tracer is 2-deoxy-2-(^{18}F)fluoro-D-glucose (FDG). Fluorine-18 has a half-life of 110 minutes and so is normally available from commercial radiopharmacies without the need for an on-site cyclotron. FDG is a glucose analog that is transported, phosphorylated and trapped in cells in proportion to their glucose metabolism. It is widely used in oncology to detect malignancy. The normal myocardium in the fasting states obtains its energy by fatty acid metabolism, but when glucose-loaded or when metabolically challenged by ischaemia or inflammation it switches to glucose metabolism. Abnormalities are therefore either increased uptake in the fasting state or reduced uptake when glucose-loaded. FDG is most commonly used in the

heart to image myocardial viability, but it can also be used to detect tumours and myocardial inflammation in sarcoidosis (see Plate 16). Other PET tracers are rubidium-82 as shown in Plate 16 (Le Guludec *et al.* 2008), ^{13}N-ammonia and ^{15}O-water for myocardial viability and perfusion imaging, and ^{11}C-acetate for myocardial metabolism (Ishida *et al.* 1998).

Okumura and colleagues used FDG PET to detect myocardial sarcoidosis (Okumura *et al.* 1999). Ten of 16 patients with sarcoidosis had cardiac abnormalities suggesting cardiac involvement, and all of them had abnormal myocardial FDG uptake, whereas 80 percent had abnormal MIBI scans and only 50 percent had abnormal gallium uptake. The regions with abnormal glucose metabolism did not necessarily correspond with scarring indicated by MIBI defects, consistent with the different processes imaged by each tracer.

Yamagishi and colleagues investigated whether combined ammonia perfusion imaging and FDG metabolic imaging could identify cardiac involvement in patients with sarcoidosis (Yamagishi *et al.* 2003). The FDG imaging was performed under fasting conditions so that uptake was only seen in abnormal areas. Fourteen of 17 patients had areas of abnormal FDG uptake and 13 had perfusion abnormalities by ammonia PET, but only 6 had myocardial scarring by thallium imaging and 3 had myocardial inflammation by gallium imaging. The ammonia perfusion abnormalities were observed most frequently in the basal anteroseptal myocardium and FDG uptake most frequently in the basal and mid-anteroseptal and lateral myocardium with apical involvement being rare. In seven patients who had follow-up imaging one month after steroid treatment, the ammonia defects did not change but the FDG abnormalities were decreased or abolished. The authors concluded that combined ammonia and FDG PET was the most useful method for both the detection and monitoring of myocardial involvement.

Twenty-two patients with systemic sarcoidosis, half of whom had cardiac involvement according to the Japanese guidelines (see Box 19.1) although not including the scintigraphic criteria, were studied with fasting FDG PET, MIBI SPECT and gallium scintigraphy. The sensitivity of FDG PET for detecting myocardial involvement was 100 percent, compared with 64 percent for MIBI and 36 percent for gallium, and the overall accuracy of FDG was higher than that of gallium. It was concluded that FDG is able to detect myocardial inflammation at an earlier stage than gallium, and that detecting inflammation is more sensitive than detecting scarring (Okumura *et al.* 2004).

The period of fasting before FDG imaging may be relevant, since brief overnight fasting may not adequately suppress myocardial glucose utilization. Langah and colleagues reviewed 76 patients with suspected cardiac sarcoidosis who had either FDG PET after an 18-hour fast or gallium scintigraphy (Langah *et al.* 2009). Using the Japanese guidelines as the reference standard (see Box 19.1) the sensitivity, specificity and accuracy of PET were 85, 90 and 87 percent, respectively, compared with 15, 80 and 43 percent for gallium; and the authors highlighted the importance of revising the guidelines to incorporate PET and the importance of adequate fasting before myocardial FDG PET.

Table 19b.1   Imaging characteristics in cardiac sarcoidosis

Imaging technique	Physiological process	Strengths	Weaknesses
Gallium-67	Inflammation	Widely available; whole-body imaging with little confounding uptake; easily combined with CT, monitoring treatment response	High radiation exposure, 48- to 72-hour imaging
Thallium-201	Myocardial viability and perfusion	Widely available	Intermediate radiation exposure; low resolution; hence insensitive for scarring
Technetium-99m-sestamibi and tetrofosmin	Myocardial viability and perfusion	Widely available; LV function	Intermediate radiation exposure; low resolution; hence insensitive for scarring
Iodine-123 mIBG	Sympathetic innervation and tone	No simple alternative, more sensitive than viability imaging	Cost; limited experience
FDG	Glucose metabolism and inflammation	Whole-body imaging with little confounding uptake; easily combined with CT; sensitive	Cost; prolonged fasting
Nitrogen-13 ammonia	Myocardial viability and perfusion	Easily combined with FDG	Cost; on-site cyclotron
Magnetic resonance imaging	Cardiac function, oedema and fibrosis	High contrast and resolution; monitoring treatment response	Incompatible with pacemakers

FDG, 2-deoxy-2-(^{18}F)fluoro-d-glucose; mIBG, meta-iodo-benzyl guanidine

COMPARISON WITH MAGNETIC RESONANCE IMAGING

Magnetic resonance imaging (MRI) is another valuable technique for the diagnosis and monitoring of cardiac sarcoidosis (Matsuki and Matsuo 2000; Shimada et al. 2001; Smedema et al. 2005,2006). Active myocardial lesions are seen with increased signal on T_2-weighted imaging because of oedema, and increased signal on late gadolinium enhancement imaging (LGE) because of fibrosis (Vignaux et al. 2002; Slater et al. 2003; Vignaux 2005).The oedema signal can be used to monitor the effect of corticosteroid treatment but the fibrosis signal does not change with treatment (Matoh et al. 2008).

A disadvantage of MRI is the difficulty of imaging patients with pacemakers, which are implanted in a significant proportion of patients with cardiac sarcoidosis, although MRI-compatible pacemakers will become more common in the future.

FDG imaging and MRI provide complementary diagnostic information (Ishimaru et al. 2005), and the characteristics of the various imaging options are summarized in Table 19b.1.

CONCLUSION

Rapid advances in radionuclide imaging techniques from planar imaging to SPECT and PET and the development of new tracers have enhanced the diagnosis, assessment of prognosis and monitoring of treatment response in cardiac sarcoidosis. Although a specific tracer for cardiac involvement has not yet been developed, the combination of conventional clinical assessment with imaging can be very valuable (Sharma 2009). Assuming that prospective clinical trials confirm the evidence already available, revised diagnostic criteria and guidelines can be expected to include imaging in the routine assessment of patients with known or suspected cardiac sarcoidosis.

REFERENCES

Eguchi M, Tsuchihashi K et al. (2000). Technetium-99m sestamibi/tetrofosmin myocardial perfusion scanning in cardiac and non-cardiac sarcoidosis. Cardiology 94(3): 193–9.

Futamatsu H, Suzuki J, Adachi S et al. (2006). Utility of gallium-67 scintigraphy for evaluation of cardiac sarcoidosis with ventricular tachycardia. Int J Cardiovasc Imaging 22: 443–8.

Hoitsma E, Faber CG et al. (2005). Association of small fiber neuropathy with cardiac sympathetic dysfunction in sarcoidosis. Sarcoid Vasc Diff Lung Dis 22: 43–50.

Ishida Y, Fukuchi K et al. (1998). Imaging of myocardial perfusion and metabolism with positron emission tomography. Nippon Rinsho 56: 813–23.

Ishimaru S, Tsujino I et al. (2005). Combination of ^{18}F-fluoro-2-deoxyglucose positron emission tomography and magnetic resonance imaging in assessing cardiac sarcoidosis. Sarcoid Vasc Diff Lung Dis 22: 234–5.

Jacobson AF, Senior R et al. (2010). Myocardial iodine-123 meta-iodobenzylguanidine imaging and cardiac events in heart failure: results of the prospective ADMIRE-HF (AdreView Myocardial Imaging for Risk Evaluation in Heart Failure) study. J Am Coll Cardiol 55: 2212–21.

Kim YC, Brown ML et al. (1977). Scintigraphic patterns of gallium-67 uptake in the breast. Radiology 124: 169–75.

Langah R, Spicer K et al. (2009). Effectiveness of prolonged fasting ^{18}F-FDG PET-CT in the detection of cardiac sarcoidosis. J Nucl Cardiol 16: 801–10.

Le Guludec D, Lautamaki R et al. (2008). Present and future of clinical cardiovascular PET imaging in Europe: a position statement by the European Council of Nuclear Cardiology (ECNC). Eur J Nucl Med Mol Imaging 35: 1709–24.

Matoh F, Satoh H et al. (2008). The usefulness of delayed enhancement magnetic resonance imaging for diagnosis and evaluation of cardiac function in patients with cardiac sarcoidosis. J Cardiol 51(3): 179–88.

Matsuki M, Matsuo M (2000). MR findings of myocardial sarcoidosis. Clin Radiol 55: 323–5.

Misumi I, Kimura Y et al. (1996). Scintigraphic detection of regional disruption of the adrenergic nervous system in sarcoid heart disease. Jpn Circ J 60: 774–8.

Nakazawa A, Ikeda K, Ito Y et al. (2004). Usefulness of dual 67Ga and 99mTc-sestamibi single-photon-emission CT scanning in the diagnosis of cardiac sarcoidosis. Chest 126: 1372–6.

Nomura S, Funabashi N, Tsubura M et al. (2011). Cardiac sarcoidosis evaluated by multimodality imaging. Int J Cardiol 150: e81–4.

Okayama K, Kurata C et al. (1995). Diagnostic and prognostic value of myocardial scintigraphy with thallium-201 and gallium-67 in cardiac sarcoidosis. Chest 107: 330–4.

Okumura W., Iwasaki T. et al. (1999). Usefulness of ^{18}F-FDG PET for diagnosis of cardiac sarcoidosis. Kaku Igaku 36: 341–8.

Okumura W, Iwasaki T et al. (2004). Usefulness of fasting ^{18}F-FDG PET in identification of cardiac sarcoidosis. J Nucl Med 45: 1989–98.

Radulescu B, Imperiale A, Germain P, Ohlmann P (2010). Severe ventricular arrhythmias in a patient with cardiac sarcoidosis: insights from MRI and PET imaging and importance of early corticosteroid therapy. Eur Heart J 31: 400.

Sharma S. (2009). Cardiac imaging in myocardial sarcoidosis and other cardiomyopathies. Curr Opin Pulm Med 15: 507–12.

Shimada T, Shimada K et al. (2001). Diagnosis of cardiac sarcoidosis and evaluation of the effects of steroid therapy by gadolinium-DTPA-enhanced magnetic resonance imaging. Am J Med 110: 520–7.

Skye HW, Rao BR (1983). Cardiac gallium citrate concentration. Eur J Nucl Med 8: 507–8.

Slater GM, Rodriguez ER et al. (2003). A unique presentation of cardiac sarcoidosis. Am J Roentgenol 180: 1738–9.

Smedema JP, Snoep G, van Kroonenburgh MP et al. (2005). Evaluation of the accuracy of gadolinium-enhanced cardiovascular magnetic resonance in the diagnosis of cardiac sarcoidosis. J Am Coll Cardiol 45: 1683–90.

Smedema JP, Truter R, de Klerk PA et al. (2006). Cardiac sarcoidosis evaluated with gadolinium-enhanced magnetic resonance and contrast-enhanced 64-slice computed tomography. Int J Cardiol 112: 261–3.

Smulders NM, Bast A et al. (2008). Improvement of cardiac sympathetic nerve function in sarcoidosis. Sarcoid Vasc Diff Lung Dis 25: 140–2.

Tobes MC, Jaques S et al. (1985). Effect of uptake-one inhibitors on the uptake of norepinephrine and metaiodobenzylguanidine. J Nucl Med 26: 897–907.

Vignaux O (2005). Cardiac sarcoidosis: spectrum of MRI features. Am J Roentgenol 184: 249–54.

Vignaux O, Dhote R et al. (2002). Detection of myocardial involvement in patients with sarcoidosis applying T_2-weighted, contrast-enhanced, and cine magnetic resonance imaging: initial results of a prospective study. J Comput Assist Tomogr 26: 762–7.

Weiner RE (1996). The mechanism of 67Ga localization in malignant disease. Nucl Med Biol 23: 745–51.

Yamagishi H, Shirai N et al. (2003). Identification of cardiac sarcoidosis with (13)N-NH(3)/(18)F-FDG PET. J Nucl Med 44: 1030–6.

20

Pulmonary hypertension

T J CORTE AND S J WORT

DEFINITION AND CLASSIFICATION

Pulmonary hypertension (PH) is defined hemodynamically by right heart catheter (RHC) measurements of a mean pulmonary arterial pressure (mPAP) ≥ 25 mmHg at rest, with a pulmonary capillary wedge pressure ≥ 15 mmHg and pulmonary vascular resistance ≥ 3 Wood units.

The classification of pulmonary hypertension was revised at the world symposium on pulmonary arterial hypertension (PAH) at Dana Point (Box 20.1) (Simonneau et al. 2009). Pulmonary hypertension was divided into five main groups. PH associated with lung disease or hypoxemia was identified as a distinct subgroup, with subcategories including PH related to interstitial lung disease. As the pathogenesis of PH in sarcoidosis is complex and multifactorial, sarcoidosis is included in the fifth 'miscellaneous' group. However, it has been suggested that sarcoidosis fits into all five PH classes (Baughman 2007).

PREVALENCE OF PH IN SARCOIDOSIS

Pulmonary hypertension is a well-recognized complication of sarcoidosis, occurring in 5–74 percent of patients (Mayock et al. 1963; Battesti et al. 1978; Rizzato et al. 1983; Shorr et al. 2005; Shigemitsu et al. 2007). The exact prevalence of PH in sarcoidosis is unknown, and it clearly differs depending on the measurement technique and patient selection criteria used in the screening process.

In unselected sarcoidosis cohorts, 5–6 percent of patients have PH on either echocardiography or RHC (Rizzato et al. 1983; Handa et al. 2006). However, following exercise, up to 43 percent of sarcoidosis patients may develop PH (Gluskowski et al. 1984). Moreover, PH is present in 47 percent of patients with dyspnea out of proportion to their pulmonary function abnormalities (Baughman et al. 2006). PH is more common in patients with advanced sarcoidosis, and has been reported in up to 74 percent of sarcoidosis patients awaiting lung transplantation (Shorr et al. 2005). However, PH is not always associated with pulmonary sarcoidosis, with 40–60 percent of patients with sarcoid-associated PH (SAPH) having no radiographic evidence of pulmonary fibrosis (Sulica et al. 2005; Nunes et al. 2006). The severity of the PH does not correlate well with the severity of the underlying lung disease (Emirgil et al. 1971; Handa et al. 2006; Nunes et al. 2006). In fact, PH may be more severe when it occurs in the absence of fibrotic pulmonary sarcoidosis (Nunes et al. 2006). This suggests that there are other factors apart from the underlying lung disease contributing to the pathogenesis of PH.

IMPLICATIONS OF PH IN SARCOIDOSIS

Patients with SAPH have poorer functional status, and greater supplemental oxygen requirements than sarcoid patients without PH (Shorr et al. 2003). Indeed, in one study, over 70 percent of patients with SAPH required assistance with daily functional activities (Shorr et al. 2003). Little is known about the natural history of SAPH. Patients with SAPH are more likely to be listed for lung transplantation than those with isolated pulmonary sarcoidosis (Shorr et al. 2005). Moreover, SAPH in the absence of pulmonary fibrosis may be a more rapidly progressive disorder, with higher pulmonary vascular resistance levels (Nunes et al. 2006).

SAPH is usually mild to moderate in severity, with survival depending on the severity of the underlying lung disease,

Box 20.1 Dana Point classification of pulmonary arterial hypertension (PAH)

1. **Pulmonary arterial hypertension (PAH)**
    1.1   Idiopathic PAH
    1.2   Heritable
          1.2.1   BMPR2
          1.2.2   ALK1, endoglin ± hereditary hemorrhagic telangectasia)
          1.2.3   Unknown
    1.3   Drug- and toxin-induced
    1.4   Associated with:
          1.4.1   Collagen tissue diseases
          1.4.2   HIV infection
          1.4.3   Portal hypertension
          1.4.4   Congenital heart disease
          1.4.5   Schistosomiasis
          1.4.6   Chronic hemolytic anemia
    1.5   Persistent pulmonary hypertension of the newborn

1. **Pulmonary veno-occlusive disease and/or pulmonary capillary haemangiomatosis**

2. **Pulmonary hypertension with left heart disease**
    2.1   Left-sided atrial or ventricular heart disease
    2.2   Left-sided valvular heart disease

3. **Pulmonary hypertension associated with lung diseases and/or hypoxemia**
    3.1   Chronic obstructive pulmonary disease
    3.2   Interstitial lung disease
    3.3   Other pulmonary diseases with mixed restrictive and obstructive pattern
    3.4   Sleep-disordered breathing
    3.5   Alveolar hypoventilation disorders
    3.6   Chronic exposure to high altitude
    3.7   Developmental abnormalities

4. **Chronic thromboembolic pulmonary hypertension (CTEPH)**

5. **Pulmonary hypertension with unclear and/or multifactorial mechanisms**
    5.1   Hematologic disorders: myeloproliferative disorders, splenectomy
    5.2   Systemic disorders: sarcoidosis, pulmonary Langerhans cell histiocytosis, lymphangioleiomyomatosis, neurofibromatosis, vasculitis
    5.3   Metabolic disorders: glycogen storage disease, Gaucher disease, thyroid disorders
    5.4   Others: tumoral obstruction, fibrosing mediastinitis, chronic renal failure on dialysis

rather than the PH *per se*. However, PH is an independent risk factor for mortality in sarcoidosis patients awaiting lung transplantation (Arcasoy *et al.* 2001; Shorr *et al.* 2002, 2003). In one study, an elevated right atrial pressure above 15 mmHg was the strongest predictor of mortality in sarcoidosis patients listed for lung transplantation (Arcasoy *et al.* 2001). Prognosis

of SAPH is poor, with an estimated 5-year survival of only 59 percent (Nunes *et al.* 2006). These reports have led to the recommendation for early assessment for lung transplantation for patients with SAPH (Orens *et al.* 2006).

PATHOPHYSIOLOGY OF PH

The pathophysiology of PH related to sarcoidosis is complex, with multiple mechanisms contributing (Fig. 20.1).

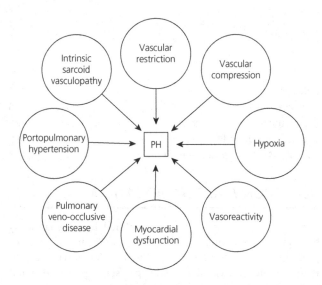

Figure 20.1   Mechanisms involved in the pathophysiology of pulmonary hypertension associated with sarcoidosis.

DESTRUCTION OF THE PULMONARY VASCULAR BED

Historically, SAPH has been attributed to the obliteration of the vascular bed by parenchymal fibrosis (Mitchell and Scadding 1974). SAPH is more common in patients with advanced pulmonary fibrosis, with the majority of patients having chest radiography in stage IV (Nunes *et al.* 2006) and impaired pulmonary function tests. However, SAPH occurs in the absence of significant pulmonary fibrosis (Smith *et al.* 1983; Shorr *et al.* 2005); and in severe SAPH there is an inverse relationship between vital capacity and mean pulmonary arterial pressures (Shorr *et al.* 2005), indicating that fibrotic ablation alone cannot account for all SAPH.

EXTRINSIC COMPRESSION OF PULMONARY VESSELS

In contrast to other interstitial lung diseases (ILDs), extrinsic compression of the large pulmonary arteries by sarcoid lymphadenopathy (Damuth *et al.* 1980; Nunes *et al.* 2006) or mediastinal fibrosis (Hamilton-Craig *et al.* 2009; Toonkel *et al.* 2010) may result in increased pulmonary vascular resistance. However, a recent Japanese study showed no relationship between SAPH and mediastinal lymphadenopathy on high-resolution CT scanning (Handa *et al.* 2006).

HYPOXIC VASOCONSTRICTION AND PULMONARY VASCULAR REMODELING

Hypoxia is a known trigger for pulmonary vasoconstriction and, over time, this may lead to pulmonary vascular remodeling. However, the role of hypoxemia is not clearly defined in SAPH. In advanced sarcoidosis, patients with SAPH have higher oxygen requirements, with patients with severe SAPH having a 7-fold increase in oxygen supplementation (Shorr *et al.* 2005). However, in this study, there was no independent relationship found between pulmonary pressures and the level of hypoxemia, suggesting strongly that, in many cases, factors other than hypoxia play a role in the development of PH in sarcoidosis.

INCREASED VASOREACTIVITY

There may be increased pulmonary vasoreactivity in sarcoidosis, as suggested by the favorable acute response to vasodilators, including nitric oxide (NO) (Preston *et al.* 2001; Fisher *et al.* 2006) and prostacyclin (Barst and Ratner 1985; Jones *et al.* 1989). The mechanism for this increase in pulmonary vasoreactivity is not clear, but it may be related to endothelial damage from sarcoid granulomas. Endothelial dysfunction may result in decreased synthesis and release of NO and prostaglandins, leading to an imbalance of endothelial-derived vasoactive mediators, with subsequent pulmonary vasoconstriction and remodeling.

PULMONARY VENO-OCCLUSIVE DISEASE

Pulmonary veno-occlusive disease (PVOD) is a recognized complication of sarcoidosis (Hoffstein *et al.* 1986; Jones *et al.* 2009). In one SAPH study, 5 of 22 patients had evidence of PVOD at biopsy, but all patients had an occlusive venopathy with intimal fibrosis and evidence of chronic hemosiderosis (Nunes *et al.* 2006), leading the authors to suggest that the contribution of PVOD to SAPH may be underestimated.

MYOCARDIAL DYSFUNCTION

Direct myocardial infiltration by sarcoid granulomas may lead to left ventricular systolic or diastolic dysfunction (Preston *et al.* 2001; Baughman *et al.* 2006). Indeed, the pulmonary capillary wedge pressure is elevated in approximately 10 percent of SAPH patients, and it is imperative to exclude left-heart dysfunction in the investigation of SAPH. However, neither the pulmonary capillary wedge pressure nor cardiac index were predictive of SAPH in sarcoidosis patients awaiting lung transplantation (Shorr *et al.* 2005), indicating that myocardial dysfunction probably plays a minor role in the pathogenesis of SAPH.

PORTOPULMONARY HYPERTENSION

Hepatic sarcoid infiltration and subsequent cirrhosis is not an uncommon complication of sarcoidosis, and, consequently, portopulmonary hypertension may develop (Salazar *et al.* 1994). Although portopulmonary hypertension is rare in sarcoidosis, hepatic ultrasound is recommended in the investigation of SAPH.

INSTRINSIC SARCOID VASCULOPATHY

Granulomatous invasion of the pulmonary vessel wall is common in SAPH, occurring in 69–100 percent of cases (Rosen *et al.* 1977; Takemura *et al.* 1992). Sarcoid granulomas are preferentially located in the pulmonary lymphatics that are adjacent to the pulmonary vessels. This may explain how vascular involvement may occur in the absence of pulmonary fibrosis. All layers of the vessel wall are involved in this granulomatous 'vasculitis', with resultant occlusive vasculopathy occurring in the small pulmonary aretrioles and venules (Shigemitsu *et al.* 2007; Plate 14 and Fig. 20.2). The occlusive venous changes may mimic PVOD hemodynamically.

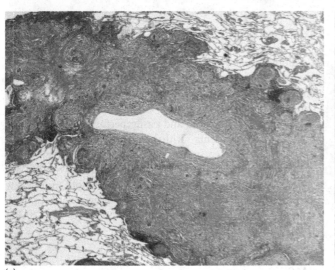

(a)

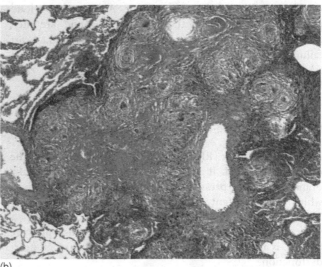

(b)

Figure 20.2   (a–b) Histopathology of the pulmonary artery in sarcoid-associated pulmonary hypertension. Expansion of all three layers of the pulmonary artery is present in SAPH. Reprinted with permission from Corte TJ *et al.* (2011). Pulmonary hypertension in sarcoidosis: a review. *Respirology* 16: 69–77.

POSSIBLE MEDIATORS INVOLVED IN PH

Endothelin-1 (ET-1) is produced mainly by endothelial cells, but also by leukocytes, macrophages and smooth muscle cells (Luscher and Barton 2000), and its production is induced by hypoxia, shear stress, and various growth factors and cytokines (Galie et al. 2004). ET-1 acts directly on smooth muscle cells, binding to ETA and ETB receptors, leading to vasoconstriction (Pollock et al. 1995), cytokine and growth-factor production (Luscher and Barton 2000) and increased inflammation and platelet aggregation (Jozsef et al. 2002). It also binds to ETB receptors on endothelial cells, stimulating nitric oxide (NO) and prostacyclin release, leading to endothelium-dependent vasodilation. ET-1 thus has a bimodal effect, with an initial mild vasodilation, followed by prolonged vasoconstriction (Eddahibi et al. 1993). ET-1 may, therefore, have an acute vasoconstrictive effect, or a longer-term effect of pulmonary vascular remodeling.

ET-1 has been implicated in the pathogenesis of idiopathic pulmonary arterial hypertension. In some patients with sarcoidosis, ET-1 levels are increased in the urine, plasma and bronchoalveolar lavage fluid (Letizia et al. 2001; Reichenberger et al. 2001; Terashita et al. 2006). ET-1 may play a role in the development of SAPH. However, it is unclear whether ET-1 is an inflammatory marker or a marker for pulmonary vascular remodeling in sarcoidosis (Diaz-Guzman et al. 2008).

DIAGNOSIS OF PH

Recognition of SAPH may be delayed, as it is often confounded by the clinical features of underlying pulmonary sarcoidosis. Symptoms, including dyspnea, cough, reduced exercise capacity and fatigue, are common to both SAPH and pulmonary sarcoidosis (Baughman et al. 2006, 2007). One study reported no difference in the presenting symptoms of sarcoidosis patients with and without PH (Sulica et al. 2005). Physical signs reflective of SAPH (such as a loud pulmonary component of the second heart sound) are often difficult to hear in respiratory disease. Signs of right heart failure (including peripheral edema) occur in 21 percent of SAPH patients, and are generally late findings (Sulica et al. 2005).

RIGHT HEART CATHETER

Right heart catheter (RHC) remains the gold standard for the diagnosis of SAPH. It allows the direct measurement of the pulmonary artery pressure and right atrial pressure, both of which are important prognostic indicators (Arcasoy et al. 2001; Shorr et al. 2003). An estimation of either left ventricular pressure or pulmonary arterial wedge pressure at RHC is also important to exclude the presence of left heart dysfunction.

RHC is a moderately invasive procedure, requiring hospital admission, and so a number of non-invasive investigations are often used to screen for disease in the assessment for PH.

ECHOCARDIOGRAPHY

Continuous Doppler flow echocardiography allows estimation of the systolic pulmonary arterial pressure (PAP) from the maximal velocity of the tricuspid regurgitation jet. It is not possible to estimate the systolic PAP in the absence of tricuspid regurgitation. Although echocardiography is the most reliable non-invasive method to diagnose SAPH – with good correlation between systolic pulmonary arterial pressure measurements on echocardiography and RHC (Baughman et al. 2006) – its accuracy is lower in patients with chronic lung disease (Arcasoy et al. 2003). However, echocardiography does complement RHC in the assessment of PH as it provides other, structural cardiac information.

NATRIURETIC PEPTIDES

Brain natriuretic peptide (BNP) is released in response to atrial and ventricular wall stretch. Plasma BNP concentrations are elevated in pulmonary arterial hypertension. There is some evidence to suggest that elevated BNP is also a marker of poor prognosis in patients with chronic lung diseases (Leuchte et al. 2006).

PULMONARY FUNCTION

Sarcoidosis patients with SAPH have lower Pao_2 and diffusion capacity for carbon monoxide (DLco) levels than those without PH (Handa et al. 2005). In fact, sarcoidosis patients with DLco levels below 60 percent have a 7-fold risk of having SAPH (Bourbonnais and Samavati 2008). Patients with SAPH have lower lung volumes, however, so there is poor correlation between spirometric volumes and PAP, as PH can develop at any stage of the underlying disease (Sulica et al. 2005). In fact, an inverse relationship between vital capacity and mean pulmonary artery pressure is present in patients with severe SAPH (Shorr et al. 2005).

EXERCISE TESTING

Cardiopulmonary exercise tests (CPETs) may be useful to identify early, or exercise-induced PH, as a cause of exercise-limitation in these patients with sarcoidosis. However, if patients are unable to perform CPET, 6-minute walk testing (6MWT), a reproducible and easily performed test, may be used instead. Patients with SAPH have lower 6MWT distance, and lower end-exercise Spo_2 (Baughman et al. 2007; Bourbonnais and Samavati 2008). Patients with 6MWT oxygen desaturation below 90 percent are 12-fold more likely to have SAPH, and thus 6MWT has been suggested as a screening test to identify high-risk patients for SAPH (Bourbonnais and Samavati 2008).

IMAGING

Patients with SAPH are more likely to have advanced chest radiography stages (stage III and IV) (Sulica et al. 2005; Handa et al. 2006). However, fibrosis is not always evident on

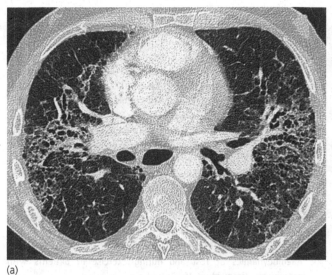
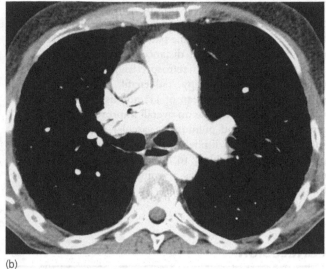

(a)   (b)

Figure 20.3   (a, b) CT scans of a patient with sarcoidosis and pulmonary hypertension, with dilatation of the main pulmonary artery compared to the aorta. Reprinted with permission from Corte TJ *et al.* (2011). Pulmonary hypertension in sarcoidosis: a review. *Respirology* 16: 69–77.

chest radiography, and the absence of fibrotic changes should not preclude further evaluation for SAPH (Nunes *et al.* 2006).

The main and segmental pulmonary artery size may be measured on computerized tomography (Fig. 20.3). There is little data to support the use of CT in the diagnosis of PH in patients with lung disease (Zisman *et al.* 2007; Devaraj *et al.* 2008). However, CT scans provide additional important structural information, including central compression of the pulmonary vessels by mediastinal lymphadenopathy, or evidence suggestive of PVOD (Nunes *et al.* 2006).

Cardiac MRI provides the most accurate measurement of right ventricular mass and ejection fraction. Its role in the diagnosis of PH in this patient group is promising, but requires further study.

MANAGEMENT OF SARCOID-ASSOCIATED PH

Management of SAPH is controversial, and is based on limited evidence. Hypoxemia correlates to some extent with the severity of PH, and supplemental oxygen is thus recommended to reverse resting hypoxemia. Full assessment and treatment of co-morbidities (including left ventricular systolic or diastolic heart failure, pulmonary emboli and obstructive sleep apnea) is also important.

There are conflicting reports regarding the use of corticosteroids, with some describing improvement (Davies *et al.* 1982; Mangla *et al.* 1985; Rodman and Lindenfeld 1990), and others worsening of SAPH (Damuth *et al.* 1980; Barst and Ratner 1985; Gluskowski *et al.* 1990). One study describes an improvement following corticosteroid treatment in patients with limited pulmonary fibrosis, but no effect in patients with stage IV disease (Nunes *et al.* 2006). These results suggest that corticosteroids may be useful in a subset of SAPH patients. It is difficult to predict which patients will benefit from corticosteroid therapy. Patients with active inflammation, or PH associated with compression of the proximal pulmonary

vessels by mediastinal lymphadenopathy, may be more likely to benefit from corticosteroid therapy.

Specific PH therapy is not routinely recommended in SAPH as there are no successful placebo-controlled trials of disease-targeted PH therapies in this patient group. Several studies have reported an acute improvement in pulmonary hemodynamics following the administration of pulmonary vasodilators, including intravenous epoprostenol and inhaled NO (Preston *et al.* 2001; Fisher *et al.* 2006). In one study of six SAPH patients, intravenous epoprostenol was given for a mean of 29 months. Five patients had an improvement in functional class, and there was one death. In another study of eight patients receiving longer-term inhaled NO, five patients had an improvement of 6-minute walking distance and three had an improvement in functional class (Preston *et al.* 2001). There is concern over pulmonary vasodilators leading to increased pulmonary shunting and worsened ventilation–perfusion mismatch, with subsequent hypoxia. Furthermore, in patients with post-capillary PH (including PVOD), vasodilators may lead to acute pulmonary edema, and sudden death. Vasodilators must therefore be used with caution in SAPH.

ET-1 is thought to play an important role in the pathophysiology of SAPH. There have been a number of recent publications of case reports of successful therapy with the ET-1 receptor antagonist bosentan (Foley and Metersky 2005; Sharma *et al.* 2005; Pitsiou *et al.* 2009). Baughman and associates treated five patients with a mean mPAP of 50 mmHg with bosentan for at least 4 months, and found that the mPAP fell significantly to 35 mmHg in the three patients with repeat RHC (Baughman *et al.* 2006). A randomized, placebo-controlled study with bosentan is currently under way in SAPH patients.

Sildenafil, a phosphodiesterase type-5 inhibitor, is a pulmonary vasodilator with an antiproliferative effect on vascular smooth muscle cells. Sildenafil may be a more selective pulmonary vasodilator, thus leading to less ventilation–perfusion mismatch and hypoxia than other vasodilators. A recent Danish study of 12 SAPH patients receiving sildenafil for a median of 4 months showed an improvement in mPAP and cardiac output in the nine patients with repeat RHC, but no improvement in 6MWT distance (Milman *et al.* 2008).

Barnett and associates retrospectively studied 22 SAPH patients receiving therapy (sildenafil, 9; bosentan, 12; epoprostenol, 1) for a mean of 11 months. In this group of treated patients, there was an overall improvement in 6MWT distance, mPAP and pulmonary vascular resistance. In this study, patients with limited pulmonary fibrosis (FVC >50 percent) were most likely to benefit from treatment. However, the overall prognosis remained poor, with a 3-year transplant-free survival of only 74 percent (Barnett *et al.* 2009).

CONCLUSION

It has been suggested that carefully selected SAPH patients already treated with anti-inflammatory therapy may benefit from specific PH therapy (Heresi and Dweik 2009). Placebo-controlled studies are under way to determine the effect of PH-specific therapies in SAPH. In the absence of an effective, approved therapy, pulmonary transplantation remains an important consideration. Patients with SAPH have a high mortality rate, and thus evaluation for pulmonary transplantation should be considered early.

REFERENCES

Arcasoy SM, Christie JD, Pochettino A *et al.* (2001). Characteristics and outcomes of patients with sarcoidosis listed for lung transplantation. *Chest* **120**: 873–80.

Arcasoy SM, Christie JD, Ferrari VA *et al.* (2003). Echocardiographic assessment of pulmonary hypertension in patients with advanced lung disease. *Am J Respir Crit Care Med* **167**: 735–40.

Barnett CF, Bonura EJ, Nathan SD *et al.* (2009) Treatment of sarcoidosis-associated pulmonary hypertension: a two-center experience. *Chest* **135**: 1455–61.

Barst RJ, Ratner SJ (1985). Sarcoidosis and reactive pulmonary hypertension. *Arch Intern Med* **145**: 2112–14.

Battesti JP, Georges R, Basset F, Saumon G (1978). Chronic cor pulmonale in pulmonary sarcoidosis. *Thorax* **33**: 76–84.

Baughman RP (2007). Pulmonary hypertension associated with sarcoidosis. *Arthritis Res Ther* **9**(Suppl. 2): S8.

Baughman RP, Engel PJ, Meyer CA *et al.* (2006). Pulmonary hypertension in sarcoidosis. *Sarcoid Vasc Diff Lung Dis* **23**: 108–16.

Baughman RP, Sparkman BK, Lower EE (2007). Six-minute walk test and health status assessment in sarcoidosis. *Chest* **132**: 207–13.

Bourbonnais JM, Samavati L (2008). Clinical predictors of pulmonary hypertension in sarcoidosis. *Eur Respir J* **32**: 296–302.

Damuth TE, Bower JS, Cho K, Dantzker DR (1980). Major pulmonary artery stenosis causing pulmonary hypertension in sarcoidosis. *Chest* **78**: 888–91.

Davies J, Nellen M, Goodwin JF (1982). Reversible pulmonary hypertension in sarcoidosis. *Postgrad Med J* **58**: 282–5.

Devaraj A, Wells AU, Meister MG *et al.* (2008). The effect of diffuse pulmonary fibrosis on the reliability of CT signs of pulmonary hypertension. *Radiology* **249**: 1042–9.

Diaz-Guzman E, Farver C, Parambil J, Culver D (2008). Pulmonary hypertension caused by sarcoidosis. *Clin Chest Med* **29**: 549–63.

Eddahibi S, Springall D, Mannan M *et al.* (1993). Dilator effect of endothelins in pulmonary circulation: changes associated with chronic hypoxia. *Am J Physiol* **265**: L571–80.

Emirgil C, Sobol BJ, Herbert WH, Trout K (1971). The lesser circulation in pulmonary fibrosis secondary to sarcoidosis and its relationship to respiratory function. *Chest* **60**: 371–8.

Fisher KA, Serlin DM, Wilson KC *et al.* (2006). Sarcoidosis-associated pulmonary hypertension: outcome with long-term epoprostenol treatment. *Chest* **130**: 14818.

Foley RJ, Metersky ML (2005). Successful treatment of sarcoidosis-associated pulmonary hypertension with bosentan. *Respiration* **75**: 211–14.

Galie N, Manes A, Branzi A (2004). The endothelin system in pulmonary arterial hypertension. *Cardiovasc Res* **61**: 227–37.

Gluskowski J, Hawrylkiewicz I, Zych D *et al.* (1984). Pulmonary haemodynamics at rest and during exercise in patients with sarcoidosis. *Respiration* **46**: 26–32.

Gluskowski J, Hawrylkiewicz I, Zych D, Zielinski J (1990). Effects of corticosteroid treatment on pulmonary haemodynamics in patients with sarcoidosis. *Eur Respir J* **3**: 403–7.

Hamilton-Craig CR, Slaughter R, McNeil K *et al.* (2009). Improvement after angioplasty and stenting of pulmonary arteries due to sarcoid mediastinal fibrosis. *Heart Lung Circ* **18**: 222–5.

Handa T, Nagai S, Shigematsu M *et al.* (2005). Patient characteristics and clinical features of Japanese sarcoidosis patients with low bronchoalveolar lavage CD4/CD8 ratios. *Sarcoid Vasc Diff Lung Dis* **22**: 154–60.

Handa T, Nagai S, Miki S *et al.* (2006). Incidence of pulmonary hypertension and its clinical relevance in patients with sarcoidosis. *Chest* **129**: 1246–52.

Heresi GA, Dweik RA (2009). Sarcoidosis-associated pulmonary hypertension: one size does not fit all. *Chest* **135**: 1410–12.

Hoffstein V, Ranganathan N, Mullen JB (1986). Sarcoidosis simulating pulmonary veno-occlusive disease. *Am Rev Respir Dis* **134**: 809–11.

Jones K, Higenbottam T, Wallwork J (1989). Pulmonary vasodilation with prostacyclin in primary and secondary pulmonary hypertension. *Chest* **96**: 784–9.

Jones RM, Dawson A, Jenkins GH *et al.* (2009). Sarcoidosis-related pulmonary veno-occlusive disease presenting with recurrent haemoptysis. *Eur Respir J* **34**: 517–20.

Jozsef L, Khreiss T, Fournier A *et al.* (2002). Extracellular signal-regulated kinase plays an essential role in endothelin-1-induced homotypic adhesion of human neutrophil granulocytes. *Br J Pharmacol* **135**: 1167–74.

Letizia C, Danese A, Reale MG *et al.* (2001). Plasma levels of endothelin-1 increase in patients with sarcoidosis and fall after disease remission. *Panminerva Med* **43**: 257–61.

Leuchte HH, Baumgartner RA, Nounou ME *et al.* (2006). Brain natriuretic peptide is a prognostic parameter in chronic lung disease. *Am J Respir Crit Care Med* **173**: 744–50.

Luscher TF, Barton M (2000). Endothelins and endothelin receptor antagonists: therapeutic considerations for a novel class of cardiovascular drugs. *Circulation* **102**: 2434–40.

Mangla A, Fisher J, Libby DM, Saddekni S (1985). Sarcoidosis, pulmonary hypertension, and acquired peripheral pulmonary artery stenosis. *Cathet Cardiovasc Diagn* **11**: 69–74.

Mayock RL, Bertrand P, Morrison CE, Scott JH (1963). Manifestations of sarcoidosis: analysis of 145 patients, with a review of nine series selected from the literature. *Am J Med* **35**: 67–89.

Milman N, Burton CM, Iversen M *et al.* (2008). Pulmonary hypertension in end-stage pulmonary sarcoidosis: therapeutic effect of sildenafil? *J Heart Lung Transplant* **27**: 329–34.

Mitchell DN, Scadding JG (1974). Sarcoidosis. *Am Rev Respir Dis* **110**: 774–802.

Nunes H, Humbert M, Capron F *et al.* (2006). Pulmonary hypertension associated with sarcoidosis: mechanisms, haemodynamics and prognosis. *Thorax* **61**: 68–74.

Orens JB, Estenne M, Arcasoy S *et al.* (2006). International guidelines for the selection of lung transplant candidates: 2006 update. A consensus report from the Pulmonary Scientific Council of the International Society for Heart and Lung Transplantation. *J Heart Lung Transplant* **25**: 745–55.

Pitsiou GG, Spyratos D, Kioumis I *et al.* (2009). Sarcoidosis-associated pulmonary hypertension: a role for endothelin receptor antagonists? *Ther Adv Respir Dis* **3**: 99–101.

Pollock DM, Keith TL, Highsmith RF (1995). Endothelin receptors and calcium signaling. *FASEB J* **9**: 1196–204.

Preston IR, Klinger JR, Landzberg MJ *et al.* (2001). Vasoresponsiveness of sarcoidosis-associated pulmonary hypertension. *Chest* **120**: 866–72.

Reichenberger F, Schauer J, Kellner K *et al.* (2001). Different expression of endothelin in the bronchoalveolar lavage in patients with pulmonary diseases. *Lung* **179**: 163–74.

Rizzato G, Pezzano A, Sala G *et al.* (1983). Right heart impairment in sarcoidosis: haemodynamic and echocardiographic study. *Eur J Respir Dis* **64**: 121–8.

Rodman DM, Lindenfeld J (1990). Successful treatment of sarcoidosis-associated pulmonary hypertension with corticosteroids. *Chest* **97**: 500–2.

Rosen Y, Moon S, Huang CT *et al.* (1977). Granulomatous pulmonary angiitis in sarcoidosis. *Arch Pathol Lab Med* **101**: 170–4.

Salazar A, Mana J, Sala J *et al.* (1994). Combined portal and pulmonary hypertension in sarcoidosis. *Respiration* **61**: 117–19.

Sharma S, Kashour T, Philipp R (2005). Secondary pulmonary arterial hypertension: treated with endothelin receptor blockade. *Tex Heart Inst J* **32**: 405–10.

Shigemitsu H, Nagai S, Sharma OP (2007). Pulmonary hypertension and granulomatous vasculitis in sarcoidosis. *Curr Opin Pulm Med* **13**: 434–8.

Shorr AF, Davies DB, Nathan SD (2002). Outcomes for patients with sarcoidosis awaiting lung transplantation. *Chest* **122**: 233–8.

Shorr AF, Davies DB, Nathan SD (2003). Predicting mortality in patients with sarcoidosis awaiting lung transplantation. *Chest* **124**: 922–8.

Shorr AF, Helman DL, Davies DB, Nathan SD (2005). Pulmonary hypertension in advanced sarcoidosis: epidemiology and clinical characteristics. *Eur Respir J* **25**: 783–8.

Simonneau G, Robbins BM *et al.* (2009). Updated clinical classification of pulmonary hypertension. *J Am Coll Cardiol* **54**: S43–54.

Smith LJ, Lawrence JB, Katzenstein AA (1983). Vascular sarcoidosis: a rare cause of pulmonary hypertension. *Am J Med Sci* **285**: 38–44.

Sulica R, Teirstein AS, Kakarla S *et al.* (2005). Distinctive clinical, radiographic, and functional characteristics of patients with sarcoidosis-related pulmonary hypertension. *Chest* **128**: 1483–9.

Takemura T, Matsui Y, Saiki S, Mikami R (1992). Pulmonary vascular involvement in sarcoidosis: a report of 40 autopsy cases. *Hum Pathol* **23**: 1216–23.

Terashita K, Kato S, Sata M *et al.* (2006). Increased endothelin-1 levels of BAL fluid in patients with pulmonary sarcoidosis. *Respirology* **11**: 145–51.

Toonkel RL, Borczuk AC, Pearson GD *et al.* (2010). Sarcoidosis-associated fibrosing mediastinitis with resultant pulmonary hypertension: a case report and review of the literature. *Respiration* **79**: 341–5.

Zisman DA, Karlamangla AS, Ross DJ *et al.* (2007). High-resolution chest computed tomography findings do not predict the presence of pulmonary hypertension in advanced idiopathic pulmonary fibrosis. *Chest* **132**: 773–9.

21

The upper respiratory tract

HESHAM SALEH, STEPHEN R DURHAM AND GURPREET SANDHU

HISTORICAL PERSPECTIVE

Cesar Boeck of Christiania, Denmark, was the first to use the word sarcoid and described the multisystem nature of the disease in 1899 (Black 1973). He mentioned the clinical similarity to a previous case described by Jonathan Hutchinson of London in 1898 as Mortimer's Malady where a female patient, Mrs Mortimer, had generalized skin lesions and swelling of the bridge of the nose. In 1905 Boek recorded infiltration of the nasal mucosa in a case of multiple benign sarcoid (Boeck 1905). Kreibich and Kraus described a patient in 1908 with sarcoid of the skin of the nose and forehead who also had nasal symptoms (Kreibich and Kraus 1908). The involvement of the tonsils was documented by Shaumann in 1914 who reported that, in two out of three cases of lupus pernio, the tonsils showed specific histological features (Shaumann 1936). In 1918 Ulrich reported the involvement of the larynx (Ulrich 1918). Subsequently many reports of upper respiratory tract involvement were published but it was not until recently that epidemiological studies attempted to define the incidence of various organ involvement.

CLINICAL FEATURES OF SARCOIDOSIS OF THE UPPER RESPIRATORY TRACT

The nose

Patients with systemic sarcoidosis commonly develop nasal symptoms and are referred to the ear, nose and throat (ENT) clinic for evaluation of possible nasal sarcoidosis. Nasal symptoms affect more than 20 percent of the general population (Bauchau and Durham 2004), whereas involvement of the nose and upper respiratory tract in sarcoidosis

occurs in approximately 6 percent of cases (James et al. 1982; Panselinas et al. 2010) such that it is far more common that nasal symptoms are unrelated to the underlying sarcoidosis. In these circumstances it is important to diagnose nasal sarcoid in the minority since nasal involvement is frequently associated with insidious onset, and more systemic involvement and progression of the disease with the frequent requirement for treatment with oral corticosteroids with/ without other immunosuppressive therapies. Equally, it is important to exclude nasal sarcoid in the majority of sarcoidosis sufferers for whom an accurate alternative diagnosis is reassuring and frequently amenable to effective management.

Nasal involvement in sarcoidosis is insidious and typically involves nasal congestion that is bilateral and varies from mild stuffiness to severe congestion and rarely complete nasal obstruction. Unlike non-granulomatous disorders, crusting is a prominent feature and may be the only symptom although frequently associated with intermittent nasal bleeding and/or anosmia (Reed et al. 2010). Facial discomfort/pain may accompany obstruction of sinus ostia and/or cartilaginous involvement. Nasal swellings may result in deformity and rarely cartilaginous ulceration and perforation with collapse of the bridge and a typical 'saddle nose' (Fig. 21.1). This particularly occurs in those who have had previous surgery (Reed et al. 2010). Secondary infection of the lesions following sinus obstruction is not uncommon and results in mucopurulent anterior and posterior nasal discharge and cacosmia. Involvement of the nasolacrimal duct may lead to excessive tearing. Perforation of the palate is a rare and distressing complication that leads to an unpleasant taste and halitosis.

Two out of three patients with nasal sarcoidosis will have skin involvement, the severity of which seems to be parallel to that of the severity of nasal sarcoidosis (Neville et al. 1976).

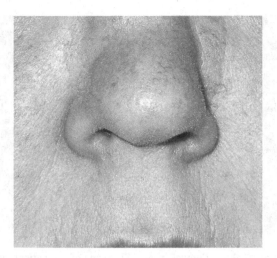

Figure 21.1   Sarcoidosis with saddling of the nasal bridge.

Typically this appears as 'lupus pernio' with brawny red or brown indurated raised lesions around the nares extending to the external nasal surface and surrounding facial skin (Fig. 21.2). Sarcoid skin lesions may be apparent elsewhere as painless, discolored, smooth indurated papules or raised plaques (Plate 17). In a distinct small group of patients the nasal bones are involved and present with symmetrical hard swelling over the bridge of the nose (Plate 18).

There are commonly features of other systemic involvement, particularly pulmonary sarcoid that may be associated with cough or breathlessness but may be asymptomatic and manifest only on chest X-ray or CT scan. The diagnosis should also be considered in patients with a previous diagnosis of chronic sinusitis who have responded poorly to usual treatment.

On examination, there may be local skin lesions of lupus pernio. Nasal sarcoidosis almost always involves the anterior nasal cavity and may be seen through an ophthalmoscope with auriscopic attachment. There is often narrowing of the nasal cavities. The nasal mucosa is often red, swollen and friable with crusts that may contribute to nasal obstruction. There may be typical raised 1–4 mm pale nodules or rounded superficial submucosal swellings (equivalent to 'apple jelly' nodules of skin sarcoid) (Fig. 21.3).

At endoscopy, mucosal swelling and crusting may be seen to contribute to obstruction of the ostiomeatal complex. In more advanced disease there may be distortion and scarring of

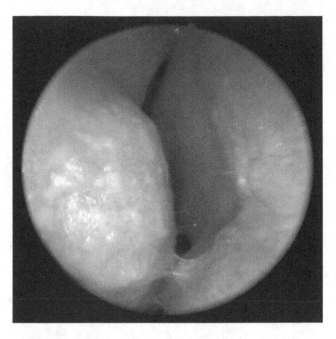

Figure 21.3   Typical 'apple-jelly' nodule affecting the right inferior turbinate. Note the inflammation of the remaining nasal mucosa and the associated crusting.

the normal architecture with a more fibrotic and dry appearance of the mucosa with pronounced crusting and marked narrowing of the nasal cavities. Scarring and adhesions are a common occurrence after surgery, which should be avoided if possible in patients with nasal sarcoidosis (Fig. 21.4). Mucopurulent discharge or secondary infection is a not an uncommon finding. 'Burnt out' appearances with a dry atrophic mucosa and crusting may be a feature of longstanding disease (Fig. 21.5).

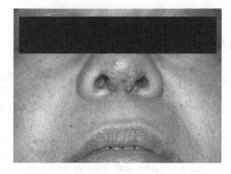

Figure 21.2   Lupus pernio of the nasal skin in a patient with severe nasal sarcoidosis.

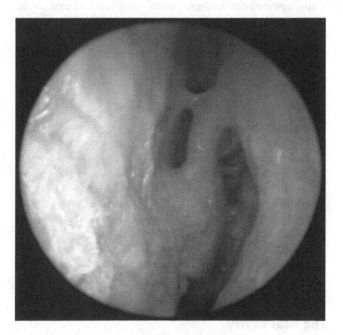

Figure 21.4   Endoscopic view of the left nasal cavity showing multiple adhesions and crusting in a patient with nasal sarcoidosis who had previous endoscopic sinus surgery.

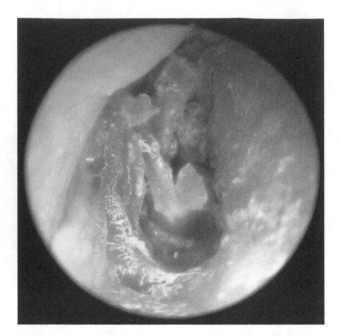

Figure 21.5   Endoscopic view of the left nasal cavity in a patient with longstanding nasal sarcoidosis and atrophic rhinitis.

The paranasal sinuses

Patients with nasal sarcoidosis often present with symptoms of chronic sinusitis such as postnasal drip, facial pressure/pain and congestion. This can be secondary to obstruction of the ostiomeatal complex by the sarcoid disease and not necessarily due to sinus mucosal involvement with the granulomatous inflammation. The incidence of sinus mucosal involvement in patients with nasal sarcoidosis is unclear, and biopsies do not always show granulomas (van den Boer *et al.* 2010).

It is extremely rare for patients to present with isolated sinus involvement without nasal symptoms (Fergie *et al.* 1999; Zeitlin *et al.* 2000; Braun *et al.* 2004). Only a small number of such cases have been reported and certainly this reflects the authors' experience. Findings on CT scanning of the sinuses are non-specific with uniform opacity and occasional bony erosion (Fig. 21.6).

The nasopharynx

Several historic case reports suggest the involvement of nasopharynx in patients with sarcoidosis of the upper respiratory tract (Carasso 1974; Kirschner and Holinger 1976; Braun *et al.* 2004). These patients present with enlargement of the adenoid tissue causing nasal obstruction and/or symptoms of Eustachian tube dysfunction. This has been uncommon in the authors' experience; we find that the majority of patients with nasal sarcoidosis have a normal nasopharynx on endoscopy.

The oral cavity

Oral involvement in sarcoidosis is uncommon. Multiple case reports have been published and a review in 2005 reported 68

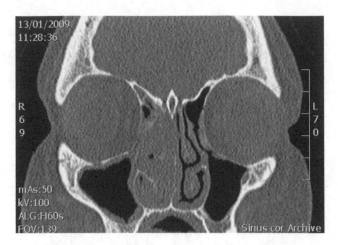

Figure 21.6   Coronal sinus CT scan of a patient with predominantly right-sided nasal sarcoidosis. The patient presented with secondary maxillary sinusitis on the same side and histology of the sinus mucosa did not show sarcoid changes.

well-documented cases in the world literature (Suresh and Radfar 2005). Areas involved include jaw bones, buccal mucosa, lips, floor of the mouth, tongue, salivary glands and palate. Clinical presentations include localized swelling or nodules, ulcers, swelling with multiple ulcers, gingivitis, gingival hyperplasia and gingival recession. Rarely ulceration of the palate has led to the development of a perforation.

The tonsils

Tonsil involvement with sarcoidosis has been reported frequently, albeit being very uncommon. Because of its easy accessibility, random tonsillar biopsies have been advocated to diagnose sarcoidosis but there is a low diagnostic yield (Karma *et al.* 1980). In a retrospective review of the histopathology of 26386 tonsils, sarcoidosis appeared in only 0.03 percent of all examined specimens (Kardon and Thompson 2000). Sarcoidosis of the tonsil may present as a unilateral mass lesion with accompanying cervical lymphadenopathy mimicking malignancy, so that histological examination of the tonsil in this clinical setting is mandatory (Kardon and Thompson 2000).

Parotid/salivary glands

Parotid and minor salivary gland involvement has been reported in sarcoidosis, and whole-body gallium scanning has demonstrated increased uptake in asymptomatic patients (Judson 1999). In one large series, 3.9 percent of patients had enlarged parotids and many of them had bilateral swellings (Baughman *et al.* 2001). Heerfordt's syndrome refers to patients who have symmetrical parotid swelling, uveitis and facial palsy (Baughman *et al.* 2010). Patients with salivary gland involvement often present with dry mouth. If the lacrimal glands are also involved, the patient ultimately develops secondary Sjögren's syndrome.

The larynx and trachea

Otorhinolaryngologic manifestations are rare, with laryngeal involvement accounting for fewer than 1 percent of presentations (Bower *et al.* 1980). Laryngeal involvement is typically supraglottic and presents initially with hoarseness or sensation of throat swelling and may progress to dysphagia, stridor and progressive breathlessness. Choking episodes due to acute upper airway obstruction may occur and may occasionally lead to respiratory arrest that requires urgent tracheostomy.

Laryngeal involvement most commonly involves the epiglottis, ary-epiglottic folds and arytenoids. The macroscopic appearance of laryngeal sarcoid is considered pathognomonic with a supraglottis that is diffusely thick, edematous and pale or pink. Appearances may also vary from marked general edematous swelling to more localized and asymmetric rounded or nodular swellings of the supraglottic region with extension towards – but typically not involving – the vocal folds (Fig. 21.7). Endotracheal lesions / endobronchial sarcoid may appear as a red swollen mucosa and/or the presence of pale nodules and swellings with/without associated narrowing of the airway lumen (Fig. 21.8).

DIAGNOSIS

The diagnosis of sarcoidosis depends on the presence of typical clinical features and non-caseating granulomatous inflammation on biopsy of an affected organ with the exclusion of other known causes of granulomas, including tuberculosis, leprosy, syphilis and fungal disease (Baughman *et al.* 2003). Biopsy may not be necessary with the typical subacute presentation that occurs in young female adults,

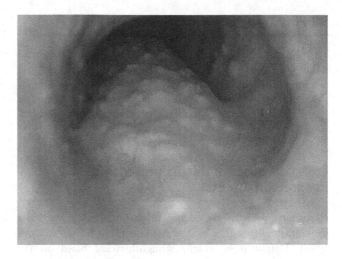

Figure 21.8   Tracheal sarcoidosis showing nodules in the lumen of the trachea.

with malaise, erythema nodosum of the lower limbs and bilateral hilar lymphadenopathy and that carries a good prognosis. By contrast, upper respiratory involvement in sarcoidosis is associated with the more usual insidious onset and protracted course of the disease. For such patients – and in view of the possible need for long-term immunosuppressive therapy – biopsy is required for confirmation of the diagnosis and exclusion of other treatable causes, including infectious causes.

INVESTIGATIONS

The full blood count may be normal or reveal a normocytic anemia of chronic disease with an elevated erythrocyte sedimentation rate. There may be lymphopenia with a reduction in the CD4/CD8 T-cell ratio (Sweiss *et al.* 2010). The serum angiotensin-converting enzyme (ACE) level is typically elevated but may be within the normal range. Serum antineutrophil cytoplasmic antibody (ANCA) is normal. Biopsy of an affected organ is used to confirm granulomatous inflammation and for special stains to exclude known infectious causes including tuberculosis, leprosy, syphilis and fungi and other granulomatous diseases and vasculitis (Baughman *et al.* 2010). On the other hand, if the mucosa appears macroscopically normal then biopsy is seldom positive (Wilson *et al.* 1988).

In patients presenting for the first time with nasal symptoms suggestive of sarcoid, investigations to detect systemic involvement are performed. Chest radiography may reveal hilar lymphadenopathy with/without pulmonary infiltrates or evidence of pulmonary fibrosis (if the chest X-ray appears normal, a CT scan of the chest may be required). Serum calcium may be elevated, and a 24 h urine collection should be obtained to exclude elevated urinary calcium excretion. A gallium scan may show enhanced uptake in the lacrimal and parotid glands due to granulomatous inflammation. ECG and echocardiogram is usual in order to exclude cardiac involvement.

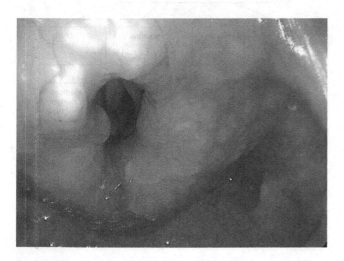

Figure 21.7   Generalized supraglottic swelling and multiple nodules with inflammation in a patient with laryngeal sarcoidosis.

DIFFERENTIAL DIAGNOSIS

This involves the identification of common but unrelated nasal conditions in patients with sarcoidosis (Saleh and Durham 2007) as well as distinction from other granulomatous disorders that may mimic the symptoms and findings on examination in sarcoidosis (Baughman *et al.* 2010).

Common nasal problems presenting in sarcoid patients

Common problems are allergy, infection or structural nasal problems along with a host of less common disorders (Lund 1994). Diagnosis is usually straightforward based on the history, examination and targeted skin/RAST testing.

Twenty-five per cent of the population, and likely 25 percent of patients with sarcoidosis, may present with typical symptoms of allergic rhinitis that comprise itching, sneezing, anterior nasal watery discharge and associated eye symptoms (Scadding *et al.* 2008a). Symptoms occur after exposure to the provoking allergen and seasonality (pollens, moulds), so the relationship of symptoms to exposure to potential sensitizers in the workplace should be established. Perennial symptoms may result from exposures to domestic pets, whereas there may not be such a close association with house-dust mite where exposure is continuous. The appearances of the mucosa are either pale or swollen watery discharge or normal if patient is asymptomatic at examination. Skin/RAST testing provides/excludes objective confirmation of IgE sensitivity and should be performed/interpreted only in the context of the clinical history. Treatment involves avoidance where possible and symptomatic treatment with antihistamines and/or topical nasal steroids (Bousquet *et al.* 2001). Treatment failure is usually due to failure of regular use or poor technique with the nasal spray, whereas allergen immunotherapy via the subcutaneous or sublingual route may be beneficial in selected patients who fail to respond to antiallergic drugs (Bousquet *et al.* 1998).

Chronic rhinosinusitis may complicate or occur independently from sarcoidosis (Fokkens *et al.* 2005; Scadding *et al.* 2008b). Symptoms comprise mucopurulent discharge, which may be anterior or typically posterior, facial discomfort, congestion and constitutional upset. Appearances are of redness, swelling and mucopurulent discharge in the absence of the crusting and bleeding that is typical of sarcoidosis. Treatment involves attention to any underlying immune deficiency, nasal douching with isotonic, warmed saline and bicarbonate of soda solution, and a prolonged course of antibiotics (generally for 10–14 days) with adjustment according to antibiotic sensitivities of nasal discharge following culture. Nasal corticosteroids are prescribed but in general are not helpful for chronic rhinosinusitis in the absence of polyps or associated nasal eosinophilia.

Structural problems typically present with nasal obstruction and/or concerns about the cosmetic appearance of the nose. Deflected nasal septum is frequently seen in asymptomatic individuals. There may be a history of nasal trauma, but frequently no such history is obtained. If symptoms are consistently worse on the side of the deflection and interfere with sleep and/or quality of life, then surgical referral is indicated. Unusually, structural problems of the anterior nasal valve area may present with nasal blockage. Careful explanation of the nature of the problem is needed with advice for use of 'Easibreath' nasal bridge plasters. In general, surgical procedures for treating obstruction due to nasal valve abnormalities have been disappointing. Nasal polyps present with nasal obstruction and absence of smell. Endoscopy usually reveals typical appearances of grayish rounded polyps protruding from and obstructing the orifice of the ostiomeatal complex inferior and lateral to the middle turbinate. Treatment involves topical steroids and often a requirement for courses of systemic oral corticosteroids. Surgery is indicated for recurrent nasal polyps that fail to respond to these measures (Fokkens *et al.* 2005).

Other causes of nasal symptoms in patients with sarcoidosis include drugs (beta-blockers, angiotensin-converting enzyme inhibitors, aspirin) and so-called rhinitis medicamentosa due to prolonged and excessive use of over-the-counter topical decongestants (Lund 1994). Hormonal causes include pregnancy, menopause, premenstrual rhinitis and thyroid disorders. So-called 'idiopathic' rhinitis involves symptoms of discharge or congestion on exposure to irritants, typically changes in temperature or air conditioning, in the absence of other underlying predisposing causes. Unilateral symptoms of obstruction, pain or bleeding in an older patient should raise the possibility of an underlying tumor, whereas persistent unilateral clear nasal discharge, particularly in females, should raise the possibility of cerebrospinal fluid rhinorrhea, usually idiopathic but possibly following trauma or surgery. Treatment involves identifying and avoidance or treating the underlying cause and specialist referral when indicated.

Figure 21.9 gives a summary of differential diagnoses and approaches to therapy (Lund 1994).

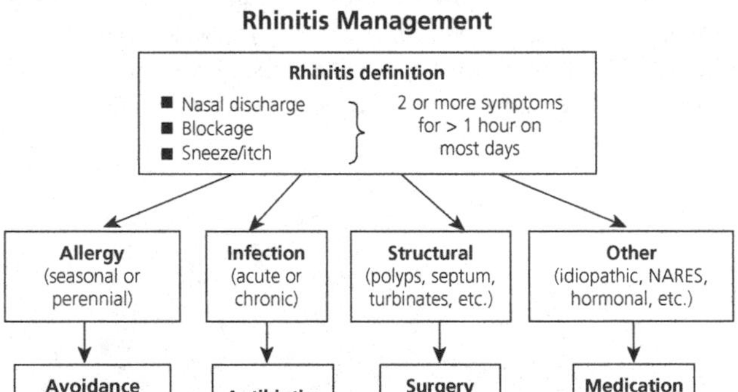

Rhinitis Management

Figure 21.9   Summary of the differential diagnosis and approach to therapy for patients with nasal symptoms.

Differentiation of nasal sarcoid from other granulomatous disorders

As mentioned above, cardinal features of nasal sarcoid include an insidious onset, bilateral nasal crusting, bleeding and obstruction (Baughman *et al.* 2010; Reed *et al.* 2010). The typical appearances, together with other systemic manifestations of sarcoidosis including skin, lung, ocular, cardiac, neurological, joint or renal involvement, may be diagnostic (de Shazo *et al.* 1999; Braun *et al.* 2004). However, crusting, bleeding and obstruction may occur in the vasculitides, particularly Wegener's granulomatosis, and in atrophic rhinitis which may rarely be primary (Chand and Macarthur 1997) but more commonly occurs following extensive surgery or prolonged infective chronic rhinosinusitis (Ly *et al.* 2009). Drug abuse, particularly of cocaine, may mimic granulomatous disease (Rachapalli and Kiely 2008), as occasionally may habitual nose-picking. It cannot be over-emphasized that unilateral pain, crusting or bleeding should raise the need to exclude an underlying malignancy.

In practice, the most important differential diagnosis of nasal sarcoidosis is Wegener's granulomatosis. A comparison has recently been published by Baughman (Table 21.1).

Whereas the nose is affected in around 6 percent of patients with systemic sarcoidosis (James *et al.* 1982; Panselinas *et al.* 2010), it is extremely common in Wegener's (Kornblutt *et al.* 1980). Whereas crusting and obstruction are common to both, the nasal mucosal lesions of Wegener's tend to be subacute rather than insidious, more progressive and more destructive, and if untreated may progress rapidly to destruction of cartilage with saddle-nose deformity and

perforation of the nasal septum. Local necrosis in advanced Wegener's has a characteristic unpleasant odor of which the patient is frequently unaware. Whereas sarcoid classically involves the anterior nasal cavity extending to the ethmoids and maxillary sinuses, both sarcoid and Wegener's may extend posteriorly and involve the choanae, nasopharynx, palate and palatine tonsil.

Both may affect the larynx and trachea. Sarcoid more commonly affects the supraglottis and occasionally the pharynx and palatine tonsils, whereas Wegener's typically involves the subglottic region and trachea and may rapidly progress to stridor and breathlessness and episodes of acute upper airway obstruction due to occlusion by crusting, particularly with secondary bacterial infection of the lesions. Long-term effects include subglottic fibrosis and stenosis that may require repeated dilatation and/or permanent tracheostomy.

Pulmonary involvement in Wegener's gives rise to multiple mass lesions throughout the lungs which cavitate and give rise to infection and hemoptysis, whereas pulmonary sarcoid may be asymptomatic with hilar lymphadenopathy or progress insidiously with pulmonary infiltrates typically involving the mid and upper zones and pulmonary fibrosis. Renal vasculitis is very common in Wegener's and detectable as micro-albuminuria, microscopic hematuria, and the presence of red cell and granular casts on urine microscopy as well as progressive decline in creatinine clearance, whereas

Table 21.1   Comparison between sarcoidosis and Wegener's granulomatosis.

	Sarcoidosis	Wegener's granulomatosis
Clinical presentation		
Upper airway	Occurs in <10% of cases	Extremely common
Lung	Common	Common
	Adenopathy	Nodular infiltrates, sometimes with cavities
	Diffuse infiltrates, usually upper lobes	Infiltrates localized to areas of hemorrhage, often lower lobe
Eye	Uveitis, retinitis, optic neuritis	Episcleritis
Skin	Maculopapular lesions	Vasculitic lesions
	Lupus pernio	Occasionally seen
Kidney	Glomerulonephritis rare, renal failure usually due to hypercalcemia	Focal necrotizing glomerulitis in >50% of cases
Neurological disease	10% of patients; often mass seen on MRI	Up to 30% of cases will have lesions; usually due to vasculitic lesions
Joints	Uncommon; can see specific bone cysts	Uncommon
Tracheal/proximal airway stenosis	Rare	Common
ANCA	Negative	Positive in >80% of cases
ACE	Positive in >60% of cases	Negative
Treatment		
Corticosteroids	Drug of choice for initial management	Supportive but not used for maintenance
Methotrexate	Effective	Effective
Azathioprine	Effective	Effective
Cyclophosphamide	Reserved for refractory cases	Treatment for extensive disease
Anti-TNF therapy	Effective for refractory disease	Not effective for most patients
Ritixumab	Effectiveness unknown	Effective for refractory cases

ANCA, antineutrophil cytoplasmic antibody; TNF, tumor necrosis factor
Reproduced with permission from Baughman RP, Lower EE, Tami T (2010). Upper airway. 4: Sarcoidosis of the upper respiratory tract (SURT). *Thorax* 65: 181–6.

renal involvement in sarcoid is rare and usually secondary to nephrocalcinosis, recurrent renal calculi or rarely the presence of granuloma (without vasculitis or necrosis) on renal biopsy.

An elevated serum antineutrophil cytoplasmic antibody (ANCA) and accompanying elevated serum antiproteinase 3 occurs in most cases of Wegener's (Baughman *et al.* 2010); and is absent in sarcoid (Aubart *et al.* 2006) whereas angiotensin-converting enzyme level is increased in the majority (60 percent) of new cases of sarcoid and absent in Wegener's. Other systemic manifestations including ocular, joint, and neurologic involvement are considered elsewhere and summarized in Table 21.1 (Baughman *et al.* 2010), along with a comparison of the response to treatment of the two conditions.

A positive ANCA is also seen in a minority of patients presenting with Churg Strauss syndrome that also has prominent nasal manifestations (Baldini *et al.* 2010). This syndrome occurs in asthmatics with an atopic history and is associated with rhinosinusitis and nasal polyps rather than granulomata, with dominant nasal obstruction and *absence* of sense of smell as typical features. There is blood eosinophilia and frequently episodes of pulmonary eosinophilia that masquerade as recurrent infective exacerbations of asthma although are distinguishable by the presence of peripheral eosinophilia rather than neutrophilia alone. Other systemic manifestations of Churg Strauss syndrome include arthralgia, arthritis and cutaneous vasculitis. Less common but important manifestations include cardiac involvement (particularly endomyocarditis) and neurological involvement (mononeuritis multiplex).

Habitual cocaine abuse results in intense anterior rhinitis which leads to mucosal ulceration, crusting and bleeding. Ultimately there is perforation and destruction of the cartilaginous septum. Patients frequently deny substance abuse, whereas performance of a urine test for cocaine metabolites is diagnostic with high predictive value (Rachapalli and Kiely 2008). There should be a high index of suspicion for cocaine abuse in patients presenting with nasal crusting and bleeding in the absence of systemic disease such that permission should always be sought to obtain urine for toxicology studies. In the authors' clinic (and as previously reported) we have seen several cases presenting with clinical and histological features suggestive of *isolated* nasal Wegener's granuloma, including a positive ANCA and raised antiproteinase 3 level whereas positive urine cocaine metabolites subsequently confirmed cocaine abuse as the underlying cause.

MANAGEMENT OF UPPER RESPIRATORY TRACT SARCOIDOSIS

The consequences of sarcoidosis can be divided into local effects and general effects on health and wellbeing. In the absence of known underlying causes, the management of upper respiratory tract sarcoidosis (as with other systemic involvement) can only be symptomatic with/without suppression of underlying disease activity. Principles of effective management include:

- monitoring of symptoms and disease activity;
- control of symptoms in order to improve quality of life;
- interventions to prevent disease progression;
- interventions to prevent or treat life-threatening complications;
- balancing such interventions against treatment-related side-effects.

An overall treatment strategy according to disease severity has been elegantly summarized by Baughman's group (Baughman *et al.* 2010) and is reproduced here with permission (Fig. 21.10).

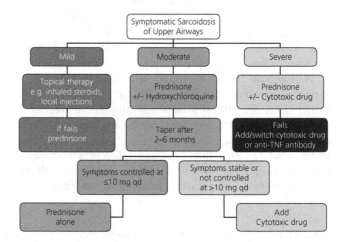

Figure 21.10   Summary of treatment strategy for SURT.

Monitoring disease activity

Outpatient follow-up is required to monitor subjective severity of nasal symptoms, and the presence or absence of mucopurulent discharge that might indicate secondary bacterial infection. Hoarseness is an early sign of laryngeal involvement with/without progressive stridor or breathlessness. Feeling non-specifically unwell is a particular feature of sarcoid and may occur in the absence of progressive organ involvement and reduce work and social performance. Such general malaise may be accompanied by objective features such as weight loss, elevated ESR and raised liver enzymes.

Endoscopy of the nose, pharynx and larynx allows direct inspection of sarcoid lesions. General examination of the chest, cardiovascular system, skin, eyes, salivary glands, lymph nodes and abdomen for signs of hepatosplenomegaly should be routine. Ophthalmic and neurologic examination should be performed if indicated. Inspection for possible corticosteroid side-effects, including measurement of blood pressure, blood glucose and bone density every 2–3 years, should be performed if oral corticosteroids are to be continued. Blood count, ESR, C-reactive protein and ACE levels should be requested. Other investigations are spirometry, including flow–volume loop, chest X-ray for lung involvement, and ECG if there is a history of palpitations, syncope or dyspnea that is unexplained by or disproportionate to any pulmonary involvement.

Control of symptoms

Treatment may be local or systemic. Nasal crusting is a major problem that responds well to regular use of a warmed, isotonic, pH-adjusted salt and bicarbonate nasal douche. Use of a large-volume nasal douche 1–3 times daily or as needed may be combined with topical antibacterial nasal creams applied to the nasal vestibule on the tip of the finger. Rotation of topical antibiotics every 2 weeks reduces the emergence of antibiotic resistance. Steam inhalations may provide symptomatic relief for laryngeal involvement.

Intranasal corticosteroids are a logical and frequently used choice, although there are no controlled trials that confirm or exclude efficacy and nasal steroids may cause/exacerbate nasal bleeding in up to 10 percent of subjects.

Such measures alone or in combination may be highly effective in controlling symptoms. Intralesional corticosteroids by injection may provide temporary relieve of lupus pernio lesions, although they often need to be repeated and there is a risk of skin atrophy. Intranasally injected steroids are rarely used because of extremely rare reports of associated blindness. We have used them sporadically in patients not responding to maximal systemic therapy, especially those with sarcoidosis of the nasal bones (Plate 19). An intralesional injection of 40 mg of triamcinolone with a maximum dose of 100 mg can be used up to three times a year.

Oral antibiotics should be prescribed if bacterial infection is suspected, and therapy guided by culture sensitivities. Empirical, more prolonged courses for at least 2 weeks are often needed. Furthermore, if there is a history of repeated mucopurulent discharge with response to antibiotics, then it is reasonable to prescribe regular prophylactic antibiotics. The combination of trimethoprim and sulfamethoxazole has been shown to be effective (Kaluza 1991). However, this combination is associated with increased incidence of side-effects such as nephrotoxicity and blood dyscrasias. Although there are no controlled trials, we have as an alternative used a macrolide antibiotic such as azithromycin on 3 days per month (or more frequently as needed) with apparent benefit.

If the above measures fail then treatment with oral corticosteroids, prednisolone 30–60 mg either daily or on alternate days, is generally effective with tapering after symptom control (generally after at least 4 weeks), with maintenance therapy up to 10–20 mg daily with monitoring for systemic side-effects and gradual further tapering as symptoms permit (Baughman et al. 2010). Such doses are often very effective at controlling the general malaise that may accompany sarcoidosis. In such a chronic disease, when oral steroids are used to treat symptoms and quality of life in the absence of disease progression, the benefits should be weighed very carefully against the associated inevitable consequences of steroid side-effects.

Prevention of disease progression

Where symptoms of upper respiratory tract sarcoid are severe and/or there is relapse following intermittent short-course prednisolone therapy and/or there is objective evidence of progression and organ damage, then treatment with long-term corticosteroids is indicated with or without various steroid sparing strategies (Zeitlin et al. 2000; Aubart et al. 2006). There are no controlled trials to guide dosing. Initially 30–40 mg daily or 60 mg on alternate days, taken in the morning to minimize adrenal suppression, may be given and continued for 4 weeks or longer until symptoms and objective findings improve, with tapering thereafter to 10–20 mg daily or on alternate days while monitoring for relapse. If the patient is severely symptomatic, consideration may be given to using methylprednisolone (either 500–1000 g daily for 3 days or 1 g weekly for 6 weeks), with concomitant oral prednisolone (initially 15–20 mg daily) that is maintained during the timing of the intravenous course and gradually tapered thereafter.

If symptoms fail to respond or relapse when the prednisolone dose is reduced to 10 mg daily, then an additional immunosuppressant is indicated. Hydroxychloroquine (less oculotoxic than chloroquine) is given orally in daily doses of 200–400 mg (Aubart et al. 2006). Hydroxychloroquine has been shown to be effective for lupus pernio and other sarcoid skin lesions whereas there is poor documentation for efficacy for upper or lower respiratory tract sarcoid (Hassid et al. 1998).

Methotrexate, although more toxic, is the preferred steroid sparing agent for systemic disease other than skin involvement and may be given instead of, or in addition to, hydroxychloroquine (Zeitlin et al. 2000; Aubart et al. 2006). After an initial single dose of 2.5–5 mg, methotrexate is increased at 1–2 weekly intervals by 2.5 mg, with repeated monitoring of blood count and liver function, to a maximum of 15–20 mg once weekly; and if tolerated it is continued in the long term while repeating a gradual taper of prednisolone dose. Folic acid 5 mg rescue is given orally on the day following methotrexate. Malaise, nausea, vomiting, rash and stomatitis are common side-effects. Marrow suppression may occasionally occur. Methotrexate is highly teratogenic and contraindicated in women who are at risk of pregnancy. Potential long-term complications are hepatitis that may lead to cirrhosis and progressive interstitial lung disease, which unchecked may lead to pulmonary fibrosis. Thus long-term use of methotrexate requires monitoring of blood count, chest X-ray, lung and liver function. Even less is known concerning use of alternative immunosuppressives such as azathioprine and leflunomide for sarcoidosis involving the upper respiratory tract.

In rare cases where corticosteroids alone or in combination with methotrexate and/or hydroxychloroquine fail, there is a rationale for use of strategies against tumor necrosis factor-alpha (TNF-α) (Antoniu 2010) which is known to be involved in granuloma formation, although at present there is very little evidence for or against their use in patients with predominant upper respiratory tract sarcoid.

Drugs that either inhibit TNF-α synthesis (thalidomide; Baughman et al. 2002) or release (pentoxifylline; Tong et al. 2003) may be considered. In an open study of thalidomide in patients with lupus pernio, thalidomide was associated with improved sinus symptoms in four of eight patients with sinus disease (Baughman et al. 2002). The recombinant TNF-α receptor fusion protein etanercept has been used in a prospective double-blind study of ocular sarcoid (Baughman *et al.* 2005) and in a prospective open study in pulmonary sarcoid (Utz *et al.* 2003), both with disappointing results. Monoclonal antibodies directed against TNF-α (infliximab, adalimumab) have also been used. In a double-blind phase II trial in patients with chronic pulmonary sarcoidosis, infliximab was effective in improving forced vital capacity at 24 weeks, although there was no effect on secondary end-points including symptoms and quality of life indices (Baughman *et al.* 2006). There are only anecdotal reports of efficacy of adalimumab in pulmonary sarcoid (Callejas-Rubio *et al.* 2006), and in general little information on the effects of anti-TNF-α therapy specifically for sarcoidosis of the upper airway. Further controlled trials are needed (Baughman *et al.* 2008).

Interventions to prevent or treat life-threatening complications

Hoarseness in sarcoidosis is commonly a side-effect of inhaled corticosteroids, whereas the larynx should be inspected in every case to exclude laryngeal involvement, particularly in the presence of nasal sarcoidosis. Progression to stridor with airway narrowing and the risk of upper airway obstruction is an indication for aggressive intervention. In the presence of advanced or progressive disease elsewhere, high-dose methyl-prednisolone (1 g daily for 3 days) with introduction of high-dose oral prednisolone (60 mg daily) with or without initiation of methotrexate therapy is justified.

A recently introduced alternative approach has been local intervention with intralesional steroid, and laser therapy (Butler *et al.* 2010). Up to 3 mL of methylprednisolone acetate at a concentration of 40 mg/mL (Pharmacia Ltd, Kent, England) is injected at multiple sites in the lesion using a standard microlaryngoscopy injection needle. The lesion is reduced using the CO_2 laser at a continuous setting of 8–10 watts. Any pedunculated lesions encroaching into the airway are excised with a small arc using the laser. Multiple narrow pits are created with the CO_2 laser, separated by approximately 2 mm, and extending to the depth of the lesion. This 'pepper-pot' pattern is mucosal sparing but reduces the volume of the disease both immediately and as healing takes place by scarring and contracture (Fig. 21.11).

Occasionally a tracheostomy is inserted electively to bypass airway compromise due to laryngeal disease. Emergency tracheostomy may be indicated if there is acute airway obstruction due to excessive laryngeal crusting or secondary to bacterial infection.

Balancing interventions against treatment-related side-effects

The principle is to neither overtreat nor undertreat the disease. The *threshold* for treating upper respiratory tract sarcoid *in order to improve symptoms and quality of life* with toxic therapies including high-dose, or even continuous low-dose corticosteroids is much higher than for reasons of progressive local disease (deformity and progressive nasal obstruction) or life-threatening laryngeal obstruction. This is because of the poor evidence base for this rare form of sarcoid and the serious side-effects of prolonged treatment with even low-dose steroids that may be required for this chronic disease.

For local disease much can be achieved by careful explanation of the need for vigorous nasal douching, topical local antibiotics and intranasal steroids, particularly beta-methasone drops prescribed in the 'head upside down position', together with antibiotic therapy.

Careful monitoring is needed to detect progressive and potentially irreversible disease in the nose, pharynx or larynx, in order to initiate steroid therapy with/without immuno-suppressive therapy. The decision to initiate aggressive regimens where there is a risk of upper airway obstruction or other concomitant severe systemic involvement in the disease requires considerable skill and experience.

In these circumstances, ENT surgeons and physicians familiar with nasal and laryngeal sarcoid need to work closely with respiratory physicians with expert knowledge of pulmonary and systemic disease and broader experience with the use and side-effects of cytotoxic therapies. A combined medical/surgical ENT clinic is particularly relevant for the management of such patients.

Finally, it should be acknowledged that little is known to guide effective therapy for advanced upper respiratory tract sarcoidosis, as illustrated by the following case report.

A 58-year-old woman had a secure diagnosis of sarcoidosis based on bilateral hilar lymphadenopathy and the presence of non-caseating granulomas on biopsy of her supraglottis and a palatal lesion. She presented with a one-year history of progressive nasal crusting and bleeding with sinusitis, septal perforation and a perforation of the posterior palate. ACE and ANCA levels were negative. Over the preceding 6 months she had failed to respond to prednisolone 40 mg daily, methotrexate 15 mg weekly, several courses of antibiotics and the performance of regular local nasal toilet by her ENT surgeon. She was referred to our hospital for review and consideration of anti-TNF-α therapy. In view of the history of recurrent nasal mucopurulent discharge and quiescence of disease in other organs there was reluctance to initiate anti-TNF-α, and instead the patient was advised to discontinue methotrexate and to slowly reduce her prednisolone back to 10 mg over 3 months, with monitoring of her chest X-ray, carbon monoxide transfer factor and serum ACE level. She was prescribed a 3-month course of rifampicin and doxycycline (although culture of nasal discharge on several occasions had proved negative for bacteria, fungi and tubercle bacilli). Ciprofloxacin was substituted for rifampicin after 2 weeks because of intractable nausea associated with this drug. Inadvertently the patient discontinued her prednisolone completely on discharge from hospital. At review 3 months later she was dramatically improved. The mucopurulent discharge was gone and, although she had continued nasal crusting, this was controlled by regular nasal douching. On examination the nasal airways were patent with minimal crusting, there was a healthy appearance of the mucosa and the previous palatal perforation had healed. She remained

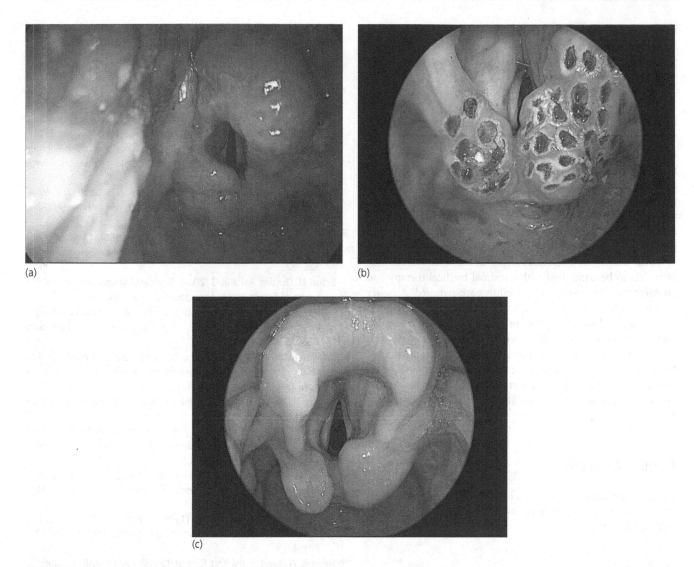

Figure 21.11   Laryngeal sacoidosis: (a) pre-treatment; (b) following steroid injection and 'pepper-pot' CO_2 laser photoreduction; (c) appearance of larynx 3 weeks later.

well for 6 months, deteriorated when one or other antibiotic was stopped, and has subsequently remained well for 2 years on both antibiotics and no immunosuppressive treatment. More important, having discontinued corticosteroids she lost about 13 kg in weight and her usual sleep pattern and mood were restored.

We are unsure of the etiology of this woman's granulomatous disease, whereas it seems that bacterial infection may have been prominent at review possibly resulting in an infected secondary atrophic rhinitis. With the benefit of hindsight, the avoidance of a regimen of anti-TNF-α on top of aggressive immunosuppressive therapy that had failed to make an impact on her upper airway disease was in her case the best course of action. By the accident of complete withdrawal of her corticosteroids we were also able to confirm the lack of benefit of continued immunosuppression, the devastating side-effects of corticosteroid on her quality of life, as well as her convincing response to antibiotics and local toilet.

THE ROLE OF SURGERY

A biopsy for histological confirmation of the diagnosis is the most common surgical procedure to be performed in patients with sarcoidosis. Biopsies taken from clinically inflamed upper respiratory tract lesions will usually be supportive of the diagnosis but those from otherwise normal-looking mucosa are mostly negative (Wilson *et al.* 1988).

Nasal surgery is generally to be discouraged in the presence of active disease as experience shows that it is fraught with complications such a septal perforation, saddling and extensive intranasal adhesions (see Figs 21.1 and 21.4). In patients with these deformities surgery should be postponed until the disease is in remission; our experience shows that cartilage and mucosal grafts will be involved by an active disease with the resultant resorption (Sachse and Stoll 2010).

Surgery is indicated only in the presence of active disease in certain situations, such as managing acute or chronic sinusitis that is not responding to medical treatment and in the treatment of complications such as orbital infections and laryngeal obstruction (Kay and Harl-El 2001). In these situations the authors have performed endoscopic sinus surgery on selected patients.

CONCLUSION

Upper airway involvement is an uncommon manifestation of multisystem sarcoidosis. The most common region involved is the nasal mucosa, followed by the larynx and the salivary glands. Although patients can present with minor symptoms, many have severe disease with significant reduction in their quality of life. Life-threatening airway obstruction is also a possibility in patients with laryngeal sarcoidosis.

Local therapy is usually effective in nasal sarcoidosis but often has to be combined with maximal medical therapy and on some occasions surgical procedures are required. A policy of monitoring disease activity, controlling the symptoms, prevention of disease progression and treating life-threatening complications may be achieved via meticulous follow-up with combined efforts of ENT specialists and chest physicians. Nonetheless, there is much to be learned and there will be no substitute for randomized controlled trials of available and novel medications that include strategies against TNF-α.

Acknowledgment

We are very grateful to Professor Robert Baughman for his advice and for giving us permission to reproduce Table 21.1 and Fig. 21.10.

REFERENCES

Antoniu SA (2010). Targeting the TNF-alpha pathway in sarcoidosis. *Expert Opin Ther Targets* 14: 21–9.

Aubart FC, Ouayoun M, Brauner M *et al.* (2006). Sinonasal involvement in sarcoidosis: a case–control study of 20 patients. *Medicine (Baltimore)* 85: 365–71.

Baldini C, Talarico R, Della Rossa A, Bombardieri S (2010). Clinical manifestations and treatment of Churg–Strauss syndrome. *Rheum Dis Clin North Am* 36: 527–43.

Bauchau V, Durham SR (2004). Prevalence and rate of diagnosis of allergic rhinitis in Europe. *Eur Respir J* 24: 758–64.

Baughman RP, Teirstein AS, Judson MA *et al.* (2001). Clinical characteristics of patients in a case control study of sarcoidosis. *Am J Respir Crit Care Med* 5; 164(10 Pt 1): 1885–9.

Baughman RP, Judson MA, Teirstein AS *et al.* (2002). Thalidomide for chronic sarcoidosis. *Chest* 122: 227–32.

Baughman RP, Lowe EE, du Bois RM (2003). Sarcoidosis. *Lancet* 361: 1111–18.

Baughman RP, Lower EE, Bradley DA (2005). Etanercept for refractory ocular sarcoidosis: results of a double-blind randomized trial. *Chest* 128: 1062–47.

Baughman RP, Drent M, Kavuru M (2006). Infliximab therapy in patients with chronic sarcoidosis and pulmonary involvement. *Am J Respir Crit Care Med* 174: 795–802.

Baughman RP, Lower EE, Drent M (2008). Inhibitors of tumor necrosis factor (TNF) in sarcoidosis: who, what, and how to use them. *Sarcoid Vasc Diff Lung Dis* 25: 76–89.

Baughman RP, Lower EE, Tami T (2010). Upper airway. 4: Sarcoidosis of the upper respiratory tract (SURT). *Thorax* 65: 181–6.

Black JI (1973). Sarcoidosis of the nose. *Proc R Soc Med* 66: 669–75.

Boeck C (1905). Fortgesetzte Untersuchungenuber das multiple benigne Sarkoid. *Archiv fur Dermatologie und Syphilis* 73: 301.

Bousquet J, Lockey R, Malling HJ (1998). WHO position paper: Allergen immunotherapy – therapeutic vaccines for allergic diseases. *Allergy* 53: 1–42.

Bousquet J, van Cauwenberge P, Khaltaev N (2001). The WHO initiative: Allergic rhinitis and its impact on asthma (ARIA). *J Allergy Clin Immunol* 108: 147–334.

Bower JS, Belen JE, Weg JG, Dantzker DR (1980). Manifestations and treatment of laryngeal sarcoidosis. *Am Rev Respir Dis* 122: 325–32.

Braun JJ, Gentine A, Pauli G (2004). Sinonasal sarcoidosis: review and report of fifteen cases. *Laryngoscope* 114: 1960–3.

Butler CR, Nouraei SAR, Mace AD *et al.* (2010). Endoscopic management of laryngeal sarcoidosis. *Arch Otolaryngol Head Neck Surg* 136: 251–5.

Callejas-Rubio JL, Ortego-Centeno N, Lopez-Perez L, Benticuaga MN (2006). Treatment of therapy-resistant sarcoidosis with adalimumab. *Clin Rheumatol* 25: 596–7.

Carasso B (1974). Sarcoidosis of the larynx causing airway obstruction. *Chest* 65: 693–5.

Chand MS, Macarthur CJ (1997). Primary atrophic rhinitis: a summary of four cases and review of the literature. *Otolaryngol Head Neck Surg* 116: 554–8.

de Shazo RD, O'Brien MM, Justice WK. (1999). Diagnostic criteria for sarcoidosis of the sinuses. *J Allergy Clin Immunol* 103: 789–95.

Fergie N, Jones NS, Havlat MF (1999). The nasal manifestations of sarcoidosis: a review and report of eight cases. *J Laryngol Otol* 113: 893–8.

Fokkens W, Lund V, Bachert C *et al.* (2005). EAACI position paper on rhinosinusitis and nasal polyps executive summary. *Allergy* 60: 583–601.

Hassid S, Choufani G, Saussez S *et al.* (1998). Sarcoidosis of the paranasal sinuses treated with hydroxychloroquine. *Postgrad Med J* 74: 172–4.

James DG, Barter S, Mackinnon DM, Carstairs LS (1982). Sarcoidosis of the upper respiratory tract (SURT). *J Laryngol Otol* 96: 711–18.

Judson MA, Baughman RP, Teirstein AS (1999). Defining organ involvement in sarcoidosis: the ACCESS proposed instrument. ACCESS Research Group: a case–control etiologic study of sarcoidosis. *Sarcoid Vasc Diff Lung Dis* 16: 75–8.

Kaluza CL (1991). Use of trimethoprim and sulfamethoxazole in the treatment of nasal sarcoidosis. *Ear Nose Throat J* 70: 470.

Kardon DE, Thompson LD (2000). A clinicopathologic series of 22 cases of tonsillar granulomas. *Laryngoscope* 110(3 Pt1): 476–81.

Karma A, Sutinen S, Karma P (1980). Conjunctival and tonsillar biopsies in sarcoidosis [letter]. *Chest* 78: 900–1.

Kay DJ, Har-El G (2001). The role of endoscopic sinus surgery in chronic sinonasal sarcoidosis. *Am J Rhinol* 15: 249–54.

Kirschner BS, Holinger PH (1976). Laryngeal obstruction in children with sarcoidosis. *J Pediatr* 88: 263–5.

Kornblutt AD, Wolff SM, deFries HO, Fauci AS (1980). Wegener's granulomatosis. *Laryngoscope* 90: 1453–65.

Kreibich C, Kraus A (1908). Beitragezur Kenntniss des Boeckschen benignen Miliarlupoid. *Archiv Dermatologie Syphilis* 92: 173.

Lund V (1994). International Consensus Report on the Diagnosis and Management of Rhinitis. *Allergy* **49**: 1–34.

Ly TH, deShazo RD, Olivier J *et al.* (2009). Diagnostic criteria for atrophic rhinosinusitis. *Am J Med* **122**: 747–53.

Neville E, Mills RG, Jash DK *et al.* (1976). Sarcoidosis of the upper respiratory tract and its association with lupus pernio. *Thorax* **31**: 660–4.

Panselinas E, Halstead L, Schlosser RJ, Judson MA (2010). Clinical manifestations, radiographic findings, treatment options, and outcome in sarcoidosis patients with upper respiratory tract involvement. *South Med J* **103**: 870–5.

Rachapalli SM, Kiely PD (2008). Cocaine-induced midline destructive lesions mimicking ENT-limited Wegener's granulomatosis. *Scand J Rheumatol* **37**: 477–80.

Reed J, deShazo RD, Houle TT *et al.* (2010). Clinical features of sarcoid rhinosinusitis. *Am J Med* **123**: 856–62.

Rosen T, Doherty C (2007). Successful long-term management of refractory cutaneous and upper airway sarcoidosis with periodic infliximab infusion. *Dermatol Online J* **13**: 14.

Sachse F, Stoll W (2010). Nasal surgery in patients with systemic disorders. *Laryngorhinootologie* **89**(Suppl. 1): S103–15.

Saleh HA, Durham SR (2007). Perennial rhinitis. *Br Med J* **335**: 502–7.

Scadding GK, Durham SR, Mirakian R *et al.* (2008a). BSACI guidelines for the management of allergic and non-allergic rhinitis. *Clin Exp Allergy* **38**: 19–42.

Scadding GK, Durham SR, Mirakian R *et al.* (2008b). BSACI guidelines for the management of rhinosinusitis and nasal polyposis. *Clin Exp Allergy* **38**: 260–75.

Schaumann J (1936). Lymphogranulomatosis benigna in the light of prolonged clinical observations and autopsy findings. *Br J Dermatol* **48**: 399.

Suresh L, Radfar L (2005). Oral sarcoidosis: a review of literature. *Oral Dis* **11**: 138–45.

Sweiss NJ, Salloum R, Ghandi S *et al.* (2010). Significant CD4, CD8, and CD19 lymphopenia in peripheral blood of sarcoidosis patients correlates with severe disease manifestations. *PLoS One* **5**(5): 9088.

Tong Z, Dai H, Chen B *et al.* (2003). Inhibition of cytokine release from alveolar macrophages in pulmonary sarcoidosis by pentoxifylline: comparison with dexamethasone. *Chest* **124**: 1526–32.

Ulrich K (1918). Die Schleimhautverasnderungender oberen Luftwege beim Boeck'schen Sarkoid und ihreStellungzum Lupuspernio. *Archiv Laryngologie Rhinologie* **31**: 506.

Utz JP, Limper AH, Kalra S (2003). Etanercept for the treatment of stage II and III progressive pulmonary sarcoidosis. *Chest* **124**: 177–85.

van den Boer C, Brutel G, de Vries N (2010). Is routine histopathological examination of FESS material useful? *Eur Arch Otorhinolaryngol* **267**: 381–4.

Wilson R, Lund V, Sweatman M *et al.* (1988). Upper respiratory tract involvement in sarcoidosis and its management. *Eur Respir J* **1**: 269–72.

Zeitlin JF, Tami TA, Baughman R, Winget D (2000). Nasal and sinus manifestations of sarcoidosis. *Am J Rhinol* **14**: 157–61.

22

The airways

FARHANA SHORA, ANDREW MENZIES-GOW, NICOLE GOH AND ELISABETTA RENZONI

INTRODUCTION

Sarcoid granulomas tend to follow a perilymphatic distribution and are thus most abundant in the bronchiolo-arterial bundles and in the interlobular septa (Corrin and Nicholson 2006). Granulomas are also numerous in the mucosa and submucosa of the main airways. It is therefore not surprising that both large and small airways can be affected by sarcoidosis, through a variety of mechanisms.

The morphological manifestations of airway sarcoidosis include bronchial mucosa inflammatory abnormalities (edema, fine granularity, nodules, plaques), cicatricial airway stenosis, airway distortion and traction bronchiectasis caused by surrounding fibrosis, and, less frequently, extrinsic compression from enlarged lymph nodes. The frequency of airway involvement increases as the parenchymal disease progresses (Harrison et al. 1991; Lamberto et al. 1985).

Anatomical evidence of airway obstruction may or may not be associated with functional obstruction or symptoms. Conversely, there may be evidence of functional airflow limitation without identifiable anatomical abnormalities. When different types of airway assessment modalities are used, including bronchoscopy with bronchial mucosa sampling, radiology and lung function testing, airway involvement has been observed in more than two-thirds of patients with sarcoidosis, although there is limited correlation between the different modalities (Levinson et al. 1977; Sharma and Johnson 1988; Davies et al. 2000; Hunninghake et al. 1999).

ANATOMICAL SITES OF AIRWAY INVOLVEMENT

The incidence of bronchial obstruction at different anatomical sites varies widely between studies, most likely because of the differences in method of ascertainment, definition criteria, patient selection and differing ethnic mixes. Broadly speaking, airway abnormalities can be divided into those affecting the large and the small airways, with the latter being significantly more frequently involved.

Large airways

Although sarcoid granulomas are found in the trachea and main bronchi, they do not usually cause significant obstructive symptoms or physiological abnormalities. Their relative rarity is highlighted by the series reported by Sharma and co-workers, in which only 1 of 220 patients had fixed upper airway obstruction arising from abnormalities in the main bronchi (Sharma and Mohan 2004). The lobar, segmental and subsegmental airways are more frequently involved, although less often than the small airways. The stenotic lesions of the large airways can be single, multiple or diffuse; when extensive, they can present with wheezing, shortness of breath and/or stridor (Chambellan et al. 2005). Severe airway obstruction can be associated with segmental or lobar collapse, occurring in under 1 percent of sarcoidosis patients, most frequently involving the right middle lobe (Hansell et al. 2010).

Variations in patient selection are likely to partly explain the reported difference in frequency of large airway narrowing. Historical series have reported frequencies of large airway narrowing ranging from 2.5 to 9 percent (Smellie and Hoyle 1960; Olsson et al. 1979; Scadding and Mitchell 1985). By contrast, in a recent large French study of 2500 patients with sarcoidosis, in which significant obstruction of the proximal airways was defined by findings on bronchoscopy (bronchial narrowing of at least 50 percent of the lumen), only 18 cases with proximal endoluminal bronchial stenosis were identified, all with significant functional impairment. However, the series by Chambellan and co-workers excluded patients with stage IV disease, known to have a higher prevalence of airway stenosis (Chambellan *et al.* 2005).

Small airways

The small airways are the most commonly involved. Bronchiolar and peribronchiolar granulomas are very frequent in sarcoidosis, also in the absence of parenchymal involvement (Carrington 1976; Fig. 22.1). Indeed, airflow obstruction at the level of the small airways is probably one of the earliest features of sarcoidosis (Kaneko and Sharma 1977; Levinson *et al.* 1977). In the presence of active pulmonary infiltration, these changes are more marked and found in a large proportion of cases.

PATHOPHYSIOLOGY OF AIRWAY OBSTRUCTION

Narrowing of the bronchial lumen can occur through several mechanisms, the most frequent of which include:

- endobronchial and submucosa granulomatous inflammation, which can occur in airways of any size, causing narrowing, occlusion and/or bronchiectasis;
- fibrotic scarring of the bronchial lesions with stenosis of the bronchial lumen;
- extrinsic compression and distortion from surrounding fibrosis.

Although extrinsic compression of the central airways by the enlarged mediastinal and hilar lymph nodes would seem an attractive explanation, it seems to be a rarely occurring phenomenon, mostly occurring in the right middle lobe (Goldberg and Greenspan 1960; Fig. 22.2).

The most frequent mechanism appears to be endoluminal, caused by sarcoid granulomas spreading in the submucosa, associated with thickened and edematous mucosa (Sharma 1978; Corsello *et al.* 1983; Corrin and Nicholson 2006). With

time, the granulomas may be replaced by a mucosal and submucosal cicatricial process, developing into fixed fibrotic stenosis. This sequence of events, although unproven, is suggested by the finding that endobronchial proximal stenoses in stage I to III disease are reversible in the majority of patients if treatment is started early, but can develop into fixed stenoses if treatment with systemic corticosteroids is delayed (Chambellan *et al.* 2005).

Although direct obstruction of the large airways by enlarged hilar lymph nodes is rare, the perihilar conglomerate fibrosis of sarcoidosis is a frequent cause of bronchial distortion and narrowing (Hansell *et al.* 2010; Fig. 22.3). A rare cause of obstruction is the endobronchial mass lesion, likely derived from the coalescence of multiple granulomas (Corsello *et al.* 1983). Finally, airway distortion, narrowing and traction bronchiectasis and bronchiolectasis are relatively common in fibrotic sarcoidosis (Fig. 22.4 and Fig. 22.5), as the parenchymal fibrosis can constrict and distort the airways (Di Benedetto and Ribaudo 1966; Hadfield *et al.* 1982; Udwadia *et al.* 1990). Variable airflow obstruction may be caused by accumulation of secretions in larger and smaller airways, and bronchial hyper-reactivity due to released chemical mediators (Cullen *et al.* 1965; Harrison *et al.* 1991).

BRONCHOSCOPIC FINDINGS

Bronchoscopy allows the use of a variety of diagnostic modalities to assess the airways in sarcoidosis. Macroscopically, the most frequent abnormality is a friable, edematous mucosal appearance, with fine granularity. Less common sarcoid bronchial lesions include yellowish nodules, which can give a cobblestone appearance with coalescent, flat yellowish plaques, and localized papilloma-like formations (Scadding and Mitchell 1985). Occasionally, coalescent bronchial granulomas form a mass-like lesion that can obstruct the bronchial lumen, simulating a malignant lesion (Corsello *et al.* 1983).

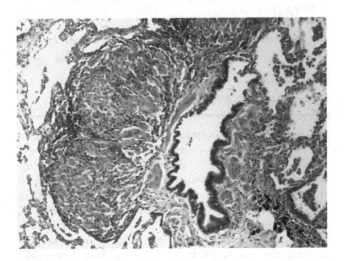

Figure 22.1   Non-necrotizing granuloma next to a bronchiole.

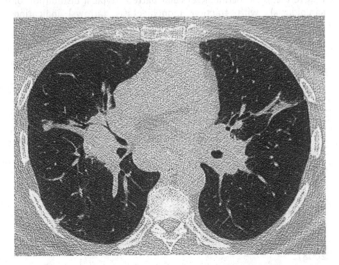

Figure 22.2   Moderate to severe compression of the right middle lobe bronchus by enlarged hilar lymph nodes (there was a similar degree of compression of the lingula in adjacent sections).

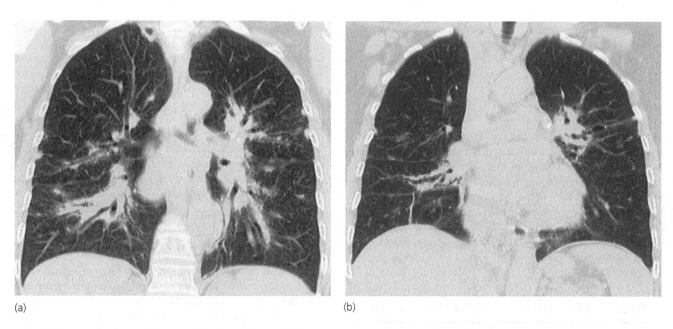

(a)   (b)

Figure 22.3   Generalized large airway distortion in conglomerate perihilar fibrosis: (a) and (b) show two different cuts of coronal images in the same patient.

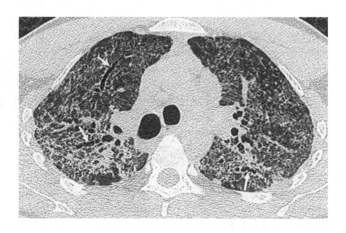

Figure 22.4   Perihilar reticular pattern (typical distribution of sarcoidosis), with traction bronchiectasis (arrows) indicating established fibrosis.

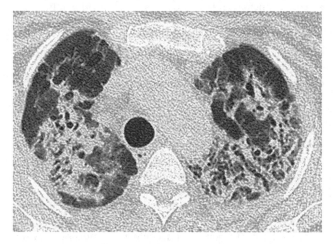

Figure 22.5   Dense peribronchial opacification and coarse reticular pattern at lung apices, with marked traction of the underlying airways.

Because of the airway-centered distribution of granulomas, even with a normal-appearing mucosa, sarcoid granulomas are identified by bronchial biopsy in approximately a third of cases, while diagnostic yield rises to 75 percent in the presence of mucosal abnormalities. Transbronchial biopsy has an even higher diagnostic yield of up to 85 percent, although it is associated with a higher rate of complications, including bleeding and pneumothorax (Shorr *et al.* 2001b; Iannuzzi *et al.* 2007). Bronchial biopsy has been shown to increase the diagnostic yield by more than 20 percent (Shorr *et al.* 2001a), and should thus always be added to transbronchial biopsy in the diagnostic work-up of sarcoidosis (Bradley *et al.* 2008).

In addition to allowing histological confirmation through biopsy procedures, bronchoscopy can provide valuable information concerning the location, extent of involvement, and the mechanism of the stenosis, as well as the degree of the endoluminal narrowing (Chambellan *et al.* 2005).

CLINICAL PRESENTATION AND FINDINGS

Sarcoidosis confined to the airway can masquerade as asthma, presenting with cough, wheezing and shortness of breath, and should be considered in the differential diagnosis when symptoms fail to resolve with conventional treatment (Olsson *et al.* 1979). As mentioned previously, bronchostenoses are detected more frequently later in the course of sarcoidosis, affecting principally the proximal parts of segmental or lobar bronchi, and only occasionally involving the main bronchi (Benatar and Clark 1974; Miller *et al.* 1985). Bronchial obstruction can be associated with dyspnea that is out of proportion to the density of any parenchymal changes evident on imaging, and often with prolongation of inspiration and faint inspiratory as well as expiratory stridor. It may also lead to recurrent or persistent collapse–consolidation in segments with narrowed bronchi.

However, significant obstruction to the large airways can also be identified earlier in disease, in association with the presence of granulomas on endobronchial biopsy, respiratory symptoms (including cough, dyspnea, wheeze and, less frequently, hemoptysis), moderate to severe obstructive defects, and good response to systemic steroids, if treatment is initiated early (Chambellan et al. 2005).

Occasionally, patients may present with a distressing cough in the absence of other symptoms, functional or imaging abnormalities. In this context, it can be difficult to assess whether the cough is related to sarcoidosis or to other common causes such as post-nasal drip, gastro-esophageal reflux or asthma, and the finding of significant BAL lymphocytosis and/or granulomas on bronchial biopsies may help in attributing the cough to sarcoidosis activity. Seasonal shortness of breath with audible wheezing mimicking asthma has also been reported as a relatively infrequent manifestation of sarcoidosis (reported in 30 of 210 biopsy-proven sarcoidosis patients) (Sharma and Mohan 2004).

On auscultation, there may be inspiratory and expiratory wheezing. Although squawks are more commonly associated with hypersensitivity pneumonitis, they can occasionally be heard in sarcoidosis, probably reflecting small airway obstruction (Earis et al. 1982; Udwadia et al. 1990).

LUNG FUNCTION

Large airways

The reported prevalence of functionally evident large airway obstruction varies widely between 4 percent and 67 percent of patients, again reflecting differences in patient selection, severity of disease, criteria used to define functional obstruction, prevalence of smoking, and ethnicity (Miller et al. 1974,1985; Levinson et al. 1977; Dines et al. 1978). An obstructive airway defect is a common finding at presentation (Dines et al. 1978; Young et al. 1980; Stjernberg and Thunell 1984; Newman et al. 1997) and was the most common presenting pulmonary function abnormality in another study, occurring at all stages (Harrison et al. 1991). On the other hand, pulmonary function testing may be normal even if imaging shows significant anatomical abnormalities.

A reduced FEV_1/FVC ratio (<80 percent) was reported in 53 percent of 736 patients with sarcoidosis within 6 months of diagnosis by Baughman et al. (2001). Lower rates were reported in a study by the British Thoracic Society (BTS) of 149 sarcoidosis patients, with a prevalence of 11 percent in 79 lifelong non-smokers (Gibson et al. 1996). At least some of the differences between these studies are likely to relate to ethnicity; in the study by Baughman and associates, 44 percent of patients were African-American and 53 percent were Caucasian, while in the BTS study only 9 of the 149 study patients were not Caucasian (Gibson et al. 1996).

A significantly higher frequency of airway obstruction in blacks was first reported in the study by Sharma and co-workers, with a ratio FEV_1/FVC ratio under 75 percent seen in 63 percent, and FEV_1/FVC under 80 percent seen in 80 percent of African-American non-smoking sarcoidosis patients compared to much lower rates in Caucasian and Japanese patients (Thunell et al. 1987; Sharma and Johnson 1988; Cieslicki et al. 1991; Handa et al. 2009).

The presence of significant airway obstruction is associated with increased mortality. Viksum and Vestbo (1993) demonstrated that patients with an FEV_1/VC less than 70 percent of the predicted value had an increased mortality risk of 1.9 compared with patients with an FEV_1/VC above 70 percent of predicted.

Small airways

Functionally evident airway obstruction is most frequently caused by small airway involvement. Indices of small airway disease include the mid-expiratory flow rate at 50 percent of FVC (MEF_{50}), mid-expiratory flow rate at 25 percent FVC (MEF_{25}), reduction in the forced expiratory flow over the middle half of the forced expiratory curve (FEF_{25-75}), forced expiratory volume at 3 seconds (FEV_3), and measures derived from the single-breath nitrogen test. Density-dependence of flow measures (e.g. ΔV_{max50}, and closing volume) are more specific measures of small airways abnormalities. There are no published data yet available on measurement of small airway function in sarcoidosis using newer techniques such as alveolar nitric oxide (NO) measurement and multiple-breath nitrogen washout.

One study of airway function in 39 patients with sarcoidosis demonstrated typical changes in lung physiology consistent with restrictive disease in four patients, but abnormal small airway function in all patients (Argyropoulou et al. 1984). The maximal expiratory flow rate at 25 or 50 percent of vital capacity was decreased in 62 percent of patients with parenchymal involvement, demonstrating that small airway dysfunction is common in early sarcoidosis in the absence of a restrictive defect.

However, functional measures of small airways abnormalities are highly variable, and not tightly linked to symptoms or imaging, and this limits their usefulness (Antic and Macklem 1976; Stanescu 1999). Having said this, most sarcoidosis patients have at least one abnormal small airway lung function parameter (Levinson et al. 1977; Rizzato et al. 1980).

The very high frequency of small airway obstruction is also compatible with HRCT findings, discussed in subsequent sections.

Airway hyper–reactivity

Airway hyper-reactivity (AHR) has been variably reported in 6 to 50 percent of patients with sarcoidosis, with the most frequently reported estimate being approximately 20 percent (Bechtel et al. 1981; Olafsson et al. 1985; Manresa et al. 1986; Marcias et al. 1994; Aggarwal et al. 2004). AHR has been associated with symptoms of dyspnea, cough and wheeze in individuals with sarcoidosis by Bechtel *et al.* (1981), although others have found no correlation between symptoms classically associated with airway disease and AHR (Shorr *et al.* 2001b). Similarly, AHR has been associated with worse pulmonary function as measured by spirometry, while others have not found a significant link between the results of pulmonary function tests and airway hyper-reactivity (Bechtel *et al.* 1981; Olafsson *et al.* 1985; Aggarwal *et al.* 2004).

The mechanisms underlying AHR in sarcoidosis have not been fully elucidated. AHR can be a transient phenomenon, most frequently seen during the acute stages of the disease, lasting only for a few months; AHR has been associated with areas of extensive epithelial damage uncovering underlying afferent nerve endings of the bronchial mucosa, suggesting a neurogenic pathway (Laitinen *et al.* 1983). In a study of 42 newly diagnosed sarcoidosis patients, Shorr *et al.* (2001b) found that all patients with AHR (20 percent) had endobronchial granulomas, compared to only 45 percent of those with a negative bronchial provocation test; higher serum ACE levels were also associated with AHR. By contrast, no association was found between AHR and abnormal airway appearances, indices of airflow obstruction or radiographic stage. The authors suggest that endobronchial granulomas may lead to AHR through a variety of pathways, including airway narrowing, disruption of cholinergic receptors and the direct effect of inflammatory mediators produced by granulomas (Shorr *et al.* 2001b). One of the difficulties in assessing AHR in sarcoid patients is related to the finding that a smaller baseline diameter of an abnormal airway, as can be seen in sarcoidosis, can potentially increase airway resistance and lead to a falsely positive bronchoprovocation test result (Polychronopoulos and Prakash 2009).

Smoking

Smoking is known to induce airway abnormalities in otherwise healthy individuals. Interestingly, most, but not all, studies have reported a protective effect of smoking on the development of sarcoidosis (Terris and Chaves 1966; Bresnitz and Strom 1983; Douglas *et al.* 1986; Hance *et al.* 1986; Harf *et al.* 1986). This effect appears to be related to a reduced likelihood of developing sarcoidosis in smokers rather than a reduced severity caused by smoking; in one study, 30 percent of sarcoidosis patients were current smokers compared to 46 percent of an age-matched normal French population, although functional severity was similar when smoking and non-smoking sarcoidosis patients were compared (Valeyre *et al.* 1988). On the other hand, the incidence of small airways disease seems to be higher in smokers than in lifelong non-smokers with sarcoidosis, and the prevalence of FEV_1/FVC ratio reduction was higher in smokers than in non-smokers in a group of Japanese sarcoidosis patients (Dutton *et al.* 1982; Terasaki *et al.* 2005).

The protective effect of smoking may be related to an inhibitory and/or immunomodulatory effect on the number and function of immune and inflammatory cells in the lung. Compared to non-smoking sarcoidosis patients, sarcoidosis smokers were found to have higher serum ACE levels, higher gallium uptake and increased numbers of BAL

CD8+ lymphocytes and alveolar macrophages. Although the pathogenetic mechanism of smoking-induced protection is not known, an alteration of the regulation between macrophages and lymphocytes appears likely (Liu *et al.* 1984; Ettensohn *et al.* 1986; Rich *et al.* 1987).

IMAGING PATTERNS OF AIRWAY INVOLVEMENT

The chest radiograph understates airway involvement. However, the much higher sensitivity of CT allows identification of large airway abnormalities (lobar up to sub-segmental airways) in up to two-thirds of patients, including smooth or nodular bronchial wall thickening, and/or regular or irregular luminal narrowing (Lenique *et al.* 1995). A frequent cause of airway narrowing is the perihilar conglomerate fibrosis (see Fig. 22.3), and the architectural distortion caused by fibrosis (Fig. 22.6), well highlighted by CT. The rare involvement of the trachea and mainstem bronchi can be identified by CT, showing a smooth, nodular, diffusely stenotic and mass-like appearance.

CT scanning can be helpful in detecting bronchial lesions, but is less accurate in the prediction of whether a given abnormality is endobronchial, submucosal or extrinsic (Chambellan *et al.* 2005). Furthermore, CT may miss significant large airways stenosis, particularly if conventional CT (transaxial) with interspaced thin sections is used. However, with the use of multiplanar reconstructions (reconstructions along the long axis of the airway in question), even subtle narrowings are unlikely to be missed, although to our knowledge this has not been specifically assessed in sarcoidosis.

On CT, areas of decreased attenuation, more obvious on expiration (termed 'mosaic attenuation'), suggest obstruction

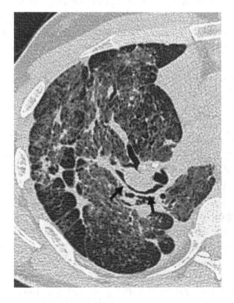

Figure 22.6   HRCT section through the middle and lower lobes shows marked architectural distortion by established fibrosis. Note the abnormal course and narrowing of the apical segmental bronchus of the right lower lobe (arrows).

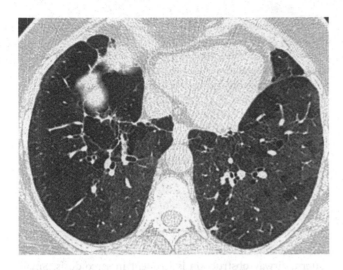

Figure 22.7   Inspiratory HRCT through lower lobes showing a limited reticular pattern and a background mosaic attenuation pattern (areas of blacker lung) reflecting small airway involvement.

of peripheral airways (Fig. 22.7). Gleeson and associates first described the finding that CT scanning at end-exhalation in patients with sarcoidosis identified lobular air trapping, presumed to be secondary to granulomas in small airways (Gleeson et al. 1996). Subsequent studies have confirmed the very high frequency of mosaic attenuation on expiratory images seen in sarcoidosis patients with rates of up to 95 percent reported by Davies and co-workers (Stern et al. 1994; Hansell et al. 1998; Davies et al. 2000; Magkanas et al. 2001). Areas of low attenuation on expiratory HRCT have been demonstrated not only at the secondary lobule level, but also in sublobular-sized areas and at the sub-segmental and segmental levels, suggesting air trapping can occur in either multiple confluent pulmonary lobules, larger airways, or both (Bartz and Stern 2000).

Interestingly, the prevalence of mosaic attenuation does not differ according to stage of disease or to region of the lung, nor is there a correlation with any of the radiological patterns of sarcoidosis (Bartz and Stern 2000; Davies et al. 2000; Magkanas et al. 2001). Expiratory evidence of air trapping can be the only radiological feature present, and while non-specific, it is a common feature in patients with pulmonary sarcoidosis, which can support the diagnosis (Gleeson et al. 1996; Davies et al. 2000; Magkanas et al. 2001).

STRUCTURE–FUNCTION CORRELATION

Sarcoid granulomas have a preferential distribution along the peribronchial and peribronchiolar structures, following the distribution of lymphatics. Histologically, both the large and small airways are involved in relatively early stages of the disease (Friedman et al. 1963; Dines et al. 1978; Lenique et al. 1995). However, the functional correlates between histology and lung function are tenuous at best. Young and associates described a lack of correlation between histological evidence of small airway involvement and substantial airflow limitation (Young et al. 1980). Carrington (1976) suggested that a smaller number of strategically located granulomas may

cause narrowing of the small airways, resulting in significant functional impairment, whereas larger numbers of less critically located granulomas may cause minimal or no dysfunction. This could at least partially explain the poor correlation between the profusion of nodules revealed by CT scans and pulmonary function tests, especially the indexes of airflow obstruction (Mayse et al. 2004).

Bronchoscopically evident bronchostenosis or extrinsic bronchial compression are associated with an obstructive pattern (Mendelson et al. 1983; Stjernberg and Thunell 1984; Harrison et al. 1991). Other studies have shown that pulmonary fibrosis due to sarcoidosis also results in an obstructive pattern (Miller et al. 1974; Bergin et al. 1989).

Varying degrees of correlation have been found between a CT pattern of mosaic attenuation more obvious on expiration and functional evidence of small airways disease. One report found a significant correlation between air trapping on CT and percentage predicted maximal mid-expiratory flow rate between 25 and 75 percent of the vital capacity (Davies et al. 2000), while another found a correlation only with RV/TLC and RV in 30 sarcoidosis patients, but not with FEV_1/FVC or FEF_{25-75} (Magkanas et al. 2001). By contrast, Hansell and co-authors reported that CT features compatible with small airways disease are common but contribute little to airflow obstruction (Hansell et al. 1998), while extent of reticulation was the CT feature most strongly associated with indices of large and small airways obstruction, including FEV_1/FVC ratio, MEF_{50} and MEF_{25} as well as RV/TLC, independently of disease severity. This study concluded that the obstructive component in sarcoidosis is mainly related to the extent of reticular pattern on CT scans, suggesting that the development of significant airway obstruction is more closely related to the progression towards fibrosis. Interestingly, extent of reticulation was also correlated with a history of wheezing, suggesting that the major determinant of 'asthma-like' symptoms may be linked to airway-centered fibrosis rather than to concomitant asthma or AHR (Hansell et al. 1998). In this study, the association between thickness and diameter of the large airways and indices of airway obstruction was not assessed. However, in another study a decreased luminal area of the central airways was correlated with peak expiratory flow in 43 Japanese sarcoidosis patients (the majority with stage 0 and I disease) (Handa et al. 2009).

THERAPEUTIC OPTIONS

A comprehensive approach to the treatment of sarcoidosis is outside the scope of this chapter. Although evidence-based characterization of the symptoms and/or findings that necessitate treatment is lacking, the decision to treat a patient with airway obstruction essentially depends on severity and rate of progression of symptoms. As is the case for other patterns of sarcoidosis, corticosteroids are recognized as the initial preferred treatment, while immunosuppressive agents including methotrexate, azathioprine, and hydroxychloroquine are used as steroid sparing agents and/or in case of contraindications to steroid use. Although most clinicians would agree that steroid treatment is often effective in the treatment of significant airway obstruction, there are a few studies reporting little or no improvement in a handful of patients with severe obstruction (Olsson et al. 1979; Miller et al. 1985; Lewis and Horak 1987). Olsson and co-workers described a handful of patients with single or multiple segmental stenosis with poor response to steroids (Olsson et al. 1979). Lewis and Horak observed continued progression in a patient with very severe obstruction, despite maintenance steroid therapy (Lewis and Horak 1987). Miller and co-authors described two patients with severe airway obstruction; one experienced no improvement, whereas the other improved only after prolonged treatment with high-dose oral corticosteroids (Miller et al. 1985).

By contrast, there are several reports indicating at least partial reversibility of obstructive symptoms and physiology on steroid treatment. One reported improvement of FEV_1 in three out of six patients with low baseline FEV_1 (Smellie et al. 1961). Another reported substantial improvement in 72 percent of cases following treatment of airway obstruction due to bronchial wall involvement by sarcoid granulomas (Lavergne et al. 1999). A few other case reports describe improvement of airway obstruction with treatment (Benatar and Clark 1974; Corsello et al. 1983).

The reported differences in treatment responsiveness are likely to be at least partially related to the timing of treatment, which is more likely to be successful if instituted before irreversible fibrotic obstruction of the airways has developed (Chambellan et al. 2005). However, it is possible that in a very small proportion of patients, the mechanisms underlying airway stenosis are not steroid responsive from the start, possibly because of a striking early predominance of pro-fibrotic over inflammatory pathways. In severe cases, it is worth considering pulsed intravenous methylprednisolone treatment, which can be more effective than high-dose oral steroids. Furthermore, pulsed therapy has been associated with fewer side-effects than continuous oral steroids (in particular, reduced bone mass loss and Cushingoid features in the IV-treated groups), in other immune-mediated diseases, including rheumatoid arthritis and Graves' disease (Marcocci et al. 2001; Frediani et al. 2004).

Treatment with inhaled steroids seems intuitively attractive in the context of endobronchial sarcoidosis. However, when compared to placebo, several controlled clinical trials have not suggested a significant benefit from inhaled steroids on functional or imaging parameters, although patients with airway obstruction were not specifically selected (Milman et al. 1994; Alberts et al. 1995; Paramothayan and Jones 2002). On the other hand, a few placebo controlled trials suggest potential benefits in symptom control; in particular, Alberts and co-workers reported a significant improvement in symptoms following inhaled budesonide treatment in newly diagnosed pulmonary sarcoidosis (Alberts et al. 1995). In a separate study, a trend towards symptomatic improvement, not reaching statistical significance, was observed following the use of fluticasone in stable sarcoidosis patients (du Bois et al. 1999). The use of systemic glucocorticosteroids, followed by inhaled corticosteroids, has been shown to be more effective than placebo in stage II pulmonary disease (Pietinalho et al. 1999; Mixides and Guy 2003). A trial with inhaled corticosteroids may be beneficial in patients who present with cough,

wheezing and/or bronchial hyper-reactivity (Paramothayan and Jones 2000).

Sarcoidosis complicated by proximal endobronchial stenosis should be treated early to avoid the development of fixed stenotic lesions and irreversible pulmonary function impairment (Chambellan et al. 2005). Bronchoscopic dilatation by balloon dilatation or laser phototherapy can be attempted to relieve airway obstruction in severe stenosis; placement of a mechanical stent may subsequently be necessary to maintain airway patency (Iles 1981; Putnam 1993; Chan et al. 2003).

CONCLUSION

Despite being traditionally associated with a restrictive pattern, airway obstruction is frequent in sarcoidosis. Small airway involvement is common and appears to occur early in the course of the disease; reduction in FEF_{25-75} and RV/TLC and/or a CT pattern of mosaic attenuation on expiration may be the only abnormalities pointing towards the airways. Large airway obstruction, characterized by a reduced FEV_1/FVC ratio, is less frequent, and tends to develop later in the course of the disease, in the fibrotic stages of sarcoidosis. Wide ethnic variability is seen, with the highest frequencies of large airway obstruction reported in African-American patients. The presence of large airway obstruction is associated with an almost 2-fold increased mortality. Sarcoidosis complicated by proximal endobronchial obstruction should be treated early to avoid the development of fixed stenotic lesions and irreversible pulmonary function impairment.

REFERENCES

Aggarwal AN, Gupta D, Chandrasekhar G, Jindal SK (2004). Bronchial hyperresponsiveness in patients with sarcoidosis. J Assoc Physicians India 52: 21–3.

Alberts C, van der Mark TW, Jansen HM (1995). Dutch Study Group on Pulmonary Sarcoidosis: Inhaled budesonide in pulmonary sarcoidosis: a double-blind, placebo-controlled study. Eur Respir J 8: 682–8.

Antic R, Macklem PT (1976). The influence of clinical factors on site of airway obstruction in asthma. Am Rev Respir Dis 114: 851–9.

Argyropoulou PK, Patakas DA, Louridas GE (1984). Airway function in stage I and stage II pulmonary sarcoidosis. Respiration 46: 17–25.

Bartz RR, Stern EJ (2000). Airways obstruction in patients with sarcoidosis: expiratory CT scan findings. J Thorac Imaging 15: 285–9.

Baughman RP, Teirstein AS, Judson MA et al. (2001). Clinical characteristics of patients in a case control study of sarcoidosis. Am J Respir Crit Care Med 164: 1885–9.

Bechtel JJ, Starr T, Dantzker DR, Bower JS (1981). Airway hyperreactivity in patients with sarcoidosis. Am Rev Respir Dis 124: 759–61.

Benatar SR, Clark TJ (1974). Pulmonary function in a case of endobronchial sarcoidosis. Am Rev Respir Dis 110: 490–6.

Bergin CJ, Bell DY, Coblentz CL et al. (1989). Sarcoidosis: correlation of pulmonary parenchymal pattern at CT with results of pulmonary function tests. Radiology 171: 619–24.

Bradley B, Branley HM, Egan JJ et al. (2008). Interstitial lung disease guideline: the British Thoracic Society in collaboration with the

Thoracic Society of Australia and New Zealand and the Irish Thoracic Society. *Thorax* **63**(Suppl. 5): 1–58.

Bresnitz EA, Strom BL (1983). Epidemiology of sarcoidosis. *Epidemiol Rev* **5**: 124–56.

Carrington CB (1976). Structure and function in sarcoidosis. *Ann NY Acad Sci* **278**: 265–83.

Chambellan A, Turbie P, Nunes H *et al.* (2005). Endoluminal stenosis of proximal bronchi in sarcoidosis: bronchoscopy, function, and evolution. *Chest* **127**: 472–81.

Chan AL, Yoneda KY, Allen RP, Albertson TE (2003). Advances in the management of endobronchial lung malignancies. *Curr Opin Pulm Med* **9**: 301–8.

Cieslicki J, Zych D, Zielinski J (1991). Airways obstruction in patients with sarcoidosis. *Sarcoidosis* **8**: 42–4.

Corrin B, Nicholson AG (2006). *Pathology of the Lungs*, 2nd edn. Churchill Livingstone Elsevier, Philadelphia, pp. 285–90.

Corsello BF, Lohaus GH, Funahashi A (1983). Endobronchial mass lesion due to sarcoidosis: complete resolution with corticosteroids. *Thorax* **38**: 157–8.

Cullen JH, Katz HL, Kaemmerlen JT (1965). Chronic diffuse pulmonary infiltration and airway obstruction. *Am Rev Respir Dis* **92**: 775–80.

Davies CW, Tasker AD, Padley SP *et al.* (2000). Air trapping in sarcoidosis on computed tomography: correlation with lung function. *Clin Radiol* **55**: 217–21.

Di Benedetto RJ, Ribaudo C (1966). Bronchopulmonary sarcoidosis. *Am Rev Respir Dis* **94**: 952–5.

Dines DE, Stubbs SE, McDougall JC (1978). Obstructive disease of the airways associated with stage I sarcoidosis. *Mayo Clin Proc* **53**: 788–91.

Douglas JG, Middleton WG, Gaddie J *et al.* (1986). Sarcoidosis: a disorder commoner in non-smokers? *Thorax* **41**: 787–91.

du Bois RM, Greenhalgh PM, Southcott AM *et al.* (1999). Randomized trial of inhaled fluticasone propionate in chronic stable pulmonary sarcoidosis: a pilot study. *Eur Respir J* **13**: 1345–50.

Dutton RE, Renzi PM, Lopez-Majano V, Renzi GD (1982). Airway function in sarcoidosis: smokers versus nonsmokers. *Respiration* **43**: 164–73.

Earis JE, Marsh K, Pearson MG, Ogilvie CM (1982). The inspiratory 'squawk' in extrinsic allergic alveolitis and other pulmonary fibroses. *Thorax* **37**: 923–6.

Ettensohn DB, Lalor PA, Roberts NJ (1986). Human alveolar macrophage regulation of lymphocyte proliferation. *Am Rev Respir Dis* **133**: 1091–6.

Frediani B, Falsetti P, Bisogno S *et al.* (2004). Effects of high-dose methylprednisolone pulse therapy on bone mass and biochemical markers of bone metabolism in patients with active rheumatoid arthritis: a 12-month randomized prospective controlled study. *J Rheumatol* **31**: 1083–7.

Friedman OH, Blaugrund SM, Siltzbach LE (1963). Biopsy of the bronchial wall as an aid in diagnosis of sarcoidosis. *J Am Med Assoc* **183**: 646–50.

Gibson GJ, Prescott RJ, Muers MF *et al.* (1996). British Thoracic Society Sarcoidosis study: effects of long term corticosteroid treatment. *Thorax* **51**: 238–47.

Gleeson FV, Traill ZC, Hansell DM (1996). Evidence of expiratory CT scans of small-airway obstruction in sarcoidosis. *Am J Roentgenol* **166**: 1052–4.

Goldberg GJ, Greenspan RH (1960). Middle-lobe atelectasis due to endobronchial sarcodosis, with hypercalcemia and renal impairment. *New Engl J Med* **262**: 1112–16.

Hadfield JW, Page RL, Flower CD, Stark JE (1982). Localised airway narrowing in sarcoidosis. *Thorax* **37**: 443–7.

Hance AJ, Basset F, Saumon G *et al.* (1986). Smoking and interstitial lung disease: the effect of cigarette smoking on the incidence of pulmonary histiocytosis X and sarcoidosis. *Ann NY Acad Sci* **465**: 643–56.

Handa T, Nagai S, Hirai T *et al.* (2009). Computed tomography analysis of airway dimensions and lung density in patients with sarcoidosis. *Respiration* **77**: 273–81.

Hansell DM, Milne DG, Wilsher ML, Wells AU (1998). Pulmonary sarcoidosis: morphologic associations of airflow obstruction at thin-section CT. *Radiology* **209**: 697–704.

Hansell D, Lynch DA, McAdams HP (2010). *Imaging of Diseases of the Chest*, 5th edn. Elsevier Mosby, New York, pp. 653–7.

Harf RA, Ethevenaux C, Gleize J *et al.* (1986). Reduced prevalence of smokers in sarcoidosis: results of a case–control study. *Ann NY Acad Sci* **465**: 625–31.

Harrison BD, Shaylor JM, Stokes TC, Wilkes AR (1991). Airflow limitation in sarcoidosis: a study of pulmonary function in 107 patients with newly diagnosed disease. *Respir Med* **85**: 59–64.

Hunninghake GW, Costabel U, Ando M *et al.* (1999). ATS/ERS/WASOG statement on sarcoidosis. *Sarcoid Vasc Diff Lung Dis* **16**: 149–73.

Iannuzzi MC, Rybicki BA, Teirstein AS (2007). Sarcoidosis. *New Engl J Med* **357**: 2153–65.

Iles PB (1981). Multiple bronchial stenoses: treatment by mechanical dilatation. *Thorax* **36**: 784–6.

Kaneko K, Sharma OP (1977). Airway obstruction in pulmonary sarcoidosis. *Bull Eur Physiopathol Respir* **13**: 231–40.

Laitinen LA, Haahtela T, Kava T, Laitinen A (1983). Non-specific bronchial reactivity and ultrastructure of the airway epithelium in patients with sarcoidosis and allergic alveolitis. *Eur J Respir Dis Suppl* **131**: 267–84.

Lamberto C, Saumon G, Loiseau P *et al.* (1985). Respiratory function in recent pulmonary sarcoidosis with special reference to small airways. *Bull Eur Physiopathol Respir* **21**: 309–15.

Lavergne F, Clerici C, Sadoun D *et al.* (1999). Airway obstruction in bronchial sarcoidosis: outcome with treatment. *Chest* **116**: 1194–9.

Lenique F, Brauner MW, Grenier P *et al.* (1995). CT assessment of bronchi in sarcoidosis: endoscopic and pathologic correlations. *Radiology* **194**: 419–23.

Levinson RS, Metzger LF, Stanley NN *et al.* (1977). Airway function in sarcoidosis. *Am J Med* **62**: 51–9.

Lewis MI, Horak DA (1987). Airflow obstruction in sarcoidosis. *Chest* **92**: 582–4.

Liu MC, Proud D, Schleimer RP, Plaut M (1984). Human lung macrophages enhance and inhibit lymphocyte proliferation. *J Immunol* **132**: 2895–903.

Magkanas E, Voloudaki A, Bouros D *et al.* (2001). Pulmonary sarcoidosis: correlation of expiratory high-resolution CT findings with inspiratory patterns and pulmonary function tests. *Acta Radiol* **42**: 494–501.

Manresa PF, Romero CP, Rodriguez SB (1986). Bronchial hyperreactivity in fresh stage I sarcoidosis. *Ann NY Acad Sci* **465**: 523–9.

Marcias S, Ledda MA, Perra R *et al.* (1994). Aspecific bronchial hyperreactivity in pulmonary sarcoidosis. *Sarcoidosis* **11**: 118–22.

Marcocci C, Bartalena L, Tanda ML *et al.* (2001). Comparison of the effectiveness and tolerability of intravenous or oral glucocorticoids associated with orbital radiotherapy in the management of severe Graves' ophthalmopathy: results of a prospective, single-blind, randomized study. *J Clin Endocrinol Metab* **86**: 3562–7.

Mayse ML, Greenheck J, Friedman M, Kovitz KL (2004). Successful bronchoscopic balloon dilation of nonmalignant tracheobronchial obstruction without fluoroscopy. *Chest* **126**: 634–7.

Mendelson DS, Norton K, Cohen BA *et al.* (1983). Bronchial compression: an unusual manifestation of sarcoidosis. *J Comput Assist Tomogr* 7: 892–4.

Miller A, Brown LK, Teirstein AS (1985). Stenosis of main bronchi mimicking fixed upper airway obstruction in sarcoidosis. *Chest* 88: 244–8.

Miller A, Teirstein AS, Jackler I *et al.* (1974). Airway function in chronic pulmonary sarcoidosis with fibrosis. *Am Rev Respir Dis* 109: 179–89.

Milman N, Graudal N, Grode G, Munch E (1994). No effect of high-dose inhaled steroids in pulmonary sarcoidosis: a double-blind, placebo-controlled study. *J Intern Med* 236: 285–90.

Mixides G, Guy E (2003). Sarcoidosis confined to the airway masquerading as asthma. *Can Respir J* 10: 114–16.

Newman LS, Rose CS, Maier LA (1997). Sarcoidosis. *New Engl J Med* 336: 1224–34.

Olafsson M, Simonsson BG, Hansson SB (1985). Bronchial reactivity in patients with recent pulmonary sarcoidosis. *Thorax* 40: 51–3.

Olsson T, Bjornstad-Pettersen H, Stjernberg NL (1979). Bronchostenosis due to sarcoidosis: a cause of atelectasis and airway obstruction simulating pulmonary neoplasm and chronic obstructive pulmonary disease. *Chest* 75: 663–6.

Paramothayan NS, Jones PW (2000). Corticosteroids for pulmonary sarcoidosis. *Cochrane Database Syst Rev : C* 4: D001114.

Paramothayan S, Jones PW (2002). Corticosteroid therapy in pulmonary sarcoidosis: a systematic review. *J Am Med Assoc* 287: 1301–7.

Pietinalho A, Tukiainen P, Haahtela T *et al.* (1999). Finnish Pulmonary Sarcoidosis Study Group: Oral prednisolone followed by inhaled budesonide in newly diagnosed pulmonary sarcoidosis: a double-blind, placebo-controlled multicenter study. *Chest* 116: 424–31.

Polychronopoulos VS, Prakash UB (2009). Airway involvement in sarcoidosis. *Chest* 136: 1371–80.

Putnam JB (1993). Palliation of central airway stenoses with the Dumon silicone stent. *Chest* 104: 1651–2.

Rich EA, Tweardy DJ, Fujiwara H, Ellner JJ (1987). Spectrum of immunoregulatory functions and properties of human alveolar macrophages. *Am Rev Respir Dis* 136: 258–65.

Rizzato G, Brambilla I, Bertoli L (1980). Impaired airway function and pulmonary haemodynamics in sarcoidosis. In: Jones Williams W, Davies BH (eds). *Proceedings of the Eighth International Conference on Sarcoidosis.* Alpha Omega Publishing, Cardiff, pp. 349–59.

Scadding JG, Mitchell D (1985). *Sarcoidosis*, 2nd edn. Chapman and Hall, London, pp. 140–3.

Sharma OP (1978). Airway obstruction in sarcoidosis. *Chest* 73: 6–7.

Sharma OP, Johnson R (1988). Airway obstruction in sarcoidosis: a study of 123 nonsmoking black American patients with sarcoidosis. *Chest* 94: 343–6.

Sharma SK, Mohan A (2004). Uncommon manifestations of sarcoidosis. *J Assoc Physicians India* 52: 210–14.

Shorr AF, Torrington KG, Hnatiuk OW (2001a). Endobronchial biopsy for sarcoidosis: a prospective study. *Chest* 120: 109–14.

Shorr AF, Torrington KG, Hnatiuk OW (2001b). Endobronchial involvement and airway hyperreactivity in patients with sarcoidosis. *Chest* 120: 881–6.

Smellie H, Hoyle C (1960). The natural history of pulmonary sarcoidosis. *Q J Med* 29: 539–59.

Smellie H, Apthorp GH, Marshall R (1961). The effect of corticosteroid treatment on pulmonary function in sarcoidosis. *Thorax* 16: 87–90.

Stanescu D (1999). Small airways obstruction syndrome. *Chest* 116: 231–3.

Stern EJ, Webb WR, Gamsu G (1994). Dynamic quantitative computed tomography: a predictor of pulmonary function in obstructive lung diseases. *Invest Radiol* 29: 564–9.

Stjernberg N, Thunell M (1984). Pulmonary function in patients with endobronchial sarcoidosis. *Acta Med Scand* 215: 121–6.

Terasaki H, Fujimoto K, Muller NL *et al.* (2005). Pulmonary sarcoidosis: comparison of findings of inspiratory and expiratory high-resolution CT and pulmonary function tests between smokers and nonsmokers. *Am J Roentgen* 185: 333–8.

Terris M, Chaves AD (1966). An epidemiologic study of sarcoidosis. *Am Rev Respir Dis* 94: 50–5.

Thunell M, Stjernberg N, Rosenhall L, Backman C (1987). Pulmonary function in patients with sarcoidosis: a three-year follow-up. *Sarcoidosis* 4: 129–33.

Udwadia ZF, Pilling JR, Jenkins PF, Harrison BD (1990). Bronchoscopic and bronchographic findings in 12 patients with sarcoidosis and severe or progressive airways obstruction. *Thorax* 45: 272–5.

Valeyre D, Soler P, Clerici C *et al.* (1988). Smoking and pulmonary sarcoidosis: effect of cigarette smoking on prevalence, clinical manifestations, alveolitis, and evolution of the disease. *Thorax* 43: 516–24.

Viskum K, Vestbo J (1993). Vital prognosis in intrathoracic sarcoidosis with special reference to pulmonary function and radiological stage. *Eur Respir J* 6: 349–53.

Young RC, Sahetya GK, Hassan SN *et al.* (1980). Chronic airways obstruction in pulmonary sarcoidosis: its poor response to bronchodilators. *J Natl Med Assoc* 72: 965–72.

23

Pulmonary fibrosis

TOBY M MAHER AND ROBIN J McANULTY

INTRODUCTION

The lung is the most frequently affected organ in patients with sarcoidosis (Scadding 1961; Mitchell *et al.* 1977; Neville *et al.* 1983; Hillerdal *et al.* 1984; Baughman *et al.* 2001). Pulmonary sarcoidosis exhibits a wide range of clinical and radiological phenotypes. The most frequent of these is a predominantly bronchocentric, and often self-limiting, granulomatous inflammation. Up to 10 percent of patients however, even at first presentation have irreversible fibrotic or fibrobullous change (Scadding 1961; Baughman *et al.* 2001). This is generally associated with ongoing granulomatous inflammation. Furthermore, as many as 10–20 percent of the patients who present with initially inflammatory lesions alone subsequently develop chronic disease that progresses to fibrosis.

In 1956, Scadding proposed a four-part staging system for pulmonary sarcoidosis based on the appearance of the presenting chest radiograph. Despite considerable advances in imaging technology over the last half century this staging system has yet to be superseded. Subsequent to Scadding's seminal paper, a further stage has been added to the chest radiograph classification. The accepted classification is now:

- stage 0, normal radiograph;
- stage I, hilar adenopathy alone;
- stage II, hilar adenopathy with associated parenchymal inflammatory change;
- stage III, inflammatory parenchymal change but no adenopathy;
- stage IV, evidence of fibrotic change, i.e. loss of lung volume, tenting of diaphragms, fibrobullous destruction or parenchymal bands.

In a subsequent longitudinal study, Scadding was able to demonstrate that initial chest X-ray stage predicted subsequent prognosis (Scadding 1961). After 5 years, 84 percent of patients presenting with a stage I radiograph had normal X-ray appearances and 97 percent were symptom-free. By contrast, of 26 patients with a stage IV X-ray, 6 had died as a consequence of pulmonary fibrosis and only 7 of the remaining 20 had shown any improvement in respiratory symptoms or radiographic appearance. Furthermore, 43 percent and 57 percent of the patients with stage II and III disease, respectively, demonstrated evidence of radiographic progression with the development of some degree of sarcoidosis-related fibrotic lung disease. Subsequent studies have replicated this pattern of sarcoidosis disease behavior (Siltzbach *et al.* 1974; Baughman *et al.* 1997; Baughman *et al.* 2006b). Developments in cross-sectional thoracic imaging have provided important insights into both the frequency with which pulmonary fibrosis occurs in sarcoidosis and the different patterns of fibrotic lung disease encountered in this ever-challenging condition.

This chapter will review the clinical features and treatment of fibrotic sarcoidosis and will overview the current understanding of key pathogenetic mechanisms involved in the evolution of granulomatous inflammation to irreversible fibrosis.

EPIDEMIOLOGY

Sarcoidosis is more common in early adulthood and middle age, and it varies in incidence according to gender, ethnicity and geographic location (Milman and Selroos 1990; Pietinalho *et al.* 1995; Baughman *et al.* 2001; Behbehani *et al.* 2007; Morimoto *et al.* 2008). Although the condition has been reported to occur in all age groups, it is most common between 25 and 40 years with, in some studies, an apparent second peak of incidence in the over-50s (Baughman *et al.* 2001; Byg *et al.* 2003).

In American and European populations, the incidence of sarcoidosis is approximately three times higher in blacks than in Caucasians (Rybicki *et al.* 1997). Furthermore, in blacks the disease is more frequently disseminated, is more severe and follows a more chronic course than sarcoidosis occurring in other ethnic groups (Baughman *et al.* 2001; Reich 2001; Rabin *et al.* 2004).

Although sarcoidosis is generally considered to be a sporadic disease, in 1.7–17 percent of cases the condition shows familial clustering, supporting a possible genetic influence in disease pathogenesis (McGrath *et al.* 2000; Rybicki *et al.* 2001). Interestingly, sarcoidosis has also been reported in temporal and spatial clusters and shows a seasonal variation in incidence, being more common in spring (Hiraga *et al.* 1977; Hills *et al.* 1987; Hosoda *et al.* 1997). This, together with the reported occurrence of sarcoidosis in previously unaffected individuals following the transplantation of an affected organ, suggests a role for transmissible agents in the pathogenesis of the disease (Padilla *et al.* 2002).

At presentation, most affected individuals have stage I or II pulmonary disease on chest radiography (Scadding 1961; Neville *et al.* 1983; Baughman *et al.* 2001). A significant minority of patients with biopsy-confirmed sarcoidosis have evidence of pulmonary fibrosis at presentation with 5–10 percent having a stage IV appearance on radiography (Scadding 1961; Baughman *et al.* 2001). In the US ACCESS report, the occurrence of pulmonary involvement in patients with sarcoidosis was, on multivariate analysis, independent of age, gender and ethnicity (Baughman *et al.* 2001). Stage IV disease is associated with a worse prognosis than disease in stages 0–II, with a lower likelihood of disease regression and increased likelihood of chronicity and disease progression (Scadding 1961; Siltzbach *et al.* 1974; Neville *et al.* 1983; Pietinalho *et al.* 2000; Judson *et al.* 2003; Baughman *et al.* 2006b). Furthermore, patients with sarcoidosis who have pulmonary fibrosis have greater symptoms with worse dyspnea and greater fatigue and an increased likelihood of depression. Similarly, patients with sarcoidosis-related pulmonary fibrosis have a greater incidence of disease complications, including pulmonary hypertension, respiratory failure and mycetomas (Pietinalho *et al.* 2000; Judson *et al.* 2003).

In a number of retrospective studies the mortality rate from sarcoidosis has been reported to lie between 1 and 5 percent, with the majority of deaths being related to chronic pulmonary disease and pulmonary fibrosis (Gideon and Mannino 1996; Reich 2002).

CLINICAL FEATURES OF FIBROTIC PULMONARY SARCOIDOSIS

Sarcoidosis is a notorious mimic of other diseases and this remains true even in patients with fibrotic pulmonary sarcoidosis, in which there is no single defining clinical phenotype at disease presentation. Similarly, the radiographic appearance of pulmonary fibrosis in sarcoidosis is very variable and in a proportion of cases mirrors the appearance of other interstitial lung diseases. Clinicians need to be alert to the possibility of sarcoidosis as a diagnosis in any patient with fibrotic lung disease of unknown etiology.

History and examination

The majority of patients with pulmonary involvement have dyspnea and a dry cough. The frequency and severity of these two symptoms tends to be greater in patients with fibrotic lung disease. Very few patients with sarcoidosis complain of chest pain. In keeping with the systemic nature of the disease, patients with pulmonary sarcoidosis frequently have associated symptoms of lethargy and fatigue (Gvozdenovic *et al.* 2008; de Kleijn *et al.* 2009). In the ACCESS study the severity of lung disease in sarcoidosis, as determined by FVC at presentation, was significantly associated with symptoms of depression (Yeager *et al.* 2005).

Even in patients with severe pulmonary fibrosis due to sarcoidosis, clinical signs are often absent. This contrasts with patients with other forms of fibrosing lung disease who frequently present with finger clubbing and fine, Velcro-like crepitations on auscultation. Patients with sarcoidosis almost never have finger clubbing, described in the disease in only a handful of case reports (Yancey *et al.* 1972; West *et al.* 1981). Equally, crepitations are heard only in a minority of individuals with sarcoidosis-associated pulmonary fibrosis. In a small case series, Baughman's group noted crepitations in only 17 percent of patients with fibrotic sarcoidosis, compared to 100 percent of patients with idiopathic pulmonary fibrosis (Baughman *et al.* 1991). The reason for the lack of clinical signs in pulmonary sarcoidosis remains to be elucidated.

Lung function

The characteristic lung function abnormality in fibrotic pulmonary sarcoidosis is a restrictive defect on spirometry with impairment of DLco. In general, reduction in VC correlates with the severity of fibrosis as assessed by CT (Bergin *et al.* 1989; Abehsera *et al.* 2000). FVC has also been shown in a number of small series to predict mortality in fibrotic pulmonary sarcoid (Baughman *et al.* 1997; Handa *et al.* 2006b). A proportion of patients with fibrotic sarcoidosis also display airflow obstruction and, thus, have a reduced FEV_1/FVC ratio on spirometry (Harrison *et al.* 1991; Handa *et al.* 2006a).

Airflow obstruction in sarcoidosis may arise through a number of mechanisms, including endobronchial disease, extraluminal airway compression by nodal disease or conglomerate fibrosis, or bronchostenosis. In a study linking HRCT appearances to lung function, Hansell and co-workers demonstrated that airflow obstruction was most frequently associated with a reticular pattern of fibrosis on CT (Hansell *et al.* 1998). Patients with conglomerate perihilar fibrosis also tend to present with airflow obstruction (Handa *et al.* 2006a). The small proportion of sarcoidosis patients with fibrobullous destruction often have a lung function pattern that mimics severe emphysema, with airflow obstruction and evidence of gas trapping with an increased residual volume (Judson and Strange 1998).

Radiology

The spectrum of radiographical abnormalities seen in patients with pulmonary sarcoidosis is described in Chapter 8. As has been noted, patients with sarcoid-related pulmonary fibrosis will have a stage IV chest X-ray appearance (Fig. 23.1). Most commonly, fibrosis in sarcoidosis results in loss of volume, particularly in the upper lobes, thus resulting in tenting of the diaphragm. Ancillary evidence of sarcoidosis may be evident in the form of mediastinal and/or hilar adenopathy, and in individuals with mixed inflammatory and fibrotic disease there may be widespread parenchymal nodularity evident on the chest radiograph. In a small proportion of patients, upper-lobe fibrosis may progress to fibrobullous destruction with cavitation that may be complicated by mycetoma formation. Conglomerate areas of fibrosis may result in apparent mass lesions on chest X-ray.

High-resolution CT scanning has enabled a greater appreciation of the spectrum of structural pulmonary abnormalities that may occur in sarcoidosis. Furthermore, CT scanning enables the appreciation of lesions that may not be evident on plain imaging. As with chest X-ray, the distribution of abnormalities on CT tends to be in the upper lobes. Although the pattern of distribution of parenchymal lesions tends to be bronchovascular, diffuse lesions and peripherally based abnormalities may also be observed (Nishimura *et al.* 1993; Abehsera *et al.* 2000; Nakatsu *et al.* 2002). Many of the parenchymal lesions seen on CT in sarcoidosis are reversible and will resolve with time and therapy (Brauner *et al.* 1992; Akira *et al.* 2005). A number of important CT changes, however, correlate with the development of irreversible fibrosis. These include fibrous bands, architectural distortion of the lung, thickening of the intralobular septae, hilar retraction, traction bronchiectasis, cysts, bullae, and paracicatrical emphysema (Abehsera *et al.* 2000; Akira *et al.* 2005).

In a study assessing serial CT in 40 patients with pulmonary sarcoidosis, Akira and associates demonstrated that parenchymal nodules tended to reduce in size or disappear over follow-up (Akira *et al.* 2005). Conglomerate nodules, although shrinking, tended to lead to bronchial distortion and the evolution of airflow obstruction. Ground-glass attenuation and consolidation frequently evolved into reticular or honeycomb change, resulting in restrictive spirometry.

In studies of the radiographic appearance of patients with fibrotic pulmonary sarcoidosis, a number of distinct patterns of fibrosis emerge (Remy-Jardin *et al.* 1994; Abehsera *et al.* 2000; Hennebicque *et al.* 2005). The principal appearance is one of upper-lobe predominant fibrosis or fibrocavitatory change with destruction of normal lung parenchyma and architectural distortion (Fig. 23.2). A significant proportion of patients have confluent perihilar fibrosis, often with associated reticular change in a bronchovascular distribution centered around the hila, a change reminiscent of the progressive massive fibrosis seen in pneumoconiosis (Fig. 23.3). Much smaller numbers of patients present with widespread bullous destruction of the lung (Fig. 23.4) or with widespread fine fibrosis characterized by diffuse ground-glass attenuation associated with traction bronchiectasis (Fig. 23.5).

A very small proportion of patients with sarcoidosis have a radiographic appearance on CT that is indistinguishable from that seen in idiopathic pulmonary fibrosis, with subpleural, predominantly basal, reticular change and honeycombing (Padley *et al.* 1996; Nobata *et al.* 2006; Fig. 23.6).

Although these different CT manifestations of sarcoid-related fibrosis have been shown to relate to different patterns of physiological impairment on lung function testing, it is not clear whether any individual pattern of disease confers a worse prognosis, over and above that encountered in chronic fibrotic sarcoidosis overall. In a number of studies, CT, although correlating with symptoms and disease severity as judged by physiological impairment, has failed to provide any further prognostic information to that gained from the chest radiograph and full lung function studies (Bergin *et al.* 1989; Brauner *et al.* 1989; Remy-Jardin *et al.* 1994).

Bronchoscopy and lavage

Bronchoscopy with endobronchial or transbronchial biopsy is frequently useful in confirming a suspected diagnosis of sarcoidosis through the demonstration of non-caseating granulomatous inflammation. Bronchoalveolar lavage (BAL) can also be useful in discriminating sarcoidosis from other forms of interstitial lung disease.

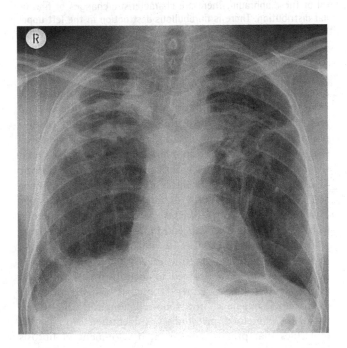

Figure 23.1 Plain chest X-ray of a 44-year-old man with stage IV fibrotic pulmonary sarcoid. There is bilateral upper-zone fibrosis with loss of upper-lobe volume and tenting of the diaphragms.

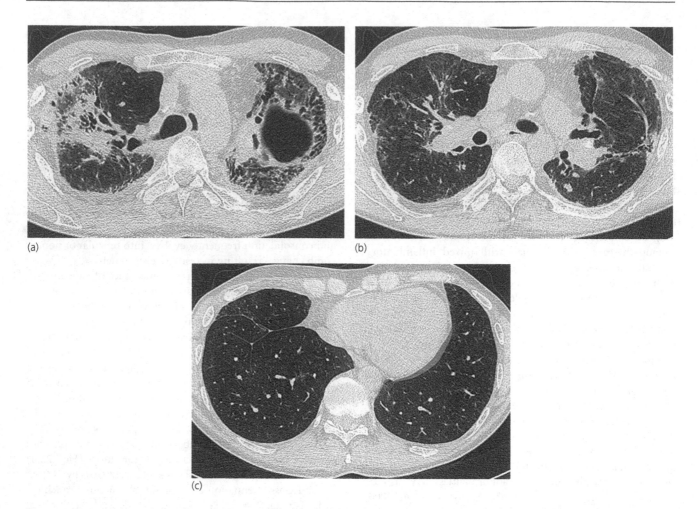

(a)

(b)

(c)

Figure 23.2   High-resolution CT scan of a 53-year-old man with biopsy-proven fibrotic pulmonary sarcoid showing sections at (a) the level of the aortic arch, (b) below the carina, and (c) just above the level of the diaphragm. There are characteristic changes of fibrotic pulmonary sarcoid with fibrosis streaming off the hila in a bronchovascular distribution. There is fibrobullous destruction in the left upper lobe (a). Notably, the fibrosis predominantly affects the upper lobes with sparing of the lower lobes (c).

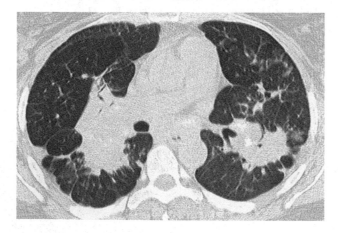

Figure 23.3   High-resolution CT scan of a 68-year-old female with pulmonary sarcoid and extensive, conglomerate perihilar fibrosis reminiscent of progressive massive fibrosis.

The characteristic BAL finding in sarcoidosis is a lymphocytosis with an increased CD4 to CD8 ratio (Verstraeten *et al.* 1990). In patients with fibrotic pulmonary

sarcoidosis, however, BAL findings can be indistinguishable from those encountered in other fibrosing lung diseases and may show a neutrophilia with or without a mild eosinophilia. Probably for this reason, the finding of increased BAL neutrophils and eosinophils in sarcoidosis has been shown to associate with the development of chronic fibrotic disease (Lin *et al.* 1985; Drent *et al.* 1999; Ziegenhagen *et al.* 2003; Prasse *et al.* 2008). A range of pro-inflammatory cytokines as well as pro-collagen peptides have been shown to be found in elevated concentrations in BAL from patients with sarcoidosis (Lammi *et al.* 1997; Miotto *et al.* 2001; Roberts *et al.* 2005; Ozdemir *et al.* 2007). However, the majority of studies performed to identify BAL biomarkers in sarcoidosis have either contained small numbers of patients or have not followed longitudinal disease behavior. Therefore, no study has identified any specific molecules that predict subsequent development of fibrosis in sarcoidosis.

In future, it is to be hoped that the application of novel proteomic methodologies to BAL fluid obtained from large populations of patients with well-phenotyped pulmonary

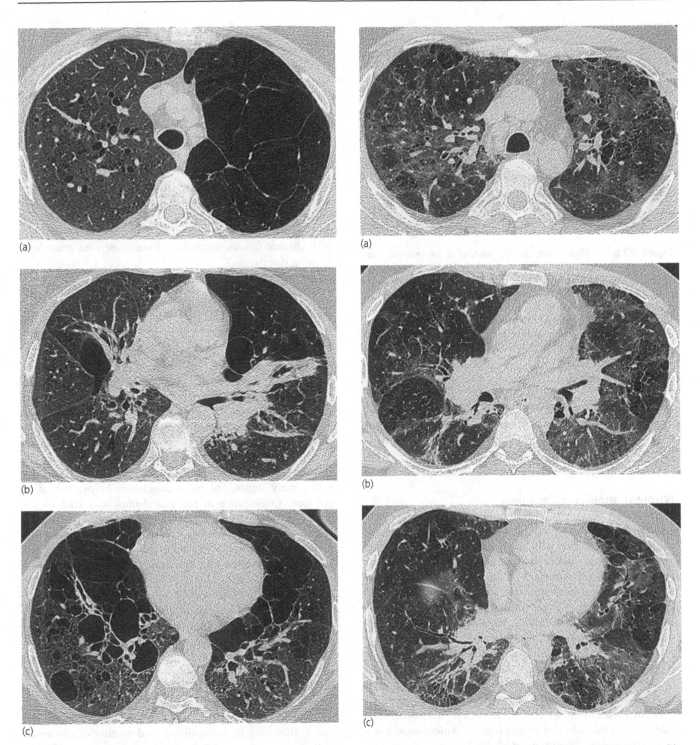

Figure 23.4   High-resolution CT scan of a 52-year-old woman with progressive bullous destruction due to sarcoidosis. Sections taken through (a) upper, (b) mid and (c) lower zones demonstrate evidence of perihilar fibrosis in a bronchovascular distribution. This is associated with extensive bullous destruction affecting both lungs but that is most extensive in the left upper lobe. The apparent increase in attenuation of the lung parenchyma is likely to represent redistribution of pulmonary blood flow through areas of uninvolved lung tissue.

Figure 23.5   High-resolution thoracic CT scan of a 37-year-old man with lung biopsy-proven sarcoidosis. Sections are shown at levels (a) just below the aortic arch, (b) below the carina, and (c) above the diaphragm. The predominant pattern is of diffuse ground-glass change with no clear pattern of distribution. Within the ground-glass change there is evidence of traction bronchiectasis, reticular change and, in subpleural regions, honeycomb change suggesting that the ground glass represents extensive fine fibrosis.

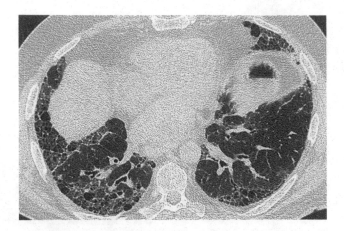

Figure 23.6 High-resolution CT scan of a 64-year-old man diagnosed 20 years earlier with sarcoidosis following a mediastinal lymph node biopsy. CT shows subpleural, predominantly basal honeycomb change with minimal ground glass — an appearance more usually associated with a diagnosis of idiopathic pulmonary fibrosis. Surgical lung biopsy confirmed bronchocentric granulomas on a background of fibrotic change reminiscent of usual interstitial pneumonitis (UIP).

sarcoidosis followed longitudinally, will enable the discovery of novel biomarkers and at the same time shed light on key pathogenetic mechanisms responsible for the progression of this enigmatic disease (Kriegova *et al.* 2006).

Nuclear medicine imaging

Gallium-67 citrate scanning is frequently used as an adjunct to diagnosis in patients with suspected sarcoidosis. Gallium uptake has been shown to correlate with areas of active granulomatous inflammation in sarcoidosis, so gallium-67 scanning has been used both as an adjunct to diagnosis and to distinguish between 'active' and 'inactive' disease (Rizzato *et al.* 1983; Abe *et al.* 1984). Baseline gallium activity at diagnosis has been shown to correlate with subsequent disease progression at 2 years in one small study (Baughman *et al.* 1987). However, this finding was not replicated (Hollinger *et al.* 1985). In a cohort of patients with chronic pulmonary sarcoidosis, Beaumont and associates were able to discriminate between fixed fibrotic lesions and inflammatory parenchymal infiltrates on the basis that fibrotic regions demonstrated a lack of gallium uptake (Beaumont *et al.* 1982).

Intuitively, one might expect that gallium scanning would provide a useful measure of disease activity when making decisions to wean therapy in patients with chronic sarcoid. However, probably because corticosteroid therapy is effective in suppressing gallium uptake, studies evaluating the use of gallium scanning as part of an algorithm for deciding changes in pharmacotherapy in chronic sarcoidosis have produced mixed results (Line *et al.* 1981; Kohn *et al.* 1982; Rizzato and Blasi 1986; Turner-Warwick *et al.* 1986).

Positron emission tomography (PET) with fluorine-18-flurodeoxyglucose (FDG) has shown increased uptake in active sarcoid lesions with regression of uptake following corticosteroid therapy (Lewis and Salama 1994). It has been postulated that FDG-PET with CT fusion may provide a more sensitive method for discriminating fixed fibrotic change from active parenchymal inflammation in patients with chronic pulmonary sarcoidosis (Mana and van Kroonenburgh 2005). Interestingly, it has been shown in a retrospective review of 77 patients with sarcoidosis that high SUV values in lung parenchyma following FDG PET scanning correlated with BAL neutrophilia, a cell profile that correlates with sarcoid-associated pulmonary fibrosis (Keijsers *et al.* 2010). Unfortunately, the authors were unable to evaluate their cohort longitudinally, so it remains to be determined whether baseline PET scanning is capable of discriminating patients with chronic fibrotic sarcoidosis from those with acute self-limiting disease.

PATHOGENESIS OF PULMONARY FIBROSIS

The characteristic histological feature of pulmonary sarcoidosis is the presence of non-caseating granulomas localized to the lymphatics of the pleura, interlobular septa and bronchovascular bundles, generally sparing the alveolar structures (Cavazza *et al.* 2009). The granulomas consist of macrophages, epithelioid cells and multinucleated giant cells surrounded by lymphocytes with a preponderance of CD4 over CD8 T-lymphocytes. The granulomas may be surrounded by loose cellular connective tissue, particularly in the early stages, but more commonly by dense hyaline collagen. Coalescence of the granulomas may lead to the formation of large fibrogranulomatous masses. As the lesions mature, the hyaline collagen penetrates and fragments the granulomas. In many cases, the granulomatous lesions may resolve and the lung heals, leaving only a residual mild scarring. In 10–30 percent of individuals the disease may develop with progressive fibrosis, traction bronchiectasis and honeycombing. This progressive disease, which expands into the lung parenchyma, results in significant morbidity and mortality. The etiopathogenesis of sarcoidosis is poorly understood but the current evidence supports the view that a genetic or epigenetic predisposition results in a chronic immunological response to an environmental antigenic stimulus.

Evidence for a genetic component includes familial and ethnic clustering in susceptibility and severity of disease as well as associations with human leukocyte antigen (HLA) and other genes to disease susceptibility and in some cases, persistence or progression. Genes associated with sarcoidosis and pertinent to the pathogenesis of fibrosis will be discussed in more detail below. A more extensive review of sarcoid genetics can be found elsewhere in this book. The most consistent association is with HLA genes and is consistent with antigen presentation playing a central role in the disease process. In addition, the fact that non-HLA genetic associations have often been found to be variable or inconsistent is indicative of a complex disease pattern with multiple genes and/or environmental factors contributing to susceptibility and progression.

The role of epigenetics in the pathogenesis of sarcoidosis has not been investigated. However, alterations in the chemical modifications to DNA, their associated proteins and miRNAs which regulate gene expression without altering gene sequence, are increasingly recognized to play critical roles in the pathogenesis of complex disease including pulmonary fibrosis (Sanders *et al.* 2008).

Evidence for an environmental stimulus is also supported by familial and spatial as well as seasonal clustering of cases. Considerable circumstantial evidence exists for non-infectious and infectious agents including mycobacteria and propionibacteria, but none has been proven to be a stimulus. The most likely explanation is that multiple environmental stimuli may initiate the onset of sarcoidosis and that each may subtly influence disease phenotype including progression.

Immunopathogenesis of granuloma formation

Immunological studies suggest that granuloma formation results from interaction of an, as yet unidentified, antigen with antigen-presenting cells such as macrophages or dendritic cells that exhibit enhanced expression of MHC class II molecules. The antigens are internalized and processed to form MHC–peptide complexes which can be recognized by and interact with α/β T-cell receptors on CD4+ T-lymphocytes that differentiate into T-helper 1 (Th1) cells and initiate granuloma formation.

Activated antigen-presenting cells secrete high levels of cytokines and chemokines including tumor necrosis factor TNF-α, interleukin (IL)-1, IL-6, IL-12, IL-15, IL-18, macrophage inflammatory protein (MIP)-1α (CCL3), MIP-1β/CCL4, monocyte chemotactic protein 1 (MCP-1), RANTES (regulated on activation, normal T-cell expressed and secreted/CCL5), granulocyte macrophage colony stimulating factor (GMCSF), interferon (IFN)-inducible protein 10 (IP-10/CXCL10), monokine induced by IFN-γ (Mig/CXCL9), and IFN-inducible T-cell α chemoattractant (I-TAC/CXCL11) (Agostini and Semenzato 1998; Tsiligianni *et al.* 2005; Antoniou *et al.* 2006; Nishioka *et al.* 2007).

A characteristic of CD4+ lymphocytes that differentiate into Th1 cells is their expression of CXCR3 and CCR5 chemokine receptors. The production of CXCR3 ligands, IP-10, Mig and I-TAC, in combination with IL-12 and IL-18 therefore plays an important role in the recruitment and differentiation of Th1 cells. These Th1 cells produce IFN-γ, IL-2 and increase macrophage TNF-α production. IFN-γ activates and induces macrophage transformation into giant cells, and TNF-α induces the proliferation of monocytes and differentiation of macrophages into epithelioid cells which together aggregate to form the granulomas. With time, these become surrounded by dense hyaline collagen. Matrix metalloproteinases 8, 9 and 12 are increased in sarcoid lung in the absence of increased levels of tissue inhibitor of metalloproteinase (TIMP)-1, which is indicative of extracellular matrix breakdown and remodeling (Fireman *et al.* 2002; Henry *et al.* 2002; Crouser *et al.* 2009). In addition, analysis of type I and type III procollagen expression and aminoterminal peptides in sarcoid lung provides evidence of active type I and III collagen synthesis in the areas surrounding and occasionally within granulomas (Kaarteenaho-Wiik *et al.* 2005). In addition to their chemokine activity, CXCR3 ligands also exhibit angiostatic properties. Although there is currently little experimental evidence, this would be consistent with the hypovascular nature of sarcoid granulomas (Tzouvelekis *et al.* 2006).

In addition to the uncertainty as to the initiating stimuli, the reasons why sarcoid lesions resolve or progress are unknown. One possible explanation, for which there is evidence in experimental models, is that granulomatous inflammation is down-regulated and resolves when the antigen is removed. Such a mechanism could feasibly explain the waxing and waning nature of disease activity in many patients with sarcoidosis. In contrast, failure to clear antigen, in experimental models, results in persistent antigenic stimulation leading to a hybrid Th1/Th2 phenotype with Th2 cytokines activating fibroblasts to proliferate, synthesize and deposit extracellular matrix proteins, including collagens, in a response to generate a protective barrier against the inciting agent. There is little evidence for an increase in Th2 cytokines in sarcoidosis, although these have not been selectively evaluated in fibrotic sarcoidosis (Taniguchi *et al.* 2000; Mollers *et al.* 2001; Hauber *et al.* 2003). Further studies are required to investigate this potential mechanism of disease progression in sarcoidosis.

Alternatively, aberrant control of mechanisms involved in the ordered production, 'encasement' and resolution of granuloma, possibly due to additional genetic or epigenetic factors, could lead to progressive fibrosis. There is evidence that polymorphisms in a number of genes that are known to influence the development of fibrosis are also associated with either susceptibility to or persistence/severity of sarcoidosis.

Evidence for genetic susceptibility to pulmonary fibrosis

A number of non-HLA gene polymorphisms have been found to associate either with the risk of or protection from disease persistence/progression. However, the findings have often been difficult to replicate. This may, in part, be due to the small size of many studies but also likely reflects the extensive heterogeneity in the disease phenotype related to combined complex genetic and environmental exposures. Nevertheless, where associations are found, these may provide important clues to pathogenesis in subgroups such as those with progressive pulmonary fibrosis.

Angiotensin-converting enzyme (ACE)

In the ACE gene, an insertion (I)/deletion (D) polymorphism has been identified that influences ACE levels with the DD genotype related to higher levels. The DD genotype has been associated with sarcoidosis and more advanced chest

X-ray stage or poorer prognosis (Maliarik *et al.* 1998; Pietinalho *et al.* 1999). In sarcoidosis, epithelioid cells produce ACE and, consistent with studies in other diseases, the DD genotype is associated with higher levels of ACE and X-ray stage (Papadopoulos *et al.* 2000). ACE controls the key regulatory step in the synthesis of angiotensin II (Ang II) which, in addition to its vasoconstrictor effects, stimulates fibroblast proliferation and production of cytokines including TGF-β1 (Marshall *et al.* 2000). In addition, in animal models, ACE inhibitors inhibit lung fibrogenesis (Marshall *et al.* 2004). Thus increased levels of ACE in sarcoidosis could contribute to the development and progression of fibrosis.

CCR5

CCR5 is a receptor for lymphocyte and monocyte chemokines including MIP-1α, MIP-1β, RANTES, and CCL8 (monocyte chemotactic protein 2). Despite this, there is no firm association with susceptibility to sarcoidosis (Petrek *et al.* 2000; Spagnolo *et al.* 2005). However, an association has been observed in British and Dutch patient groups between a CCR5 haplotype (HHC) and with persistent lung involvement of radiographic stage II and above, reduced FEV_1 and FVC (Spagnolo *et al.* 2005; Sato *et al.* 2010). The functional consequences of the genetic polymorphisms investigated are poorly understood. However, several of the polymorphisms are present within promoter regions predicted to alter transcription factor binding and potentially increase transcription. In animal models of pulmonary fibrosis, CCR5 has been shown to play an important role in pulmonary fibrogenesis through MIP-1α-mediated recruitment and activation of bone marrow-derived cells including fibrocytes (Smith *et al.* 1994; Ishida *et al.* 2007). Increased MIP-1α localized to macrophages and fibroblasts has been reported in sarcoid lung, and additionally, MIP-1α production by BAL immune cells from sarcoidosis patients with progressing disease are higher than from those with stable disease (Standiford *et al.* 1993; Ziegenhagen *et al.* 1998). Furthermore, CCR5 expression is increased in lymphocytes and macrophages, with higher numbers of CCR5-positive cells in sarcoidosis patients, with a trend towards further increases with radiographic stage (Capelli *et al.* 2002; Petrek *et al.* 2002). Thus, high levels of MIP-1α, increased CCR5 expression and recruitment of CCR5-positive cells could potentially contribute to fibrotic progression in sarcoidosis.

Clara cell 10 kD protein (CC10)

The G38A polymorphism in the non-coding region of exon 1 of CC10 has been shown to be functional with lower levels associated with the A/A genotype. Ohchi and co-workers found that the 38A allele frequency was significantly increased in a Japanese population of patients with progressive sarcoidosis compared with controls and that those with

CC10 38A polymorphism exhibited lower levels of BAL CC10 (Ohchi *et al.* 2004). Furthermore, in reporter assays, the 38A construct showed lower transcriptional activity in response to IFN-γ compared with the 38G construct. Levels of CC10 in another study were also found to be lower in serum and BALF of individuals with progressive sarcoidosis than in resolving disease (Shijubo *et al.* 2000). CC10 has potent anti-inflammatory properties including inhibition of IL-2 mediated release of TNF-α, IL-1β and IFN-1γ (Pilon 2000). In addition, bleomycin exposure in mice results in a loss of CC10 expressing Clara cells (Daly *et al.* 1997) but its role in the development of fibrosis has not been fully investigated.

Inhibitor kappa B-alfa

Potentially functional IκBβ promoter polymorphisms have been demonstrated to associate with susceptibility to sarcoidosis and with increasing severity based on radiographic staging in UK and Dutch white populations, with carriage of the −826C allele appearing to associate with fibrotic disease (Abdallah *et al.* 2003). IκBα is a member of the IκB family of proteins which hold NF-κB in an inactive form in the cytoplasm, preventing its translocation to the nucleus, transcriptional activation and limiting inflammatory and immune responses. NF-κB expression has been shown to be greater in the more severe stages of sarcoidosis (Rutherford *et al.* 2001). Furthermore, pharmacological inhibition of IκBα has recently been shown to inhibit inflammation and fibrosis in an animal model of silicosis (Di *et al.* 2009). Therefore, if IκBα polymorphisms affect its expression, they could modulate the inflammatory response and potential to progress to fibrosis in sarcoidosis.

Prostaglandin endoperoxide synthase 2 (PTGS2)

We have shown that a promoter polymorphism, −765G > C, in PTGS2 (also known as cyclooxygenase-2, COX-2) that reduces PTGS2 expression via altered transcription factor binding is strongly associated with susceptibility to sarcoidosis and with risk of developing pulmonary fibrosis (Papafili *et al.* 2002; Hill *et al.* 2006). In a second smaller study, with limited numbers of samples from patients with persistent/progressive disease, this polymorphism was found to be of borderline significance; but association with another polymorphism in the 3′ untranslated region of the gene, PTGS2 8473T > C, was found, reinforcing the association of a potential pathophysiological role for PTGS2 in sarcoidosis (Lopez-Campos *et al.* 2009).

PTGS2 is a rate-limiting enzyme in the conversion of arachidonic acid to prostanoids. The major prostanoid synthesized in the lung is PGE2 which is an important regulator of tissue homeostasis and inflammation. It has important antifibrotic properties, including limiting fibroblast chemotaxis, proliferation, differentiation into myofibroblasts, extracellular matrix protein synthesis, as well as limiting epithelial cell and promoting fibroblast apoptosis

(McAnulty *et al.* 1995,1997; Keerthisingam *et al.* 2001; Kohyama *et al.* 2001; Kolodsick *et al.* 2003; Maher *et al.* 2010). In sarcoidosis and other fibrotic lung diseases, PTGS2 expression is reduced. Immunolocalization of PTGS2 in sarcoid lung has demonstrated reduced levels associated with bronchial epithelial cells and macrophages compared with controls (Petkova *et al.* 2003). Consistent with this, either no change or decreased levels of PGE2 in BALF or cultured macrophages from sarcoidosis patients have been reported compared with controls (Baughman *et al.* 1984; Bachwich *et al.* 1987; De *et al.* 1997). In other fibrotic lung diseases, decreased levels of PTGS2 have been shown to be due to a decreased capacity to up-regulate PTGS2 expression (Keerthisingam *et al.* 2001). Furthermore, in animal models PTGS2 deficiency results in a more profound fibrotic response in the lung due to reduced levels of PGE2 (Keerthisingam *et al.* 2001; Hodges *et al.* 2004); and conversely, over-expression of PTGS2 limits fibroproliferation (Copeman *et al.* 2004).

There is, therefore, strong evidence in man and animals to support a role for reduced expression of PTGS2 in progressive fibrotic phenotypes of sarcoidosis.

Transforming growth factor-beta

Members of the TGF-β family of polypeptide mediators play critical roles in both immunomodulatory and fibroproliferative processes (Howell and McAnulty 2006; Wahl 2007). TGF-β isoforms also exhibit a combination of shared and specific functions (Bottoms *et al.* 2010). Therefore, it is not surprising that apparently contradictory findings have been reported in relation to TGF-β and sarcoidosis, a disease with strong immune and fibroproliferative components.

For example, levels of TGF-β1 have been shown to be increased in patients with sarcoidosis with impaired pulmonary function (Salez *et al.* 1998), while others have shown increased TGF-β production by BAL cells in patients who underwent spontaneous remission compared with those with more progressive disease (Zissel *et al.* 1996). It is therefore critical to consider the stage of disease, cellular localization and TGF-β isoform when assessing the functional roles of TGF-β in the pathogenesis of sarcoidosis. Polymorphisms in TGF-β isoforms β1, β2 and β3 have been reported to affect protein expression and function. TGF-β1 polymorphisms, −509CC, codon 10TT or haplotypes containing these variants have been shown to associate with more severe disease assessed by radiographic score (Jonth *et al.* 2007). Interestingly these are genotypes that associate with lower levels of TGF-β1, suggesting the association with greater severity may be linked to reduced immunomodulatory effects of TGF-β1 rather than its fibroproliferative effects. Consistent with these data, Kruit *et al.* (2006) did not find an association with TGF-β1 polymorphisms and fibrotic sarcoidosis. However, the TGF-β2 59941 G, TGF-β3 4875 A and TGF-β3 17369 C alleles were found to be more abundant in fibrotic patients assessed by radiographic staging, although the association with TGF-β2 was lost after correction. TGF-β3 has been reported to have antifibrotic effects in the skin and lung (Shah *et al.* 1995; Ask *et al.* 2008). The association of

TGF-β3 variants with fibrotic disease would be consistent with reduced functionality of this isoform in fibrotic sarcoidosis. However, the functional nature of these polymorphisms has yet to be elucidated.

Toll-like receptor 4

Mutations in the TLR4 coding region (Asp299Gly and Thr399Ile) have been associated with chronic persistent disease in sarcoidosis (Pabst *et al.* 2006). These TLR4 polymorphisms have been shown to reduce the response to LPS challenge in humans and also impair LPS-mediated signal transduction through NF-κB *in vitro* (Arbour *et al.* 2000). Conversely, TLR4 activation enhances TGF-β signaling and induces collagen synthesis and deposition; thus, down-regulation of TLR4 responses in sarcoidosis could conceivably lead to deficient 'encasement' of granuloma and disease progression (Seki *et al.* 2007; He *et al.* 2009). Furthermore, Ang II induces TLR4 expression and signaling through NF-κB (Wu *et al.* 2009). Therefore, the effects of TLR4 mutations on progression and fibrosis in sarcoidosis will probably depend on the combined genotype of many genes.

Vascular endothelial growth factor

Several VEGF polymorphisms have been associated with altered production of VEGF, including VEGF +813C/T where the T allele results in the loss of an AP-4 transcription factor binding site in association with reduced serum levels of VEGF in healthy individuals (Renner *et al.* 2000; Watson *et al.* 2000). The VEGF + 813T allele is under-represented in sarcoidosis and therefore associated with protection (Morohashi *et al.* 2003). In addition, a recent investigation of single nucleotide polymorphisms (SNPs) in VEGF and VEGF receptors (VEGFR)-1 and -2 identified three VEGF SNPs that were associated with acute remitting sarcoidosis, three VEGFR-1 SNPs that were associated with sarcoidosis, one VEGFR-2 SNP that was associated with acute remitting sarcoidosis, and two VEGFR-2 SNPs that were associated with persistent/chronic sarcoidosis (Pabst *et al.* 2010). Further analysis identified a VEGF haplotype associated with both sarcoidosis and a persistent/chronic disease course.

VEGF and VEGFR expression in sarcoidosis appears to be complex. Increased VEGF expression and protein production as well as over-expression of VEGF receptor-2 has been reported in activated macrophages, epithelioid cells and giant cells of sarcoid granulomas (Tolnay *et al.* 1998). In addition, increased VEGF levels have been observed in serum of sarcoidosis patients requiring steroid treatment compared with those with spontaneous remission (Sekiya *et al.* 2003). In contrast, decreased levels of VEGF have been reported in BALF and induced sputum from sarcoidosis patients and were further decreased in patients with stage III and IV disease (Koyama *et al.* 2002; Fireman *et al.* 2009). Furthermore, VEGF genotypes and haplotypes have been associated with lower serum levels of VEGF and increased mortality in ARDS patients (Zhai *et al.* 2007).

The complex interactions between VEGF, its signaling and decoy receptors and multiple other genes in the regulation of vascular permeability, angiogenesis, inflammation and fibrosis provides considerable challenges in identifying the role of VEGF in sarcoidosis pathogenesis. However, several in-vitro and in-vivo studies may provide some clues. VEGF inhibitors are capable of inhibiting TGF-β production (Lee et al. 2008), and TGF-β1 can induce VEGF and VEGFR-1 expression by macrophages, suggesting a complex interplay between VEGF and TGF-β. In animals, over-expression of soluble VEGF receptor-1, which acts as a decoy, inhibits the development of bleomycin-induced lung inflammation and fibrosis independently (Hamada et al. 2005). In contrast, pharmacological inhibition of VEGF receptor-2 only inhibits bleomycin-induced fibrosis if administered in the early inflammatory phase and not when dosed in the fibrotic phase and appears to act, at least partly, by reducing VEGF and VEGFR-2 expression, TGF-β1 levels and Smad 3 phosphorylation (Ou et al. 2009). These studies suggest an important role for VEGFR-2 in the early inflammatory and angiogenic phases of bleomycin-induced fibrosis and a more important role for VEGFR-1 signaling in the fibroproliferative phase. Thus, polymorphisms which lead to increased VEGF, decreased soluble VEGFR-1 or increased VEGFR-1 signaling may potentially play important roles in the progression of sarcoidosis to fibrosis.

Gene sets

From the analysis of the potential involvement of the foregoing few genes in the pathogenesis of pulmonary fibrosis associated with sarcoidosis, it is clear that unravelling the complex interplay between the environmental stimuli, genes and pathways that determine whether sarcoid granulomas resolve or progress to fibrosis remains an enormous challenge. In a recent study, Lockstone and co-workers used gene expression profiling in combination with gene-set enrichment analysis to identify functionally related sets of genes that distinguish self-limiting from persistent sarcoidosis, based on disease status at two years (Lockstone et al. 2010). These studies identified a group of gene sets enriched in the persistent group that were consistent with stronger immune activation. Application of such an approach to a more severe fibrotic sarcoidosis group could be useful in identifying groups of functionally related genes related to fibrogenesis.

PROGNOSIS AND COMPLICATIONS

Chronic sarcoidosis often follows a relapsing and remitting course. Patients with fibrotic pulmonary sarcoidosis may enter into long-term remission with stabilization of their disease and associated symptoms. A small proportion of individuals, however, suffer with inexorably progressive disease that ultimately leads to respiratory failure and, without lung transplantation, death. Over half of all sarcoid-related deaths occur as a consequence of end-stage fibrosing lung disease

(Gideon and Mannino 1996; Baughman et al. 1997). Besides disease progression, individuals with sarcoid-related pulmonary fibrosis are prone to other disease-related complications including pulmonary hypertension, secondary lung cancer and infection.

Pulmonary hypertension

Clinically significant pulmonary hypertension occurs in 1–5 percent of individuals with sarcoidosis (Smith et al. 1983; Barst and Ratner 1985; Takemura et al. 1992; Shigemitsu et al. 2007). Sarcoid-related pulmonary hypertension results in significant morbidity, including worsening dyspnea, reduced exercise tolerance and increased oxygen requirement, and mortality.

The etiology of pulmonary hypertension in sarcoidosis is, however, multifactorial and differs between patients (Nunes et al. 2006). Potential causes include sarcoid angiitis, infiltration and/or obliteration of small pulmonary vessels and the alveolar capillary bed by granulomatous inflammation, extrinsic compression of main pulmonary arteries by enlarged nodes, obliteration of the pulmonary vascular bed due to pulmonary fibrosis or hypoxic vasoconstriction. In a study of the causes of sarcoid-related pulmonary hypertension in two US centers, half of patients had developed the condition in the context of severe fibrotic or fibrocystic lung disease (Barnett et al. 2009). Furthermore, in a study conducted in the USA, the incidence of cardiac catheter-proven hypertension in patients with fibrotic pulmonary sarcoidosis listed for transplantation was 74 percent (Shorr et al. 2005). In this cohort of patients with fibrotic pulmonary sarcoidosis, pulmonary hypertension is an independent predictor of mortality (Shorr et al. 2002, 2003).

There is a lack of clinical evidence to guide the treatment of pulmonary hypertension arising in individuals with fibrotic pulmonary sarcoidosis. A pragmatic approach to management involves optimization of therapy for sarcoidosis and correction of any resting, exertional or nocturnal hypoxia. Small uncontrolled studies or case reports suggest that therapies with proven efficacy in primary pulmonary hypertension, such as endothelin antagonists or phosphodiesterase inhibitors, may also be effective in the management of sarcoid-related pulmonary hypertension (Preston et al. 2001; Fisher et al. 2006; Milman et al. 2008; Barnett et al. 2009).

Lung cancer

Fibrotic lung disease, particularly idiopathic pulmonary fibrosis, has, in some cohort studies, been associated with an increased incidence of primary lung cancer (Turner-Warwick et al. 1980; Hubbard et al. 2000; Harris et al. 2010). Whether fibrotic pulmonary sarcoidosis is truly associated with an increased incidence of lung cancer remains unclear: one of the challenges in interpreting any study into the association of sarcoidosis with lung malignancy is that approximately 1–3 percent of primary lung tumors give rise to a 'sarcoid-like' non-caseating granulomatous reaction in mediastinal nodes (Hunsaker et al. 1996).

Brincker and Wilbeck (1974) retrospectively studied 2544 patients with pulmonary sarcoidosis in a Danish registry. They found 48 patients who went on to develop a subsequent malignancy. This compared to their estimate of 33.8 cases of cancer that might have been expected to have occurred in an age-matched population. The most frequently occurring cancers were lymphoma and primary lung cancer. The authors estimated that lymphoma occurred 11 times and lung cancer 3 times more frequently than expected. They did not relate the development of cancer to the radiographic stage or extent of pulmonary disease. They did, however, note that the increased risk of cancer was greatest during the first 4 years following the diagnosis of the sarcoidosis.

In a similar study, utilizing a Swedish registry of just over 9000 patients, Askling *et al* (1999) found an increased incidence of lung cancer, lymphoma, cancer of the gastro-intestinal tract, melanoma and liver cancer in patients with a pre-existing diagnosis of sarcoidosis. As with the earlier study, they found that the increase in incidence was most marked in the first 4 years following diagnosis. However, in their cohort, patients with sarcoidosis remained at increased risk of cancer for up to 9 years after diagnosis. Interestingly, in this study, the vast majority of cases of lung cancer occurred in patients with pre-existing parenchymal disease, suggesting that confounding by a granulomatous response to malignancy may not account for the association.

Fungal disease

Mycetomas, typically due to *Aspergillus* species, may develop in areas of cystic lung damage. Patients with sarcoidosis seem to be especially prone to the development of mycetomas when compared to other groups of patients with cystic lung disease (e.g. emphysema and lymphangieolyomyomatosis). In sarcoid, mycetomas most usually occur in upper-lobe cavities in patients with radiographic stage III or IV disease (Israel and Ostrow 1969; Wollschlager and Khan 1984; Tomlinson and Sahn 1987). Mycetomas may be asymptomatic and detected incidentally on chest X-ray or thoracic CT (Fig. 23.7). A proportion of patients present with recurrent hemoptysis which, in a minority, may be life-threatening.

Other clinical complications include supra-added bacterial infection within the cavity containing the mycetoma and, occasionally, pleuritic pain. Ipsilateral pleural thickening has been reported to precede the development of radiographic signs of mycetoma formation on plain chest X-ray (Libshitz *et al*. 1974).

Until relatively recently, the mainstay of therapy for symptomatic mycetomas has been surgical resection. Other treatment approaches that have been tried include bronchial artery embolization and intracavitatory instillation of amphotericin. The development of antifungal agents with true fungicidal activity (including the newer azoles and the echinocandins) has resulted in a move away from surgical intervention to medical management of pulmonary fungal disease (Camuset *et al*. 2007). Resolution of aspergillomas with protracted voriconazole therapy has been reported in lung transplant recipients (Zoumot *et al*. 2006). Whether similar success can be achieved in mycetomas complicating sarcoidosis is uncertain.

The presence of a mycetoma complicating fibrotic pulmonary sarcoidosis conveys a relatively poor prognosis.

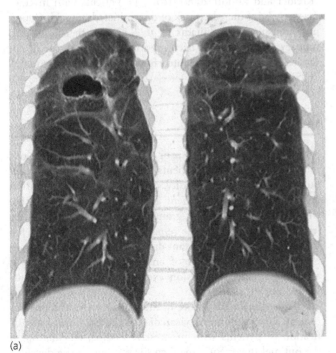
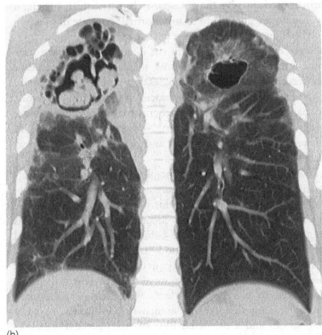

(a) (b)

Figure 23.7 Coronal reconstructions of thoracic CT scans obtained 3 years apart, from a 32-year-old female with sarcoidosis. (a) The earlier scan demonstrates fibrocavitatory disease in the right upper lobe with parenchymal change suggestive of sarcoidosis in the left upper lobe. (b) Three years later there has been considerable progression of the fibrocavitatory destruction with the new finding of two well-demarcated mycetomas within the right upper lobe cavity.

Tomlinson and Sahn (1987) reported a median survival of only 12 months in 14 patients with symptomatic aspergillomas on a background of chronic sarcoidosis. This contrasted with a one-year mortality of 20 percent in a similar number of patients with symptomatic aspergillomas due to previous tuberculosis. In this study, the major difference between the two groups that appeared to affect both choice of treatment and subsequent outcome was that patients with sarcoidosis often had multifocal cavities and, therefore, more extensive aspergillomas. Hadjiliadis et al. (2002) found that patients with sarcoidosis complicated by mycetomas who underwent lung transplantation had worse outcomes than sarcoidosis patients without mycetomas. Although they had only small numbers in their study, the authors felt that the use of post-transplant antifungal therapy might be effective in obviating the increased risk posed by pre-transplant fungal colonization.

TREATMENT

The philosophy of treatment in sarcoidosis, together with the spectrum of available pharmacotherapies, is discussed in detail elsewhere in this book. It is, however, worth considering a number of key principles when approaching the therapy of fibrotic pulmonary sarcoidosis.

The evolution of fibrosis or fibrobullous disease in sarcoidosis, in keeping with changes seen in other destructive lung diseases such as emphysema and idiopathic pulmonary fibrosis, is typically accompanied by distortion and architectural destruction of the underlying alveolar structure. For this reason, even if it proved possible to reverse the fibrotic process and dissolve the collagen-rich extracellular matrix, it would not be possible to restore normal structure or function to the lung. Consequently, in patients with fibrotic pulmonary sarcoid, the aim of treatment is not to restore lost lung function and improve symptoms. Instead, the aim should be to prevent further disease progression and the development of additional symptoms and associated morbidity. Therefore, in patients with previously progressive fibrotic disease, the attainment of disease stability with treatment *should be viewed as a therapeutic success* and not, as is often the case, as a treatment failure.

Keeping in mind this principle, the approach to treatment of fibrotic pulmonary sarcoidosis is similar to that of other manifestations of sarcoidosis. Corticosteroids form the mainstay of therapy with second-line agents such as methotrexate or azathioprine being used to reduce steroid exposure. There is no good trial evidence to guide therapeutic decisions in this patient cohort. Infliximab has been shown to result in a small improvement in FVC compared to placebo in patients with chronic pulmonary sarcoidosis (as defined by parenchymal infiltrates on chest radiograph and a predicted FVC of <85 percent) (Baughman et al. 2006a). For 103 patients receiving 6-weekly infusions of infliximab (at doses of either 3 or 5 mg/kg), mean FVC improved by 2.5 percent from baseline after 24 weeks. This compared to no change in the placebo group of 44 patients ($p = 0.38$). Hence, infliximab should be considered in patients with progressive disease refractory to other interventions.

The dose and duration of therapy in patients with chronic fibrotic sarcoidosis can be difficult to gauge. In the absence of any clear biomarker with which to measure underlying disease activity, the prolonged use of corticosteroids and immunosuppressants in individuals with chronic disease has to be balanced against the risk of disease progression following de-escalation of therapy. In patients with marginal lung function as a consequence of fibrotic pulmonary sarcoidosis, the risks of disease progression on withdrawing treatment often outweigh the potential risks associated with protracted exposure to low-dose steroids and second-line immunosuppressants.

For patients with progressive, treatment-refractory, sarcoid-related pulmonary fibrosis or fibrobullous disease resulting in respiratory failure, lung transplantation remains an important therapeutic option. Timing of referral for transplantation in patients with sarcoidosis is frequently challenging as there are few reliable clinical indicators of prognosis. Data derived from transplant waiting-list patients with sarcoidosis suggest that pulmonary hypertension is the best predictor of mortality (Shorr et al. 2002, 2003). Consequently, the International Society for Heart and Lung Transplant (ISHLT) guidelines recommend that patients with sarcoidosis who have the following characteristics be considered for listing for lung transplantation: NYHA functional class III–IV with hypoxemia, pulmonary hypertension, and/or right atrial pressure exceeding 15 mmHg (Orens et al. 2006).

Outcomes for patients with sarcoidosis following transplantation are comparable to those of other disease groups (Kreider and Kotloff 2009). However, patients with mycetomas may be at increased risk of disseminated fungal infection post-transplant (Hadjiliadis et al. 2002). Furthermore, pulmonary sarcoidosis has been reported to recur in the donor organs of patients transplanted for sarcoidosis (Ionescu et al. 2005).

CONCLUSION

Although irreversible fibrotic or fibrobullous change develops in only a minority of patients, it contributes a significant burden in terms of morbidity, chronic healthcare utilization and mortality in this patient group. The mechanisms that trigger the switch from granulomatous inflammation to irreversible fibrotic change remain poorly understood. That inflammation is an important driver of the fibrotic process is exemplified by the effect of anti-inflammatory therapy in arresting disease progression even in individuals with advanced fibrotic disease.

Challenges for the future in the management and prevention of fibrotic pulmonary sarcoidosis include earlier identification of patients with progressive disease, elucidation of the optimal therapeutic regimen for preventing the development of fibrotic change, and improving understanding of the role played by infectious agents, especially fungi, in driving the progression of disease in patients with chronic pulmonary sarcoidosis.

REFERENCES

Abdallah A, Sato H, Grutters JC et al. (2003). Inhibitor kappa B-alpha (IkappaB-alpha) promoter polymorphisms in UK and Dutch sarcoidosis. Genes Immun 4: 45–4.

Abe S, Munakata M, Nishimura M et al. (1984). Gallium-67 scintigraphy, bronchoalveolar lavage, and pathologic changes in patients with pulmonary sarcoidosis. Chest 85: 650–5.

Abehsera M, Valeyre D, Grenier P et al. (2000). Sarcoidosis with pulmonary fibrosis: CT patterns and correlation with pulmonary function. Am J Roentgen 174: 1751–7.

Agostini C, Semenzato G (1998). Cytokines in sarcoidosis. Semin Respir Infect 13: 184–96.

Akira M, Kozuka T, Inoue Y, Sakatani M (2005). Long-term follow-up CT scan evaluation in patients with pulmonary sarcoidosis. Chest 127: 185–91.

Antoniou KM, Tzouvelekis A, Alexandrakis MG et al. (2006). Different angiogenic activity in pulmonary sarcoidosis and idiopathic pulmonary fibrosis. Chest 130: 982–8.

Arbour NC, Lorenz E, Schutte BC et al. (2000). TLR4 mutations are associated with endotoxin hyporesponsiveness in humans. Nat Genet 25: 187–91.

Ask K, Bonniaud P, Maass K et al. (2008). Progressive pulmonary fibrosis is mediated by TGF-beta isoform 1 but not TGF-beta3. Int J Biochem Cell Biol 40: 484–95.

Askling J, Grunewald J, Eklund A et al. (1999). Increased risk for cancer following sarcoidosis. Am J Respir Crit Care Med 160: 1668–72.

Bachwich PR, Lynch JP, Kunkel SL (1987). Arachidonic acid metabolism is altered in sarcoid alveolar macrophages. Clin Immunol Immunopathol 42: 27–37.

Barnett CF, Bonura EJ, Nathan SD et al. (2009). Treatment of sarcoidosis-associated pulmonary hypertension: a two-center experience. Chest 135: 1455–61.

Barst RJ, Ratner SJ (1985). Sarcoidosis and reactive pulmonary hypertension. Arch Intern Med 145: 2112–14.

Baughman RP, Gallon LS, Barcelli U (1984). Prostaglandins and thromboxanes in the bronchoalveolar lavage fluid: possible immunoregulation in sarcoidosis. Am Rev Respir Dis 130: 933–6.

Baughman RP, Shipley R, Eisentrout CE (1987). Predictive value of gallium scan, angiotensin-converting enzyme level, and bronchoalveolar lavage in two-year follow-up of pulmonary sarcoidosis. Lung 165: 371–7.

Baughman RP, Shipley RT, Loudon RG, Lower EE (1991). Crackles in interstitial lung disease: comparison of sarcoidosis and fibrosing alveolitis. Chest 100: 96–101.

Baughman RP, Winget DB, Bowen EH, Lower EE (1997). Predicting respiratory failure in sarcoidosis patients. Sarcoid Vasc Diff Lung Dis 14: 154–8.

Baughman RP, Teirstein AS, Judson MA et al. (2001). Clinical characteristics of patients in a case control study of sarcoidosis. Am J Respir Crit Care Med 164: 1885–9.

Baughman RP, Drent M, Kavuru M et al. (2006a). Infliximab therapy in patients with chronic sarcoidosis and pulmonary involvement. Am J Respir Crit Care Med 174: 795–802.

Baughman RP, Judson MA, Teirstein A et al. (2006b). Presenting characteristics as predictors of duration of treatment in sarcoidosis. Q J Med 99: 307–15.

Beaumont D, Herry JY, Sapene M et al. (1982). Gallium-67 in the evaluation of sarcoidosis: correlations with serum angiotensin-converting enzyme and bronchoalveolar lavage. Thorax 37: 11–18.

Behbehani N, JayKrishnan B, Khadadah M et al. (2007). Clinical presentation of sarcoidosis in a mixed population in the Middle East. Respir Med 101: 2284–8.

Bergin CJ, Bell DY, Coblentz CL et al. (1989). Sarcoidosis: correlation of pulmonary parenchymal pattern at CT with results of pulmonary function tests. Radiology 171: 619–24.

Bottoms SE, Howell JE, Reinhardt AK et al. (2010). Tgf-Beta isoform specific regulation of airway inflammation and remodelling in a murine model of asthma. PloS One 5: e9674.

Brauner MW, Grenier P, Mompoint D et al. (1989). Pulmonary sarcoidosis: evaluation with high-resolution CT. Radiology 172: 467–71.

Brauner MW, Lenoir S, Grenier P et al. (1992). Pulmonary sarcoidosis: CT assessment of lesion reversibility. Radiology 182: 349–54.

Brincker H, Wilbek E (1974). The incidence of malignant tumours in patients with respiratory sarcoidosis. Br J Cancer 29: 247–51.

Byg KE, Milman N, Hansen S (2003). Sarcoidosis in Denmark 1980–1994: a registry-based incidence study comprising 5536 patients. Sarcoid Vasc Diff Lung Dis 20: 46–52.

Camuset J, Nunes H, Dombret MC et al. (2007). Treatment of chronic pulmonary aspergillosis by voriconazole in non-immunocompromised patients. Chest 131: 1435–41.

Capelli A, Di SA, Lusuardi M et al. (2002). Increased macrophage inflammatory protein-1 alpha and macrophage inflammatory protein-1 beta levels in bronchoalveolar lavage fluid of patients affected by different stages of pulmonary sarcoidosis. Am J Respir Crit Care Med 165: 236–41.

Cavazza A, Harari S, Caminati A et al. (2009). The histology of pulmonary sarcoidosis: a review with particular emphasis on unusual and underrecognized features. Int J Surg Pathol 17: 219–30.

Copeman DM, Hodges RJ, Bottoms SE et al. (2004). Effect of upregulating cyclooxygenase-2 and prostaglandin E2 on the development of bleomycin-induced lung fibrosis. Am J Respir Crit Care Med 169: A300.

Crouser ED, Culver DA, Knox KS et al. (2009). Gene expression profiling identifies MMP-12 and ADAMDEC1 as potential pathogenic mediators of pulmonary sarcoidosis. Am J Respir Crit Care Med 179: 929–38.

Daly HE, Baecher-Allan CM, Barth RK et al. (1997). Bleomycin induces strain-dependent alterations in the pattern of epithelial cell-specific marker expression in mouse lung. Toxicol Appl Pharmacol 142: 303–10.

de Kleijn WP, De VJ, Lower EE et al. (2009). Fatigue in sarcoidosis: a systematic review. Curr Opin Pulm Med 15: 499–506.

De RV, Trentin L, Crivellari MT et al. (1997). Release of prostaglandin E2 and leukotriene B4 by alveolar macrophages from patients with sarcoidosis. Thorax 52: 76–83.

Di GM, Gambelli F, Hoyle GW et al. (2009). Systemic inhibition of NF-kappaB activation protects from silicosis. PLoS One e 4: 5689.

Drent M, Jacobs JA, De VJ et al. (1999). Does the cellular bronchoalveolar lavage fluid profile reflect the severity of sarcoidosis? Eur Respir J 13: 1338–44.

Fireman E, Kraiem Z, Sade O et al. (2002). Induced sputum-retrieved matrix metalloproteinase 9 and tissue metalloproteinase inhibitor 1 in granulomatous diseases. Clin Exp Immunol 130: 331–7.

Fireman E, Gilburd D, Marmor S (2009). Angiogenic cytokines in induced sputum of patients with sarcoidosis. Respirology 14: 117–23.

Fisher KA, Serlin DM, Wilson KC et al. (2006). Sarcoidosis-associated pulmonary hypertension: outcome with long-term epoprostenol treatment. Chest 130: 1481–8.

Gideon NM, Mannino DM (1996). Sarcoidosis mortality in the United States 1979–1991: an analysis of multiple-cause mortality data. *Am J Med* 100: 423–7.

Gvozdenovic BS, Mihailovic-Vucinic V, Ilic-Dudvarski A *et al.* (2008). Differences in symptom severity and health status impairment between patients with pulmonary and pulmonary plus extrapulmonary sarcoidosis. *Respir Med* 102: 1636–42.

Hadjiliadis D, Sporn TA, Perfect JR *et al.* (2002). Outcome of lung transplantation in patients with mycetomas. *Chest* 121: 128–34.

Hamada N, Kuwano K, Yamada M *et al.* (2005). Anti-vascular endothelial growth factor gene therapy attenuates lung injury and fibrosis in mice. *J Immunol* 175: 1224–31.

Handa T, Nagai S, Fushimi Y *et al.* (2006a). Clinical and radiographic indices associated with airflow limitation in patients with sarcoidosis. *Chest* 130: 1851–6.

Handa T, Nagai S, Miki S *et al.* (2006b). Incidence of pulmonary hypertension and its clinical relevance in patients with sarcoidosis. *Chest* 129: 1246–52.

Hansell DM, Milne DG, Wilsher ML, Wells AU (1998). Pulmonary sarcoidosis: morphologic associations of airflow obstruction at thin-section CT. *Radiology* 209: 697–704.

Harris JM, Johnston ID, Rudd R *et al.* (2010). Cryptogenic fibrosing alveolitis and lung cancer: the BTS study. *Thorax* 65: 70–6.

Harrison BD, Shaylor JM, Stokes TC, Wilkes AR (1991). Airflow limitation in sarcoidosis: a study of pulmonary function in 107 patients with newly diagnosed disease. *Respir Med* 85: 59–64.

Hauber HP, Gholami D, Meyer A, Pforte A (2003). Increased interleukin-13 expression in patients with sarcoidosis. *Thorax* 58: 519–24.

He Z, Zhu Y, Jiang H (2009). Toll-like receptor 4 mediates lipopolysaccharide-induced collagen secretion by phosphoinositide3-kinase-Akt pathway in fibroblasts during acute lung injury. *J Recept Signal Transduct Res* 29: 119–25.

Hennebicque AS, Nunes H, Brillet PY *et al.* (2005). CT findings in severe thoracic sarcoidosis. *Eur Radiol* 15: 23–30.

Henry MT, McMahon K, Mackarel AJ *et al.* (2002). Matrix metalloproteinases and tissue inhibitor of metalloproteinase-1 in sarcoidosis and IPF. *Eur Respir J* 20: 1220–7.

Hill MR, Papafili A, Booth H *et al.* (2006). Functional prostaglandin-endoperoxide synthase 2 polymorphism predicts poor outcome in sarcoidosis. *Am J Respir Crit Care Med* 174: 915–22.

Hillerdal G, Nou E, Osterman K, Schmekel B (1984). Sarcoidosis: epidemiology and prognosis. A 15-year European study. *Am Rev Respir Dis* 130: 29–32.

Hills SE, Parkes SA, Baker SB (1987). Epidemiology of sarcoidosis in the Isle of Man. 2: Evidence for space-time clustering. *Thorax* 42: 427–30.

Hiraga Y, Hosoda Y, Zenda I (1977). A local outbreak of sarcoidosis in Northern Japan. *Z Erkr Atmungsorgane* 149: 38–43.

Hodges RJ, Jenkins RG, Wheeler-Jones CP *et al.* (2004). Severity of lung injury in cyclooxygenase-2-deficient mice is dependent on reduced prostaglandin E (2) production. *Am J Pathol* 165: 1663–76.

Hollinger WM, Staton GW, Jr., Fajman WA *et al.* (1985). Prediction of therapeutic response in steroid-treated pulmonary sarcoidosis: evaluation of clinical parameters, bronchoalveolar lavage, gallium-67 lung scanning, and serum angiotensin-converting enzyme levels. *Am Rev Respir Dis* 132: 65–9.

Hosoda Y, Yamaguchi M, Hiraga Y (1997). Global epidemiology of sarcoidosis. What story do prevalence and incidence tell us? *Clin Chest Med* 18: 681–94.

Howell JE, McAnulty RJ (2006). TGF-beta: its role in asthma and therapeutic potential. *Curr Drug Targets* 7: 547–65.

Hubbard R, Venn A, Lewis S, Britton J (2000). Lung cancer and cryptogenic fibrosing alveolitis: a population-based cohort study. *Am J Respir Crit Care Med* 161: 5–8.

Hunsaker AR, Munden RF, Pugatch RD, Mentzer SJ (1996). Sarcoid-like reaction in patients with malignancy. *Radiology* 200: 255–61.

Ionescu DN, Hunt JL, Lomago D, Yousem SA (2005). Recurrent sarcoidosis in lung transplant allografts: granulomas are of recipient origin. *Diagn Mol Pathol* 14: 140–5.

Ishida Y, Kimura A, Kondo T *et al.* (2007). Essential roles of the CC chemokine ligand 3-CC chemokine receptor 5 axis in bleomycin-induced pulmonary fibrosis through regulation of macrophage and fibrocyte infiltration. *Am J Pathol* 170: 843–54.

Israel HL, Ostrow A (1969). Sarcoidosis and aspergilloma. *Am J Med* 47: 243–50.

Jonth AC, Silveira L, Fingerlin TE *et al.* (2007). TGF-beta 1 variants in chronic beryllium disease and sarcoidosis. *J Immunol* 179: 4255–62.

Judson MA, Strange C (1998). Bullous sarcoidosis: a report of three cases. *Chest* 114: 1474–8.

Judson MA, Baughman RP, Thompson BW *et al.* (2003). Two-year prognosis of sarcoidosis: the ACCESS experience. *Sarcoid Vasc Diff Lung Dis* 20: 204–11.

Kaarteenaho-Wiik R, Lammi L, Lakari E *et al.* (2005). Localization of precursor proteins and mRNA of type I and III collagens in usual interstitial pneumonia and sarcoidosis. *J Mol Histol* 36: 437–46.

Keerthisingam CB, Jenkins RG, Harrison NK *et al.* (2001). Cyclooxygenase-2 deficiency results in a loss of the anti-proliferative response to transforming growth factor-beta in human fibrotic lung fibroblasts and promotes bleomycin-induced pulmonary fibrosis in mice. *Am J Pathol* 158: 1411–22.

Keijsers RG, Grutters JC, van Velzen-Blad H *et al.* (2010). 18)F-FDG PET patterns and BAL cell profiles in pulmonary sarcoidosis. *Eur J Nucl Med Mol Imaging* 37: 1181–8.

Kohn H, Klech H, Mostbeck A, Kummer F (1982). 67Ga scanning for assessment of disease activity and therapy decisions in pulmonary sarcoidosis in comparison to chest radiography, serum ACE and blood T-lymphocytes. *Eur J Nucl Med* 7: 413–16.

Kohyama T, Ertl RF, Valenti V *et al.* (2001). Prostaglandin E (2) inhibits fibroblast chemotaxis. *Am J Physiol Lung Cell Mol Physiol* 281: L1257–63.

Kolodsick JE, Peters-Golden M, Larios J *et al.* (2003). Prostaglandin E2 inhibits fibroblast to myofibroblast transition via E prostanoid receptor 2 signaling and cyclic adenosine monophosphate elevation. *Am J Respir Cell Mol Biol* 29: 537–44.

Koyama S, Sato E, Haniuda M *et al.* (2002). Decreased level of vascular endothelial growth factor in bronchoalveolar lavage fluid of normal smokers and patients with pulmonary fibrosis. *Am J Respir Crit Care Med* 166: 382–5.

Kreider M, Kotloff RM (2009). Selection of candidates for lung transplantation. *Proc Am Thorac Soc* 6: 20–7.

Kriegova E, Melle C, Kolek V *et al.* (2006). Protein profiles of bronchoalveolar lavage fluid from patients with pulmonary sarcoidosis. *Am J Respir Crit Care Med* 173: 1145–54.

Kruit A, Grutters JC, Ruven HJ *et al.* (2006). Transforming growth factor-beta gene polymorphisms in sarcoidosis patients with and without fibrosis. *Chest* 129: 1584–91.

Lammi L, Kinnula V, Lahde S *et al.* (1997). Propeptide levels of type III and type I procollagen in the serum and bronchoalveolar lavage fluid of patients with pulmonary sarcoidosis. *Eur Respir J* 10: 2725–30.

Lee KS, Park SJ, Kim SR et al. (2008). Inhibition of VEGF blocks TGF-beta1 production through a PI3K/Akt signalling pathway. Eur Respir J 31: 523–31.

Lewis PJ, Salama A (1994). Uptake of fluorine-18-fluorodeoxyglucose in sarcoidosis. J Nucl Med 35: 1647–9.

Libshitz HI, Atkinson GW, Israel HL (1974). Pleural thickening as a manifestation of Aspergillus superinfection. Am J Roentgen Radium Ther Nucl Med 120: 883–6.

Lin YH, Haslam PL, Turner-Warwick M (1985). Chronic pulmonary sarcoidosis: relationship between lung lavage cell counts, chest radiograph, and results of standard lung function tests. Thorax 40: 501–7.

Line BR, Hunninghake GW, Keogh BA et al. (1981). Gallium-67 scanning to stage the alveolitis of sarcoidosis: correlation with clinical studies, pulmonary function studies, and bronchoalveolar lavage. Am Rev Respir Dis 123: 440–6.

Lockstone HE, Sanderson S, Kulakova N et al. (2010). Gene-set analysis of lung samples provides insight into pathogenesis of progressive, fibrotic pulmonary sarcoidosis. Am J Respir Crit Care Med 181: 1367–75.

Lopez-Campos JL, Rodriguez-Rodriguez D, Rodriguez-Becerra E et al. (2009). Cyclooxygenase-2 polymorphisms confer susceptibility to sarcoidosis but are not related to prognosis. Respir Med 103: 427–33.

Maher TM, Evans IC, Bottoms SE et al. (2010). Diminished prostaglandin E2 contributes to the apoptosis paradox in idiopathic pulmonary fibrosis. Am J Respir Crit Care Med 182: 73–82.

Maliarik MJ, Rybicki BA, Malvitz E et al. (1998). Angiotensin-converting enzyme gene polymorphism and risk of sarcoidosis. Am J Respir Crit Care Med 158: 1566–70.

Mana J, van Kroonenburgh M (2005). Nuclear imaging techniques in sarcoidosis. Eur Respir Mon 32: 284–300.

Marshall RP, McAnulty RJ, Laurent GJ (2000). Angiotensin II is mitogenic for human lung fibroblasts via activation of the type 1 receptor. Am J Respir Crit Care Med 161: 1999–2004.

Marshall RP, Gohlke P, Chambers RC et al. (2004). Angiotensin II and the fibroproliferative response to acute lung injury. Am J Physiol Lung Cell Mol Physiol 286: L156–64.

McAnulty RJ, Chambers RC, Laurent GJ (1995). Regulation of fibroblast procollagen production: transforming growth factor-beta 1 induces prostaglandin E2 but not procollagen synthesis via a pertussis toxin-sensitive G-protein. Biochem J 307(Pt 1): 63–8.

McAnulty RJ, Hernandez-Rodriguez NA, Mutsaers SE et al. (1997). Indomethacin suppresses the anti-proliferative effects of transforming growth factor-beta isoforms on fibroblast cell cultures. Biochem J 321(Pt 3): 639–43.

McGrath DS, Daniil Z, Foley P et al. (2000). Epidemiology of familial sarcoidosis in the UK. Thorax 55: 751–4.

Milman N, Selroos O (1990). Pulmonary sarcoidosis in the Nordic countries 1950–1982: epidemiology and clinical picture. Sarcoidosis 7: 50–7.

Milman N, Burton CM, Iversen M et al. (2008). Pulmonary hypertension in end-stage pulmonary sarcoidosis: therapeutic effect of sildenafil? J Heart Lung Transplant 27: 329–34.

Miotto D, Christodoulopoulos P, Olivenstein R et al. (2001). Expression of IFN-gamma-inducible protein; monocyte chemotactic proteins 1, 3, and 4; and eotaxin in TH1- and TH2-mediated lung diseases. J Allergy Clin Immunol 107: 664–70.

Mitchell DN, Scadding JG, Heard BE, Hinson KF (1977). Sarcoidosis: histopathological definition and clinical diagnosis. J Clin Pathol 30: 395–408.

Mollers M, Aries SP, Dromann D et al. (2001). Intracellular cytokine repertoire in different T-cell subsets from patients with sarcoidosis. Thorax 56: 487–93.

Morimoto T, Azuma A, Abe S et al. (2008). Epidemiology of sarcoidosis in Japan. Eur Respir J 31: 372–9.

Morohashi K, Takada T, Omori K et al. (2003). Vascular endothelial growth factor gene polymorphisms in Japanese patients with sarcoidosis. Chest 123: 1520–6.

Nakatsu M, Hatabu H, Morikawa K et al. (2002). Large coalescent parenchymal nodules in pulmonary sarcoidosis: 'sarcoid galaxy' sign. Am J Roentgen 178: 1389–93.

Neville E, Walker AN, James DG (1983). Prognostic factors predicting the outcome of sarcoidosis: an analysis of 818 patients. Q J Med 52: 525–33.

Nishimura K, Itoh H, Kitaichi M et al. (1993). Pulmonary sarcoidosis: correlation of CT and histopathologic findings. Radiology 189: 105–9.

Nishioka Y, Manabe K, Kishi J et al. (2007). CXCL9 and 11 in patients with pulmonary sarcoidosis: a role of alveolar macrophages. Clin Exp Immunol 149: 317–26.

Nobata K, Kasai T, Fujimura M et al. (2006). Pulmonary sarcoidosis with usual interstitial pneumonia distributed predominantly in the lower lung fields. Intern Med 45: 359–62.

Nunes H, Humbert M, Capron F et al. (2006). Pulmonary hypertension associated with sarcoidosis: mechanisms, hemodynamics and prognosis. Thorax 61: 68–74.

Ohchi T, Shijubo N, Kawabata I et al. (2004). Polymorphism of Clara cell 10-kD protein gene of sarcoidosis. Am J Respir Crit Care Med 169. 180–6.

Orens JB, Estenne M, Arcasoy S et al. (2006). International guidelines for the selection of lung transplant candidates: 2006 update – a consensus report from the Pulmonary Scientific Council of the International Society for Heart and Lung Transplantation. J Heart Lung Transplant 25: 745–55.

Ou XM, Li WC, Liu DS et al. (2009). VEGFR-2 antagonist SU5416 attenuates bleomycin-induced pulmonary fibrosis in mice. Int Immunopharmacol 9: 70–9.

Ozdemir OK, Celik G, Dalva K et al. (2007). High CD95 expression of BAL lymphocytes predicts chronic course in patients with sarcoidosis. Respirology 12: 869–73.

Pabst S, Baumgarten G, Stremmel A et al. (2006). Toll-like receptor (TLR) 4 polymorphisms are associated with a chronic course of sarcoidosis. Clin Exp Immunol 143: 420–6.

Pabst S, Karpushova A, az-Lacava A et al. (2010). VEGF gene haplotypes are associated with sarcoidosis. Chest 137: 156–63.

Padilla ML, Schilero GJ, Teirstein AS (2002). Donor-acquired sarcoidosis. Sarcoid Vasc Diff Lung Dis 19: 18–24.

Padley SP, Padhani AR, Nicholson A, Hansell DM (1996). Pulmonary sarcoidosis mimicking cryptogenic fibrosing alveolitis on CT. Clin Radiol 51: 807–10.

Papadopoulos KI, Melander O, Orho-Melander M et al. (2000). Angiotensin converting enzyme (ACE) gene polymorphism in sarcoidosis in relation to associated autoimmune diseases. J Intern Med 247: 71–7.

Papafili A, Hill MR, Brull DJ et al. (2002). Common promoter variant in cyclooxygenase-2 represses gene expression: evidence of role in acute-phase inflammatory response. Arterioscler Thromb Vasc Biol 22: 1631–6.

Petkova DK, Clelland CA, Ronan JE et al. (2003). Reduced expression of cyclooxygenase (COX) in idiopathic pulmonary fibrosis and sarcoidosis. Histopathology 43: 381–6.

Petrek M, Drabek J, Kolek V et al. (2000). CC chemokine receptor gene polymorphisms in Czech patients with pulmonary sarcoidosis. Am J Respir Crit Care Med 162: 1000–3.

Petrek M, Kolek V, Szotkowska J, du Bois RM (2002). CC and C chemokine expression in pulmonary sarcoidosis. Eur Respir J 20: 1206–12.

Pietinalho A, Hiraga Y, Hosoda Y et al. (1995). The frequency of sarcoidosis in Finland and Hokkaido, Japan: a comparative epidemiological study. Sarcoidosis 12: 61–7.

Pietinalho A, Furuya K, Yamaguchi E et al. (1999). The angiotensin-converting enzyme DD gene is associated with poor prognosis in Finnish sarcoidosis patients. Eur Respir J 13: 723–6.

Pietinalho A, Ohmichi M, Lofroos AB et al. (2000). The prognosis of pulmonary sarcoidosis in Finland and Hokkaido, Japan: a comparative five-year study of biopsy-proven cases. Sarcoid Vasc Diff Lung Dis 17: 158–66.

Pilon AL (2000). Rationale for the development of recombinant human CC10 as a therapeutic for inflammatory and fibrotic disease. Ann NY Acad Sci 923: 280–99.

Prasse A, Katic C, Germann M et al. (2008). Phenotyping sarcoidosis from a pulmonary perspective. Am J Respir Crit Care Med 177: 330–6.

Preston IR, Klinger JR, Landzberg MJ et al. (2001). Vasoresponsiveness of sarcoidosis-associated pulmonary hypertension. Chest 120: 866–72.

Rabin DL, Thompson B, Brown KM et al. (2004). Sarcoidosis: social predictors of severity at presentation. Eur Respir J 24: 601–8.

Reich JM (2001). Course and prognosis of sarcoidosis in African-Americans versus Caucasians. Eur Respir J 17: 833.

Reich JM (2002). Mortality of intrathoracic sarcoidosis in referral vs population-based settings: influence of stage, ethnicity, and corticosteroid therapy. Chest 121: 32–9.

Remy-Jardin M, Giraud F, Remy J et al. (1994). Pulmonary sarcoidosis: role of CT in the evaluation of disease activity and functional impairment and in prognosis assessment. Radiology 191: 675–80.

Renner W, Kotschan S, Hoffmann C et al. (2000). A common 936 C/T mutation in the gene for vascular endothelial growth factor is associated with vascular endothelial growth factor plasma levels. J Vasc Res 37: 443–8.

Rizzato G, Blasi A (1986). A European survey on the usefulness of 67Ga lung scans in assessing sarcoidosis: experience in 14 research centers in seven different countries. Ann NY Acad Sci 465: 463–78.

Rizzato G, Spinelli F, Tansini G et al. (1983). Assessment of sarcoidosis activity by 67gallium lung scan: a study with follow-up. Respiration 44: 360–7.

Roberts SD, Kohli LL, Wood KL et al. (2005). CD4 + CD28-T cells are expanded in sarcoidosis. Sarcoid Vasc Diff Lung Dis 22: 13–19.

Rutherford RM, Kehren J, Staedtler F et al. (2001). Functional genomics in sarcoidosis: reduced or increased apoptosis? Swiss Med Wkly 131: 459–70.

Rybicki BA, Major M, Popovich J et al. (1997). Racial differences in sarcoidosis incidence: a 5-year study in a health maintenance organization. Am J Epidemiol 145: 234–41.

Rybicki BA, Iannuzzi MC, Frederick MM et al. (2001). Familial aggregation of sarcoidosis: a case–control etiologic study of sarcoidosis (ACCESS). Am J Respir Crit Care Med 164: 2085–91.

Salez F, Gosset P, Copin MC et al. (1998). Transforming growth factor-beta1 in sarcoidosis. Eur Respir J 12: 913–19.

Sanders YY, Pardo A, Selman M et al. (2008). Thy-1 promoter hypermethylation: a novel epigenetic pathogenic mechanism in pulmonary fibrosis. Am J Respir Cell Mol Biol 39: 610–18.

Sato H, Williams HR, Spagnolo P et al. (2010). CARD15/NOD2 polymorphisms are associated with severe pulmonary sarcoidosis. Eur Respir J 35: 324–30.

Scadding JG (1956). Clinical problems of diffuse pulmonary fibrosis. Br J Radiol 29: 633–41.

Scadding JG (1961). Prognosis of intrathoracic sarcoidosis in England: a review of 136 cases after five years' observation. Br Med J 2: 1165–72.

Seki E, De MS, Osterreicher CH et al. (2007). TLR4 enhances TGF-beta signaling and hepatic fibrosis. Nat Med 13: 1324–32.

Sekiya M, Ohwada A, Miura K et al. (2003). Serum vascular endothelial growth factor as a possible prognostic indicator in sarcoidosis. Lung 181: 259–65.

Shah M, Foreman DM, Ferguson MW (1995). Neutralisation of TGF-beta 1 and TGF-beta 2 or exogenous addition of TGF-beta 3 to cutaneous rat wounds reduces scarring. J Cell Sci 108(Pt 3): 985–1002.

Shigemitsu H, Nagai S, Sharma OP (2007). Pulmonary hypertension and granulomatous vasculitis in sarcoidosis. Curr Opin Pulm Med 13: 434–8.

Shijubo N, Itoh Y, Shigehara K et al. (2000). Association of Clara cell 10-kDa protein, spontaneous regression and sarcoidosis. Eur Respir J 16: 414–19.

Shorr AF, Davies DB, Nathan SD (2002). Outcomes for patients with sarcoidosis awaiting lung transplantation. Chest 122: 233–8.

Shorr AF, Davies DB, Nathan SD (2003). Predicting mortality in patients with sarcoidosis awaiting lung transplantation. Chest 124: 922–8.

Shorr AF, Helman DL, Davies DB, Nathan SD (2005). Pulmonary hypertension in advanced sarcoidosis: epidemiology and clinical characteristics. Eur Respir J 25: 783–8.

Siltzbach LE, James DG, Neville E et al. (1974). Course and prognosis of sarcoidosis around the world. Am J Med 57: 847–52.

Smith LJ, Lawrence JB, Katzenstein AA (1983). Vascular sarcoidosis: a rare cause of pulmonary hypertension. Am J Med Sci 285: 38–44.

Smith RE, Strieter RM, Phan SH et al. (1994). Production and function of murine macrophage inflammatory protein-1 alpha in bleomycin-induced lung injury. J Immunol 153: 4704–12.

Spagnolo P, Renzoni EA, Wells AU et al. (2005). C-C chemokine receptor 5 gene variants in relation to lung disease in sarcoidosis. Am J Respir Crit Care Med 172: 721–28.

Standiford TJ, Rolfe MW, Kunkel SL et al. (1993). Macrophage inflammatory protein-1 alpha expression in interstitial lung disease. J Immunol 151: 2852–63.

Takemura T, Matsui Y, Saiki S, Mikami R (1992). Pulmonary vascular involvement in sarcoidosis: a report of 40 autopsy cases. Hum Pathol 23: 1216–23.

Taniguchi H, Katoh S, Kadota J et al. (2000). Interleukin 5 and granulocyte-macrophage colony-stimulating factor levels in bronchoalveolar lavage fluid in interstitial lung disease. Eur Respir J 16: 959–64.

Tolnay E, Kuhnen C, Voss B et al. (1998). Expression and localization of vascular endothelial growth factor and its receptor flt in pulmonary sarcoidosis. Virchows Arch 432: 61–5.

Tomlinson JR, Sahn SA (1987). Aspergilloma in sarcoid and tuberculosis. Chest 92: 505–8.

Tsiligianni I, Antoniou KM, Kyriakou D et al. (2005). Th1/Th2 cytokine pattern in bronchoalveolar lavage fluid and induced sputum in pulmonary sarcoidosis. BMC Pulm Med 5: 8.

Turner-Warwick M, Lebowitz M, Burrows B, Johnson A (1980). Cryptogenic fibrosing alveolitis and lung cancer. Thorax 35: 496–9.

Turner-Warwick M, McAllister W, Lawrence R *et al.* (1986). Corticosteroid treatment in pulmonary sarcoidosis: do serial lavage lymphocyte counts, serum angiotensin converting enzyme measurements, and gallium-67 scans help management? *Thorax* **41**: 903–13.

Tzouvelekis A, Anevlavis S, Bouros D (2006). Angiogenesis in interstitial lung diseases: a pathogenetic hallmark or a bystander? *Respir Res* **7**: 82.

Verstraeten A, Demedts M, Verwilghen J *et al.* (1990). Predictive value of bronchoalveolar lavage in pulmonary sarcoidosis. *Chest* **98**: 560–7.

Wahl SM (2007). Transforming growth factor-beta: innately bipolar. *Curr Opin Immunol* **19**: 55–62.

Watson CJ, Webb NJ, Bottomley MJ, Brenchley PE (2000). Identification of polymorphisms within the vascular endothelial growth factor (VEGF) gene: correlation with variation in VEGF protein production. *Cytokine* **12**: 1232–5.

West SG, Gilbreath RE, Lawless OJ (1981). Painful clubbing and sarcoidosis. *J Am Med Assoc* **246**: 1338–9.

Wollschlager C, Khan F (1984). Aspergillomas complicating sarcoidosis: a prospective study in 100 patients. *Chest* **86**: 585–8.

Wu J, Yang X, Zhang YF *et al.* (2009). Angiotensin II upregulates Toll-like receptor 4 and enhances lipopolysaccharide-induced CD40 expression in rat peritoneal mesothelial cells. *Inflamm Res* **58**: 473–82.

Yancey J, Luxford W, Sharma OP (1972). Clubbing of the fingers in sarcoidosis. *J Am Med Assoc* **222**: 582.

Yeager H, Rossman MD, Baughman RP *et al.* (2005). Pulmonary and psychosocial findings at enrollment in the ACCESS study. *Sarcoid Vasc Diff Lung Dis* **22**: 147–53.

Zhai R, Gong MN, Zhou W *et al.* (2007). Genotypes and haplotypes of the VEGF gene are associated with higher mortality and lower VEGF plasma levels in patients with ARDS. *Thorax* **62**: 718–22.

Ziegenhagen MW, Schrum S, Zissel G *et al.* (1998). Increased expression of proinflammatory chemokines in bronchoalveolar lavage cells of patients with progressing idiopathic pulmonary fibrosis and sarcoidosis. *J Invest Med* **46**: 223–31.

Ziegenhagen MW, Rothe ME, Schlaak M, Muller-Quernheim J (2003). Bronchoalveolar and serological parameters reflecting the severity of sarcoidosis. *Eur Respir J* **21**: 407–13.

Zissel G, Homolka J, Schlaak J *et al.* (1996). Anti-inflammatory cytokine release by alveolar macrophages in pulmonary sarcoidosis. *Am J Respir Crit Care Med* **154**: 713–19.

Zoumot Z, Carby M, Hall AV (2006). Radiological resolution of cavitating *Aspergillus fumigatus* infection following treatment with oral voriconazole in two lung transplant recipients. *Transplant Int* **19**: 688–90.

THE LIVER AND GI TRACT, SPLEEN, BLOOD AND BONE MARROW, NERVOUS SYSTEM, RENAL AND CALCIUM METABOLISM, AND PSYCHIATRIC ASPECTS

24

Hepatobiliary sarcoidosis

PATRICK KENNEDY, PRIYAJIT BOBBY PRASAD AND JAMES BOYER

INTRODUCTION

A minority of patients with sarcoidosis show clinically evident involvement of the liver, although both biopsy and necropsy studies usually show that the liver contains granulomas. Clinically significant hepatic dysfunction is rare, but up to one-third of patients have hepatomegaly or a cholestatic pattern of deranged liver function, with minimal change in aminotransferase levels. Typically this mild derangement in liver parameters is asymptomatic; however, hepatic sarcoid has been associated with recognized clinical syndromes, such as portal hypertension, chronic intrahepatic cholestasis, and even Budd–Chiari syndrome. Such a clinical presentation in a patient in whom the diagnosis of sarcoidosis was not readily evident, from involvement of other organs, would require the exclusion of a wide range of liver diseases where granulomatous changes can also be present on liver histology.

INCIDENCE OF HISTOLOGICAL INVOLVEMENT OF THE LIVER

The causes of hepatic granulomas are numerous and their identification can be difficult. However, sarcoidosis remains the leading cause of hepatic granulomas, with granulomatous change reported on liver biopsy in 40–70 percent of patients (Newman et al. 1997) and as high as 94 percent (Klatskin 1977).

The best available evidence of the frequency of symptomless granulomas in the liver in sarcoidosis comes from historical data, when aspiration liver biopsy was central to confirming a histological diagnosis of sarcoidosis. In 1943, Van Beek and Haex were the first to report the use of aspiration liver biopsy in sarcoidosis. They found typical non-caseating granulomas in biopsies from two of four cases with clinical features of sarcoidosis, although there was no other evidence of liver involvement. These findings were supported by Van Buchem (1946) who reported specific changes in liver biopsies in all of 14 cases of sarcoidosis. Later studies reported the presence of sarcoid tubercles in liver biopsies in 16 of 21 cases in which the diagnosis of sarcoidosis seemed likely on other grounds (Shay et al. 1951). Mather et al. (1955) studied 93 patients with sarcoidosis, of whom 59 (63 percent) showed tuberculoid granulomas on liver biopsy; 11 had had erythema nodosum, and of these 10 showed specific changes. Among patients with intrathoracic changes, the liver showed granulomas in a higher proportion of those with hilar lymph-node enlargement (up to 75 percent), with or without lung infiltration, compared with lung infiltration only (38 percent).

The data are consistent across the historical studies in which large series have been reported. This includes a study of 275 patients by Scadding with a confirmed diagnosis of sarcoidosis. Liver biopsy was performed as part of the diagnostic work-up in 73 patients; hepatic granulomas were reported in 48 (66 percent) of these patients, and notably this finding was more frequently reported in the earlier stages of the disease. Where intrathoracic changes consisted of hilar lymph-node enlargement only, 87 percent of patients had hepatic granulomas; when there was concomitant infiltration of the lungs, 67 percent had hepatic granulomas; infiltration of the lungs without hilar node enlargement was associated with hepatic granulomas in 59 percent of patients.

Liver biopsies from patients with sarcoidosis demonstrate the presence of granulomas within the lobule or in the portal zone, but more commonly these granulomas are reported to be small and localized to the portal spaces (Blich and Edoute 2004). It is recognized that there is some heterogeneity in the size and shape of these lesions, the lower limit being set by the need to have sufficient cells in a recognizable arrangement to give a specific appearance and the upper limit for a non-confluent lesion being about 1 mm. Sarcoid tubercles are clearly demarcated from the liver cells and surrounding cellular reaction is rare. Sherlock described this in 1958, when a clear distinction between granuloma and the surrounding liver cells on a glycogen-stained section was demonstrated. These lesions have the classical appearance of a non-caseating epithelioid cell tubercle; occasionally there may be lymphocytes, CD4 and CD8, and to a lesser extent B-lymphocytes, scattered at the periphery, forming a rim around the granuloma (Tsuda and Kita 1994). Giant cells were also reported in the early description of the lesion, but are variable in number (Klatskin and Yesner 1950; Maddrey et al. 1970). Asteroids are only occasionally seen and Schaumann bodies are rarely reported on liver histology. In older, more mature lesions, there is a variable amount of hyaline fibrosis. In this context, the number of epithelioid cells decreases and that of lymphocytes increases; in some cases groups of hyalinizing tubercles become confluent and in extreme instances can give rise to extensive fibrosis, which may give rise to irreversible organ destruction and physiological dysfunction (Inoue et al. 1996).

When serial sections are routinely performed in a patient suspected of sarcoid, the yield of positive granulomas is greater than 90 percent. Klatskin (1977) calculated that, if one granuloma was seen in a 5 μm section of a 30 mg biopsy specimen, then a 1500 g liver would contain 15 000 000 granulomas.

HEPATIC GRANULOMAS

Hepatic granulomas are frequently encountered on liver biopsy and may represent a primary hepatic process, a manifestation of a systemic illness, or in some instances be an incidental finding of no clinical relevance. Therefore, the demonstration of granulomas on liver biopsy, like that of other biopsy procedures, must be considered in the context of historical and clinical data in order to reach an accurate diagnosis and guide further management. Thus, the whole spectrum of etiologies for hepatic granulomas must be considered: bacterial, fungal, viral or parasitic infection; a manifestation of drug-induced liver injury; a manifestation of underlying malignancy; or in some instances idiopathic cases (Bhardwaj et al. 2009).

The most frequently encountered granulomas in the liver are 'lipogranulomas' which contain lipid droplets surrounded by macrophages. They were seen in about 3 percent of livers in a series of 5500 liver biopsies (Klatskin 1977) and as high as 48 percent of autopsy specimens (Wanless and Geddie 1985). Their morphological features are distinctive, consisting of a sharply circumscribed group of vacuolated histiocytes mostly attached to the wall of central veins – although some may be found in portal triads. They are easily distinguished from epithelioid granulomas characteristic of sarcoid (Klatskin 1977).

Among infective agents, those causing predominantly granulomatous inflammation, notably Mycobacterium tuberculosis, and in endemic areas histoplasmosis and coccidioides, are most likely to cause hepatic granulomas resembling those of sarcoidosis. In the 1940s, Van Beek reported tubercles on liver histology in patients with erythema nodosum attributed to primary tuberculosis (TB), all of whom had acute hematogenous TB. Subsequently Klatskin and Yesner (1950) reported tuberculoid granulomas in liver biopsies from 7 of 18 patients with tuberculosis, only one of whom showed caseation.

Tuberculosis remains the most important infectious agent as the cause for hepatic granulomas. There is a clear geographic variation in its incidence, with rates reported at 20 and 34 percent in Turkey and Saudi Arabia, respectively. Diagnosis has improved significantly since these early descriptions of TB-related hepatic granulomas with the development of polymerase chain reaction (PCR) in addition to Ziehl–Nielsen staining for the identification and confirmation of Mycobacterium tuberculosis. However, it is remarkable that TB as an etiology for hepatic granulomas reported in studies from the West – namely Greece, the USA, Ireland and Scotland – does not exceed 4 percent (Wainwright 2007).

Other infectious agents accounted for a wide variation in the incidence of the hepatic granulomas seen in different patient populations. Parasitic infestation with Schistosomiasis accounted for 54 percent of the hepatic granulomas reported in one study from Saudi Arabia (Satti et al. 1990). In the same study it was reported that the presence of fever was associated with either TB or brucellosis, while other infectious agents included hydatid disease and typhoid fever. Prior to this, a Spanish study had reported Mediterranean exanthematous fever, toxoplasmosis and leprosy as potential causes for hepatic granulomas outside the better recognized infectious agents listed above (Vilaseca et al. 1979).

The literature also reports the demonstration of hepatic granulomas in other rare infectious diseases, such as actinomycosis, blastomycosis and tularemia. However, reports of hepatic granulomas in more common viral infections such as influenza B and infectious mononucleosis also exist. In Klatskin's personal series of 742 biopsy-documented hepatic granulomas, 565 were distinguished as epithelioid as opposed to lipogranulomas. Three hundred and nineteen had granulomatous diseases, 174 were associated with underlying hepatic disease, and 72 were seen in miscellaneous disorders (Klatskin 1977). Sarcoid, tuberculosis and schistosomiasis were the major diagnoses in patients with granulomatous diseases with the highest incidence found in patients with sarcoid (94 percent).

The discovery of hepatitis C virus (HCV) and the subsequent widespread availability of serological testing from 1991 led to the recognition of hepatic granulomas associated with the virus. Significant variability has been reported with the incidence of HCV-related hepatic granulomas. It has been reported up to 13 percent in Italy (Guglielmi et al. 1994), but a later and more comprehensive prevalence study reported a 1.3 percent incidence (Ozaras et al. 2004).

Autoimmune disease, primarily primary biliary cirrhosis (PBC), has accounted for a large proportion of hepatic granulomas in the recent literature. Comparison of the data from different studies reflecting the diversity of disease between countries has demonstrated a high incidence of PBC-related hepatic granulomas in Greece (68 percent), Ireland (55 percent), Scotland (36 percent) and the USA (4.5 percent) (Sartin and Walker 1991; McCluggage and Sloan 1994; Wainwright 2007).

Drugs are the most likely etiology when eosinophils are demonstrated in association with granulomas, and a history of exposure to agents associated with the development of granulomas is confirmatory. Studies report the incidence of drug-associated granulomas to be between 1 and 9 percent (Wainwright 2007). The list of culprit drugs has remained unchanged over the years, with allopurinol, nitrofurantoin, phenylbutazone and sulphonamides the most likely agents.

In chronic beryllium disease there may be granulomas in the liver. Agate (1948) reported a patient with epithelioid cell granulomas on liver biopsy, and Hardy (1951) referred to similar findings without detailing the frequency of granulomas. There are conflicting data regarding the presence of hepatic granulomas in berylliosis.

Granulomas in the liver may also be a response to malignant or inflammatory disease. Bagley et al. (1972) reported hepatic granulomas in patients with Hodgkin's disease. Klatskin (1976) reported non-caseating granulomas in patients with intra-abdominal lymphoma, carcinoma and inflammatory bowel disease.

Owing to the now extensive investigation of patients with hepatic granulomas, the percentage of idiopathic cases should be low. However, this is likely to vary from institution to institution and the level of liver expertise within each institution.

CLINICAL EVIDENCE OF SARCOIDOSIS OF THE LIVER

The liver is frequently involved in sarcoidosis, but it rarely gives rise to symptoms. Liver involvement can be associated with hepatomegaly, which historically was difficult to measure objectively – relying largely on clinical signs (Mayock et al. 1963; Lehmuskallio et al. 1977). However, with the benefit of imaging modalities, hepatomegaly is objectively reported in up to 30 percent of patients with liver involvement, but even in this group severe hepatic dysfunction is rare (Newman et al. 1997).

The proportions of patients in historical unselected series showing abnormalities in biochemical tests of liver function also showed some variation (Maddrey et al. 1970; Lehmuskallio et al. 1977). It is now considered that up to one-third of patients have a cholestatic pattern of biochemical alterations, with minimal augmentation in aminotransferase levels (Newman et al. 1997). These numbers are supported by recent studies, including one of 131 consecutive patients with a proven diagnosis of sarcoidosis, in whom 31 percent were reported to have abnormal liver biochemistry – primarily elevated alkaline phosphatase and γ-glutamyl transaminase activity – attributable to liver involvement (Kennedy et al. 2006).

While liver involvement in sarcoidosis is largely considered to be asymptomatic, progressive disease can occur and lead to the development of the rarer hepatic manifestations of sarcoid which include jaundice and chronic cholestasis, portal hypertension or Budd–Chiari syndrome. Since these cases usually present with one predominant feature, it is more convenient to consider these presentations individually, notwithstanding that there may be considerable overlap with the development of end-stage liver disease. Maddrey et al. (1970) reported portal hypertension in patients with hepatic sarcoid, giving rise to esophageal variceal bleeding and one death after an operation for a portosystemic shunt. This was an early insight into the potential gravity of hepatic sarcoid and indeed its propensity to the development of end-stage chronic liver disease, albeit in the minority of cases.

PORTAL HYPERTENSION

The earliest reports in the literature of sarcoidosis and portal hypertension were published by Mino et al. (1948) and Klatskin and Yesner (1950). Since then it has been widely reported, but more importantly a clear distinction has emerged between cirrhotic and non-cirrhotic portal hypertension (Cheitlin et al. 1960; Mistilis and Schiff 1964; Nelson and Schwabe 1966; Maddrey et al. 1970; Vilinskas et al. 1970; Berger and Katz 1973; Moreno-Merlo et al. 1997). Bleeding from esophageal varices, presenting with hematemesis and melena, was an important symptom in approximately half of these reported cases; ascites was reported in a smaller proportion of them; and in a minority of patients the diagnosis of portal hypertension was established without either of these presentations and was confirmed by measurement of splenic pulp or wedged hepatic vein pressures. Portal hypertension can occur without pathological evidence of cirrhosis (Nelson and Sears 1968; Berger and Katz 1973; Moreno-Merlo et al. 1997).

Conversely, some patients were found to have macronodular cirrhosis, biliary cirrhosis (with a predominantly micronodular biliary pattern at autopsy) or periportal fibrosis (Maddrey et al. 1970; Vilinskas et al. 1970; Berger and Katz 1973).

The etiology of portal hypertension in sarcoidosis is likely to involve different mechanisms. Maddrey et al. (1970) reported that small arteriovenous shunts may be formed in the region of the granulomas in the liver and spleen, resulting in increased portal blood flow with a compensatory increase in intrahepatic resistance. This leads to portal hypertension, as portal pressure is a function of portal blood flow and resistance. Large and confluent granulomas can be associated with healing of the parenchyma in a haphazard distribution, resulting in elevated resistance in the intrahepatic sinusoids. The subsequent development of portal central bridging fibrosis can then progress to cirrhotic remodeling with consequent portal hypertension. Bile duct destruction by granulomas gives rise to a biliary type of cirrhosis (Valla et al. 1987; Murphy et al. 1990). Mistilis and Schiff (1964) reported that granulomas in the portal areas restrict portal flow, resulting in a pre-sinusoidal portal hypertension. Another theory is that cirrhosis and focal fibrosis are a consequence of ischemia secondary to primary granulomatous phlebitis of the portal and hepatic veins, which can result in pre- and post-sinusoidal resistance (Moreno-Merlo *et al.* 1997).

Corticosteroid treatment has no role in the treatment of hepatic sarcoid unless in association with constitutional symptoms usually related to sarcoid in other organs. In this case, pancytopenia, liver biochemistry and constitutional symptoms may all improve. Portosystemic shunts with (Mino *et al.* 1948; Vilinskas *et al.* 1970) or without (Klatskin 1976; Maddrey *et al.* 1970;) splenectomy has in the past given satisfactory results, and can be considered in patients with portal hypertension due to sarcoidosis without serious hepatocellular dysfunction; in those with enlarged spleens and hypersplenism, splenectomy and splenorenal shunt may be the operation of choice. Transjugular intrahepatic porto-systemic shunt (TIPS) may also be considered. However, in some individuals with portal hypertension and end-stage chronic liver disease, orthotopic liver transplantation is both a safe and feasible treatment option (Kennedy *et al.* 2006).

Cholestasis

Chronic cholestasis is a rare manifestation of hepatic sarcoid and usually signals advanced disease with limited treatment options. Cases of sarcoidosis of the liver in which jaundice and/or liver failure were the main clinical presentation have been reported (Goeckerman 1928; Klatskin and Yesner 1950; Shay *et al.* 1951; Dagradi *et al.* 1952; Wagoner *et al.* 1953; Porter 1961; Nelson and Sears 1968; Bass *et al.* 1982). In such advanced disease, portal hypertension is often present, increasing further the risk of liver complications.

Chronic cholestasis can be intra- or extrahepatic, with intrahepatic disease resulting in a clinical and biochemical picture similar to that of primary biliary cirrhosis. Fox-worthy and Freeman (1952) reported briefly the case of a young black man with jaundice, hepatosplenomegaly, cuta-neous xanthomas, high serum lipids and granulomas in the liver and lymph nodes; all these features improved on treatment with ACTH and cortisone. Rudzki *et al.* (1975) reported on another small cohort of patients with advanced chronic cholestasis and biopsy-proven sarcoidosis. Portal hypertension was reported in this group with the develop-ment of ascites and bleeding esophageal varices, which resulted in death in one individual. A further three patients in this cohort died over the course of follow-up, as a consequence of complications relating to their sarcoid liver disease. Histologically, the livers showed granulomas, in-trahepatic cholestasis, diminishing numbers of interlobular bile ducts, periportal fibrosis leading to micronodular cirrhosis, and high copper levels in hepatocytes. Hepatotoxic drugs, environmental factors and other etiologies of liver disease including autoimmune liver disease were excluded in all cases. Typically, response to corticosteroid treatment was limited to temporary reduction in bilirubin levels and cholestatic enzymes and the relief of pruritus in one individual. In some instances it may be difficult to distinguish cholestatic sarcoidosis from primary biliary cirrhosis (Keeffe 1987).

DIFFERENTIAL DIAGNOSIS BETWEEN PRIMARY BILIARY CIRRHOSIS AND HEPATIC SARCOIDOSIS

Cases with features leading to combined diagnoses of sarcoidosis and primary biliary cirrhosis were reported by Holtzman (1961) and Karlish *et al.* (1969). Subsequent to this, hepatic sarcoidosis and chronic cholestasis with clinical and histological features resembling primary biliary cirrhosis were described in a number of reports (Rudzki *et al.* 1975; Bass *et al.* 1982; Nakanuma *et al.* 2001). Sarcoidosis was confirmed in patients prior to or after the onset of jaundice, based on the presence of granulomatous disease in two or more organs and the exclusion of other identifiable causes. Clinical manifestation of disease consisted of jaundice, pruritus, right upper quadrant pain and hepatosplenomegaly. Biopsy demonstrated classical non-caseating granulomas, a reduction in the number of interlobular bile ducts, evidence of epithelial damage, fibrous tissue linking the portal areas, chronic non-specific inflammatory infiltrate and chronic cholestasis (Blich and Edoute 2004). While corticosteroids led to improvement in jaundice in one patient, corticoster-oids had no effect on the progression of liver disease (Bass *et al.* 1982). In the same publication, Bass also describes a key differentiating feature of sarcoidosis: unlike with PBC, bile duct damage is less conspicuous, while granulomas are abundant and well-formed, which is the reverse of the histological finding in PBC.

DIFFERENTIAL DIAGNOSIS BETWEEN PRIMARY SCLEROSING CHOLANGITIS AND HEPATIC SARCOIDOSIS

Primary sclerosing cholangitis (PSC) is characterized by inflammation and progressive fibrosis of the intra- and extrahepatic biliary tree leading to chronic cholestatic liver disease (Lee and Kaplan 1995). Sarcoidosis has been reported in the literature to present with severe cholestasis and cholangiographic features of sclerosing cholangitis (Devaney *et al.* 1993; Alam *et al.* 1997; Manuel *et al.* 1998). However, the diagnosis of sarcoidosis was made in these reports on the basis of the presence of non-caseating granulomas in more than two organs or in one organ combined with classical respiratory symptoms. Clinical manifestations included jaundice, anorexia and abdominal pain. Biochemical para-meters demonstrated elevations in the alkaline phosphatase activity and serum neutrophil cytoplasmic antibodies (ANCA) were negative in all patients. Liver biopsy revealed focal portal and lobular non-caseating epithelioid cell granulomas surrounded by extensive fibrosis and bile duct proliferation with cholestasis.

While it has been reported that sarcoidosis can co-exist with PSC (Ilan *et al.* 1993), key features allow the two conditions to be differentiated. These include the absence of clinical evidence of inflammatory bowel disease; narrowing of the bile ducts being restricted to a specific site within the biliary tree; lack of histological features of PSC – such as concentric periductal fibrosis; absence of serum ANCA autoantibodies; normal IgM titers; and improvement with corticosteroid therapy. All support a diagnosis of sarcoidosis resembling sclerosing cholestasis and make a diagnosis of a fibrotic sclerosing process less likely.

EXTRAHEPATIC CHOLESTASIS

Obstructive jaundice secondary to sarcoid granuloma obstructing the common hepatic duct is extremely rare but has been reported (Bloom *et al.* 1978). This was reportedly due to narrowing of the common bile duct by granulomatous infiltration of its wall and a mass of surrounding granulomatous lymph nodes in a young black woman aged 29. She presented initially with bronchopulmonary and hilar lymph node sarcoidosis and 18 months later developed jaundice. Temporary biliary drainage by T-tube followed by corticosteroid therapy provided relief of her jaundice. Similar cases were reported in the literature subsequent to this report (Baughman 1998; Rezeig and Fashir 1997). However, the biochemical pattern was consistent across all cases with raised serum angiotensin-converting enzyme (ACE), elevated alkaline phosphatase activity, and elevated glutamic and hepatic transaminase levels. Autoantibodies were negative in all cases. Clinical manifestations included jaundice, pruritus, anorexia and abdominal pain. Axial imaging, where available, and ERCP confirmed narrowing of the common hepatic duct with intrahepatic biliary dilatation.

Intra-abdominal lymphadenopathy is common in sarcoidosis and, while it may involve nodes in the hepatic hilum or surrounding the extrahepatic biliary tree, obstructive complications are rarely observed (Becker and Coleman 1961). This is likely to be a consequence of the capsular surface of the node remaining intact, while obstructive symptoms appear to arise when the granuloma involves the biliary tract, resulting in narrowing of the common hepatic duct as described in the cases above.

Budd–Chiari syndrome

There are reported cases of hepatic venous thrombosis as a complication of sarcoidosis in the literature (Natalino *et al.* 1978; Russi *et al.* 1986), but this is considered a rare complication. In the reported cases, the diagnosis of sarcoidosis was made on the basis of the detection of granulomatous disease in two or more organs with no other identifiable cause. Both patients presented with ascites, jaundice and hepatosplenomegaly. Biochemical parameters demonstrated an elevated alkaline phosphatase activity. Granulomas were detected on liver biopsy and there was considerable dilatation and congestion of the centrilobular veins and paracentral sinusoids of the hepatic parenchyma. Scattered hepatocytes within these areas were reported to be undergoing early coagulative necrosis. The intrahepatic veins, both large and medium sized, were reportedly narrowed by granulomas or were occluded by thrombotic masses. One patient was treated with a mesocaval shunt and steroids

and the other patient responded to a combination of anticoagulation and steroids.

The development of Budd–Chiari syndrome in sarcoidosis is considered the result of extrinsic compression on hepatic veins by inflammation and edema from sarcoid granulomas with resultant narrowing of venous channels, venous stasis and subsequent thrombosis.

DIAGNOSIS OF LIVER DISEASE WITH GRANULOMATOUS FEATURES

Although some present diagnostic difficulties, most patients with granulomas in the liver undergo extensive investigations and the clinicopathologic features of the presentation allow a diagnosis to be reached in the majority of cases.

Iversen *et al.* (1970) reported on 2813 liver biopsies in a general hospital practice. They found 19 patients with epithelioid cell granulomas; the final diagnosis was sarcoidosis in six, miliary tuberculosis in one, acute hepatitis in three, cirrhosis in two, chronic alcoholism in three, fatty liver in one, hepatomegaly (with no further categorization) in one, fever of unknown origin in one, and malignancy in one. Two further patients with less well formed lipogranulomas were considered to have infectious mononucleosis and acute hepatitis. The authors emphasized that if epithelioid cell granulomas were present in an otherwise normal or near-normal liver, the most likely diagnosis was either sarcoidosis or tuberculosis. This conclusion remains unchanged today, but further consideration may need to be given to cases arising in areas of differing prevalence of infectious diseases prior to reaching a diagnosis, as discussed earlier. Referral bias and the general level of expertise of a specific unit investigating the cause of hepatic granulomas should also be considered.

The recognition of mycobacterial infection as the cause of a granulomatous hepatitis may be difficult if the liver is the only evidently involved organ. However, TB remains the most important infectious agent to be excluded as the cause for hepatic granulomas. Acid-fast bacilli are found only in very few cases, but the combination of now widely available PCR for *M. tuberculosis* DNA, in addition to Ziehl–Nielsen stain and culture, have markedly improved the diagnosis of TB. A therapeutic trial of antimycobacterial chemotherapy is now reserved for only a minority of patients where an unequivocal diagnosis cannot be reached.

Diagnostic problems of patients presenting with granulomatous hepatitis have been discussed by Klatskin (1977), Israel and Goldstein (1973) and Simon and Wolff (1973). Israel's team reported on 30 patients with granulomas on liver biopsy and normal chest radiographs. In 16 there was clinical and/or biopsy evidence of changes in other organs consistent with a diagnosis of sarcoidosis. Kveim tests (see Chapter 16) were performed in 15 of these, but only one was positive, indicating that this test has no value in excluding a diagnosis of sarcoidosis. Four patients improved spontaneously and ten improved on corticosteroid treatment; one died of an unrelated cause, and the outcome in one was unknown. Of the 14 patients with no evidence, direct or indirect, of granulomas in other organs, one was found at postmortem to have Hodgkin's disease, and the liver granulomas were thought to be a response to this. The remaining 13 cases in which there was no clear evidence of systemic disease or infection were left with no final diagnosis, beyond granulomatous hepatitis; seven recovered spontaneously, three after tetracycline given on an unsubstantiated suspicion of Q fever.

Simon and Wolff (1973) analyzed 13, among 200 patients investigated for prolonged fever, who were found to have granulomas on liver biopsy. Of these, one had had bilateral hilar lymph node enlargement, and in spite of some central necrosis in the granulomas was thought to have sarcoidosis. One responded to antimycobacterial chemotherapy, and in one the final diagnosis was Hodgkin's disease. In the remaining ten patients, the changes in the liver could not be associated with any systemic disease or causal factor.

Klatskin (1977), in his personal series of 5500 liver biopsies, described epithelial granulomata in 10 percent, the majority of which were patients with documented granulomatous disease. Granulomas were identified in 94 percent of patients with sarcoid, 43 percent with tuberculosis, and 76 percent with schistosomiasis. Brucellosis, berylliosis, temporal arteritis, visceral larval migrans and starch granuloma of peritoneum made up the rest. The morphological appearance in most of these disorders was essentially the same so that diagnosis was dependent on other clinical criteria. Only occasionally did acid-fast bacilli in tuberculosis, ova in schistosomiasis, larvae in visceral larva migrans or birefringent granules in starch granuloma enable the diagnosis to be made on histological grounds. Granulomas, associated with biopsy-documented liver disorders, were also seen in 4 percent of cases overall, with 40 percent in primary biliary cirrhosis and 3–12 percent in various forms of acute or chronic viral hepatitis.

It is evident that there are cases in which diagnostic categorization can be carried no further than granulomatous hepatitis, a category that should be regarded, at least initially, as provisional.

Gallbladder

Lloyd-Davies and Forbes (1965) reported the case of a man who, at the age of 21 years, presented with a history of vomiting and pain in the right hypochondrium. An adherent fibrotic gallbladder was removed; non-caseating granulomas of epithelioid cells and a few giant cells were present in the fibrotic wall and mucosa of the gallbladder and in the adherent liver. No other evidence of sarcoidosis was found, and a Kveim test was negative; but two years earlier, he was reported to have had had unexplained transient enlargement of the submandibular glands and a Mantoux test was negative. Although the evidence is incomplete, it seems likely that this was a case of sarcoidosis with disease localized to the gallbladder.

In cases of obstructive jaundice due to involvement of the common bile duct as reported by Bloom et al. (1978) and

discussed earlier, the gallbladder was removed and found to be infiltrated with sarcoid granulomas.

Ascites

The presence of ascites in sarcoidosis does not always imply hepatic disease. The most common etiology is right-sided heart failure as a consequence of pulmonary hypertension (Ebert and Nagar 2008). However, significant liver involvement leading to severe or end-stage disease – independent of lung or other organ involvement – is likely to cause portal hypertension with resultant ascites (Blich and Edoute 2004). In these cases the ascites is typically a transudate and is managed symptomatically. In some cases, however, ascites can be diuretic-resistant and, in the most challenging cases, all options must be considered including orthotopic liver transplantation for end-stage liver disease (Kennedy et al 2006).

Sarcoidosis can also be associated with an exudate and there are reports in the literature of the development of chylous ascites (Provenza and Bacon 1991). In this case, ascites was considered to have developed secondary to the complete replacement of the mesenteric and para-aortic lymph nodes with non-caseating granulomas. A further report by Cappell et al. (1993) documented chyloperitoneum; this was believed to be a consequence of intrathoracic nodal fibrosis and lymphatic obstruction, or alternatively, studding of the peritoneum with nodules.

TREATMENT OF HEPATIC SARCOID

Almost all patients with sarcoid will have evidence of liver involvement, yet the majority will have very mild disease. The use of corticosteroids should be limited to cases where there is significant cholestatic injury and when there are constitutional symptoms, where the criteria for treatment are more clearly related to non-hepatic involvement. Ursodeoxycholic acid therapy (15 mg/kg daily) is also recommended in such cases (Iannuzzi et al. 2007). Fewer than 1 percent of liver transplants are performed in patients with sarcoidosis.

REFERENCES

Agate JN (1948). Delayed pneumonitis in a beryllium worker. *Lancet* ii: 530.

Alam I, Levenson SD, Ferrell LD, Bass NM (1997). Diffuse intrahepatic biliary strictures in sarcoidosis resembling sclerosing cholangitis: case report and review of the literature. *Dig Dis Sci* 42: 1295–301.

Bagley CM, Roth JA, Thomas LB et al. (1972). Liver biopsy in Hodgkin's disease: clinicopathologic correlations in 127 patients. *Ann Intern Med* 76: 219–22.

Bass NM, Burroughs AK, Scheuer PJ et al. (1982). Chronic intrahepatic cholestasis due to sarcoidosis. *Gut* 23: 417–21.

Baughman RP (1998). Can tuberculosis cause sarcoidosis? [editorial]. *Chest* 114: 363–4.

Becker WF, Coleman WO (1961). Surgical significance of abdominal sarcoidosis. *Ann Surg* 153: 987–95.

Berger I, Katz M (1973). Portal hypertension due to hepatic sarcoidosis. *Am J Gastroenterol* **59**: 147–51.

Bhardwaj SS, Saxena R, Kwo PY (2009). Granulomatous liver disease. *Curr Gastroenterol Rep* **11**: 42–9.

Blich M, Edoute Y (2004). Clinical manifestations of sarcoid liver disease. *J Gastroenterol Hepatol* **19**: 732–7.

Bloom R, Sybert A, Mascatello VJ (1978). Granulomatous biliary tract obstruction due to sarcoidosis: report of a case and review of the literature. *Am Rev Respir Dis* **117**: 783–7.

Cappell MS, Friedman D, Mikhail N (1993). Chyloperitoneum associated with chronic severe sarcoidosis. *Am J Gastroenterol* **88**: 99–101.

Cheitlin MD, Sullivan BH, Myers JE, Hench RF (1960). Portal hypertension in hepatic sarcoidosis. *Gastroenterology* **38**: 60–9.

Dagradi AE, Sollod N, Friedlander JH (1952). Sarcoidosis with marked hepatosplenomegaly and jaundice: a case report with biopsy findings. *Ann Intern Med* **36**: 1317–23.

Devaney K, Goodman ZD, Epstein MS et al. (1993). Hepatic sarcoidosis: clinicopathologic features in 100 patients. *Am J Surg Pathol* **17**: 1272–80.

Ebert EC, Nagar M (2008). Gastrointestinal manifestations of amyloidosis. *Am J Gastroenterol* **103**: 776–87.

Foxworthy DT, Freeman S (1952). Biliary cirrhosis with cutaneous xanthomatosis due to sarcoidosis: treatment with low cholesterol diet, ACTH and cortisone. *J Lab Clin Med* **40**: 799.

Goeckerman WH (1928). Sarcoids and related lesions: report of 17 cases; review of recent literature. *Arch Derm Syphilol* **18**: 237–62.

Guglielmi V, Manghisi OG, Pirrelli M, Caruso ML (1994). Granulomatous hepatitis in a hospital population in southern Italy. *Pathologica* **86**: 271–8.

Hardy HL (1951). The toxicity of beryllium. *Lancet* **258**: 448.

Holtzman IN (1961). Sarcoidosis followed by biliary cirrhosis and xanthomatosis. *NY State J Med* **61**: 1757–64.

Iannuzzi MC, Rybicki BA, Teirstein AS (2007). Sarcoidosis. *New Engl J Med* **357**: 2153–65.

Ilan Y, Rappaport I, Feigin R, Ben-Chetrit E (1993). Primary sclerosing cholangitis in sarcoidosis. *J Clin Gastroenterol* **16**: 326–8.

Inoue Y, King TE, Tinkle SS (1996). Human mast cell basic fibroblast growth factor in pulmonary fibrotic disorders. *Am J Pathol* **149**: 2037–54.

Israel HL, Goldstein RA (1973). Hepatic granulomatosis and sarcoidosis. *Ann Intern Med* **79**: 669–78.

Iversen K, Christoffersen P, Poulsen H (1970). Epithelioid cell granulomas in liver biopsies. *Scand J Gastroenterol Suppl* **7**: 61–7.

Karlish AJ, Thompson RP, Williams R (1969). A case of sarcoidosis and primary biliary cirrhosis. *Lancet* **2**: 599.

Keeffe EB (1987). Sarcoidosis and primary biliary cirrhosis: literature review and illustrative case. *Am J Med* **83**: 977–80.

Kennedy PT, Zakaria N, Modawi SB et al. (2006). Natural history of hepatic sarcoidosis and its response to treatment. *Eur J Gastroenterol Hepatol* **18**: 721–6.

Klatskin G (1976). Hepatic granulomata: problems in interpretation. *Ann NY Acad Sci* **278**: 427–32.

Klatskin G (1977). Hepatic granulomata: problems in interpretation. *Mt Sinai J Med* **44**: 798–812.

Klatskin G, Yesner R (1950). Hepatic manifestations of sarcoidosis and other granulomatous diseases; a study based on histological examination of tissue obtained by needle biopsy of the liver. *Yale J Biol Med* **23**: 207–48.

Lee Y-M, Kaplan MM (1995). Primary sclerosing cholangitis. *New Engl J Med* **332**: 924–933.

Lehmuskallio E, Hannuksela M, Halme H (1977). The liver in sarcoidosis. *Acta Med Scand* **202**: 289–93.

Lloyd-Davies RW, Forbes GB (1965). Sarcoidosis of the gall bladder. *Gastroenterology* **49**: 287–90.

Maddrey WC, Johns CJ, Boitnott JK et al. (1970). Sarcoidosis and chronic hepatic disease: a clinical and pathologic study of 20 patients. *Medicine* **49**: 375–95.

Manuel RG, Emilio SG, Angeles OM et al. (1998). Sarcoidosis sclerosing cholangitis and chronic atrophic autoimmune gastritis: a case of infiltrative sclerosing cholangitis. *J Clin Gastroenterol* **27**: 162–5.

Mather G, Dawson J, Hoyle C (1955). *Q J Med* **48**: 331.

Mayock RL, Bertrand P, Morrison CE, Scot JH (1963). Manifestations of sarcoidosis: analysis of 145 patients, with a review of nine series selected from the literature. *Am J Med* **35**: 67–89.

McCluggage WG, Sloan JM (1994). Hepatic granulomas in Northern Ireland: a thirteen year review. *Histopathology* **25**: 219–28.

Mino RA, Frelick RW et al. (1948). Severe systemic sarcoidosis with ascites and splenomegaly. *Del Med J* **20**(4): 65–75.

Mistilis SP, Schiff L (1964). Steroid therapy in chronic hepatitis. *Arch Intern Med* **113**: 54–62.

Moreno-Merlo F, Wanless IR, Shimamatsu K et al. (1997). The role of granulomatous phlebitis and thrombosis in the pathogenesis of cirrhosis and portal hypertension in sarcoidosis. *Hepatology* **26**: 554–60.

Murphy JR, Sjögren MH, Kikendall JW et al. (1990). Small bile duct abnormalities in sarcoidosis. *J Clin Gastroenterol* **12**: 555–61.

Nakanuma Y, Tsuneyama K, Harada K (2001). Pathology and pathogenesis of intrahepatic bile duct loss. *J Hepato Pancreat Surg* **8**: 303–15.

Natalino MR, Goyette RE, Owensby LC, Rubin RN (1978). The Budd–Chiari syndrome in sarcoidosis. *J Am Med Assoc* **239**: 2657–8.

Nelson RS, Sears ME (1968). Massive sarcoidosis of the liver: report of two cases. *Am J Dig Dis* **13**: 95–106.

Nelson S, Schwabe AD (1966). Progressive hepatic decompensation with terminal hepatic coma in sarcoidosis: report of a case. *Am J Dig Dis* **11**: 495–501.

Newman LS, Rose CS, Maier LA (1997). Sarcoidosis. *New Engl J Med* **336**: 1224–34.

Ozaras R, Tahan V, Mert A, Uraz S (2004). The prevalence of hepatic granulomas in chronic hepatitis C. *J Clin Gastroenterol* **38**: 449–52.

Porter GH (1961). Hepatic sarcoidosis: a cause of portal hypertension and liver failure; review. *Arch Intern Med* **108**: 483–95.

Provenza JM, Bacon BR (1991). Chylous ascites due to sarcoidosis. *Am J Gastroenterol* **86**: 92–5.

Rezeig MA, Fashir BM (1997). Biliary tract obstruction due to sarcoidosis: a case report. *Am J Gastroenterol* **92**: 527–8.

Rudzki C, Ishak KG, Zimmerman HJ (1975). Chronic intrahepatic cholestasis of sarcoidosis. *Am J Med* **59**: 373–87.

Russi EW, Bansky G, Pfaltz M et al. (1986). Budd–Chiari syndrome in sarcoidosis. *Am J Gastroenterol* **81**: 71–5.

Sartin JS, Walker RC (1991). Granulomatous hepatitis: a retrospective review of 88 cases at the Mayo Clinic. *Mayo Clin Proc* **66**: 914–18.

Satti MB, Hussein AF, Ibrahim J et al. (1990). Hepatic granuloma in Saudi Arabia: a clinicopathological study of 59 cases. *Am J Gastroenterol* **85**: 669–74.

Shay H, Berk JE, Sones M et al. (1951). The liver in sarcoidosis. *Gastroenterology* **19**: 441–61.

Simon HB, Wolff SM (1973). Granulomatous hepatitis and prolonged fever of unknown origin: a study of 13 patients. *Medicine* **52**: 1–21.

Tsuda T, Kita S (1994). Histochemical study of sarcoid granulomatous lesions. *Nippon Rinsho* **52**: 1456–61.

Valla D, Pessegueiro-Miranda H, Degott C et al. (1987). Hepatic sarcoidosis with portal hypertension: a report of seven cases with a review of the literature. *Q J Med* **63**: 531–44.

Van Beek C, Haex AJC (1943). *Ned Tijdschr Geneesk* **87**: 1264.

Van Buchem FSP (1946). *Acta Med Scand* **124**: 168.

Vilaseca J, Guardia J, Cuxart A *et al.* (1979). Granulomatous hepatitis: etiologic study of 107 cases. *Med Clin (Barcelona)* **72**: 272–5.

Vilinskas J, Joyeuse R, Serlin O (1970). Hepatic sarcoidosis with portal hypertension. *Am J Surg* **120**: 393–6.

Wagoner G, Freiman DG, Schiff L (1953). An unusual case of jaundice in a patient with sarcoidosis. *Gastroenterology* **25**: 574–81.

Wainwright H (2007). Hepatic granulomas. *Eur J Gastroenterol Hepatol* **19**: 93–5.

Wanless IR, Geddie WR (1985). Mineral oil lipogranulomata in liver and spleen. *Arch Pathol Lab Med* **109**: 283–6.

25

The gastrointestinal tract

AMEET DHAR, NISHA PATEL AND PRIYAJIT BOBBY PRASAD

INTRODUCTION

Autopsy studies of sarcoid patients have demonstrated that scattered granulomas in the gastrointestinal (GI) tract are not an unusual finding. Conversely, symptomatic sarcoidosis in the GI tract is rare and occurs in fewer than 1 percent of cases (Tinker *et al.* 1984; Sprague *et al.* 1984; Chinitz *et al.* 1985; Morretti *et al.* 1993; Fireman *et al.* 1997). The diagnosis of gastrointestinal sarcoid can be difficult to make, even in patients with pre-existing sarcoidosis, and it can be initially mistaken for malignancy. Case reports provide the bulk of the evidence.

ETIOLOGY AND PATHOGENESIS

The etiology of sarcoidosis is unknown. There are a number of potential etiological factors including occupational, genetic and environmental risk factors. A wide variety of potential antigens have been hypothesized as the trigger, such as pollen, wood smoke, exposure to animals and pets, plants, soil and exposure to wood milling and lumbering.

After beryllium exposure was found to be the cause of 'Salem sarcoid' in the 1940s, several studies have explored the possibility of an occupational risk factor. Exposure to fumes, dusts and metals have been found to cause similar granulomatous disease of the lung that prove difficult to differentiate from sarcoidosis. None of these potential risk factors has been found to cause sarcoidosis of the large bowel, pancreas, spleen or peritoneum specifically.

Familial clustering of the disease in the USA, Japan and Ireland suggests polygenic inheritance. Class I HLA-A1 and -B8 and class II HLA-DR3 are common genotypes found in patients. This genetic predisposition to the disease is likely to trigger an immune reaction when a provoking antigen is presented, resulting in granulomatous disease (Powell *et al.* 2005; Gajbhiye *et al.* 2008; Iyer *et al.* 2008). Approximately 40 percent of patients with GI tract sarcoidosis have been shown to have subtle changes in their GI immune responses, the significance of which is unknown (McCormick *et al.* 1988a; Papadopoulous *et al.* 1999). Elevated T-helper cell type 1 (Th1) immune response reactions and a depressed cutaneous delayed-type hypersensitivity reaction have been observed at the site of active disease. Circulating immune complexes and hyperactivity of B-cells may also be seen. The ratio of CD4+ to CD8 cells in the blood is reduced while the reverse is found in active tissues. A higher level of activated CD4+ cells in infiltrated tissue leads to the release of cytokines and other factors that result in an influx of monocytes, causing granuloma formation and fibrosis. It has been suggested that monocytes that circulate have a granulomagenic factor prior to differentiation into an organ-specific macrophage, explaining the multisystem distribution of disease. Autoimmunity may also play a role as there have been case reports of sarcoidosis in conjunction with rheumatoid arthritis, celiac disease, scleroderma and endometriosis in which autoimmunity may play a developmental role (Gajbhiye *et al.* 2008).

HISTOLOGY

Characteristic histology includes multiple non-caseating granulomas containing epithelioid cells, multinucleated giant cells and lymphocytes. In pancreatic disease, inter- and intralobular fibrosis surrounding the granulomas may be detected both in the tissue and in peri-pancreatic lymph nodes. Splenic sarcoid histology shares similar basic features: hyalinization around splenic granuloma frequently begins at the periphery and progresses to the center of the granuloma. A diffuse lymphoreticular histocytosis preceding granuloma formation has been reported although this has not been widely described (Takahasi *et al.* 1970). Large areas composed of intertwined eosinophilic material that stain brightly with Masson's trichrome stain have been described in splenic disease. This is not a feature that has been found readily in other organs infiltrated with sarcoid (Papowitz and Li 1971). In peritoneal disease, granulomas are usually surrounded by a lattice of stromal tissue containing plasma cells, lymphocytes and eosinophils.

Sarcoidosis infiltrating the large bowel can be differentiated from Crohn's disease histologically by the presence of prominent intramucosal granulomas (rather than sparse submucosal granulomas found in the latter), Schaumann bodies (intracellular concentric calcifications), and a lack of fistulas. Granulomas are surrounded by fibroblasts, lymphocytes and plasma cells with little crypt abscess formation. Vacuoles and asteroid bodies may be demonstrated in giant cells and nuclei are randomly distributed throughout the cytoplasm, unlike tuberculous giant cells.

As seen occasionally in gastric sarcoidosis, histological evidence of sarcoidosis in the colon has been found in grossly normal mucosa (Tobi *et al.* 1982; Sprague *et al.* 1984). Gallbladder neck and biliary duct specimens usually retrieved at surgery show non-caseating epithelioid granulomas with multinucleated giant cells causing stenosis of the duct and nodularity of the gallbladder mucosa.

LABORATORY TESTS

Angiotensin-converting enzyme (ACE) is synthesized in epithelioid cells and macrophages of sarcoid granulomas by ACE-inducing factor. It is elevated in 60–90 percent of patients with active sarcoidosis, although a normal serum ACE does not exclude the diagnosis, particularly if the disease is in its early stages or localized to a small area. Elevated levels of serum ACE are not specific to sarcoidosis: it is not a diagnostic serum test. It is normally present in macrophages and the vascular endothelium of a number of organs including the lungs, small bowel, adrenals, kidneys, thyroid and prostate. Other conditions associated with elevated serum ACE levels include tuberculosis, diabetes mellitus, histoplasmosis, rheumatoid arthritis, Gaucher's disease, hyperthyroidism and primary biliary cirrhosis. Patients who have had chemotherapy, radiotherapy or who are taking prescribed ACE inhibitors may have falsely low serum ACE levels and it cannot be reliably used in some patients with ACE gene polymorphisms. Chronically elevated levels of amylase and lipase may also be seen in patients with pancreatic sarcoid infiltration.

Hypercalcemia has been reported in 10–15 percent of patients with sarcoidosis. 1,25-Dihydroxyvitamin D3 (calcitriol) is produced at sites of active disease by macrophages and possibly T-lymphocytes. Elevated serum levels of calcitriol in patients with sarcoidosis leads to increased absorption of calcium and phosphate from the GI tract, resulting in hypercalcemia and hypercalciuria. Hypercalcemia may be present in cases of splenic, hepatic and bone marrow infiltration (the abdominal 'triad').

Raised levels of serum lysozyme have been reported in patients with sarcoidosis. Lysozyme is an enzyme normally secreted by monocytes and polymorphonuclear leukocytes, but it is thought epithelioid histiocytes which comprise sarcoid granulomas are the source for both lysozyme and ACE. Raised lysozyme levels have been reported in parallel to raised serum ACE levels and hence may relate to disease activity.

Patients with hepatosplenomegaly, acute, chronic or subacute cholecystitis may have elevated transaminase levels, a cholestatic picture, or a combination of both.

Elevated serum levels of cancer antigen 125 (CA125) produced by mesothelial cells have been described in peritoneal granulomatous disease. This is not a specific test: elevated levels are found in peritoneal inflammation, although malignant disease needs to be excluded with subsequent peritoneal biopsy (Fuchs *et al.* 2007).

THE ESOPHAGUS

Sarcoidosis involving the esophagus is uncommon. It was first described as a case over 50 years ago, with sporadic case reports since (Lukens *et al.* 2002) and no large case series. In individual case reports, it has become apparent that sarcoidosis may affect both the proximal and distal esophagus, with symptoms proportional to the area affected.

CLASSIFICATION

Vahid *et al.* (2007) have suggested that esophageal sarcoid can be classed as four distinct subgroups based on pathological involvement:

- *superficial mucosal involvement*, which can present as discrete plaque-like lesions 3–10 mm in size, or as mucosal erythema and nodularity (Levine *et al.* 1989; Lukens *et al.* 2002);
- *myopathic involvement*, caused by a granulomatous myositis involving the skeletal muscle portion of esophagus and posterior pharynx (Siegal *et al.* 1961);
- *extrinsic esophageal compression* from mediastinal lymphadenopathy (Hardy *et al.* 1967; Cook *et al.* 1970; Cappell 1995);
- *direct infiltration of the distal esophagus* by granulomatous inflammation with direct involvement of enteric nervous system, which can result in esophageal dysfunction mimicking an achalasia-like condition (Polachek *et al.* 1964; Weisner *et al.* 1971; Dufrense *et al.* 1983; Aronson *et al.* 1985; Nidiry *et al.* 1991; Boruchowicz *et al.* 1996).

CLINICAL SYMPTOMS

Esophageal dysmotility often gives rise to dysphagia, with ensuing weight loss. Dysmotility has been attributed to neuropathy and myopathy, as well as extrinsic compression (Ebert *et al.* 2008). Infiltration of the wall of the esophagus, secondary to granulomas, can result in complications including stricturing and ulceration (Ebert *et al.* 2008), which can present also as dysphagia and pain.

INVESTIGATIONS

Imaging techniques including contrast swallow and CT scanning can demonstrate stricturing, esophageal dilatation and mediastinal lymphadenopathy (Cappell 1995; Lukens *et al.* 2002). Esophageal manometry can show an abnormal lower sphincter pressure with absent relaxation of the lower esophageal sphincter on swallowing, and diminished peristalsis (Dufrense *et al.* 1983; Aronson *et al.* 1985; Nidiry *et al.* 1991; Boruchowicz *et al.* 1996). Endoscopic evaluation and mucosal biopsy also have an important role in establishing the diagnosis.

TREATMENT

Treatment of esophageal sarcoidosis is similar to other sites of involvement and needs to be guided by the patient's overall symptomatology. In practice, acid suppression has initially already been prescribed. First-line therapy where appropriate can involve the use of corticosteroids and has been reported to be successful. In particular, infiltration of the lower esophagus has been reported to be very responsive to steroid treatment (Hardy *et al.* 1967; Cook *et al.* 1970; Cappell 1995). If the proximal esophagus or cricopharyngeus are involved, surgery such as myotomy may sometimes be required (Siegel *et al.* 1961).

THE STOMACH

Gastric sarcoidosis was first described over 80 years ago and is the most common GI manifestation of sarcoidosis (Chinitz *et al.* 1985). Up to 10 percent of pulmonary sarcoid patients have gastric granulomas, but the vast majority of these will not exhibit gastric symptoms and they are often found incidentally. The antrum is most commonly involved, and in some variants endoscopic appearances can resemble gastric carcinoma.

CLASSIFICATION

Four different types of gastric sarcoid have been described (Vahid *et al.* 2007).

Subclinical gastric sarcoidosis

Gastric sarcoid is often diagnosed incidentally. Endoscopic evaluation can be normal, or demonstrate a patchy erythematous or nodular gastritis, with non-caseating granulomas seen on gastric mucosal biopsy. Atrophic gastritis has also been described. This type of presentation often follows a benign course, and rarely develops extra-GI manifestations of sarcoidosis (Palmer 1958).

Ulcerative gastric sarcoidosis

Gastric ulceration can result following granulomatous infiltration. Any part of the stomach can be involved, but most commonly sarcoid-related ulceration occurs in the gastric antrum, pylorus and lesser curvature of the stomach (Kremer and William 1970; Panella *et al.* 1998). In keeping with any form of ulceration, it can present as epigastric pain or upper GI bleeding (Ona 1981). Pyloric ulceration can additionally result in gastric outflow obstruction. Endoscopically these ulcers can be confused with gastric malignancy, and hence biopsy and follow-up endoscopy to ensure healing are vital in confirming the diagnosis, confirming the presence of non-caseating granulomas and the absence of neoplasia (Levine *et al.* 1989).

Infiltrative gastric sarcoidosis

Infiltrative gastric sarcoidosis can be localized or diffuse (Vahid *et al.* 2007). Localized gastric infiltration occurs more frequently in the distal stomach and can result in a smooth narrowing (Konda *et al.* 1980; Levine *et al.* 1989; Kaneki *et al.* 2001). It arises as a result of granulomatous infiltration of the muscle layers of the stomach (Konda *et al.* 1980; Chinitz *et al.* 1985; Panella *et al.* 1988) and hence can result in reduced peristalsis and gastroparesis (Farman *et al.* 1997). Diffuse infiltration endoscopically may look similar to segmental linitis plastica, and indeed cases have been reported following gastric resection for presumed gastric carcinoma (Apell 1951; Newton *et al.* 1998). Mucosal biopsies are usually required to differentiate between the two. If granulomatous infiltration is confined to the submucosa and deeper layers of the stomach, superficial biopsies may miss the diagnosis of gastric sarcoidosis, and endoscopic ultrasound should be considered (Levine *et al.* 1989), which can also be of value in evaluating and obtaining a tissue diagnosis of perigastric and celiac lymphadenopathy (Liang *et al.* 2010).

Polypoid gastric sarcoidosis

Polypoidal lesions secondary to sarcoid are the least common form of gastric sarcoid. Case reports have described patients with multiple gastric polypoid lesions secondary to sarcoidosis (Panella *et al.* 1998; Kaneki *et al.* 2001; Liang *et al.* 2010). This form may be a precursor for a form of diffuse infiltrative gastric sarcoidosis (Kaneki *et al.* 2001).

CLINICAL SYMPTOMS

Symptoms relate to both the anatomical distribution of gastric involvement and the severity of granulomatous inflammation (Ebert *et al.* 2008). Common symptoms include epigastric pain, which is often post-prandial, and symptoms relating to gastric outflow obstruction, such as nausea, vomiting and bloating. Gastric outflow tract obstruction can arise from either ulceration or direct infiltration of the gastric mucosa in the region of the gastric antrum or pylorus. Both result in fibrotic scarring and subsequent limitation of gastric emptying. Extrinsic compression to the lower stomach caused by localized lymphadenopathy can result in a similar scenario.

Sarcoid-related gastric ulceration should be considered when upper GI bleeding occurs in sarcoid patients, and can be life-threatening (Fung *et al.* 1975; Ona 1981; Ebert *et al.* 2008). Indeed, up to a quarter of cases of symptomatic gastric sarcoid can present with upper GI bleeding (Ona 1981). Weight loss can occur and may be profound (Adler *et al.* 2007). A single case report has reported gastrointestinal functional symptoms secondary to sarcoidosis, with the authors suggesting that sarcoidosis may be a rare differential for irritable bowel syndrome (Leeds *et al.* 2006).

INVESTIGATIONS

Endoscopic evaluation is the mainstay of establishing a diagnosis of gastric sarcoidosis, and should be considered in any patient with pre-existing sarcoidosis and upper GI symptoms. Mucosal biopsies complement endoscopy by demonstrating non-caseating granulomas, and confirm the diagnosis. Gastric aspirates can demonstrate elevated ACE levels, but are rarely used in clinical practice (Okamura *et al.* 1991). Endoscopic ultrasound and radiological investigations have a role in excluding neoplastic disease, especially when diffuse infiltrative disease is mistaken for a gastric carcinoma. Pernicious-type anemia has been described with positive anti-parietal cell antibodies (Romero-Gomez *et al.* 1998), as well as elevated gastrin levels and antibodies against H^+/K^+ ATPase pump in up to 25 percent of patients (Papadopoulos *et al.* 1999).

TREATMENT

Acid suppression may often have been initiated prior to referral. Corticosteroid treatment is the mainstay of treatment of symptomatic gastric sarcoid. Despite no randomized controlled trials, it is well documented that corticosteroid therapy can produce a significant response in symptomatic disease (Siegel *et al.* 1961; Vahid *et al.* 2007). The length of treatment is related to the clinical response; if steroids are stopped prematurely symptoms often reoccur. In refractory cases methotrexate, chlorambucil, azathioprine, infliximab and ciclosporin have all be tried in isolated cases (Vahid *et al.* 2007). Surgery is indicated if there is refractory gastric outflow tract obstruction or massive GI hemorrhage which cannot be controlled by endoscopic measures.

THE SMALL INTESTINE

Sarcoidosis of the small bowel is the least common form of GI sarcoidosis (Ebert *et al.* 2008). It was first described over 30 years ago (Miyamoto *et al.* 1972). It mainly occurs in partnership with disseminated GI sarcoidosis, but isolated small bowel involvement has been described (Douglas *et al.* 1984; Sprague *et al.* 1984; Bulger *et al.* 1988).

CLINICAL MANIFESTATIONS

Presentation with diarrhea, malabsorption, protein-losing enteropathy, periumbilical or epigastric pain, and hemorrhage has been reported (Fleming *et al.* 1994; MacRury *et al.* 1992). There may be associated folate deficiency, vitamin B_{12} malabsorption with terminal ileal disease or achlorhydria (Sprague *et al.* 1984; Tinker *et al.* 1984).

An association between sarcoidosis and celiac disease has been found (Douglas *et al.* 1984). A higher prevalence of celiac disease in sarcoidosis patients has been noted (Rutherford *et al.* 2004). Antigliadin antibodies have been detected in 15–41 percent of patients with sarcoidosis, of which 1–4 percent are positive for endomysial antibodies (McCormick *et al.* 1988a; Papadopoulos *et al.* 1999). Screening of sarcoid patients for celiac disease has been recommended in some countries (Rutherford *et al.* 2004). Tissue transglutaminase antibodies are increasingly used as part of the serological testing for celiac disease. Sarcoidosis of the distal small intestine can mimic Crohn's disease, with stricturing. The two different pathologies may be differentiated by a raised ACE level and less prominent inflammatory infiltrates on histology in sarcoidosis. Small bowel intestinal obstruction from external compression by lymphadenopathy may also occur.

INVESTIGATIONS

Small bowel enteroscopy with mucosal biopsies is the investigation of choice. Crohn's disease, Whipple's disease, intestinal tuberculosis and fungal infections may also result in similar histological changes to small bowel sarcoidosis, hence clinical evidence of other sarcoid activity will aid with establishing a diagnosis, and should be actively sought.

TREATMENT

Steroids are the mainstay in keeping with other forms of gastrointestinal sarcoid. The anti-TNF-α antibody infliximab has been reported to be efficacious in steroid-resistant cases of small bowel sarcoidosis (Yee *et al.* 2001).

THE PANCREAS

Nickerson and associates reported the first case of pancreatic sarcoid tubercles in 1937. Primary pancreatic sarcoidosis is limited to individual reports and small case series. Most cases are asymptomatic and are discovered on autopsy. A Japanese autopsy case series over a period of 28 years reported a 2.1 percent incidence of pancreatic involvement of sarcoidosis in patients with systemic disease, although a number of autopsy studies report a 1–5 percent prevalence of pancreatic involvement with sarcoid in patients with systemic disease (Longcope and Freiman 1952; Mayock *et al.* 1963; Iwai *et al.* 1988; McCormick *et al.* 1998b; Romboli *et al.* 2004).

CLINICAL MANIFESTATIONS

Symptomatic patients often complain of general symptoms such as fatigue, weight loss, myalgia and fever. Organ-specific symptoms often relate to infiltration of pancreatic tissue and pancreatic masses masquerading as pancreatic malignancy. More than half of these are reported in the head of the pancreas resulting in abdominal pain, obstructive jaundice, weight loss and vomiting. Presentations with acute pancreatitis, pancreatic insufficiency and biliary obstruction have been described. Approximately 75 percent of patients with pancreatic sarcoidosis have also been found to have bilateral hilar lymphadenopathy.

INVESTIGATIONS

Computerized tomography (CT) scan is an important diagnostic modality and can demonstrate a diffusely nodular pancreas with abnormal signal pattern, hypodense lesions or a soft tissue mass usually in the head of the pancreas. Biliary obstruction mimicking a pancreatic malignancy or pancreatitis is not uncommon. An autoimmune cholangiopancreatitis can also mimic a pancreatic malignancy. CT-guided pancreatic biopsy can be used to obtain pancreatic tissue. Magnetic resonance imaging (MRI) can be useful to further determine infiltration to surrounding tissues, lymphadenopathy, vascular invasion and exclusion of malignancy. Features suggestive of sarcoid-related disease include masses with low T1-weighted signal intensity and mild high T2-weighted signal intensity with reduced gadolinium enhancement. Magnetic resonance cholangiopancreatography (MRCP) may be carried out if a patient presents with biliary obstruction and may be useful in determining biliary or pancreatic duct filling defects and stenosis. Endoscopic ultrasound can be used to identify smaller pancreatic lesions, and further define extent of involvement, and is often used with fine-needle aspiration (FNA) or Tru-Cut biopsy to obtain tissue for histology.

Histology is mandatory, given the high clinical index of suspicion for pancreatic cancer in most patients (based on clinical symptoms and radiology which are not specific to sarcoidosis). Endoscopic retrograde cholangiopancreatography (ERCP) with biliary and pancreatic duct brushings for diagnosis and stent therapy may be necessary to relieve biliary obstruction.

TREATMENT

Pharmacotherapy with corticosteroids forms the basis of treatment. There are no established guidelines for the treatment of pancreatic involvement with sarcoidosis. The duration of treatment usually depends on the severity of the disease and symptomatology. Recurrence in severe symptomatic cases after discontinuation of steroids has been reported. Long-term steroids are often required mainly to relieve symptoms such as abdominal pain, although these are often discontinued due to multiple side-effects.

In general there is a good prognosis in patients with mild pancreatic involvement with high spontaneous remission rates. Surgery is confined to cases in which a firm diagnosis cannot be made and malignancy needs to be excluded. A pylorus-preserving partial pancreaticoduodenectomy may be indicated in masses of the head of the pancreas.

THE SPLEEN

Primary splenic sarcoidosis is rare and accompanies systemic disease, often in association with granulomatous hepatic inflammation.

CLINICAL MANIFESTATIONS

Splenomegaly may cause abdominal pain and laboratory abnormalities such as anemia, leukopenia and thrombocytopenia. Fifteen percent of patients with splenic sarcoid are symptomatic and 20 percent are hypersplenic, often with gross splenomegaly. The spleen is palpable in 5–14 percent of patients with systemic disease and is related to extrathoracic involvement and serum ACE levels. It may occur as part of the 'abdominal triad' with bone marrow and hepatosplenic infiltration.

INVESTIGATIONS

Discrete low-attenuation splenic nodules, homogeneous splenomegaly and calcification may be seen on CT, MRI, positron emission tomography (PET) and occasionally ultrasound scan. Hypodense nodules seen on dynamic CT may coalesce as they increase in size, resulting in a speckled appearance of the spleen due to multiple lacunae. T2-weighted fat-suppressed MRI provides valuable radiological evidence of disease, including abnormal splenic signal patterns, irregular organ contour and nodularity. A definitive diagnosis is reached by splenic biopsy using either CT or US guidance, or at surgery with a diagnostic laparoscopy or splenectomy.

TREATMENT

Splenomegaly does not usually require treatment unless symptomatic or at risk of splenic rupture, in which case splenectomy is indicated.

Corticosteroids can be used to treat splenic sarcoid. Methotrexate and antimalarials have also been used. Rebound splenomegaly has been reported if steroids are stopped prematurely. In patients with isolated splenic sarcoid, long-term follow-up is required to monitor for systemic disease.

THE PERITONEUM

One of the earliest reports of peritoneal sarcoidosis was by Robinson and Ernst (1954). To date, approximately 20 cases have been reported in the UK literature. Serosal sarcoidosis has rarely been described. Peritoneal sarcoidosis is a rare manifestation of the disease in isolation, usually occurring as part of systemic disease.

CLINICAL MANIFESTATIONS

Ascites and abdominal pain are the most common symptoms and intractable hiccups and intraperitoneal masses have also been described (Hackworth et al. 2009). Ascites commonly results as a consequence of hepatic infiltration, biliary cirrhosis and ensuing portal hypertension. Sclerosing peritonitis has also been described in conjunction with exudative ascites (Ngo *et al.* 2009). Transudative ascites may also develop as a result of myocardial infiltration leading to pulmonary hypertension and right-sided heart failure. Intraperitoneal masses causing extrinsic compression of bowel have been reported and have to be differentiated from malignancies such as ovarian cancer (Brown *et al.* 2010).

INVESTIGATIONS

CT is an excellent imaging modality to investigate and detect peritoneal disease. The findings are non-specific and hence further histology, in combination with clinical and radiological findings, are required for the diagnosis. Findings on CT often simulate tuberculous disease especially if there is pulmonary disease. Abdominal fluid collections, a nodular peritoneum, soft tissue masses mimicking malignancies or secondary spread may be seen. If peritoneal disease is part of systemic disease, in the abdomen there may be thickening of bowel wall, encasement of abdominal vessels with a soft tissue mass or hepatosplenic disease. The diagnosis may be suggested clinically, radiologically or at surgery in the presence of established disease. A histological specimen should be obtained to differentiate from malignancy and infective causes such as tuberculosis.

A lymphocytic exudative ascites is suggestive of peritoneal sarcoidosis although there is a broad differential diagnosis. Sarcoidosis should be included in the differential diagnosis of exudative ascites of unknown etiology. At laparotomy the peritoneum and omentum may be studded with nodules which may not have been seen on CT scan. Ascites, intraperitoneal masses and thickening of the bowel wall may also be found with features of sclerosing peritonitis such as a dense off-white membrane and granulomas around scar sites.

TREATMENT

Peritoneal sarcoidosis has reportedly been successfully treated with corticosteroids. Most cases of exudative ascites appear to resolve with therapy in a period of several months. There are reported cases, however, of subsequent relapse of peritoneal disease and with a more fulminant disease course and severe intractable ascites (Gajbhiye *et al.* 2008). Sclerosing peritonitis has also been treated with corticosteroid therapy and may help maintain remission, although it is not clear whether steroids help resolution of the disease.

THE COLON

The first case of possible colonic sarcoidosis was reported in 1949 with the finding of non-caseating granulomas at laparotomy (Raven 1949). Approximately 10 percent of patients with known sarcoidosis have submucosal granulomas in the GI tract (Mayock *et al.* 1963).

CLINICAL MANIFESTATIONS

The sigmoid colon is the most common site of involvement, although symptoms are rare. Chronic abdominal pain appears to be the predominant symptom in large bowel sarcoidosis (Gould *et al.* 1973). Lower abdominal pain is also a prominent feature in rectal disease and proctocolitis secondary to sarcoidosis. Infiltration may cause symptoms such as diarrhea, hematochezia, urgency and tenesmus (Davies 1972). Large bowel obstruction may occur due to colonic narrowing or stricture formation due to infiltrative disease or result from extrinsic compression by enlarged lymph nodes. This may lead to vomiting, weight loss, abdominal pain and distension. Colonic polyposis and rectal masses due to sarcoidosis have also been described in individual case reports (Zech *et al.* 1993; Veitch and Badger 2004).

INVESTIGATIONS

Lower gastrointestinal endoscopy is the mainstay of investigation. Colonic features of sarcoidosis can be non-specific and simulate inflammatory, infective, ischemic and neoplastic causes of colitis. Endoscopic appearances include colonic ulcers, friable mucosa, polyps, colonic narrowing and stricturing seen at colonoscopy or sigmoidoscopy. Plaque-like lesions, large bowel mucosal nodularity and thickening of the folds may be seen (Beniwal *et al.* 2003; Nchimi *et al.* 2003), as well as areas of small punctuate bleeding.

There is an extensive list of differential diagnoses of lower GI tract sarcoidosis. Colonic carcinoma and lymphoma can be excluded on histology, although microbiological tests need to be undertaken to exclude infectious causes. Granulomatous infectious diseases such as *Mycobacterium tuberculosis* can be excluded using Ziehl–Nielsen staining for acid-fast bacilli and should be cultured using Lowenstein–Jensen medium. Schistosome ova may be present in intestinal venules and large bowel mucosa, and foreign bodies may be seen in the mucosa causing granulomatous disease (Sachar and Rochester 2004).

Inflammatory bowel disease can be excluded histologically and by serum ACE levels which are normally within range in IBD. There have been cases, however, where ulcerative colitis and sarcoidosis of the colon have co-existed (Silverstein *et al.* 1981; Theodoropoulos *et al.* 1981; Fries *et al.* 1995; Fellerman *et al.* 1997).

Whipple's disease should be excluded prior to the diagnosis with the absence of mucosal macrophage infiltration, large lysosomes and PAS-positive particles. Microscopic colitis can be excluded by the absence of an increased number of intra-epithelial lymphocytes and well-preserved crypt architecture. Non-necrotizing pericryptal granulomas can be seen in microscopic colitis. Radiation colitis histology includes subendothelial accumulation of macrophages, crypt abscesses and increased eosinophils.

TREATMENT

Despite the lack of clinical trial data, corticosteroid therapy is well documented as effective in the treatment of large bowel sarcoidosis. However, steroids should not be started without careful exclusion of other forms of granulomatous disease such as colonic tuberculosis. Large bowel sarcoidosis responds more rapidly compared to Crohn's disease although they can be present together. Steroid sparing agents such as methotrexate, azathioprine and ciclosporin have been used. Infliximab may be used although only a few cases have been reported and outcomes have been variable. Large bowel obstruction usually responds to conservative treatment with steroids (Hilzenrat et al. 1995; Beniwal et al. 2003). Large bowel hemorrhage or obstruction that does not respond to pharmacotherapy, or large bowel perforation, may require surgical intervention.

THE GALLBLADDER

Sarcoidosis involvement of the gallbladder occurs very rarely and usually in association with extrapulmonary disease, commonly gastric infiltration (Barillari et al. 1995; Maamouri et al. 2010).

CLINICAL MANIFESTATIONS

Acute cholecystitis was described in a case report from 1983 due to sarcoidosis (Freed and Reiner 1983). More commonly patients present insidiously with non-specific symptoms such as right upper-quadrant abdominal pain, fever, sweats, fatigue and deranged liver function tests suggesting chronic or subacute cholecystitis. This may occur due to extrinsic compression of the cystic duct by granulomatous inflammation of the gallbladder or surrounding adenopathy. Obstructive jaundice with a serum cholestatic picture may occur due to extrahepatic lymph node enlargement or stenosis of the common hepatic duct.

INVESTIGATIONS

Features suggestive of acute or chronic cholecystitis may be evident on ultrasound, CT or MRI. In keeping with other forms of gastrointestinal sarcoidosis, the diagnosis is usually made histologically, following cholecystectomy. In isolated sarcoidosis of the gallbladder, more often than not histological evidence of sarcoidosis is found after cholecystectomy (which was performed without prior diagnosis) (Lloyd-Davies and Forbes 1965). Evolution into systemic disease on follow-up investigations usually ensues if not already present at the time of diagnosis.

TREATMENT

Spontaneous resolution of gallbladder disease has been reported, as has improvement with corticosteroids. In many cases the gallbladder is removed, although this clearly will not cause remission of disease elsewhere.

GRANULOMATOUS APPENDICITIS

Appendiceal sarcoid involvement is extremely rare and has been described only in patients with systemic disease. Only one case of granulomatous appendicitis was reported in a study of 50 000 appendicectomy pathology samples (Collins 1995). Other causes of granulomatous appendicitis include Crohn's disease, *Mycobacterium tuberculosis*, idiopathic granulomatous appendicitis and foreign bodies such as fecoliths. Infective causes of granulomas in the appendix include brucellosis, yersiniosis, actinomycosis and fungal infections including histoplasmosis, candidiasis and blastomycosis. Solitary granulomatous disease of the appendix without systemic disease is thought of as a separate clinical entity.

CONCLUSION

Although sarcoid has been described in virtually every organ of the gastrointestinal system, it is a rare finding even in those with established sarcoidosis. It can be described in isolation although more commonly is part of systemic disease. Diagnosis is often challenging and requires a combination of clinical, serum, radiological and histological findings. Despite the absence of randomized clinical trials, treatment with corticosteroids is recognized as having therapeutic benefit. Large case series and well-designed clinical trials are required to evaluate further treatment options.

REFERENCES

Adler M, Burroughs A, Beynon H (2007). Gastrointestinal sarcoid: a review. *Sarcoid Vasc Diff Lung Dis* 24: 3–11.

Apell AA (1951). Pyloric obstruction due to sarcoid of the stomach. *Arch Surg* 62: 140–4.

Aronson PJ, Fretzin DF, Morgan NE (1985). A unique case of sarcoidosis with coexistent collagen vascular disease: possible result of a compatible disease-sustaining immunologic environment. *J Am Acad Dermatol* 13: 886–89.

Barillari G, Manazzone O, Pasquadibisceglie A et al. (1995). Sarcoidosis of the gallbladder and of the quadriceps muscle. *Riv di Nuero* 41: 725–9.

Beniwal RS, Cummings OW, Cho WK (2003). Symptomatic gastrointestinal sarcoidosis: case report and review of the literature. *Dig Dis Sci* 48: 174–8.

Boruchowicz A, Canva-Celcambre V, Guillemot F et al. (1996). Sarcoidosis and achalasia: a fortuitous association? *Am J Gastroenterol* 91: 413–14.

Brown JV, Epstein HD, Chang M, Goldstein HG (2010). Sarcoidosis presenting as an intraperitoneal mass. *Case Rep Oncol* 3: 9–13.

Bulger K, O'Riodaron M, Purdy S et al. (1988). Gastrointestinal sarcoidosis resembling Crohn's disease. *Am J Gastroenterol* 83: 1415–17.

Cappell MS (1995). Endoscopic, radiographic, and manometric findings in dysphagia associated with sarcoid due to extrinsic esophageal compression from subcarinal lymphadenopathy. *Am J Gastroenterol* 90: 489–92.

Chinitz MA, Brandt LJ, Frank MS et al. (1985). Symptomatic sarcoidosis of the stomach. *Dig Dis Sci* 30: 682–8.

Collins DCS (1995). A study of 50,000 specimens of the human vermiform appendix. *Surg Gynecol Obstet* 101: 437–45.

Cook DM, Dines DE, Dycus DS (1970). Sarcoidosis: report of a case presenting as dysphagia. *Chest* 57: 84–6.

Davies RJ (1972). Dysphagia, abdominal pain, and sarcoid granulomata. *Br Med J* 3: 564–5.

Douglas JG, Gillon J, Logan RF et al. (1984). Sarcoidosis and celiac disease: an association? *Lancet* ii: 13–15.

Dufrense CR, Jeyasingham K, Baker KK (1983). Achalasia of the cardia associated with pulmonary sarcoidosis. *Surgery* 94: 32–5.

Ebert EC, Kierson M, Hagspiel KD (2008). Gastrointestinal and hepatic manifestations of sarcoidosis. *Am J Gastroenterol* 103: 3184–92.

Farman J, Ramirez G, Rybak B et al. (1997). Gastric sarcoidosis. *Abdom Imaging* 22: 248–52.

Fellermann K, Stahl M, Dahlhoff K et al. (1997). Crohn's disease and sarcoidosis: systemic granulomatosis? *Eur J Gastroenterol Hepatol* 9: 1121–4.

Fireman Z, Sternberg A, Yarchovsky Y et al. (1997). Multiple antral ulcers in gastric sarcoid. *J Clin Gastroenterol* 24: 97–9.

Fleming RH, Nuzek M, McFadden DW (1994). Small intestinal sarcoidosis with massive hemorrhage: report of a case. *Surgery* 115: 127–31.

Freed JS, Reiner MA (1983). Acute cholecystitis as a complication of sarcoidosis. *Arch Int Med* 143: 2188–9.

Fries W, Grassi SA, Leone L et al. (1995). Association between inflammatory bowel disease and sarcoidosis: report of two cases and review of the literature. *Scand J Gastroenterol* 30: 1221–3.

Fuchs F, Le Tohic A, Raynal P et al. (2007). Ovarian and peritoneal sarcoidosis mimicking an ovarian cancer. *Gynecol Obstet Fertil* 35: 41–4.

Fung WP, Foo KT, Lee YS (1975). Gastric sarcoid presenting with haematemesis. *Med J Aust* 12(2): 47–9.

Gajbhiye R, Suryawanshi A, Khan S et al. (2008). Multiple endometrial antigens are targeted in autoimmune endometriosis. *Reprod Biomed Online* 16: 817–24.

Gould SR, Handley AJ, Barnardo DE (1973). Rectal and gastric involvement in a case of sarcoidosis. *Gut* 14: 971–3.

Hackworth WA, Kimmelshue KN, Stravitz RT (2009). Peritoneal sarcoidosis: a unique cause of ascites and intractable hiccups. *Gastro Hep* 5: 859–61.

Hardy WE, Tulgan H, Haidak G et al. (1967). Sarcoidosis: a case presenting with dysphagia and dysphonia. *Ann Intern Med* 66: 353–7.

Hilzenrat N, Spanier A, Lamoureux E et al. (1995). Colonic obstruction secondary to sarcoidosis: nonsurgical diagnosis and management. *Gastroenterology* 108: 1556–9.

Iwai K, Tachibana T, Hosoda Y, Matsui Y (1988). Sarcoidosis autopsies in Japan: frequency and trend in the last 28 years. *Sarcoidosis* 5: 60–5.

Iyer S, Afshar K, Sharma OP (2008). Peritoneal and pleural sarcoidosis: an unusual association – review and clinical report. *Curr Opin Pulm Med* 14: 481–7.

Kaneki T, Kizumi T, Yamamoto H et al. (2001). Gastric sarcoidosis: a single polypoid appearance in the involvement. *Hepato-gastroenterology* 48: 1209–10.

Konda J, Ruth M, Sassaris M, Hunter FM (1980). Sarcoidosis of stomach and rectum. *Am J Gastroenterol* 73: 516–18.

Kremer RM, William JS (1970). Gastric sarcoidosis: a difficult diagnosis. *Am Surg* 36: 686–90.

Leeds J, McAlindon E, Lorenz E et al. (2006). Gastric sarcoidosis mimicking irritable bowel syndrome: cause not association? *World J Gastroenterol* 12: 4754–6.

Levine MS, Ekberg O, Rubesin SE, Gatenby RA (1989). Gastrointestinal sarcoidosis: radiographic findings. *Am J Roentgenol* 153: 293–5.

Liang DB, Price JC, Ahmed H et al. (2010). Gastric sarcoidosis: case report and literature review. *J Natl Med Assoc* 102: 348–5.

Lloyd-Davies RW, Forbes GB (1965). Sarcoidosis of the gall bladder. *Gastroenterology* 49: 287–90.

Longcope WT, Freiman DG (1952). A study of sarcoidosis. *Medicine* 31: 1–132.

Lukens FJ, Machicao VI, Woodward TA, DeVault KR (2002). Esophageal sarcoidosis: an unusual diagnosis. *J Clin Gastroenterol* 34: 54–6.

Maamouri N, Guellouz S, Ben Hariz F et al. (2010). Gastrointestinal sarcoidosis. *Rev Med Int* 31: 262–7.

MacRury SM, McQuaker G, Morton R, Hume R (1992). Sarcoidosis: association with small bowel disease and folate deficiency. *J Clin Pathol* 45: 823–5.

Mayock LR, Bertrand P, Morrison CE, Scott JH (1963). Manifestations of sarcoidosis. *Am J Med* 35: 67–89.

McCormick PA, Feighery C, Dolan C et al. (1988a). Altered gastro-intestinal immune response in sarcoidosis. *Gut* 29: 1628–31.

McCormick PA, O'Donnell M, McGeeney K (1988b). Sarcoidosis and the pancreas. *Ir J Med Sci* 157: 181–3.

Miyamoto C, Nomura S, Kudo E, Hamamoto Y (1972). An autopsy case of sarcoidosis in the intestinal canal. *Bull Osaka Med School* 18: 48–55.

Moretti AM, Sallustio G, Attimonelli R et al. (1993). Gastric localization of sarcoidosis. *Recent Prog Med* 84: 750–5.

Nchimi A, Francotter N, Rausin L, Khamis J (2003). Ileocecal sarcoidosis. *Radiology* 228: 452–5.

Newton C, Nochomovitz L, Sackier JM (1998). Gastric adenocarcinoma associated with isolated granulomatous gastritis. *Ann Surg Oncol* 5: 407–10.

Ngo Y, Messing B, Marteau P et al. (2009). Peritoneal sarcoidosis: an unrecognized cause of sclerosing peritonitis. *Int J Surg Pathol* 17: 219–30.

Nickerson DA (1937). Boeck's sarcoid. *Arch Pathol Lab Med* 24: 19–29.

Nidiry JJ, Mines S, Hackney R et al. (1991). Sarcoidosis: a unique presentation of dysphagia, myopathy, and photophobia. *Am J Gastroenterol* 86: 1679–82.

Okamura S, Iesaki K, Muramatsu S (1991). Gastric-aspirate angiotensin-converting enzyme in gastrosarcoidosis. *Lancet* 338: 121.

Ona FV (1981). Gastric sarcoid: unusual cause of upper gastrointestinal hemorrhage. *Am J Gastroenterol* 75: 286–8.

Palmer ED (1958). Note on silent sarcoidosis of the gastric mucosa. *J Lab Clin Med* 52: 231–4.

Panella VS, Katz S, Kahn E, Ulberg R (1988). Isolated gastric sarcoidosis: unique remnant of disseminated disease. *J Clin Gastroenterol* 10: 327–31.

Papadopoulos KI, Sjoberg K, Lindgren S et al. (1999). Evidence of gastrointestinal immune reactivity in patients with sarcoidosis. *J Int Med* 245: 525–31.

Papowitz AJ, Li JK (1971). Abdominal sarcoidosis with ascites. *Chest* 59: 692–5.

Polachek AA, Matre WJ (1964). Gastrointestinal sarcoidosis: report of a case involving the esophagus. *Am J Dig Dis* 9: 429.

Powell JL, Cunill ES, Gajewski WH, Novotny DB (2005). Sarcoidosis mimicking recurrent endometrial cancer. *Gynecol Oncol* 99: 770–3.

Raven RW (1949). The surgical manifestations of sarcoidosis. *Ann R Coll Surg Engl* 5: 3–28.

Robinson EK, Ernst RW (1954). Boeck's sarcoid of the peritoneal cavity: a case report. *Surgery* 36: 986–91.

Romboli E, Campana D, Piscitelli L et al. (2004). Pancreatic involvement in systemic sarcoidosis: a case report. *Dig Liver Dis* 36: 222–7.

Romero-Gomez M, Suarez-Garcia E, Otero MA et al. (1998). Sarcoidosis, sclerosing cholangitis, and chronic atrophic autoimmune gastritis: a case of infiltrative sclerosing cholangitis. *J Clin Gastroenterol* **27**: 162–5.

Rutherford RM, Brutsche MH, Kearns M *et al.* (2004). Prevalence of coeliac disease in patients with sarcoidosis. *Eur J Gastroenterol Hepatol* **16**: 911–15.

Sachar DB, Rochester J (2004). The myth of gastrointestinal sarcoidosis: a case of guilt by association. *Inflamm Bowel Dis* **10**: 441–3.

Siegel CI, Honda M, Salik J *et al.* (1961). Dysphagia due to granulomatous myositis of the cricopharyngeus muscle: physiological and cineradiographic studies prior to and following successful surgical therapy. *Trans Assoc Am Phys* **74**: 342–52.

Silverstein E, Fierst SM, Simon MR *et al.* (1981). Angiotensin converting enzyme in Crohn's disease and ulcerative colitis. *Am J Clin Pathol* **75**: 175–8.

Sprague R, Harper P, McClain S *et al.* (1984). Disseminated gastrointestinal sarcoidosis: case report and review of the literature. *Gastroenterology* **87**: 421–5.

Takahashi M (1970). Histopathology of sarcoidosis and its immunological bases. *Pathol Int* **20**: 171–82.

Theodoropoulos G, Archimandritis A, Davaris P *et al.* (1981). Ulcerative colitis and sarcoidosis: a curious association report of a case. *Dis Colon Rectum* **24**: 308–10.

Tinker MA, Viswanathan B, Laufer H, Margolis IB (1984). Acute appendicitis and pernicious anemia as complications of gastrointestinal sarcoidosis. *Am J Gastroenterol* **79**: 868–72.

Tobi M, Kobrin I, Ariel I (1982). Rectal involvement in sarcoidosis. *Dis Colon Rectum* **25**: 491–3.

Vahid B, Spodik M, Braun KN *et al.* (2007). Sarcoidosis of gastrointestinal tract: a rare disease. *Dig Dis Sci* **52**: 3316–20.

Veitch AM, Badger I (2004). Sarcoidosis presenting as colonic polyposis: report of a case. *Dis Colon Rectum* **47**: 937–9.

Yee AM, Pochapin MB (2001). Treatment of complicated sarcoidosis with infliximab anti-tumour necrosis factor alpha therapy. *Ann Intern Med* **135**: 27–31.

Wiesner PJ, Kleinman MS, Condemi JJ *et al.* (1971). Sarcoidosis of esophagus. *Am J Dig Dis* **16**: 943–51.

Zech JR, Kroger E, Bonnin AJ, Richmond GW (1993). Sarcoidosis: unusual cause of a rectal mass. *South Med J* **86**: 1054–5.

26

The spleen, bone marrow and blood

JOANNA C PORTER, ESTELLA MATUTES AND DONALD N MITCHELL

THE SPLEEN

The spleen is often involved in sarcoidosis but the true incidence is not known, as splenic involvement is not always specifically looked for. The normal human spleen weighs approximately 150–250 g, and becomes palpable beyond the costal margin if it has doubled in size. Massive splenomegaly is defined as a splenic weight of greater than 1 kg, or four to six times the normal weight. The proportion of patients with sarcoid with a palpable spleen varies from 1.4 to 42 percent. Spleen size is related to angiotensin-converting enzyme (ACE) levels and to extrathoracic sarcoidosis but not to pulmonary involvement (Ebert et al. 2008). Increased cases of sarcoid splenomegaly are picked up radiologically with ultrasound scanning, CT, MRI and PET scan. At postmortem, 38–78 percent of sarcoid patients are found to have an enlarged spleen (Selroos 1976a,b).

There are cases in the literature of isolated sarcoidosis of the spleen, with no extrasplenic involvement, but these are rare. Zia et al. (2005) report the case of a 47-year-old female who presented with nausea and abdominal pain. An abdominal ultrasound revealed normal biliary and pancreatic anatomy and multiple splenic lesions. Computed tomography of the abdomen confirmed the multiple hypodense lesions within the spleen. The patient underwent a diagnostic laparoscopy with splenectomy. No other intra-abdominal pathology was found. Pathology revealed multiple non-caseating splenic granulomas.

The sarcoid granulomas typically produce macroscopically visible nodules on the surface of the spleen. The nodules are usually hypovascular and most are discrete, but may coalesce as they become bigger (Ebert et al. 2008).

Folz and associates retrospectively analyzed abdominal CT scans in 49 patients with tissue-proven sarcoidosis, that had been performed between 1987 and 1993 (Folz et al. 1995). They found splenic abnormalities in 26 (53 percent) of patients, with no correlation to stage of thoracic sarcoidosis. Fifty-four percent of those with spleen abnormalities had liver or lymph node abnormalities as well. The splenic abnormalities on CT were diffuse splenomegaly (mild in 10 percent, moderate in 20 percent and massive in 2 percent), single or multiple low-density lesions (6 percent), or punctate calcifications (14 percent). In a more recent study, Ebert and co-workers found nodules in the spleen in 15 percent of those patients with sarcoid who underwent CT scanning of the abdomen (Ebert et al. 2008).

There are sparse data reporting FDG-PET/CT imaging for splenic sarcoidosis, but reports describe abnormal focal, or less commonly, diffuse splenic uptake of the tracer (Lewis and Salama, 1994; Kaira et al. 2007; Chundru et al. 2008). In either case, correlation with additional anatomic imaging (calcified nodes, hepatic lesions, etc.) and laboratory findings (ACE elevation) is necessary to establish the diagnosis, as reviewed by Liu (2009).

Massive splenomegely may mimic malignancy, so pathological evidence is mandatory for differentiation of sarcoidosis from malignancy, such as lymphoma, especially if FDG-PET is positive. There is some early evidence that sarcoidosis can be distinguished from malignancy using PET scanning with (18)F-FMT as a tracer. FMT is taken up by malignant cells but not by sarcoid granulomas, so this may be a useful way to distinguish the two (Kaira et al. 2007).

Histology (either by aspiration of biopsy) is usually required to confirm the diagnosis of sarcoid. Selroos advocates fine-needle aspiration of the spleen as a safe diagnostic procedure (Selroos 1976a; Selroos and Koivunen 1983). This was carried out in 557 patients. In 381 cases, the aspiration was performed because of suspected sarcoidosis. The sensitivity of the technique was 59 percent and the specificity 97 percent. The cytological picture of the spleen was abnormal in 184 patients with sarcoidosis and in 7 patients with extrinsic allergic alveolitis. No major complications occurred. The method provides a simple, safe, quick and reliable way of producing evidence of a granulomatous process in patients with suspected sarcoidosis, and may prevent the need for more invasive techniques. However, despite these findings, splenic aspiration is seldom performed because of fears of complications. More recently there has been some resurgence of interest in this technique in other settings where it is claimed to be safe and efficacious (Kang *et al.* 2007; Mantur *et al.* 2008). We would urge caution despite this recent interest.

Common symptoms of splenic infiltration occur in only 2 percent of patients with sarcoidosis and are usually confined to those with massive splenomegaly. These symptoms include fever, weight loss, early satiety, left upper-quadrant fullness, and ache and severe pain because of splenic infarct secondary to gastric compression (Liu 2009). Functional impairments in patients with splenic infiltration include anemia, leukopenia, thrombocytopenia and splenic rupture (Roberts and Rang 1958).

Asymptomatic, mild enlargement of the spleen requires no treatment. However, massive splenomegaly and associated hematological and immunological complications may require therapeutic intervention if there is no sign of spontaneous regression. It should be noted that even a massive spleen may regress spontaneously. In an interesting but unusual case, Ogiwara and associates describe a patient with hypoglycemia due to ectopic secretion of insulin-like growth factor-I arising from a spleen involved with sarcoid (Ogiwara *et al.* 2010); the hypoglycemia responded to splenectomy.

In general, the primary management of uncomplicated splenic sarcoidosis consists of medical therapy with prednisone, methotrexate and/or antimalarial drugs, to good effect (Aide *et al.* 2009; Kitamura *et al.* 2009). However, if the splenomegaly is associated with portal hypertension then response is of course unlikely unless the hepatic pathology is reversed. Response can be measured clinically, radiologically and with FDG-PET (Aide *et al.* 2009). Patel describes a patient with systemic sarcoidosis and bone marrow involvement who was intolerant to prednisolone but responded to the TNF antagonist adalimumab with recovery of hemoglobin, and reduction in splenomegaly to normal levels over a 2-year period (Patel 2009).

Occasionally splenectomy is required. Indications for surgery include symptomatic splenomegaly, severe hypersplenism, prophylaxis for splenic rupture, and neoplastic exclusion. However, rupture of the spleen is fortunately rare in sarcoid with just one report (James and Sharma 1967), and a second case in the literature of fatal rupture of a splenic artery due to sarcoid (Barton *et al.* 2010).

Penna and Deroide describe a 45-year-old woman with a history of mediastinal sarcoidosis, who had been treated with oral corticosteroids 6 years previously, and now presented with pain in the left upper quadrant of her abdomen. Computerized tomography revealed heterogeneous splenomegaly with multiple hypovascular nodules (Penna and Deroide 2003; Fig. 26.1 and Plate 20). After two years of follow-up, the patient still reported abdominal pain, and the spleen had increased in size from 16 to 20 cm. A laparoscopic splenectomy was performed. Pathological examination

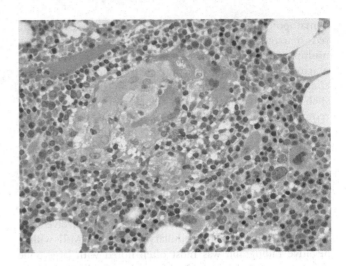

Figure 26.1   Granuloma in the bone marrow of a patient with sarcoidosis (× 40). With thanks to, and permission from, Dr Andrew Wotherspoon, Department of Histopathology, Royal Marsden Hospital, London. See also plate 20.

confirmed the presence of sarcoidosis in the spleen and the lymph nodes of the splenic hilum. The patient did well with no further treatment and had no sign of recurrence on thoracoabdominal CT at two years of follow-up.

THE BONE MARROW

Sarcoidosis is acknowledged to affect the bone marrow but in many cases this is probably asymptomatic and not specifically recognized. In a recent study from Istanbul (Yanardag *et al.* 2002), of 92 patients diagnosed with sarcoid, 50 consented to a bone marrow biopsy. In 10 percent of the patients there were non-caseating granulomas on biopsy. Anemia was detected in 22 percent and anemia with leukopenia in 6 percent. Patients with bone marrow involvement had increased extrapulmonary involvement, as well as more hematological abnormalities (leukopenia, lymphopenia and anemia) than those without bone marrow involvement. Of the 11 patients with anemia, 3 had bone marrow involvement and 8 had iron-deficiency anemia, emphasizing that the cause of anemia in the majority of cases is not due to marrow infiltration.

In severe cases, sarcoidosis of the bone marrow may present as a fever of unknown origin, localized bone pains, or with associated blood abnormalities that can mimic a number of infectious, inflammatory or neoplastic processes (Miller *et al.* 2007). Diagnosis in such patients can be difficult. If bone marrow involvement is suspected clinically even when plain radiographs and bone scans are normal, MRI may be helpful. MRI has been shown to reveal multiple small nodular lesions within the marrow, and can help localize sarcoid lesions for diagnostic marrow biopsy. In a prospective study, 42 patients over 3.5 years with a diagnosis of sarcoid were referred for MRI because of musculoskeletal complaints (Moore *et al.* 2005). The criterion used for the diagnosis of marrow infiltration was intramedullary signal alteration compared with the adjacent fatty and/or hematopoietic marrow. Differentiation of bone lesions from red marrow deposition was based on morphology (e.g. multiple, discrete cannonball-like foci not characteristic of marrow replacement, in contrast to patchy areas more characteristic of red marrow) and location (not characteristic, such as proximal phalanges, as compared to characteristic of red marrow residua, such as the proximal femurs). The lesions were described as confined to the medullary space or with extraosseous extension, and as violating the cortex or not. In 17 subjects, MRI showed intramedullary lesions ranging in size from < 1 to 3–4 cm, of which 13 were in the large bones or axial. Nine of these were biopsied, of which one biopsy was not diagnostic and eight showed non-caseating granulomas, characteristic of sarcoid involvement. The association of intramedullary lesions on MRI with a negative radiograph was most often noted with large-bone lesions ($n = 5$). Using standard musculoskeletal protocols, the MRI appearance of these lesions is not specific and needs to be differentiated from metastatic disease, multiple myeloma, lymphoma, osseous hemangioma, and disseminated granulomatous infection. Some of the patients had background changes of red marrow replacement in the pelvis and spine, which made distinguishing their marrow lesions more difficult. Dedicated sequences such as opposed-phase gradient-echo sequences might be more accurate for distinguishing hematopoietic from pathological bone marrow (Moore et al. 2005). It should be noted that the patients in this MRI study were highly selected, and were all known to have sarcoid with musculoskeletal involvement. In our experience, MRI results must be treated with caution as such imaging may be exquisitely sensitive and detect abnormalities that are not clinically significant, in patients who are asymptomatic.

Another modality that can detect bone marrow involvement in sarcoidosis is whole-body (18)F-FDG PET. This is known to pick up activity in sarcoidosis, and one team looked at whether such a scan could help in patients with sarcoidosis and symptomatic anemia (de Prost et al. 2010). This study looked at ten patients with proven sarcoid who had had FDG-PET scanning. Of these, three had anemia and FDG-PET showed bone involvement. Bone marrow biopsies in all three showed granulomas and confirmed the diagnosis of bone marrow sarcoid. In seven control patients with sarcoid but no anemia, FDG-PET did not show bone marrow involvement. The percentage of anemic patients with bone marrow involvement was 100 percent in the group, which is much higher than in previous studies. This may reflect their presentation, in that two of the three patients had bone pain. Interestingly, in all three patients (one of whom was heterozygous for beta-thalassemia trait), the anemia was microcytic but only partly responded to iron.

From these studies it is estimated that as many as 10 percent of patients known to have sarcoid can be shown, on biopsy, to have bone marrow involvement. However, there are many other possible etiologies when granulomas are found on bone marrow biopsy (a finding in less than 3 percent of bone marrow biopsies). The spectrum of underlying etiology depends on the geographical area and the reason for performing a bone marrow examination (Bodem

et al. 1983; Bhargava and Farhi 1988). In Bhargava and Farhi's study from Ohio, they looked at 6988 bone marrow biopsies seen from 1973 to 1986. Granulomas were identified in 72 specimens (1.03 percent). In this period, biopsies doubled, but the yearly incidence of granulomas increased from 0.3 to 2.2 percent. The granulomas were associated with infectious disease (30 percent), hematological disorders (25 percent), sarcoidosis (11 percent), non-hematological malignancies (10 percent), drug reaction (5 percent), other diseases (6 percent), and no final diagnosis (6 percent). Over this time the incidence of sarcoidosis dropped from 32 to 3 percent. Patients with fever of unknown origin were 15 times more likely to have marrow granulomas than patients biopsied for other reasons. In an English study, 58 cases of bone marrow granuloma were seen over a 20-year period (Bodem et al. 1983).

There are no morphological features that allow reliable differentiation between the causes of bone marrow granulomas. By combining careful histological, microbiological and serological techniques, an etiology can be documented in most patients (87 percent) with marrow granulomas. Vijnovich Baron et al. (1994) studied 2250 bone marrow biopsies taken from March 1983 to March 1991 from patients in Argentina. Granulomas and/or granulomatous lesions were found in 24 of them (1.06 percent). In general sarcoid is probably responsible for 3–30 percent of granulomas on bone marrow biopsy with an average of <10 percent. Of these, 90–95 percent have lung involvement. This number is, of course, dependent on the incidence of sarcoid in, and the ethnicity of, the population. For example, in an ACCESS study (Baughman et al. 2001), 3.9 percent of 736 patients were documented to have bone marrow involvement and this was more common in black than in white subjects (chi-squared $= 18.8$, $p < 0.001$). However, as bone marrow involvement was not specifically sought in this study, many cases would have been missed.

Although granulomas in the bone marrow may be a rather non-specific manifestation of other disease, and are seldom enough to establish a confident diagnosis of sarcoidosis on their own, there are several examples in the literature of the value of bone marrow biopsy as an adjunct to diagnosis. To take just two:

A 27-year-old black man presented with renal failure and hypercalcemia (Ponce and Gujral 2004). A renal biopsy showed interstitial nephritis and membranous glomerulopathy thought to be secondary to non-steroidal anti-inflammatory drugs. His renal function and symptoms improved with short-term prednisone therapy. Discontinuation of steroids led to a recurrence of renal failure and severe hypercalcemia. On the basis of an elevated ACE level of 160 U/L and anemia, a bone marrow biopsy was performed. Acid-fast, bacillus-negative, non-caseating granulomas suggested the diagnosis of sarcoidosis. The patient recovered after restarting prednisone.

In another study (Miller et al. 2007), a patient with a PUO and lymphopenia, but no lymphadenopathy and a normal chest radiograph for 2 months, was found to have non-caseating granulomas on bone marrow biopsy. A diagnosis of sarcoid was made and the patient responded very well to steroids.

The take-home message from all these studies is that bone marrow biopsy may be a useful adjunct to diagnosis, and radiological investigation of patients, both with and without symptoms of bone marrow involvement. Radiological investigations, such as plain films, MRI and PET, can reveal bone marrow involvement that was not anticipated, and guide bone marrow biopsy to specific involved sites. It should be emphasized that it is extremely rare for sarcoid to present as a granuloma in the bone marrow, and isolated extra-pulmonary sarcoidosis, although described (Browne et al. 1978; Miller et al. 2007), accounts for fewer than 5 percent of such cases.

Although sarcoid involvement of the bone marrow is probably under-reported and may be as high as 10 percent of cases, the effects of sarcoid on bone marrow function may be even higher. Bone marrow toxicity can result from mechanical disruption of the marrow by granulomas as well as by an indirect effect from the variety of cytokines released.

BLOOD

Several studies of adult patients with sarcoidosis have shown one or more hematologic abnormalities in over half of the cases, only some of which will be due to bone marrow involvement. Various hematologic abnormalities described include anemia (which may be hemolytic or non-hemolytic), lymphopenia, monocytosis, eosinophilia and thrombocytopenia. More unusual are leukemoid reactions and secondary polycythemia in response to the hypoxia of chronic lung disease. In many of these cases treatment is with immunosuppression, such as prednisolone. Patel describes a patient with systemic sarcoidosis and bone marrow involvement who was intolerant to prednisolone but responded to the TNF antagonist adalimumab with recovery of hemoglobin (and reduction of concomitant splenomegaly) to normal levels over a 2-year period (Patel 2009).

Anemia affects up to about one-third of patients with sarcoidosis for which there are various underlying causes in addition to bone marrow involvement: the anemia of chronic disease, anemia associated with autoimmune activity, hypersplenism, and concomitant hemoglobinopathies. In addition, anemia may result from nutritional deficiencies such as iron (Veitch and Badger 2004); and megaloblastic anemia due to folate or vitamin B_{12} deficiency as a consequence of gastric and small bowel involvement by sarcoid has been described (MacRury et al. 1992). Lower and associates studied 75 patients with active pulmonary sarcoid, 28 percent of whom had anemia (Lower et al. 1988). Of these, 17 patients had bone marrow investigation and this showed non-caseating granulomas in 9 and absent iron stores in 8. In the 'majority of unexplained' anemia cases, hemoglobin normalized with prednisolone.

There are only a few reports of hemolytic anemia secondary to sarcoid, and in at least one case the anemia

preceded the appearance of overt sarcoid (Semple, 1975). The direct antiglobulin Coombs test has been found to be both positive (Lebacq et al. 1956; Yasuda et al. 1996) and negative (West, 1959), and response to treatment has been variable. In general steroids have improved the anemia and in some cases led to lasting remission (Lebacq et al. 1956; Yasuda et al. 1996), but in others there has been no response (Johansson, 1958). In the same way splenectomy may (West, 1959) or may not (Johansson, 1958) lead to remission; on the other hand hemolytic anemia may develop after removal of the spleen for pancytopenia (Lebacq et al. 1956) or thrombocytopenia (Thadani et al. 1975). There have also been cases in which the spleen has been removed for hemolytic anemia in sarcoid and shown no changes (Cox and Donald 1964).

Leukopenia occurs in as many as 55 percent of patients but is rarely severe (Lower et al. 1988). In the absence of splenomegaly, leukopenia may reflect bone marrow involvement. Lymphopenia is common and patients often have fewer than 1500 cells per microliter, with a reduction in T-lymphocytes while B-lymphocyte numbers are normal (Kataria et al. 1976; Wurm and Lohr, 1986). Secondary polycythemia may occur secondary to chronic lung disease. Other hematological abnormalities such as eosinophilia and chronic immune thrombocytopenia (Hisada et al. 1990; Kondo et al. 1993; Chakrabarti et al. 1997) have been described but are thought to be rare. One report documented the utility of high-dose steroids to treat immune thrombocytopenia associated with sarcoidosis (Chakrabarti et al. 1997). However, a review of 31 cases of thrombocytopenia (Mahevas et al. 2006), followed by a series of 20 cases of sarcoid and immune thrombocytopenia from the same group (Mahevas et al. 2009), suggests that the association may be more common than realized. They conclude that hypersplenism and bone marrow infiltration account for many of the cases of a low platelet count, but if these are excluded an immune mechanism may be responsible as was the case in 17 of 31 cases (Mahevas et al. 2006). In the same authors' review of patients with autoimmune thrombocytopenia in the context of sarcoid, 19 of the 20 were treated with prednisone at 1 mg/kg daily for at least three consecutive weeks, with additional intravenous immunoglobulin (IVIg) in 10 patients. Twelve patients achieved a complete response, six a partial response and only one failed to respond. The course of ITP was chronic in four patients; two of these underwent splenectomy with complete response, and two were treated with rituximab (375 mg/m^2, four infusions) and achieved a partial response at one year.

One possible association is between sarcoid and hematological malignancy as well as other cancers. Epidemiological studies have suggested an increased incidence of lymphoma in patients with sarcoidosis. Brickner and Wilbeck estimated an incidence of lymphoid diseases 11.5 times higher than expected in a cohort of 2544 patients with sarcoidosis (Brincker and Wilbek 1974). However, a subsequent study on the 18 percent of the Danish population documented that the incidence was 5.5 higher than expected, with a 3.5 higher frequency of lung cancer (Brincker, 1986). The sarcoid–lymphoma syndrome refers to the development of lymphoma at least 1–2 years after the diagnosis of sarcoid (Cohen and

Kurzrock 2007). Other main features of the 'sarcoidosis–lymphoma syndrome' are:

- the median age of the onset of sarcoidosis in these patients tends to be 10 years above that of unselected sarcoidosis patients;
- Hodgkin's lymphoma is more frequent than non-Hodgkin's lymphoma.

In addition, it has been suggested that the chronic form of sarcoidosis and treatment with steroids are predisposing factors. The majority of lymphoma cases are of B-cell origin and development of a T-cell leukemia/lymphoma is exceedingly rare but has been documented (Karakantza et al. 1996). Considering that there is an impairment of the immune system in patients with sarcoidosis, it is reasonable to speculate that this is the major contributing factor for the predisposition to develop lymphoma. In tissues from patients with sarcoidosis there is an increase of activated $CD4^+$ ($CD25^+$, HLA-DR$^+$) T-lymphocytes while there is a decrease on the regulatory suppressor $CD8^+$ T-cells. The decreased number of the latter lymphocytes may allow the escape of a B-cell favoring the emergence of a B-cell clone, resulting in a lymphoma.

Sarcoid may also be linked to other hematological malignancies, in particular leukemia. There are several cases in the literature of acute myeloid leukemia (AML) and sarcoidosis. In some cases the sarcoid preceeded the AML by some years and AML occurred after sarcoid became quiescent (Leymarie et al. 2005); in others the diseases were diagnosed at the same time (Pagano et al. 1998), or sarcoid developed after a cure of AML. As for lymphomas, the impairment of the T-cell response is postulated to either predispose to the development of AML or lead to a smoldering form of the disease (Leymarie et al. 2005); alternatively, the development of sarcoidosis during AML may reflect a sarcoid-like reaction to tumor antigens (Reich 1985). In other cases it has been postulated that the AML may be a leukemoid-like response to sarcoid (Bordelon et al. 1977). AML is characterized by chromosomal translocations that lead to the fusion of selected genes, resulting in the production of a chimeric protein which acts as a transcription factor or has tyrosine kinase activity.

Cytogenetic studies in sarcoidosis have shown evidence of aneuploidy in the granuloma cells as well as in peripheral blood lymphocytes. Therefore, this genetic instability in myeloid cells may predispose to the development of acute myeloid leukemias (Nordenson et al. 1989).

In general, the possible association between sarcoid and hematological malignancy is poorly characterized, and the numbers of cases are really too small to draw conclusions.

REFERENCES

Aide N, Allouache D, Ollivier Y et al. (2009). Early 2′-deoxy-2′-[18F]fluoro-D-glucose PET metabolic response after corticosteroid therapy to differentiate cancer from sarcoidosis and sarcoid-like lesions. Mol Imaging Biol 11: 224–8.

Barton JH, Tavora F, Farb A et al. (2010). Unusual cardiovascular manifestations of sarcoidosis, a report of three cases: coronary artery aneurysm with myocardial infarction, symptomatic mitral valvular disease, and sudden death from ruptured splenic artery. Cardiovasc Pathol 19(4): 119–23.

Baughman RP, Teirstein AS, Judson MA et al. (2001). Clinical characteristics of patients in a case control study of sarcoidosis. Am J Respir Crit Care Med 164: 1885–9.

Bhargava V, Farhi DC (1988). Bone marrow granulomas: clinicopathologic findings in 72 cases and review of the literature. Hematol Pathol 2: 43–50.

Bodem CR, Hamory BH, Taylor HM, Kleopfer L (1983). Granulomatous bone marrow disease: a review of the literature and clinicopathologic analysis of 58 cases. Medicine (Baltimore) 62: 372–83.

Bordelon J, Stone MJ, Frenkel EP (1977). Probable myeloblastic leukemoid reaction with disseminated sarcoidosis. South Med J 70: 1378–80.

Brincker H (1986). The sarcoidosis–lymphoma syndrome. Br J Cancer 54: 467–73.

Brincker H, Wilbek E (1974). The incidence of malignant tumours in patients with respiratory sarcoidosis. Br J Cancer 29: 247–51.

Browne PM, Sharma OP, Salkin D (1978). Bone marrow sarcoidosis. J Am Med Assoc 40: 2654–5.

Chakrabarti S, Behera D, Varma S, Bambery P (1997). High-dose methyl prednisolone for autoimmune thrombocytopenia in sarcoidosis. Sarcoid Vasc Diff Lung Dis 14: 188.

Chundru S, Wong CY, Wu D et al. (2008). Granulomatous disease: is it a nuisance or an asset during PET/computed tomography evaluation of lung cancers? Nucl Med Commun 29: 623–7.

Cohen PR, Kurzrock R (2007). Sarcoidosis and malignancy. Clin Dermatol 25: 326–33.

Cox WL, Donald JM (1964). Acquired hemolytic anemia and Boeck's sarcoidosis: review of the literature. Am Surg 30: 199–202.

de Prost N, Kerrou K, Sibony M et al. (2010). Fluorine-18 fluorodeoxyglucose with positron emission tomography revealed bone marrow involvement in sarcoidosis patients with anaemia. Respiration 79: 25–31.

Ebert EC, Kierson M, Hagspiel KD (2008). Gastrointestinal and hepatic manifestations of sarcoidosis. Am J Gastroenterol 103: 3184–92 quiz: 3193.

Folz SJ, Johnson CD, Swensen SJ (1995). Abdominal manifestations of sarcoidosis in CT studies. J Comput Assist Tomogr 19: 573–9.

Hisada M, Okamoto S, Nakajima H et al. (1990). Chronic immune thrombocytopenia in sarcoidosis. Keio J Med 39: 261–4.

James DG, Sharma OP (1967). Neurosarcoidosis. Proc R Soc Med 60: 1169–70.

Johansson R (1958). Sarcoidosis (Schaumann's disease) and hemolytic anemia. Nord Med 60: 1746–9.

Kaira K, Ishizuka T, Yanagitani N et al. (2007). Value of FDG positron emission tomography in monitoring the effects of therapy in progressive pulmonary sarcoidosis. Clin Nucl Med 32: 114–16.

Kang M, Kalra N, Gulati M et al. (2007). Image guided percutaneous splenic interventions. Eur J Radiol 64: 140–6.

Karakantza M, Matutes E, MacLennan K et al. (1996). Association between sarcoidosis and lymphoma revisited. J Clin Pathol 49: 208–12.

Kataria YP, LoBuglio AF, Bromberg PA, Hurtubise PE (1976). Sarcoid lymphocytes: B- and T-cell quantitation. Ann NY Acad Sci 278: 69–79.

Kitamura A, Takiguchi Y, Sugiura T et al. (2009). Symptomatic splenomegaly in a young Japanese man with sarcoidosis accompanied by spleen, liver, kidney, lung and lymph node lesions. Nihon Kokyuki Gakkai Zasshi 47: 742–5.

Kondo H, Sakai S, Sakai Y (1993). Autoimmune haemolytic anaemia, Sjögren's syndrome and idiopathic thrombocytopenic purpura in a patient with sarcoidosis. *Acta Haematol* **89**: 209–12.

Lebacq E, Tirzmalis A, Mairiaux E, Pluygers E (1956). Besnier–Boeck–Schaumann sarcoidosis with hemolytic anemia caused by auto-immunization. *Bull Mem Soc Med Hop Paris* **72**: 614–20.

Lewis PJ, Salama A (1994). Uptake of fluorine-18-fluorodeoxyglucose in sarcoidosis. *J Nucl Med* **35**: 1647–9.

Leymarie V, Galoisy AC, Falkenrodt A et al. (2005). Latent acute promyelocytic leukemia t(15;17)(q22;q12-21) and sarcoidosis: long-term cohabitation. *Eur J Intern Med* **16**: 598–600.

Liu Y (2009). Clinical significance of diffusely increased splenic uptake on FDG-PET. *Nucl Med Commun* **30**: 763–69.

Lower EE, Smith JT, Martelo OJ, Baughman RP (1988). The anemia of sarcoidosis. *Sarcoidosis* **5**: 51–5.

MacRury SM, McQuaker G, Morton R, Hume R (1992). Sarcoidosis: association with small bowel disease and folate deficiency. *J Clin Pathol* **45**: 823–5.

Mahevas M, Le Page L, Salle V et al. (2006). Thrombocytopenia in sarcoidosis. *Sarcoid Vasc Diff Lung Dis* **23**: 229–35.

Mahevas M, Chiche L, Khellaf M et al. (2009). Characteristics of sarcoidosis-associated immune thrombocytopenia: a consecutive study of 20 cases In: *Proceedings of 51st ASH Annual Meeting*, New Orleans, LA, p. 2407.

Mantur BG, Mulimani MS, Bidari L et al. (2008). Splenic puncture: diagnostic accuracy and safety in infectious diseases. *Int J Infect Dis* **12**: 446–7.

Miller AC, Chacko T, Rashid RM, Ledford DK (2007). Fever of unknown origin and isolated noncaseating granuloma of the marrow: could this be sarcoidosis? *Allergy Asthma Proc* **28**: 230–5.

Moore SL, Teirstein A, Golimbu C (2005). MRI of sarcoidosis patients with musculoskeletal symptoms. *Am J Roentgen* **185**: 154–9.

Nordenson I, Bjermer L, Holmgren G et al. (1989). t(6;9) in bone marrow cells in two patients with sarcoidosis and acute myeloid leukemia. *Cancer Genet Cytogenet* **38**: 297–300.

Ogiwara Y, Mori S, Iwama M et al. (2010). Hypoglycemia due to ectopic secretion of insulin-like growth factor-I in a patient with an isolated sarcoidosis of the spleen. *Endocr J* **57**: 325–30.

Pagano L, Visani G, Ferrara F et al. (1998). Contemporaneous acute myeloid leukaemia and sarcoidosis: report of three cases. *Sarcoid Vasc Diff Lung Dis* **15**: 67–70.

Patel SR (2009). Systemic sarcoidosis with bone marrow involvement responding to therapy with adalimumab: a case report. *J Med Case Reports* **3**: 8573.

Penna C, Deroide GA (2003). Images in clinical medicine: splenic sarcoidosis. *New Engl J Med* **349**: e16.

Ponce C, Gujral JS (2004). Renal failure and hypercalcemia as initial manifestations of extrapulmonary sarcoidosis. *South Med J* **97**: 590–2.

Reich JM (1985). Acute myeloblastic leukemia and sarcoidosis: implications for pathogenesis. *Cancer* **55**: 366–9.

Roberts JC, Rang MC (1958). Sarcoidosis of liver and spleen. *Lancet* **2**: 296–9.

Selroos O (1976a). Fine-needle aspiration biopsy of the spleen in diagnosis of sarcoidosis. *Ann NY Acad Sci* **278**: 517–21.

Selroos O (1976b). Sarcoidosis of the spleen. *Acta Med Scand* **200**: 337–40.

Selroos O, Koivunen E (1983). Usefulness of fine-needle aspiration biopsy of spleen in diagnosis of sarcoidosis. *Chest* **83**: 193–5.

Semple P (1975). Thrombocytopenia, haemolytic anaemia and sarcoidosis. *Br Med J* **4**: 440–1.

Thadani U, Aber CP, Taylor JJ (1975). Massive splenomegaly, pancytopenia and haemolytic anaemia in sarcoidosis. *Acta Haematol* **53**: 230–40.

Veitch AM, Badger I (2004). Sarcoidosis presenting as colonic polyposis: report of a case. *Dis Colon Rectum* **47**: 937–9.

Vijnovich Baron IA, Barazzutti L, Tartas N et al. (1994). Bone marrow granulomas. *Sangre* (Barcelona) **39**: 35–8.

West WO (1959). Acquired hemolytic anemia secondary to Boeck's sarcoid: report of a case and review of the literature. *New Engl J Med* **261**: 688–90.

Wurm K, Lohr G (1986). Immunocytological blood tests in cases of sarcoidosis. *Sarcoidosis* **3**: 52–9.

Yanardag H, Pamuk GE, Karayel T, Demirci S (2002). Bone marrow involvement in sarcoidosis: an analysis of 50 bone marrow samples. *Haematologia* (Budapest) **32**: 419–25.

Yasuda N, Kohda M, Nomura M et al. (1996). Sarcoidosis in a patient with autoimmune hemolytic anemia. *Nihon Kyobu Shikkan Gakkai Zasshi* **34**: 931–6.

Zia H, Zemon H, Brody F (2005). Laparoscopic splenectomy for isolated sarcoidosis of the spleen. *J Laparoendosc Adv Surg Tech A* **15**: 160–2.

27

Neurosarcoidosis

GAVIN GIOVANNONI, VIQUAR CHAMOUN, JOHN SCADDING AND EDWARD THOMPSON

INTRODUCTION

The first historical account of neurosarcoidosis can be ascribed to Winkler who described peripheral neuropathy with sarcoid lesions in peripheral nerves in 1905 (Winkler, cited by Salvesen in 1935 and Colover in 1948). Heerfordt described cranial neuropathy in association with uveo-parotid fever in 1909. His patients included a man in his twenties and boys of 11 and 14, who complained of lassitude and had the three cardinal signs of fever, parotid swelling and uveitis. Two had optic neuritis with papilledema and facial palsy; one had paralysis of the vagus and scattered sensory signs suggestive of mononeuritis multiplex. Dysphagia was another transient symptom. The man had thirst and polyuria which gradually lessened and his spinal fluid showed mild pleocytosis. Heerfordt found that the prognosis was good, although at follow-up two years later one of the boys had developed acute retrobulbar neuritis (Urban 1910, cited by Colover 1948).

DEFINITION OF SARCOIDOSIS

The study of any disease requires an unambiguous definition of the condition, which allows diagnostic criteria to be developed. From this standpoint, it is immaterial whether a disease is defined on the basis of symptoms, signs, radiology, immunology, biochemistry, histology, genetics or natural history; the definition must, however, aim to be unambiguous. Sarcoidosis has been a particularly difficult disorder to define. In 1976 the subcommittee of the Seventh International Conference on Sarcoidosis proposed that the definition should be formulated as a short paragraph, which is quoted here (James et al. 1976):

Sarcoidosis is a multisytem granulomatous disorder of unknown etiology most commonly affecting young adults and presenting with bilateral hilar lymphadenopathy, pulmonary infiltration, and skin or eye lesions. The diagnosis is established most securely when clinical or radiographic findings are supported by histologic evidence of widespread non-caseating epithelioid granulomas in more than one organ or by a positive Kveim–Siltzbach skin test. Immunologic features are depression of delayed-type hypersensitivity suggesting impaired cell-mediated immunity and raised or abnormal immunoglobulins. There may also be hypercalcuria with or without hypercalcemia. The course and prognosis may correlate with mode of onset. An acute onset with erythema nodosum heralds a self-limited course and spontaneous resolution, whereas an insidious onset may be followed by relentless progression or fibrosis. Corticosteroids relieve symptoms and suppress inflammation and granuloma formation.

This definition has been roundly criticized (Scadding and Mitchell 1985):

One of the few unequivocal statements in it is that sarcoidosis is of unknown cause, which entails the logical difficulties in the study of causation... It includes one statement, concerning cell-mediated immunity (as opposed to hypersensitivity) that is probably incorrect... It provides no indication of the way in which, in the final analysis, agreement might be reached in a case over which informed observers disagree.

In the absence of a recent consensus definition, sarcoidosis is best considered as a multiorgan granulomatosis, without central caseation or other pathology complicating the granulomas.

Granulomas are aggregates of epithelioid cells, interspersed with multinucleate giant cells and surrounded by a ring of lymphocytes. The giant cells can be of the 'foreign-body' or Langerhans type, and may contain inclusion bodies that are not specific for sarcoidosis. There is no caseation within the granuloma, although a small amount of granular eosinophilic necrosis is allowable in the center of occasional granulomas in an otherwise typical case. This definition distinguishes sarcoidosis from other conditions that can mimic it. These include:

- other inflammatory conditions that are not associated with granulomas;
- granulomatosis that exhibits significant central necrosis, whether caseous or suppurative;
- non-caseating granulomatosis that exhibits additional histological abnormalities such as vasculitis, eosinophilic or neoplastic infiltration, non-commensal organisms or inorganic foreign bodies.

Granulomatosis that does not exhibit a multisystem natural history, but is identical in other respects, is described as 'focal granulomatosis'.

Tuberculosis, for instance, causes granulomatosis with a multisystem predilection, but the granulomas have characteristic central caseation – the so-called 'classical' granuloma. Mycobacteria, fungi, helminths, other bacteria, and foreign bodies may also be visualized with appropriate staining when present and responsible for the granulomatosis. In Wegener's granulomatosis and the Churg–Strauss syndrome, the granulomas are less well defined, less compact and may show central necrosis. However it is again the additional abnormalities that are most striking: tissue necrosis, often extensive and liquefactive, granulomatous and non-granulomatous necrotizing vasculitis, alveolar capillaritis and focal segmental necrotizing glomerulonephritis. The Churg–Strauss syndrome exhibits an infiltration of eosinophils, the necrotic areas in the center of granulomas containing granular eosinophilic debris and Charcot–Leyden crystals. In focal granulomatosis the granulomas remain confined to one organ and often to a particular site within the organ. The best documented cause of focal granulomatosis is an imbedded foreign body, be that microbial or inorganic in nature. Foreign bodies or other causes of a focal granulomatosis may, of course, be present in several different organs, but not be detectable. If this is indeed the case, they would be an unidentified cause of sarcoidosis.

Some have included the absence of a known cause as part of the definition of sarcoidosis. However, there are logical difficulties with this approach: How does one investigate the cause of a disease that is defined by the absence of a cause? There are also practical disadvantages to any definition that incorporates idiopathy as one of its features. It leads to an ongoing reclassification of diseases. It would mean that if an agent were discovered to be responsible for some of the cases presently classified as sarcoidosis, the original diagnosis of sarcoidosis would become incorrect. This occurs despite the fact that histological changes will have implications for diagnosis, management and prognosis, regardless of the etiology. The value inherent in a histological classification will fail

to be utilized. Thus vasculitis has distinct diagnostic and management implications, whether idiopathic or associated with systemic lupus erythematosus or polyarteritis nodosa (PAN).

We adopt the alternative view that a multiorgan granulomatosis, without central caseation or other pathology complicating the granulomas, is sarcoidosis irrespective of etiology or other findings. Sarcoidosis is defined here solely by histological changes and by the bodily distribution of these changes. There is no reference to inoculants, genetic factors, biochemical or physiological findings, or to clinical features. If information on any of these becomes available, this simply adds to our knowledge of the condition. If, for instance, a particular agent such as *Mycobacterium tuberculosis* is discovered as a cause of some or all of the cases, these may become reclassified as tuberculosis under a formal classification system (e.g. the International Classification of Diseases), but could still continue to be called sarcoidosis. One label would describe the condition in terms of its histological changes and the other in terms of its infective etiology. The situation would be analogous to the manner in which, for example, head injury, intracranial hematoma, raised intracranial pressure and coma can all describe different aspects of the same condition.

DEFINITION OF NEUROSARCOIDOSIS

Neurosarcoidosis can be defined as:

> a multiorgan granulomatosis, without central caseation or other pathology complicating the granulomas, that involves the neurological tissue of either brain, spinal cord, meninges, cranial nerve or peripheral nerve.

Sarcoidosis may therefore have neurological features and not be neurosarcoidosis; these features may reflect the neurological effects of damage in other organs. For neurosarcoidosis to be diagnosed there must be reason to believe that the relevant histological changes have occurred within nervous tissue. Equally, typical sarcoid histology restricted to the nervous system should not constitute neurosarcoidosis in the absence of evidence of multisystem involvement. It should also be noted that neurosarcoidosis, as defined here, embraces both central nervous system (meningeal and parenchymal) sarcoidosis and peripheral neurosarcoidosis.

EPIDEMIOLOGY OF NEUROSARCOIDOSIS

An epidemiological study to directly assess the incidence or prevalence of neurosarcoidosis has yet to be performed. Information about this has to be derived by estimating the proportion of patients with sarcoidosis who develop neurological complications, and applying them to incidence and prevalence data for sarcoidosis in general. The figures obtained for sarcoidosis have depended on the geographical area studied and methodology used. The majority of patients with sarcoidosis are either asymptomatic or have such minor symptoms that they do not bother to consult a doctor (Sartwell and Edwards 1974).

Data from mass radiographic screening carried out in European countries over two decades to detect pulmonary tuberculosis suggest prevalence in the order of 10–50 per 100 000 (Bauer and Löfgren 1964). The incidence of sarcoid varied from 0.04 case per 100 000 population in Spain to 64 cases per 100 000 in Sweden. However, postmortems on 6707 individuals in Malmo, Sweden, from 1957 to 1962, comprising 60 percent of all deaths in the town over the period, found evidence of sarcoidosis in 43 cases (Bauer and Wijkstrom 1964). Only three cases had been diagnosed as having sarcoidosis during life. This would suggest a prevalence value of 641 per 100 000 – a figure that is about ten times higher than the figure obtained from mass radiographic screening in Sweden. If this ratio of the prevalence value detected by postmortem to that detected by mass radiographic screening is assumed for the other countries, the true prevalence of sarcoidosis may be between 100 and 500 per 100 000, depending on the region.

Neurosarcoidosis is detected in about 5 percent of sarcoidosis cases during life (Siltzbach et al. 1974; Delaney 1977). Postmortem series suggest that about 10 percent of sarcoidosis cases have neurological involvement which remains undetected (Ricker and Clark 1949; Waxman and Sher 1979). Subclinical optic nerve involvement has been detected in 24 percent of sarcoidosis cases (Streletz et al. 1981). Allowing for the lack of accurate (and up-to-date) information, prevalences of 100 per 100 000 for sarcoidosis and 10 per 100 000 for neurosarcoidosis would not seem unreasonable.

CLINICAL PRESENTATIONS

See Table 27.1 for a summary.

Peripheral nervous system

Skeletal muscle is commonly involved in sarcoidosis, and myopathy is a well-described primary presentation (Zisman et al. 2002) (see Chapter 32). In the peripheral nervous system neurosarcoidosis typically presents as a neuropathy – either a mononeuropathy, a mononeuritis multiplex (Garg et al. 2005) or a polyneuropathy. The most common cranial nerve involvement is a facial palsy, which can be unilateral or bilateral. When the facial palsy is associated with fever, uveitis and swelling of the parotid gland it is referred to as Heerfordt's syndrome. Other cranial nerves are less commonly involved and typically occur in association with meningeal involvement. Peripheral mononeuropathies are rare but well described, so they should be included in the differential diagnosis of any mononeuropathy or mononeuritis multiplex.

Sarcoid peripheral neuropathy is relatively rare. The presentations are variable, with motor, sensory, sensorimotor and small-fiber involvement (Vital et al. 2008). Neuropathic sensory symptoms, especially pain and dysethesias, are typically more prominent than weakness and sensory loss. Pain appears to be the main cause of disability and can be refractory to treatment. Almost always the pattern of peripheral nerve involvement is asymmetric and not length-dependent; this helps distinguish it from other distal polyneuropathies. Symmetric presentations are typically pseudo-symmetric in that the nerve conduction studies and electromyography show a multifocal pattern (Said et al. 2002). As with all neurosarcoid presentations, systemic symptoms such as fatigue, malaise, arthralgia, fever and weight loss aid in the diagnosis. The clinical course is typically subacute in onset although acute presentations have been described (Said et al. 2002; Vital et al. 2008; Fahoum et al. 2009).

Sarcoid neuropathies are predominantly axonal although demyelinating features occur. In a large series on the natural history of limb-onset sarcoid neuropathies, only 3 out of 57 cases (5 percent) were demyelinating (Burns et al. 2006). Small-fiber neuropathy including autonomic neuropathy has also been described (Bakkers et al. 2010). Surprisingly, there is even an isolated report of a peripheral nervous system presentation of neurosarcoidosis with a multifocal motor presentation with conduction block (Sawai et al. 2010). Meningeal involvement can present as polyradiculopathy, but this is usually in conjunction with intrinsic spinal cord disease (Atkinson et al. 1982).

Central nervous system

Sarcoid involvement of the CNS has a predilection for the hypothalamus and pituitary gland (Bihan et al. 2007), anterior visual pathways (Myers et al. 2004), cerebral cortex, cerebellum (Wani et al. 1999) and spinal cord (Saleh et al. 2006). Patients with pituitary involvement typically present with polydipsia and polyuria, indicative of diabetes insipidus (Miyoshi et al. 2007). Other symptoms of pituitary and/or hypothalamic involvement may be present, and these include: changes in appetite, hyperphagia with obesity (Kleine–Levine–Critchley syndrome; Afshar et al. 2008); alterations in sleep pattern (hypersomnolence, insomnia, sleep cycle reversal); narcolepsy (Rubinstein et al. 1988); impaired temperature regulation, particularly hypothermia (Lipton et al. 1977); amenorrhea (Porter et al. 2003); galactorrhea (Bihan et al. 2007); and impotence (Porter et al. 2003).

Optic neuritis and optic neuropathy is a common manifestation and is typically associated with infiltration of the optic nerve in the anterior visual pathways (Myers et al. 2004). Patients typically present with blurred vision or loss of vision. When unilateral there will be an afferent pupillary defect. Color vision is abnormal and visual field defects are common and typical of those associated with optic nerve involvement, namely central or paracentral scotomas. Co-morbid anterior and posterior uveitis is common and may result in patients complaining of floaters, pain and redness of the eye. Par planitis or intermediate uveitis is not common in sarcoidosis, and when it does occur it should raise the diagnostic possibility of multiple sclerosis (Jakob et al. 2009). Dry and gritty eyes are common and are due to conjunctival, scleral and/or lacrimal gland involvement (Menezo et al. 2009).

Focal hemispheric syndromes are common and include various lobe syndromes: frontal (Mendez and Zander 1992; Grand et al. 1996); temporal (Uruha et al. 2009); parietal

Table 27.1   Spectrum of clinical presentations attributed to neurosarcoidosis.

Syndrome	Description	References
Peripheral nervous system		
Myopathy	Proximal and focal myopathies	Covered in Chapter 32
Mononeuropathies, mononeuritis multiplex, cranial neuropathies	Facial palsy, which can be unilateral or bilateral When associated with fever, uveitis and swelling of the parotid gland it is referred to as Heerfordt's syndrome	Heerfordt 1909; Garg et al. 2005
Polyneuropathy	Motor, sensory, sensorimotor and small-fiber involvement Acute to subacute in onset. Predominantly axonal, although demyelinating features occur Autonomic neuropathy and multifocal motor neuropathy with conduction block also described	Vital et al. 2008; Said et al. 2002; Fahoum et al. 2009; Bakkers et al. 2010; Sawai et al. 2010
Radiculopathy and plexopathies	Meningeal involvement can rarely present as polyradiculopathy	Atkinson et al. 1982
Central nervous system		
Hypothalamus and pituitary gland	Diabetes insipidus, hypopituitarism, hyperphagia with obesity, hypersomnolence, insomnia, sleep cycle reversal, narcolepsy, hypothermia, amenorrhea, galactorrhea, impotence, cavernous sinus syndromes	Bihan et al. 2007; Miyoshi et al. 2007; Afshar et al. 2008; Rubinstein et al. 1988; Lipton et al. 1977; Porter et al. 2003; Chang et al. 2009; Zarei et al. 2002
Anterior visual pathways	Optic neuritis	Myers et al. 2004
Cerebral cortex, brainstem and cerebellar syndromes	Focal hemispheric syndromes, generalized confusion and raised intracranial pressure, pseudotumoral lesions, Parinaud's or dorsal mid-brain syndromes, amnesia, psychosis, psychiatric syndromes, dementia, hiccups	Kanemitsu et al. 2008; Mendez and Zander 1992; Grand et al. 1996; Uruha et al. 2009; Griggs et al. 1973; Powers 1985; Oishi et al. 2008; Makino et al. 2009; Westhout and Linskey 2008; Benzagmout et al. 2007; Willigers and Koehler 1993; Friedman and Gould 2002; Sabaawi et al. 1992; Morita and Ikeda 2004; Lin and Huang 2010
Meningeal	Sarcoid meningitis, meningoencephalitis	Ginsberg and Kidd 2008; Yuasa et al. 2000; Abrey et al. 1998
Seizures	Focal and generalized seizures, status epilepticus	Delaney 1980
Vascular and hemorrhagic syndromes	Ischemic stroke secondary to angiitis, cardiac thromboembolic disease, transient ischemic attacks, intracerebral hemorrhage, subarachnoid hemorrhage, subdural hematoma, venous sinus thrombosis	Wani et al. 1999; Navi and DeAngelis 2009; Hodge et al. 2007; Brisman et al. 2006; Peison and Padleckas 1964; Gonzalez-Aramburu et al. 2011; Yamaguchi et al. 2006; Berek et al. 1993; de Tribolet and Zander 1978; Selvi et al. 2009
Headache	Meningitic, vasculitic, space occupying with raised intracranial pressure, hydrocephalic, neuralgias	La Mantia and Erbetta 2004; Quinones-Hinojosa et al. 2003; Kraemer and Berlit 2010
Hydrocephalus	Obstructive hydrocephalus	
Spinal cord	Hypyeracute (vascular), acute (necrotizing), subacute and chronic myelopathies Diffuse or focal involvement Intra- and extra-medullary involvement	Saleh et al. 2006; Newman et al. 1997; Caccamo et al. 1992; Terunuma et al. 1988; Espinosa et al. 1985; Erickson et al. 1942; Vrbica et al. 2010; Markert et al. 2007
Conus and cauda equina syndromes	Distal spinal cord with sphincter involvement Lumbar sacral	Shah and Lewis 2003; Marra 1982; Kaiboriboon et al. 2005; Zajicek 1990
Olfaction	Anosmia	Reed et al. 2010; Kieff et al. 1997
Extrapyramidal syndromes	Tremor, opsoclonus, focal and hemidystonia	Ogawa et al. 2008; Henriet et al. 1991; Ellefsen 1970a,b; Caviness and Knox 1996
Fatigue	Chronic fatigue syndrome	Greim et al. 2007

(Griggs et al. 1973); and occipital (Powers 1985). Brainstem and cerebellar involvement are also well-described (Oishi et al. 2008; Makino et al. 2009). Generalized confusion is less common and may be due to raised intracranial pressure from hydrocephalus (Westhout and Linskey 2008; Benzagmout et al. 2007) or pseudotumoral lesions (Grand et al. 1996), sarcoid meningitis (Ginsberg and Kidd 2008), meningoencephalitis (Yuasa et al. 2000) or seizures (Delaney 1980).

Confusion due to seizures occurs post-ictally or due to focal non-convulsive status.

Cerebrovascular involvement is rare, but includes transient ischemic attacks (Gonzalez-Aramburu et al. 2011), ischemic stroke syndromes (Brisman et al. 2006; Hodge et al. 2007; Navi and DeAngelis 2009), intracerebral hemorrhage (Yamaguchi et al. 2006), subarachnoid hemorrhage (Berek et al. 1993), subdural hematoma (de Tribolet and Zander 1978) and venous sinus thrombosis (Selvi et al. 2009; Degardin et al. 2010). Ischemic stroke is presumably due to granulomatous angiitis (Peison and Padleckas 1964) or cardiac thromboembolic disease – the latter being due to cardiac involvement (Kanemitsu et al. 2008).

Headache is a common, albeit non-specific, manifestation of sarcoidosis occurring in up to 30 percent of patients with neurosarcoidosis (La Mantia and Erbetta 2004). Headache needs to be interpreted in the context of the history, examination and investigations. Headache typically occurs with meningeal involvement, hydrocephalus, cranial nerve involvement (Quinones-Hinojosa et al. 2003) or rarely granulomatous angiitis (Kraemer and Berlit 2010).

Meningeal involvement is one of the most common CNS manifestations of neurosarcoidosis. The presentations are protean and vary from chronic meningitis with headache, photophobia and neck stiffness, cranial nerve palsies, obstructive hydrocephalus with or without visual symptoms, spinal nerve root and cauda equina syndromes (Abrey et al. 1998), and very rarely pseudotumoral presentations due to mass effect from large granulomas. A good example of meningeal sarcoid granulomas mistaken for a tumor is the striking case of Jackson and colleagues presenting with headache, decreased memory, personality changes and incoordination and found to have parafalcine and bilateral convexity meningeal involvement that was thought initially to be a meningioma (Jackson et al. 1998).

Obstructive hydrocephalus due to meningeal involvement can be a difficult problem to manage. The hydrocephalus is frequently associated with extensive meningeal disease and a high cerebrospinal fluid (CSF) protein level. In addition to immunomodulation, CSF diversion procedures, for example lumbar peritoneal and ventricular peritoneal shunts, are effective in reducing the raised pressure. The relief is often temporary with a tendency of the shunts to malfunction as a result of blockages due to the high levels of CSF protein. These patients typically develop chronic papilledema, with enlarged blind spots and constricted visual fields. If not managed aggressively the chronic papilledema will lead to optic atrophy with reduced central visual acuities and ultimately blindness. In this setting it may be worth trying acetazolamide, a carbonic anhydrase inhibitor, to reduce the production of CSF. Other surgical procedures, such as optic nerve sheath fenestration (Ramsey et al. 2006) and the largely abandoned subtemporal craniotomy (Papadakis and Epstein 1975), may be tried in patients who fail to respond to standard measures.

Myelopathy is one of the 'classic' presentations of neurosarcoidosis and is widely believed to more common in patients with African ancestry (Newman et al. 1997). The presentations can be very protean with hyperacute vascular (Caccamo et al. 1992), acute or more commonly subacute to chronic presentations. Clinically patients present with paraparesis (Terunuma et al. 1988), triparesis or quadriparesis (Espinosa et al. 1985), spinal cord sensory syndromes, sphincter involvement, occasionally with autonomic spinal dysreflexia (Erickson et al. 1942) and with conus and cauda equina syndromes (Marra 1982; Zajicek 1990; Shah and Lewis 2003; Kaiboriboon et al. 2005). Although the cervical cord appears to be affected more than other segments (Nagai et al. 1985), no part of the cord is spared and in almost a third of cases there is diffuse involvement (Saleh et al. 2006). The distribution can be intramedullary (Beros et al. 2008) or secondary to meningeal or vascular involvement. Rarely, the involvement may be compressive due to pachymeningitis (Mehta et al. 2006). The prognosis is variable and relates to the tempo of the onset of the myelopathy. In acute necrotizing granulomatous myelopathy, the prognosis is invariably poor (Markert et al. 2007; Vrbica et al. 2010), presumably due to vascular involvement. In comparison, a gradual-onset myelopathy, with minimal disability, diagnosed and managed appropriately, usually has a favorable outcome.

Rarer CNS manifestations include hypopituitarism, narcolepsy (Rubinstein et al. 1988), cavernous sinus syndromes (Zarei et al. 2002; Chang et al. 2009), Parinaud's or dorsal midbrain syndrome (Oishi et al. 2008), amnesia (Willigers and Koehler 1993), psychosis (Friedman and Gould 2002), psychiatric syndromes (Sabaawi et al. 1992), dementia (Morita and Ikeda 2004), hiccups (Lin and Huang 2010), anosmia (Kieff et al. 1997; Reed et al. 2010), tremor (Ogawa et al. 2008), opsoclonus (Henriet et al. 1991), and focal dystonia (Ellefsen 1970a,b) or hemidystonia (Caviness and Knox 1996).

Fatigue is common in patients with neurosarcoidosis and other immune-mediated diseases of the CNS (Greim et al. 2007). It is rarely the primary presentation of neurosarcoidosis but is often resistant to treatment.

DIAGNOSIS

Diagnostic criteria for neurosarcoidosis

The aim of a diagnostic work-up is to increase one's diagnostic confidence of the person having the disease in question and to exclude other conditions in the differential diagnosis, which in some cases is extensive.

Ideally one should aim for a diagnosis of *definite* or *probable* neurosarcoidosis (Chamoun et al. 2011; Box 27.1). These two diagnostic categories require the diagnosis of neurosarcoidosis to be confirmed histologically, which is very important to exclude other infectious etiologies and sarcoid mimics. If a biopsy is not possible or desirable because of the site involved, a diagnosis of possible neurosarcoidosis can be made based on the clinical picture. The Kveim test, which is now not used owing to the risk of transmitting an infectious agent, was commonly used to support the diagnosis and is referred to mainly for historical reasons in Box 27.1.

The clinical support for the diagnosis needs two or more findings, such as typical chest X-ray, or gallium or FDG-PET scan findings, or elevated serum angiotensin-converting enzyme (ACE) levels. Hypercalcemia and/or hypercalciuria

Box 27.1 New diagnostic criteria for neurosarcoidosis (Chamoun *et al.* 2011)

Essential criteria to be fulfilled by all cases

i. Multisystem disease with neurological involvement compatible with sarcoidosis
ii. Neurological and systemic involvement must be temporally related with evidence of disease activity occurring within 5 years of each other
iii. No occupational or surgical exposure to inorganic foreign bodies
iv. No alternative diagnoses

1. **Possible** neurosarcoidosis – clinically supported
    1a: Clinically supported without Kveim testing*
        Clinical picture compatible with sarcoidosis
    1b: Clinically supported with Kveim testing
        Clinical picture compatible with sarcoidosis and histological evidence of granulomatous reaction on Kveim testing*
2. **Probable** neurosarcoidosis – histologically supported by non-nervous tissue biopsy
    Histological evidence of sarcoid granulomas on a non-nervous tissue biopsy.
3. **Definite** neurosarcoidosis – histologically supported by nervous tissue biopsy
    Histological evidence of sarcoid granulomas on nervous tissue biopsy

Notes

● Multisystem disease: There must be definite evidence of symptomatic or asymptomatic involvement of at least two organ systems using clinical, paraclinical (radiological, radionucleotide scanning or biochemically) or histological (organ biopsy) criteria. If not confirmed histologically the pattern of organ involvement should be compatible with sarcoidosis.
● Neurological involvement. This must be definite evidence of symptomatic or asymptomatic involvement of the central or peripheral nervous systems using clinical, paraclinical (radiological, neurophysiological) or histological (nervous tissue biopsy) criteria.
● * Kveim testing is not used now but is included for historical reasons to allow the retrospective application of these criteria.

are *not* sufficient to be used in isolation to support the diagnosis as they rarely if ever occur in the absence of easily identifiable systemic disease or a raised serum ACE. We emphasize the importance in all cases of demonstrating that:

● that the disease is a multisystem disease with neurological involvement compatible with sarcoidosis;
● the neurological and systemic involvement is temporally related, with evidence of disease activity occurring within 5 years of each other;
● there is no occupational or surgical exposure to inorganic foreign bodies that can result in granulomatous disease;
● there is no alternative diagnosis.

The proposal that neurosarcoidosis can be a single-organ disease, as some have suggested (e.g. Hoitsma *et al.* 2004), is incompatible with the current definitions of sarcoidosis (James 1976). The temporal association between neurological and systemic disease is very important. In our experience it is not uncommon for clinicians to label patients presenting with neurological symptoms as having neurosarcoidosis, when they simply have a past or remote history of sarcoidosis. Sarcoidosis is often monophasic and resolves spontaneously (Scadding and Mitchell 1985), so the assumption that the contemporary neurological presentation is due to neurosarcoidosis is flawed, particularly if the history of previous sarcoidosis is remote. Unless there is evidence of active systemic sarcoidosis within the last 5 years the diagnosis of neurosarcoidosis is unlikely and the patient should have an appropriate diagnostic work-up, to investigate alternative conditions.

The differential diagnosis

See Table 27.2.

Sarcoidosis is a multifocal disease, so its involvement of the nervous system is often protean. Neurosarcoidosis has been associated with virtually all known neurological presentations and should therefore be considered as a potential diagnosis for any neuro-inflammatory condition, particularly when there are associated signs of systemic disease.

Neurosarcoidosis is notorious for mimicking a number of more common conditions. In fact in the modern era sarcoidosis and not syphilis should be referred to as the great mimicker (Brinar and Habek 2008; Walid *et al.* 2008). Almost all neurological syndromes have been described with sarcoidosis. When a neurological presentation occurs in the setting of systemic sarcoidosis the diagnosis is usually easily made. In neurological practice in the developed world the main differential is between neurosarcoidosis, other granulomatous conditions (particularly isolated CNS vasculitis; Younger *et al.* 1988), multiple sclerosis (Scott *et al.* 2010) and the uveomeningeal syndromes (Lueck *et al.* 1993).

LYMPHOMA AND HISTIOCYTOSIS

Lymphoma (Santos and Scolding 2010) and the histiocytic syndromes (Sheu *et al.* 2004) can be notoriously difficult to distinguish clinically from neurosarcoidosis, but are easily differentiated histologically. Erdheim–Chester disease, a non-Langerhan's cell histiocytosis, frequently presents with CNS involvement and is typically misdiagnosed as neurosarcoidosis.

Table 27.2   Differential diagnosis of neurosarcoidosis.

Disease	Clinical scenario	References
Multiple sclerosis and neuromyelitis optica	Particularly when associated with uveitis. The uveitis can be posterior, intermediate (par planitis) or anterior	Scott et al. 2010; Walid et al. 2008; Brinar and Habek 2008; Kasp et al. 1989; Graham et al. 1989
CNS vasculitis	Non-granulomatous and granulomatous Wegner's granulomatosis, polyarteritis nodosa, Churg–Strauss syndrome	Younger et al. 1988
Uveo-meningeal syndromes	Behçet's disease, Vogt–Koyanagi–Harada syndrome, Wegener's granulomatosis, autoimmune overlap syndromes	Lueck et al. 1993; Ideguchi et al. 2010; Keino et al. 2009; Brazis et al. 2004
CNS lymphoma	Can be isolated CNS lymphoma or systemic lymphoma with CNS involvement	Santos and Scolding 2010
Histiocytic syndromes	Focal and generalized histiocytosis, Erdheim–Chester disease, Rosai–Dorfman disease	Sheu et al. 2004; Kidd et al. 2006
Other granulomatous conditions	Vasculitis, lymphoma and tumor-related	Newman et al. 1997
Infections	Tuberculosis, brucellosis, histoplasmosis, paracoccidioidomycosis, cryptococcosis, Nocardia, Lyme disease, neurosyphilis, cysticercosis, schistosomiasis, toxoplasmosis, herpes infection in immunocompromised hosts	Buitrago et al. 2011; Marie et al. 2010; Favre et al. 1998; Jain et al. 2006; Ishihara et al. 1998; Ito et al. 1998; Cohen-Gadol et al. 2003; Perez Olivan et al. 2002; Ideguchi et al. 2010; Keino et al. 2009; Brazis et al. 2004

Rosai–Dorfman disease, which is characterized by histiocytic infiltration of lymphoid tissue, is a systemic disease that frequently involves the orbit and nasopharynx and on rare occasions presents with neurological manifestations that can mimic neurosarcoidosis (Kidd et al. 2006). These particular conditions are very difficult to distinguish from neurosarcoidosis without a tissue diagnosis. The rule is: 'if in doubt, a biopsy should be performed'.

INFECTIONS

In the developing countries it is particularly important to exclude infectious diseases, particularly tuberculosis, neurosyphilis and brucellosis. Other infectious mimics include systemic fungal infections such as histoplasmosis and paracoccidioidomycosis (Buitrago et al. 2011), cryptococcosis (Marie et al. 2010), Nocardia (Favre et al. 1998) and Lyme disease (Ishihara et al. 1998; Jain et al. 2006). Fungal and nocardial infections are particularly pertinent in the setting of systemic immunosuppression.

In the immunocompromised host, viral infections may also need to be considered. For example, the presentation and course of herpes infections are often atypical; they tend to be subacute in onset, with a more indolent course and frequently with multisystem involvement, particularly of the retina and uveal tract. The main parasitic infections that need to be excluded in relation to neurosarcoidosis are cysticercosis (Ito et al. 1998), schistosomiasis (Cohen-Gabol et al. 2003) and toxoplasmosis (Perez Olivan et al. 2002). The presence of blood eosinophilia should alert one to consider the possibility of parasitosis or the Churg–Strauss syndrome.

UVEOMENINGITIC SYNDROMES

The uveomeningitic syndromes are often confused with neurosarcoidosis. These include Behçet's disease (Ideguchi et al. 2010), Vogt–Koyanagi–Harada syndrome (Keino et al. 2009), Wegener's granulomatosis (Brazis et al. 2004), overlap autoimmune syndromes, lymphoma and the various infections referred to above. In our experience, however, the occurrence of uveitis in association with multiple sclerosis remains the most common indication for a diagnostic work-up to exclude the diagnosis of neurosarcoidosis (Graham et al. 1989; Kasp et al. 1989).

MULTIPLE SCLEROSIS

Distinguishing neurosarcoidosis from multiple sclerosis can be particularly difficult and vexed (Ketonen et al. 1986; Oksanen and Salmi 1986; Oksanen 1986,1987,1994; Ketonen et al. 1987; McLean et al. 1990). There is no easy way to confirm or exclude neurosarcoidosis and we would therefore urge clinicians to be very cautious when making the diagnosis. It is clear that most existing diagnostic criteria have been formulated incorrectly (Chamoun et al. 2011) and have allowed patients with other disease to be inadvertently classified as having neurosarcoidosis (James et al. 1976; Zajicek et al. 1999). The risks inherent in managing neurosarcoidosis with long-term corticosteroids or immunosuppressive agents are well known (Zajicek et al. 1999; Zajicek 2000; Hoitsma et al. 2004,2010; Schwendimann et al. 2009; Terushkin et al. 2010), but the implications of diagnostic uncertainty are particularly pertinent with the emergence of effective disease-modifying therapies for multiple sclerosis (Giovannoni 2011).

Proposed new criteria

Our limited understanding of neurosarcoidosis has arisen for several reasons. The number of patients in most collected series is simply too small to allow reliable generalizations. This is not just because neurosarcoidosis is uncommon; diagnostic criteria that could be expected to be accurate are normally too impractical for routine clinical use. The most commonly cited criterion for definite disease requires 'a compatible clinical picture of a multisystem disease and histological confirmation of sarcoid tissue' (James and Sharma 1967; Hoitsma *et al.* 2004). An organ biopsy, especially brain biopsy, is often unjustifiable.

Whatever selection criterion is used, its predictive value is likely to be unknown. The numbers of false diagnoses within such series cannot be assumed to be negligible. Consequently, features of other diseases have become associated with neurosarcoidosis, while the statistical significance of genuine relationships become eroded. Small series are particularly vulnerable to the biasing effects of false diagnoses.

Finally, the risk of circular analysis appears when selection criteria are not explicit (Hoitsma *et al.* 2010). The findings observed within a series may thus simply reflect the initial basis for case selection.

To address these problems we applied an evidence-based approach and proposed the new set of diagnostic criteria for neurosarcoidosis presented in Box 27.1.

INVESTIGATIONS

Neuroimaging: CT and MRI

Computerized tomography (CT) and magnetic resonance imaging (MRI) can both be used to localize pathology in neurosarcoidosis, but MRI has become the investigation of choice with its better anatomical localization of lesions (Pickuth and Heywang-Kobrunner 2000; Pickuth *et al.* 2000). MRI is safer than CT with regard to the repeat imaging that is usually required to monitor the response of the disease to therapy.

Lesions in neurosarcoidosis typically enhance after the administration of gadolinium (Gd) and may be associated with edema and mass effect. However, late in the disease course and when patients are receiving corticosteroid or other immunosuppressive therapy, the enhancement may be suppressed (Pickuth and Heywang-Kobrunner 2000; Pickuth *et al.* 2000). Gd-enhanced imaging in combination with CSF analysis is helpful in documenting meningeal involvement. MRI shows thickening and enhancement of the leptomeninges and nerve-root thickening. Dural enhancement also occurs (Lury *et al.* 2004). CT and MRI are particularly useful in excluding other conditions and for detecting complications of sarcoidosis, for example hydrocephalus (Benzagmout *et al.* 2007; Westhout and Linskey 2008) and cerebral infarction as a result of granulomatous angiitis (Peison and Padleckas 1964), or cardio-thromboembolic disease (Kanemitsu *et al.* 2008). Pseudotumoral lesions detected on MRI from granulomatous masses also occur (Grand *et al.* 1996). Rarely neurosarcoidosis can present with hemorrhage: intracerebral (Yamaguchi *et al.* 2006), subarachnoid (Berek *et al.* 1993) or subdural (de Tribolet and Zander (1978). Venous sinus thrombosis as a complication of neurosarcoidosis has also been described (Degardin *et al.* 2010; Selvi *et al.* 2009).

Spinal cord atrophy is seen early in necrotizing disease or as a late-stage phenomenon in chronic disease (Junger *et al.* 1993). The MRI appearances are not specific and can be highly variable. Enhancement can typically be seen to start or be more prominent on the meningeal surface and extend into the cord parenchyma, which has led some to claim that it starts at the meninges and affects the cord secondarily (Nesbit *et al.* 1989).

Junger and colleagues have classified the MRI manifestations of the intramedullary lesions into the following four stages, on the premise that the gadolinium enhancement is associated with active inflammation (Junger *et al.* 1993):

- Stage 1 presents as linear leptomeningeal enhancement and is a sign of early inflammation.
- In stage 2 the inflammation spreads through the perivascular or Virchow–Robin spaces leading to parenchymal involvement and is seen as diffusely enhancing lesions within the cord parenchyma.
- Stage 3 presents with a relatively normal-sized cord with focal or multifocal areas of enhancement.
- Stage 4 occurs when there is relative atrophy of the cord and no gadolinium enhancement.

The suppression of gadolinium enhancement on MRI is very helpful in detecting and monitoring a response to treatment (Christoforidis *et al.* 1999; Dumas *et al.* 2000) and is a useful marker to monitor subclinical recurrence (Koike *et al.* 2000; Ravaglia *et al.* 2003).

Gallium and PET scanning

A whole-body gallium (Ga) scan may show increased uptake. Gallium uptake may be related to CNS disease in fewer than 5 percent of patients with neurosarcoidosis, but may give evidence of the presence of systemic disease in 45 percent of patients with CNS involvement. Gallium-67 citrate, which is injected intravenously, is not only taken up by sites of active sarcoid, but also localizes other inflammatory and neoplastic processes such as tuberculosis and lymphoma.

The introduction of whole-body (18)F-fluoro-2-deoxy-D-glucose positron emission tomography, particularly in combination with computed tomography (so-called (18)F-FDG PET/CT), has effectively replaced gallium scanning because of its increased sensitivity (Braun *et al.* 2008; Seve *et al.* 2009; Kim *et al.* 2010; Morgenthau and Iannuzzi 2011). The lack of specificity limits the utility of the gallium and (18)F-FDG PET scanning as a primary diagnostic test (Johns and Michele 1999; Braun *et al.* 2008). However, both these investigations are helpful in identifying systemic sites of involvement for potential biopsy (Johns and Michele 1999; Braun *et al.* 2008; Balan *et al.* 2010). In the case of (18)F-FDG PET/CT, focal areas of pathological tracer uptake have been shown to regress with treatment and increase during recurrence (Braun *et al.* 2008). (18)F-FDG PET is therefore a potentially useful modality to assess the efficacy of treatment in patients with neurosarcoidosis (Aide *et al.* 2007; Bolat *et al.* 2009).

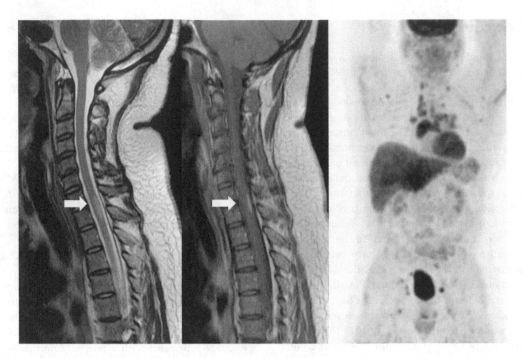

Figure 27.1   MRI of the cervical spine of a 45-year-old male presenting with a 2-month history of tingling in his toes, positive Lhermitte's phenomenon, perineal hypoesthesia and sexual dysfunction. T2-weighted MRI on the left shows a high signal lesion in the posterior cord, extending from lower body of C7 to T1, associated with some mild cord swelling. The middle image, a T1-weighted MRI done after the administration of gadolinium, demonstrates linear enhancement of the lesion. The FDG-PET/CT on the right shows numerous areas of increased tracer uptake in small nuchal, posterior triangle and in the left supraclavicular, mediastinal, hilar and subcarinal lymph nodes. Moderate uptake is noted in the axillary lymph nodes bilaterally and in a nodular pattern in both lungs. The liver demonstrates heterogeneous, intensely increased tracer uptake and multiple foci are also seen in the spleen and porta hepatis, left common iliac and external iliac lymph nodes bilaterally. Liver biopsy demonstrated non-caseating granulomas compatible with sarcoidosis.

Cerebrospinal fluid analysis

Spinal fluid analysis is a useful adjunct in the investigation of a patient presenting with symptoms and signs of possible neurosarcoidosis. Importantly, CSF analysis is an essential investigation in helping exclude other potential diagnoses. The majority of patients with CNS disease (>75 percent) will have elevated CSF total protein levels, i.e. ≥0.5 g/L (Zajicek *et al.* 1999). Occasionally, when there is a CSF block, the total protein is markedly raised; this typically occurs with severe pachymeningitis of the spinal cord. CSF examination typically shows a lymphocytic pleocytosis, an increase in total protein and hypoglycorrhachia.

In approximately 50 percent of patients there is a raised leukocyte count (≥5 cells/mm^3), which is usually a lymphocytosis (Zajicek *et al.* 1999). A neutrophilia and/or eosinophilia should alert one to alternative diagnoses, for example Behçet's disease or parasitic infections, respectively.

CSF glucose may be depressed, usually associated with a pleocytosis. Very low glucose levels as are seen in tuberculous meningitis and CNS lymphomas are rarely if ever associated with neurosarcoidosis. ACE in the cerebrospinal fluid is raised in the minority of cases (see below). Local synthesis of CSF oligoclonal bands is rare and if found should alert one to an alternative diagnosis (Chamoun *et al.* 2011), particularly multiple sclerosis or infection.

Angiotensin-converting enzyme in CSF

In 1975, Lieberman measured serum ACE concentrations in 200 patients with chronic lung disease and 200 healthy controls. Enzyme levels were either normal or depressed in the vast majority of patients with lung disease, but were elevated in 15 of 17 cases of active sarcoidosis. Patients with sarcoidosis who were receiving corticosteroid treatment did not have raised levels. Lieberman's test has since been used in the diagnosis of sarcoidosis and in monitoring disease activity.

It was therefore natural to consider CSF levels of activity of the enzyme in the diagnosis and monitoring of neurosarcoidosis. The development of a particularly specific and sensitive inhibitor binding assay (Fyhrquist *et al.* 1984) afforded the opportunity to examine the ACE activity in CSF. Oksanen and associates examined the CSF and serum ACE activity in 20 patients with neurosarcoidosis, 9 of whom were taking corticosteroids; these were compared to three sets of controls: 12 patients with sarcoidosis devoid of neurological involvement, 49 patients with neurological diseases other than neurosarcoidosis, and 38 patients who underwent a lumbar puncture but in whom disease was excluded (Oksanen *et al.* 1985). The findings demonstrated that the mean CSF ACE (CACE) level was significantly higher in neurosarcoidosis than in healthy controls or in patients with non-neurological sarcoidosis. The mean level was also higher than in demyelinating diseases, cerebrovascular attacks and polyneuropathies – provided corticosteroids were not being administered. Importantly, a significant difference in CACE levels was not evident between patients with neurosarcoidosis and those with brain tumors or CNS infections.

A recently published critical appraisal of the literature reveals that CACE levels are very insensitive (24–55 percent), but if elevated are reasonably specific for CNS neurosarcoidosis

(94–95 percent; Khoury *et al.* 2009). However, the authors concluded that CACE cannot replace tissue diagnosis. We would agree with their conclusions and would not rely on a normal level of ACE in cerebrospinal fluid to exclude a diagnosis of neurosarcoidosis, nor would we recommend a raised CACE level as the only paraclinical test to support a diagnosis of possible neurosarcoidosis.

The Kveim skin test

The Kveim (or Nickerson–Kveim or Kveim–Siltzbach) skin test was widely used in the investigation of sarcoidosis. It was performed by injecting a splenic extract from a patient with known sarcoidosis into the skin of a patient suspected of having sarcoidosis. If granulomas were found on a biopsy, 4–6 weeks later, the test was regarded as positive. If the patient had been taking treatment, particularly a corticosteroid, the test give a false negative result. The test is not now performed in the UK. There is a concern that certain infections, such as bovine spongiform encephalopathy, could be transmitted through a Kveim test and as a result there has been no testing in the UK since 1996. Although the Kveim test has high sensitivity and specificity in systemic sarcoidosis, its performance in neurosarcoidosis has never been formerly assessed.

An immunoblotting technique, for the detection of antigen-specific immunoglobulin G (IgG), using Kveim material as antigen was developed and applied to paired sera and cerebrospinal fluid from patients with neurosarcoidosis (McLean *et al.* 1990). Only patients whose CSF showed local synthesis of oligoclonal total IgG were likely to have local synthesis of 'Kveim-specific IgG'. These results have not been reproduced. In the light of our findings that indicate that CSF oligoclonal IgG bands are uncommon or rare in neurosarcoidosis (Chamoun *et al.* 2011), we now interpret the binding of oligoclonal IgG bands to Kveim antigen as being non-specific. In conclusion, we would not recommend using the Kveim antigen-specific immunoblotting test to aid in the diagnosis of neurosarcoidosis.

TREATMENT

As neurosarcoidosis is a relatively uncommon disease there are no double-blind placebo-controlled trials to guide therapy. Most therapeutic decisions are empirical based on experience with immunosuppressive drugs in systemic sarcoidosis.

A general principle is that most experts recommend earlier and more aggressive treatment than with systemic sarcoidosis (see Chapter 42). Aggressive early immunosuppression appears to be associated with a more favorable course. When inflammation is left to 'smolder', due to suboptimal treatment, it tends to result in progressive accumulation of neurological deficits and ultimately a poorer prognosis. These comments are based on our collective experience in a tertiary setting with a high likelihood of referral bias.

Prior to starting immunosuppressive therapy it is essential to predefine treatment responses and obtain objective baseline assessments in order to be in a position to monitor disease activity. Gd-enhanced MRI, FDG-PET, CSF analysis and systemic markers of inflammation – for example, serum ACE and C-reactive protein levels – are important adjuncts for monitoring a response to treatment, in addition to clinical measures of improvement.

Immunosuppression

Corticosteroids, typically in combination with a steroid sparing agent, remain the cornerstone of therapy. Recommendations for initial therapy are typically in the order of 1–2 mg/kg daily of oral prednisolone (Hoitsma *et al.* 2004). This is higher than the typical dose advised for the treatment of systemic sarcoidosis.

On the assumption that patients will need to remain on corticosteroids for longer than 6 months, it is advisable to initiate a steroid sparing agent simultaneously. Typically this would be methotrexate at a dose of 7.5–15 mg per week (Kaliszky *et al.* 2002). An alternative option is azathioprine (Baughman *et al.* 2008). It is important to measure the patient's red cell thiopurine methyl transferase (TPMT) activity prior to starting azathioprine. It is generally advised that azathioprine should be avoided in slow azathioprine metabolizers, because of the risk of bone marrow suppression. The majority of subjects will be normal metabolizers and will require a maintenance dose of 2–3 mg/kg daily. In comparison, approximately 4 percent of the population who are rapid azathioprine metabolizers will require a higher dose, typically in the range 4–5 mg/kg daily. It is advisable to monitor the lymphocyte count with the aim of inducing a mild lymphopenia of $0.8–1.2 \times 10^9$/L; this is a relatively good indicator that the dose of azathioprine is in the required therapeutic range. Starting azathioprine at 50 mg per day in adults and increasing by 25 mg per day every two weeks, provided the liver function tests and blood counts remain normal, reduces the chance of patients stopping the therapy due to gastrointestinal side-effects.

In patients unable to tolerate either methotrexate or azathioprine, other options include mycophenolate mofetil (Androdias *et al.* 2011), leflunomide (Baughman *et al.* 2008) or ciclosporin A (Patel *et al.* 2007).

Once patients have been established on daily prednisolone and a maintenance dose of a steroid sparing agent for at least 6–12 weeks, the alternate-day dose of prednisolone can be tapered. The dose can typically be tapered by 10 mg alternate day every 1–2 weeks until the patient is only taking alternate-day prednisolone. Provided the patient has responded to treatment and there are no signs of a flare-up in disease activity, the alternate-day steroids can then be tapered as well. This should be done slowly; initially by 10 mg alternate days every 2–4 weeks until the patient is on 40 mg alternate days and then by 5 mg alternate days every 2–4 weeks.

Tapering the prednisone slowly allows one to get an idea of the minimal effective maintenance dose of prednisolone the patient requires should a flare-up in disease activity occur. From experience, the maintenance dose is variable and difficult to predict in individual patients. When being weaned from the relatively high doses of prednisolone, patients should be made aware of the possibility of developing

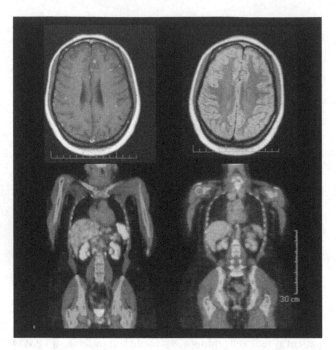

Figure 27.2   A 35-year-old female presented with parotid and lacrimal gland swelling and erythema nodosum. Sarcoidosis was diagnosed after a minor salivary gland biopsy. Despite treatment with oral prednisone and azathioprine therapy her disease progressed with eye involvement. She developed monocular blindness after neovascularization of her left optic disk. She was unable to tolerate ciclosporin A, mycophenolate mofetil or methotrexate. Her disease was stabilized with 6-weekly intravenous methylprednisolone and cyclophosphamide infusions. She subsequently presented with headaches and meningeal symptoms. Neurological involvement was confirmed by MR studies of the brain and spinal cord. After switching her onto infliximab with concurrent azathioprine therapy her symptoms resolved. On the left is a gadolinium-enhanced T1-weighted MRI of the head matched with a whole body FDG-PET/CT prior to treatment with infliximab. Multiple contrast enhancing nodules are seen throughout the meninges and are associated with extensive tracer uptake in the periphery. Twelve months after infliximab therapy there is almost complete resolution of disease.

pseudo-rheumatism – typically the occurrence of generalized arthralgias and myalgias. This should not be interpreted as a flare-up of their sarcoidosis (Hargreave et al. 1969).

It is important that when a patient is started on prednisolone he or she has blood glucose levels and blood pressures checked on a regular basis; this should be weekly initially, and then monthly once the patient is established on a maintenance dose. If a patient develops diabetes or hypertension, these should be managed appropriately. All patients should also have a baseline bone densitometry done and should be started on osteoporosis prophylaxis. This will typically include a combination of bisphosphonate, vitamin D and calcium supplements. The uninterrupted long-term use of bisphosphonates, for periods of longer than 5 years, has been called into question, in view of the potential for inducing brittle bone disease and osteonecrosis (Friedrich and Blake 2007). It is recommended that patients needing to be maintained on long-term corticosteroids should be referred to a metabolic bone clinic for supervision of the management of their osteoporosis prophylaxis. In addition, all patients should be counseled about the side-effects of long-term steroid

therapy, provided with a steroid card, and specifically warned about the potential for developing rare serious adverse events – particularly Addisonian crises (Jacobs et al. 1988), opportunistic infections and avascular necrosis of the hip, long bones and vertebrae (Ito et al. 2005; Powell et al. 2010).

In addition to the 'standard' steroid sparing immunosuppressive agents there have been favorable reports of chloroquine phosphate and hydroxychloroquine sulfate as adjunctive treatment to prednisolone. Chloroquine is typically prescribed at 250 mg twice daily and hydroxychloroquine at 200 mg twice daily. In one small retrospective series, only 2 out of 12 patients failed to respond to the addition of chloroquine and hydroxychloroquine (Sharma 1998). The recommended doses are generally safe, but at higher doses both drugs can cause irreversible ototoxicity and retinopathy (Bernstein et al. 1963). For patients receiving long-term chloroquine therapy it is advised that that they are monitored every 3–6 months for these retinal and neurological complications.

The practice of using pulsed high-dose intravenous methylprednisolone, once weekly or monthly, as induction therapy or in patients refractory to oral steroids, is based on empirical observations in systemic sarcoidosis. Intravenous methylprednisolone allows more rapid suppression of inflammation and is also particularly useful in patients with space-occupying lesions and marked cerebral or spinal cord edema. The effects of high-dose corticosteroids on edema are due to membrane rather than their anti-inflammatory effects (Andersson and Goodkin 1998).

In patients refractory to the combination of prednisolone and a steroid sparing agent, the response to infliximab has been very promising (Keijsers et al. 2008; Moravan and Segal 2009; Sodhi et al. 2009; Chintamaneni et al. 2010; Vargas and Stern 2010). Infliximab is a monoclonal antibody that neutralizes soluble TNF-α and targets macrophages expressing TNF-α on their surface. In the past these patients would have been treated with pulsed cyclophosphamide (Doty et al. 2003). Infliximab has to be given in combination with either methotrexate or azathioprine to prevent the development of neutralizing antibodies that are responsible for some of the infusion reactions seen with infliximab (Ebert et al. 2008). Infliximab is associated with an increased incidence of opportunistic infections, particularly tuberculosis, so patients should be screened for latent disease. If there is evidence of previous TB, the person should either receive TB prophylaxis or be treated simultaneously for TB.

Radiation therapy

There are reports of radiation therapy in patients with refractory neurosarcoidosis with focal disease of the spine (Kang and Suh 1999; Menninger et al. 2003) or more extensive disease of the brain (Bejar et al. 1985; Rubinstein et al. 1988). These patients are usually very disabled and it is difficult to know, without randomized trials, whether or not radiotherapy is effective. Our local experience with localized radiotherapy to the spinal cord has been disappointing; neurological deficits have continued to progress despite there being no signs of ongoing inflammation in the spinal cord. Without better evidence we are reluctant to recommend radiotherapy.

Surgery

Occasionally neurosurgical intervention is necessary to treat life-threatening complications, for example resection of pseudotumoral granulomatous tissue masses compressing the spinal cord, optic nerve or brainstem (Fried *et al.* 1993). It is not uncommon for a diagnosis of neurosarcoidosis to be made after histological analysis of tissue removed as part of emergency neurosurgery. The most frequent indication for surgical intervention is CSF diversion procedures to manage hydrocephalus in patients with chronic granulomatous meningitis (Foley *et al.* 1989).

CONCLUSION

Neurosarcoidosis has supplanted neurosyphilis as the great mimicker. As it is a multifocal disease it is highly variable in its clinical presentations. However, it has a predilection for the meninges, particularly the basal and spinal meninges, and therefore often presents with involvement of the anterior visual pathways, hypothalamus, pituitary gland, posterior fossa structures and spinal cord. As it is a multisystem disease it usually presents in association with systemic disease.

Thorough investigation is always required to make the diagnosis. Histological confirmation is usually necessary to exclude other conditions that mimic sarcoidosis, particularly the generalized histiocytosis syndromes, infections, malignancies and uveomeningitic syndromes. Neuroimaging, radionucleotide metabolic imaging (gallium and FDG-PET imaging), CSF analysis, ACE and other blood tests are not specific enough to make a confident diagnosis of neurosarcoidosis, but may provide important supportive information.

Corticosteroids, typically in combination with a steroid sparing agent, remain the cornerstone of therapy. More recently, in patients refractory to corticosteroids, the response to anti-TNF-α therapies appears promising. Gd-enhanced MRI, FDG-PET and repeat CSF analysis are important for monitoring response to treatment.

The prognosis is variable and depends on the clinical site of involvement and the tempo of the disease onset. Clinical presentations that are hyperacute in onset imply vascular involvement due a granulomatous angiitis, and have the poorest prognosis. In general, aggressive early immunosuppression is associated with a more favorable course. When inflammation is left to 'smolder' due to suboptimal immunosuppression, it tends to result in progressive accumulation of neurological deficits and a poorer prognosis. Long-term immunosuppression is frequently associated with secondary complications.

Neurosarcoidosis is a rare disease and as a result there are as yet no large well-controlled trials of treatment. One option would be to enrol patients in an international register so that prospective high-quality observational data could be collected, to improve the management of this enigmatic disease.

REFERENCES

Abrey LE, Rosenblum MK, DeAngelis LM (1998). Sarcoidosis of the cauda equina mimicking leptomeningeal malignancy. *J Neurooncol* 39: 261–5.

Afshar K, Engelfried K, Sharma OP (2008). Sarcoidosis: a rare cause of Kleine–Levine–Critchley syndrome. *Sarcoid Vasc Diff Lung Dis* 25: 60–3.

Aide N et al. (2007). Impact of [18F]-fluorodeoxyglucose ([18F]-FDG) imaging in sarcoidosis: unsuspected neurosarcoidosis discovered by [18F]-FDG PET and early metabolic response to corticosteroid therapy. *Br J Radiol* 80(951): e67–71.

Andersson PB, Goodkin DE (1998). Glucocorticosteroid therapy for multiple sclerosis: a critical review. *J Neurol Sci* 160: 16–25.

Androdias G et al. (2011). Mycophenolate mofetil may be effective in CNS sarcoidosis but not in sarcoid myopathy. *Neurology* 76: 1168–72.

Atkinson R et al. (1982). Sarcoidosis presenting as cervical radiculopathy: a case report and literature review. *Spine* (Philadelphia) 7: 412–16.

Bakkers M et al. (2010). Pain and autonomic dysfunction in patients with sarcoidosis and small fibre neuropathy. *J Neurol* 257: 2086–90.

Balan A et al. (2010). Multi-technique imaging of sarcoidosis. *Clin Radiol* 65: 750–60.

Bauer HJ, Löfgren S (1964). International study of pulmonary sarcoidosis in mass chest radiography. *Acta Med Scand Suppl* 425: 103–5.

Bauer HJ, Wijkstrom S (1964). The prevalence of pulmonary sarcoidosis in Swedish mass radiography surveys. *Acta Med Scand Suppl* 425: 112–14.

Baughman RP, Costabel U, du Bois RM (2008). Treatment of sarcoidosis. *Clin Chest Med* 29: 533–48 ix–x.

Bejar JM et al. (1985). Treatment of central nervous system sarcoidosis with radiotherapy. *Ann Neurol* 18: 258–60.

Benzagmout M et al. (2007). Neurosarcoidosis which manifested as acute hydrocephalus: diagnosis and treatment. *Intern Med* 46: 1601–4.

Berek K et al. (1993). Subarachnoid hemorrhage as presenting feature of isolated neurosarcoidosis. *Clin Investig.* 71: 54–6

Bernstein H et al. (1963). The ocular deposition of chloroquine. *Invest Ophthalmol* 2: 384–92.

Beros V et al. (2008). Thoracic intramedullary sarcoidosis mimicking an intramedullary tumor. *Coll Antropol* 32: 645–7.

Bihan H et al. Sarcoidosis: clinical, hormonal, and magnetic resonance imaging manifestations of hypothalamic-pituitary disease in 9 patients and review of the literature. *Medicine (Baltimore)* 86: 259–68.

Bolat S et al. (2009). Fluorodeoxyglucose positron emission tomography (FDG-PET) is useful in the diagnosis of neurosarcoidosis. *J Neurol Sci* 287: 257–9.

Braun JJ et al. (2008). 18F-FDG PET/CT in sarcoidosis management: review and report of 20 cases. *Eur J Nucl Med Mol Imaging* 35: 1537–43.

Brazis PW, Stewart M, Lee AG (2004). The uveo-meningeal syndromes. *Neurologist* 10: 171–84.

Brinar VV, Habek M (2008). Isolated central nervous system sarcoidosis: a great mimicker. *Clin Neurol Neurosurg* 110: 939–42.

Brisman JL et al. (2006). Successful emergent angioplasty of neurosarcoid vasculitis presenting with strokes. *Surg Neurol* 66: 402–4.

Buitrago MJ et al. (2011). Histoplasmosis and paracoccidioidomycosis in a non-endemic area: a review of cases and diagnosis. *J Travel Med* 18(1): 26–33.

Burns TM, Dyck PJ, Aksamit AJ (2006). The natural history and long-term outcome of 57 limb sarcoidosis neuropathy cases. *J Neurol Sci* 244: 77–87.

Caccamo DV, Garcia JH, Ho KL (1992). Isolated granulomatous angiitis of the spinal cord. *Ann Neurol* 32: 580–2.

Caviness JN, Knox CA (1996). Hemidystonia occurring in a patient with sarcoidosis. *Mov Disord* 11: 340–1.

Chamoun V *et al.* (2011). Evidence-based diagnostic criteria for neurosarcoidosis based on cerebrospinal fluid analysis. *J Neurol Neurosurg Psychiatry* (submitted).

Chang C. *et al.* (2009). Cavernous sinus syndrome due to sarcoidosis: a case report. *Acta Neurol Taiwan* 18: 37–41.

Chintamaneni S *et al.* (2010). Dramatic response to infliximab in refractory neurosarcoidosis. *Ann Indian Acad Neurol* 13: 207–10.

Christoforidis GA *et al.* (1999). MR of CNS sarcoidosis: correlation of imaging features to clinical symptoms and response to treatment. *Am J Neuroradiol* 20: 655–69.

Cohen-Gadol AA *et al.* (2003). Spinal cord biopsy: a review of 38 cases. *Neurosurgery* 52: 806–15; discussion 815–16.

Colover J (1948). Sarcoidosis with involvement of the nervous system. *Brain* 71(Pt. 4): 451–75.

de Tribolet N, Zander E (1978). Intracranial sarcoidosis presenting angiographically as a sub-dural hematoma. *Surg Neurol* 9: 169–71.

Degardin A *et al.* (2010). Cerebrovascular symptomatic involvement in sarcoidosis. *Acta Neurol Belg* 110: 349–52.

Delaney P (1977). Neurologic manifestations in sarcoidosis: review of the literature, with a report of 23 cases. *Ann Intern Med* 87: 336–45.

Delaney P (1980). Seizures in sarcoidosis: a poor prognosis. *Ann Neurol* 7: 494.

Doty JD, Mazur JE, Judson MA (2003). Treatment of corticosteroid-resistant neurosarcoidosis with a short-course cyclophosphamide regimen. *Chest* 124: 2023–6.

Dumas JL *et al.* (2000). Central nervous system sarcoidosis: follow-up at MR imaging during steroid therapy. *Radiology* 214: 411–20.

Ebert EC *et al.* (2008). Non-response to infliximab may be due to innate neutralizing anti-tumor necrosis factor-alpha antibodies. *Clin Exp Immunol* 154: 325–31.

Ellefsen P (1970a). [Tracheal dystony and Boeck sarcoidosis]. *Nord Med* 84: 1054.

Ellefsen P (1970b). Tracheal dystonia and sarcoidosis. *Acta Otolaryngol* 70: 438–42.

Erickson T, Odom G, Stern K (1942). Boeck's disease (sarcoid) of the central nervous system: report of a case with complete clinico-pathological study. *Arch Neurol Psychiatry* 48: 613–21.

Espinosa GA *et al.* (1985). Spinal cord sarcoidosis. *Mil Med* 150: 309–13.

Fahoum F *et al.* (2009). Neurosarcoidosis presenting as Guillain–Barré-like syndrome: case report and review of the literature. *J Clin Neuromuscul Dis* 11: 35–43.

Favre J *et al.* (1998). Recurrent nocardial brain abscesses treated by repeated stereotactic aspirations. *J Clin Neurosci* 5: 97–100.

Foley K, Howell JD, Junck L (1989). Progression of hydrocephalus during corticosteroid therapy for neurosarcoidosis. *Postgrad Med J* 65: 481–4.

Fried ED *et al.* (1993). Spinal cord sarcoidosis: a case report and review of the literature. *J Assoc Acad Minor Phys* 4: 132–7.

Friedman SH, Gould DJ (2002). Neurosarcoidosis presenting as psychosis and dementia: a case report. *Int J Psychiatry Med* 32: 401–3.

Friedrich RE, Blake FA (2007). Avascular mandibular osteonecrosis in association with bisphosphonate therapy: a report on four patients. *Anticancer Res* 27: 1841–5.

Fyhrquist F *et al.* (1984). Inhibitor binding assay for angiotensin-converting enzyme. *Clin Chem* 30: 696–700.

Garg S *et al.* (2005). Mononeuritis multiplex secondary to sarcoidosis. *Clin Neurol Neurosurg* 107: 140–3.

Ginsberg L, Kidd D (2008). Chronic and recurrent meningitis. *Pract Neurol* 8: 348–61.

Giovannoni G (2011). Promising emerging therapies for multiple sclerosis. *Neurol Clin* 29: 435–48.

Gonzalez-Aramburul *et al.* (2011). Sarcoidosis presenting as transient ischemic attack status. *J Stroke Cerebrovasc Dis* (in press).

Graham EM *et al.* (1989). A point prevalence study of 150 patients with idiopathic retinal vasculitis. 1: Diagnostic value of ophthalmological features. *Br J Ophthalmol* 73: 714–21.

Grand S *et al.* (1996). Case report: pseudotumoral brain lesion as the presenting feature of sarcoidosis. *Br J Radiol* 69: 272–5.

Greim B *et al.* (2007). Fatigue in neuroimmunological diseases. *J Neurol* 254(Suppl. 2): II102–6.

Griggs RC, Markesbery WR, Condemi J (1973). Cerebral mass due to sarcoidosis: regression during corticosteroid therapy. *Neurology* 23: 981–9.

Hargreave FE, McCarthy DS, Pepys J (1969). Steroid 'pseudorheumatism' in asthma. *Br Med J* 1: 443–4.

Heerfordt C (1909). On febris uveo parotidea subchronica localized in the parotid gland and uvea of the eye, frequently complicated by paralysis of the cerebrospinal nerves. *Ugeskr Laeger* 71: 417–21.

Henriet M *et al.* (1991). [Opsoclonus associated with multisystemic sarcoidosis]. *Rev Neurol (Paris)* 147: 674–5.

Hodge MH, Williams RL, Fukui MB (2007). Neurosarcoidosis presenting as acute infarction on diffusion-weighted MR imaging: summary of radiologic findings. *Am J Neuroradiol* 28: 84–6.

Hoitsma E *et al.* (2004). Neurosarcoidosis: a clinical dilemma. *Lancet Neurol* 3: 397–407.

Hoitsma E, Drent M, Sharma O (2010). A pragmatic approach to diagnosing and treating neurosarcoidosis in the 21st century. *Curr Opin Pulm Med* 16: 472–9.

Ideguchi H *et al.* (2010). Neurological manifestations of Behçet's disease in Japan: a study of 54 patients. *J Neurol* 257: 1012–20.

Ishihara M *et al.* (1998). Seroprevalence of anti-Borrelia antibodies among patients with confirmed sarcoidosis in a region of Japan where Lyme borreliosis is endemic. *Graefes Arch Clin Exp Ophthalmol* 236: 280–4.

Ito A *et al.* (1998). Novel antigens for neurocysticercosis: simple method for preparation and evaluation for serodiagnosis. *Am J Trop Med Hyg* 59: 291–4.

Ito M *et al.* (2005). Vertebral osteonecrosis associated with sarcoidosis: case report. *J Neurosurg Spine* 2: 222–5.

Jackson RJ *et al.* (1998). Parafalcine and bilateral convexity neurosarcoidosis mimicking meningioma: case report and review of the literature. *Neurosurgery* 42: 635–8.

Jacobs TP *et al.* (1988). Addisonian crisis while taking high-dose glucocorticoids: an unusual presentation of primary adrenal failure in two patients with underlying inflammatory diseases. *J Am Med Assoc* 260: 2082–4.

Jain V, Deshmukh A, Gollomp S (2006). Bilateral facial paralysis: case presentation and discussion of differential diagnosis. *J Gen Intern Med* 21: C7–10.

Jakob E *et al.* (2009). Uveitis subtypes in a German interdisciplinary uveitis center: analysis of 1916 patients. *J Rheumatol* 36: 127–36.

James DG (1976). The centenary of sarcoidosis. *Ann NY Acad Sci* 278: 736–41.

James DG, Sharma O (1967). Extrathoracic sarcoidosis. *Proc R Soc Med* 60: 992–4.

James DG *et al.* (1976). Description of sarcoidosis: report of the Subcommittee on Classification and Definition. *Ann NY Acad Sci* 278: 742.

Johns CJ, Michele TM (1999). The clinical management of sarcoidosis: a 50-year experience at the Johns Hopkins Hospital. *Medicine (Baltimore)* 78: 65–111.

Junger SS et al. (1993). Intramedullary spinal sarcoidosis: clinical and magnetic resonance imaging characteristics. Neurology 43: 333–7.

Kaiboriboon K, Olsen TJ, Hayat GR (2005). Cauda equina and conus medullaris syndrome in sarcoidosis. Neurologist 11: 179–83.

Kaliszky Z, Walker A, Tyor WR (2002). Therapeutic options in neurosarcoidosis. Expert Rev Neurother 2: 703–8.

Kanemitsu S, Miyake Y, Okabe M (2008). Surgical removal of a left ventricular thrombus associated with cardiac sarcoidosis. Interact Cardiovasc Thorac Surg 7: 333–5.

Kang S, Suh JH (1999). Radiation therapy for neurosarcoidosis: report of three cases from a single institution. Radiat Oncol Investig 7: 309–12.

Kasp E et al. (1989). A point prevalence study of 150 patients with idiopathic retinal vasculitis. 2: Clinical relevance of antiretinal autoimmunity and circulating immune complexes. Br J Ophthalmol 73: 722–30.

Keijsers RG et al. (2008). 18F-FDG PET in sarcoidosis: an observational study in 12 patients treated with infliximab. Sarcoid Vasc Diff Lung Dis 25: 143–9.

Keino H et al. (2009). Frequency and clinical features of intraocular inflammation in Tokyo. Clin Experiment Ophthalmol 37: 595–601.

Ketonen L et al. (1986). Hypodense white matter lesions in computed tomography of neurosarcoidosis. J Comput Assist Tomogr 10: 181–3.

Ketonen L, Oksanen V, Kuuliala I (1987). Preliminary experience of magnetic resonance imaging in neurosarcoidosis. Neuroradiology 29: 127–9.

Khoury J et al. (2009). Cerebrospinal fluid angiotensin-converting enzyme for diagnosis of central nervous system sarcoidosis. Neurologist 15: 108–11.

Kidd DP, Revesz T, Miller NR (2006). Rosai–Dorfman disease presenting with widespread intracranial and spinal cord involvement. Neurology 67: 1551–5.

Kieff DA et al. (1997). Isolated neurosarcoidosis presenting as anosmia and visual changes. Otolaryngol Head Neck Surg 117: S183–6.

Kim SK et al. (2010). F-18 fluorodeoxyglucose and F-18 fluorothymidine positron emission tomography/computed tomography imaging in a case of neurosarcoidosis. Clin Nucl Med 35: 67–70.

Koike H et al. (2000). Differential response to corticosteroid therapy of MRI findings and clinical manifestations in spinal cord sarcoidosis. J Neurol 247: 544–9.

Kraemer M, Berlit P (2010). Systemic, secondary and infectious causes for cerebral vasculitis: clinical experience with 16 new European cases. Rheumatol Int 30: 1471–6.

La Mantia L, Erbetta A (2004). Headache and inflammatory disorders of the central nervous system. Neurol Sci 25(Suppl. 3): S148–53.

Lieberman J (1975). Elevation of serum angiotensin-converting-enzyme (ACE) level in sarcoidosis. Am J Med 59: 365–72.

Lin LF, Huang PT (2010). An uncommon cause of hiccups: sarcoidosis presenting solely as hiccups. J Chin Med Assoc 73: 647–50.

Lipton JM, Kirkpatrick J, Rosenberg RN (1977). Hypothermia and persisting capacity to develop fever: occurrence in a patient with sarcoidosis of the central nervous system. Arch Neurol 34: 498–504.

Lueck CJ et al. (1993). Ocular and neurological Behçet's disease without orogenital ulceration? J Neurol Neurosurg Psychiatry 56: 505–8.

Lury KM et al. (2004). Neurosarcoidosis: review of imaging findings. Semin Roentgenol 39: 495–504.

Makino T et al. (2009). Diffuse neurosarcoidosis involving only the leptomeninges of the brainstem and spinal cord. Intern Med 48: 1909–13.

Marie I et al. (2010). Cryptococcosis in sarcoidosis. South Med J 103: 1275–6.

Markert JM et al. (2007). Necrotizing neurosarcoid: three cases with varying presentations. Clin Neuropathol 26: 59–67.

Marra TR (1982). Sarcoid polyradiculoneuropathy with myelographic confirmation. Wis Med J 81(3): 21–4.

McLean BN, Mitchell DN, Thompson EJ (1990). Local synthesis of specific IgG in the cerebrospinal fluid of patients with neurosarcoidosis detected by antigen immunoblotting using Kveim material. J Neurol Sci 99(2/3): 165–75.

Mehta A, Duggal R, Nema SK (2006). Hypertrophic spinal pachymeningitis presenting as compressive myelopathy: a case report. Indian J Pathol Microbiol 49: 286–8.

Mendez MF, Zander B (1992). Frontal lobe dysfunction from meningeal sarcoidosis. Psychosomatics 33: 215–17.

Menezo V et al. (2009). Ocular features in neurosarcoidosis. Ocul Immunol Inflamm 17: 170–8.

Menninger MD, Amdur RJ, Marcus RB (2003). Role of radiotherapy in the treatment of neurosarcoidosis. Am J Clin Oncol 26(4): e115–18.

Miyoshi T et al. (2007). An elderly patient with sarcoidosis manifesting panhypopituitarism with central diabetes insipidus. Endocr J 54: 425–30.

Moravan M, Segal BM (2009). Treatment of CNS sarcoidosis with infliximab and mycophenolate mofetil. Neurology 72: 337–40.

Morgenthau AS, Iannuzzi MC (2011). Recent advances in sarcoidosis. Chest 139: 174–82.

Morita H, Ikeda S (2004). [Dementia due to sarcoidosis]. Nippon Rinsho 62(Suppl): 441–4.

Myers TD et al. (2004). Use of corticosteroid sparing systemic immunosuppression for treatment of corticosteroid dependent optic neuritis not associated with demyelinating disease. Br J Ophthalmol 88: 673–80.

Nagai H, Ohtsubo K, Shimada H (1985). Sarcoidosis of the spinal cord: report of an autopsy case and review of the literature. Acta Pathol Jpn 35: 1007–22.

Navi BB, DeAngelis LM (2009). Sarcoidosis presenting as brainstem ischemic stroke. Neurology 72: 1021–2.

Nesbit GM et al. (1989). Spinal cord sarcoidosis: a new finding at MR imaging with Gd-DTPA enhancement. Radiology 173: 839–43.

Newman LS, Rose CS, Maier LA (1997). Sarcoidosis. New Engl J Med 336: 1224–34.

Ogawa Y, Tominaga T, Ikeda H (2008). Neurosarcoidosis manifesting as tremor of the extremities and severe hypopituitarism: case report. Neurol Med Chir (Tokyo) 48: 314–17.

Oishi A, Miyamoto K, Yoshimura N (2008). Dorsal midbrain syndrome induced by midbrain neurosarcoidosis. Jpn J Ophthalmol 52: 236–8.

Oksanen V (1986). Neurosarcoidosis: clinical presentations and course in 50 patients. Acta Neurol Scand 73: 283–90.

Oksanen V (1987). New cerebrospinal fluid, neurophysiological and neuroradiological examinations in the diagnosis and follow-up of neurosarcoidosis. Sarcoidosis 4: 105–10.

Oksanen V (1994). Neurosarcoidosis. Sarcoidosis 11: 76–9.

Oksanen V, Salmi T (1986). Visual and auditory evoked potentials in the early diagnosis and follow-up of neurosarcoidosis. Acta Neurol Scand 74: 38–42.

Oksanen V et al. (1985). Angiotensin converting enzyme in cerebrospinal fluid: a new assay. Neurology 35: 1220–3.

Papadakis N, Epstein F (1975). Subtemporal craniectomy for recurrent shunt obstruction [letter]. J Neurosurg 42: 115–17.

Patel AV, Stickler DE, Tyor WR (2007). Neurosarcoidosis. Curr Treat Options Neurol 9: 161–8.

Peison B, Padleckas R (1964). Granulomatous angiitis of the central nervous system. *Ill Med J* 126: 330–4.

Perez Olivan S *et al.* (2002). [A case of primary toxoplasmosis in an immunocompetent patient]. *Arch Soc Esp Oftalmol* 77: 107–10.

Pickuth D, Heywang-Kobrunner SH (2000). Neurosarcoidosis: evaluation with MRI. *J Neuroradiol* 27: 185–8.

Pickuth D, Spielmann R, Heywang-Kobrunner SH (2000). Role of radiology in the diagnosis of neurosarcoidosis. *Eur Radiol* 10: 941–4.

Porter N, Beynon HL, Randeva HS (2003). Endocrine and reproductive manifestations of sarcoidosis. *Q J Med* 96: 553–61.

Powell C *et al.* (2010). Steroid-induced osteonecrosis: an analysis of steroid dosing risk. *Autoimmun Rev* 9: 721–43.

Powers JM (1985). Sarcoidosis of the tentorium with cortical blindness. *J Clin Neuroophthalmol* 5(2): 112–15.

Quinones-Hinojosa A *et al.* (2003). Isolated trigeminal nerve sarcoid granuloma mimicking trigeminal schwannoma: case report. *Neurosurgery* 52: 700–5; discussion 704–5.

Ramsey CN *et al.* (2006). Prevention of visual loss caused by shunt failure: a potential role for optic nerve sheath fenestration – report of three cases. *J Neurosurg* 104(2 Suppl): 149–51.

Ravaglia S *et al.* (2003). Clinical MRI dissociation in myelopathy: a clue to sarcoidosis? *J Neurol Neurosurg Psychiatry* 74: 1122.

Reed J *et al.* (2010). Clinical features of sarcoid rhinosinusitis. *Am J Med* 123: 856–62.

Ricker W, Clark M (1949). Sarcoidosis; a clinicopathologic review of 300 cases, including 22 autopsies. *Am J Clin Pathol* 19: 725–49.

Rubinstein I *et al.* (1988). Neurosarcoidosis associated with hypersomnolence treated with corticosteroids and brain irradiation. *Chest* 94: 205–6.

Sabaawi M, Gutierrez-Nunez J, Fragala MR (1992). Neurosarcoidosis presenting as schizophreniform disorder. *Int J Psychiatry Med* 22: 269–74.

Said G *et al.* (2002). Nerve granulomas and vasculitis in sarcoid peripheral neuropathy: a clinicopathological study of 11 patients. *Brain* 125(Pt 2): 264–75.

Saleh S *et al.* (2006). Sarcoidosis of the spinal cord: literature review and report of eight cases. *J Natl Med Assoc* 98: 965–76.

Salvesen H (1935). The sarcoid of Boeck, a disease of importance to internal medicine. *Acta Med Scand Suppl* 86: 127.

Santos E, Scolding NJ (2010). Neurolymphomatosis mimicking neurosarcoidosis: a case report. *J Med Case Reports* 4: 5.

Sartwell PE, Edwards LB (1974). Epidemiology of sarcoidosis in the US Navy. *Am J Epidemiol* 99: 250–7.

Sawai S *et al.* (2010). Multifocal conduction blocks in sarcoid peripheral neuropathy. *Intern Med* 49: 471–4.

Scadding J, Mitchell D (1985). *Sarcoidosis.* Chapman & Hall, London.

Schwendimann RN *et al.* (2009). Neurosarcoidosis: clinical features, diagnosis, and management. *Am J Ther* (Epub ahead of print).

Scott TF *et al.* (2010). Neurosarcoidosis mimicry of multiple sclerosis: clinical, laboratory, and imaging characteristics. *Neurologist* 16: 386–9.

Selvi A *et al.* (2009). Cerebral venous thrombosis in a patient with sarcoidosis. *Intern Med* 48: 723–5.

Seve P *et al.* (2009). Fluorodeoxyglucose positron emission tomography for the diagnosis of sarcoidosis in patients with unexplained chronic uveitis. *Ocul Immunol Inflamm* 17: 179–84.

Shah JR, Lewis RA (2003). Sarcoidosis of the cauda equina mimicking Guillain–Barré syndrome. *J Neurol Sci* 208(1/2): 113–17.

Sharma OP (1998). Effectiveness of chloroquine and hydroxychloroquine in treating selected patients with sarcoidosis with neurological involvement. *Arch Neurol* 55: 1248–54.

Sheu SY *et al.* (2004). Erdheim–Chester disease: case report with multisystemic manifestations including testes, thyroid, and lymph nodes, and a review of literature. *J Clin Pathol* 57: 1225–8.

Siltzbach LE *et al.* (1974). Course and prognosis of sarcoidosis around the world. *Am J Med* 57: 847–52.

Sodhi M *et al.* (2009). Infliximab therapy rescues cyclophosphamide failure in severe central nervous system sarcoidosis. *Respir Med* 103: 268–73.

Streletz LJ *et al.* (1981). Visual evoked potentials in sarcoidosis. *Neurology* 31: 1545–9.

Terunuma H *et al.* (1988). Sarcoidosis presenting as progressive myelopathy. *Clin Neuropathol* 7: 77–80.

Terushkin V *et al.* (2010). Neurosarcoidosis: presentations and management. *Neurologist* 16: 2–15.

Urban O (1910). *Arch Derm Syph Wien* 101: 175.

Uruha A, Koide R, Taniguchi M (2009). Unusual presentation of sarcoidosis: solitary intracranial mass lesion mimicking a glioma. *J Neuroimaging* 21(2): e180–2.

Vargas DL, Stern BJ (2010). Neurosarcoidosis: diagnosis and management. *Semin Respir Crit Care Med* 31: 419–27.

Vital A *et al.* (2008). Sarcoid neuropathy: clinico-pathological study of 4 new cases and review of the literature. *Clin Neuropathol* 27: 96–105.

Vrbica Z *et al.* (2010). Necrotising sarcoid granulomatosis of the spinal cord: case report. *Coll Antropol* 34: 713–17.

Walid MS, Ajjan M, Grigorian AA (2008). Neurosarcoidosis: the great mimicker. *J Natl Med Assoc* 100: 859–61.

Wani MK *et al.* (1999). Neurosarcoidosis: an unusual case presenting as a cerebellopontine angle tumor. *Otolaryngol Head Neck Surg* 121: 301–2.

Waxman JS, Sher JH (1979). The spectrum of central nervous system sarcoidosis: a clinical and pathologic study. *Mt Sinai J Med* 46: 309–17.

Westhout FD, Linskey ME (2008). Obstructive hydrocephalus and progressive psychosis: rare presentations of neurosarcoidosis. *Surg Neurol* 69: 288–92; discussion 292.

Willigers H, Koehler PJ (1993). Amnesic syndrome caused by neurosarcoidosis. *Clin Neurol Neurosurg* 95: 131–5.

Winkler M (1905). *Arch Derm Syph Wien* 77.

Yamaguchi S *et al.* (2006). [CNS sarcoidosis presenting with intracerebral hemorrhage: case report]. *No Shinkei Geka* 34: 839–42.

Younger DS *et al.* (1988). Granulomatous angiitis of the brain: an inflammatory reaction of diverse etiology. *Arch Neurol* 45: 514–18.

Yuasa H *et al.* (2000). [A case of sarcoid meningoencephalitis with an isolated supratentorial lesion]. *Rinsho Shinkeigaku* 40: 900–5.

Zajicek J (1990). Sarcoidosis of the cauda equina: a report of three cases. *J Neurol* 237: 424–6.

Zajicek JP *et al.* (1999). Central nervous system sarcoidosis: diagnosis and management. *Q J Med* 92: 103–17.

Zajicek JP (2000). Neurosarcoidosis. *Curr Opin Neurol* 13: 323–5.

Zarei M *et al.* (2002). Cavernous sinus syndrome as the only manifestation of sarcoidosis. *J Postgrad Med* 48: 119–21.

Zisman DA, Shorr AF, Lynch J (2002). Sarcoidosis involving the musculoskeletal system. *Semin Respir Crit Care Med* 23: 555–70.

28

The kidneys, calcium metabolism and vitamin D

OM P SHARMA, VIOLETA VUCINIC AND DONALD MITCHELL

INTRODUCTION

The kidneys are less frequently affected by sarcoidosis than other organs. Nevertheless, physicians taking care of sarcoidosis patients need to be aware of the possibility of renal involvement in order to diagnose this potentially fatal complication early and treat it effectively. The kidneys may be affected primarily by sarcoid granulomas or secondarily from hypercalcemia, hypercalciuria, and nephrocalcinosis. Hypercalcemia, an important complication of sarcoidosis, results from over-production of 1,25-dihydroxyvitamin D3 (calcitriol) by activated macrophages and sarcoidosis granulomas. Calcitriol, in turn, causes increased absorption of calcium from the gut. Hypercalcemia is not specific to sarcoidosis: it is found in other granulomatous disorders including tuberculosis, coccidioidomycosis, histoplasmosis, leprosy, and granulomatous necrotizing vasculitis. Hyperparathyroidism and malignancy are two common non-granulomatous causes of hypercalcemia.

RENAL SARCOIDOSIS

Clinically manifest renal involvement is rare in sarcoidosis (Longcope and Freiman 1952; Siltzbach et al. 1974; Scadding and Mitchell 1985; Baughman et al. 2001; Lower 2006; see also Table 28.1).

The reported prevalence of renal disease ranges widely due to the enormous variation in study designs and enrolled patient populations. Several small series of biopsy findings suggest that some degree of renal involvement occurs in approximately 35–50 percent of patients with chronic sarcoidosis, but rarely in those with acute sarcoidosis (Muther et al. 1981; Hagege et al. 1983; Guenel and Chevet

1990; Lower 2006). Lebacq and associates performed 25 percutaneous kidney biopsies in 25 selected cases of sarcoidosis with suspected renal involvement; ten (40 percent) showed non-caseating granulomas (Lebacq et al. 1970). MacSerraigh and colleagues investigated 90 patients with sarcoidosis; renal functions were abnormal in nine patients and epithelioid granulomas were seen in five of eight (68 percent) who had a renal biopsy (MacSearraigh et al. 1978). Löfgren reported the occurrence of transient interstitial nephritis in association with bilateral hilar adenopathy and erythema nodosum (Löfgren et al. 1957).

Postmortem analysis reports indicate that 20 percent of patients have histological changes in the kidneys (Baughman et al. 2001). These studies, carried out retrospectively on patients of different ethnic backgrounds and habits, were open to sampling errors. Autopsy studies in the Japanese patients revealed an incidence of 26 percent (Taneo and Kobayashi 1994). In a series of 46 patients studied by Bergener and colleagues between 1995 and 2002, 15 (32 percent) exhibited renal function abnormalities, of whom 10 underwent kidney biopsy; 6 of 10 showed nephrocalcinosis, of whom two showed granulomatous interstitial nephritis, one interstitial nephritis without granulomas and one immunoglobulin-A (IgA) glomerulonephritis. In two patients they found a combination of granulomatous interstitial nephritis with either nephrocalcinosis or with IgA nephritis (Bergner et al. 2003).

The frequency of clinically significant disease remains low. In the ACCESS study (A Case–Control Etiologic Study of Sarcoidosis), clinical involvement of the kidneys was observed in only 0.7 percent of patients (see Table 28.1). Renal involvement may be the initial manifestation of sarcoidosis. It may appear during the course of the illness and follow the onset of the disease after many years. Occasionally,

Table 28.1   Organ involvement in sarcoidosis (percentages).

	Siltzbach et al. 1974 International study	James et al. (1976) UK study	Baughman et al. (2001) ACCESS study, USA
Lungs	87	88	95
Skin (chronic)	9	18	15.9
Erythema nodosum	17	34	8.3
Lymph nodes	28	39	11.8
Eyes	–	27	11.5
Liver	–	10	8.3
Nervous system	4	9	4.6
Cardiac	–	3	2.3
Calcium abnormality	11	18	3.7
Renal disease	–	1	0.7

nephrolithiasis is the only presenting feature of sarcoidosis (Rizzato and Colombo 2003).

Diagnosis of renal disease

The criteria for establishing the diagnosis of sarcoidosis are:

- compatible clinical or radiographic evidence of multi-system involvement;
- histological evidence of non-caseating granulomas;
- the absence of acid-fast bacilli, fungi, other bacteria in sputum, body fluids, and tissue biopsy specimens;
- negative complement fixation test for coccidioidomycosis (endemic in San Joaquin Valley in California), histoplasmosis (endemic in Central and South America), brucellosis (Middle East and India), and negative PCR for Whipple's disease (Hunninghake et al. 1999).

A diagnosis based on only one of the features is misleading since clinical and radiological features present too wide a spectrum of differential diagnoses, whereas non-caseating granulomas may be caused by many bacteria, fungi, viruses, inhaled (organic and inorganic) agents, and drugs (prescribed and over-the-counter).

A presumptive diagnosis of renal sarcoidosis is justified in cases where typical non-caseating granulomas are found in the kidneys, corticosteroid treatment leads to resolution, and attempts to discover evidence of other causes of granulomatous reaction are unsuccessful. Occasionally, lymphoma and malignancy can produce granulomas (Sharma and Lamb 2003).

Clinical features of renal disease

Renal disease in sarcoidosis may be divided into the following clinical categories (Box 28.1).

> **Box 28.1 Types of renal involvement in sarcoidosis**
>
> - Granulomatous interstitial nephritis
> - Glomerulonephritis
> - IgA nephropathy (Berger's disease)
> - Renal cell carcinoma
> - Granulomatous vasculitis or renal angiitis
> - Nephrocalcinosis and nephrolithiasis

GRANULOMATOUS INTERSTITIAL NEPHRITIS

Although about 20 percent of patients with sarcoidosis may show granulomas in the kidneys, development of the clinical syndrome of granulomatous interstitial nephritis is unusual. Utas and associates described a patient who had developed mild proteinuria (Utas et al. 1999). Creatinine clearance was 60 mL/min, while renal biopsy showed typical non-caseating granulomas with normal glomeruli. A chest X-ray film and whole-body gallium scan showed no abnormality. The patient had uveitis and thus most probably had sarcoidosis. Nevertheless, a review of 1010 renal biopsy specimens found only six instances of granulomatous interstitial nephritis, all of which were caused by drugs (Schwarz et al. 2000). In another study of 76 cases of granulomatous nephritis, drugs were the main causative agent (Schwarz et al. 1988).

Marie and co-workers described a 60-year-old man with diffuse joint pains, albuminuria and hematuria (Marie et al. 2000). Serum angiotensin-converting enzyme (ACE) and autoantibody screening were normal. A renal biopsy specimen showed interstitial and granulomatous nephritis, direct immunofluorescence and negative Zeil–Nelson test results. Thoracic and abdominal computerized tomography, echocardiography and accessory salivary gland and duodenal biopsy results were normal. Despite corticosteroid therapy, the patient's general condition and renal function deteriorated. Biopsy of the ileum revealed the changes of Whipple's disease, and PCR analysis of ribosomal RNA demonstrated the presence of Tropheryma whipplei. This patient not only did not have clinical or radiological evidence of sarcoidosis, but also failed to response to corticosteroid therapy. The unusual presentation necessitated a further evaluation, which confirmed the presence of a rare illness. This case is an excellent example showing that, if all the criteria recommended for diagnosing sarcoidosis are not met, a diagnostic error is likely to occur.

Manes and co-workers described a 59-year-old man with acute renal failure, hypercalcemia, anaemia and unilateral facial palsy (Manes et al. 2000). Renal biopsy revealed interstitial granulomatous nephritis. Corticosteroid therapy normalized the calcium level, improved renal failure and subdued facial palsy. In this patient renal failure appeared with the advent of other features of sarcoidosis and he responded accordingly.

GLOMERULONEPHRITIS

The histological changes of focal segmental sclerosis, membranous glomerulonephritis, mesangioproliferative glomerulonephritis, IgA nephropathy and crescentic glomerulonephritis have been described sporadically. Most such patients have either proteinuria or clinical nephrotic syndrome. Hypertension is frequent, but rarely a serious problem.

Membranous glomerulonephritis (nephropathy) associated with nephritic syndrome is seen in sarcoidosis. Renal biopsy shows membranous nephropathy with or without granulomas, and electron microscopy may reveal typical subepithelial deposits. Corticosteroids are effective (Khan et al. 1994; Mundlein et al. 1996; Parry and Falk 1997; Dimitriades et al. 1999). Glomerular involvement is rare. The mechanism of glomerular injury is not known, but IgG complement deposits have been observed (Quismorio et al. 1977). In a reported patient with crescentic glomerulonephritis and granulomas, antineutrophilic cytoplasmic antibodies (ANCA) were found (Auinger et al. 1977). In another patient with glomerulonephritis, the diagnosis of Wegener's granulomatosis was entertained (Ahuja et al. 1996). These patients do not meet the diagnostic criteria for sarcoidosis and most likely belong to a vasculitis group.

IGA NEPHROPATHY (BERGER'S DISEASE) AND GLOMERULAR DISEASE

Membranous and proliferative abnormalities have been described in sarcoidosis. In 1968, Burger and Hinglais first described IgA nephropathy. The histological appearance consists of mesangial deposits of IgA, variable amounts of complement component 3, IgM and IgG associated with proliferative glomerulonephritis. Although the cause remains unknown, clinical exacerbations follow a viral illness. In 1996, Taylor and Ansell reported a sarcoidosis patient with IgA nephropathy and nephritic syndrome. Nishiki and associates observed a similar patient who also had thyroiditis (Nishiki et al. 1999). Both these patients responded to corticosteroid therapy.

Schmidt and associates described a 39-year-old man who developed end-stage renal failure due to IgA nephropathy and received a renal transplant (Schmidt et al. 1999). After 17 months the patient developed a massive pleural effusion and finger clubbing. Lung and pleural biopsy specimens showed non-caseating granulomas. He responded to corticosteroids. Hamada and co-workers reported one definite and two subclinical cases of IgA nephropathy during the course of sarcoidosis (Hamada et al. 2003). These anecdotal reports do not reveal precisely the incidence or nature of the relationship between sarcoidosis and IgA nephropathy.

INTERSTITIAL NEPHRITIS AND UVEITIS

A curious clinically entity, occurring mainly in women, has been described. It is called TINU or tubulointestinal nephritis and uveitis syndrome (Cacoub et al. 1989; Vidal et al. 1992; Gafter et al. 1993; Takemura et al. 1999; Sessa et al. 2000). Although its cause is not known, these patients should be evaluated for signs of both sarcoidosis and Sjögren's syndrome (such as xerostomia) (Vidal et al. 1992). Regardless of the cause, this disorder responds to corticosteroid therapy, while lack of treatment may allow progression to chronic

renal failure. Recurrent uveitis can occur, but the renal disease is usually cured by the initial course of therapy (Gafter et al. 1993).

RENAL CELL CARCINOMA

It is well known that sarcoid granulomas may be found in regional lymph nodes draining carcinomas or lymphomas. Granulomas have also been found in cancerous or lymphoma tissue. This limited or local granulomatous response should not be confused with multisystem sarcoidosis (Table 28.2). Occasionally a neoplasm, particularly breast, renal or testicular, may cause bilateral hilar adenopathy. Rarely, sarcoidosis and neoplasm may co-exist. By applying strict diagnostic criteria, most cases can be separated into a limited granulomatous response or multisystem sarcoidosis.

A 53-year old man was found to have microalbuminuria. A renal biopsy showed perivascular granulomas. Renal ultrasonography suggested renal cell carcinoma. At operation, a papillary adenocarcinoma of the right kidney was found. The chest radiograph, eye examination and serum ACE levels were normal. This represents a local sarcoid reaction to renal cancer and not systemic sarcoidosis (Gobel et al. 2001). Marinides and associates described a renal papillary adenocarcinoma and associated granulomatous reaction in the same kidney (Marinides et al. 1994). Hypernephroma has also been described as causing or co-existing with a granulomatous response (Moder et al. 1990; Campbell and Douglas-Jones 1991; Hoffbrand 1994).

Table 28.2 Differences between a non-specific local sarcoid reaction due to cancer or trauma and multisystem sarcoidosis.

	Local sarcoidosis	Multisystem sarcoidosis
Number of organs involved	Usually one	More than one
Age (years)	Any	20–50
Chest radiograph	Usually normal	Abnormal in 90% Most have typical features
HRCT scan	May suggest tumor, cancer or localized infiltrate	May suggest sarcoidosis
Elevated serum ACE	<5%	>60%
Kveim–Siltzbach test	Negative	Positive in active sarcoidosis
Bronchoalveolar lymphocytes	Absent	Present
Slit-lamp examination	Normal	Positive in 15–20%
Hypercalcemia	May be present in some cancers	Present in >10% of sarcoid patients
Whole-body gallium scan	Localized uptake	Multisystem uptake

ACE, angiotensin-converting enzyme

GRANULOMATOUS VASCULITIS

Although hyaline deposits in arterial walls occur frequently in sarcoidosis, true obliterative granulomatous involvement of the renal artery is uncommon.

URINARY TRACT DISEASE

Retroperitoneal lymph node involvement, retroperitoneal fibrosis, renal stones, and ureteral involvement may cause ureteral obstruction in sarcoidosis patients. The renal artery can become enmeshed in retroperitoneal fibrosis (Godin et al. 1980; Gross et al. 1986; Fraioli et al. 1990; Mariano and Sussman 1998). Obstructive uropathy due to retroperitoneal involvement responds to corticosteroids.

HYPERCALCEMIA, HYPERCALCIURIA, NEPHROCALCINOSIS AND RENAL STONES

The relationship between renal function impairment and hypercalcemia was studied by Löfgren and colleagues in the 1950s. They carried out biochemical studies and renal biopsies in 16 patients with pulmonary sarcoidosis (Löfgren et al. 1957). Six of the patients who had hypercalcemia showed evidence of renal function impairment. Renal biopsies revealed scattered calcium deposits in tubules and interstitial connective tissue; three specimens showed non-caseating granulomas. On the other hand, among the ten patients with normal serum calcium, only one showed small granulomas and non-calcium deposits in a renal biopsy specimen. MacSerraigh and co-workers studied 90 patients with sarcoidosis and found close correlation between nephrocalcinosis, hypercalcemia and creatinine clearance (MacSerraigh et al. 1978). Of the eight patients with impaired renal function, granulomas were found in four, nephrocalcinosis in five, and both in one.

Hypercalcemia has long been recognized as a complication of sarcoidosis, but the importance of hypercalciuria has been less thoroughly realized. Hypercalciuria, however, is three times more common than hypercalcemia (Sharma et al. 1967; see Table 28.2). Hypercalciuria has been reported to be more common in males than females and, in London (UK), in Caucasian rather than in West Indian patients. In patients with abnormal renal function, hypercalciuria is present when the patient has sarcoidosis-related hypercalcemia.

The mechanism of hypercalciuria appears to be threefold:

- absorptive, associated with elevated calcitriol levels and abnormal urinary calcium:creatinine ratio;
- resorptive, associated with excessive dissemination of sarcoidosis involving the bones and high serum ACE level;
- associated with osteoclast-activating factor, a bone-resorbing substance (Mundy et al. 1974).

According to Broulik and colleagues, the urinary excretion rate of calcium is based on the filtered load of calcium when corrected for urinary calcium excretion. The tubular maximum resorptive rate for calcium is not increased. These results suggest that calcitriol has no direct effect on renal calcium handling, and hypercalciuria is due to the flow of calcium from the gut and bone (Broulik et al. 1990).

Persistent hypercalciuria may lead to nephrocalcinosis, renal stones, obstruction of the collecting tubules and finally renal failure. Renal stones were the presenting feature of sarcoidosis in 4 of 116 of consecutive Italian patients with histologically proven sarcoidosis, followed at a sarcoidosis clinic in Milan (Rizzato et al. 2004). Hamada and colleagues found renal impairment mostly in patients with hypercalcemia; nephrocalcinosis was absent in all cases (Hamada et al. 2003).

Renal transplantation

End-stage renal disease requiring renal transplant is most often caused by hypercalcemic nephropathy rather than granulomatous nephritis or a glomerulonephropathy. The outcome in five patients who had undergone renal transplantation for end-stage renal disease due to sarcoidosis has been published (Padilla et al. 1997). One patient with granulomatous nephritis developed symptomatic recurrent sarcoidosis six years after transplant. Treatment with increased doses of glucocorticoid resulted in improved renal function and long-term graft survival. Similar events occurred in another patient 11 months after renal transplantation. Graft loss due to disease recurrence has not been reported.

VITAMIN D AND CALCIUM METABOLISM

Vitamin D

Vitamin D, a hormone and a vitamin, is ingested from the diet or synthesized in the skin. It is metabolized in the liver to a biologically inactive 25-hydroxyvitamin D, or 25(OH)D, the major circulating form of vitamin D. Through hydroxylation by 1α-hydroxylase it is converted to the biologically active 1,25-dihydroxyvitamin D, or 1,25(OH)2D, primarily in the kidneys. In 1983, Adams and colleagues first showed that monocyte/macrophages from sarcoidosis patients synthesized the active form of vitamin D, 1-25-dihydroxyvitamin D, from precursor 25-hydroxyvitamin D (25(OH)D) (Adams et al. 1983). At about the same time, the receptor for 1–25(OH)(2)D (vitamin D receptor, VDR) on proliferating lymphocytes was recognized. That vitamin D has two functions is now common knowledge: the hormonal function of regulating mineral and skeletal homeostasis, and the evolutionary function of protecting the inside environment of the host. The latter is conducted by 1,25(OH)2D cytokine, generated by monocyte/macrophage, interacting with VDR and modulating the innate immune system to deal with the invading microbes (Adams and Hewison 2010). Increased production of 1,25(OH)2D by activated macrophages is a common finding in many cases of granulomatous inflammation.

Throughout antiquity it was commonly believed that patients suffering from tuberculosis (TB) improved in response to sunlight and good nutrition. In times long gone, before the advent of isoniazid and other effective anti-tuberculosis drugs, every hospitalized TB patient received a daily dose of cod liver oil, a rich source of vitamin D, which was considered an essential part of TB therapy. This was indirect evidence of the protective mechanism of vitamin D. Liu and colleagues have offered a biochemical explanation for such a hypothesis (Liu et al. 2006). These researchers have shown that the human macrophages produce a large amount of the antimicrobial peptide cathelicidin (LL-37) which, when stimulated by TLR2/1L in the presence of 1,25(OH2)D3, shows intense mycobactericidal activity. Rook and colleagues observed that 1,25(OH2)D3 directly inhibited the growth of *Mycobacterium tuberculosis* in cultured macrophages (Rook et al. 1986). Multiple studies now show that hypovitaminosis-D is a risk factor for the development of active tuberculosis (Nnoaham and Clarke 2008; Ginde et al. 2009).

Sarcoidosis occurs most frequently in the winter months, when vitamin D levels are low. Sarcoidosis is also more prevalent in areas that are farther from the equator (Benatar 1977; Edmondstone and Wilson 1985; Ginde et al. 2009).The disease is also common in dark pigmented individuals, and is particularly high in African-Americans living in the south-eastern United States, who have a higher incidence of vitamin D deficiency (Rybicki et al. 1997). Cathelicidin mRNA is present in lower amounts in the bronchoalveolar lavage fluid (BALF) of sarcoidosis patients; it is much lower in patients with severe sarcoidosis as compared to patients with mild disease (Kanchwala et al. 2009). It has been suggested that the presence of cathelicidin mRNA in the innate immune system may be relevant in persons who are susceptible to vitamin D deficiency (Agerberth et al. 1999).

Production of calcitriol, the most active metabolite of vitamin D, in the kidney is closely regulated by parathyroid hormone and serum phosphate. Calcitriol functions like a steroid hormone by binding to specific receptors and initiating expression of various proteins. The binding to specific receptors in the intestine and generation of calcium-binding proteins increases calcium absorption. Calcitriol, by binding to specific receptors on bone cells, stimulates osteoblasts to make osteocalcin, the specific protein involved in bone mineralization and differentiation of stem cells in the bone marrow. It increases the formation of cells in the hematopoietic system and B-lymphocyte function. It inhibits proliferation of cancer cells.

In three sarcoidosis patients with hypercalcemia, plasma levels of calcitriol were high when calcium levels were raised and fell when calcium levels returned to normal either spontaneously or after prednisone treatment (Bell et al. 1979). Further evidence that abnormally high levels of calcitriol occur in hypercalcemic sarcoidosis patients was provided by Mitchell and co-workers who reported a 28-year-old female with hypoparathyroidism who had required vitamin D therapy since the age of 19 years. She developed sarcoidosis and became hypercalcemic. On cessation of vitamin D therapy her calcium level returned to normal, but the administration of hydrocortisone caused hypocalcemia. Her plasma calcitriol level was three times the highest level recorded in a patient with hypoparathyroidism undergoing

treatment with vitamin D (Mitchell et al. 1983). Another patient studied by Zimmerman and co-workers had hypoparathyroidism but was able to discontinue the vitamin D treatment with maintenance of normal calcium levels when sarcoidosis developed (Zimmerman et al. 1983). An elevated concentration of calcitriol, a metabolite synthesized solely in normal non-pregnant human subjects, occurred in a hypercalcemic anephric male patient with sarcoidosis (Barbour et al. 1981). These observations support the original contention of Henneman and co-workers in 1956 that the hypercalcemia of sarcoidosis is a form of vitamin D intoxication and also establish that the hormone is produced at an extrarenal site.

Adams and colleagues showed that calcitriol causes hypercalcemia in sarcoidosis and that macrophages from patients with active sarcoidosis are the synthetic source of the hormone (Singer and Adams 1986). A similar metabolite was identified in preparations of sarcoid granulomas incubated with calcitriol (Mason et al. 1984).

The identity of the hormone and its origin are now known, but the question remains as to why nature bothers to produce this hormone. Is the reason behind production to cause damage to tissue? Is it produced to protect the body from an uncontrolled wild immunological response? Of course, there is the third possibility that the hormone is a harmless bystander.

Role of 1,25–dihydroxyvitamin D3

The following evidence supports an immunoregulatory role for calcitriol:

- the presence of high-affinity intracellular receptors for calcitriol (vitamin D receptors or VDRs) on lymphocytes, macrophages, and dendritic cells (Bhalla et al. 1983; Cadranel 1995);
- the inhibition by calcitriol of mitogen-induced lymphocyte proliferation and immunoglobulin production (Rigby et al. 1985);
- the reduction by calcitriol of interleukin-2 (IL-2) by lymphocytes (Haq 1986);
- enhancement by calcitriol of the ability of macrophages to inhibit proliferation of M. tuberculosis, in vitro (Adams et al. 1989b; Barnes et al. 1989).

Thus the hormonal form of vitamin D seems to possess a role similar to that of cytokines. The precise lesion that controls the abnormal regulation of calcitriol synthesis is obscure, but it may be due to a defective feedback control of calcitriol at the site of synthesis in macrophages or in target cells for calcitriol such as lymphocytes. Production of the hormone may thus be part of the normal immune response to retaliation to antigenic stimulation, and may induce secretion of other mediators. Calcitriol modulates the cytotoxic and antibody-producing functions of lymphocytes. The action depends on the threshold of VDR expression, and is mediated through inhibition of the T-cell cytokine IL-2. Calcitriol retards interferon-γ synthesis by T-cells, and this may act as part of the control of calcitriol synthesis by macrophages that produce the hormone when stimulated by interferon-γ. The inhibition of immunoglobulin production is due to direct suppression of T-helper cells or macrophages (Provvedini et al. 1986). The presence of VDRs in T-cell-mediated natural killer cells indicates that calcitriol may modulate the immune response to viral and neoplastic processes (Rigby et al. 1987; McFadden et al. 1991).

Hypercalcemia: its clinical significance

Hypercalcemia is one of the most common biochemical abnormalities found in clinical practice. It may be discovered when the serum calcium level is measured as a screening test or as part of the evaluation for fatigue, unexplained weakness, neuromuscular disability, renal stones or osteopenia (Box 28.2).

The three common causes of hypercalcemia are primary hyperparathyroidism, granulomatous disorders, and malignancy. Disturbance of vitamin D metabolism contributes to a state of disordered calcium homeostasis in these diseases. In granulomatous disorders, including sarcoidosis, Crohn's disease, tuberculosis, leprosy and coccidioidomycosis, the inappropriate endogenous overproduction of the metabolite calcitriol by activated macrophages and granulomas is responsible for hypercalcemia.

The reported incidence of hypercalcemia in sarcoidosis ranges from 2 to 63 percent. The frequency with a few exceptions tends to be higher in North American series: the highest, 63 percent, was reported by McCort et al. (1947). Cummings (1959) found calcium levels of more than 11 mg/ dL in 35 percent of his patients. Mayock et al. (1963) in their review of 509 patients recorded a frequency of 17 percent. Only 6 of 62 patients at the Brompton Hospital, London, showed serum calcium levels >11 mg/dL (Scadding and Mitchell 1985). Mather reported a still lower prevalence: only 4 of 86 untreated patients with sarcoidosis exhibited hypercalcemia (Mather 1957). In Finland, Putkonen and colleagues could find only two patients with high calcium levels in a series of 60 (Putkonen et al. 1965). There is no conclusive evidence that race, age, sex, occupation or area of residence consistently influence the development of hypercalcemia.

Although hypercalcemia appears to be a feature of sarcoidosis, the studies showing an excessively high frequency of occurrence need to be revised. It is reasonable to accept the

Box 28.2 Signs and symptoms of hypercalcemia

- Polyuria and polydipsia
- Renal colic
- Lethargy
- Dyspepsia
- Peptic ulceration
- Constipation
- Depression
- Drowsiness and impaired cognition
- Weight loss in malignancy and lymphoma

incidence of 11 percent noted in a worldwide review of 3676 patients with sarcoidosis (James et al. 1976).

Hypercalcemia is usually transient in subacute sarcoidosis and persistent and fluctuating in chronic disease, depending on the activity of the disease. Furthermore, hypercalcemia may occur only at a certain phase during the long course of chronic sarcoidosis (James et al. 1976). In order to get a true picture of calcium abnormality, serum calcium levels should be measured regularly over a long period. It has been reported that hypercalcemia is more frequent during the summer months when exposure to the sun is at its peak. However, this is not always the case (Webb et al. 1988; Cronin et al. 1990). Hypercalcemia occurs frequently in London and Reading (UK), New York (USA) and Lisbon (Portugal), and does not correlate with summer temperatures. Besides, Putkonen's group found lower levels of serum calcium in summer months and slightly higher mean levels in late autumn (Putkonen et al. 1965).

Harrell and Fisher were the first to recognize the relationship between sarcoidosis and vitamin D. In 1939 they described the presence of hypercalcemia in 6 of 11 patients with sarcoidosis. In one of their patients, serum calcium level rose from 9.6 to 14.2 mg/dL after consumption of cod liver oil (Harrell and Fisher 1939). These authors made three important clinical observations:

- hypercalcemia is a feature of sarcoidosis;
- consuming a diet rich in vitamin D results in worsening of hypercalcemia;
- vitamin D might be related to calcium abnormality in sarcoidosis.

Soon after, Henneman's group postulated that the disordered calcium homeostasis in sarcoidosis patients was strikingly similar to that seen in patients with vitamin D intoxication (Henneman et al. 1956). In 1963, Taylor and associates observed that, in 345 patients with sarcoidosis in North Carolina (USA), mean serum calcium in the winter months was 9.89 mg/dL, but rose to 10.26 mg/dL in summer months; whereas, among 12027 controls the levels during the winter and summer months remained unchanged (Taylor et al. 1963). In two hypercalcemic patients at the University College Hospital, London, further rises in serum calcium level occurred after whole-body ultraviolet irradiation (Dent 1970). Hendrix, conversely, gave two hypercalcemic and hypercalciuric patients with sarcoidosis a diet deficient in vitamin D and shielded them from sunlight; in 8 weeks serum calcium levels became normal, hypercalciuria subsided, and fecal excretion of calcium increased (Hendrix 1922). These observations strengthened the belief that the development of hypercalcemia in sarcoidosis was due to enhanced target responsiveness to vitamin D, increasing calcium absorption in the intestine, increasing resorption in the bones, and increased excretion in the kidneys.

TREATMENT OF HYPERCALCEMIA

Persistently high serum and high urinary excretion require treatment (Rizzato 2006). Severe hypercalcemia, defined as a serum calcium concentration >14 mg/dL, is unusual for sarcoidosis. The therapeutic goals are as follows:

- reduction of oral and intravenous intake of calcium and vitamin D, and curtailment of dietary calcium;
- maintenance of an expanded intravascular volume;
- reduction of the inappropriate production of calcitriol from sarcoid macrophages and granulomas;
- reduction of calcitriol-induced calcium absorption and bone resorption.

Prednisone 20–40 mg daily is the drug of choice for reducing the endogenous production of calcitriol. Corticosteroids cause a swift decrease in circulating calcitriol and serum calcium falls within 3–5 days. A decrease in urinary calcium excretion soon follows within 7–10 days. Failure to normalize serum calcium after 2 weeks should lead the clinician to exclude the possibility of a co-existing disorder, which might be hyperparathyroidism, lymphoma, carcinoma or myeloma. Once the serum calcium is brought down to normal, the prednisone dose can be reduced over a period of 4–6 weeks. Serum calcium and urinary calcium excretion need to be monitored frequently. If the patient develops unbearable side-effects of corticosteroid therapy or fails to respond, chloroquine or hydroxychloroquine (200 mg twice a day) should be given; both these drugs reduce serum calcitriol and serum calcium levels (O'Leary et al. 1986; Barré et al. 1987; Adams et al. 1989a). The antifungal drug ketoconazole, a known inhibitor of cytochrome P450 steroid oxidase, lowers circulating calcitriol and serum calcium levels; however, efficacy of the drug is not widely known (Adams et al. 1990; Ejaz et al. 1994).

The patient should be instructed to avoid sunlight, curtail intake of major dietary sources of vitamin D and calcium, and drink plenty of fluids. The major sources of vitamin D are fish (sardine, salmon, cod), liver, and egg yolk. In the USA and Scandinavia, dairy products are fortified with 400 IU of either vitamin D_2 or vitamin D_3, but in other countries milk is not supplemented.

Normocalcemic patients with sarcoidosis may develop hypercalcemia, renal stones and renal failure. Urinary stones due to persistent hypercalciuria can be pulverized by extracorporeal lithotripsy (Sharma and Alfaro 1986; Table 28.3).

Vitamin D deficiency

Vitamin D deficiency is worldwide. In the USA alone, vitamin D inadequacy occurs in about 36 percent of otherwise healthy adults and in up to 57 percent of general medicine patients, with even higher numbers in Europe. Severe vitamin D deficiency may lead to osteomalacia, muscle weakness, fatigue, and non-specific body pains. Many of these features are common to patients with sarcoidosis with or without associated chronic fatigue and depression. In a large population-based study, depression and severity of depression were strongly associated with low serum 25(OH)D levels. It is essential to the overall general health and wellbeing of sarcoidosis patients to have their serum

Table 28.3   Prevention of nephrocalcinosis/nephrolithiasis.

Diet	
Fluid	>3–4 L in 24 h
Sodium	Restricted intake
Protein	Moderate
Calcium/vitamin D	Avoid
Oxalate	Avoid (e.g. rhubarb)
Drugs	
Diuretics (thiazides)	Reduces calcium excretion; helpful in hypercalciuria and recurrent stone formation
Allopurinol	If serum urate or urate excretion is high
Vitamin D supplements	Avoid

25(OH)D levels measured. It is important for physicians to counsel sarcoidosis patients to ensure adequate intake in order to avoid chronic debilitating and harmful effects of vitamin D deficiency.

CONCLUSION

The spectrum of multisystem sarcoidosis also encompasses renal sarcoidosis, a relatively uncommon but dangerous complication of the disease. Renal involvement may be primary, due to granulomatous involvement of the kidney tissue, or secondary to altered calcium metabolism. Although hypercalcemia and hypercalciuria may both occur in sarcoidosis, the latter is about three times more common than the former. Renal disease if diagnosed early can be subdued by judicious use of corticosteroids, immunosuppressive drugs, antimalarials, and anti-tumor necrosis factor agents.

REFERENCES

Adams J, Hewison M (2010). Update in vitamin D. *J Clin Endocrinol Metab* **95**: 471–8.

Adams J, Sharma O, Gacad M, Singer F (1983). Metabolism of 25-hydroxyl vitamin-D 3 by cultured pulmonary alveolar macrophages in sarcoidosis. *J Clin invest* **72**: 1856–60.

Adams J, Diz M, Sharma O (1989a). Effective reduction in the serum 1,25-dihydroxy vitamin D and calcium concentration in sarcoidosis associate hypercalcemia with short course of chloroquine therapy. *Ann Intern Med* **111**: 437–8.

Adams J, Modlin R, Diz M et al. (1989b). Potentiation of the macrophage 25-hydroxyl-vitamin D-1 hydroxylation reaction by human tuberculous effusion fluid. *J Clin Endocrinol Metab* **69**: 457–60.

Adams J, Sharma O, Diz M et al. (1990). Ketoconazole decreases the serum 1,25-dihydroxy vitamin D and calcium concentration in sarcoidosis associated hypercalcemia. *J Clin Endocrinol Metab* **70**: 1090–5.

Agerberth B, Grunewald J, Castanos-Velez E et al. (1999). Antibacterial components in bronchoalveolar lavage fluid from healthy individuals and sarcoidosis patients. *Am J Respir Crit Care Med* **160**: 283–90.

Ahuja T, Mattana J, Valerraman E et al. (1996). Wegener's granulomatosis followed by development of sarcoidosis. Am J Kidney Dis 28: 893–8.

Auinger M, Irsigler K, Breiteneder S et al. (1977). Normocalcemic hepato-renal sarcoidosis with crescentic glomerulonephritis. Nephron Dial Transplant 12: 1474–7.

Barbour G, Coburn J, Slatopolsky E et al. (1981). Hypercalcemia in an anephric patient with sarcoidosis: evidence for an extra-renal generation of 1,25-dihtdroxy vitamin-D. New Engl J Med 305: 440–3.

Barnes P, Modlin R, Bikle D et al. (1989). Transpleural gradient of 1,25-dihydroxy vitamin D in tuberculous pleuritis. J Clin Invest 83: 1527–32.

Barré P, Gascon-Barré M, Meakins J et al. (1987). Hydroxychloroquine treatment of hypercalcemia in a patient with sarcoidosis undergoing hemodialysis. Am J Med 82: 1259–62.

Baughman R, Teirstein A, Judson M et al. (2001). Clinical characteristics of patients in a case control study of sarcoidosis (ACCESS). Am J Respir Crit Care Med 164: 1885–9.

Bell N, Stern P, Pantzer E et al. (1979). Evidence of increased circulating 1,25-dihydroxy vitamin D as the probable cause of abnormal calcium metabolism in sarcoidosis. J Clin Invest 64: 218–25.

Benatar SR (1977). Sarcoidosis in South Africa: a comparative study in Whites, Blacks, and Coloureds. S Afr Med J 52: 602–6.

Bergner R, Hoffmann M, Waldherr R, Uppenkamp M (2003). Frequency of kidney disease in chronic sarcoidosis. Sarcoid Vasc Diff Lung Dis 20: 126.

Bhalla A, Ameno E, Clemens T et al. (1983). Specific high-affinity receptors for 1,25-dihydroxy vitamin-D3 in human peripheral blood mononuclear cells, presence in monocytes and induction in T-lymphocytes following activation. J Clin Endocrinol Metab 57: 1308–10.

Broulik P, Votava V, Packovsky V (1990). The tubular maximum for calcium absorption in patients with chronic active sarcoidosis. Eur Respir J 3: 747–9.

Burger J, Hinglais N (1968). Intracapillary deposits of IgA and IgM. J Urol Nephrol (Paris) 74: 694–5.

Cacoub P, Deray G, Le Hoang P et al. (1989). Idiopathic acute interstitial nephritis associated with anterior uveitis in adults. Clin Nephrol 31: 307.

Cadranel J (1995). Vitamin D, endocrine and paracrine mediators in cases of pulmonary granulomatosis. Rev Med Respir 12: 119–20.

Campbell F, Douglas-Jones A (1991). Sarcoid-like granulomas in primary renal-cell carcinoma. Sarcoidosis 10: 128–31.

Cronin C, Dimnear S, O'Mahony D et al. (1990). Precipitation of hypercalcemia in sarcoidosis by foreign sun holiday: report of four cases. Postgrad Med 66: 307–9.

Cummings M (1959). Epidemiologic and clinical observations in sarcoidosis. Ann Intern Med 50: 879–90.

Dent C (1970). Calcium metabolism in sarcoidosis. Postgrad Med 46: 471–3.

Dimitriades C, Shetty A, Vehaskari M et al. (1999). Membranous nephropathy associated with childhood sarcoidosis. Pediatr Nephrol 13: 444–7.

Edmondstone WM, Wilson AG (1985). Sarcoidosis in Caucasians, Blacks and Asians. Br J Dis Chest 79(1): 27–36.

Ejaz A, Zbanch R, Tiwari P et al. (1994). Ketoconazole in the treatment of recurrent nephrolithiasis associated with sarcoidosis. Nephrol Dial Transplant 9: 1492–4.

Fraioli P, Montemurro L, Castrignano L, Rizzato G (1990). Retroperitoneal involvement in sarcoidosis. Sarcoidosis 7: 101.

Gafter U, Kalechman Y, Zevin D et al. (1993). Tubulointerstitial nephritis and uveitis: association with suppressed cellular immunity. Nephrol Dial Transplant 8: 821.

Ginde AA, Liu MC, Camargo CA (2009). Demographic differences and trends of vitamin D insufficiency in the US population, 1988–2004. Arch Intern Med 169: 626–32.

Gobel V, Kettritz R, Schneider W et al. (2001). The protean face of renal sarcoidosis. J Am Soc Nephrol 12: 616–23.

Godin M, Fillastre JP, Ducastelle T et al. (1980). Sarcoidosis: retroperitoneal fibrosis, renal arterial involvement, and unilateral focal glomerulosclerosis. Arch Intern Med 140: 1240.

Gross KR, Malleson G, Lirenman DS et al. (1986). Vasculopathy with renal artery stenosis in a child with sarcoidosis. J Pediatr 108: 724.

Guenel J, Chevet D (1990). Interstitial nephritis in sarcoidosis. Presse Med 19: 1215–17.

Hagege A, Baglin J, Prinseau J et al. (1983). Sarcoidosis disclosed by renal insufficiency (three cases). Sem Hop 59: 2823–6.

Hamada H, Nagai S, Ono T et al. (2003). Sarcoidosis complicated with IgA nephropathy. Sarcoid Vasc Diff Lung Dis 20: 69–73.

Haq A (1986). 1,25-dihydroxy vitamin-D (calcitriol) suppresses IL-2 murine thymocytic proliferation. Thymus 8: 195–306.

Harrell G, Fisher S (1939). Blood chemical changes in Boeck's sarcoid with particular reference to protein, calcium, and phosphorus values. J Clin Invest 18: 687–93.

Hendrix J (1922). The remission of hypercalcemia and hypercalciuria in systemic sarcoidosis by vitamin D depletion. Clin Res 11: 220–5.

Henneman P, Dempsey E, Carol E et al. (1956). The cause of hypercalcemia in sarcoidosis and its treatment with cortisone and sodium phytate. J Clin Invest 35: 1229–42.

Hoffbrand B (1994). The kidney in sarcoidosis. In: James DG (ed.). Sarcoidosis and Other Granulomatous Disorders. Marcel Dekker, New York, pp. 335–43.

Hunninghake G, Costabel U, Ando M et al. (1999). American Thoracic Society/European Respiratory Society/World Association of Sarcoidosis and Other Granulomatous Disorders: statement on sarcoidosis. Sarcoid Vasc Diff Lung Dis 16: 149–73.

James DG, Neville E, Siltzbach L et al. (1976). A worldwide view of sarcoidosis. Ann NY Acad Sci 278: 321–34.

Kanchwala AA, Barna BP, Singh RJ et al. (2009). Deficiencies of cathelicidin and vitamin D accompany disease severity in sarcoidosis. Am J Respir Crit Care Med 179: A3997.

Khan I, Simpson J, Catto G et al. (1994). Membranous nephropathy and granulomatous nephritis in sarcoidosis. Nephron 66: 459–61.

Lebacq E, Desmet V, Verhaegen H (1970). Renal involvement in sarcoidosis. Postgrad Med J 46: 526.

Liu PT, Stenger S, Li H et al. (2006). Toll-like receptor triggering of a vitamin D-mediated human antimicrobial response. Science 311: 1770–3.

Löfgren S, Snellman B, Lindgren AH (1957). Renal complications in sarcoidosis: functional and biopsy studies. Acta Med Scand 295: 305.

Longcope W, Freiman D (1952). A study of sarcoidosis. Medicine (Baltimore) 31: 1.

Lower E (2006). Renal sarcoidosis. In: Baughman R (ed.). Sarcoidosis. Taylor & Francis, New York, p. 651.

MacSearraigh ET, Doyle CT, Twomey M, O'Sullivan DJ (1978). Sarcoidosis with renal involvement. Postgrad Med J 54: 528.

Manes M, Molino A, Gaiter A et al. (2000). Isolated renal failure secondary to sarcoidosis. Recent Prog Med 91: 441–3.

Mariano R, Sussman S (1998). Sarcoidosis of the ureter [letter]. Am J Roentgen 171: 1431.

Marie I, Lecomte F, Leveque H (2000). Granulomatous nephritis as the first manifestation of Whipple's disease. *Ann Intern Med* 132: 94–5.

Marinides G, Hajdu G, Grans R (1994). Unique association of renal carcinoma and sarcoid reaction in the kidney. *Nephron* 67: 477–80.

Mason R, Frankel J, Chan Y *et al.* (1984). Vitamin-D conversion by sarcoid lymph node homogenate. *Ann Intern Med* 100: 59–61.

Mather G (1957). Calcium metabolism and bone changes in sarcoidosis. *Br Med J* 1: 248–53.

Mayock R, Bertrand P, Morrison C *et al.* (1963). Manifestations of sarcoidosis: an analysis with a review of nine series from the literature. *Am J Med* 35: 67–89.

McCort J, Wood R, Hamilton J *et al.* (1947). Sarcoidosis: a clinical study of 28 proven cases. *Arch Intern Med* 80: 293–321.

McFadden R, Vickers K, Fraher L (1991). Lymphocyte chemokinetic factors derived from human tonsils: modulation by 1,25-dihydroxy vitamin-D (calcitriol). *Am J Respir Cell Mol Biol* 4: 42–9.

Mitchell T, Stamp T, Jenkins J (1983). Hypercalcemic sarcoidosis in hypoparathyroidism. *Br Med J* 1: 764–5.

Moder K, Litin S, Gaffey T (1990). Renal-cell carcinoma associated like tissue reaction. *Mayo Clin Proc* 65: 1498–501.

Mundlein E, Green T, Ritz E *et al.* (1996). Grave's disease and sarcoidosis in a patient with minimal glomerulonephritis. *Nephrol Dial Transplant* 11: 860–2.

Mundy G, Raisz A, Cooper R *et al.* (1974). Evidence for secretion of an osteoclast stimulating factor in myeloma. *New Engl J Med* 291: 1041–6.

Muther R, McMarron D, Bennett W (1981). Renal manifestations of sarcoidosis. *Arch Intern Med* 141: 643–6.

Nishiki M, Murakama Y, Yamane Y *et al.* (1999). Steroid sensitive nephritic syndrome sarcoidosis and thyroiditis. *Nephron Dial Transplant* 14: 2008–10.

Nnoaham KE, Clarke A (2008). Low serum vitamin D levels and tuberculosis: a systematic review and meta-analysis. *Int J Epidemiol* 37(1): 113–19.

O'Leary T, Jones G, Yip A *et al.* (1986). The effects of chloroquine on serum 1,25-dihydroxy vitamin D and calcium metabolism in sarcoidosis. *New Engl J Med* 315: 727–30.

Padilla ML, Schilero GJ, Teirstein AS (1997). Sarcoidosis and transplantation. *Sarcoid Vasc Diff Lung Dis* 14: 16.

Parry R, Falk C (1997). Minimal change disease associated with sarcoidosis. *Nephrol Dial Transplant* 12: 2159–60.

Provvedini D, Tsoukas C, Deftos I *et al.* (1986). 1(α,25-dihydroxy vitamin-D binding molecules in human B-lymphocytes: effects on immunoglobulin production. *J Immunol* 136: 2734–40.

Putkonen T, Hannuksela N, Hahme H (1965). Calcium and phosphorus metabolism in sarcoidosis. *Acta Med Scand* 177: 327–35.

Quismorio F, Sharma O, Chandor S (1977). Immunopathological studies on the cutaneous lesions in sarcoidosis. *Br J Dermatol* 97: 637–42.

Rigby W, Denome S, Fanger M (1987). Regulation of lymphokine production and human T lymphocyte activation by 1,25-dihydroxy vitamin-D3. *J Clin Invest* 79: 1659–64.

Rigby W, Noelle R, Krause K *et al.* (1985). The effect of 1α25-dihydroxy vitamin-D on human lymphocyte activation and proliferation: a cycle analysis. *J Immunol* 135: 2279–86.

Rizzato G (2006). Calcium metabolism. In: Baughman R (ed.). *Sarcoidosis*. Taylor & Francis, New York, p. 635.

Rizzato G, Colombo P (2003). Nephrolithiasis as a presenting feature of chronic sarcoidosis. *Sarcoid Vasc Diff Lung Dis* 20: 118–25.

Rizzato G, Palmieri G, Agrati AM, Zanussi C (2004). The organ-specific extrapulmonary presentation of sarcoidosis: a frequent occurrence but a challenge to an early diagnosis – a 3-year-long prospective observational study. *Sarcoid Vasc Diff Lung Dis* 21: 119.

Rook GA, Steele J, Fraher L *et al.* (1986). Vitamin D3, interferon, and control of proliferation of *Mycobacterium tuberculosis* by human monocytes. *Immunology* 57: 159–63.

Rybicki BA, Major M, Popovich J *et al.* (1997). Racial differences in sarcoidosis incidence: a 5-year study in a health maintenance organization. *Am J Epidemiol* 148: 234–41.

Scadding J, Mitchell D (1985). The kidney and calcium in sarcoidosis. In: Scadding J, Mitchell D (eds). *Sarcoidosis*. Chapman & Hall, London, pp. 390–413.

Schmidt R, Bender F, Change W *et al.* (1999). Sarcoidosis after renal transplant. *Transplantation* 68: 1420–3.

Schwarz A, Krause P, Kelter F *et al.* (1988). Granulomatous interstitial nephritis after non-steroidal anti-inflammatory drugs. *Am J Nephrol* 8: 410–16.

Schwarz A, Krause P, Kunzendorf V *et al.* (2000). The current outcome of interstitial nephritis: risk factors for the transition from acute to chronic nephritis. *Clin Nephrol* 52: 179–90.

Sessa A, Meroni M, Battini G *et al.* (2000). Acute renal failure due to idiopathic tubulo-intestinal nephritis and uveitis: 'TINU syndrome'. Case report and review of the literature. *J Nephrol* 13: 377.

Sharma O, Alfaro C (1986). Hypercalciuria and renal stones in a patient treated by extracorporeal shockwave lithotripsy. *Sarcoidosis* 3: 7–9.

Sharma O, Lamb C (2003). Cancer in interstitial lung disease and sarcoidosis. *Curr Opin Pulm Med* 9: 396–401.

Sharma O, Trowell J, Cohen N *et al.* (1967). Abnormal calcium metabolism in sarcoidosis. In: Turiaf J, Chabot J (eds). *La Sarcoidose: Rapports de IV Conference Internationale* [Proceedings of the IV International Conference on Sarcoidosis]. Maison et Cie, Paris, pp. 627–31.

Siltzbach L, James D, Neville E *et al.* (1974). Course and prognosis of sarcoidosis around the world. *Am J Med* 37: 847–52.

Singer FR, Adams JS (1986). Abnormal calcium homeostasis in sarcoidosis. *New Engl J Med* 315: 755.

Takemura T, Okada M, Hino S *et al.* (1999). Course and outcome of tubulointerstitial nephritis and uveitis syndrome. *Am J Kidney Dis* 34: 1016.

Taneo S, Kobayashi Y (1994). Renal manifestations of sarcoidosis: a review. *Nippon Rinsho* 52: 1613–18.

Taylor J, Ansell I (1996). Sarcoid sensitive nephritis syndrome and renal impairment in a patient with sarcoidosis. *Nephrol Dial Transplant* 11: 355–6.

Taylor R, Lynch H, Winsor W (1963). Seasonal influence of sunlight on the hypercalcemia of sarcoidosis. *Am J Med* 35: 67–9.

Utas C, Dogukan A, Patriroghu T *et al.* (1999). Granulomatous interstitial nephritis in extrapulmonary sarcoidosis. *Clin Nephrol* 51: 252–4.

Vidal E, Rogues AM, Aldigier JC (1992). The Tinu syndrome or the Sjögren syndrome? [letter]. *Ann Intern Med* 116: 93.

Webb AR, Kline L, Hollick MF (1988). Influence of season and latitude on the cutaneous synthesis of vitamin D3: exposure to winter sunlight in Boston and Edmonton will not promote vitamin D3 synthesis in human skin. *J Clin Endocrinol Metab* 67: 371–8.

Zimmerman J, Hollick M, Silver J (1983). Normocalcemia in a hypothyroid patient with sarcoidosis: evidence for parathyroid hormone independent synthesis of 1,25-dihydroxy vitamin-D. *Ann Intern Med* 98: 338–40.

29

Psychiatric aspects

PAUL E PFEFFER AND JEREMY M PFEFFER

INTRODUCTION

Sarcoidosis is a disease with variable clinical course and often spontaneous remission, so the decision to actively treat is based on clinical judgment that treatment will improve the patient's quality of life. Understanding the psychological and psychiatric aspects is paramount. It is important to consider several topics: the psychosocial burden secondary to the disease, patients presenting with psychiatric illness as a primary manifestation of sarcoidosis, and the side-effects of treatment.

Research in this field has two major limitations: tertiary center bias, and being cross-sectional rather than longitudinal. Most research is conducted at tertiary care units where the patient population may be skewed towards patients with more persistent and/or severe disease; studies may overstate the psychosocial morbidity in sarcoidosis. The second limitation refers to the fact most studies compare clinical markers of sarcoidosis severity to quality of life at a fixed moment in time, rather than changes over time.

QUALITY-OF-LIFE AND PSYCHIATRIC MORBIDITY

Several studies have shown a decreased quality of life in sarcoidosis. Cox et al. (2004) used the Medical Outcomes Study 36-Item Short Form Survey (SF-36) and St George's Respiratory Questionnaire (SGRQ) with 111 patients, 80 percent of whom were African-American, with a median of two organs involved. There was reduced quality of life in patients with sarcoidosis as shown by lower scores across all domains of the SF-36 and worse scores on SGRQ as compared to historical healthy controls. However, the validity of this control population is questionable.

Antoniou et al. (2006) compared 75 patients with active sarcoidosis to unmatched controls in a European Caucasian population. They used three instruments – the Quality of

Well-Being (QWB) questionnaire, the Hospital Anxiety and Depression Questionnaire (HADS), and SGRQ – and found worse psychosocial health status in the patients using all three questionnaires.

Wirnsberger et al. (1998) compared 64 patients with sarcoidosis to matched controls in Holland using the World Health Organization's Quality of Life Assessment Instrument 100 (WHOQOL-100). The patients had a significantly worse score on Overall Quality of Life and General Health, and a worse score on the Physical Health domain, compared to the healthy control group. Interestingly, these scores were similar in the symptomatic and asymptomatic patient groups. Symptomatic patients scored significantly worse on several facets, particularly in Level of Independence, compared to asymptomatic patients. Drent et al. (1998) investigated the same study population using the Sickness Impact Profile (SIP) questionnaire. Symptomatic patients had worse scores on multiple SIP subscales compared to asymptomatic patients. Both patients with and without symptomatic complaints had worse scores on the SIP subscale of sleep and rest compared to healthy controls.

Interestingly, Cox et al. (2004) found significantly worse quality of life in patients treated with oral corticosteroids even after adjustment for confounding variables. Goracci et al. (2008) found that subjects taking steroids had worse scores on several domains of the Quality of Life Enjoyment and Satisfaction Questionnaire (Q-LES-Q).

Lung function and quality of life

Cox et al. (2004) found no significant relationship between spirometry or organ burden and SF-36 or SGRQ scores. Antoniou et al. (2006) found both worse spirometry and duration of disease were associated with worse score on SGRQ, but not with the other two quality-of-life measures. Goracci et al. (2008) found correlations between spirometry and Q-LES-Q domains of Physical Health and General Activities. Wirnsberger *et al.* (1998) found no correlations between WHOQOL-100 scores and lung function tests. Drent *et al.* (1998) found patients with decreased gas transfer (DLco) had more symptomatic complaints.

The ACCESS multicenter study used the SF-36 tool and compared this to spirometry with 736 patients (Yeager *et al.* 2005). They found an association between worse lung function and SF-36 scores. However the associations, although significant, showed weak correlation. The correlation was stronger between SF-36 scores and patient-reported dyspnea (using the Medical Research Council dyspnea scale).

There are many reasons to explain the lack of a consistent relationship between measures of lung function and quality of life. Wirnsberger *et al.* (1997) investigated in 18 sarcoid patients whether other measures of respiratory muscle function may be better than spirometry or gas transfer. There was a correlation between respiratory muscle endurance time and two subscales on the SIP quality-of-life questionnaire. FEV_1 did not show a similar relationship. Spruit *et al.* (2005) studied 22 sarcoid patients reporting fatigue using measures of muscle strength (such as quadriceps peak torque), the SF-36 and HADS tools. Worse quadriceps peak torque correlated with higher levels of depression and worse scores on several SF-36 subscales.

Although breathlessness is a major symptom for many patients, constitutional symptoms – particularly fatigue – predominate. Michielsen *et al.* (2006) compared fatigue measured with the Fatigue Assessment Scale (FAS) and scores on WHOQOL-100 in 145 sarcoid patients. Fatigue correlated well with worse quality of life across multiple domains of WHOQOL-100. However, fatigue did not correlate strongly with DLco or spirometry. Baughman *et al.* (2007) investigated the relationship between the 6-minute walk test, lung function, fatigue and health status in 142 patients. Psychosocial health status as measured by SGRQ showed a strong correlation to FAS score and MRC dyspnea score. Causality is difficult to interpret: many aspects of sarcoidosis could cause a reduction in a patient's daily activities leading to deconditioning, secondary muscle weakness and fatigue. Alternatively, fatigue and muscular weakness may be a direct part of the pathophysiology of sarcoidosis.

Depression

One difficulty in diagnosing depression in sarcoidosis is that fatigue is a primary symptom of both sarcoidosis and depression. This problem affects both research studies and the doctor in clinic. One advantage of including a psychiatrist with specialist knowledge of sarcoidosis in the care team is the awareness of this problem, allowing more accurate psychiatric examination.

Chang *et al.* (2001) studied the prevalence of depression in sarcoidosis, using a shortened form of the Center for Epidemiological Studies' Depression Scale (CES-D). They found 60 percent of 144 study patients were depressed. More organ systems involved and dyspnea on exertion were both associated with higher prevalence of depression. Steroid

therapy was not associated with increased depression. Reduced ability to pay for medical care was associated with depression, and 44 percent of the study population fell below the mean poverty level. Their study population was predominantly female, African-American with an average of more than one organ system involved. The ACCESS study also used the CES-D tool. They found 46 percent of sarcoidosis cases had a CES-D score of ≥9, compared to 27 percent of controls – higher scores indicating more depressive symptoms. However, a score of ≥16 on CES-D is usually taken as suggestive of depression, rather than ≥9, making this result hard to interpret.

Goracci *et al.* (2008) used the Mini International Neuropsychiatric Interview (MINI-PLUS) in 80 Italian patients with sarcoidosis to evaluate the prevalence of psychiatric disease (DSM-IV axis I diagnoses). Criteria for diagnosis of Major Depressive Disorder were met in 25 percent of patients, Panic Disorder in 6.3 percent, Bipolar Disorder in 6.3 percent, and Generalized Anxiety Disorder in 5 percent. Criteria for at least one psychiatric disorder were met in 44 percent of study patients. Patients meeting the criteria for psychiatric disease had significantly worse scores on multiple domains of the Q-LES-Q measure.

Wirnsberger *et al.* (1998) and Drent *et al.* (1998) used the Beck Depression Inventory (BDI). Twelve of the 64 patients had scores above the threshold associated with significant depression. All but one of these cases were from the group of patients reporting ongoing symptoms. Comparing symptomatic and asymptomatic patients, the former had significantly worse BDI scores. This group also had significantly higher Cognitive Depression Index scores (a reduced inventory removing items directly affected by the physical effects of illness).

Discussion

The studies highlighted are cross-sectional, comparing clinical markers of sarcoidosis severity to psychosocial health at a fixed moment in time. What may well be more important in determining psychosocial health is dynamic changes in disease severity. For example, the rate of decline in lung function can be more important than absolute lung function because a patient's lifestyle can become adjusted to a static reduced lung function. Alternatively there may be a threshold effect: the patient's quality of life may start to become affected only when lung function falls below a certain level and becomes limiting.

Most depression in patients with sarcoidosis is reactive or coincidental. However, depression and other psychiatric symptoms can feature as a side-effect of pharmacotherapy and as a direct effect of neurosarcoidosis. Psychiatric disease due to neurosarcoidosis (in the absence of symptoms of other organ involvement) can be the initial presentation of sarcoidosis, although this is rare. Cases of depression, delusions and hallucinations, paranoia, and abnormal behavior due to neurosarcoidosis with no other neurological or pulmonary symptoms have been described in the literature (Stiller *et al.* 1984; Bona *et al.* 1998; Bourgeois *et al.* 2005). Chest imaging is often abnormal and suggestive of sarcoidosis. Investigation is as for neurosarcoidosis. The psychiatric presentation may be atypical with cognitive dysfunction and other neurological signs (Sabaawi et al. 1992). Neurosarcoidosis with psychiatric symptoms may present many years after treatment of sarcoidosis without previous neuropsychiatric involvement (O'Brien et al. 1994). There may be considerable delay in making the correct diagnosis of underlying neurosarcoidosis; there are some patients with psychiatric disease due to neurosarcoidosis in which the correct diagnosis will never be reached.

Treatment to successfully stabilize the disease and psychiatric symptoms may be achieved with corticosteroids, though antidepressants and antipsychotics may be needed.

PSYCHIATRIC EFFECTS OF STEROIDS

The cornerstone of treatment of sarcoidosis is corticosteroids, which can have psychiatric side-effects. The Boston Collaborative Drug Surveillance Program (1972) studied 718 patients started on prednisolone in hospital. They found 21 patients to have an acute psychiatric reaction, principally psychosis and inappropriate euphoria, while receiving an average dose of 59.5 mg prednisolone daily. Psychiatric reactions accounted for approximately one-quarter of the acute reactions to prednisolone. Unlike acute gastrointestinal and other reactions, the incidence of acute psychiatric reactions was dose-related. However, psychiatric reactions still occurred in 6 of 463 patients receiving 40 mg or less prednisolone daily. With reduction of the prednisolone dose and brief psychopharmacotherapy there was remission in psychiatric pathology.

A review of psychiatric changes during corticosteroid therapy by Brown and Chandler (2001) noted an increased level of mood disorders in these patients. The mood changes occurred early after starting corticosteroids and there was a predominance of manic symptoms. They also found evidence of cognitive impairment, for example in declarative memory, while patients were taking corticosteroids. Management of these changes is principally by corticosteroid dose reduction.

Although patients may need to take many tablets each day, the physical treatment burden and consequent interference with daily life is less than in other lung diseases such as cystic fibrosis, where nebulizers and daily chest physiotherapy are necessary. However, the need to regularly take medications can still have a profound psychological effect, acting as a constant reminder of their disease and that they are 'different', even when the disease is in remission and they feel well.

PSYCHIATRIC TREATMENT

Psychiatric treatment can be divided into three different areas: physical, psychological and social. Physical methods are mainly medication. Psychological treatments are most commonly cognitive behavioral therapy (CBT) and psychodynamic therapy. In CBT the patient learns how to alter his/her thinking from negative to objective and thereby alter

behavior and mood. In psychodynamic therapy the patient talks about his/her background and issues with a therapist interpreting what the patient says; this is a much less directive form of treatment. In social treatment, the patient's environment is manipulated to remove the problem causing his/her psychological symptoms.

The most commonly seen problems that one will need to treat in sarcoidosis are reactive mood disorders, acute organic brain syndromes e.g. an acute confusional state and acute psychoses, and psychiatric disorders secondary to treatment, such as steroid psychoses. Mood disorders can most commonly be divided into anxiety and depression although the two often co-exist.

The treatment of anxiety disorder is generally CBT with occasionally medication being given both in acute cases, where benzodiazepines or small doses of antipsychotics can be used, and in chronic anxiety, where drugs such as pregabalin or the selective serotonin-reuptake inhibitors (SSRIs) would be favored.

For depression the treatment of choice depends on the severity of the disorder. In mild to moderate depressive disorder, CBT or psychodynamic therapy would be the treatment of choice; in more severe disorders, antidepressant medication is indicated. The most commonly used antidepressants are the SSRIs as they have fewer side-effects. Different SSRIs vary slightly in their side-effect profiles and as to whether they stimulate or sedate. Tricyclic antidepressants are also used but tend to have more side-effects; they are less safe in patients with cardiac disorders, prostate disease or glaucoma. Sedative antidepressants should be avoided where possible when there are severe respiratory problems.

In steroid-induced psychosis, most commonly manic in type, major tranquilizers are used, usually the newer atypical antipsychotics with better side-effect profiles. Mood stabilizers are usually not needed as these are generally short-lived disorders unless patients need long-term steroids. When a patient has a history of steroid-induced mania it would be wise to cover high doses of steroids with an atypical antipsychotic.

In an acute confusional state the treatment is of the underlying medical disorder. General nursing measures should be used including, where necessary, keeping a nurse with a patient at all times because of the risks of both suicide and homicide secondary to paranoid ideation. It is best to use the same nurse wherever possible so the patient gets used to that nurse. The patient should be nursed in a side-room with lighting, as the more normal cues he/she is able to pick up the better. Medication is used only when the patient is unmanageable without, and our personal preference is small doses of antipsychotic drugs such as haloperidol.

CONCLUSION

Sarcoidosis can impose a considerable health burden and have a deleterious effect on psychosocial health. Limitations in the current literature mean an accurate picture of quality of life in sarcoidosis is difficult to discern. There is no clear relationship between lung function and quality of life. Fatigue is a prominent symptom and may be more important in determining patient quality of life than any other symptom. The incidence of psychiatric disease in sarcoidosis in similarly unclear but can occur in a reactive manner, secondary to corticosteroid therapy and also as a primary manifestation of neurosarcoidosis.

REFERENCES

Antoniou KM, Tzanakis N, Tzouvelekis A *et al.* (2006). Quality of life in patients with active sarcoidosis in Greece. *Eur J Intern Med* **17**: 421–6.

Baughman RP, Sparkman BK, Lower EE (2007). Six-minute walk test and health status assessment in sarcoidosis. *Chest* **132**: 207–13.

Bona JR, Fackler SM, Fendley MJ, Nemeroff CB (1998). Neurosarcoidosis as a cause of refractory psychosis: a complicated case report. *Am J Psychiatry* **155**: 1106–8.

Boston Collaborative Drug Surveillance Program (1972). Acute adverse reactions to prednisolone in relation to dosage. *Clin Pharm Therapeut* **13**: 694–8.

Bourgeois JA, Maddock RJ, Rogers L *et al.* (2005). Neurosarcoidosis and delirium. *Psychosomatics* **46**: 148–50.

Brown ES, Chandler PA (2001). Mood and cognitive changes during systemic corticosteroid therapy. *Primary Care Comp J Clin Psychiatry* **3**: 17–21.

Chang B, Steimel J, Moller DR *et al.* (2001). Depression in sarcoidosis. *Am J Respir Crit Care Med* **163**: 329–34.

Cox CE, Donohue JF, Brown CD *et al.* (2004). Health-related quality of life of persons with sarcoidosis. *Chest* **125**: 997–1004.

Drent M, Wirnsberger RM, Breteler MHM *et al.* (1998). Quality of life and depressive symptoms in patients suffering from sarcoidosis. *Sarcoid Vasc Diff Lung Dis* **15**: 59–66.

Goracci A, Fagiolini A, Martinucci M *et al.* (2008). Quality of life, anxiety and depression in sarcoidosis. *Gen Hosp Psychiatry* **30**: 441–5.

Michielsen HJ, Drent M, Peros-Golubicic T, De Vries J (2006). Fatigue is associated with quality of life in sarcoidosis patients. *Chest* **130**: 989–94.

O'Brien GM, Baughman RP, Broderick JP *et al.* (1994). Paranoid psychosis due to neurosarcoidosis. *Sarcoidosis* **11**: 34–6.

Sabaawi M, Gutierrez-Nunez J, Fragala MR (1992). neurosarcoidosis presenting as schizophreniform disorder. *Int J Psychiatry Med* **22**: 269–74.

Spruit MA, Thomeer MJ, Gosselink R *et al.* (2005). Skeletal muscle weakness in patients with sarcoidosis and its relationship with exercise intolerance and reduced health status. *Thorax* **60**: 32–8.

Stiller J, Goodman A, Kamhi LM *et al.* (1984). Neurosarcoidosis presenting as major depression. *J Neurol Neurosurg Psychiatry* **47**: 1050–1.

Wirnsberger RM, Drent M, Hekelaar N *et al.* (1997). Relationship between respiratory muscle function and quality of life in sarcoidosis. *Eur Respir J* **10**: 1450–5.

Wirnsberger RM, de Vries J, Breteler MHM *et al.* (1998). Evaluation of quality of life in sarcoidosis patients. *Respir Med* **92**: 750–6.

Yeager H, Rossman MD, Baughman RP *et al.* (2005). Pulmonary and psychosocial findings at enrollment in the ACCESS study. *Sarcoid Vasc Diff Lung Dis* **22**: 147–53.

PART **VI**

SKIN, EYES, JOINTS AND SKELETAL MUSCLES, SUPERFICIAL LYMPHADENOPATHY, AND ENDOCRINE GLANDS

30

The skin

NILESH MORAR AND RICHARD STAUGHTON

INTRODUCTION

Sarcoidosis began life as a dermatological disease, and it remains salutary today to marvel how early observers without histology or X-rays delineated it as a separate entity. It remains a matter of debate who recorded the first case, but many credit Sir Jonathan Hutchinson. He observed a girl with skin lesions and eye problems and followed her from 1865 to 1875 under the title of 'relapsing iritis of inherited gout'. In 1898 he reported another probable case of cutaneous sarcoidosis as 'Mortimer's malady'. Meanwhile in Paris, Besnier first used the term 'lupus pernio'. Further cases were described but it remained until 1914 for Schaumann to recognize that these skin lesions were part of a systemic disease. This was only fully acknowledged at the first international conference on sarcoidosis in 1934.

Perhaps a contemporary parallel could be drawn with the observation by New York dermatologists of young men with Kaposi's sarcoma as the first signal of a new systemic disease, at first thought to be immunological. The story progressively unfolded until the causative retrovirus was found, and the 'immunology' was explained.

The cause of sarcoidosis continues to elude us, but there is certainly much immunology and consideration of the skin allows us to observe its several somewhat confusing aspects. The sarcoid antigen seems to be able to trigger vast antibody globulin production resulting in an acute immune complex disease, witnessed in the skin as erythema nodosum. It seems also to be able to lodge in the various tissues of the body, where it is pinioned by groups of macrophages ('naked granulomas'), giving rise to a whole variety of longer lasting skin lesions such as papules, plaques, nodules and lupus pernio. The Kveim reaction to intradermally injected material derived from sarcoid patients engenders, in the majority of patients, a histological picture identical to that seen in such cutaneous sarcoidosis. A further effect of the antigen is to quell the whole body's cell mediated immunity – witnessed by the dermatologist as cutaneous anergy (e.g. a negative Mantoux reaction).

FREQUENCY OF CUTANEOUS MANIFESTATIONS

Approximately 25 percent of patients with chronic systemic sarcoidosis will present with one or more cutaneous lesions. Erythema nodosum occurs in 25–50 percent with acute presentations characterized by associated bihilar lymphadenopathy and arthralgia (Löfgren's syndrome) (Newman et al. 1997) and 80 percent of patients show cutaneous anergy. Historically, 80 percent of patients showed a positive Kveim reaction. Cutaneous sarcoidosis can also occur without systemic disease. (Collin et al. 2010).

Since so many varieties of lesion can be caused by sarcoidosis, and the skin is so much more accessible to biopsy than lung or lymph nodes, it is always preferable to biopsy even questionable lesions if the diagnosis is suspected. Skin lesions in sarcoid patients can easily be overlooked or misinterpreted given the challengingly variable morphologies that can occur. They often appear at the onset of systemic illness, providing a valuable opportunity for early diagnosis (Hanno et al. 1981; Samtsov 1992; Mana et al. 1997; English et al. 2001). Hence, clinicians treating sarcoid patients should be taught how to carry out the simple speedy procedure of punch biopsy under local anesthesia. With practice the procedure takes less than five minutes and is no more painful than venepuncture.

Sarcoidosis is a rare condition and direct presentation to the skin department is an uncommon event probably amounting to 1 in every 5000 patients seen. There is certainly geographical and racial susceptibility which greatly influences the incidence from hospital to hospital. In Europe it is more common in northern countries (30–40 per 100000) (Djuric 1985; Milman and Selroos 1990; Rybicki *et al.* 1997). American blacks (36–64 per 100000) are more commonly affected that whites (10–14 per 100000). The Indian subcontinent is reported as having a high incidence of sarcoidosis (61–150 per 100000) (Gupta and Gupta 1990). Observations from Africa are sparse, but in South Africa there is a much higher incidence in the black population than white (Benatar 1977). Chong *et al.* (2005) reported a series from The National Skin Centre in Singapore, where over a 23-year period only 24 cases of histologically proven cutaneous sarcoidosis was found. Thirteen patients were Indian, 11 Chinese and one Eurasian. In 13, sarcoidosis was confined to the skin and the sex ratio was unusual (15 males to 10 females). Infiltration of scars occurred in three patients.

CLASSIFICATION

A sharp distinction must be drawn between the infiltrations of the skin by sarcoid granulomas and erythema nodosum that occurs in only a proportion of patients, usually at the onset, and is indistinguishable histologically from erythema nodosum associated with other diseases. Eruptions are generally classified as 'specific' (when a typical granulomatous infiltrate is present on skin biopsy) or 'non-specific'. Specific lesions include macules, papules, plaques, nodules, infiltrated scars, subcutaneous lesions and lupus pernio. The most common cutaneous presentation is with papules and nodules. Such lesions are flesh-colored and typically asymptomatic.

Non-specific manifestations include erythema nodosum and other rarities including calcification, erythema multiforme, prurigo and nail clubbing.

CLINICAL SPECTRUM OF CUTANEOUS LESIONS

Erythema nodosum

The characteristic inflamed subcutaneous nodules on the anterior legs are acutely tender and present more often to the family practitioner or the accident and emergency department rather than to dermatology departments. Erythema nodosum is a non-specific finding that occurs in association with numerous underlying etiologies. The majority of patients with erythema nodosum have conditions other than sarcoidosis (Box 30.1).

The histological pattern is identical in erythema nodosum from all causes and shows septal panniculitis. This cannot confirm or negate a diagnosis of sarcoidosis. Lesions can be accompanied by arthritis, ankle edema and low-grade fever. Löfgren's syndrome is more prevalent in young females of Nordic ancestry and in the Irish (Löfgren and Lundback 1952). The prognosis is good: many patients heal within 6 months, and 85 percent within 2 years of onset of symptoms. The treatment includes bedrest and non-steroidal anti-inflammatory drugs if necessary.

Box 30.1 Causes of erythema nodosum

- Bacterial infections
  - *Streptococcus*
  - *Mycoplasma pneumoniae*
  - Tuberculosis
  - *Salmonella*
  - *Campylobacter*
  - *Yersinia enterocolitica*
- Systemic fungal infections
  - Coccidioidomycosis
  - Blastomycosis
  - Histoplasmosis
- Inflammatory conditions
  - Inflammatory bowel disease
  - Sarcoidosis
  - Behçet's disease
- Drugs
  - Sulfonamides
  - Oral contraceptive pills
- Pregnancy
- Lymphoma

Papular sarcoidosis

This is the characteristic primary lesion of sarcoidosis. The papules are akin to the more common lichen planus papules but less violaceous, more flesh-colored or reddish brown and never itchy (Fig. 30.1 and 30.2). The oral mucosa should be checked for the characteristic lacy white changes of lichen planus. The sarcoid papules are often crowded on the upper shoulders and on the back of the neck. On the face, the upper eyelids, nasal alae and lips are affected (Plate 21). Unlike rosaceous papules they are never pustular. They must be distinguished from syringomas which are usually below the eye and yellowish in color, or xanthelasmas which are even more yellow, flatter and larger. They may be found on extensor aspects of the limbs. Less commonly they are seen on the trunk and buttocks. They can be telangiectatic. Annular lesions occur composed of rings of small papules

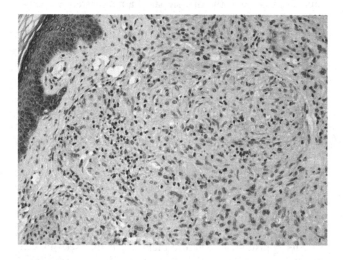

Figure 30.1   Confluent superficial dermal granulomas.

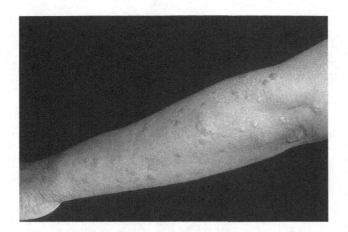

Figure 30.2   Disseminated papular lesions.

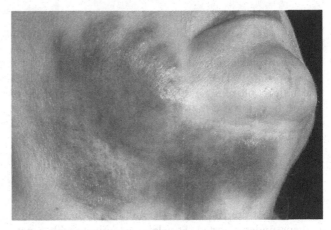

Figure 30.3   Tumid plaques with erythema and pigmentation.

with paler atrophic centers (Plate 22). Sometimes the circles are not complete and lesions form serpiginous granulomas reminiscent of tertiary syphilis. On diascopy, drained of blood, they have an apple-jelly color. A punch biopsy settles the matter and mostly shows characteristic naked granulomas. As they involute their centers become depressed, and lesions eventually flatten to brown stains with residual telangiectasia. They are pigmented when active and paler when healed. There is seldom scaling and they never have the Whickham's striae seen in lichen planus.

Nodular sarcoidosis

Nodules are larger than 5 mm and usually much sparser (Plate 23). The lesions are firm, skin-colored at first, becoming violaceous or purplish brown later, mostly on the proximal part of limbs, trunk and face. Telangiectasia may be seen on the surface of lesions. They may show follicular indentation, and diascopy reveals an apple-jelly color. Rarely the nodules can ulcerate.

Plaque sarcoidosis

Plaques of sarcoidosis are rounded or oval in shape, with slightly raised darker rims (Plate 24). They may be single or more commonly multiple, distributed on face, back, buttocks and extremities. Lesions can appear in sun-exposed areas (Truchot *et al.* 2003). Clearing may occur from the center, giving annular or serpiginous forms. Large telangiectatic vessels may be seen coursing over the surface of plaques or of lupus pernio, and some authors use the term 'angio-lupoid' lesions. Certainly many resolving sarcoid skin lesions can leave behind permanent telangiectasia in the gradually fading post-inflammatory pigmentary patches (Fig. 30.3). Such plaques on the legs can resemble necrobiosis lipoidica or morphea.

Lupus pernio

This characteristic and infamous form of sarcoidosis is a cosmetic disaster and can be emotionally devastating. These

are the lesions originally described as chilblain-like by Hutchinson in 1887 and Besnier in 1889. They are more frequently seen in older patients, mostly women, particularly in black Americans and West Indian patients, but even more striking in the fair-skinned (Plate 25).

Lupus pernio is associated with chronic disease and extrapulmonary involvement (Yanardag *et al.* 2003). It attacks and swells the nose and presents with violaceous infiltrations sometimes with pronounced dilated blood vessels. It is extremely difficult to cover or camouflage and often accompanied by destruction of the underlying nasal bones. Exuberant swollen violaceous plaques and papules may spread over the cheekbones, forehead and ears. Lesions feel firm and there may be sparse superficial erosions. Involvement of the fingers and toes is associated with destructive lesions of the underlying digital bones with multiple lattice-like rare fraction on X-ray. There may be associated sarcoid skin plaques on the arms, buttocks and thighs.

Lupus pernio may be the first overt evidence of sarcoidosis and is typically persistant, slowly evolving and challenging to treat. Thirty-five such patients were described by Spiteri *et al.* (1985), 95 percent of whom had sarcoid granulomas in the nasal mucosal biopsies, 74 percent pulmonary involvement and 43 percent bone cysts on radiography of the digits of hands and feet. Thirty-seven percent had ocular involvement. In their series there was a preponderance of West Indian women aged over 45 years.

Scar sarcoidosis

There are many reports of patients where changes occur in scars, often on the knees. Trivial childhood accidents have led to the diagnosis of sarcoidosis. Previously atrophic scars suddenly become purple and livid and skin biopsy reveals active sarcoid tissue. The diagnosis should thus be suspected when scars change. Keloids and hypertrophic scars usually develop soon after surgery. Scar sarcoidosis usually occurs in old or forgotten scars. Such changes may be seen accompanying the acute eruptive phase following erythema nodosum when a biopsy of a changing scar may well provide the diagnosis. In later stages of sarcoidosis, scar infiltration may signal pulmonary or systemic progression. Scar sarcoid may appear at sites of new injury such as venepuncture, razor bumps, tuberculin tests or tattoos. It was noted by Olumide in 7 of the 13 patients with cutaneous sarcoidosis he described after scarification from native herbalists in Nigeria (Ong *et al.* 2002).

In Scadding's (1972) series of 500 patients reviewed, 24 had infiltration of scars at some time during the observed course. In 14 this was the only form of skin infiltration. James (1959) recorded scar sarcoid in 6 of 33 patients with cutaneous sarcoidosis.

Subcutaneous sarcoidosis

This was first described by Darier and Roussy in 1904 and is perhaps under-reported. Females predominate with a peak incidence in the fifth and sixth decades. The lesions themselves are usually multiple and characteristically on the forearms, where they resemble multiple lipomas being skin-colored subcutaneous nodules 1–4 cm in diameter. They may coalesce to form linear bands. Of 10 such patients reported from Barcelona by Marcoval *et al.* (2005), these occurred on the forearms, coalescing in linear bands in five patients. In six of their patients lesions remitted spontaneously in less than two years. Although rare, when it does occur, it usually heralds systemic involvement (Higgins *et al.* 1993). The lesions differ from erythema nodosum in that they are non-tender, the epidermis is not discolored, and the lesions present for a long time.

Rarer cutaneous forms of sarcoidosis

If sarcoidosis is seriously suspected, any unusual skin lesion should be biopsied. In experienced hands, a 4 mm punch is an almost painless and cosmetically acceptable investigation. The finding of naked granulomas will prove sarcoidosis as the cause.

SCALP ALOPECIA

A sarcoid granuloma on the scalp usually starts as a flesh-colored plaque. The hair is lost and a patch of alopecia develops which subsequently shrinks to form a telangiectatic pigmented scar. Lesions simulate discoid lupus erythematosus, lichen planopilaris or scleroderma. Lesions sometimes expand to cover large areas of scalp and can result in permanent hair loss (Katta *et al.* 2000; Cho *et al.* 2004; Fig. 30.4).

FOREHEAD SARCOIDOSIS

Hyperpigmented areas with or without a central indurated lesion have been seen in patients with sarcoidosis, particularly on the limbs. Unlike leprosy, such lesions are not anesthetic. A biopsy usually, but not always, reveals sarcoid granulomas (Plate 26).

HYPOPIGMENTED SARCOIDOSIS

Sarcoid can present as depigmented patches. These are less symmetrical and less starkly white than vitiligo, and

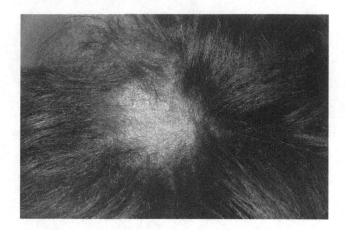

Figure 30.4   Scalp alopecia.

sometimes with an obliging red plaque centrally (the 'fried egg' configuration). Unlike in tuberculoid leprosy, lesions are not anesthetic. They are almost exclusively seen in patients with pigmented skin (Alexis 1994). Such lesions were reported in 8 of 145 American patients with sarcoidosis (Mayock *et al.* 1963).

ERYTHRODERMIC SARCOIDOSIS

This is an extremely rare cause of erythroderma and clinically challenging to diagnose. Red plaques and patches extend to cover most of the skin surface. Diascopy may reveal apple-jelly changes, most commonly observed after the histological report has been read. As resolution occurs the erythroderma breaks up into plaques and nodules.

ICHTHYOSIFORM SARCOIDOSIS

Rarely some well-documented patients with systemic sarcoidosis have developed large, thick, polygonal, adherent, fish-like scales on the lower legs with underlying dark-red patches or nodules. Biopsy shows epidermal changes consistent with ichthyosis overlying dermal epithelioid granulomas (Cather and Cohen 1999; Young *et al.* 2001; Plate 27).

MUCOSAL SARCOIDOSIS

The nasal mucosa is most often affected particularly in lupus pernio patients. Biopsy reveals granulomas and there may be difficulty in breathing and purulent catarrh. Nasal bones show porosity on X-ray and the nasal cartilage can collapse. The larynx can be involved, presenting with a hoarse voice.

NAIL SARCOIDOSIS

This is rare but may be seen when underlying bone cysts cause swelling of terminal phalanges, accompanied by over-lying nail abnormalities with thickening, fragility and reddish brown discoloration of nail beds. Eventual nail loss can occur (Cox and Gawkrodger 1988; Fig. 30.5).

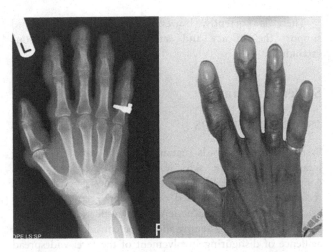

Figure 30.5 (a, b) Sarcoid dactylitis with swelling of the fingers and lysis of bone seen on the X-ray.

CHILDHOOD SARCOIDOSIS

Childhood sarcoidosis is rare. In older children, full-blown systemic sarcoidosis can occur, preceded by erythema nodosum and accompanied by progressive eye and joint involvement. Younger children present predominantly with skin lesions, uveitis, arthritis and stage I changes on chest X-ray (Hoffmann *et al.* 2004).

ULCERATED SARCOIDOSIS

Although rare, more than 35 cases have now been described – mostly in black women with punched-out ulcers on their posterior legs (Plate 28) (Neill *et al.* 1984; Hruza and Kerdel 1986). Occasionally, patients with lupus pernio can develop ulceration of the ears or nose. Ulceration may follow over-enthusiastic treatment with intralesional steroid injections.

TREATMENT

Remission of sarcoidosis occurs in more than 50 percent of patients within 3 years of disease onset (Iannuzzi *et al.* 2007). The decision to treat cutaneous sarcoidosis will depend on the extent of lesions and the degree of disfigurement or if there is associated systemic involvement, especially of the lungs. While skin lesions are largely asymptomatic, patients with subcutaneous sarcoidosis may experience functional impairment and discomfort with application of pressure.

To date, however, there are no objective indices of disease severity and there is lack of uniformity of clinical end-points of treatment. There are no randomized controlled trials on any therapy for cutaneous sarcoidosis (Izikson and English 2008). Recommendations for treatment are therefore anec-dotal and based on clinical experience, case series and non-randomized trials. For limited skin disease, topical therapy will suffice, and sometimes camouflage (Plate 29 and Fig. 30.6).

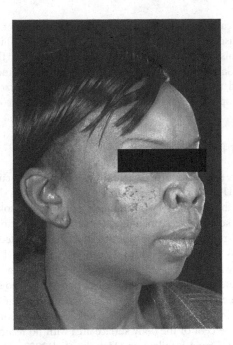

Figure 30.6 Cosmetic camouflage for disfiguring facial lesions.

Topical therapy

TOPICAL STEROIDS

Corticosteroids suppress inflammation by binding to the glucocorticoid receptor, hence suppressing transcription factors, notably nuclear factor kappa-B (NFκB), which mediates the expression of inflammatory genes (Hayashi *et al.* 2004).

There are limited data on the use of potent topical steroids in the treatment of cutaneous lesions. Halobetasol has been used to treat lupus pernio when applied twice weekly (Khatri *et al.* 1995). Once weekly application of clobetasol propionate lotion left under a hydrocolloid occlusive patch (Duoderm) resulted in remission of skin lesions in the three patients studied after 3–5 weeks (Volden 1992). Intralesional triamci-nolone (10 mg/mL) resulted in resolution of palpebral lesions when administered three times a week over a 4-week period (Bersani and Nichols 1985). The main side-effects of topical steroids in this context are atrophy and hypopigmentation.

TACROLIMUS

Tacrolimus is a macrolide immunosuppressive that inhibits T-cell responses via inhibition of transcription factor NF-AT (Sawada *et al.* 1987). It is licensed for treating moderate to severe atopic dermatitis (Ruzicka *et al.* 1997). Th1 cytokines are important in sarcoid granuloma formation (Agostini *et al.* 1998) and tacrolimus has been demonstrated to inhibit hapten-induced production of Th1 cytokines by T-cells (Nagai *et al.* 1997; Homey *et al.* 1998; Katoh *et al.* 2002). A patient who failed topical steroids and had a minimal response to low-dose prednisolone had markedly improved after a 3-month course of 0.01% tacrolimus; the response was noticed 2 weeks after initiating therapy (Katoh *et al.* 2002). A patient with sarcoidosis affecting the alar nasae and lungs responded to a 3-month course of twice weekly applications of 0.01% tacrolimus after failing mometasone furoate ointment (Green 2007). Lichenoid sarcoidois has also successfully been treated in this way (Vano-Galvan *et al.* 2008). Further controlled studies are required to compare the effectiveness of topical tacrolimus versus topical steroids in the treatment of skin sarcoid.

PHOTOTHERAPY

There are several reports on light sources used to treat cutaneous lesions. UVA-1 irradiation, similar to UVB, has been shown to induce the expression of immunosuppressive cytokines in human keratinocytes, including tumor necrosis factor-α and IL-10 (Krutmann and Morita 2001). Hypopigmented sarcoidosis has been treated with psoralen-UVA therapy (Patterson and Fitzwater 1982). Medium-dose UVA-1 therapy has successfully treated cutaneous sarcoidosis in a patient with no systemic involvement: 50 treatments with a total dose of 2.640 J/cm^2 resulted in clearance of extensive trunk lesions involving more than 70 percent of the body surface area with no recurrence of lesions at 5-month follow-up (Mahnke *et al.* 2003).

Photodynamic therapy has been successfully used to treat facial and lower limb lesions in patients who had failed or had a minimal response to topical corticosteroids, tacrolimus and oral immunosuppressive agents (Karrer *et al.* 2002; Wilsmann-Theis *et al.* 2008; Patterson 2009). The treatment resulted in remission periods ranging from 6 to 18 months. The mechanism of action is postulated at present. It has been suggested that the immunomodulatory cytokines released after phototherapy inhibit granuloma formation (Karrer *et al.* 2002; Patterson 2009). The most frequent side-effect is burning and stinging of the treated area which may continue after treatment. Caution is advised in pigmented skin as post-inflammatory hyperpigmentation may occur (Patterson 2009).

The flashlamp-pumped pulsed dye laser (FPDL) works by selective destruction of blood vessels. Vascular endothelial growth factor (VEGF) and other angiogenic factors play a role in granulomatous conditions and may provide a therapeutic target (Roos *et al.* 2009). Nodular cutaneous sarcoidosis lesions on the back were treated using a FPDL which resulted in clearance of lesions at 4-week follow-up. *Varicella zoster* virus-induced scar sarcoidosis in a 10-year-old boy improved with PDL (Holzmann *et al.* 2008). Post-inflammatory hyper- or hypopigmentation may occur as a side-effect. Lupus pernio has also been treated successfully with FPDL (Goodman and Alpern 1992; Cliff *et al.* 1999). A report suggested that the laser therapy improved the cosmetic appearance of the lesions but not the underlying disease process as granulomatous inflammation was still evident in the post-treatment skin biopsy (Cliff *et al.* 1999).

Ablative lasers such as the CO$_2$ laser have been used to treat disfiguring lupus pernio (Stack *et al.* 1996; Young *et al.* 2002; O'Donoghue and Barlow 2006). In one series, the debulking effect of the laser resulted in a favorable cosmetic response which remained in two out of three patients at 16-month follow-up (O'Donoghue and Barlow 2006). The non-ablative Q-switched ruby laser has been used to treat scar sarcoidosis resulting from traumatic tattoos in a patient who failed FPDL (Grema *et al.* 2002).

There is currently, however, insufficient evidence to support the efficacy and safety of lasers in cutaneous sarcoidosis.

Systemic therapy

ORAL CORTICOSTEROIDS

Systemic corticosteroids remain the 'gold standard' for the treatment of severe skin lesions, although randomized controlled trials are lacking for extrapulmonary disease and recommendations are based on anecdotal reports and the track record of clinical experience (Badgwell and Rosen 2007; Lodha *et al.* 2009). Therapy should be considered if there is evidence of disfiguring involvement of the face, widespread cutaneous lesions, if monotherapy with topical agents has failed, and if there is concomitant systemic involvement. Oral corticosteroids do not result in a sustained remission.

The initial dose ranges from 40 to 80 mg per day which is gradually tapered depending on the clinical response (Veien 1986; Badgwell and Rosen 2007).

The side-effects of long-term steroid treatment must be borne in mind. These include the development of Cushingoid features, osteoporosis, hypertension, hyperglycemia, acne and pyschosis (Badgwell and Rosen 2007). As a result, second-line systemic agents are often required to prevent a relapse when oral steroids are tapered or stopped.

ANTIMALARIAL AGENTS

Chloroquine, hydroxychloroquine and mepacrine are anti-malarials. The drugs inhibit antigen processing and presentation by antigen-presenting cells to CD4 + T-cells (Doherty and Rosen 2008). In a review examining the published evidence on the efficacy of antimalarials in cutaneous sarcoidosis, 82 of the 103 patients who were treated with antimalarials had a positive response (Izikson and English 2008). The authors concluded that, while none of the studies was a randomized controlled trial, this was reasonable evidence to recommend this treatment option. A single randomized trial of chloroquine for pulmonary sarcoidosis showed improvement in pulmonary function (Baltzan *et al.* 1999).

The long-term use of antimalarials can lead to ocular complications, the most serious of which is irreversible retinopathy and blindness. This risk is lower with hydroxychloroquine, though its efficacy in cutaneous sarcoidosis is less than that of chloroquine (Zic *et al.* 1991) While universal consensus is lacking, baseline ophthalmological assessment is necessary with a repeat review 6–12 monthly, or sooner if symptoms such as blurred vision occur (King and Kelly 2009). Other side-effects include gastrointestinal upsets, central nervous system toxicity, neuromuscular reactions, cutaneous pigmentation, and rarely agranulocytosis (Izikson and English 2008; King and Kelly 2009).

METHOTREXATE

Methotrexate inhibits the enzyme dihydrofolate reductase, and this prevents purine synthesis. The drug has an antiproliferative effect at high doses and is anti-inflammatory in low doses. It is used as an adjunctive therapy in steroid-resistant sarcoidosis and in patients who have not responded to antimalarials.

Usage is based on non-randomized and uncontrolled clinical trials. The first study by Veien (1986) reported that 12 of 16 patients had clearing of skin lesions after a starting dose of 25 mg per week which was tapered to 5–15 mg per week. There was no long-term follow-up in this study. In another study, methotrexate had a steroid sparing effect in 9 of 11 patients with refractory pulmonary sarcoidosis. Of these, four patients with primarily cutaneous lesions had a 50 percent reduction in skin lesions (Lower and Baughman 1990). The same group investigated the use of methotrexate over a 2-year period in 50 patients who received a 10 mg weekly dosage. Sixteen of 17 patients with skin involvement improved, but relapse was rapid after discontinuation of treatment.

The drug may be associated with nausea and vomiting, bone marrow suppression, hepatotoxicity and hypersensitivity pneumonitis, which may be difficult to differentiate from a sarcoidosis exacerbation.

THALIDOMIDE

Thalidomide inhibits TNF-α and interferon-γ which are the key cytokines that drive granulomatous processes. In 10 patients with refractory sarcoidosis treated with 1.84 mg/kg of thalidomide for 2.8 months, three patients had a complete response, four had a partial response, and three showed no response (Estines et al. 2001). In an open-label, dose-escalation study of thalidomide to treat 15 patients with lupus pernio with dosages ranging from 50 to 200 mg per day, all patients experienced subjective improvement and 10 of 12 patients experienced improvement with clinical photography (Baughman et al. 2002). In a retrospective analysis of thalidomide in dosages ranging from 100 to 200 mg per day, in 12 patients cutaneous lesions regressed in an average time of 2–3 months in 10 patients; 4 patients experienced a complete response. Systemic symptoms were also attenuated (Nguyen et al. 2004). The most serious side-effect is peripheral neuropathy which usually resolves with decreasing the dose or stopping medication (Baughman and Lower 2004a).

There is inconsistency across trials with regard to the populations studied, dosage used and clinical end-points measured, suggesting that, while this is a useful alternative, a large randomized controlled trial is required.

TETRACYCLINES

Tetracyclines are broad-spectrum antibiotics that inhibit granuloma formation by inhibition of protein kinase C (Sapadin and Fleischmajer 2006). In a non-randomized, open study of cutaneous sarcoidosis, 12 patients were treated with minocycline 200 mg per day for a median duration of 12 months. The median follow-up was 26 months. Complete responses in eight patients with papulonodular and plaque type lesions and partial responses in two patients was noted. Three patients relapsed after discontinuation of treatment but cleared when doxycycline 200 mg per day was introduced

(Bachelez et al. 2001). A 6-month course of doxycycline at a dose of 200 mg per day led to complete remission in a single case reported (El Sayed et al. 2006). A 4-month course of doxycycline 200 mg per day with mid-potency topical steroids resulted in clearance of sarcoidosis resulting from a cosmetic tattoo (Antonovich and Callen 2005).

Side-effects of tetracyclines include photosensitivity and gastrointestinal upsets. Minocycline may be associated with hypersensitivity and pigmentation. Nevertheless, tetracyclines represent an easy alternative to other systemic treatments associated with a higher side-effect profile (Izikson and English 2008). Further studies are required.

ISOTRETINOIN

Isotretinoin is a retinoid which has an immunomodulatory effect. Retinoids exert this effect directly on epidermal cells and inhibit lymphocyte activation (Dupuy et al. 1989). A female patient with cutaneous lesions achieved remission at 15-month follow-up after an 8-month course of 1 mg/kg daily of isotretinoin (Georgiou et al. 1998). The beneficial effects of isotretinoin for cutaneous lesions are described in case reports (Waldinger et al. 1983; Mosam and Morar 2004; Chong et al. 2005).

The role of oral retinoids in sarcoidosis requires further study. The most serious side-effect is teratogenicity and the most common side-effect is cheilitis.

TNF-ALPHA ANTAGONISTS

The TNF-α antagonists include monoclonal antibodies (infliximab, adalimumab) and the soluble receptor against TNF-α (etanercept). The most widely studied agent is infliximab. There are no randomized controlled trials on either of these agents, nor is there a comparison between the different agents in sarcoidosis.

TNF-α is important in granuloma formation, and variations in the TNF-α gene are important in determining the clinical subtypes of sarcoidosis (Seitzer et al. 2002).

There are several reports emerging on the rapid response of progressive cutaneous lesions to infliximab (Mallbris et al. 2003; Meyerle and Shorr 2003; Haley et al. 2004; Rosen and Doherty 2007). In one study, infliximab was administered together with prednisolone which was tapered gradually over the infliximab course (Haley et al. 2004). The longest follow-up period to date is described for a patient with lupus pernio who remained clear with continued 8–10 weekly infusions for three and a half years after initiation of treatment (Rosen and Doherty 2007). In a retrospective study of 10 patients with refractory systemic and cutaneous involvement, including five with lupus pernio, all patients experienced objective improvement over the treatment period over 6 weeks to 2.5 years. The drug was well tolerated and resulted in a steroid sparing effect.

The drug is given as a slow infusion ranging from 3 to 10 mg/kg per dose at weeks 0, 2 and 6, and then 8–10 weekly thereafter depending on the clinical response. The typical starting dose is 5 mg/kg per infusion. Low-dose methotrexate is often combined with infliximab to prevent the development of anti-infliximab blocking antibodies (Baughman and Lower 2001).

Adalimumab has been effective in treating ulcerated cutaneous sarcoidosis on the shins unresponsive to conventional therapy (Philips *et al.* 2005) and in a patient with nodules on her shins and nose (Heffernan and Smith 2006). The drug was given at a dose of 40 mg subcutaneously weekly.

A patient with progressive cutaneous lesions who had failed therapy with systemic steroids and immunosuppressive agents responded to etanercept as monotherapy (Tuchinda and Wong 2006). The dosage used is 50 mg subcutaneously weekly. A patient with lupus pernio and sarcoid arthropathy who failed systemic steroids and disease-modifying anti-rheumatism agents responded when etanercept was added (Khanna *et al.* 2003).

Anti-TNF-α drugs are immunosuppressive, so infections such as tuberculosis or the reactivation of latent tuberculosis are a risk. The long-term side-effects such as malignancies must also be borne in mind. Notably, a series of 10 patients is described who, when treated with etanercept, infliximab and adalimumab for rheumatoid arthritis and spondyloarthritis, developed sarcoidosis after a median period of 18 months. This suggests that the effect of anti-TNF-α agents on cytokine modulation and Th1 responses is complex. Sarcoid-like granulomatosis is thought to be rare, occurring in 1 in 2800 patients, and remits with discontinuation of the anti-TNF-α agent (Daien *et al.* 2009).

Based on the current evidence, it is recommended that biologics are useful as alternative or additional therapy in extremely recalcitrant cases (Izikson and English 2008).

OTHER DRUGS

Several other drugs have been used to treat cutaneous sarcoidosis. The data on these drugs, however, are not sufficient to make unequivocal recommendations for their use.

Leflunomide is a cytotoxic drug that inhibits pyrimidine and hence DNA synthesis and suppresses TNF-α. Current evidence of efficacy in cutaneous diseases is limited and can be inferred only from case series of patients with both systemic and skin involvement. A loading dose of 100 mg per day given for 3 days followed by 20 mg per day improved refractory skin lesions (Majithia *et al.* 2003). It is well tolerated and has been recommended either as a good alternative if methotrexate toxicity develops, or as adjunctive therapy as, when used in combination with methotrexate, the response rate was better (Baughman and Lower 2004b). The most common adverse effect is gastrointestinal upsets. The drug has rarely been associated with Stevens–Johnson syndrome and toxic epidermal necrolysis.

A patient with pulmonary sarcoidosis who developed ulcerative sarcoidosis of her lower legs responded well to a tapering course of oral prednisolone and a low dose (50 mg per day) of the cytotoxic drug azathioprine (Poonawalla *et al.* 2008). A patient with recalcitrant cutaneous sarcoidosis also responded to azathioprine (Mosam and Morar 2004). However, there are limited data on the beneficial effects of azathioprine to treat cutaneous sarcoidosis.

Mycophenolate mofetil (MMF) inhibits inosine monophosphate dehydrogenase and attenuates lymphocyte proliferation (Kouba *et al.* 2003). In a case series of five patients with recalcitrant skin disease who failed oral steroids and immunosuppressive drugs, MMF at a dose of 1.5 mg twice daily resulted in significant improvement when used together with hydroxychloroquine and a tapered course of oral prednisolone (Kouba *et al.* 2003). The authors recommend MMF as an adjunctive agent.

There are several cases reported to have responded to allopurinol (Antony and Layton 2000; Mosam and Morar 2004; Bregnhoej and Jemec 2005; Martin *et al.* 2007). This includes a granulomatous reaction in a cosmetic tattoo (Martin *et al.* 2007) and responses noted in recalcitrant cases (Mosam and Morar 2004; Bregnhoej and Jemec 2005). The drug inhibits multinucleate giant cell formation (Bregnhoej and Jemec 2005).

Pentoxifylline inhibits TNF-α. There are anecdotal reports on its use as a corticosteroid sparing agent at a dose of 400 mg three times daily (Mosam and Morar 2004).

Chlorambucil is an alklyating agent that inhibits T-cells. It is used at a dose of 4–12 mg per day. There is limited evidence of efficacy in cutaneous sarcoidosis (Kataria 1980; Israel and McComb 1991).

Melatonin at a dose of 20 mg daily cleared skin lesions in two patients after 5 months of therapy (Cagnoni *et al.* 1995) and in three patients after a 24-month treatment course (Pignone *et al.* 2006). The drug has an anti-inflammatory and immunomodulatory effect.

There are two reports on the efficacy of mepacrine for skin lesions (Hughes and Pembroke 1994; Yesudian and Azurdia 2004). Mepacrine has an antimalarial and antihelminthic action. It may be used together with hydroxychloroquine or serves as an option if the patient is intolerant to antimalarials. A yellow discoloration of the skin may result (Fig. 30.7).

A review describes results of 12 of 17 patients who responded to fumaric acid esters and concludes that the current evidence is insufficient to recommend routine use (Izikson and English 2008). Fumaric acid esters are immunomodulatory and inhibit granuloma formation.

CONCLUSION

Based on the current literature it is recommended that, for moderate to severe cutaneous sarcoidosis, antimalarials can be used as a first-line agent, followed by – or in combination with – corticosteroids or methotrexate if indicated. A literature review on non-steroidal systemic therapy revealed that only antimalarials, methothrexate and thalidomide have sufficient published evidence to show benefit. The review recommends that anti-TNF-α agents, tetracyclines and allopurinol need additional study but may be considered in difficult cases (Izikson and English 2008).

Patients with recalcitrant cutaneous sarcoidosis often benefit from rotational therapy using potent drugs for short periods to minimize side-effects (Mosam and Morar 2004).

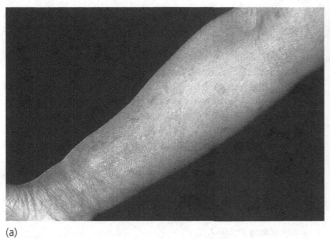 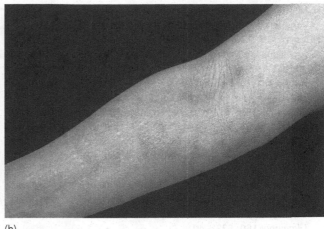

(a)   (b)

Figure 30.7   (a) Yellow discoloration of skin on mepacrine therapy. (b) Flattening of plaques after 4 months of therapy.

REFERENCES

Agostini C, Costabel U *et al.* (1998). Sarcoidosis news: immunologic frontiers for new immunosuppressive strategies. *Clin Immunol Immunopathol* **88**: 199–204.

Alexis JB (1994). Sarcoidosis presenting as cutaneous hypopigmentation with repeatedly negative skin biopsies. *Int J Dermatol* **33**: 44–5.

Antonovich DD, Callen JP (2005). Development of sarcoidosis in cosmetic tattoos. *Arch Dermatol* **141**: 869–72.

Antony F, Layton AM (2000). A case of cutaneous acral sarcoidosis with response to allopurinol. *Br J Dermatol* **142**: 1052–3.

Bachelez H, Senet P *et al.* (2001). The use of tetracyclines for the treatment of sarcoidosis. *Arch Dermatol* **137**: 69–73.

Badgwell C, Rosen T (2007). Cutaneous sarcoidosis therapy updated. *J Am Acad Dermatol* **56**: 69–83.

Baltzan M, Mehta S *et al.* (1999). Randomized trial of prolonged chloroquine therapy in advanced pulmonary sarcoidosis. *Am J Respir Crit Care Med* **160**: 192–7.

Baughman RP, Judson MA *et al.* (2002). Thalidomide for chronic sarcoidosis. *Chest* **122**: 227–32.

Baughman RP, Lower EE (2001). Infliximab for refractory sarcoidosis. *Sarcoid Vasc Diff Lung Dis* **18**: 70–4.

Baughman RP, Lower EE (2004a). Newer therapies for cutaneous sarcoidosis: the role of thalidomide and other agents. *Am J Clin Dermatol* **5**: 385–94.

Baughman RP, Lower EE (2004b). Leflunomide for chronic sarcoidosis. *Sarcoid Vasc Diff Lung Dis* **21**: 43–8.

Benatar SR (1977). Sarcoidosis in South Africa. A comparative study in Whites, Blacks and Coloureds. *S Afr Med J* **52**: 602–6.

Bersani TA, Nichols CW (1985). Intralesional triamcinolone for cutaneous palpebral sarcoidosis. *Am J Ophthalmol* **99**: 561–2.

Bregnhoej A, Jemec GB (2005). Low-dose allopurinol in the treatment of cutaneous sarcoidosis: response in four of seven patients. *J Dermatolog Treat* **16**: 125–7.

Cagnoni ML, Lombardi A *et al.* (1995). Melatonin for treatment of chronic refractory sarcoidosis. *Lancet* **346**: 1229–30.

Cather JC, Cohen PR (1999). Ichthyosiform sarcoidosis. *J Am Acad Dermatol* **40**(5 Pt 2): 862–5.

Cho HR, Shah A *et al.* (2004). Systemic sarcoidosis presenting with alopecia of the scalp. *Int J Dermatol* **43**: 520–2.

Chong WS, Tan H *et al.* (2005). Cutaneous sarcoidosis in Asians: a report of 25 patients from Singapore. *Clin Exp Dermatol* **30**: 120–4.

Cliff S, Felix RH *et al.* (1999). The successful treatment of lupus pernio with the flashlamp pulsed dye laser. *J Cutan Laser Ther* **1**: 49–52.

Collin B, Rajaratnam R *et al.* (2010). A retrospective analysis of 34 patients with cutaneous sarcoidosis assessed in a dermatology department. *Clin Exp Dermatol* **35**(2): 131–4.

Cox NH, Gawkrodger DJ (1988). Nail dystrophy in chronic sarcoidosis. *Br J Dermatol* **118**: 697–701.

Daien CI, Monnier A *et al.* (2009). Sarcoid-like granulomatosis in patients treated with tumor necrosis factor blockers: 10 cases. *Rheumatology* (Oxford) **48**: 883–6.

Djuric B (1985). Sarcoidosis in Eastern Europe. *Sarcoidosis* **2**(1): 35–7.

Doherty CB, Rosen T (2008). Evidence-based therapy for cutaneous sarcoidosis. *Drugs* **68**: 1361–83.

Dupuy P, Bagot M *et al.* (1989). Synthetic retinoids inhibit the antigen presenting properties of epidermal cells *in vitro*. *J Invest Dermatol* **93**: 455–9.

El Sayed F, Dhaybi R *et al.* (2006). Subcutaneous nodular sarcoidosis and systemic involvement successfully treated with doxycycline. *J Med Liban* **54**: 42–4.

English JC, Patel PJ *et al.* (2001). Sarcoidosis. *J Am Acad Dermatol* **44**: 725–43; quiz 744–6.

Estines O, Revuz J *et al.* (2001). [Sarcoidosis: thalidomide treatment in ten patients]. *Ann Dermatol Venereol* **128**: 611–13.

Georgiou S, Monastirli A *et al.* (1998). Cutaneous sarcoidosis: complete remission after oral isotretinoin therapy. *Acta Derm Venereol* **78**: 457–9.

Goodman MM, Alpern K (1992). Treatment of lupus pernio with the flashlamp pulsed dye laser. *Lasers Surg Med* **12**: 549–51.

Green CM (2007). Topical tacrolimus for the treatment of cutaneous sarcoidosis. *Clin Exp Dermatol* **32**: 457–8.

Grema H, Greve B *et al.* (2002). Scar sarcoidosis: treatment with the Q-switched ruby laser. *Lasers Surg Med* **30**: 398–400.

Gupta SK, Gupta S (1990). Sarcoidosis in India: a review of 125 biopsy-proven cases from eastern India. *Sarcoidosis* **7**: 43–9.

Haley H, Cantrell W *et al.* (2004). Infliximab therapy for sarcoidosis (lupus pernio). *Br J Dermatol* **150**: 146–9.

Hanno R, Needelman A *et al.* (1981). Cutaneous sarcoidal granulomas and the development of systemic sarcoidosis. *Arch Dermatol* **117**: 203–7.

Hayashi R, Wada J et al. (2004). Effects of glucocorticoids on gene transcription. Eur J Pharmacol 500(1/3): 51–62.

Heffernan MP, Smith DI (2006). Adalimumab for treatment of cutaneous sarcoidosis. Arch Dermatol 142: 17–19.

Higgins EM, Salisbury JR et al. (1993). Subcutaneous sarcoidosis. Clin Exp Dermatol 18: 65–6.

Hoffmann AL, Milman N et al. (2004). Childhood sarcoidosis in Denmark 1979–1994: incidence, clinical features and laboratory results at presentation in 48 children. Acta Paediatr 93: 30–6.

Holzmann RD, Astner S et al. (2008). Scar sarcoidosis in a child: case report of successful treatment with the pulsed dye laser. Dermatol Surg 34: 393–6.

Homey B, Assmann T et al. (1998). Topical FK506 suppresses cytokine and costimulatory molecule expression in epidermal and local draining lymph node cells during primary skin immune responses. J Immunol 160: 5331–40.

Hruza GJ, Kerdel FA (1986). Generalized atrophic sarcoidosis with ulcerations. Arch Dermatol 122: 320–2.

Hughes JR, Pembroke AC (1994). Cutaneous sarcoid treated with mepacrine. Clin Exp Dermatol 19: 448.

Iannuzzi MC, Rybicki BA et al. (2007). Sarcoidosis. New Engl J Med 357: 2153–65.

Israel HL, McComb BL (1991). Chlorambucil treatment of sarcoidosis. Sarcoidosis 8: 35–41.

Izikson L, English JC (2008). Cutaneous sarcoidosis. In: Williams H et al. (eds). Evidence-based Dermatology, 2nd edn. Blackwell/BMJ Books, Oxford, pp. 595–607.

James DG (1959). Dermatological aspects of sarcoidosis. Q J Med 28: 108–24.

Karrer S, Abels C et al. (2002). Successful treatment of cutaneous sarcoidosis using topical photodynamic therapy. Arch Dermatol 138: 581–4.

Kataria YP (1980). Chlorambucil in sarcoidosis. Chest 78: 36–43.

Katoh N, Mihara H et al. (2002). Cutaneous sarcoidosis successfully treated with topical tacrolimus. Br J Dermatol 147: 154–6.

Katta R, Nelson B et al. (2000). Sarcoidosis of the scalp: a case series and review of the literature. J Am Acad Dermatol 42: 690–2.

Khanna D, Liebling MR et al. (2003). Etanercept ameliorates sarcoidosis arthritis and skin disease. J Rheumatol 30: 1864–7.

Khatri KA, Chotzen VA et al. (1995). Lupus pernio: successful treatment with a potent topical corticosteroid. Arch Dermatol 131: 617–18.

King CS, Kelly W (2009). Treatment of sarcoidosis. Dis Mon 55: 704–18.

Kouba DJ, Mimouni D et al. (2003). Mycophenolate mofetil may serve as a steroid-sparing agent for sarcoidosis. Br J Dermatol 148: 147–8.

Krutmann JSH, Morita A (2001). UVA1 Phototherapy: Indications and Mode of Action. Springer, New York.

Lodha S, Sanchez M et al. (2009). Sarcoidosis of the skin: a review for the pulmonologist. Chest 136: 583–96.

Löfgren S, Lundback H (1952). The bilateral hilar lymphoma syndrome; a study of the relation to tuberculosis and sarcoidosis in 212 cases. Acta Med Scand 142: 265–73.

Lower EE, Baughman RP (1990). The use of low dose methotrexate in refractory sarcoidosis. Am J Med Sci 299: 153–7.

Mahnke N, Medve-Koenigs K et al. (2003). [Medium-dose UV-A1 phototherapy. Successful treatment of cutaneous sarcoidosis]. Hautarzt 54: 364–6.

Majithia V, Sanders S et al. (2003). Successful treatment of sarcoidosis with leflunomide. Rheumatology (Oxford) 42: 700–2.

Mallbris L, Ljungberg A et al. (2003). Progressive cutaneous sarcoidosis responding to anti-tumor necrosis factor-alpha therapy. J Am Acad Dermatol 48: 290–3.

Mana J, Marcoval J et al. (1997). Cutaneous involvement in sarcoidosis: relationship to systemic disease. Arch Dermatol 133: 882–8.

Marcoval J, Mana J et al. (2005). Subcutaneous sarcoidosis: clinico-pathological study of 10 cases. Br J Dermatol 153: 790–4.

Martin JM, Revert A et al. (2007). Granulomatous reactions to permanent cosmetic tattoos successfully treated with topical steroids and allopurinol. J Cosmet Dermatol 6: 229–31.

Mayock RL, Bertrand P et al. (1963). Manifestations of sarcoidosis: analysis of 145 patients, with a review of nine series selected from the literature. Am J Med 35: 67–89.

Meyerle JH, Shorr A (2003). The use of infliximab in cutaneous sarcoidosis. J Drugs Dermatol 2: 413–14.

Milman N, Selroos O (1990). Pulmonary sarcoidosis in the Nordic countries 1950–1982: epidemiology and clinical picture. Sarcoidosis 7: 50–7.

Mosam A, Morar N (2004). Recalcitrant cutaneous sarcoidosis: an evidence-based sequential approach. J Dermatolog Treat 15: 353–9.

Nagai H, Hiyama H et al. (1997). FK-506 and cyclosporin A potentiate the IgE antibody production by contact sensitization with hapten in mice. J Pharmacol Exp Ther 283: 321–7.

Neill SM, Smith NP et al. (1984). Ulcerative sarcoidosis: a rare manifestation of a common disease. Clin Exp Dermatol 9: 277–9.

Newman LS, Rose CS et al. (1997). Sarcoidosis. New Engl J Med 336: 1224–34.

Nguyen YT, Dupuy A et al. (2004). Treatment of cutaneous sarcoidosis with thalidomide. J Am Acad Dermatol 50: 235–41.

O'Donoghue NB, Barlow RJ (2006). Laser remodelling of nodular nasal lupus pernio. Clin Exp Dermatol 31: 27–9.

Ong PY, Ohtake T et al. (2002). Endogenous antimicrobial peptides and skin infections in atopic dermatitis. New Engl J Med 347: 1151–60.

Patterson C (2009). Successful treatment of cutaneous sarcoid by photodynamic therapy with minimal discomfort using a fractionated dosing regime. Photodermatol Photoimmunol Photomed 25: 276–7.

Patterson JW, Fitzwater JE (1982). Treatment of hypopigmented sarcoidosis with 8-methoxypsoralen and long-wave ultraviolet light. Int J Dermatol 21: 476–80.

Philips MA, Lynch J et al. (2005). Ulcerative cutaneous sarcoidosis responding to adalimumab. J Am Acad Dermatol 53: 917.

Pignone AM, Rosso AD et al. (2006). Melatonin is a safe and effective treatment for chronic pulmonary and extrapulmonary sarcoidosis. J Pineal Res 41: 95–100.

Poonawalla T, Colome-Grimmer MI et al. (2008). Ulcerative sarcoidosis in the legs with granulomatous vasculitis. Clin Exp Dermatol 33: 282–6.

Roos S, Raulin C et al. (2009). Successful treatment of cutaneous sarcoidosis lesions with the flashlamp pumped pulsed dye laser: a case report. Dermatol Surg 35: 1139–40.

Rosen T, Doherty C (2007). Successful long-term management of refractory cutaneous and upper airway sarcoidosis with periodic infliximab infusion. Dermatol Online J 13(3): 14.

Ruzicka T, Bieber T et al. (1997). European Tacrolimus Multicenter Atopic Dermatitis Study Group: A short-term trial of tacrolimus ointment for atopic dermatitis. New Engl J Med 337: 816–21.

Rybicki BA, Major M et al. (1997). Racial differences in sarcoidosis incidence: a 5-year study in a health maintenance organization. Am J Epidemiol 145: 234–41.

Samtsov AV (1992). Cutaneous sarcoidosis. Int J Dermatol 31: 385–91.

Sapadin AN, Fleischmajer R (2006). Tetracyclines: nonantibiotic properties and their clinical implications. *J Am Acad Dermatol* **54**: 258–65.

Sawada S, Suzuki G *et al.* (1987). Novel immunosuppressive agent, FK506: in-vitro effects on the cloned T-cell activation. *J Immunol* **139**: 1797–803.

Scadding JG (1972). Skin infiltrations in 500 cases of sarcoidosis. *Praxis* **61**: 133–6.

Seitzer U, Gerdes J *et al.* (2002). Genotyping in the MHC locus: potential for defining predictive markers in sarcoidosis. *Respir Res* **3**: 6.

Spiteri MA, Matthey F *et al.* (1985). Lupus pernio: a clinico-radiological study of thirty-five cases. *Br J Dermatol* **112**: 315–22.

Stack BC, Hall PJ *et al.* (1996). CO_2 laser excision of lupus pernio of the face. *Am J Otolaryngol* **17**: 260–3.

Truchot F, Skowron F *et al.* (2003). [Photo-induced sarcoidosis]. *Ann Dermatol Venereol* **130**(1 Pt 1): 40–2.

Tuchinda C, Wong HK (2006). Etanercept for chronic progressive cutaneous sarcoidosis. *J Drugs Dermatol* **5**: 538–40.

Vano-Galvan S, Fernandez-Guarino M *et al.* (2008). Lichenoid type of cutaneous sarcoidosis: great response to topical tacrolimus. *Eur J Dermatol* **18**: 89–90.

Veien NK (1986). Cutaneous sarcoidosis: prognosis and treatment. *Clin Dermatol* **4**(4): 75–87.

Volden G (1992). Successful treatment of chronic skin diseases with clobetasol propionate and a hydrocolloid occlusive dressing. *Acta Derm Venereol* **72**: 69–71.

Waldinger TP, Ellis CN *et al.* (1983). Treatment of cutaneous sarcoidosis with isotretinoin. *Arch Dermatol* **119**: 1003–5.

Wilsmann-Theis D, Hagemann T *et al.* (2008). Facing psoriasis and atopic dermatitis: are there more similarities or more differences? *Eur J Dermatol* **18**: 172–80.

Yanardag H, Pamuk ON *et al.* (2003). Lupus pernio in sarcoidosis: clinical features and treatment outcomes of 14 patients. *J Clin Rheumatol* **9**: 72–6.

Yesudian PD, Azurdia RM (2004). Scar sarcoidosis following tattooing of the lips treated with mepacrine. *Clin Exp Dermatol* **29**: 552–4.

Young HS, Chalmers RJ *et al.* (2002). CO_2 laser vaporization for disfiguring lupus pernio. *J Cosmet Laser Ther* **4**(3/4): 87–90.

Young RJ, Gilson RT *et al.* (2001). Cutaneous sarcoidosis. *Int J Dermatol* **40**: 249–53.

Zic JA, Horowitz DH *et al.* (1991). Treatment of cutaneous sarcoidosis with chloroquine: review of the literature. *Arch Dermatol* **127**: 1034–40.

31

Ocular changes

CLAIRE HOOPER AND SUE LIGHTMAN

INTRODUCTION

Ocular involvement in sarcoidosis is not only common and potentially vision-threatening but may also be the initial presentation of sarcoidosis (Rothova *et al.* 1989; Matsuo *et al.* 2005). Intraocular inflammation of the uveal tract, or uveitis, is the most frequent manifestation (Obenauf *et al.* 1978; Jabs and Johns 1986; James 1986; Rothova *et al.* 1989), making sarcoidosis the leading systemic cause of uveitis, accounting for 3–7 percent of non-infectious cases in specialist clinics. (Jones 2002; James *et al.* 1976; Rothova *et al.* 1992). However, a wide spectrum of inflammatory lesions involving the external eye, orbit and adnexae is additionally associated with sarcoidosis.

EPIDEMIOLOGY

Frequency of ocular involvement

The reported frequency of ocular involvement in sarcoidosis varies considerably, from 11.8 to 79 percent (Iwata *et al.* 1976; Ohara *et al.* 1992; Baughman *et al.* 2001). This variation is attributable to the extent of the ophthalmic examination and duration of follow-up as well as to referral bias and the demographics of the population studied. The ACCESS (A Case Control Etiologic Study of Sarcoidosis) trial found an incidence of ocular sarcoidosis of 11.8 percent (Baughman *et al.* 2001). They enrolled 736 patients with sarcoidosis within 6 months of the first positive biopsy from ten clinical centers in the USA. The study population was suitably heterogeneous but the study investigators were all pulmonologists and no details were provided regarding the extent of the ocular

examination performed. Hence it is likely that this study underestimated the true prevalence of ocular involvement in sarcoidosis (Judson *et al.* 1999).

In contrast, two Japanese studies have reported intraocular manifestations in 79 percent of cases (Iwata *et al.* 1976; Ohara *et al.* 1992). Both studies were conducted by ophthalmologists and involved a full examination including gonioscopy. Iwata and co-workers noted ocular changes in 55 out of 70 patients who were routinely examined over 1–11 years. Ohara and co-workers described evidence of intraocular involvement in 126 out of 159 patients. (Ohara *et al.* 1992). However, both are limited by the fact that only a minority of cases had histological confirmation of systemic sarcoidosis. A recent Japanese retrospective review, of 123 patients with a histopathological diagnosis of sarcoidosis, detected ocular inflammation in 60 patients (50 percent) during a mean follow-up period of 6 years (Matsuo *et al.* 2005). Of biopsy-proven cases of sarcoidosis, approximately 25–60 percent of patients worldwide present with or develop ocular manifestations (Crick *et al.* 1961; Mayock *et al.* 1963; Karma 1979; Jabs and Johns 1986; James 1986; Rothova *et al.* 1989; Matsuo *et al.* 2005; Khanna *et al.* 2007).

Notwithstanding the lack of histopathological corroboration, studies have consistently documented higher rates of ocular sarcoidosis, in particular uveitis, in the Japanese population. The majority of European and North American studies have reported uveitis rates between 20 and 40 percent (Crick *et al.* 1961; Mayock *et al.* 1963; Jabs and Johns 1986; James 1986; Rothova *et al.* 1989; Evans *et al.* 2007), whereas studies in Japan have revealed that the rates of sarcoid-associated uveitis are as high as 60–80 percent (Uyama 1971; Yamada *et al.* 1971; Ohara *et al.* 1992). In addition to Japanese patients, a higher prevalence of ocular sarcoidosis is observed in black patients (Jabs and

Johns 1986; Rothova *et al.* 1989; Baughman *et al.* 2001; Khalatbari *et al.* 2004). Rothova and co-workers reviewed 121 consecutive patients with biopsy-proven sarcoidosis who were seen at the sarcoidosis clinic of a university teaching hospital. Eye involvement was found to occur in 30 out of 52 (58 percent) of black patients compared with 20 out of 69 (29 percent) of white patients ($p < 0.005$) (Rothova *et al.* 1989). Similarly, the ACCESS study reported that eye involvement was more likely among black patients (17 percent) than among white patients (7.5 percent; $p < 0.0001$) (Baughman *et al.* 2001).

However, this apparent predilection for ocular involvement in pigmented races may not necessarily occur across the board. Large series from the Indian subcontinent have revealed ocular involvement rates of only 8–16 percent, although one small series did report an incidence of 40 percent (Sharma and Mohan 2002). A recent study from a university teaching hospital in India is probably the most representative (Khanna *et al.* 2007). In this study, 48 consecutive patients with histologically confirmed sarcoidosis underwent a detailed ophthalmic examination and ocular involvement was noted in 14 cases (29 percent).

A female preponderance has also reported in many studies (Obenauf *et al.* 1978; Jabs and Johns 1986; James 1986; Rothova *et al.* 1989; Yamaguchi *et al.* 1989; Baughman *et al.* 2001), but not in all studies (Karma 1979; Gupta and Gupta 1990; Atmaca *et al.* 2009). Rothova and co-workers found the frequency of ocular sarcoidosis was significantly higher in the Netherlands for female patients (38 out of 68, 56 percent) than for male patients (12 out of 53, 23 percent; $p < 0.001$) (Rothova *et al.* 1989). The ACCESS trial in the USA also found that women were more likely to have eye involvement than men ($p < 0.05$) (Baughman *et al.* 2001). Similarly, 30 percent of women compared with 23 percent of men had ocular sarcoidosis in a large London series of 818 histologically confirmed cases of sarcoidosis (James 1986). A slight female bias is also seen in reports from Japan (Yamaguchi *et al.* 1989), but in India ocular sarcoidosis seems to be equally common or more common in men (Gupta and Gupta 1990; Atmaca *et al.* 2009).

Two peaks of incidence have been described for age at onset of ocular sarcoidosis, the first at 20–30 years and the second at 50–60 years (Rothova 2000). This mirrors the bimodal age distribution observed by some in the onset of sarcoidosis, with the second peak being particularly common in women (Hillerdal *et al.* 1984; Yamaguchi *et al.* 1989) and has been widely quoted. Another study investigating demographic-related variations in posterior-segment ocular sarcoidosis noted that white females had the highest mean age at initial examination (58 years compared with 37 years for all others; $p < 0.005$) (Khalatbari *et al.* 2004). Other studies, however, have failed to demonstrate these peaks. On the contrary, age at onset of ocular sarcoidosis was between 32 and 53 years in 47 percent of patients in one study and between 31 and 50 years in 48 percent of patients in another study (Khalatbari *et al.* 2004; Tugal-Tutkun *et al.* 2007). Recognition that ocular sarcoidosis in children and the elderly is rare but can occur is important.

The presence of ocular sarcoidosis has generally not been found to correlate with any specific extraocular manifestations (Dresner *et al.* 1986; Rothova *et al.* 1989; Evans *et al.* 2007; Atmaca *et al.* 2009). One study noted that the majority of patients (72 percent) with ocular involvement had stage II pulmonary sarcoidosis, but no significant relationship between radiological grading and ocular involvement was detected (Atmaca *et al.* 2009). This confirmed previous analyses by Rothova *et al.* (1989) and Evans *et al.* (2007). Another study by Karma (1979), with a high proportion of conjunctival and lacrimal ocular sarcoidosis cases, did detect a significant association between ocular sarcoidosis and skin changes, peripheral lymphadenopathy and hypercalcemia but these findings have not been replicated.

Likewise, the type of ocular involvement has generally not been found to correlate with any specific extraocular manifestations. Uveitis patients do not differ from non-uveitis patients with ocular sarcoidosis with respect to systemic symptoms, radiological staging of pulmonary disease or presence of a positive gallium scan (Jabs and Johns 1986; Rothova *et al.* 1989). No difference has been found in the systemic manifestations of patients with acute compared with chronic anterior uveitis (Crick *et al.* 1961; Jabs and Johns 1986; Rothova *et al.* 1989). One possible exception is the reported increased risk of central nervous system involvement in patients with posterior uveitis (20–35 percent compared with 5–10 percent of all cases) (Gould and Kaufman 1961; Obenauf *et al.* 1978). However, subsequent reports have not confirmed an association (Spalton and Sanders 1981; Edelsten *et al.* 1999).

Heerfordt's syndrome, also known as uveoparotid fever, is characterized by low fever, parotid gland enlargement and uveitis sometimes accompanied by cranial nerve palsy, especially the facial nerve. However, the syndrome merely represents a rare combination of sarcoidosis features, with each component occurring more frequently alone than in association with the others. A large London series of 388 patients with histologically confirmed sarcoidosis found parotid gland enlargement in 23 patients (6 percent), parotid involvement and uveitis in 8 (2 percent), and parotid involvement, uveitis and facial nerve palsy in only 1 (0.03 percent) (Greenberg *et al.* 1964). Conversely, if Heerfordt's syndrome does occur it is virtually pathognomonic for sarcoidosis.

Löfgren's syndrome is another well-recognized clinical entity of sarcoidosis. The first reports (Löfgren 1946; Löfgren and Lundback 1952) described patients with an acute onset of erythema nodosum and bilateral hilar lymphadenopathy although subsequent reports have variously included fever or ankle arthritis or periarticular inflammation in the definition (Mana *et al.* 1996,1999; Baughman *et al.* 2001; Ohta *et al.* 2006). Only 6 percent of the 212 patients in the original series by Löfgren were found to have uveitis, but in all cases it was an acute anterior uveitis (Löfgren and Lundback 1952) and other authors have confirmed this pattern of association (James 1986; Rothova 2000).

Ocular involvement as the presenting feature

The reported frequency with which ocular disease is the initial clinical manifestation of sarcoidosis varies greatly, from 1.5 to 87 percent (Dana *et al.* 1996; Rizzato *et al.* 1996). This variation is attributable to the medical specialty of the investigators and clinic referral bias as well as the demographics of the population studied. Rizzato and co-workers retrospectively reviewed the medical records of 1156 white patients with histologically proven sarcoidosis who were seen at the sarcoid clinic or the lung department of two Italian hospitals. In only 9 patients (0.8 percent) was uveitis documented as the reason for seeking medical attention, which led to the discovery of systemic sarcoidosis. In a further 8 patients (0.7 percent) uveitis preceded the diagnosis of systemic sarcoidosis by between 1 and 11 years (Rizzato *et al.* 1996).

On the other hand, series involving ophthalmologists have demonstrated much higher rates of ocular sarcoidosis as the presenting feature. Rothova and co-workers reported that 17 out of 121 patients (14 percent) in their series in the Netherlands (69 whites and 52 blacks) presented to an ophthalmologist first (Rothova *et al.* 1989). Obenauf and co-workers reviewed 532 cases of sarcoidosis in North Carolina, USA, of whom three-quarters were in black patients, and found 19 percent had ocular symptoms on presentation (Obenauf *et al.* 1978). Similarly, eye symptoms were the presenting feature in 29 out of 185 patients (16 percent) in an English series (Crick *et al.* 1961). A review of 123 Japanese patients found that eye symptoms accounted for 26 percent of presentations resulting in a diagnosis of sarcoidosis (Matsuo *et al.* 2005).

If uveitis series are considered, the rates of subsequent diagnosis of systemic sarcoidosis are even higher. Development of non-ocular manifestations of sarcoidosis may be delayed, emphasizing the need for periodic re-evaluation of uveitis patients for sarcoidosis. In the series by Rothova and co-workers, 15 of 29 patients (52 percent) consulted an ophthalmologist first before their diagnosis was later established by a pulmonologist. In 9 of the 29 cases (31 percent), uveitis preceded the development of non-ocular signs by more than one year (Rothova *et al.* 1989). In another retrospective university hospital review, 27 of 44 cases (61 percent) were seen first with uveitis before a diagnosis of systemic sarcoidosis was established. The interval between onset of uveitis and diagnosis was between 2 and 15 years in 52 percent of these cases (Tugal-Tutkun *et al.* 2007). In a prospective study of 865 patients with uveitis, the diagnosis was established after the onset of the uveitis in 44 of the 59 cases (75 percent) of biopsy-proven sarcoidosis. In five cases initial work-up for sarcoidosis was negative and the diagnosis was not proved until more than one year later (Rothova *et al.* 1992).

UVEITIS

Classification

Uveitis is a general term for inflammation of the uveal tract, the pigmented vascular middle coat of the eye, which comprises the iris, ciliary body and choroid. The classification of uveitis entities is on the basis of the anatomical location of the inflammation (Jabs *et al.* 2005):

- 'anterior' refers to iris or ciliary body involvement (iritis or iridocyclitis);
- 'intermediate' applies when inflammation is centered on the vitreous, pars plana and peripheral retina (vitritis or pars planitis);
- 'posterior' signifies inflammation of the choroid or, by extension, the retina (choroiditis, retinitis or retinal vasculitis).

The term 'panuveitis' is employed when there is no predominant site of inflammation, but inflammation is observed in the anterior chamber, vitreous and retina and/or choroid.

Sarcoidosis is considered to be one of the great mimickers in uveitis and is a differential diagnosis for any form of intraocular inflammation. There are no pathognomonic signs in sarcoid-associated uveitis, but certain patterns of inflammation occur more frequently than others, such as isolated acute or chronic anterior uveitis, vitritis with 'snowball' opacities, panuveitis, peripheral retinal vasculitis and multifocal chorioretinal lesions. Other signs that are infrequent but suggestive of sarcoidosis include choroidal and optic nerve granulomas (Herbort *et al.* 2009). Race, gender and age may also increase the likelihood of a particular pattern; for example, anterior uveitis is more common presentation in black patients and multifocal choroiditis occurs more frequently in older white females (Rothova 2000; Thorne and Brucker 2000; Khalatbari *et al.* 2004).

Anterior uveitis

Anterior uveitis is classified as either acute, of sudden onset and limited duration of less than 3 months, or chronic, of insidious onset and persistent duration greater than 3 months (Herbort *et al.* 2009). Granulomatous and non-granulomatous are descriptive terms, based on appearance rather than histology: they are frequently employed but do not form part of the standardized uveitis nomenclature. Anterior uveitis is regarded as granulomatous when medium-to-large 'mutton fat' keratic precipitates (Fig. 31.1) or iris nodules are observed. Keratic precipitates are deposits of epithelioid cell conglomerates on the endothelial surface of the cornea. Koeppe iris 'nodules' (Plate 30) are also precipitates of inflammatory debris either at the pupillary margin or on the iris surface and occur infrequently. Busacca nodules, true nodules consisting of granulomatous inflammation within the iris stroma, are rare (Smith and Foster 1996; Herbort *et al.* 2009). Busacca nodules are usually accompanied by anterior uveitis in a patient with systemic sarcoidosis (Cohen and Peyman 1986; Finger *et al.* 2007) but very rarely may be the only manifestation and require biopsy for diagnosis (Maca *et al.* 2004). Gonioscopy may reveal trabecular meshwork nodules or tent-shaped peripheral anterior synechiae which are thought to be a result of the scarring and resolution of these nodules (Iwata *et al.* 1976; Kawaguchi *et al.* 2007; Herbort *et al.* 2009). Inflammation is described as non-granulomatous when keratic precipitates are small or absent.

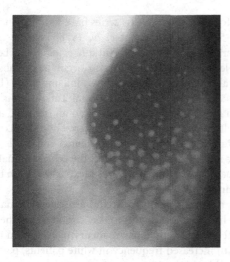

Figure 31.1 'Mutton fat' keratic precipitates: deposits of epithelioid cell conglomerates on the endothelial surface of the cornea.

Anterior chamber cells and proteinaceous flare are present in acute and chronic disease but circumcorneal ciliary injection may be absent in chronic cases. There may be evidence of past episodes of inflammation such as posterior and peripheral anterior synechiae formation. Other complications, such as cystoid macular edema, glaucoma, cataract and band keratopathy, are more common in chronic disease (Rothova 2000). The symptoms of anterior uveitis are similar regardless of etiology and do not help to differentiate the cause. These include discomfort or aching, redness and watering of the eye as well as photophobia, blurring of vision and floaters. Usually both eyes are affected although this may be asymmetrical or consecutive. Not all symptoms will be present and patients with chronic disease may be asymptomatic.

Acute or chronic granulomatous anterior uveitis is considered classical of ocular sarcoidosis, although many other non-infectious (multiple sclerosis, sympathetic ophthalmia, Vogt–Koyanagi–Harada syndrome) and infectious (tuberculosis, herpetic disease, toxoplasmosis, syphilis, Lyme disease) etiologies can present in the same way. The series by Obenauf and co-workers, of whom three-quarters were black patients, found chronic granulomatous uveitis to be the most common ocular abnormality (52.5 percent) (Obenauf et al. 1978). Another US series, of which 77 percent of patients were white, determined that 81 percent of the 112 eyes evaluated had granulomatous uveitis (Dana et al. 1996). However, other series have reported that non-granulomatous uveitis is more common (Jones 2002; Evans et al. 2007); Jones found it to be twice as common in Manchester, UK. A tertiary referral center in Southern California also reported that 22 out of the 33 biopsy-proven uveitis cases had non-granulomatous inflammation, although it was acknowledged that many had received prior treatment (Evans et al. 2007).

Intermediate uveitis

A predominantly intermediate pattern of uveitis is only seen in a minority (10–20 percent) of patients with ocular

sarcoidosis (Jones 2002; Lobo et al. 2003; Tugal-Tutkun et al. 2007). However, vitreous inflammation, or vitritis, in combination with anterior or posterior uveitis is a major manifestation. The vitritis may consist of a fine cellular reaction, but vitreous 'snowball' opacities are more typical. Snowballs appear as grayish white globoid opacities and vary in size from small particles to one-third of a disc diameter (Plate 31). They are usually located in the inferior vitreous anterior to the equator and often occur in chains, for which the term 'string of pearls' has been used to describe them. They may also occasionally coalesce to form a 'snowbank'. Snowballs have been documented in 35–69 percent of cases of sarcoid-associated uveitis (Khalatbari et al. 2004; Matsuo et al. 2005; Kawaguchi et al. 2007; Tugal-Tutkun et al. 2007), but although characteristic of ocular sarcoidosis they are not exclusive to it and occur in other conditions such as pars planitis and multiple sclerosis.

Posterior uveitis

The proportion of cases in which the posterior segment of the eye has been found to be involved varies greatly between reported series. This may in part be due to differing racial profiles (Rothova 2000). It has been noted that high frequencies of sarcoid-associated anterior uveitis (70–75 percent) were seen mainly in the studies where the majority of patients were black (Obenauf et al. 1978; Dresner et al. 1986; Jabs and Johns 1986); whereas posterior or panuveitis was more commonly observed in white patients (65–85 percent), specifically in elderly female patients (Karma 1979; Rothova et al. 1989, 1992; Dana et al. 1996; Stavrou et al. 1997). However, two recent studies have found the prevalence of posterior uveitis does not differ significantly between races. One was a US university hospital study which reported posterior-segment disease in 85 percent of black patients and 100 percent of white patients (Khalatbari et al. 2004). The other was a UK tertiary referral hospital study which documented posterior uveitis in 89 percent of black patients and 85 percent of white patients (Lobo et al. 2003).

Differences in the definition of posterior-segment involvement, extent of ophthalmic assessment and referral bias may also partly account for the variation observed among studies. Studies that report posterior uveitis as a fraction of the total ocular sarcoidosis cases, rather than as a fraction of the total uveitis cases, will appear to have less posterior-segment disease (Obenauf et al. 1978). In addition, investigators who classify intermediate uveitis as a separate entity will also seem to have lower rates of posterior-segment involvement (Dana et al. 1996). Studies that include cystoid macular edema as a posterior-segment finding may report diverse rates, depending on whether the diagnosis is based on clinical, fluorescein angiography or optical coherence tomography findings. Tertiary referral centers also tend to have a higher representation of posterior-segment disease as these cases are usually the more complex ones (Lobo et al. 2003; Khalatbari et al. 2004).

Posterior uveitis in the absence of anterior-segment inflammation was noted to be rare (5 percent) in the US series by Obenauf et al. (1978). However other studies have documented higher rates of posterior-segment disease as the sole manifestation of ocular sarcoidosis (Spalton and Sanders 1981; Bienfait and Baarsma 1986; Matsuo *et al.* 2005; Khanna *et al.* 2007; Atmaca *et al.* 2009). Three European studies, of whom the majority or all of the patients were white, reported between 11 and 22 percent of their cases having disease limited to the posterior segment of the eye (Spalton and Sanders 1981; Bienfait and Baarsma 1986; Atmaca *et al.* 2009). Matsuo and co-workers found isolated posterior uveitis developed in 20 out of 60 Japanese patients (33 percent) with a diagnosis of histologically confirmed ocular sarcoidosis (Matsuo *et al.* 2005). Moreover, a recent small study from India detected posterior-segment involvement only in 9 out of 14 patients (63 percent) with biopsy-confirmed ocular sarcoidosis (Khanna *et al.* 2007).

Posterior-segment inflammation, and particularly that in association with minimal or chronic anterior uveitis, may be asymptomatic. Alternatively, patients may present with floaters or decreased vision due to vitritis or due to complications of the inflammation. Complications include cystoid macular edema, epiretinal membrane, retinal hemorrhage and exudation secondary to retinal vasculitis, vitreous hemorrhage resulting from neovascularization, and optic nerve involvement. These are general findings that are not specific to ocular sarcoidosis. Fundus findings which are suggestive of ocular sarcoidosis include retinal vascular changes, in particular periphlebitis and retinal macroaneurysm, multifocal chorioretinal lesions, choroidal nodules and optic disc granulomas.

Retinal vasculature changes

Periphlebitis is the most common fundus finding in ocular sarcoidosis, and sarcoidosis is among the most common causes of retinal vasculitis. It occurs in up to 60 percent of patients with posterior-segment involvement (Spalton and Sanders 1981) and, as with all other ocular signs of sarcoidosis, the manifestations are protean. However, characteristic appearances occur that are suggestive of sarcoidosis. The typical pattern is segmental areas of sheathing along the small branch veins at the equatorial fundus. This inflammation may be very subtle and demonstrable only by leakage on fluorescein angiography. Alternatively, it may result in large, creamy yellow exudates which appear to drip from the involved area of vein (Plate 32). The latter are known as 'candle wax drippings', the best recognized lesion of retinal sarcoidosis, although not pathognomonic.

Acute periphlebitis may be accompanied by retinal hemorrhage and edema, and retinal pigment epithelial atrophy may subsequently develop beneath these lesions (Spalton and Sanders 1981). Severe inflammation at involved sites may also occasionally result in peripheral or branch retinal vein occlusions or peripheral capillary closure. Large vein occlusions secondary to ocular sarcoidosis are very rare. Capillary non-perfusion may lead to neovascularization of the optic disc or the periphery. In one English study, neovascularization was reported in 8 out of 36 patients (22 percent) with fundus involvement (Spalton and Sanders

1981). However, most uveitis series have found the incidence to be 4–5 percent (Obenauf *et al.* 1978; Lobo *et al.* 2003; Khalatbari *et al.* 2004; Tugal-Tutkun *et al.* 2007; Lee *et al.* 2009). Neovascularization can also occur in the absence of peripheral closure as a direct effect of inflammation (Doxanas *et al.* 1980; Miyao *et al.* 1999; Tugal-Tutkun *et al.* 2007), although most cases are attributable to an ischemic mechanism (Spalton and Sanders 1981; Duker *et al.* 1988; Lobo *et al.* 2003). Rarely, optociliary shunts, dilated collateral veins on the optic nerve head which connect the central retinal vein to the peripapillary choroidal venous plexus, have been reported (Mansour 1986).

Until relatively recently, sarcoid-associated retinal vasculopathy had been thought to be confined to the retinal venules. However, retinal macroaneuryms have been noted to occur with increased frequency in white patients, particularly women, older than 60 years of age with active multifocal choroiditis, the majority of whom had biopsy-proven or presumed ocular sarcoidosis (Rothova and Lardenoye 1998; Verougstraete *et al.* 2001). A review of 48 cases, of peripheral multifocal choroiditis and vitritis seen at a university hospital in the Netherlands, identified eight patients (17 percent) with arterial macroaneurysms. Three of the eight patients had histologically confirmed sarcoidosis, one had bilateral hilar lymphadenopathy and a further two had elevated serum ACE. All patients with macroaneurysms were white females older than 60 years of age, with a mean age of 76 years. Three of them did not suffer from hypertension (Rothova and Lardenoye 1998).

A subsequent report from a university hospital in Belgium confirmed these findings (Verougstraete *et al.* 2001). Seven cases (6 percent of their adult ocular sarcoidosis patients) of multiple macroaneurysms, vitritis and multifocal peripheral punched-out chorioretinal scars were identified. Of these seven cases, three patients had biopsy-proven sarcoidosis; two had a positive bronchoalveolar lavage as well as other investigations highly suggestive of sarcoidosis; and the remaining two had a raised serum ACE in one case and anergy in the other. Six of the seven patients were women and all were older than 60 years. Six of them also had hypertension. This study also observed the formation of new macroaneurysms and found that a retrospective analysis of prior fluorescein angiograms suggested previous focal inflammation or circulatory perturbations at the site where new ectasias developed.

Fluorescein angiography is invaluable in assessing the retinal vasculature status. Venule wall staining and leakage enables the detection of subclinical periphlebitis. It can also differentiate between diffuse optic nerve head leakage due to inflammation and focal leakage due to granulomatous infiltration. Neovascularization is readily visualized and the presence and extent of peripheral capillary closure can be determined, which guides the need for laser photocoagulation. Fluorescein angiography also reveals cystoid macular edema that is not obvious clinically. Optical coherence tomography has only recently become widely available and is a non-invasive method of detecting and quantifying cystoid macular edema. It is used for monitoring the progression or resolution of macular edema as it is quick and easy to perform and risk-free.

Cystoid macular edema

It is crucial to ascertain the presence and extent of cystoid macular edema as it is the most frequent cause of visual loss and is often reversible. Inflammation renders the retinal capillaries more permeable, which allows fluid to leak into the outer plexiform and inner nuclear layers of the retina. Initially there is a characteristic cystoid pattern, but with greater leakage or chronicity the edema may become diffuse. Cystoid macular edema may occur as a result of anterior uveitis, particularly chronic anterior uveitis, but is more commonly seen as a complication of posterior-segment involvement. Cystoid macular edema has been reported to occur in between 7 and 58 percent of patients with sarcoid-associated uveitis (Bienfait and Baarsma 1986; Dana et al. 1996; Smith and Foster 1996; Thorne and Brucker 2000; Khalatbari et al. 2004; Matsuo et al. 2005; Khanna et al. 2007; Tugal-Tutkun et al. 2007; Lee et al. 2009). This substantial variation is predominantly due to the differing demographics of the population studied as well as the length of follow-up and, to a lesser degree, the availability of fluorescein angiography and optical coherence tomography.

The majority of US and European sarcoid-related uveitis series with follow-up report cystoid macular edema prevalence rates between 27 and 58 percent (Bienfait and Baarsma 1986; Dana et al. 1996; Smith and Foster 1996; Tugal-Tutkun et al. 2007). However, cystoid macular edema does not appear to be a prominent feature in Japanese studies (Iwata et al. 1976; Ohara et al. 1992; Matsuo et al. 2005). Matsuo and co-workers found that cystoid macular edema occurred in only 8 out of 112 eyes (7 percent) of patients with biopsy-proven sarcoid-related uveitis who were followed for a mean period of 6 years (Matsuo et al. 2005). A Korean series also revealed that only 3 of 39 eyes (8 percent) of patients with histologically confirmed sarcoid uveitis developed cystoid macular edema over a 4-year follow-up (Lee et al. 2009). These differences appear to be attributable to race. Possible confounders include age and proportion of cases with posterior-segment involvement. However, the mean patient age, 49 years in the Japanese study and 43 years in the Korean study, is comparable to other studies. Furthermore, posterior-segment involvement, which is associated with higher rates of macular edema, occurred in the majority of cases (88 and 59 percent, respectively) (Matsuo et al. 2005; Lee et al. 2009).

Several studies have demonstrated that cystoid macular edema occurs with significantly higher frequency in older individuals (Smith and Foster 1996; Khalatbari et al. 2004). One study observed that 27 percent of patients older than 35 years developed cystoid macular edema, compared with 3 percent in the under-35 age group (Smith and Foster 1996). Another study looked at demographic-related variations in biopsy-proven posterior-segment ocular sarcoidosis (Khalatbari et al. 2004). They found an overall incidence of cystoid macular edema of 31 percent but observed its presence in only 5 percent of patients younger than 32 years compared with 65 percent of patients greater than 53 years of age ($p < 0.001$). This study also compared differences in race and gender. White patients were noted to have higher rates of cystoid macular edema than black patients ($p = 0.005$).

Females also had higher rates than males but the difference was not statistically significant ($p = 0.1$). When race/sex groups were compared, white females had the highest rate of cystoid macular oedema (61 percent) versus all others ($p = 0.002$) (Khalatbari et al. 2004).

Posterior-segment inflammation, in particular peripheral multifocal choroiditis with vitritis, has been consistently associated with much higher rates of cystoid macular edema (Lardenoye et al. 1997; Thorne and Brucker 2000; Lobo et al. 2003; Abad et al. 2004). Lobo and co-workers found cystoid macular edema occurred more frequently in multifocal choroiditis (2/7, 29 percent) and in panuveitis with retinal vasculitis (3/28, 11 percent) compared with anterior uveitis (1/24, 4 percent) (Lobo et al. 2003). In a series of patients with peripheral multifocal choroiditis, 15 of 25 (60 percent) biopsy-proven or presumed sarcoidosis cases had cystoid macular edema (Abad et al. 2004). In another series of 53 patients with peripheral multifocal choroiditis, 48 percent were found to have cystoid macular edema on initial examination and this increased to 72 percent after more than 2 years' follow-up. Of these patients, 25 percent were diagnosed with sarcoidosis and an additional 29 percent had an elevated serum ACE (Lardenoye et al. 1997).

Peripheral multifocal choroiditis

Choroidal lesions associated with sarcoidosis may be single or multifocal and located anywhere in the fundus (Fig. 31.2). However, the classical picture is of multiple, small (less than half a disc diameter), round, white, 'punched out' lesions which are located predominately post-equatorial and more commonly in the inferior half of the fundus (Jones 2002). In 1949, Franceschetti and Babel coined the term 'taches de bougie', which translates as 'candle wax spots', to describe these lesions but the original meaning was lost and 'candle wax drippings' have now come to mean the exudates associated with the periphlebitis of sarcoidosis. To avoid ambiguity, most ophthalmologists reserve the phrase 'candle wax drippings' for the perivenous exudates and describe the punched-out peripheral lesions as 'multifocal choroiditis',

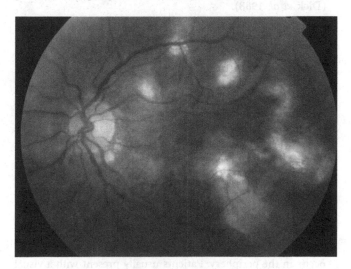

Figure 31.2 Active multifocal choroiditis.

although this is a generic term that is not specific to sarcoidosis.

Multifocal choroiditis has been detected in between 9 and 45 percent of patients with sarcoid-associated uveitis (Karma 1979; Bienfait and Baarsma 1986; Lardenoye et al. 1997; Lobo et al. 2003) and in 35–56 percent of patients with posterior-segment involvement (Gould and Kaufman 1961; Spalton and Sanders 1981; Khalatbari et al. 2004). Several studies have noted that this pattern of inflammation is more common in white patients, particularly females, who have an older age of onset of disease (Hershey et al. 1994; Vrabec et al. 1995; Lardenoye et al. 1997; Thorne and Brucker 2000; Lobo et al. 2003; Abad et al. 2004; Khalatbari et al. 2004). In a small series of seven patients, with peripheral multifocal choroiditis and panuveitis and a positive conjunctival biopsy, six were women and were 58 years of age or older (Hershey et al. 1994). In another series of peripheral multifocal choroiditis, of the 25 patients with biopsy-proven or presumed sarcoidosis, 22 (88 percent) were white, 19 (76 percent) were female and the mean age was 62 years (Abad et al. 2004). The median age at which multifocal choroiditis was first diagnosed in two other studies was 52 and 54 years (Vrabec et al. 1995; Lobo et al. 2003). Another study confirmed that white patients had significantly higher rates of choroidal punched-out lesions than black patients ($p = 0.005$) (Khalatbari et al. 2004). Conversely, a study investigating causes of uveitis in women first presenting over the age of 60, found 16 of 30 patients had multifocal choroiditis and of these 11 had positive chest CT scans and 9 had a positive biopsy for sarcoidosis (Kaiser et al. 2002).

The multiple chorioretinal lesions of ocular sarcoidosis have also been described as mimicking birdshot chorioretinopathy, appearing as larger, pale yellow–orange streaks located more posteriorly. One series described 16 patients with multifocal choroiditis-type lesions and 6 patients with lesions indistinguishable from those of birdshot chorioretinopathy who were subsequently diagnosed with sarcoidosis (Vrabec et al. 1995). In addition, there are two case reports of ocular sarcoidosis presenting as serpiginous choroiditis (Edelsten et al. 1994) and a report of an association with acute posterior multifocal placoid pigment epitheliopathy (Dick et al. 1988).

Choroidal nodules

Choroidal nodules are uncommon but highly suggestive of sarcoidosis, although tuberculosis may also present in this way and must always be excluded. Very rarely, they may be the sole ocular manifestation of sarcoidosis, in which case the differential diagnosis includes metastatic choroidal tumor (Campo and Aaberg 1984). Obenauf and co-workers reported choroidal nodules in 5.5 percent of patients (Obenauf et al. 1978). They are typically solitary, creamy-white elevated lesions, ranging in size from 0.5 to 4 disc diameters, which are located in the macular or peripapillary region (Desai et al. 2001) (Plate 33). However, they may also be multiple or occur in the periphery. Patients usually present with a visual field scotoma or reduced or distorted vision due to the mass and/or associated subretinal fluid (Marcus et al. 1982; Olk et al. 1983; Wolfensberger and Tufail 2000). Retinal pigment epithelial detachment has also been described in association with choroidal nodules (Bourcier et al. 1998) and without obvious choroidal involvement (Salchow and Weiss 2006).

Accompanying anterior uveitis is uncommon. Nor does there appear to be an increased risk of intracranial lesions (Tingey and Gonder 1992; Desai et al. 2001). Desai and co-workers have published the largest case series of choroidal nodules. They reviewed the records of all patients with a diagnosis of sarcoidosis who underwent an ophthalmic examination at a Michigan hospital over a 5-year period. They identified nine patients with choroidal nodules, all of whom were African-American. Eight of the nine had a pre-existing diagnosis of sarcoidosis. Eight patients had a solitary granuloma. Although four cases had a past history of anterior uveitis, only one had concurrent inflammation. None of the nine patients had non-ocular neurological symptoms. Eight underwent gadolinium-enhanced MRI of the head. No intracranial lesions and specifically no intracranial granulomas were detected.

Optic nerve involvement

Optic nerve head abnormalities occur in up to 40 percent of patients with posterior-segment involvement (Spalton and Sanders 1981). These changes range from mild leakage on fluorescein angiography to clinically apparent swelling. Visible edema can result either directly from severe posterior inflammation, presumably by inducing local vascular leakage in the optic nerve head, or indirectly due to hypotony resulting from ciliary body shutdown. Focal swelling indicates granulomatous infiltration of the optic nerve. Optic nerve head granuloma is an uncommon but important complication of sarcoidosis, which may lead to a substantial nerve-fiber bundle defect or rarely retinal vascular occlusion (Suresh and Jones 1999). Optic nerve head edema may also represent papilledema consequent to raised intracranial pressure from neurosarcoidosis. In addition, optic atrophy or neovascularization may be noted. Optic nerve involvement is considered in greater detail in Chapter 27.

SCLERA AND EPISCLERA

Episcleritis and scleritis are rare complications of ocular sarcoidosis (Jabs and Johns 1986; Tuft and Watson 1991; Matsuo et al. 2005). In a series of 183 patients with chronic sarcoidosis who were followed for a mean of 13 years, 47 patients (26 percent) had ocular involvement. Of these, one was found to have scleral disease, which was described as a scleral plaque (Jabs and Johns 1986). Another series of 123 patients with sarcoidosis followed for a mean of 6 years reported ocular sarcoidosis in 61 patients, one of whom had bilateral episcleritis (Matsuo et al. 2005). In a study of 281 patients with sarcoidosis, Karma reported five cases of episcleritis occurring early in the disease, coinciding with the appearance of erythema nodosum in four of them (Karma

1979). Conversely, Tuft and Watson reviewed the clinical features of 290 patients with scleral disease and found only one patient with sarcoidosis (Tuft and Watson 1991).

CONJUNCTIVA AND CORNEA

Granulomatous inflammation of the conjunctiva is a not uncommon manifestation of ocular sarcoidosis. Many studies have reported the presence of conjunctival nodules in approximately 7–17 percent of patients with ocular sarcoidosis (Obenauf et al. 1978; Karma et al. 1980; Jabs and Johns 1986; James 1986; Atmaca et al. 2009). Others have reported much higher rates of conjunctival involvement (Rothova et al. 1989). Rothova and co-workers observed conjunctival involvement in 23 patients, 19 percent of the overall series and 46 percent of the patients with ocular sarcoidosis (Rothova et al. 1989). It is difficult to know the true incidence, as most conjunctival nodules are not biopsied and they can closely resemble normal lymphoid follicles. Karma biopsied 218 patients with sarcoidosis and granulomas were detected in 17 percent of the biopsy specimens (Karma 1979). Only 41 percent of 66 cases in which nodules were thought to be suspicious of sarcoidosis were positive. This may indicate a tendency to overestimate conjunctival involvement clinically or may reflect histopathological false negatives.

Typical granulomas have been described as small elevations, just visible to the naked eye. They are translucent and slightly yellow and are located most frequently in the fornices, particularly the inferior fornix, but occasionally in the bulbar conjunctiva. They are usually scanty but may be confluent (Crick et al. 1961). Conjunctival granulomas are usually asymptomatic but occasionally cause conjunctival injection or edema and extremely rarely result in symblepharon (Kelmenson et al. 2008). The conjunctiva may also be affected by non-granulomatous changes. Keratoconjunctivitis sicca, or dry eye, may lead to degeneration of the epithelial cells of the cornea and conjunctiva. Hypercalcemia may result in deposition of calcium salts, especially in the exposed areas of the conjunctiva and cornea (Crick et al. 1961). Conjunctival involvement has not been found to correlate with any other form of ocular sarcoidosis (Bornstein et al. 1962; Karma 1979).

ORBIT AND ADNEXAE

The lacrimal gland accounts for the majority of cases of orbital involvement in sarcoidosis (Collison et al. 1986; Mavrikakis and Rootman 2007). Reported rates of lacrimal involvement vary greatly between series because only a minority of cases have histological confirmation of sarcoid infiltration of the gland. The diagnosis of lacrimal involvement is therefore mainly based on clinically evident lacrimal gland enlargement or on the presence of dry-eye symptoms or objective evidence of reduced lacrimal secretion. The latter is identified by a positive Schirmer test (tear production <5 mm after 5 minutes). Variable utilization of fluorescein or rose Bengal solutions to assess corneal and conjunctival staining also contributes to differences in the detection of dry eye and hence reported rates of lacrimal involvement in sarcoidosis.

Crick and co-workers examined 88 patients with sarcoidosis and observed rose Bengal staining in 66 percent of them compared with 6 percent of control patients and concluded that sarcoid infiltration of the lacrimal glands must be more frequent than suspected (Crick et al. 1961). Evans and co-workers diagnosed keratoconjunctivitis sicca secondary to sarcoidosis in 25 of 81 patients (31 percent) on the basis of a positive Schirmer test, but acknowledged that other causes of dry eye were not excluded (Evans et al. 2007). Using similar diagnostic criteria, Rothova and co-workers detected evidence of lacrimal gland involvement in 38 percent of patients with eye involvement and in 16 percent of the overall series (Rothova et al. 1989); whereas the large series of 532 patients by Obenauf and co-workers identified lacrimal gland involvement, on the basis of clinical enlargement or dry-eye symptoms, in 15.8 percent of patients with ocular sarcoidosis and in 6 percent of the overall series (Obenauf et al. 1978).

The correlation between dry-eye symptoms and objective evidence of tear deficiency is poor. Karma reported decreased lacrimation in 32 of 254 patients with sarcoidosis who underwent a Schirmer test but only 12 were symptomatic (Karma 1979). A poor correlation between tear deficiency and clinical enlargement of the lacrimal gland is also noted (Crick et al. 1961; Jabs and Johns 1986; Evans et al. 2007). In the series by Evans and associates, only 1 of the 25 patients found to have keratoconjunctivitis sicca also had clinically enlarged lacrimal glands. They postulated that there may be low-grade lacrimal gland inflammation significant enough to cause dry eyes but insufficient to cause clinical enlargement (Evans et al. 2007). This theory is supported by the finding that asymptomatic lacrimal gland involvement can be demonstrated on gallium scanning in 60–75 percent of sarcoidosis patients (Crick et al. 1961; Karma 1979; Jabs and Johns 1986). On the other hand, in a series of 11 patients with biopsy-proven lacrimal infiltration reported only 4 had dry-eye symptoms and only 1 had a positive Schirmer test (Prabhakaran et al. 2007).

Symptomatic lacrimal gland enlargement usually presents as bilateral palpable superolateral orbital swellings, of acute or subacute onset. It may be associated with variable amounts of eyelid swelling, ptosis and globe displacement (Mavrikakis and Rootman 2007; Prabhakaran et al. 2007; Lutt et al. 2008). Extralacrimal involvement may also present as a slowly expanding mass or as an orbital inflammatory syndrome but it is usually unilateral (Lutt et al. 2008). If the orbital mass is posterior or there is optic nerve sheath involvement, loss of vision may be the presenting feature. Extraocular muscle involvement will present with diplopia (Mavrikakis and Rootman 2007). Extralacrimal orbital soft tissue involvement is rare, occurring in fewer than 1 percent of patients with ocular sarcoidosis (Obenauf et al. 1978; Karma 1979; Jabs and Johns 1986). A multicenter retrospective study reported on 10 cases of biopsy-proven extralacrimal involvement (Prabhakaran et al. 2007). It was noted that it is more commonly seen in the fifth to seventh decades and is more frequent in women. Furthermore, there appear to be two forms: a discrete form with a predilection for the anterior inferior quadrants of the orbit, and a diffuse form. Extra-ocular muscle involvement is more common with the latter and and may mimic thyroid eye disease (Cornblath *et al.* 1993; Prabhakaran *et al.* 2007).

Eyelid skin manifestations are similar to cutaneous sarcoidosis involvement elsewhere. The most common manifestations are small papules, although large nodules, lupus pernio and plaques have all been reported (Pessoa de Souza Filho *et al.* 2005). However, sarcoid granulomas within the eyelid are an uncommon finding (Pessoa de Souza Filho *et al.* 2005; Prabhakaran *et al.* 2007). Pessoa de Souza Filho and co-workers reviewed the published literature on eyelid involvement in sarcoidosis. Of 13 cases, 10 occurred in women and 8 were the initial manifestation of sarcoidosis. One was associated with psoriasis vulgaris, one was associated with a symblepharon and one occurred in a blepharoplasty scar (Pessoa de Souza Filho *et al.* 2005). A further three cases were subsequently related (Prabhakaran *et al.* 2007). All three patients were female and in two of the cases the eyelid involvement was the initial feature of systemic disease. This report suggested that eyelid sarcoidosis may have a predilection for the lower lid.

Sarcoidosis of the lacrimal sac and nasolacrimal duct is also an uncommon finding. In the series by Karma and co-workers, 6 of 281 patients (2.1 percent) with sarcoidosis were found to have clinical evidence for lacrimal passage involvement, although only two patients had this confirmed histologically with an additional patient having sarcoidosis confirmed histologically in the nasal mucosa (Karma 1979). A retrospective review of the pathological diagnosis of 377 dacryocystorhinostomy lacrimal sac biopsy specimens revealed sarcoidosis in 8 cases (2.1 percent) (Anderson *et al.* 2003). Lacrimal sac sarcoidosis usually presents with epiphora or chronic dacryocystitis. Although most patients have a known history of sarcoidosis, in some this may be the initial presentation and lacrimal sac biopsy at the time of surgery leads to the diagnosis. In one series of 12 patients, only 3 had a prior diagnosis of sarcoidosis and the remaining 9 presented with epiphora as the sole initial symptom. Eight of the 12 patients were women and the mean age at diagnosis was 50 years (Chapman *et al.* 1999).

PEDIATRIC OCULAR SARCOIDOSIS

The manifestations of sarcoidosis in children are discussed in detail in Chapter 40. Briefly, pediatric sarcoidosis can be divided into two subgroups based on age at the time of onset of disease and relative frequencies of different organ involvement. The younger group comprises those aged <5 years and the older group includes those up to 15 years (Hoover *et al.* 1986). Older children have rates and patterns of ocular sarcoidosis similar to those of adults but younger children exhibit a different profile of eye involvement.

Younger children have much higher rates of uveitis (Hoover *et al.* 1986; Lindsley and Petty 2000; Hoffmann *et al.* 2004). Hoover and co-workers reviewed the literature on children with sarcoidosis aged 5 years and under and found that 20 out

of 26 (77 percent) reported cases had uveitis. Anterior uveitis only occurred in 15 cases (75 percent) and anterior and posterior uveitis occurred in 5 cases (25 percent) (Hoover *et al.* 1986). An international registry of sarcoid arthritis in childhood prospectively collected 53 cases of biopsy-proven pediatric sarcoidosis from 14 countries in North America, Europe and Asia (Lindsley and Petty 2000). Of these, 38 patients (72 percent) had onset of disease at ≤5 years of age. Uveitis was detected in 44 of 53 children (83 percent). It was bilateral in 43 cases (98 percent), anterior only in 21 cases (48 percent), anterior and posterior in 21 cases (48 percent) and posterior only in 2 cases (4 percent). In contrast, a retrospective review of childhood sarcoidosis in Denmark, in which 42 out of 48 cases (92 percent) were aged 8–15 years, reported uveitis in only 25 percent of patients (Hoffmann *et al.* 2004).

In both the younger and older age groups, anterior uveitis may be acute or chronic, granulomatous or non-granulomatous. Multifocal chorioretinal granulomas, vitritis and disc edema have been described in both groups but retinal periphlebitis appears to be much less common than in adults (Hoover *et al.* 1986). Uncommon ocular manifestations in adults, such as conjunctival, lacrimal or eyelid involvement, are rarely reported in children (Hoover *et al.* 1986; Pattishall *et al.* 1986; Lindsley and Petty 2000). However, complications are quite frequently recounted. Complications, including synechiae, glaucoma, cataracts and band keratopathy, developed in 14 out of 20 cases (70 percent) reviewed by Hoover *et al.* (1986). Of the 53 children described in the international registry study, 13 had glaucoma, 16 had cataracts and 5 had band keratopathy at the time of report. Eight were described as having 'diminished vision' and an additional three were described as 'blind' (Lindsley and Petty 2000). Another study reported that 2 of 28 children became blind (Kendig and Brummer 1976).

OCULAR COMPLICATIONS

Posterior–segment complications

Cystoid macular edema and retinal neovascularization have already been mentioned. Choroidal neovascularization may also occur. Optic nerve damage is usually secondary to glaucoma (see below) but is occasionally due to direct involvement of the nerve by sarcoidosis (see Chapter 27). Cystoid macular edema is present in up to 58 percent of patients with sarcoid-associated uveitis (Dana *et al.* 1996). Risk factors for its development include older age, white race, female sex, and posterior-segment involvement, particularly multifocal choroiditis with vitritis (Lardenoye *et al.* 1997; Khalatbari *et al.* 2004). Retinal neovascularization is reported in 4–5 percent of patients in the majority of series. Vitreous hemorrhage and traction retinal detachment may result. While most cases are due to ischemia, some appear to be inflammatory-driven (Lobo *et al.* 2003; Khalatbari *et al.* 2004; Tugal-Tutkun *et al.* 2007; Lee *et al.* 2009). Younger age is a possible risk factor. All three cases in one study were less than 32 years old (Khalatbari *et al.* 2004). Another study reported four cases with a mean age of 33 years (range 26–44 years) (Brown *et al.* 1987). Subretinal/choroidal neovascularization, either peripapillary or macular, is very rare with only a few case reports in the literature (Pellegrini *et al.* 1986; Inagaki *et al.* 1996; Abe *et al.* 2002; Cheung *et al.* 2002).

Anterior–segment complications

Cataract formation is a well-recognized complication of sarcoid-associated uveitis, with reported rates varying from 14 to 30 percent (Rothova *et al.* 1989; Akova and Foster 1994; Dana *et al.* 1996; Lindsley and Petty 2000; Lobo *et al.* 2003; Tugal-Tutkun *et al.* 2007; Lee *et al.* 2009). Cataract occurs either as a result of the inflammation itself or secondary to corticosteroid treatment or both. Lobo and co-workers revealed that cataract developed in 2 of 24 (8 percent) of anterior uveitis cases compared with 8 of 28 (29 percent) panuveitis with vasculitis cases and 5 of 7 (71 percent) of multifocal choroiditis cases (Lobo *et al.* 2003). Similarly, Rothova and co-workers described cataract formation in 1 of 14 (7 percent) of anterior uveitis cases compared with 5 of 15 (33 percent) of posterior and panuveitis cases (Rothova *et al.* 1989). Other studies have documented an increased risk of cataractogenesis with chronic anterior uveitis but this subgroup may have been under-represented in the anterior uveitis cases of both studies. The cataract potential of corticosteroids is dose-related and accelerated cataract progression occurs with any route of administration; however it is more common with topical and intravitreal routes.

In general, cataract surgery in sarcoid-associated uveitis is relatively straightforward and has a good outcome provided absolute control of the inflammation is achieved preoperatively and there is no permanent ocular structural damage from retinal pathology or glaucoma (Akova and Foster 1994; Jones 2002).

Band keratopathy refers to the deposition of calcium salts in a band across the exposed (interpalpebral) region of the cornea. This occurs either as a consequence of chronic inflammation or in association with hypercalcemia or, in the case of sarcoidosis, potentially both. Band keratopathy occurs in 40–50 percent of children with chronic anterior uveitis but most cases are due to juvenile idiopathic uveitis rather than sarcoidosis (Cunningham 2000). Sarcoidosis is the most common cause of hypercalcemia-associated band keratopathy. However, although hypercalcemia occurs in 17 percent of patients with ocular sarcoidosis, band keratopathy is present in only 4–5 percent of cases (Obenauf *et al.* 1978). Patients may be asymptomatic or complain of reduced vision or glare. Ocular surface discomfort can result if the calcium breaks through the corneal epithelium.

Keratoconjunctivitis sicca, or dry eye, occurs as a result of lacrimal gland infiltration and has been discussed in detail above.

Glaucoma

The term 'glaucoma' is reserved for progressive optic nerve damage with corresponding field defect and is mainly due to increased intraocular pressure (IOP). Raised IOP without optic nerve damage is referred to as 'ocular hypertension'.

There are a number of ways in which sarcoid-related uveitis can lead to increased IOP. Aqueous is produced by the ciliary body, flows between the lens and the iris through the pupil then out through the trabecular meshwork into the Schlemm canal of the drainage angle located peripherally in the anterior segment. Posterior synechiae between the posterior iris and the lens can block aqueous flow through the pupil (pupil block) causing the iris to bow forwards (iris bombe) and obstruct the drainage angle. Alternatively, the anterior iris stroma can become attached to the trabecular meshwork of the drainage angle, so-called peripheral anterior synechiae formation. A special subset is neovascular glaucoma in which new blood vessels result in obliteration of the drainage angle. These mechanisms are known as 'angle closure glaucoma'.

If the angle appears open at the macroscopic level, that is on slit-lamp examination, then the glaucoma is termed 'open angle glaucoma'. This accounts for 80 percent or more of cases (Iwata *et al.* 1976; Merayo-Lloves *et al.* 1999). Acutely, increased IOP with an open angle may be caused by:

- microscopic outflow obstruction due to inflammatory proteins, debris and cells clogging the trabecular meshwork (Merayo-Lloves *et al.* 1999);
- nodular infiltration of the trabecular meshwork (Iwata *et al.* 1976);
- inflammation of the canal of Schlemm (Hamanaka *et al.* 2002).

Fibrotic tissue replacement of the canal and other structural changes in the aqueous outflow pathway can lead to glaucoma (Hamanaka *et al.* 2002). Corticosteroids are another important cause of an acute increase in IOP or glaucoma. Any route of administration may cause IOP rise but it is more common with topical and intravitreal routes. Approximately 30 percent of the population will experience an IOP rise with steroids (Armaly and Becker 1965), and such individuals are termed 'steroid responders'.

A large US series, of 119 patients with sarcoid-associated uveitis, reported that 15 patients (13 percent) developed glaucoma and an additional 14 patients (12 percent) ocular hypertension over a mean follow-up period of 2.3 years (Merayo-Lloves *et al.* 1999). This study investigated the prevalence of glaucoma secondary to many different causes of uveitis. Overall, the predominant clinical phenotype associated with glaucoma was chronic or recurrent (90 percent), anterior (67 percent), granulomatous (76 percent) uveitis. However, both Rothova *et al.* (1989) and Lobo *et al.* (2003) found that glaucoma secondary to sarcoidosis was more common with posterior-segment involvement. Lobo theorized that this may be due to a lower prevalence of chronic anterior uveitis cases in their series.

OCULAR COURSE

The course of sarcoid-associated uveitis can be described as monophasic, relapsing/recurrent or chronic. No correlation has been noted between the course of the uveitis and the course of the systemic sarcoidosis (Karma 1979; Jabs and Johns 1986). In one US series, despite all patients having chronic systemic sarcoidosis of 5 years or longer, the anterior uveitis did not pursue a chronic course in 15 out of 33 cases (45 percent) and was generally characterized by a single episode at the onset of disease (Jabs and Johns 1986). Karma reported a similar proportion of sarcoid-related uveitis cases (8/21, 38 percent) to have a monophasic course, while 43 percent were recurrent and 19 percent were chronic (Karma 1979). A Turkish study found 28 of 44 patients (64 percent) had a monophasic course, 23 percent were recurrent and 13 percent were chronic (Tugal-Tutkun et al. 2007). In contrast, Dana and co-workers identified 55 of 60 cases (91 percent) as chronic, 7 percent as recurrent and only 2 percent as monophasic (Dana et al. 1996). This considerable variation is due to referral bias as well as variable follow-up and differing racial profiles.

The course of other ocular manifestations is not well-characterized as these are rarely vision-threatening. Karma and co-workers undertook a follow-up study of 71 of 79 patients with ocular sarcoidosis a mean of 9 years after initial presentation. Of the 71 patients, 33 (46 percent) showed chronic ophthalmic changes at the follow-up examination. Aside from 4 cases of chronic uveitis, 13 patients had conjunctival granulomas, 22 patients had lacrimal gland involvement and 3 patients had lacrimal passage involvement (Karma 1979). No correlation has been observed between the course of the uveitis and the course of other ocular manifestations, with the exception that band keratopathy only occurs with chronicity (Karma 1979; Rothova et al. 1989).

OCULAR PROGNOSIS

Several studies have reported on the visual prognosis for sarcoid-associated uveitis and there is a high concordance in the observed rates of legal blindness. Legal blindness is usually defined as a best corrected visual acuity of less than 6/60 Snellen equivalent and is found in at least one eye of 10–16 percent of patients (Rothova et al. 1989,1996; Smith and Foster 1996; Lobo et al. 2003). Another study reported that about 5 percent of 75 patients followed up for a median of 4 years had a visual acuity of less than 6/36 in both eyes (Edelsten et al. 1999). In a review of 582 cases of uveitis, sarcoidosis was found to be the systemic disease which most frequently caused blindness (Rothova et al. 1996). Reports of visual loss are more varied due to differing definitions and follow-up periods. A large series of 217 eyes in 118 patients with sarcoid-associated uveitis found that 37 percent of patients lost vision at final analysis (Smith and Foster 1996). Another study observed a similar rate of vision loss (46 percent) (Edelsten et al. 1999). Two other studies, which defined vision loss as 2 or more Snellen lines, reported rates of 13 percent (Lobo et al. 2003) and 18 percent (Tugal-Tutkun et al. 2007).

It is noteworthy that the majority of reported uveitis series are generated from university or tertiary referral hospitals, where a higher proportion of complex cases are seen.

Therefore, the above figures may not be representative of the community and may be biased towards a poorer prognosis. Nonetheless uveitis, or its sequelae, has a substantial impact on visual acuity outcomes in ocular sarcoidosis. Optic nerve involvement can also have a significant impact on ocular prognosis and is discussed in Chapter 27. Band keratopathy may cause mild visual impairment but is reversible. Other ocular manifestations do not cause vision loss except in rare instances of orbital granulomata compressing the optic nerve or severe keratoconjunctivitis sicca.

OCULAR PROGNOSTIC FACTORS

The extent of systemic disease does not affect the ocular prognosis. Patients with extraocular manifestations fare no differently from those with isolated ocular disease (Edelsten et al. 1999). The chief determinant of a poor visual outcome is the presence of uveitis complications, in particular cystoid macular edema (Jabs and Johns 1986; Rothova et al. 1996; Smith and Foster 1996; Stavrou et al. 1997; Lobo et al. 2003; Khalatbari et al. 2004) and glaucoma (Obenauf et al. 1978; Jabs and Johns 1986; Dana et al. 1996; Smith and Foster 1996; Lobo et al. 2003). Cystoid macular edema is the most important cause of vision loss. One study determined the median visual acuity for eyes with cystoid macular edema (6/18) and for eyes without cystoid macular edema (6/7.5; $p < 0.001$) (Khalatbari et al. 2004). Glaucoma occurs less frequently than cystoid macular edema but can be associated with a very poor visual prognosis. One series, with a mean follow-up of 13 years, reported 8 out of 11 patients (73 percent) with glaucoma suffered severe visual loss of 6/60 or less (Jabs and Johns 1986), although this study was in the pre-prostaglandin era and prior to the use of adjunctive antifibrotic agents in trabeculectomy surgery.

A chronic uveitis course (Karma 1979; Jabs and Johns 1986) and posterior-segment involvement (Dana et al. 1996; Lobo et al. 2003; Lee et al. 2009) are poor prognostic factors. Karma reported that the 8 patients with a monophasic course had a favorable outcome whereas severe visual loss occurred in 5 eyes of the 13 patients with a relapsing or chronic course (Karma 1979). Lobo and co-workers compared the risk of poor outcome, defined as a visual acuity of 6/12 or worse, for the various patterns of sarcoid-related uveitis. Poor outcome occurred more frequently in multifocal choroiditis (5/7, 71 percent) and in panuveitis with retinal vasculitis (13/28, 46 percent) compared with anterior uveitis (3/24, 13 percent). The excess risks remained significant after adjusting for other potential confounders, including age and sex (Lobo et al. 2003). Lee and co-workers also found poor visual outcome to be significantly more frequent in patients with panuveitis and multifocal choroiditis or retinal vasculitis compared to patients with anterior/intermediate uveitis ($p < 0.05$) (Lee et al. 2009). Similarly, another study reported 7 of 13 eyes (54 percent) with sarcoid-associated multifocal choroiditis had visual acuities worse than 6/12 (Hershey et al. 1994).

The poor visual outcome associated with multifocal choroiditis has been noted previously and is chiefly due to the development of chronic cystoid macular edema and glaucoma (Lardenoye *et al.* 1997; Lobo *et al.* 2003). In the study by Lobo's group, 2 of 7 eyes (29 percent) and 3 of 7 eyes (43 percent) with multifocal choroiditis developed cystoid macular edema and glaucoma, respectively (Lobo *et al.* 2003). Cystoid macular edema has also been reported to occur more commonly with older age at presentation, female sex, and white race (Rothova *et al.* 1989; Smith and Foster 1996; Khalatbari *et al.* 2004). Older age at presentation has been found to be a risk factor for poor outcome independently of its association with cystoid macular edema (Edelsten *et al.* 1999; Lobo *et al.* 2003; Lee *et al.* 2009). This can be explained by the observation that older patients are more likely to suffer a chronic uveitis course, with its inherent worse prognosis, whereas younger patients are more likely to experience an acute monophasic course (Karma 1979; Jabs and Johns 1986).

Females have been noted to have a worse visual prognosis than males in some series. In some cases this can be attributed to a higher prevalence of cystoid macular edema (Rothova *et al.* 1989), but other studies have found that the association remains even after adjusting for that edema (Khalatbari *et al.* 2004). Other studies have not observed any gender difference (Dana *et al.* 1996; Lobo *et al.* 2003; Lee *et al.* 2009). Similarly, there are conflicting reports regarding the impact of race on final visual acuity. While white patients, particularly older females with multifocal choroiditis, have higher rates of cystoid macular edema, some series have found vision loss is more common in black patients. Dana and co-workers reported that black race was correlated with a final visual acuity of worse than 6/12, irrespective of the acuity at initial presentation (Dana *et al.* 1996). Another study found only black females had a significantly lower visual acuity (Khalatbari *et al.* 2004).

DIAGNOSIS OF OCULAR SARCOIDOSIS

SUGGESTIVE INTRAOCULAR SIGNS

The association of uveitis with parotid gland enlargement and sometimes facial nerve palsy (Heerfordt's syndrome) is virtually diagnostic for sarcoidosis but ocular signs alone are not pathognomonic. However, a Japanese group identified five intraocular signs that occur with significantly higher incidence in biopsy-proven sarcoidosis patients than in controls (Kawaguchi *et al.* 2007). These were expanded on by the first International Workshop on Ocular Sarcoidosis (Herbort *et al.* 2009), which has recently published international criteria for the diagnosis of ocular sarcoidosis. The signs are:

- mutton-fat/granulomatous keratic precipitates and/or iris nodules (Koeppe/Busacca);
- trabecular meshwork nodules and/or tent-shaped peripheral anterior synechiae;
- snowballs/string-of-pearls vitreous opacities;
- multiple chorioretinal peripheral lesions (active or atrophic);
- nodular and/or segmental periphlebitis (± candlewax drippings) and/or retinal macroaneurysm in an inflamed eye;

- optic disc nodule(s)/granuloma(s) and/or solitary choroidal nodule;
- bilaterality.

The IWOS has also specified four investigations that are regarded to be of value in supporting the diagnosis of ocular sarcoidosis in patients having suggestive intraocular signs:

- negative tuberculin test in a patient who is BCG vaccinated or had a positive PPD (or Mantoux) skin test previously;
- elevated serum ACE and/or elevated serum lysozyme;
- bilateral hilar lymphadenopathy on chest X-ray;
- positive chest CT scan in patients with negative chest X-ray.

The presence of one or more suggestive intraocular signs in combination with one or more positive tests enables a standardized approach to the definitions of presumed, probable or possible ocular sarcoidosis in the absence of histological confirmation. Biopsy-proven sarcoidosis with compatible uveitis is termed 'definite ocular sarcoidosis'. Studies validating these diagnostic criteria are under way.

CONJUNCTIVAL BIOPSY

Conjunctival biopsy for histological confirmation of sarcoidosis is a quick, simple procedure performed at the slit-lamp. Three studies, totalling 116 patients, have demonstrated that it is 100 percent specific with no false positives, even in patients with other granulomatous diseases (Crick *et al.* 1955; Bornstein *et al.* 1962; Khan *et al.* 1977). No serious complications have been reported, in particular any symblepharon formation. It is also less costly and less invasive than other procedures performed to obtain a tissue sample. If conjunctival granulomas are clinically evident, the benefit of a conjunctival biopsy is undisputed. However, the role of 'blind' (random or non-directed) biopsies of clinically normal-appearing conjunctiva is controversial. While some believe this is a useful procedure (Karcioglu and Brear 1985; Spaide and Ward 1990; Chung *et al.* 2006), most believe the yield is too low (Crick *et al.* 1955; Karma 1979; Weinreb and Tessler 1984).

Small series that have taken large (10–12 mm × 3 mm) bilateral random conjunctival biopsies and, in some cases, performed extensive serial sectioning have reported success rates of up to 55 percent (Nichols *et al.* 1980; Karcioglu and Brear 1985; Spaide and Ward 1990; Chung *et al.* 2006). Interestingly, in one small series, 7 of 10 patients with multifocal choroiditis were found to have a positive non-directed conjunctival biopsy (Hershey *et al.* 1994). However, large documented series of random conjunctival biopsies have generally yielded positive results in fewer than 10 percent of cases in patients with confirmed sarcoidosis (Crick *et al.* 1955; Karma 1979). Karma and co-workers found granulomas in 17 percent of conjunctival biopsies taken from 218 patients with ocular sarcoidosis. Of the 66 cases in which nodules thought suspicious of sarcoidosis had been seen, 41 percent were positive. In the remaining

152 cases in which a random biopsy was performed, only 6.6 percent were positive (Karma 1979).

LACRIMAL GLAND BIOPSY

In known sarcoidosis, a characteristic granulomatous dacryoadenitis may be seen in 25 percent of patients with clinically normal glands and 75 percent of patients with clinically enlarged glands (Nowinski 1998). However, biopsy of the lacrimal gland is only performed in selected cases because of potential adverse effects. There are two possible approaches. The simplest approach is to biopsy part of the palpebral lobe via a conjunctival approach (Weinreb and Tessler 1984). However, sometimes the specimen predominantly comprises conjunctiva and there is insufficient lacrimal tissue for adequate pathologic inspection. On the other hand, large tissue specimens should not be removed as the lacrimal gland ductules drain through this area and damage can further exacerbate dry-eye symptoms. The alternative is an anterior transeptal approach with the potential complication of ptosis (Nowinski 1998).

PRINCIPLES OF TREATMENT

Any degree of anterior uveitis requires treatment as untreated anterior inflammation is likely to result in complications including posterior synechiae, cataract, glaucoma, and cystoid macular edema. The mainstay of treatment is topical corticosteroid drops. When anterior uveitis is severe and does not respond to drops, subconjunctival injections of corticosteroids may be efficacious. Subconjunctival corticosteroids achieve and maintain higher concentrations in the aqueous for longer periods than drops (Awan et al. 2009). Short-acting mydriatics (e.g. tropicamide or cyclopentolate) administered three times daily for severe inflammation or at night for mild inflammation are needed to keep the pupil mobile and prevent posterior synechiae formation. Atropine, a long-acting mydriatic, should not be prescribed as it can result in the pupil becoming fixed and forming posterior synechiae in the mid-dilated position.

Topical or subconjunctival corticosteroids have no effect on intermediate or posterior uveitis. Intermediate uveitis without any associated anterior uveitis or cystoid macular edema may be observed, although peri- or intraocular corticosteroid injections or systemic corticosteroids can be given if the vitreous floaters are causing deterioration in vision. Systemic corticosteroid treatment for ocular disease is also indicated in cystoid macular edema, occlusive vasculitis and optic nerve involvement. Severe anterior uveitis not controlled topically and patients whose intraocular pressure increases with topical corticosteroids are other indications. Approximately 40–50 percent of patients with sarcoid-associated uveitis require systemic corticosteroid treatment for ocular disease at some point (Edelsten et al. 1999; Jones 2002; Lobo et al. 2003). The dose depends on the severity of disease, but frequently a high dose (up to 1 mg/kg oral prednisolone) is required initially to induce remission with a slow tapering and prolonged low-dose treatment to maintain quiescence.

Sarcoid-associated uveitis is usually rapidly responsive to oral corticosteroids, but up to 15 percent of patients require additional immunosuppression owing to refractory disease, or because an unacceptably high dose of corticosteroid is required to maintain quiescence (Edelsten et al. 1999; Jones 2002; Lobo et al. 2003). Methotrexate has been shown to be efficacious in treating sarcoid-associated panuveitis in a small retrospective study (Dev et al. 1999). Nine of 11 patients (82 percent) stabilized or improved visual acuity, and of the 7 patients on oral corticosteroids, 6 were able to discontinue and the remaining patient was able to reduce the dose. Another small retrospective series demonstrated that mycophenolate mofetil is effective in the management of sarcoidosis-related intraocular inflammation (Bhat et al. 2009). Mycophenolate mofetil maintained disease quiescence and enabled cessation of systemic corticosteroids and other immunosuppressive agents in 6 of 7 patients. In another study, 6 out of 8 patients, with sarcoid-associated uveitis and who had failed or were intolerant of methotrexate, achieved control with mycophenolate mofetil (Sobrin et al. 2008).

There is mounting evidence that infliximab is effective in sarcoid-associated uveitis. In a case series of seven patients with refractory sarcoid-related chronic uveitis, all experienced a marked improvement in ocular inflammation (Baughman et al. 2005a). There have also been numerous case reports (Roberts et al. 2003; Pritchard and Nadarajah 2004; Benitez-del-Castillo et al. 2005; Doty et al. 2005; Cruz et al. 2007). However, etanercept has not been found to be effective. A small double-masked randomized controlled trial evaluated the effect of adding etanercept or placebo to a regime of methotrexate and oral corticosteroids for 18 patients with active sarcoid-associated uveitis. At the end of the 6-month follow-up period, three of the etanercept group and one from the placebo group required lower doses of corticosteroids; however, three of the etanercept group and one of the placebo group required larger doses (Baughman et al. 2005b). This is in line with reports of the minimal efficacy of etanercept in the treatment of other forms of uveitis as well as a report from a national database registry which found that etanercept was associated with a significantly greater number of uveitis cases compared with infliximab or adalimumab (Lim et al. 2007).

Symptomatic lacrimal gland or orbital involvement is another indication for systemic corticosteroids (Mavrikakis and Rootman 2007; Prabhakaran et al. 2007). An alternative is an intralesional injection of corticosteroids. In a series of 20 patients with orbital sarcoid (11 lacrimal, 9 extralacrimal orbital involvement), 8 were managed with intralesional corticosteroids alone. Twelve required oral corticosteroids, with adjunctive intralesional injections in three. Combined ciclosporin and azathioprine was used on one patient with skeletal muscle and skin involvement and hydroxychloroquine was used in a patient with neurosarcoidosis (Mavrikakis and Rootman 2007). In contrast, a multicenter study of 21 patients with orbital sarcoid (11 lacrimal, 10 extralacrimal orbital involvement) reported systemic corticosteroid use in 18 and intralesional steroid injection in only one patient. Four patients received methotrexate and five underwent surgical debulking (Prabhakaran et al. 2007).

REFERENCES

Abad S, Meyssonier V et al. (2004). Association of peripheral multifocal choroiditis with sarcoidosis: a study of thirty-seven patients. Arthritis Rheum 51: 974–82.

Abe K, Shiraki K et al. (2002). Peripapillary subretinal neovascularization in sarcoidosis: remission and exacerbation during oral corticosteroid therapy. Jpn J Ophthalmol 46: 95–9.

Akova YA, Foster CS (1994). Cataract surgery in patients with sarcoidosis-associated uveitis. Ophthalmology 101: 473–9.

Anderson NG, Wojno TH et al. (2003). Clinicopathologic findings from lacrimal sac biopsy specimens obtained during dacryocystorhinostomy. Ophthal Plast Reconstruct Surg 19(3): 173–6.

Armaly MF, Becker B (1965). Intraocular pressure response to topical corticosteroids. Fed Proc 24: 1274–8.

Atmaca LS, Atmaca-Sonmez P et al. (2009). Ocular involvement in sarcoidosis. Ocular Immunol Inflamm 17: 91–4.

Awan MA, Agarwal PK et al. (2009). Penetration of topical and subconjunctival corticosteroids into human aqueous humour and its therapeutic significance. Br J Ophthalmol 93: 708–13.

Baughman RP, Bradley DA et al. (2005a). Infliximab in chronic ocular inflammation. Int J Clin Pharm Therap 43: 7–11.

Baughman RP, Lower EE et al. (2005b). Etanercept for refractory ocular sarcoidosis: results of a double-blind randomized trial. Chest 128: 1062–47.

Baughman RP, Teirstein AS et al. (2001). Clinical characteristics of patients in a case control study of sarcoidosis. Am J Respir Crit Care Med 164 (10 Pt 1): 1885–9.

Benitez-del-Castillo JM, Martinez-de-la-Casa JM et al. (2005). Long-term treatment of refractory posterior uveitis with anti-TNFalpha (infliximab). Eye 19: 841–5.

Bhat P, Cervantes-Castaneda RA et al. (2009). Mycophenolate mofetil therapy for sarcoidosis-associated uveitis. Ocular Immunol Inflamm 17: 185–90.

Bienfait MF, Baarsma GS (1986). Sixteen cases of uveitis associated with sarcoidosis. Int Ophthalmol 9: 243–6.

Bornstein JS, Frank MI et al. (1962). Conjunctival biopsy in the diagnosis of sarcoidosis. New Engl J Med 267: 60–4.

Bourcier T, Lumbroso L et al. (1998). Retinal pigment epithelial detachment: an unusual presentation in ocular sarcoidosis. Br J Ophthalmol 82: 585.

Brown GC, Brown RH et al. (1987). Peripheral proliferative retinopathies. Int Ophthalmol 11: 41–50.

Campo RV, Aaberg TM (1984). Choroidal granuloma in sarcoidosis. Am J Ophthalmol 97: 419–27.

Chapman KL, Bartley GB et al. (1999). Lacrimal bypass surgery in patients with sarcoidosis. Am J Ophthalmol 127: 443–6.

Cheung CMG, Durrani OM et al. (2002). Peripapillary choroidal neovascularisation in sarcoidosis. Ocular Immunol Inflamm 10: 69–73.

Chung Y-M, Lin Y-C et al. (2006). Conjunctival biopsy in sarcoidosis. J Chin Med Assoc 69: 472–7.

Cohen SB, Peyman GA (1986). Sarcoid granuloma simulating amelanotic melanoma of the iris. Ann Ophthalmol 18: 343–5.

Collison JM, Miller NR et al. (1986). Involvement of orbital tissues by sarcoid. Am J Ophthalmol 102: 302–7.

Cornblath WT, Elner V et al. (1993). Extraocular muscle involvement in sarcoidosis. Ophthalmology 100: 501–5.

Crick R, Hoyle C et al. (1955). Conjunctival biopsy in sarcoidosis. Br Med J 2: 1180–1.

Crick RP, Hoyle C et al. (1961). The eyes in sarcoidosis. Br J Ophthalmol 45: 461–81.

Cruz BA, Reis DD et al. (2007). Refractory retinal vasculitis due to sarcoidosis successfully treated with infliximab. Rheumatol Int 27: 1181–3.

Cunningham ET (2000). Uveitis in children. Ocular Immunol Inflamm 8: 251–61.

Dana MR, Merayo-Lloves J et al. (1996). Prognosticators for visual outcome in sarcoid uveitis. Ophthalmology 103: 1846–53.

Desai UR, Tawansy KA et al. (2001). Choroidal granulomas in systemic sarcoidosis. Retina 21: 40–7.

Dev S, McCallum RM et al. (1999). Methotrexate treatment for sarcoid-associated panuveitis. Ophthalmology 106: 111–18.

Dick DJ, Newman PK et al. (1988). Acute posterior multifocal placoid pigment epitheliopathy and sarcoidosis. Br J Ophthalmol 72: 74–7.

Doty JD, Mazur JE et al. (2005). Treatment of sarcoidosis with infliximab. Chest 127: 1064–71.

Doxanas MT, Kelley JS et al. (1980). Sarcoidosis with neovascularization of the optic nerve head. Am J Ophthalmol 90: 347–51.

Dresner MS, Brecher R et al. (1986). Ophthalmology consultation in the diagnosis and treatment of sarcoidosis. Arch Intern Med 146: 301–4.

Duker JS, Brown GC et al. (1988). Proliferative sarcoid retinopathy. Ophthalmology 95: 1680–6.

Edelsten C, Pearson A et al. (1999). The ocular and systemic prognosis of patients presenting with sarcoid uveitis. Eye 13(Pt 6): 748–53.

Edelsten C, Stanford MR et al. (1994). Serpiginous choroiditis: an unusual presentation of ocular sarcoidosis. Br J Ophthalmol 78: 70–1.

Evans M, Sharma O et al. (2007). Differences in clinical findings between Caucasians and African Americans with biopsy-proven sarcoidosis. Ophthalmology 114: 325–33.

Finger PT, Narayana K et al. (2007). Giant sarcoid tumor of the iris and ciliary body. Ocular Immunol Inflamm 15: 121–5.

Franceschetti A, Babel J (1949). La chorio-retinie en taches de bougie, manifestation de la maladie de Besnier–Boeck. Ophthalmologica 118: 701–10.

Gould H, Kaufman HE (1961). Sarcoid of the fundus. Arch Ophthalmol 65: 453–6.

Greenberg G, Anderson R et al. (1964). Enlargement of parotid gland due to sarcoidosis. Br Med J 2: 861–2.

Gupta SK, Gupta S (1990). Sarcoidosis in India: a review of 125 biopsy-proven cases from eastern India. Sarcoidosis 7: 43–9.

Hamanaka T, Takei A et al. (2002). Pathological study of cases with secondary open-angle glaucoma due to sarcoidosis. Am J Ophthalmol 134: 17–26.

Herbort CP, Rao NA et al. (2009). International criteria for the diagnosis of ocular sarcoidosis: results of the first International Workshop on Ocular Sarcoidosis (IWOS). Ocular Immunol Inflamm 17: 160–9.

Hershey JM, Pulido JS et al. (1994). Non-caseating conjunctival granulomas in patients with multifocal choroiditis and panuveitis. Ophthalmology 101: 596–601.

Hillerdal G, Nou E et al. (1984). Sarcoidosis, epidemiology and prognosis: a 15-year European study. Am Rev Respir Dis 130: 29–32.

Hoffmann AL, Milman N et al. (2004). Childhood sarcoidosis in Denmark 1979–1994: incidence, clinical features and laboratory results at presentation in 48 children. Acta Paediatr 93: 30–6.

Hoover DL, Khan JA et al. (1986). Pediatric ocular sarcoidosis. Survey Ophthalmol 30: 215–28.

Inagaki M, Harada T et al. (1996). Subfoveal choroidal neovascularization in uveitis. Ophthalmologica 210: 229–33.

Iwata K, Nanba K et al. (1976). Ocular sarcoidosis: evaluation of intraocular findings. Ann NY Acad Sci 278: 445–54.

Jabs DA, Johns CJ (1986). Ocular involvement in chronic sarcoidosis. Am J Ophthalmol 102: 297–301.

Jabs DA, Nussenblatt RB et al. (2005). Standardization of uveitis nomenclature for reporting clinical data: results of the First International Workshop. Am J Ophthalmol 140: 509–16.

James DG (1986). Ocular sarcoidosis. Ann NY Acad Sci 465: 551–63.

James DG, Neville E et al. (1976). Ocular sarcoidosis. Trans Ophthalmol Soc UK 96: 133–9.

Jones NP (2002). Sarcoidosis and uveitis. Ophthalmol Clin North Am 15: 319–26.

Judson MA, Baughman RP et al. (1999). Defining organ involvement in sarcoidosis: the ACCESS proposed instrument. Sarcoid Vasc Diff Lung Dis 16: 75–86.

Kaiser PK, Lowder CY et al. (2002). Chest computerized tomography in the evaluation of uveitis in elderly women. Am J Ophthalmol 133: 499–505.

Karcioglu ZA, Brear R (1985). Conjunctival biopsy in sarcoidosis. Am J Ophthalmol 99: 68–73.

Karma A (1979). Ophthalmic changes in sarcoidosis. Acta Ophthalmol Suppl 141: 1–94.

Karma A, Sutinen S et al. (1980). Conjunctival and tonsillar biopsies in sarcoidosis. Chest 78: 900–1.

Kawaguchi T, Hanada A et al. (2007). Evaluation of characteristic ocular signs and systemic investigations in ocular sarcoidosis patients. Jpn J Ophthalmol 51: 121–6.

Kelmenson AT, Oliver SC et al. (2008). Sarcoid-induced symblepharon. Indian J Ophthalmol 56: 344–5.

Kendig EL, Brummer DL (1976). The prognosis of sarcoidosis in children. Chest 70: 351–3.

Khalatbari D, Stinnett S et al. (2004). Demographic-related variations in posterior segment ocular sarcoidosis. Ophthalmology 111: 357–62.

Khan F, Wessely Z et al. (1977). Conjunctival biopsy in sarcoidosis: a simple, safe, and specific diagnostic procedure. Ann Ophthalmol 9: 671–6.

Khanna A, Sidhu U et al. (2007). Pattern of ocular manifestations in patients with sarcoidosis in developing countries. Acta Ophthalmol Scand 85: 609–12.

Lardenoye CW, Van der Lelij A et al. (1997). Peripheral multifocal chorioretinitis: a distinct clinical entity? Ophthalmology 104: 1820–6.

Lee SY, Lee HG et al. (2009). Ocular sarcoidosis in a Korean population. J Korean Med Sci 24: 413–19.

Lim LL, Fraunfelder FW et al. (2007). Do tumor necrosis factor inhibitors cause uveitis? A registry-based study. Arthritis Rheum 56: 3248–52.

Lindsley CB, Petty RE (2000). Overview and report on international registry of sarcoid arthritis in childhood. Curr Rheumatol Rep 2: 343–8.

Lobo A, Barton K et al. (2003). Visual loss in sarcoid-related uveitis. Clin Exper Ophthalmol 31: 310–16.

Löfgren S. (1946). Erythema nodosum: studies on etiology and pathogenesis in 185 adult cases. Acta Med Scand 124(Suppl. 174): 1–197.

Löfgren S, Lundback H (1952). The bilateral hilar lymphoma syndrome; a study of the relation to age and sex in 212 cases. Acta Med Scand 142: 259–64.

Lutt JR, Lim LL et al. (2008). Orbital inflammatory disease. Semin Arthritis Rheum 37: 207–22.

Maca SM, Firbas U et al. (2004). Semicircular tumor of the iris and uveitis as unilocal manifestation of sarcoidosis. Ocular Immunol Inflamm 12: 237–40.

Mana J, Gomez-Vaquero C et al. (1996). Periarticular ankle sarcoidosis: a variant of Löfgren's syndrome. J Rheumatol 23: 874–7.

Mana J, Gomez-Vaquero C et al. (1999). Löfgren's syndrome revisited: a study of 186 patients. Am J Med 107: 240–5.

Mansour AM (1986). Sarcoid optic disc edema and optociliary shunts. J Clin Neuro-Ophth 6: 47–52.

Marcus DF, Bovino JA et al. (1982). Sarcoid granuloma of the choroid. Ophthalmology 89: 1326–30.

Matsuo T, Fujiwara N et al. (2005). First presenting signs or symptoms of sarcoidosis in a Japanese population. Jpn J Ophthalmol 49: 149–52.

Mavrikakis I, Rootman J (2007). Diverse clinical presentations of orbital sarcoid. Am J Ophthalmol 144: 769–75.

Mayock RL, Bertrand P et al. (1963). Manifestations of sarcoidosis: analysis of 145 patients, with a review of nine series selected from the literature. Am J Med 35: 67–89.

Merayo-Lloves J, Power WJ et al. (1999). Secondary glaucoma in patients with uveitis. Ophthalmologica 213: 300–4.

Miyao A, Ikeda T et al. (1999). Histopathological findings in proliferative membrane from a patient with sarcoid uveitis. Jpn J Ophthalmol 43: 209–12.

Nichols CW, Eagle RC et al. (1980). Conjunctival biopsy as an aid in the evaluation of the patient with suspected sarcoidosis. Ophthalmology 87: 287–91.

Nowinski TS (1998). Ocular manifestations of sarcoidosis. Curr Opin Ophthalmol 9: 80–4.

Obenauf CD, Shaw HE et al. (1978). Sarcoidosis and its ophthalmic manifestations. Am J Ophthalmol 86: 648–55.

Ohara K, Okubo A et al. (1992). Intraocular manifestations of systemic sarcoidosis. Jpn J Ophthalmol 36: 452–7.

Ohta H, Tazawa R et al. (2006). Acute-onset sarcoidosis with erythema nodosum and polyarthralgia (Löfgren's syndrome) in Japan: a case report and a review of the literature. Intern Med 45: 659–62.

Olk RJ, Lipmann MJ et al. (1983). Solitary choroidal mass as the presenting sign in systemic sarcoidosis. Br J Ophthalmol 67: 826–9.

Pattishall EN, Strope GL et al. (1986). Childhood sarcoidosis. J Pediatr 108: 169–77.

Pellegrini V, Ohno S et al. (1986). Subretinal neovascularisation and snow banking in a case of sarcoidosis: case report. Br J Ophthalmol 70: 474–7.

Pessoa de Souza Filho J, Martins MC et al. (2005). Eyelid swelling as the only manifestation of ocular sarcoidosis. Ocular Immunol Inflamm 13: 399–402.

Prabhakaran VC, Saeed P et al. (2007). Orbital and adnexal sarcoidosis. Arch Ophthalmol 125: 1657–62.

Pritchard C, Nadarajah K (2004). Tumour necrosis factor alpha inhibitor treatment for sarcoidosis refractory to conventional treatments: a report of five patients. Ann Rheum Dis 63: 318–20.

Rizzato G, Angi M et al. (1996). Uveitis as a presenting feature of chronic sarcoidosis. Eur Respir J 9: 1201–5.

Roberts SD, Wilkes DS et al. (2003). Refractory sarcoidosis responding to infliximab. Chest 124: 2028–31.

Rothova A (2000). Ocular involvement in sarcoidosis. Br J Ophthalmol 84: 110–16.

Rothova A, Lardenoye C (1998). Arterial macroaneurysms in peripheral multifocal chorioretinitis associated with sarcoidosis. Ophthalmology 105: 1393–7.

Rothova A, Alberts C *et al.* (1989). Risk factors for ocular sarcoidosis. *Docum Ophthalmol* 72(3/4): 287–96.

Rothova A, Buitenhuis HJ *et al.* (1992). Uveitis and systemic disease. *Br J Ophthalmol* 76: 137–41.

Rothova A, Suttorp-van Schulten MS *et al.* (1996). Causes and frequency of blindness in patients with intraocular inflammatory disease. *Br J Ophthalmol* 80: 332–6.

Salchow DJ, Weiss MJ (2006). Retinal pigment epithelial detachment in sarcoidosis. *Ocular Immunol Inflamm* 14: 245–8.

Sharma SK, Mohan A (2002). Sarcoidosis: global scenario and Indian perspective. *Indian J Med Res* 116: 221–47.

Smith JA, Foster CS (1996). Sarcoidosis and its ocular manifestations. *Int Ophthalmol Clin* 36: 109–25.

Sobrin L, Christen W *et al.* (2008). Mycophenolate mofetil after methotrexate failure or intolerance in the treatment of scleritis and uveitis. *Ophthalmology* 115: 1416–21.

Spaide RF, Ward DL (1990). Conjunctival biopsy in the diagnosis of sarcoidosis. *Br J Ophthalmol* 74: 469–71.

Spalton DJ, Sanders MD (1981). Fundus changes in histologically confirmed sarcoidosis. *Br J Ophthalmol* 65: 348–58.

Stavrou P, Linton S *et al.* (1997). Clinical diagnosis of ocular sarcoidosis. *Eye* 11(Pt 3): 365–70.

Suresh P, Jones NP (1999). Ischaemic retinal vasculitis in biopsy-proven sarcoidosis. *Eye* 13(Pt 6): 800–1.

Thorne JE, Brucker AJ (2000). Choroidal white lesions as an early manifestation of sarcoidosis. *Retina* 20: 8–15.

Tingey DP, Gonder JR (1992). Ocular sarcoidosis presenting as a solitary choroidal mass. *Can J Ophthalmol* 27: 25–9.

Tuft SJ, Watson PG (1991). Progression of scleral disease. *Ophthalmology* 98: 467–71.

Tugal-Tutkun I, Aydin-Akova Y *et al.* (2007). Referral patterns, demographic and clinical features, and visual prognosis of Turkish patients with sarcoid uveitis. *Ocular Immunol Inflamm* 15: 337–43.

Uyama M (1971). Ocular sarcoidosis as a clinical uveitis entity. *Jpn J Clin Ophthalmol* 25: 1513–22.

Verougstraete C, Snyers B *et al.* (2001). Multiple arterial ectasias in patients with sarcoidosis and uveitis. *Am J Ophthalmol* 131: 223–31.

Vrabec TR, Augsburger JJ *et al.* (1995). Taches de bougie. *Ophthalmology* 102: 1712–21.

Weinreb RN, Tessler H (1984). Laboratory diagnosis of ophthalmic sarcoidosis. *Survey Ophthalmol* 28: 653–64.

Wolfensberger TJ, Tufail A (2000). Systemic disorders associated with detachment of the neurosensory retina and retinal pigment epithelium. *Curr Opin Ophthalmol* 11: 455–61.

Yamada N, Watanabe H *et al.* (1971). Studies of ocular lesions in sarcoidosis. *Jpn J Clin Ophthalmol* 25: 1513–22.

Yamaguchi M, Hosoda Y *et al.* (1989). Epidemiological study on sarcoidosis in Japan: recent trends in incidence and prevalence rates and changes in epidemiological features. *Sarcoidosis* 6: 138–46.

32

Musculoskeletal and joint manifestations

ANISUR RAHMAN AND MICHAEL I POLKEY

INTRODUCTION

Symptoms in the bones, joints and muscles are well-recognized, albeit rare, clinical manifestations of sarcoidosis. A recent review cites the prevalence of bone, joint or muscle involvement in sarcoidosis as 0.9 percent (Dempsey et al. 2009). This low figure almost certainly refers to symptomatic disease. As shown later in this chapter, plain radiographs and magnetic resonance imaging (MRI) detect asymptomatic bony lesions in a larger proportion of patients with sarcoidosis (Neville et al. 1977; Moore et al. 2005). Nevertheless, musculoskeletal involvement is neither common nor especially troublesome in most patients with sarcoidosis.

JOINTS

There have been relatively few publications on sarcoidosis of the joints, possibly because cases are relatively rare, symptoms are typically short-lasting and there is little controversy about treatment. Many of the published descriptions are therefore small case series, often from many years ago (e.g. Gumpel et al. 1967; Spilberg et al. 1969).

There are characteristically two main presentations of sarcoid arthritis. The first is an acute generally symmetrical polyarthritis often starting in the ankles or knees, which often resolves within a few weeks after treatment with non-steroidal anti-inflammatory drugs. The second, rarer form is a more chronic arthritis with longer-lasting joint pain and arthritis. One paper from the 1950s suggested that this chronic form may be characterized by granulomas within the synovium but only five patients were studied. Synovial biopsies carried out in four cases contained granulomas (Sokoloff and Bunim 1959). The term 'Löfgren's syndrome' is used to characterize the combination of bilateral hilar lymphadenopathy, erythema nodosum and periarticular inflammation but it is not clear whether this represents true ankle arthritis in most cases. Kellner et al. (1992) addressed this question by carrying out ultrasound examination of the ankles and found effusions in only 6 of 24 patients with acute sarcoidosis who were examined. A Spanish study of 186 patients with Löfgren's syndrome reported that about 15 percent had arthritis in joints other than the ankle (Mana et al. 1999).

The first major cross-sectional study of sarcoid arthritis was carried out at the Johns Hopkins Hospital Sarcoidosis Clinic in 1967 (Gumpel et al. 1967). Of 118 patients studied, 45 had arthritis. These included 19 who had arthritis either at the time of diagnosis of sarcoidosis or within the first 9 months of the disease. In 16 of these cases, arthritis was a major clinical feature. This early arthritis was almost always symmetrical and affected multiple joint groups, with the ankles being the most common site of the first joint symptoms. The 16 patients who developed arthritis later in the course of the disease had less widespread joint involvement, but erythema nodosum and skin sarcoidosis were commonly found in both the early-onset and late-onset arthritis groups. Outcome was good with complete or partial resolution of symptoms in 32 of the 45 cases. Even in the 13 cases that had recurrent attacks of joint pain, treatment with corticosteroids was rarely required; the 4 patients who received corticosteroids did so as treatment for pulmonary sarcoidosis rather than for their joints. Radiological abnormalities were uncommon. Only 6 of 68 hand radiographs and 4 of 33 foot radiographs were abnormal. The abnormalities were mainly areas of cystic change in the bones (see section on bones below).

In a subsequent study in New York (Spilberg et al. 1969), 10 of 64 consecutive patients seen in a sarcoidosis clinic had a history of joint symptoms, giving a prevalence of 15.6 percent. The clinical features of these 10 patients were described together with a further 18 patients with sarcoid arthritis identified from an arthritis clinic. The findings were similar to those of Gumpel and associates, in that 27 of the 28 patients had polyarthritis, 24 had symmetrical involvement and 24 made a complete recovery. Only 2 of the 28 had radiological abnormalities but 25 percent had erythema nodosum.

A more recent case series from India included 29 patients with sarcoidosis who presented with articular symptoms between 1990 and 1999 (Govindarajan et al. 2001). In this series, 10 patients had an acute arthritis mainly in the lower limb joints, whereas 15 patients had arthritis lasting more than 6 months which resembled rheumatoid arthritis and was characterized by bilateral symmetrical involvement of the hands. Despite this difference in clinical characteristics compared to the older series, these Indian patients also had a good clinical outcome. At a median follow-up of 12 months, 15 patients had complete remission of symptoms and 11 had partial remission (Govindarajan et al. 2001).

BONES

In a seminal review of over 3000 cases of sarcoidosis that had been followed up in 11 centers of excellence on three continents, James et al. (1976) reported that the prevalence of bony abnormalities in sarcoidosis ranged from 1 to 13 percent in different centers, with an average of 5 percent. It was not clear whether bony sarcoidosis was being defined in the same way in all centers, which may have contributed to the variation. In particular, prevalence is likely to have been higher where asymptomatic lesions seen on radiographs were included.

In a study from a single center in London, UK, published a year later, Neville and co-workers found that 29 patients from a cohort of 537 patients with sarcoidosis had bony lesions on radiographs but these lesions were asymptomatic in about half the cases (Neville et al. 1977). The distribution of the lesions was predominantly in the hands and feet (26 cases), with three cases of nasal involvement (generally co-existing with lupus pernio) and one case each of sarcoidosis in the palate and temporal bones. Soft tissue swelling occurred in 13 (45 percent) of the patients. In the vast majority of patients bony sarcoidosis occurred in association with sarcoidosis of other tissues: 86 percent had intrathoracic involvement and 66 percent had skin sarcoidosis. In fact the authors particularly drew attention to the higher frequency of skin sarcoidosis in those with bone lesions than those without bone lesions. Only 23 percent of the 508 patients with no bony abnormalities had skin lesions.

Three different types of radiological lesion were described by Neville and associates in their study of bony sarcoidosis. The most common (occurring in 25/29 cases) were lytic lesions taking the form of rounded cysts. Biopsies (carried out in four cases) showed granuloma formation within these lesions. Nine patients had 'permeative' lesions with tunneling of the cortex and a change in shape of the bone; only three patients had destructive, rapidly advancing lesions with involvement of the joint space. It is possible that these

destructive lesions may occur more frequently in certain populations. For example, Morrison (1974) suggested that such lesions occurred more frequently in South African Bantu – though this was based on a study of only 18 selected cases and has not been confirmed.

Just as radiographs may identify sarcoid lesions in the bones of asymptomatic patients, MRI may identify lesions that are not visible on plain radiographs. Moore and co-workers studied 42 consecutive patients referred for MRI from a pulmonary sarcoidosis clinic on account of musculoskeletal symptoms (Moore et al. 2005). MRI showed bony lesions in 17 cases and these were not confined to the hands and feet. For example, 13 patients had lesions in the large bones or axial skeleton. In 6 of the 17 cases (5 in long bones) the lesions visible on MRI were not seen on plain radiographs. The authors suggested that radiographs are sufficient to detect sarcoidosis of bones in the hands or feet but that MRI may be helpful where symptoms occur in other areas.

However, one must bear in mind that additional imaging may not alter the management of the patient significantly. Bony lesions usually occur in patients whose dominant features of sarcoidosis lie in another system, which therefore dictates the treatment. For example, in the study of 29 patients reported by Neville and associates, 22 were treated with corticosteroids but in 15 of these cases the reason for treatment was outside the bones (e.g. lupus pernio, pulmonary sarcoidosis or uveitis) (Neville et al. 1977). Regardless of the reason for treatment, corticosteroids generally led to improvement in symptoms but not to resolution of the radiological changes. A more recent review (Wilcox et al. 2000) also stresses the usefulness of drugs, including corticosteroids, chloroquine and hydroxychloroquine, for reducing bony symptoms in sarcoidosis but not for reversing structural changes visible on radiographs.

PERIPHERAL MUSCLE

Skeletal muscle function is critical to an individual's quality of life. Without contraction of skeletal muscle it would be impossible to walk, talk or feed oneself. More importantly, respiration cannot occur without contraction of the inspiratory muscles, of which the most important is the diaphragm, accounting for approximately 70 percent of respiration in normal humans (Mead and Loring 1982). Sarcoidosis can cause skeletal muscle weakness either by virtue of disease involvement alone or combined with the side-effects of the drugs used for treatment – of which far the most important from the perspective of skeletal muscle weakness are corticosteroids. For the respiratory muscles there is the additional question of whether functional change, for example due to lung volume change, could cause weakness.

Numerous clinical conditions (e.g. amyotrophic lateral sclerosis, spinal cord injury) confirm that denervation can cause secondary muscle weakness. Since neuropathy is a recognized feature of sarcoidosis (Vital et al. 2008), it is pertinent to consider whether sarcoidosis itself can truly involve skeletal muscle. The hallmark of such a condition would be the finding of a granulomatous myopathy in the

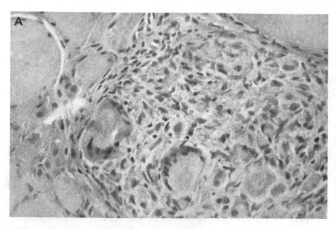
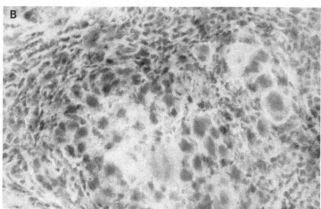

Figure 32.1   Granulomatous myositis or sarcoid myopathy. (a) In the non-necrotizing granuloma, two giant cells are apparent. Elastica van Gieson. (b) Numerous macrophages, including giant cells, marked by histochemically up-regulated acid phosphatase activity, are components of the granuloma. Reproduced with permission from Hewer and Goebel (2008).

absence of an alternative cause; even then the mechanism of injury could be by damage to the intramuscular nerve branches (Gemignani *et al.* 1998). It is well documented that granulomas can occur in muscle (Fig. 32.1), although they can also have an infectious etiology and are reportedly also a feature of graft-versus-host disease and the myopathy associated with inflammatory bowel disease (Hewer and Goebel 2008).

Case series for sarcoid myopathy are, not unexpectedly, sparse. Rothfeld and Folk (1962), in their case report, credit the first description to Licharew in 1908, though this report does not seem to be available in the English literature. Myers *et al.* (1952) described muscle granulomas in three of four cases, and Phillips and Phillips (1956) in four of five cases. Wallace *et al.* (1958) have provided the largest series: they studied random biopsies in 42 biopsies and found granulomas in 23.

While case reports of steroid responsive granulomatous myositis exist (Yamada *et al.* 2007), a true sarcoid myopathy would require a granulomatous myositis to be present with other typical features of the condition. This was elegantly demonstrated in a patient with granulomatous myositis (GM) in whom PET scanning also showed uptake in the salivary glands and mediastinal nodes (Dufour *et al.* 2007; Fig. 32.2). Similar cases have been described in which systemic disease was confirmed by gallium (Ga) scanning.

RESPIRATORY MUSCLE

Case reports exist describing respiratory muscle weakness as the presenting feature of sarcoidosis (Dewberry *et al.* 1993), but this seems to be the exception rather than the rule. Ost and associates observed a steroid responsive drop in vital capacity in a patient with sarcoidosis; granulomas were observed in a quadriceps biopsy and the presence of respiratory muscle involvement was inferred (Ost *et al.* 1995). For understandable reasons there are to our knowledge no reports of proven granulomas in diaphragm biopsy specimens obtained *in vivo*, although there is a single postmortem case report (Pandya *et al.* 1988).

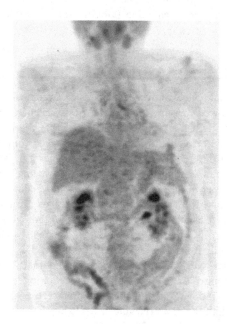

Figure 32.2   Mediastinal (solid arrow) and salivary gland (light arrows) activity demonstrated by PET scanning in a man in whom non-caseating granulomas were also observed in a quadriceps biopsy. Reproduced with permission from Dufour *et al.* (2007).

Baydur and associates compared 12 untreated patients with 12 non-smoking controls. They found few significant differences in respiratory muscle strength between patients and controls, and the data could have been confounded by alterations in lung volume, which was not measured plethysmographically. However, it should be noted that only three of nine patients who consented had demonstrable granulomas on muscle biopsy, and this cohort may by chance have had an under-representation of myopathic involvement (Baydur *et al.* 1993). A subsequent larger study showed relationships between inspiratory muscle strength and dyspnea, but again lung volumes were not measured plethysmographically (Baydur *et al.* 2001). Brancaleone and associates measured inspiratory muscle strength as maximal inspiratory mouth pressure in 34 patients with sarcoid and also did not find evidence of weakness compared with controls (Brancaleone *et al.* 2004).

TREATMENT OUTCOMES

The older literature tended not to deal with the outcome of treatment. Gardner-Thorpe in 1972 reported six cases and presented what we would now describe as a meta-analysis of preceding literature. He concluded that, in approximately 80 percent of cases, therapy with corticosteroids or ACTH had a beneficial outcome – although this was assessed after a range of treatment durations, and the outcome measures varied. Data on second-line agents are naturally more sparse. Le Roux and colleagues reported eight patients with GM and clinical features of sarcoidosis. The pattern of weakness was predominantly proximal, symmetrical and lower-limb, and only two responded to therapy – one with steroids and one with methotrexate (Le Roux *et al.* 2007).

CONCLUSION

Sarcoid granulomas can occur in bone, giving a characteristic appearance of lytic lesions which heal to form cysts. In many cases these are asymptomatic but can be detected on imaging. Severe deforming joint damage is rare and corticosteroids (often given for other co-existing manifestations of sarcoidosis) help to improve symptoms of pain and soft tissue swelling but do not alter structural damage. Arthralgia is common in Löfgren's syndrome but true arthritis is rare and usually takes the form of an acute symmetrical polyarthritis which resolves without damage to the joints. Corticosteroid treatment is not always necessary for sarcoid arthritis.

Skeletal muscle granulomas are frequent in sarcoidosis to the point where they might even be considered as a diagnostic investigation if more classical approaches fail. However, the evidence that they contribute to a worse overall outcome is sparce and the evidence of benefit following corticosteroid therapy is slender. The authors do not recommend treatment in the absence of symptoms. The involvement of respiratory muscles remains speculative; useful fruitful approaches could be sampling of non-diaphragmatic respiratory muscle (such as the intercostals) during other surgical procedures such as mediastinoscopy and the routine evaluation of the diaphragm during postmortems.

REFERENCES

Baydur A, Pandya K, Sharma OP *et al.* (1993). Control of ventilation, respiratory muscle strength, and granulomatous involvement of skeletal muscle in patients with sarcoidosis. *Chest* 103: 396–402.

Baydur A, Alsalek M, Louie SG, Sharma OP (2001). Respiratory muscle strength, lung function, and dyspnea in patients with sarcoidosis. *Chest* 120: 102–8.

Brancaleone P, Perez T, Robin S *et al.* (2004). Clinical impact of inspiratory muscle impairment in sarcoidosis. *Sarcoid Vasc Diff Lung Dis* 21: 219–27.

Dempsey OJ, Paterson EW, Kerr KM, Denison AR (2009). Sarcoidosis. *Br Med J* 339: 3206.

Dewberry RG, Schneider BF, Cale WF, Phillips LH (1993). Sarcoid myopathy presenting with diaphragm weakness. *Muscle Nerve* 16: 832–5.

Dufour JF, Billotey C, Streichenberger N *et al.* (2007). [Sarcoidosis demonstrated by fluorodeoxyglucose positron emission tomography in a case of granulomatous myopathy]. *Rev Med Intern* 28: 568–70.

Gardner-Thorpe C (1972). Muscle weakness due to sarcoid myopathy: six case reports and an evalation of steroid therapy. *Neurology* 22: 917–28.

Gemignani F, Bellanova MF, Salih S *et al.* (1998). Sarcoid neuromyopathy with selective involvement of the intramuscular nerves. *Acta Neuropathol* 95: 437–41.

Govindarajan V, Agarwal V, Aggarwal A, Misra R (2001). Arthritis in sarcoidosis. *J Assoc Physicians India* 49: 1145–7.

Gumpel JM, Johns CJ, Shulman LE (1967). The joint disease of sarcoidosis. *Ann Rheum Dis* 26: 194–205.

Hewer E, Goebel HH (2008). Myopathology of non-infectious inflammatory myopathies: the current status. *Pathol Res Pract* 204: 609–23.

James DG, Neville E, Siltzbach LE (1976). A worldwide review of sarcoidosis. *Ann NY Acad Sci* 278: 321–34.

Kellner H, Spathling S, Herzer P (1992). Ultrasound findings in Löfgren's syndrome: is ankle swelling caused by arthritis, tenosynovitis or periarthritis? *J Rheumatol* 19: 38–41.

Le Roux K, Streichenberger N, Vial C *et al.* (2007). Granulomatous myositis: a clinical study of thirteen cases. *Muscle Nerve* 35: 171–7.

Mana J, Gomez-Vaquero C, Montero A *et al.* (1999). Löfgren's syndrome revisited: a study of 186 patients. *Am J Med* 107: 240–5.

Mead J, Loring SH (1982). Analysis of volume displacement and length changes of the diaphragm during breathing. *J Appl Physiol* 53: 750–55.

Moore SL, Teirstein A, Golimbu C (2005). MRI of sarcoidosis patients with musculoskeletal symptoms. *Am J Roentgen* 185: 154–9.

Morrison JG (1974). Sarcoidosis in the Bantu: necrotizing and mutilating forms of the disease. *Br J Dermatol* 90: 649–55.

Myers GB, Gottlieb AM, Mattman PE *et al.* (1952). Joint and skeletal muscle manifestations in sarcoidosis. *Am J Med* 12: 161–9.

Neville E, Carstairs LS, James DG (1977). Sarcoidosis of bone. *Q J Med* 46: 215–27.

Ost D, Yeldandt A, Cugell D (1995). Acute sarcoid myositis with respiratory muscle involvement. *Chest* 107: 879–82.

Pandya KP, Klatt EC, Sharma OP (1988). Sarcoidosis and the diaphragm. *Chest* 94: 223.

Phillips AM, Phillips RW (1956). The diagnosis of Boeck's sarcoid by skeletal muscle biopsy; report of four cases. *Arch Intern Med* 98: 732–6.

Rothfeld B, Folk EE (1962). Sarcoid myopathy. *J Am Med Assoc* 179: 903–5.

Sokoloff L, Bunim JJ (1959). Clinical and pathological studies of joint involvement in sarcoidosis. *New Engl J Med* 260: 841–7.

Spilberg I, Siltzbach LE, McEwen C (1969). The arthritis of sarcoidosis. *Arthritis Rheum* 12: 126–37.

Vital A, Lagueny A, Ferrer X *et al.* (2008). Sarcoid neuropathy: clinicopathological study of 4 new cases and review of the literature. *Clin Neuropathol* 27: 96–105.

Wallace SL, Lattes R, Malia JP, Ragan C (1958). Muscle involvement in Boeck's sarcoid. *Ann Intern Med* 48: 497–511.

Wilcox A, Bharadwaj P, Sharma OP (2000). Bone sarcoidosis. *Curr Opin Rheumatol* 12: 321–30.

Yamada H, Ishii W, Ito S *et al.* (2007). Sarcoid myositis with muscle weakness as a presenting symptom. *Mod Rheumatol* 17: 243–6.

33

Peripheral lymphadenopathy

HELEN L BOOTH

INTRODUCTION

Of the approximately 600 lymph nodes in the body, those in the head and neck, axillary and inguinal regions are potentially palpable. With no definite size criteria for what constitutes enlargement or lymphadenopathy it has been recommended that lymph nodes outside the inguinal area present for longer than 1 month and over 1×1 cm in size without an obvious diagnosis require further investigation (Habermann and Steensma 2000). In relation to sarcoidosis, the large multicenter ACCESS study (A Case Control Etiologic Study of Sarcoidosis) standardized an assessment tool designed to define different organ involvement (Judson et al. 1999). Definite involvement was confirmed if a biopsy from the organ showed non-caseating granuloma without any other cause being identified. Criteria for other organ involvement in patients with biopsy-confirmed sarcoidosis were based on clinical criteria and classified as definite, probable and possible. The criteria for probable extrathoracic lymph node involvement in a biopsy-confirmed sarcoidosis case was defined as a new palpable lymph node above the waist and/or lymph nodes >2 cm on CT scan. Possible involvement was defined as new palpable femoral lymph node(s).

INCIDENCE

The predominant lymph node involvement in sarcoidosis is intrathoracic but, although less common, peripheral lymphadenopathy can be frequently found during the course of the illness. As with other manifestations of sarcoidosis, the proportion of cases with lymphadenopathy varies widely between series. This may reflect the underlying population surveyed, particularly the ethnic mix, the thoroughness and interpretation of clinical examination and imaging techniques used, as well as how the data were collected. In the previous edition of this book the incidence reported from an American series ranged from 69 to 100 percent with lower rates from Europe (7.7–82 percent). In a retrospective survey by Edmonstone and Wilson (1985) of 156 patients diagnosed with sarcoidosis in south London between 1969 and 1982, palpable lymphadenopathy was found significantly more commonly in blacks (33.9 percent) compared to Caucasians (8.8 percent). The more recent ACCESS study (Baughman et al. 2001) recruited 736 patients from 10 centers in the USA between November 1997 and May 1999. Patients were enrolled within 6 months of a biopsy consistent with sarcoidosis and with a compatible clinical picture. The proportion of patients with extrathoracic lymph node involvement in this large study was 15.2 percent. A higher incidence in those under 40 years (20 percent) was reported compared to those ≥ 40 years (11.2 percent, $p < 0.005$). As in the Edmonstone and Wilson study, there was a higher incidence in blacks (19.4 vs 12.2 percent, $p < 0.01$) but no differences by gender. In two cases sarcoidosis was limited to peripheral lymph nodes only. For comparison, 76.4 percent of patients recruited to the ACCESS study had intrathoracic lymphadenopathy as evidenced by Scadding chest radiograph stages I and II.

CLINICAL CHARACTERISTICS

The most common site of superficial lymph node involvement is in the neck where the posterior cervical nodes are more frequently affected. In a series reported by Yanardag and associates of 546 sarcoidosis patients seen between 1972 and 2005, 79 (14.5 percent) had clinically significant lymphadenopathy of ≥ 1 cm. Of these, 67/72 had lymph node biopsies compatible with sarcoidosis and were sampled from the cervical (21 cases, 31.3 percent), supraclavicular (20, 29.9 percent), inguinal (11, 16.4 percent), axillary (8,11.9 percent), epitrochlear (5, 7.5 percent), and submandibular (2, 3 percent) sites (Yanardag *et al.* 2007). Lymph nodes affected by sarcoidosis are characteristically discrete, firm, mobile and not tender. They do not ulcerate or form sinuses.

Peripheral lymphadenopathy is rarely the presenting symptom of sarcoidosis. In a study to examine the time to confirm a diagnosis of sarcoidosis, the initial symptoms reported by study subjects were respiratory (52 percent), skin (13 percent) and constitutional symptoms of fever, malaise and night sweats (6.3 percent). The researchers report that 16 percent had initial symptoms other than these affecting the eye, musculoskeletal and abdominal systems, but do not refer to peripheral lymphadenopathy (Judson *et al.* 2003a).

The presence of lymphadenopathy in sarcoidosis can be used as a marker of disease activity (Baughman *et al.* 2001). A cohort of 215 consecutive sarcoidosis cases recruited to the ACCESS study and followed for a median of 25 months gives some information about the natural history of peripheral lymphadenopathy in sarcoidosis (Judson *et al.* 2003b). Overall, 50 of 215 patients (23 percent) developed new organ involvement during follow-up; it was more likely in blacks and those with extrathoracic involvement at baseline (i.e. within 6 months of histologically proven sarcoidosis). Peripheral lymphadenopathy was present in 35 of the 215 (16.2 percent) at baseline, the most common extrathoracic site along with skin, and a further 8 cases arose during follow-up. Although the authors categorize spirometry, dyspnea scale and chest radiograph Scadding grade as improved, worse or unchanged improvement at the end of the 2-year follow-up period, these criteria were not used for extrathoracic involvement, including peripheral lymphadenopathy, so no data on how many peripheral lymph nodes regressed during this time are presented.

Although the presence of lymphadenopathy is not an indication *per se* for systemic treatment, patients with lymphadenopathy are often treated for other organ involvement. In a randomized double-blind placebo-controlled study of infliximab, an anti-TNF-α monoclonal antibody, Judson *et al.* (2008) developed the extrapulmonary physician organ severity tool (ePOST) to assess 17 extrapulmonary organs which included peripheral lymph nodes. At baseline, peripheral lymph node involvement was again the most common extrathoracic site affected, found in 50 of 138 cases (37 percent). After 28 weeks of treatment with infliximab there was a significant reduction in the ePOST but there was no significant change detected for any particular affected organ, including peripheral lymph nodes. This may reflect the small sample size of this subgroup analysis.

DIFFERENTIAL DIAGNOSIS

Enlarged lymph nodes are a common symptom and sign in a number of malignant, infectious and inflammatory diseases (Table 33.1). Careful history-taking and examination can help with limiting the differential diagnosis and forming an appropriate management plan. The history should include a record of exposure to animals, biting insects, risk factors for human immunodeficiency virus (HIV), and a detailed travel,

occupational and medication history. Particular attention should be paid to the age of the patient, symptoms, duration of lymphadenopathy and the site, size and pattern of lymph node involvement.

The prevalence of significant lymph node pathology varies greatly with the population studied. It has been asserted that more than 75 percent of lateral neck masses in patients older than 40 years are caused by malignant tumors, and that in the absence of overt signs of infection this situation should be considered due to metastatic squamous cell carcinoma or lymphoma until proven otherwise (Gleeson *et al.* 2000). In a review of 653 peripheral lymph node biopsies performed at one institution in the USA, 56 percent were found to be benign, 29 percent carcinoma and 15 percent lymphoma, but the proportion with malignancy was higher at 60 percent in those over the age of 50 years (Lee *et al.* 1980). In contrast, of 2556 patients who presented with unexplained lymphadenopathy to primary care, only 1.1 percent were eventually found to be due to malignancy. In those over 40 years there was a 4 percent rate of malignant lymphadenopathy versus 0.4 percent risk for those aged under 40 years (Fijten and Bliijham 1988).

Symptom enquiry is required to establish the presence of constitutional symptoms such as fever, weight loss and/or sweats suggesting infection, lymphoma, sarcoidosis or auto-immune disease.

In the primary care setting, generalized lymphadenopathy, in two or more sites, occurs in one-quarter of patients and localized lymphadenopathy of the head and neck (55 percent), inguinal (14 percent), axillary (5 percent), supraclavicular (1 percent) regions in three-quarters of cases (Ferrer 1998). Some features of the node(s) may help in indicating a possible diagnosis. Tender, erythematous and/or fluctuant nodes, especially if associated with lymphangitis of the draining area, may indicate infection. Sinus formation is associated with infections from organisms such as mycobacteria and actinomycosis. Hard, fixed asymmetrical lymph nodes are likely to be malignant.

There is a particular challenge when a patient with treated cancer develops lymphadenopathy, which with the widespread use of PET/CT scanning in the monitoring of these patients is increasingly being identified. In a study by Hunt and associates which retrospectively reviewed the results of 565 mediastinoscopies performed at their institution between 2004 and 2008, 41 sarcoidosis cases were diagnosed of which 21 (53 percent) developed after a diagnosis of cancer (48 percent breast, 10 percent each of Hodgkin's lymphoma, testicular, lung) (Hunt *et al.* 2009). There is likely to be a selection bias in that those patients with a prior malignancy are more likely to be referred for mediastinoscopy than someone with probable sarcoidosis and a stage I chest radiograph, and this is supported by the significantly older age in the former group. However, it is clear that sarcoidosis is a possible cause of lymphadenopathy in cancer patients and underlines the importance of obtaining histological confirmation as there is an obvious difference in the management of the two conditions. In the context of this chapter it is of note that, in this series, although all the patients had mediastinal adenopathy, they also had peripheral lymphadenopathy in the neck (5 percent), groin

(5 percent) and axilla (5 percent), which might have been less invasively sampled.

Even the presence of granulomas in a tissue sample is not specific to sarcoidosis and can occur in infections and rarely in response to a variety of malignant disease, including lymphoma, epitheloid carcinomas and seminomas and secondary to other causes (see Table 33.1). It has been reported that on average 4.4 percent of regional lymph nodes draining carcinomas have a sarcoidosis-like reaction (Hunninghake *et al.* 1999). Another entity, 'granulomatous lesions of unknown significance' (GLUS), describes patients with isolated granulomatous involvement of liver or lymph nodes. The lack of other organ involvement means that this is not sufficient to make a diagnosis of sarcoidosis. Interestingly, Rizzato and Montemorro (2000) describe their experience of 43 patients seen over a 20-year period with sarcoid-type granulomas identified in an isolated peripheral lymph node excision biopsy without evidence of systemic sarcoidosis clinically or on detailed initial investigation. In 33 patients a diagnosis of sarcoidosis was eventually secured, 25 pulmonary and 8 extrathoracic, after a median time of 5 years. The other 10 remained with a diagnosis of idiopathic granulomatous disease of peripheral lymph nodes compatible with GLUS.

DIAGNOSIS

The importance of confirming sarcoidosis affecting peripheral lymph nodes is to exclude malignant disease and other conditions, such as tuberculosis (TB), which need specific treatment. Furthermore, as peripheral lymph nodes are usually readily accessible for sampling, demonstration of non-caseating granulomas from these sites in the appropriate clinical setting may preclude the need for more invasive sampling to establish a diagnosis of systemic sarcoidosis. Enrollment of the 736 patients into the ACCESS study required biopsy-proven sarcoidosis. In total 776 biopsies were performed from 23 different organs. Peripheral lymph nodes were the second most common extrathoracic site sampled after skin and were biopsied in 61 cases (Teirstein *et al.* 2005).

Table 33.1   Some causes of peripheral lymphadenopathy.

		Granulomatous inflammation	Pattern of lymphadenopathy	Diagnostic testing
Infections	Tuberculosis	Yes	Localized	FNA and culture
	Mycobacteria other than TB (MOTT)	Yes	Localized	FNA and culture
	Cat scratch (*Bartonella*)	Yes	Localized	FNA/biopsy, serology
	Infectious mononucleosis	No	Cervical lymphadenopathy	Serology
	HIV	No	Generalized	HIV antibody
	Toxoplasmosis	No	Localized (usually cervical) or generalized	Serology
	Histoplasmosis	Yes	Generalized or localized	Culture, serology, antigen
	Syphilis	Yes	Generalized	Serology
Malignant	Hodgkin's lymphoma	Rarely	Generalized	Biopsy
	Non-Hodgkin's lymphoma	Rarely	Generalized	Biopsy
	Metastasis solid tumors	Rarely	Localized or generalized	FNA
	Leukemias	No	Generalized	Bone marrow
Inflammatory	Sarcoidosis	Yes	Localized or generalized	FNA/biopsy
	Sarcoid reaction in regional nodes draining carcinoma	Yes	Localized	FNA/biopsy
	Systemic lupus erythematosus	No	Generalized	Serology
	Rheumatoid arthritis	No	Generalized	Serology
	Kikuchi's disease	No	Cervical	Biopsy
	Wegener's granulomatosis	Yes	Localized	Biopsy/ANCA
	Angiofolicular lymph node hyperplasia (Castleman's disease)	No	Generalized or localized (usually cervical)	Biopsy
Other	Drugs	No	Generalized	Stop drugs
	GLUS	Yes	Localized	Biopsy
	Berylliosis	Yes	Generalized	B-lymphocyte proliferation
	Kimura's disease	No	Localized (cervical)	Biopsy

ANCA, anti-neutrophil cytoplasmic antibodies; FNA, fine-needle aspiration; GLUS, granulomatous lesions of unknown significance; HIV, human immunodeficiency virus

The node identified to sample is typically the largest. The order usually chosen is supraclavicular, cervical, axillary, epitrochlear, and then inguinal nodes. Inguinal lymph node sampling has a lower yield for pathology as most adults have some degree of inguinal lymphadenopathy. The peripheral node for sampling may be palpable or identified on CT scanning or FDG-positron emission tomography (PET). Increased uptake by head and neck nodes similar to gallium-67 scanning has been reported for FDG-PET (Prabhakar et al. 2008).

There is some controversy about the sampling technique used to investigate peripheral lymphadenopathy, particularly in the context of possible sarcoidosis, with some advocating whole lymph node excision biopsy (Judson et al. 1999) as a sarcoidosis-like reaction to lymphoma and other malignancies have been rarely reported. However, open biopsy of lymph nodes involved with metastatic cancer has been associated with worse survival, local recurrence and fungation compared to fine-needle aspiration cytology (FNA) (Gleeson et al. 2000). Even management of benign tumors is potentially made more difficult by excisional biopsy compared to FNA used to diagnose them (Gleeson et al. 2000). Biopsies of nodes in the parotid area and posterior triangle have been associated with injuries to the facial nerve and spinal accessory nerve, respectively. Compared to excision biopsy, FNA can be organized rapidly, is inexpensive, is a safer and less invasive method for sampling peripheral lymph nodes, and can be done under CT or ultrasound guidance if necessary. Furthermore, thin-needle core biopsies can often be done at the same time. Given these considerations, FNA cytology is widely used as the first investigation of choice for peripheral lymphadenopathy and has been reported as having a sensitivity of 85 percent and specificity of 99 percent (Gleeson et al. 2000). It is important to review all cells on a smear that is reported as showing granulomatous inflammation to examine for any cell atypia or malignancy. Some centers do flow cytometry on a proportion of FNA specimens to look for clonality to reduce the risk of misdiagnosis of non-Hodgkin's lymphoma (Tambouret et al. 2000). If an FNA confirms a granulomatous reaction, a judgment in the context of the clinical scenario needs to be made about whether a biopsy or even an excision biopsy then needs to be performed.

Tambouret and associates concluded that FNA was underutilized in the diagnosis of sarcoidosis as it appeared to be a reliable and cost-effective method of diagnosis (Tambouret et al. 2000). In coming to this conclusion they identified 28 patients who had had 32 FNAs performed and sarcoidosis reported as the cytological diagnosis or differential diagnosis. In nine procedures the FNA was performed on palpable peripheral lymph nodes (5 neck, 2 axillary, 2 groin). In the majority of patients in whom there was a clinical history prior to FNA, this was of, or included, sarcoidosis (14/20, 70 percent). Sixteen patients went on to have open biopsies which confirmed the FNA findings of non-necrotizing granulomatous inflammation in all cases. Four institutions involved in this study estimated that the ratio of open biopsy to FNA performed for diagnosing sarcoidois ranged from 4:1 to 19:1. The cost of diagnosing a peripheral lymph node was 2.4 times as much for a surgical biopsy compared to a FNA.

CONCLUSION

Peripheral lymphadenopathy due to sarcoidosis is are of the most common extrathoracic sites involved in sarcoidosis. It is diagnosed by confirming non-caseating granuloma on lymph node sampling in a compatible clinical setting and excluding other causes of granulomatous inflammation. The ACCESS study investigators (Judson et al. 1999) have proposed a definition for probable and possible peripheral lymph node involvement in the setting of biopsy-proven sarcoidosis from a different site. Although patients rarely present with symptomatic lymphadenopathy, it is important to examine carefully the main peripheral lymph node groups in patients with possible sarcoidosis. This may identify those with a more chronic course of the disease as it reflects extrathoracic involvement. Second, it may indicate a site for sampling. Although the 'gold standard' for diagnosing sarcoidosis is by biopsy, fine-needle aspiration is a cheaper, reliable and safe option which is probably underutilized.

REFERENCES

Baughman RP, Teirstein AS, Judson MA et al. (2001). Clinical characteristics of patients in a case control study of sarcoidosis. Am J Respir Crit Care Med 164: 1885–9.

Edmonstone WM, Wilson AG (1985). Sarcoidosis in Caucasians, Blacks and Asians in London. Br J Dis Chest 79: 27–36.

Ferrer R (1998). Lymphadenopathy: differential diagnoses and evaluation. Am Fam Physician 58: 1313–20.

Fijten GH, Blijham GH (1988). Unexplained lymphadenopathy in family practice: an evaluation of malignant causes and the effectiveness of physician's workup. J Fam Pract 27: 373–6.

Gleeson M, Herbert A, Richards A (2000). Management of lateral neck masses in adults. Br Med J 320: 1521–4.

Habermann TM, Steensma DP (2000). Lymphadenopathy. Mayo Clin Proc 75: 723–32.

Hunninghake GW, Costabel U, Ando M et al. (1999). Statement on sarcoidosis: American Thoracic Society/World Association of Sarcoidosis and other Granulomatous Disorders. Sarcoid Vasc Diff Lung Dis 16: 149–73.

Hunt BM, Vallieres E, Buduhan G et al. (2009). Sarcoidosis as a benign cause of lymphadenopathy in cancer patients. Am J Surg 197: 629–32.

Judson MA, Baughman RP, Teirstein AS et al. (1999). Defining organ involvement in sarcoidosis: the ACCESS proposed instrument. Sarcoid Vasc Diff Lung Dis 16: 75–86.

Judson MA, Thompson BW, Rabin DL et al. (2003a). The diagnostic pathway to sarcoidosis. Chest 123: 406–12.

Judson MA, Baughman RP, Thompson BW et al. (2003b). Two-year prognosis of sarcoidosis: the ACCESS experience. Sarcoid Vasc Diff Lung Dis 20: 204–11.

Judson MA, Baughman RP, Costabel U *et al.* (2008). Efficacy of infliximab in extrapulmonary sarcoidosis: results from a randomised trial. *Eur Respir J* 31: 1189–96.

Lee Y, Terry R, Lukes RJ (1980). Lymph node biopsy for diagnosis: a statistical study. *J Surg Oncol* 14: 53–60.

Prabhakar HB, Rabinowitz CB, Gibbons FK *et al.* (2008). Imaging feature of sarcoidosis on MDCT, FDG PET, and PET/CT. *Am J Radiol* 190: S1–6.

Rizzato G, Montemurro L (2000). The clinical spectrum of the sarcoid peripheral lymph node. *Sarcoid Vasc Diff Lung Dis* 17: 71–80.

Tambouret R, Geisinger KR, Powers CN *et al.* (2000). The clinical application and cost analysis of fine needle aspiration biopsy in the diagnosis of mass lesions in sarcoidosis. *Chest* 117: 1004–11.

Teirstein AS, Judson MA, Baughman RP *et al.* (2005). The spectrum of biopsy sites for the diagnosis of sarcoidosis. *Sarcoid Vasc Diff Lung Dis* 22: 139–46.

Yanardag H, Caner M, Papila I *et al.* (2007). Diagnostic value of peripheral lymph node biopsy in sarcoidosis: a report of 67 cases. *Can Respir J* 14: 209–11.

34

The endocrine glands

THEINGI AUNG, NIKI KARAVITAKI AND JOHN A H WASS

INTRODUCTION

Sarcoidosis is a multisystem disorder described more than a century ago. It can present with various manifestations, including endocrine ones and it is associated with diverse outcomes, transient or chronic. Its typical pathological findings are non-caseating granulomas in the affected tissue indicating a possible underlying immune reaction. Once mononuclear inflammatory cells accumulate in the target organ, macrophages aggregate and differentiate into epithelioid and multinucleated giant cells. Then CD4 and CD8 lymphocytes, and to a lesser extent B-lymphocytes, form a rim around the granuloma with a dense band of fibroblasts, mast cells and collagen fibers (Newman et al. 1997). The etiology is still unclear and it is most likely to be the end result of immune responses to various environmental triggers. Frequently it presents between the ages of 20 and 40 years, although cases diagnosed in childhood or in elderly subjects have been reported. The incidence of the disease has a variable distribution worldwide. Notably, its incidence and its clinical course varys in different racial groups living in the same geographical area (Porter et al. 2003). The susceptibility to sarcoidosis depends on the both genetic and environmental factors (Nowak et al. 1990; Iannuzzi 2007).

This chapter will focus on the involvement of the endocrine glands in sarcoidosis, as reported in the literature. Tables 34.1 and 34.2 provide convenient summaries of features and investigations.

VITAMIN D, PARATHYROID HORMONE AND CALCIUM METABOLISM

Metabolism and action of vitamin D

Following exposure to ultraviolet irradiation, the cutaneous precursor of vitamin D, 7-dehydrocholesterol, forms previtamin D, which is thermally labile and during a period of 48 hours undergoes a temperature-dependent molecular rearrangement leading to the production of vitamin D. Vitamin D is absorbed into the lymphatics and enters the circulation bound to a specific binding protein. On arrival in the liver, it undergoes 25-hydroxylation by a cytochrome P450 enzyme in the mitochondria and the microsomes. This is followed by 1-α hydroxylation in the proximal convoluted tubule of the kidney, making the active hormone 1,25(OH)2D. This product is metabolized to inactive ones by hydroxylation, oxidation and cleavage; 25(OH)D and 1,25(OH)2D are hydroxylated by vitamin D 24-, 23- or 26-hydroxylase in most tissues including the kidneys, cartilage and intestine to inactive forms.

The actions of vitamin D are mediated by binding to a nuclear receptor and include:

- promotion of intestinal calcium and phosphate absorption;
- an action on the parathyroid gland via a negative feedback loop to decrease parathyroid hormone (PTH) levels;

Table 34.1   Clinical features of endocrine gland involvement in sarcoidosis.

Vitamin D, PTH, calcium metabolism	Hypothalamus and pituitary	Adrenal	Pancreas	Thyroid	Others
Hypercalcemia	Hyperprolactinemia	Anorexia	Abdominal pain	Clinical and subclinical hypothyroidism	Male reproductive system
Hypercalciuria	Hypogonadism	Weight loss	Acute pancreatitis	Thyroid nodules, goiter	– Testicular mass
Long-term complications (renal stones, naphrocalcinosis, chronic renal failure, pancreatitis, osteoporosis)	SIADH	Tiredness	Chronic pancreatitis	Hyperthyroidism	– Epididymal mass
	Secondary hypothyroidism	Generalized weakness	Obstructive jaundice and abdominal mass	Graves' disease	Female reproductive system
	Secondary hypoadrenalism	Dizziness		Hashimoto's thyroiditis with hypothyroidism	– Hypogonadism
	Growth hormone deficiency	Postural hypotension	Abnormal glucose tolerance	Postpartum thyroiditis	– Menstrual irregularity (amenorrhea, menorrhagia)
	Impaired counter-regulatory mechanism to hypoglycemia	GI symptoms (nausea, vomiting, abdominal pain, diarrhea)	Pancreatic exocrine deficiency	Painful thyroid enlargement	– Postmenopausal bleeding
	Morbid obesity	Arthralgia and myalgia	Diabetes	Thyroid carcinoma	– Erosion of cervix
	Insomnia	Pyrexia of unknown origin			
	Marked somnolence	Symptomatic hypoglycemia			
	Diabetes insipidus				
	Dysregulation of body temperature				
	Personality changes				

PTH, parathyroid hormone; SIADH, syndrome of inappropriate antidiuretic hormone.

Table 34.2   Investigations.

Vitamin D, PTH, calcium metabolism	Hypothalamus and pituitary	Adrenal	Pancreas	Thyroid	Others
Plasma-corrected calcium	Pituitary function tests	9 am serum cortisol	CT/MRI of abdomen	Thyroid function test	CT/MRI of pelvis
Vitamin D, PTH, phosphate	ACE (CSF/serum)	ACTH	Histology confirmation	Thyroid antibody	Histology confirmation
Renal function	MRI of pituitary and hypothalamus	Dynamic test (short synacthen test)	Exclude other differential diagnoses	Ultrasound of thyroid/ uptake scan	Exclude other differential diagnoses
24 h urine calcium	Histology confirmation	MRI/CT of adrenals		Histology confirmation	
Renal tract ultrasound	Exclude other differential diagnoses	Histology confirmation		Exclude other differential diagnoses	
Skeletal radiograph/ BMD		Exclude other differential diagnoses			

ACE, angiotensin-converting enzyme; ACTH, adrenocorticotropic hormone; BMD, bone mineral density; CSF, cerebrospinal fluid; PTH, parathyroid hormone.

- an action on bone to escalate bone resorption by osteoclasts and raise osteoblastic bone formation;
- regulation of hematopoietic cell and probably muscle cell function.

Vitamin D and sarcoidosis

Hypercalcemia in a patient with sarcoidosis was first described in 1939 by Harrell and Fisher. Albright and associates suggested that the mechanism of the hypercalcemia is similar to the one seen in vitamin D intoxication (Albright et al. 1956). In 1963, the differences in the calcium level in patients with sarcoidosis during the summer and winter months were noted (higher in high sunlight exposure). Subsequently, raised calciferol levels were found in these patients, and macrophages (alveolar and tissue) were proposed as an origin of the increased vitamin D levels (Bell et al. 1964; Adams et al. 1983; Mason et al. 1984; Adams and Gacad 1985).

A further suggested mechanism included impairment of the feedback mechanism of calcitriol production by the macrophages. Thus, in renal tubular cells, high levels of calcitriol cause down-regulation of the 1-α hydroxylase and up-regulation of the 25(OH)D3 24-hydroxylase which converts active D3 to the metabolically inactive form 24,25(OH)2D3. In contrast, in alveolar macrophages there is no down-regulation of the 1-α hydroxylase in response to increased levels of calcitriol (Conron *et al.* 2000).

It has been proposed that the increase in vitamin D levels in sarcoidosis may be part of the immune response in this condition rather than the resulting pathology. Reports since the 1980s demontrated the expression of the intracellular receptor of 1,25 vitamin D (the vitamin D receptor; VDR) in a variety of cell types including activated lymphocytes, macrophages and dendritic cells, suggesting that it has immunomodulatory actions (Adams *et al.* 1986). In 1986, Rook and colleagues demonstrated that 1,25(OH)2D inhibits the growth of *Mycobacterium tuberculosis* (Rook 1988). It was also proposed that vitamin D enhances phagosomal bacterial killing by the host cells via an autocrine mechanism. Furthermore vitamin D shows direct effects on B-lymphocyte homeostasis and modulates T-lymphocyte proliferation with the principal target probably being T-helper cells. Therefore it has been suggested that interferon-γ stimulates 1-α hydroxylation by the alveolar macrophages, resulting in increased 1,25-dihydroxyvitamin D. This may be a compensatory mechanism to minimize inflammation. Interestingly, there is a correlation between 1-α hydroxylase gene expression in alveolar macrophages with the activity of sarcoidosis and its associated alterations in calcium metabolism (Inui *et al.* 2001).

Parathyroid hormone (PTH)

This hormone controls the minute-to-minute levels of ionized calcium in the blood and extracellular fluids. PTH release is stimulated by circulating vitamin D metabolites and by low levels of calcium. Hypercalcemia inhibits the secretion of PTH. In sarcoidosis, PTH is suppressed due to the inhibitory effects of increased vitamin D and hypercalcemia. Therefore a high PTH level in sarcoid patients should lead to the suspicion of co-existent hyperparathyroidism (Ghose *et al.* 1983; Sandler *et al.* 1984). Association with hyperparathyroidism is far less common, with 50 cases reported in the last 40 years (Tomita 1995; Porter *et al.* 2003).

PTH–RELATED PEPTIDE AND SARCOIDOSIS

Parathyroid hormone-related peptide (PTHrP) is the main mediator of humoral hypercalcemia in malignancy. The presence of PTHrP protein and mRNA in a high percentage of sarcoid lymph node biopsies suggests that PTHrP may play an important role in hypercalcemia. This was first described by Zeimer and co-workers using a polyclonal antiserum and in-situ hybridization using riboprobe on lymph node biopsies and was detected positive in 85 percent. It has been proposed that TNF-α and IL-6 stimulate PTHrP production in sarcoid macrophages (Zeimer *et al.* 1998).

A summary of the mechanisms of the hypercalcemia in sarcoidosis is show in Box 34.1.

> ## Box 34.1 Summary of mechanisms of hyper-calcemia in sarcoidosis
>
> - Increased 1,25-dihydroxyvitamin D produced by 1-α hydroxylation in the alveolar macrophages stimulated by interferon-γ
> - Defective regulation of 1-α hydroxylation in alveolar macrophages
> - Immunomodulatory actions of vitamin D in response to the inflammatory reaction
> - Increased PTHrP levels stimulated by TNF-α and IL-6 (produced by macrophages in the granuloma)
> - Genetic factors

Clinical features, investigations and treatment

CLINICAL FEATURES

Clinical manifestations are the result of hypercalcemia and hypercalciuria. The incidence of hypercalcemia is reported in a wide range between 2 and 63 percent (mostly accepted about 10 percent) and there is no association between age, race, sex, occupation or geographic distribution (James 1980; Sharma 1996,2000; Porter *et al.* 2003). The severity of hypercalcemia depends on the disease activity (transient or fluctuating). Sunlight and diet variation also have effects.

Hypercalciuria is three times more common than hypercalcemia (up to 60 percent) and it is slightly more common in men (Sharma 1996). Its mechanism is not fully understood. It has been proposed that the capacity of the tubular reabsorptive mechanisms for calcium is exceeded. Other hypotheses include absorptive hypercalciuria (1,25(OH)2D3 and the free 1,25(OH)2D3 index are raised) and resorptive hypercalciuria (where the mechanism of osteolysis is not solely accounted for by high 1,25(OH)2 vitamin D3 serum levels but related to the extent of the granulomatous process (Meyrier *et al.* 1985)).

Long-term complications of hypercalcemia and hypercalciuria include osteopenia, osteoporosis (especially with the combination of long-term treatment with steroids), pancreatitis, nephrocalcinosis, nephrolithiasis, impaired renal function and renal failure and even death (Porter *et al.* 2003). Dactylitis (inflammation of a digit, either a finger or a toe) and bone lesions are also rare complications. Skeletal involvement has been reported in 1–13 percent (average 5 percent) of the patients. Severe symptomatic hypercalcemia is uncommon. A corrected calcium level (measured Ca [mmol/L] + 0.02 × (40 − albumin [g/L])) of under 3.0 mmol/L is unlikely to cause any significant clinical manifestations.

The clinical features of hypercalcemia are well recognized, including polyuria, polydipsia, anorexia, vomiting, constipation, abdominal pain, confusion, lethargy, depression and rarely pruritus.

INVESTIGATIONS

The basic investigations include:

- plasma corrected calcium (as above);
- vitamin D, PTH, phosphate;

- renal function;
- 24-hour urinary calcium;
- renal tract ultrasound;
- skeletal radiograph / bone mineral density (BMD).

TREATMENT

Treatment is indicated in severe and persistence hypercalcemia. The therapeutic aims include symptomatic relief (although severe hypercalcemia is uncommon) and the prevention of long-term renal or bone complications. General measures comprise avoiding a high vitamin D diet (although a few epidemiological studies do not show any correlation between dietary calcium intake and the rate of nephrolithiasis) and calcium supplements, minimizing exposure to sunlight, and maintaining adequate hydration (fluid intake 2–3 L/day) (Conron et al. 2000). Medical treatment includes steroids, ketoconazole, chloroquine, hydroxycloroquine and others (e.g. diuretics). The most effective first-line treatment for hypercalcemia in sarcoidosis is corticosteroids.

Corticosteroids work through different mechanisms including:

- reduction of gastrointestinal calcium absorption and inhibition of osteoclast function;
- inhibition of 1-α hydroxylase in the macrophages;
- reduction of the production of PTHrP by macrophages by down-regulation of IL-2 and interferon-γ expression (binding to the cytokine promoter region in the macrophage nucleus).

The dose varies from 15 to 40 mg daily and stabilization of calcium levels can be expected within 3–5 days. The improvement of hypercalciuria should follow within 7–10 days. If there is no improvement following 2 weeks of treatment, other co-existing disorders should be excluded. The dose of steroid should be adjusted down according to the levels of serum and urinary calcium. Urinary calcium measurement should be repeated soon after starting the treatment, as exacerbation of hypercalcuria may be seen. Corticosteroid treatment may increase the risk of osteoporosis, but the effect is reversible if the treatment is discontinued within 6 months, especially in young patients (Rizzato and Montemurro 1998). If there are side-effects of steroids, if they cannot be tolerated or if there is no clinical response, other medications should be considered.

Ketoconazole is an inidazole antifungal agent as well as an inhibitor of cytochrome P450. Ketoconazole lowers circulating 1,25(OH)2D3 and calcium levels by inhibiting macrophage 1-α hydroxylation of the 25(OH)D. It has been used as an alternative therapy to corticosteroids with a dose of 800 mg daily. The adverse effects of ketoconazole include renal and liver function impairment. Although unlikely, when ketoconazole is used at high doses, it may cause adrenal insufficiency, a decrease in testosterone levels, and a decrease in sperm production.

Chloroquine and hydroxychloroquine are also inhibitors of 1-α hydroxylase, but they have a potential for retinal toxicity thus limiting their usefulness, especially with high doses and long-term administration. Ophthalmology follow-up is advisable in cases of long-term administration. Methotrexate and azathioprine have also been used for the treatment of hypercalcemia as adjuvant therapy.

Diuretics have different effects on the calcium concentration and excretion. Thiazide diuretics have a direct effect on the distal tubules, reducing the renal excretion of calcium. They may be used in normocalcemic patients to decrease hypercalciuria, but are contraindicated in hypercalcemic patients. Loop diuretics may be used in symptomatic hypercalcemic patients as adjuvant to other treatment options aiming to enhance the renal excretion of calcium.

THE HYPOTHALAMUS AND PITUITARY GLAND

Involvement of the pituitary and hypothalamus in sarcoidosis is caused by the infiltration by non-caseating granuloma resulting in non-tumoral, non-vascular, acquired damage. Although it is a rare clinical presentation, the diagnosis can be a challenge, as up to half of the neurosarcoidosis patients are found to have no other systemic manifestations. The frequency of neurosarcoidosis is about 5–15 percent, but subclinical and undiagnosed disease is thought to be much higher. Sarcoid granulomas have a predilection for the hypothalamus and hypothalamic involvement can be present in up to 10 percent of the neurosarcoid cases (Turkington and MacIndoe 1972). Although a pituitary defect is secondary to hypothalamic involvement, direct involvement with empty sella syndrome can also occur as a rare presentation.

CLINICAL FEATURES

The main neuroendocrine abnormalities include hyperprolactinemia, found in up to 32 percent of sarcoid patients (Barney 1992), and disturbances of water balance. Galactorrhea and menstrual disturbances may sometimes be the presenting manifestation of underlying hyperprolactinemia. Polyuria and polydipsia (17–90 percent) is the main presentation of diabetes insipidus (DI) secondary to antidiuretic hormone deficiency. DI is a presenting sign in about 40 percent of cases (Bihan et al. 2007). Dysregulation of the thirst mechanism has also been described in subjects with neurosarcoidosis. Hence, the clinical setting of DI with hypernatremia and hypovolemia in the absence of thirst can occur (Stuart et al. 1980). The syndrome of inappropriate antidiuretic hormone secretion (SIADH) in patients with systemic sarcoidosis has also been reported with hyponatremia.

Disruption of other regulatory functions of the hypothalamus can also occur. The dysregulation of body temperature in hypothalamic sarcoid was first reported in 1977 (Lipton et al. 1977) and it is associated with low metabolic rate (Braunstein 1986). Impairment of the counter-regulatory mechanisms to hypoglycemia has been described (Fery et al. 1999), though it can be under-diagnosed. Morbid obesity (due to sarcoid invasion of the ventromedial nucleus of hypothalamus) (Vesely 1989), sleep disturbances and personality changes can also be present. Other endocrine manifestations secondary to pituitary involvement may also occur including hypothyroidism, hypoadrenalism, and growth hormone deficiency. Hyperprolactinoma is found if there is stalk involvement (impairing the passage of hypothalamic dopamine due to the pituitary stalk pathology). In a recent study, all patients presented with hypogonadism and more than one-third with DI (Bihan *et al.* 2007).

Clinical features of hypothalamic and pituitary involvement in sarcoidosis are summarized in Box 34.2.

Box 34.2 Summary of clinical features of hypothalamic and pituitary involvement in sarcoidosis

Anterior and posterior pituitary
- Diabetes insipidus
- Hyperprolactinemia
- Hypogonadism
- Secondary hypothyroidism
- Secondary hypoadrenalism
- Growth hormone (GH) insufficiency

Hypothalamus
- Morbid obesity
- Insomnia
- Marked somnolence
- Dysregulation of body temperature
- Personality changes

Others
- Impaired counter-regulatory mechanisms to hypoglycemia
- Syndrome of inappropriate antidiuretic hormone (SIADH)

INVESTIGATIONS AND DIAGNOSIS

Clinical suspicion leads to the appropriate hormonal and biochemical work-up, imaging studies and pathology confirmation of granulomas. The passage of large volumes (>3 L/24 h) of dilute urine (osmolality < 300 mOsm/kg) is suggestive of diabetes insipidus. Exclusion of diabetes mellitus, renal failure, hypokalemia and hypercalcemia are included in the diagnostic work-up. In doubtful situations, the standard water deprivation is confirmatory; the diagnosis being established if there is failure to concentrate urine following fluid deprivation, in the absence of renal disease. The biochemistry will normalize after administration of desmopressin, confirming central diabetes insipidus (DI). Excessive water intake due to dysregulation of thirst in hypothalamic involvement may be present, so careful interpretation of the results is essential. The anterior pituitary function (growth hormone, thyroid stimulating hormone, gonadotrophines and prolactin) should be checked (Turner and Wass 2009).

Laboratory tests for the diagnosis of neurosarcoidosis include serum and cerebrospinal fluid (CSF) angiotensin-converting enzyme (ACE) levels and CSF examination (high protein, possible lymphocytosis). These lack sensitivity and specificity but, if positive, could support the diagnosis. Serum ACE and CSF examination may be normal in isolated neurosarcoidosis. CSF ACE is high in 50 percent of cases with neurosarcoidosis. High serum and cranial ACE suggest that the disease state is active with 50–86 percent sensitivity and 80 percent specificity (Porter *et al.* 2003). Detailed examination of CSF including lymphocyte subpopulation, oligoclonal bands and IgG index can be performed, as per clinical suspicion, aiming to differentiate other conditions such as demyelinating disorders (e.g. high lymphocytes, oligoclonal bands of IgG with CSF examination favor the demyelinating disease).

Neuroradiology including contrast-enhanced magnetic resonance imaging (MRI) may reveal either isolated thickness of the pituitary stalk (Fig. 34.1) or a sellar mass (Rubin *et al.* 2001) or, very rarely, a cystic lesion (Guoth *et al.* 1998). The presence of a sellar mass requires differential diagnosis from a pituitary adenoma (neurosarcoidosis confirmed in <1 percent of sellar masses) (Freda *et al.* 1992). Recent studies have not shown a correlation between the number of hormonal deficits and the hypothalamo-pituitary areas involved as assessed by MRI (Bihan *et al.* 2007).

If the diagnosis is still in doubt, it can be confirmed by performing a biopsy of the intracranial lesion if possible and pathological demonstration of non-caseating granulomas. In the past, the pituitary gland was not readily accessible for biopsy, so the diagnosis relied mainly on the clinical evidence of pituitary dysfunction in a patient with evidence of sarcoidosis elsewhere. Nowadays transphenoidal access to the pituitary makes this easier.

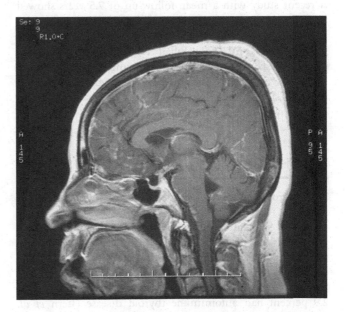

Figure 34.1 Magnetic resonance imaging (MRI) showing the thickened pituitary stalk due to granulomatous infiltration in sarcoidosis.

It should be noted that the definitive diagnosis of neurosarcoidsis requires exclusion of other granulomatous disorders (e.g. histocytosis X, giant cell granuloma). Exclusion of infection (e.g. tuberculoma, histoplasmosis, brucellosis, and coccidiomycosis), metastatic disease, CNS lymphoma and systemic vasculitis is also essential.

TREATMENT

The treatment of choice is corticosteroids continuously or in pulses. Given the long duration of treatment, the chance of having side-effects is considerabe. Other treatment options include using adjuvant radiotherapy or immunosuppressive medications (methotrexate, chloroquine, hydroxychloroquine, azathioprine, ciclosporin, cyclophosphamide).

Neurosarcoidosis sometimes needs high doses of steroid and can be a therapeutic challenge (see also Chapter 27). Patients responding to this medical treatment have a good prognosis, with 55 percent reported showing complete recovery (Bruns et al. 2004). Others may suffer from adverse side-effects of long-term high-dose steroids (glucose intolerance, cataracts, obesity). For patients resistant to or not tolerating multiple alternate immunotherapeutic drugs, some authors suggest central nervous system radiotherapy. Stelzer and colleagues suggested the possible mechanisms for radiation effects on granulomatous tissue: radiation-induced direct cytotoxicity in the macrophages, lymphocytes and plasma cells that make up the granulomatous lesions; and radiation-induced phenotypic alterations within the cellular matrix that inhibit the autocrine and paracrine signals (Stelzer et al. 1995). There are few reports in the literature showing objective responses to cranial irradiation (the dose of radiation to the whole brain varied between 12 and 30 Gy) (Bruns et al. 2004).

There are very few data on the outcome following treatment, and large prospective outcome studies are lacking. A recent study with a mean follow-up of 7.5 years showed that steroid therapy reduced the radiologic lesions, but did not reverse most endocrine defects (despite regression of the granulomatous process) (Bihan et al. 2007). There is a paucity of data on the optimal duration of treatment, but hormonal evaluation and MRI of the hypothalamus and pituitary should be performed yearly as well as after changes of therapy to monitor the response.

THE THYROID

The thyroid is an uncommon site of involvement in sarcoidosis and was first reported in 1938 by Spencer. Since then, the association between thyroid autoimmunity and sarcoidosis has been described in many reports. In autopsy series, thyroid involvement has been found within the range of 1.0 percent (Maycock 1963) to 4.2 percent (Branson 1954). In large series of patients with sarcoidosis, it was shown that 2.9 percent had autoimmune thyroid disease (Isern et al. 2007). Thyroid involvement can present either as part of other systemic symptoms in already diagnosed sarcoidosis

patients or as isolated thyroid sarcoidosis (Cabibi et al. 2006). The prevalence of overt thyroid disease in sarcoidosis is about 3.6 percent (Karlish and MacGregor 1970). High risk factors for thyroid involvement include sex (higher in females), positivity for thyroid autoantibodies, and ultrasound findings of a hypoechoic and small thyroid.

The pathogenesis of thyroid involvement is still unclear but it is generally accepted as mainly autoimmune in origin (probably related to T-helper cell type 1 lymphocytes as part of a multiple immune-mediated disorder) together with the combined effects of genetic and environmental conditions (Antonelli et al. 2006). Extensive infiltration by granuloma followed by fibrosis of the thyroid gland may result in hypothyroidism (Brun et al. 1967).

CLINICAL FEATURES, INVESTIGATIONS AND DIAGNOSIS

Thyroid involvement in sarcoidosis can manifest as hypothyroidism, subclinical hypothyroidism (with prevalence of 5 and 17 percent, respectively; Antonelli et al. 2006), thyroid nodules (Ozkan et al. 2005), goiter, hyperthyroidism including Graves' disease, Hashimoto's thyroiditis with hypothyroidism, postpartum thyroiditis, or painful thyroid enlargement. It can present as cold nodules mimicking thyroid cancer which can lead to total thyroidectomy (Ozkan et al. 2005). Clinical features depend on the type of thyroid involvement.

Thyroid function tests and the measurement of thyroid autoantibodies should be performed at a low threshold for the sarcoidosis patient. The percentage of elevated antithyroid antibodies ranges between 1.3 and 54.5 percent in different studies. Imaging should be performed according to the clinical indication.

The clinical and hormonal picture suggests the diagnosis, particularly in a patient with other systemic manifestations of the disease. Histological proof is needed if diagnosis is in doubt, especially with the presentation as cold nodule, to differentiate with the possibility of malignancy. Exclusion of other non-caseating granulomatous disease is also essential. Secondary hypothyroidism resulting from hypothalamic and pituitary involvement should also be considered.

TREATMENT

Hyperthyroidism associated with sarcoidosis may not respond well to antithyroid drugs and radioiodine. Corticosteroid treatment generally improves the symptoms but surgery seems to be a better option. In a series of patients followed-up after surgery, no disease recurrence was reported (Cabibi et al. 2006).

ADRENAL GLANDS

Adrenal involvement in sarcoidosis is rare and may be due to either hypothalamic–pituitary infiltration or adrenal infiltration/fibrosis or to autoimmunity. At least five case reports of Schmidt's syndrome (Addison's disease and autoimmune hypothyroidism) with sarcoidosis have been reported. The diagnosis of adrenal insufficiency in a sarcoid patient on corticosteroid treatment is difficult and may be delayed. The most important clue will be the presence of non-specific symptoms of adrenal insufficiency each time the dose of steroid is reduced. It is also important to exclude hypothalamo-pituitary-adrenal gland suppression due to long-term steroid treatment. Positive adrenal cortical autoantibodies favor the underlying autoimmune mechanism.

CLINICAL FEATURES

Clinical features of adrenal insufficiency include anorexia and weight loss (>90 percent of cases), tiredness, generalized weakness, dizziness and postural hypotension, gastrointestinal symptoms (nausea, vomiting, abdominal pain, diarrhea), arthralgia and myalgia. Rarely, adrenal insufficiency can present with pyrexia of unknown origin and symptomatic hypoglycemia. Other associated endocrinopathies (primary hypothyroidism and primary gonadal failure) as well as vitiligo should be looked for. Acute adrenal insufficiency can present with shock, hypotension, unexplained fever, abdominal pain (even as an acute abdomen), and those symptoms are often precipitated by major stress such as infection or surgery. There are case reports of adrenal involvement in sarcoidosis patients with adrenal crisis (Karlish and MacGregor 1970) and even death (Maycock 1963).

INVESTIGATIONS

Initial laboratory tests may show hyponatremia, hyperkalemia, elevated urea, normocytic normochromic anemia, an elevated erythrocyte sedimentation rate (ESR) and eosinophilia. Adrenal insufficiency itself can give mild hypercalcemia (because of reduced renal absorption of calcium), a finding that may be also seen related to underlying sarcoidosis. Undetectable cortisol with flat response to dynamic testing (as the short synacthen test) confirms adrenal failure. Basal adrenocorticotropic hormone (ACTH) values are important to differentiate between primary cause (adrenal) and secondary cause (pituitary or hypothalamus). The long synacthen test (depot synacthen 1 mg intramuscularly, serum cortisol measured up to 24 hours, normal response considered as an elevation in serum cortisol to >1000 nmol/L) may be required to confirm secondary adrenal failure if ACTH is equivocal. In this test, there is a progressive rise in cortisol levels in secondary adrenal insufficiency but little or no response in primary adrenal disease (Turner and Wass 2009).

Imaging may show adrenal enlargement if they are infiltrated by granulomas. They are small and atrophic if there is associated autoimmune involvement. The diagnosis can be confirmed only after excluding other possible causes of non-caseating disease.

TREATMENT

Once the diagnosis in confirmed, replacement with hydrocortisone is necessary. Fludrocortisone is also required in primary adrenal disease. Proper work-up of the adrenal reversibility is essential before stopping the replacement, aiming to be sure that the adrenals are functioning adequately. Once the patient is on 6.0 mg of prednisolone, changing to hydrocortisone should be considered (less prolonged suppression of ACTH). After 2–3 months, 9 am cortisol should be checked 24 hours after the last dose of hydrocortisone. If it is >300 nmol/L, then hydrocortisone can be stopped and a short synacthen test should be performed. If the 9 am cortisol is <300 nmol/L, then hydrocortisone should be continued for another 2–3 months and 9 am cortisol should be repeated. Once a short synacthen test shows a normal response, it is helpful to perform an insulin tolerance test to confirm the full recovery of the hypothalamo-pituitary-adrenal axis (Turner and Wass 2009).

THE PANCREAS

Pancreatic sarcoidosis is very rare and was first reported by Nickerson in an autopsy case (Nickerson 1937). A recent report demonstrates that the incidence is much higher than expected (up to 2.1 percent according to a large autopsy series in Japan with nearly half of those being asymptomatic) (Iwai 1988). In 1950, Curran and Curran reported the first case of pancreatic sarcoidosis with the initial presentation of diffuse abdominal pain needing exploratory laprotomy. There were only 26 cases of symptomatic sarcoidosis reported from 1966 to 2007 (Shukla et al. 2007).

The clinical presentation includes abdominal pain (most common), features of acute pancreatitis, hypercalcemia and chronic pancreatitis (secondary to obstruction), obstructive jaundice and an abdominal mass. Abnormal glucose tolerance with pancreatic sarcoidosis causing pancreatic exocrine deficiency (Noguchi et al. 1993) or diabetes (Papadopoulos et al. 1996) has also been described.

OVARY AND TESTES

The male reproductive system is rarely affected in sarcoidosis but there are reports involving testes and epididymis presenting as testicular or epididymal masses or hypogonadism (Murie et al. 1977). In addition to the central effects of hypogonadism, fibrosis and occlusion of the ductus epididymis can lead to oligospermia and early diagnosis with biopsy and treatment with corticosteroids is important to prevent infertility.

Menstrual irregularity in sarcoidosis is mainly due to hypogonadism secondary to hypothalamic or pituitary involvement, but very rarely can be due to the primary involvement of the female genital tract. The most common site of involvement is reported to be the uterus (presenting with menstrual irregularity, amenorrhea, menorrhagia, postmenopausal bleeding and erosion of cervix). There are seven cases reported of ovarian involvement (Wuntakal et al. 2007), 20 cases with involvement of the female genital tract including uterus, endometrial curettings and fallopian tubes

(Rosenfeld *et al.* 1989). It is clearly important to differentiate from ovarian neoplastic disease by measuring tumor markers, imaging and histology examination.

CONCLUSION

Endocrine manifestations in sarcoidosis, although rare, are important. It is central to get to the diagnosis with clinical suspicion and appropriate hormonal tests as all endocrine deficiencies are treatable. If in doubt, a referral to the endocrinologist should be made.

REFERENCES

Adams JS, Sharma OP et al. (1983). Metabolism of 25-hydroxyvitamin D3 by cultured pulmonary alveolar macrophages in sarcoidosis. *J Clin Invest* 72: 1856–60.

Adams JS, Gacad MA (1985). Characterization of 1-alpha-hydroxylation of vitamin D3 sterols by cultured alveolar macrophages from patients with sarcoidosis. *J Exp Med* 161: 755–65.

Adams JS, Gacad MA et al. (1986). Biochemical indicators of disordered vitamin D and calcium homeostasis in sarcoidosis. *Sarcoidosis* 3: 1–6.

Albright F, Carroll EL et al. (1956). The cause of hypercalcuria in sarcoid and its treatment with cortisone and sodium phytate. *J Clin Invest* 35: 1229–42.

Antonelli A, Fazzi P et al. (2006). Prevalence of hypothyroidism and Graves' disease in sarcoidosis. *Chest* 130: 526–32.

Barney BL (1992). Sarcoidosis presenting with an unusual erythematous rash and persistent hypercalcemia. *West J Med* 156: 544–7.

Bell NH, Gill JR et al. (1964). On the abnormal calcium absorption in sarcoidosis. Evidence for increased sensitivity to vitamin D. *Am J Med* 36: 500–13.

Bihan H, Christozova V et al. (2007). Sarcoidosis: clinical, hormonal, and magnetic resonance imaging (MRI) manifestations of hypothalamic-pituitary disease in 9 patients and review of the literature. *Medicine (Baltimore)* 86: 259–68.

Branson (1954). Sarcoidosis-hepatic involvement: presentation of the case with fatal liver involvement; including autopsy findings and review of the evidence for sarcoid involvement of the liver as found in the liturature. *Ann Intern Med* 40: 111–45.

Braunstein MS (1986). Sarcoidosis. *Compr Ther* 12: 36–44.

Brun J, Revol A et al. (1967). [Sarcoidosis and neuroendocrine disturbances]. *Poumon Coeur* 23: 539–68.

Bruns F, Pruemer B et al. (2004). Neurosarcoidosis: an unusual indication for radiotherapy. *Br J Radiol* 77: 777–9.

Cabibi D, Di Vita G et al. (2006). Thyroid sarcoidosis as a unique localization. *Thyroid* 16: 1175–7.

Conron M, Young C et al. (2000). Calcium metabolism in sarcoidosis and its clinical implications. *Rheumatology* (Oxford) 39: 707–13.

Curran JF, Curran JF (1950). Boeck's sarcoid of the pancreas. *Surgery* 28: 574–8.

Fery F, Plat L et al. (1999). Impaired counterregulation of glucose in a patient with hypothalamic sarcoidosis. *New Engl J Med* 340: 852–6.

Freda PU, Silverberg SJ et al. (1992). Hypothalamic-pituitary sarcoidosis. *Trends Endocrinol Metab* 3: 321–5.

Ghose RR, Woodhead JS et al. (1983). Incomplete suppression of parathyroid hormone activity in sarcoidosis presenting with hypercalcemia. *Postgrad Med J* 59: 572–4.

Guoth MS, Kim J et al. (1998). Neurosarcoidosis presenting as hypopituitarism and a cystic pituitary mass. *Am J Med Sci* 315: 220–4.

Harrell GF, Fisher S (1939). Blood chemical changes in Boeck's sarcoid with particular reference to protein, calcium, phosphate values. *J Clin Invest* 18: 687–93.

Iannuzzi MC (2007). Advances in the genetics of sarcoidosis. *Proc Am Thorac Soc* 4: 457–60.

Inui N, Murayama A et al. (2001). Correlation between 25-hydroxyvitamin D3 1-alpha-hydroxylase gene expression in alveolar macrophages and the activity of sarcoidosis. *Am J Med* 110: 687–93.

Isern V, Lora-Tamayo J et al. (2007). Sarcoidosis and autoimmune thyroid disease: a case series of ten patients. *Sarcoid Vasc Diff Lung Dis* 24: 148–52.

Iwai K (1988). Sarcoidosis autopsies in Japan: frequency and trend in the last 28 years. *Sarcoidosis* 5: 60–5.

James DG (1980). Sarcoidosis. 2: More on the differential diagnosis; the usual course; treatments of choice; prognosis. *Med Times* 108(6): 12s–16s, 21s–23s, 28s–29s.

Karlish AJ, MacGregor GA (1970). Sarcoidosis, thyroiditis, and Addison's disease. *Lancet* ii: 330–333.

Lipton JM, Kirkpatrick J et al. (1977). Hypothermia and persisting capacity to develop fever: occurrence in a patient with sarcoidosis of the central nervous system. *Arch Neurol* 34: 498–504.

Mason RS, Frankel T et al. (1984). Vitamin D conversion by sarcoid lymph node homogenate. *Ann Intern Med* 100: 59–61.

Maycock (1963). Manifestation of sarcoidosis: analysis of 145 patients with a review of nine series selected from tha literature. *Am J Med* 35: 67–89.

Meyrier A, Valeyre D et al. (1985). Resorptive versus absorptive hypercalciuria in sarcoidosis: correlations with 25-hydroxy vitamin D3 and 1,25-dihydroxy vitamin D3 and parameters of disease activity. *Q J Med* 54: 269–281.

Murie N, Hioco D et al. (1977). [The effect of sarcoidosis on calcium homeostasis]. *Probl Actuels Endocrinol Nutr* 20: 129–45.

Newman LS, Rose CS et al. (1997). Sarcoidosis. *New Engl J Med* 336: 1224–34.

Nickerson D. (1937). Boeck's sarcoid. *Arch Pathol Lab Med* 24: 19–29.

Noguchi H, Hirai K et al. (1993). Sarcoidosis accompanied by pancreatic impairment. *Intern Med* 32: 15–20.

Nowak D, Kanzow G et al. (1990). [Patients with sarcoidosis frequently have bronchial hyperreactivity]. *Pneumologie* 44(Suppl. 1): 572–3.

Ozkan Z, Oncel M et al. (2005). Sarcoidosis presenting as cold thyroid nodules: report of two cases. *Surg Today* 35: 770–3.

Papadopoulos KI, Hornblad Y et al. (1996). High frequency of endocrine autoimmunity in patients with sarcoidosis. *Eur J Endocrinol* 134: 331–6.

Porter N, Beynon HL et al. (2003). Endocrine and reproductive manifestations of sarcoidosis. *Q J Med* 96: 553–61.

Rizzato G, Montemurro L (1998). [Clinical spectrum of extrapulmonary sarcoidosis, from the onset to organ transplantation]. *Recenti Prog Med* 89(2): 82–86.

Rook (1988). Role of activated macrophages in the immunopathology of tuberculosis. *Br Med Bull* 44: 611–23.

Rosenfeld SI, Steck W et al. (1989). Sarcoidosis of the female genital tract: a case presentation and survey of the world literature. *Int J Gynaecol Obstet* 28: 373–80.

Rubin MR, Bruce JN et al. (2001). Sarcoidosis within a pituitary adenoma. *Pituitary* 4: 195–202.

Sandler LM, Winearls CG *et al.* (1984). Studies of the hypercalcaemia of sarcoidosis: effect of steroids and exogenous vitamin D3 on the circulating concentrations of 1,25-dihydroxy vitamin D3. *Q J Med* **53**: 165–80.

Sharma OP (1996). Vitamin D, calcium, and sarcoidosis. *Chest* **109**: 535–9.

Sharma OP (2000). Hypercalcemia in granulomatous disorders: a clinical review. *Curr Opin Pulm Med* **6**: 442–7.

Shukla M, Hassan MF *et al.* (2007). Symptomatic pancreatic sarcoidosis: case report and review of literature. *J Pancreas* **8**: 770–4.

Spencer J (1938). Report of a case, with clinical diagnosis confirmed at autopsy. *Arch Intern Med* **62**: 285–96.

Stelzer KJ, Thomas CR *et al.* (1995). Radiation therapy for sarcoid of the thalamus/posterior third ventricle: case report. *Neurosurgery* **36**: 1188–91.

Stuart CA, Neelon FA *et al.* (1980). Disordered control of thirst in hypothalamic-pituitary sarcoidosis. *New Engl J Med* **303**: 1078–82.

Tomita A (1995). [Primary hyperparathyroidism associated with sarcoidosis]. *Nipp Rinsho* **53**: 949–52.

Turkington RW, MacIndoe JH (1972). Hyperprolactinemia in sarcoidosis. *Ann Intern Med* **76**: 545–9.

Turner H, Wass JAH (2009). *Oxford Handbook of Endocrinology and Diabetes*. Oxford Medical Handbooks, Oxford.

Vesely DL (1989). Hypothalamic sarcoidosis: a new cause of morbid obesity. *South Med J* **82**: 758–61.

Wuntakal R, Bharathan R *et al.* (2007). Interesting case of ovarian sarcoidosis: the value of multi disciplinary team working. *World J Surg Oncol* **5**: 38.

Zeimer HJ, Greenaway TM *et al.* (1998). Parathyroid-hormone-related protein in sarcoidosis. *Am J Pathol* **152**: 17–21.

PART VII

BERYLLIUM DISEASE, HIV, AND NEOPLASMS

35

Beryllium

ANTHONY NEWMAN TAYLOR

INTRODUCTION

Beryllium compounds can cause dermatitis and acute and chronic beryllium disease. The major focus in this chapter is on chronic beryllium disease, whose clinical and pathological features can be indistinguishable from sarcoidosis.

Beryllium is of special interest as an identifiable cause of sarcoidosis, which in general is of unknown etiology. It is of clinical importance as a potential, but probably often unrecognized, cause of what is otherwise labelled 'sarcoidosis'. This may be more frequent than is usually appreciated, because the disease often manifests long after the cessation of workplace exposure to beryllium and can occur in people not exposed to beryllium at work, both in close contacts of those exposed to beryllium at work, and in those who live in the vicinity of a factory where beryllium is used.

BERYLLIUM AND ITS USES

Beryllium is a hard, light metal with atomic weight 9. Its most frequent uses are as a component of alloys, most commonly copper–beryllium alloy, and as beryllium oxide in ceramics. Its good electrical and thermal conductance and resistance to corrosion make it a stable, lightweight alloy component. Copper–beryllium alloys are used extensively in the aerospace, nuclear, telecommunication, computer, vehicle, oil and gas industries. Beryllium oxide, incorporated into ceramics, is used in electronic circuitry, ignition systems, microwave ovens and dental amalgams. The worldwide demand for beryllium is projected to increase for applications that include national defense and nuclear energy production.

Exposure to beryllium can occur in the refining of beryllium metal, the melting of beryllium-containing alloys, the grinding and machining of beryllium-containing materials, the manufacture of electronic components, and the handling of beryllium-containing materials. Because of the health hazards to the workforce caused by inhaled beryllium, the widespread use of beryllium compounds in the preparation of powdered phosphors used in the production of fluorescent lights and neon signs was discontinued by 1950.

The National Institute for Safety and Health in the USA estimated that some 44 000 workers nationally were exposed to beryllium fumes or dust in the early 1980s. In contrast, UK data from the Health and Safety Executive indicate far fewer are exposed to beryllium. In 2006, only one UK company was known to be using beryllium oxide, in the manufacture of an electronics product, although an estimated 51 firms were involved in the manufacture or machining of beryllium-containing alloys. There is no production in the UK of beryllium, its alloys or compounds: beryllium, beryllium oxide and beryllium alloys are all imported.

The important occupational circumstances in which exposure to beryllium can occur are shown in Box 35.1.

CHRONIC BERYLLIUM DISEASE

Chronic beryllium disease (CBD) was first reported in the USA by Hardy and Tabernshaw (1946). They described an outbreak of 17 cases of 'delayed chemical pneumonitis' (initially named 'Salem sarcoid'), 14 in the workforce and 3 living in the neighborhood of a company manufacturing fluorescent lights in Salem, Massachusetts. The beryllium-containing compound was zinc manganese beryllium silicate. The term 'delayed' in the description of the disease recognized that in half of the cases the disease was detected

Box 35.1 Occupations in which beryllium exposure can occur

- Beryllium metal and alloy workers
- Ceramics manufacture
- Electronics industries:
  - Transistors
  - Heat-sinks
  - X-ray windows
- Space and atomic engineering:
  - Rocket fuels
  - Heat-shields
- Laboratory workers
- Dental technicians
- Fluorescent lamp manufacture
- Recycling and disposal of beryllium-containing products (e.g. cellphones, computers)

6 months to 3 years after leaving the source of exposure. The clinical and pathological manifestations of the disease were those of sarcoidosis. The disease was characterized by severe breathlessness, considerable weight loss and a poor prognosis. One-third of patients had finger clubbing and cyanosis. Widespread nodular shadowing on the chest radiograph was accompanied in some cases by hilar lymph node enlargement. Biopsies (in three patients of skin, in one of liver; and, in 6 of the 17 patients who had died, of lung, liver, spleen and hilar lymph glands), all showed sarcoid-like granulomas without evidence of infection with tubercle bacilli. The eleven patients still alive at the end of the study remained disabled with no case of recovery.

Jackson (1950) reported the same disease in seven men who had worked in the casting shop of a metallurgy plant using copper–beryllium alloys, in which the beryllium content was on average less than 4 percent. The seven men had breathlessness and weight loss with widespread nodular shadowing on their chest radiographs. Five of the seven had postmortems, with sarcoid granulomas found in the lungs. The first death had occurred in 1938 some seven years after the first use of copper–beryllium alloy in the casting shop.

The mounting evidence of the toxicity of beryllium was not universally appreciated. An invited piece in *The Lancet* (Editorial 1951) concluded:

Beryllium seems to be the Admirable Crichton of metals. It is nearly as light as magnesium and is more elastic than steel: it is strong and hard, and it resists heat and corrosion. Being easily penetrated by X-rays, it is suitable for making X-ray tube windows, and under nuclear bombardment it is a most efficient source of neutrons. Alloyed in small proportions with other metals, it imparts to them such properties as greater strength, ductility, and conductivity; it raises their melting points and protects them from corrosion and tarnishing. It seems that if household silver contained a small percentage of beryllium housewives might no longer have to polish the silver. To charge such an admirable metal with having poisonous properties is about as

distasteful as accusing a trusted butler of stealing the family plate.

Nonetheless these early descriptions of CBD were followed by reports of CBD in virtually every circumstance in which beryllium is encountered at work, with the exception of those working with naturally occurring beryl ores, although the reported studies were undertaken before the introduction of modern tests of beryllium hypersensitivity.

The clinical and pathological manifestations of CBD are now well described and in most regards are not different from sarcoidosis, although asymptomatic bilateral hilar lymphadenopathy alone, and the ocular and neurological manifestations of sarcoidosis have not been reported. Hardy, who had first described CBD, later wrote (Hamilton and Hardy 1974):

Lead poisoning is always accompanied by some degree of anaemia due to red cell destruction. Similarly in beryllium poisoning the lung is the organ usually attacked first with varying clinical, X-ray and pathological patterns. But the lung is rarely if ever the only organ or system affected by harmful beryllium exposure.

Characteristically the disease develops after a latent interval from the onset of exposure of between 10 and 15 years, but shorter latencies of only several months have been reported, particularly since the advent of beryllium workforce surveillance using tests of beryllium sensitization. Newman (1995) described the characteristic symptoms of CBD as breathlessness on exertion of gradual onset, cough, fatigue and weight loss. More recent reports, however, have emphasized the relative paucity of symptoms in many contemporary cases, often initially identified in asymptomatic individuals from abnormalities on the chest radiograph or a positive beryllium lymphocyte proliferation test. The most common symptoms reported in these cases are of mild respiratory symptoms: breathlessness and cough (Newman *et al.* 1989).

Chronic beryllium disease can involve organs outside the lungs, including skin, lymph nodes salivary glands, liver, spleen and kidneys.

The changes on the chest radiograph are of nodular and reticular shadowing, which may be accompanied by bilateral hilar lymphadenopathy (BHL). Unlike sarcoidosis, BHL in the absence of shadowing on the chest radiograph has not been described. The characteristic changes in lung function tests are of small stiff lungs with reduced gas transfer. Total lung capacity (TLC) and forced vital capacity (FVC) are reduced, as is forced expiratory volume in one second (FEV_1) in proportion to the reduction in FVC (restrictive ventilatory defect). Measures of gas transfer, transfer factor (TLco), and gas transfer coefficient Kco (TLco adjusted for alveolar volume), can be reduced. Some cases, with predominant granulomatous inflammation of the airways, have an obstructive ventilatory defect with a disproportionate reduction of the FEV_1/FVC ratio.

Non-caseating granuloma with mononuclear cell infiltrates can be found in affected organs, now most commonly identified in lung tissue, biopsied by transbronchial lung biopsy. In addition, cells recovered at bronchoalveolar lavage (BAL) show an increase in total lymphocyte count with an increased CD4/CD8 ratio, similar to sarcoidosis.

IMMUNOPATHOLOGY OF CBD

Chronic beryllium disease is the prime example of a low-molecular-weight antigen which, in susceptible individuals, can initiate a T-lymphocyte-mediated granulomatous inflammatory reaction in the lungs and in other tissues.

Curtis (1959) showed that, in cases of CBD, patch testing with dilute solutions of soluble beryllium salts provoked a delayed-type hypersensitivity reaction in the skin after 4 hours. More recent studies have shown that lymphocytes from blood or BAL from patients with CBD proliferate when incubated with a beryllium salt. This is the basis for the beryllium lymphocyte proliferation test introduced by Rossman and colleagues (1988). They found that lung cells recovered at BAL from 14 patients who met clinical and exposure criteria for CBD all showed a proliferative response (defined as a stimulation index of more than 5 on two occasions) when incubated with dilute solutions of two beryllium salts (sulphate and fluoride), but in none of 6 normal volunteers or of 16 patients with sarcoidosis (i.e. 100 percent sensitive and specific). Subsequent studies provided evidence that blood lymphocytes from patients with CBD also proliferated when incubated with solutions of beryllium salts, although with a lower sensitivity than for BAL lymphocytes. In addition, beryllium salts stimulated the proliferation of BAL and blood lymphocytes in a number of beryllium workers without CBD.

Mroz and colleagues (1991) investigated the beryllium lymphocyte proliferation test (BeLPT) using blood of 17 cases of CBD and 18 Be-exposed controls. Sixteen (94 percent) of the 17 cases of CBD but none of the 18 Be-exposed controls had a positive blood BeLPT (as defined by a stimulation index of more than 3.5); that is, blood BeLPT was positive in 94 percent of cases with positive BAL BeLPT. BAL BeLPT was positive in all 17 cases. The test was reproducible between two separate laboratories. They concluded that blood BeLPT was a sensitive and specific test for the diagnosis of CBD. They ascribed the high sensitivity of the blood LPT, as compared to previous reports, to a number of methodological improvements in the test described in the paper.

Subsequent studies have reported a number of BeLPT-positive individuals without CBD. A number of these had 'subclinical' or 'surveillance identified' CBD, without clinical evidence of the disease, with granulomas found on lung biopsy. Newman and colleagues (1989) identified granulomas in transbronchial lung biopsies in four of five asymptomatic men exposed to beryllium, without symptoms or abnormalities on the chest radiograph, whose BeLPT was positive – suggesting, at least in some cases, that a positive BeLPT was identifying subclinical disease.

Newman and colleagues have also reported evidence of progression of beryllium sensitization to CBD (Newman *et al.* 2005). They followed, at 2-yearly intervals, 55 individuals with sensitization without evidence of disease (including abnormal BAL or granulomas in transbronchial lung biopsies) who remained exposed to beryllium. CBD developed in 17 (31 percent) after an average of 3.8 years (i.e. a rate of 6–8 percent per year from initial diagnosis); on the other hand, 38 of the 55 (69 percent) were without CBD after an average follow-up of 4.8 years.

When performed in a quality assured laboratory, BeLPT is now regarded as an acceptably specific and sensitive test for chronic beryllium disease. Lymphocytes from blood or BAL are incubated with dilute solutions of a beryllium salt (e.g. sulfate, $BeSO_4$, at 10^6, 10^5 and 10^4M). Lymphocyte proliferation is quantified by measuring the incorporation of radiolabeled thymidine. Beryllium does not provoke proliferation of blood or BAL lymphocytes in patients not exposed to beryllium or with other pulmonary granulomatous diseases, such as sarcoidosis or extrinsic allergic alveolitis (hypersensitivity pneumonitis). Beryllium lymphocyte proliferation does occur in a proportion of those exposed to beryllium without evidence of CBD, including granulomas in lung biopsy.

DIAGNOSTIC CRITERIA FOR BERYLLIUM SENSITIZATION AND CBD

The diagnosis of CBD has been transformed by the development of bronchoalveolar lavage and transbronchial lung biopsy (TBB), providing a safe access to lung tissue for the identification of non-caseating granulomas with mononuclear cell infiltrates, as well as BAL providing cells with a marginally higher sensitivity than blood for a positive BeLPT. The necessary modern diagnostic criteria for CBD are given in Box 35.2. In addition, the criteria for beryllium sensitization are (1) and (2), and subclinical CBD can be identified by the presence of (1), (2) and (3).

Box 35.2 Necessary modern diagnostic criteria for CBD (Newman et al. 1989)

1. History of beryllium exposure
2. Positive blood or BAL BeLPT with peak SI > 3 (the cut-off value varies with laboratory, based on peak stimulation index plus two standard deviations above peak stim index for a group of non-exposed normal controls run by the laboratory)
3. Pathological evidence of non-caseating granuloma, usually in transbronchial lung biopsies (Fig. 35.1)
4. Characteristic clinical findings:
   a. Respiratory symptoms or signs
   b. Reticulonodular changes on chest X-ray or HRCT (Figs 35.2, 35.3 and 35.4)
   c. Restrictive (or obstructive) ventilatory defect with impaired measures of gas transfer (TLco or Kco), O_2 desaturation at rest or with exercise

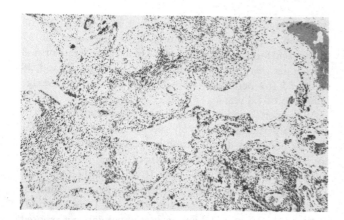

Figure 35.1   Chronic beryllium disease: lung biopsy showing numerous non-necrotizing epithelial and giant cell granulomas.

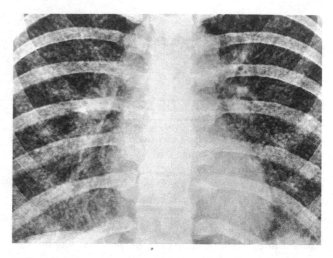

Figure 35.3   Chest radiograph show widespread nodular shadowing.

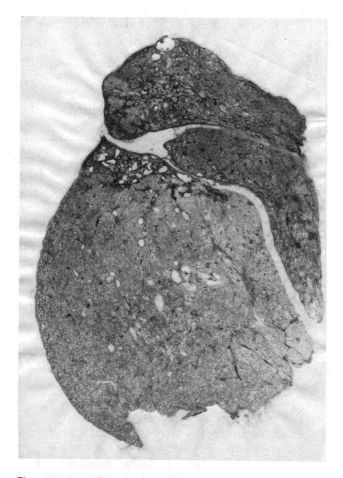

Figure 35.2   Paper-mounted whole lung section in chronic beryllium disease. The upper and middle lobes and apex of the lower lobe are contracted by extensive fibrosis.

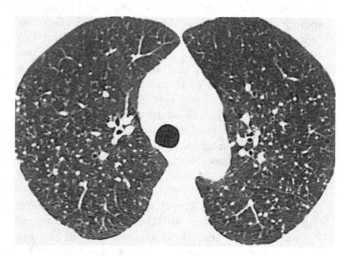

Figure 35.4   High-resolution CT scan showing nodular opacities in lung fields and subpleurally.

Richeldi and colleagues found a strong association between the development of CBD in exposed workers and the presence of glutamic acid in position 69 of the β1 chain of HLA DPB1 molecule: 31 of 32 cases (97.5 percent) of CBD were HLA DPB1* Glu69 positive as compared to 27 percent of the 44 comparably exposed referents without CBD (Richeldi *et al.* 1993). In a later study, Richeldi and colleagues (1997) investigated the risks of developing CBD in a factory workforce exposed to beryllium in relation to level of exposure (using job title as a surrogate measure) and HLA DPB1 Glu69. Six of 127 (4.7 percent) of those exposed to beryllium developed CBD, the majority of cases (5/6) occurring in the machinists who experienced higher levels of exposure (c 0.9 µg/m^3). Five cases occurred in the 41 HLA DPB1 Glu69 positive individuals and one case in the 86 HLA DPB1 Glu69 negative individuals, a 10-fold increased risk for HLA DPB1 Glu69 positive individuals. The number of the study population was small, making it difficult to interpret genetic environmental interactions with confidence; but only

IMMUNOGENETICS OF CBD

Chronic beryllium disease is a Th1 lymphocyte-dependent granulomatous response to inhaled (or cutaneous) beryllium. Th1 lymphocyte stimulation is restricted by MHC class 2 molecules on the surface of antigen-presenting cells.

one case, who was HLA DPB Glu69 positive, occurred in a non-machinist (low-exposure group) and only one case occurred in an HLA DPB Glu69 negative individual, who was a machinist (high-exposure group).

Further studies have confirmed that the risk associated with HLA DPB Glu69 is increased both for CBD and for beryllium sensitization (BeS). Between 75 and 95 percent of individuals with BeS and CBD are HLA DPB Glu69 positive (compared to 30–50 percent of referents). More recently, Snyder and colleagues have reported that Glu69 alleles with the greatest negative surface charge are associated with the greatest risk of CBD, while the risk of BeS was similar for all alleles (Snyder et al. 2008).

The mechanism of beryllium presentation by HLA DPB Glu69 remains unclear: whether Be is presented alone, linked to a peptide or through the alteration of a peptide. Following presentation, CD4 + Th1 cells proliferate (the basis of the Be LPT). In CBD, stimulated CD4+ T-cells from BAL secrete IF-γ and TNF-α, mediators which encourage the accumulation, activation and aggregation of macrophages, leading to granuloma formation. Pott and colleagues reported increased production of IF-γ, identifiable by ELISPOT in blood cells from patients with CBD, as compared to BeS, which they have proposed as a test to distinguish CBD from BeS (Pott et al. 2005).

ACUTE BERYLLIUM DISEASE

Acute beryllium disease (ABD), which was first reported in Germany and the USA in the 1930s and 40s, has been considered an example of an acute chemical pneumonitis, caused by the inhalation of beryllium in doses toxic to alveolar epithelium, causing acute pulmonary edema – similar in mechanism to that caused by inhaled phosgene, nickel carbonyl and cadmium.

However, in a recent review of the evidence, which included a description of two additional cases of ABD, Cummings and colleagues argued that ABD and CBD are two ends of a similar spectrum of a hypersensitivity-induced disease (Cummings et al. 2009). Gases, vapors and fumes that cause chemical pneumonitis are in general chemically reactive but insoluble, able to bypass dissolution in the fluid-lined airways and penetrate to the alveoli, and are toxic to alveolar epithelium, causing inflammation and edema. In general, chemical pneumonitis follows exposure to a reactive chemical in high atmospheric concentration, usually after a latent interval of between 8 and 24 hours. The condition is likely to affect all exposed to sufficient concentrations. It may cause death; but survivors, following recovery, are able to continue exposure to the chemical without the risk of a recurrence, in the absence of further exposure to airborne concentrations of the chemical in air which are toxic to alveolar epithelium. In contrast, a hypersensitivity response usually occurs only in a minority of those exposed, usually after a latent interval of weeks or months, and will recur on exposure to airborne concentrations of the cause which others, comparably exposed, can tolerate and which were previously tolerable to the affected individual.

In their review, Cummings and colleagues drew attention to a number of features of ABD that are more consistent with a hypersensitivity than a toxic response. The levels of exposure experienced by the two cases they describe were well below the $100 \, \mu g/m^3$ suggested in the 1950s as the level of beryllium exposure below which ABD would not occur. Indeed the concentrations experienced were usually below $10 \, \mu g/m^3$ and did not exceed $20 \, \mu g/m^3$. The lack of a clear exposure/response relationship in relation to ABD had been highlighted in earlier reports in the late 1940s and early 1950s (De Nardi et al. 1949; Sterner and Eisenbud 1951). The time course of ABD is also unusual for an acute chemical pneumonitis. De Nardi and colleagues described an initial dermatitis involving exposed skin in some 25 percent of new employees developing 3–10 days after first exposure to beryllium. Respiratory involvement included nasopharyngitis and tracheobronchitis. Those with tracheobronchitis who continued to work could develop pneumonitis, usually after several weeks, although a more severe disease could develop within 72 hours of massive short-lived exposure.

Pneumonitis was recognized by bilateral changes on the chest radiograph that usually developed 1–3 weeks after the onset of symptoms. Resolution of these changes occurred over the course of several months. Of particular importance, in some of the early cases reported and the two described by Cummings and colleagues, the disease recurred on re-exposure to beryllium at levels not affecting others comparably exposed.

Progression to CBD in several cases following ABD, in the absence of further exposure to beryllium, is well recognized. The review of the evidence by Cummings and colleagues is sufficient to question the usual textbook description of ABD and CBD as conditions with different underlying disease mechanisms; rather, they may represent, at least in some cases, a continuum of a hypersensitivity rather than toxic reaction with a spectrum of clinical manifestations.

POPULATION STUDIES

Beryllium register and workforce surveys

The relative difficulty of an accurate and specific case definition of CBD before the development of BeLPT limits confidence in the results of prior studies of workforces exposed to beryllium. Studies of workforces before the late 1980s defined CBD on the basis of exposure to beryllium, with appropriate clinical manifestations of disease (including abnormal chest radiographs). More recent studies have included BeLPT as a diagnostic criterion, because of the low false-positive rate and therefore high positive predictive value. BeLPT has also been used in several studies as a screening test for further case investigation, which has included BAL and TBB.

In these surveys BeS is diagnosed on the basis of beryllium exposure at work with a positive BeLPT (usually stimulation index >3) and CBD on the basis of non-caseating granulomas or mononuclear cell infiltrates in lung biopsy with a positive BeLPT and a history of beryllium exposure at work.

This sequential approach to case identification, while having the merit of efficiency, is at the potential risk of missing the few cases of CBD in whom BeLP is negative and therefore of underestimating disease prevalence (although, in the absence of a positive BeLPT, it is not possible to distinguish such cases from sarcoidosis occurring in a beryllium worker).

Harriet Hardy, who in 1946 first recognized beryllium inhalation in fluorescent light manufacturers as the cause of 'Salem sarcoid', started in 1952 a beryllium register in the USA, to which cases of disease considered by reporting physicians to be caused by beryllium were reported. The register identified a number of factors of importance. CBD occurred in all industries in which there was exposure to beryllium metal or its salts. CBD also occurred in people without direct occupational exposure, but who were in close contact with others working with beryllium (in particular, washing their clothes) or living in the vicinity of factories where beryllium was extracted or processed. The interval from first exposure to onset of disease was very variable, ranging from months to ten or more years. In many cases the disease developed after the individual had left the employment in which beryllium exposure had occurred (Hardy *et al.* 1967).

A report of the beryllium registry findings in 1974 revealed striking differences in the number of cases notified before and after 1949, when controls were instituted designed to keep levels of beryllium in air on average below $2\,\mu g/m^3$ (Hasan and Kazemi 1974; Table 35.1). Although the duration of follow-up is necessarily shorter for those exposed after 1949, with the potential for a number of long-latency cases not to have yet developed, the reduction in the number of cases reported, the very different occupations in which the majority of cases worked before and after 1949, and the great reduction in neighborhood cases is striking.

A later study of a 30-year update of the beryllium case registry to 1982 (Eisenbud and Lisson 1983) came to the conclusion, based on the marked reduction in case numbers of beryllium diseases reported, that there was substantial evidence that:

the methods of control adopted in the early 1950s have been effective in controlling occupational berylliosis. No

Table 35.1   Beryllium registry data in relation to time of onset of exposure.

Nature of exposure	Before 1949	After 1949
Extraction + smelting of Be	255 (38%)	3 (8%)
Be metal production:	90 (13%)	29 (81%)
– Alloys	36	12
– Ceramics	22	4
– X-ray tubes	8	2
– Research/electronics	24	11
Use of fluorescent powder:	256 (38%)	3 (8%)
– Fluorescent lighting tubes	213	2
– Neon lighting tubes	24	1
– Neighborhood cases	71 (11%)	1 (3%)
Totals	672	36

cases of air pollution or exposure to dust brought home on work clothes have been reported since the air quality standard in 1949 and adoption of the improved personal hygiene procedures within the production plants.

By 1982 the total number of cases reported to the registry was 622, of which 557 were occupational. Of the 65 non-occupational cases, 42 were vicinity cases and 23 household cases. All but one of the 42 vicinity cases lived close to two beryllium plants, one in Ohio, the other in Pennsylvania. The one remaining case lived across the street from a fluorescent lamp factory. The majority of occupational cases were in those exposed to phosphors (319) and beryllium extraction (101), the majority first exposed before 1943. The authors estimated the incidence of beryllium disease to have fallen from 3 per ton of beryl equivalent consumed to 0.001 per ton of beryl equivalent consumed, a reduction by a factor of 10 000. No cases had been reported to the registry who were first exposed to beryllium after 1973. Interestingly the authors reported the latent interval had fallen in some cases from more than 40 years in the 1930s to less than 10 years since 1966, probably a reflection of greater awareness and earlier identification of the disease.

In the UK, between 2002 and 2009, only two patients with CBD were reported to the voluntary reporting scheme SWORD, one working in a metal industry, the other a dental technician.

While informative, registry data are limited by the level of, and variation in, ascertainment of cases and by correct attribution of disease to beryllium, which was less certain before the introduction of a specific test (i.e. BeLPT) in the late 1980s. Nonetheless these data provide valuable information about the circumstances of beryllium exposure and their relative importance in causing disease.

The development of BeLPT, together with the introduction of fiberoptic bronchoscopy (allowing BAL and TBB), provided the basis for a number of workplace studies undertaken in the USA between 1993 and 2001. New cases of CBD were identified on the basis of beryllium exposure, positive blood BeLPT, and non-caseating granulomas found in transbronchial lung biopsy.

Kreiss and colleagues reported the findings of a prevalence survey of nuclear weapons workers in a factory that began using beryllium in 1951 and continued beryllium casting until 1979 (Kreiss *et al.* 1993a). They identified 18 individuals who were BeLPT positive, of whom 12 had chronic beryllium disease, identified by granulomas in lung biopsies, with three more developing granulomas in lung biopsy within the succeeding 2 years. The risk of being sensitized to beryllium was greatest in those engaged in machining (4.7 percent) and sawing (4.7 percent), in those who had experienced accidental over-exposure (7.4 percent), and in those whose exposure started before 1970 (3.6 percent). However, sensitization was also found in two individuals with only bystander exposure – a security guard and a secretary.

In the same year, Kreiss and colleagues reported the findings of a prevalence survey of the workforce of a factory that had manufactured beryllium oxide (beryllia) ceramics between 1958 and 1975 and subsequently metalized circuitry on to beryllia ceramics manufactured elsewhere (Kreiss *et al.* 1993b). They found 9 new cases of CBD confirmed by lung biopsy in 505 employees and ex-employees. All cases of CBD had a positive BeLPT (100 percent sensitive), but two cases of CBD with abnormal chest radiographs had a negative or inconsistent positive BeLPT (i.e. 77 percent specific for coincidental cases of sarcoidosis). The majority of newly identified cases of CBD were in the ex-employees, with a disease prevalence of 5.8 percent. The only important risk factor for the development of CBD was the level of beryllium exposure: the highest rates (11.1–15.8 percent) of newly identified CBD occurred in those engaged in dusty tasks, which were more difficult to control, such as beryllia process development and engineering. Although suggesting an exposure/response relationship, one case occurred in a man with inadvertent and seemingly 'trivial' exposure.

Kreiss and colleagues subsequently reported the prevalence of CBD in a beryllium manufacturing plant engaged in the production of beryllium metal, beryllium oxide, beryllium alloys and ceramics (Kreiss *et al.* 1997). The factory had 646 employees of whom 59 of 627 (9.4 percent) tested were BeLPT positive; 24 of the 47 of these 59, who had fiberoptic bronchoscopy and transbronchial lung biopsy, were diagnosed with CBD, on the basis of pulmonary granulomas in 20 and an increased proportion of lymphocytes among the cells recovered at BAL in 4. These 24 together with 5 previously identified cases gives a prevalence of CBD in this workforce of 4.6 percent. The prevalence of BeLPT positive cases of 9.4 percent and of CBD (4.6 percent) is the highest reported of any screened workforce. Disease prevalence was highest in those working in the ceramics plant (9 percent). Work in beryllium metal production employed after 1983 was also associated with a high prevalence of positive BeLPT (19 percent) and disease (6.4 percent), as compared to a disease prevalence of 1.3 percent in those employed in other parts of the factory in the same era. The contemporary measurements of levels of beryllium in air did not indicate higher exposure in areas of beryllium metal production than in some other areas of the plant, apparently at variance with an exposure/response relationship. However, inferences about exposure/response relationships from such cross-sectional surveys should be drawn with caution.

Newman and colleagues reported the results of three rounds of screening, undertaken at 2-yearly intervals, in a beryllium machining plant, where the median beryllium exposures during machining were 0.3 µg/m^3 (Newman *et al.* 2001). This followed the diagnosis of CBD in 1995 in an index case working in the factory. The employees (235 initially) were screened with BeLPT every 2 years and new employees within 3 months of joining. The results of the three surveys on those remaining in the factory from the 1995 study group who were without CBD and BeLPT negative at the prior test point are shown in Table 35.2.

Four of the 15 cases of CBD developed within 3 months of starting work in the factory. Only the index case had an abnormal chest X-ray or required treatment. All other cases had normal chest radiographs and lung volumes and would fulfil the criteria for subclinical CBD.

The aforementioned suggestion of Eisenbud and Lisson that CBD was a disease of the past, made in 1983 on the basis of the striking reduction in cases of CBD reported to the beryllium register, was over-optimistic. Workforce surveys in factories producing beryllium and manufacturing beryllium products have consistently shown that beryllium sensitization (identified by positive BeLPT) and CBD (identified primarily by pulmonary granulomas) – methods of investigation not available to Eisenbud and Lisson – have been found in each of these workforces. As many as 10 percent or more of these workforces have a positive BeLPT and a cumulative prevalence in 235 workers screened between 1995 and 1999 of nearly 10 percent (22 of 235) was found in a beryllium machining workforce (Newman *et al.* 2001).

Three important questions remain.

- What is the nature of 'subclinical' or 'surveillance identified' CBD, which forms the great majority of the cases identified in these later surveys? Does the presence of granulomas in the lungs herald the early stage of clinical CBD to which it may progress, or is it a separate condition with a better prognosis than classical CBD?
- Does avoidance of exposure, usually recommended in these cases, improve the prognosis, reducing the risk of progression to CBD?
- What is the nature of the exposure/response relationship?

The striking reduction in the number of cases reported to the beryllium register, both occupational and non-occupational cases, which followed the elimination of beryllium compounds from phosphors and the improved control of beryllium exposure from the 1960s, implies an exposure/response relationship. However, workforce studies reported since the late 1980s have not found clear evidence of an exposure/response relationship; in particular the job tasks associated with the highest prevalence of positive BeLPT and CBD cases do not necessarily occur in areas of the factory with the highest exposures. These surveys also report cases

Table 35.2   Results of three rounds of screening, undertaken at 2-yearly intervals, in a beryllium machining plant (Newman *et al.* 2001).

Years of screening	Workforce no. screened	BeLPT+new no.	BeLPT+cumulative no.	CBD+new no.	CBD+cumulative no.
1995–7	235	15 (6.4%)	15 (6.4%)	9	9
1997–9	187	5 (2.7%)	20 (8.5%)	4	13
1999	109	2 (1.8%)	22 (9.4%)	2	15
Totals	235	22 (9.4%)	22 (9.4%)	15	15

who seem likely to have been exposed to minimal levels of exposure. But the limitations of cross-sectional surveys for investigating exposure/response relationships should be appreciated: to investigate exposure/response relationships, disease incidence should be estimated in relation to contemporary measures of exposure in the workplace. The workplace surveys reported, while informative in relation to disease prevalence and its relationship to beryllium sensitization, suffer from the problems of cross-sectional surveys: only those who survive in work are available for study and current measurements of exposure may not reflect the levels of exposure in the past, both of which are likely to attenuate any exposure/response relationship. Investigators have endeavored to overcome these problems by including ex-employees where possible and using contemporary measures of exposure where available. Nonetheless reported studies of beryllium-exposed workforces have not overcome these problems sufficiently to exclude an exposure/response relationship modified by recognized genetic factors; that is, the potential for the susceptible genotype HLA DPB1 Glu69 not to be randomly distributed in relation to exposure (e.g. a higher proportion in lower exposure groups).

Despite these apparent anomalies, the evidence of the past 60 years does suggest that reductions in exposure to beryllium and its containment in the workplace have been associated with a marked reduction in the incidence of CBD and its severity, both inside and outside the place of work.

Non-occupational exposure to beryllium

Chronic beryllium disease has been reported both from air pollution in the residents of communities living in the vicinity of beryllium manufacturing facilities and among co-habitants of workers in the facilities from contaminated clothing brought home.

The first cases of non-occupational or community-acquired CBD were reported from Lorraine, Ohio (Eisenbud et al. 1949). The report described 11 patients with CBD of non-occupational cause who lived in the vicinity of a beryllium extraction plant. All but one of the cases lived within about 1.2 km of the plant. Ambient beryllium concentrations were, on average, $0.01\,\mu g/m^3$.

Subsequently, 21 cases of community-acquired CBD were reported in those living in the vicinity of a factory in Reading, Pennsylvania, manufacturing beryllium oxide, alloys and metal (Lieben and Metzner 1959). Those with CBD lived between about 1 km and 8.5 km from the factory. A further three cases, also living in the vicinity of this factory, were reported later.

In addition, para-occupational cases of CBD were reported in the same era. A review of the beryllium case registry in the USA of 47 non-occupational cases of CBD reported in 1961 that 24 had encountered contaminated clothing at home, 13 had lived in the vicinity of a factory using beryllium, 8 had both lived in the vicinity and had been exposed to contaminated clothing, and 2 had no known exposure. A subsequent report found that of 672 persons exposed before 1949, 11 percent were neighborhood cases, as compared to 3 percent of 36 cases exposed after 1949 (Hasan and Kazemi 1974).

No cases of community-acquired CBD had been reported after 1959 until 2008 when Maier and colleagues described eight cases of CBD, diagnosed between 1999 and 2002, who lived between about 160 m and 1600 m of the Reading, Pennsylvania, factory (Maier et al. 2008). The latent interval between potential initial exposure and the development of CBD ranged between 19 and 52 years. Four additional cases of CBD were excluded from the analysis because three had worked in the factory and one had a family member who had worked in the factory. Three of the eight had previously been given other diagnoses, two of sarcoidosis and one of silicosis. Three of the eight cases were from the same family, the mother and two sisters. All but one of the eight cases moved to the area in 1950 or after, making these seven the first cases of community-acquired CBD whose initial vicinity exposure dated from 1950 and after. Five of the eight cases had evidence of granulomas on lung biopsy. Two of the eight had died in 2000, but the remaining six had a positive BeLPT in BAL or blood or both.

CBD AND SARCOIDOSIS

Chronic beryllium disease can be difficult to diagnose if not considered. The wide and expanding modern uses of beryllium are often unknown to the physician and unrecognized by the patient. This difficulty is compounded by the length of the latent interval between initial exposure and the onset of disease, sufficiently long for the disease to develop after leaving exposure in some 50 percent of cases.

Also, the potential for non-occupational exposure, particularly among those living in the vicinity of a factory using beryllium, as a cause of CBD, long thought a thing of the past, has recently been rediscovered by Maier and colleagues.

Together these raise the question of how many cases of sarcoid may in fact be CBD attributable to an unappreciated exposure to beryllium. Few studies have investigated this question directly. Cullen and colleagues reported five cases of CBD (with positive BAL BeLPT), diagnosed and treated as sarcoidosis for several years, who had been exposed to beryllium while working for several years in a precious-metal refinery (Cullen et al. 1987). A study of 47 patients with sarcoidosis seen in a clinic in Israel identified 14 patients with a possible history of beryllium exposure (Fireman et al. 2003). Three of the 14 had a positive BeLPT, two with biopsy evidence of granulomas in the lungs and one with evidence of extrapulmonary granulomas, who did not undergo a bronchoscopic biopsy. A subsequent study of patients in two tertiary referral centers, in Germany and Israel, identified, from a detailed occupational history, 84 cases of sarcoid with known or possible beryllium exposure (Muller-Quernheim et al. 2006). These were compared with 76 healthy workers exposed to beryllium, 31 cases of sarcoid without evidence of beryllium exposure, and 13 healthy colleagues of the 84 cases of primary interest. BeLPT in blood samples was positive in 34 of the 84 exposed cases and 7 of their 13 healthy colleagues. BeLPT was negative in all of the

76 healthy workers and the 31 unexposed sarcoidosis cases. The most common occupation in the 34 cases of sarcoid with positive BeLPT was dental technician (13/34; 7 from Germany, 6 from Israel). Other occupations were evenly spread and reflected modern uses of beryllium (Table 35.3).

Table 35.3 Occupations of CBD cases initially diagnosed as sarcoidosis (Muller-Quernheim *et al.* 2006).

Occupational beryllium exposure	CBD	Exposed sensitized healthy
Individuals	34	7
Dental technician, dentist	13	1
Engine development, mechanics, automobile industry	2	2
Brass alloys, Be-containing alloys	4	1
Metallurgical factory	2	
Aircraft production and maintenance	3	
Non-sparking tools	1	
Radiation shielding	1	1
Military vehicle armor	2	
Fluorescent lamps	2	
Microelectronics/electrical relays	1	1
Chemical industry	1	
Engraving of gems	1	
Ore mining	1	
Grinding of optical lenses for precision instruments		1

WHY DISTINGUISH CBD FROM SARCOID?

The early descriptions of CBD are of a disease whose outcome was of inexorable, often rapid, progression to disabling fibrosis and death. Subsequent improvement in control of beryllium in the workplace has been associated with a condition now often only identified through screening programs of workforces exposed to beryllium, on the basis of a positive beryllium LPT and granulomata in biopsies obtained by fiberoptic bronchoscopy. First principles, based on the limited evidence available, suggest that the means most likely to prevent disease progression is early case identification and avoidance of further beryllium exposure. This is the basis of screening programs, currently more in evidence in the USA than in the UK. A similar argument applies to cases of 'sarcoidosis' found to have a positive BeLPT: the best opportunity to minimize disease progression is likely to be the avoidance of further exposure. But, how strong is the evidence for this?

Rom and colleagues found, in a prospective study of beryllium workers, miners and millers, that 8 of 11 individuals with a positive BAL lymphocyte transformation test in 1979 had a negative test in 1982, although they had changed the test method used between the two surveys (Rom *et al.* 1983). This change was concurrent with a measured reduction in levels of exposure in the workplace during the period of the study.

Sprince and colleagues in a survey of employees of a beryllium extraction and processing plant undertaken in 1971 and again in 1974 found improvements in chest radiographic abnormalities and lung function tests which were associated with a marked reduction in exposure levels (Sprince *et al.* 1989). Whereas in 1971 peak beryllium concentrations were found to be up to 50 times the contemporary allowable limit of $25\,\mu g/m^3$, in 1974 peak concentrations were all less than $25\,\mu g/m^3$. Of 31 men with evidence in 1971 of 'interstitial disease' on the chest radiograph, in 1974, 13 were lost to follow-up, 9 remained abnormal and 9 were considered normal. Arterial po_2 in 13 of 20 men in whom it was less than 80 mmHg in 1971 improved from an average po_2 in the 13 men of 72 mmHg to 91 mmHg. Seven of these 13 had abnormal chest radiographs in 1971, which were considered normal in 1974. This study suggests the potential for disease resolution with reduction in exposure to beryllium.

In contrast, a follow-up study of 55 individuals with a positive BeLPT, of whom 31 percent developed biopsy or BAL evidence of CBD, found that continuing exposure to beryllium did not influence the risk of progressing to CBD (Newman *et al.* 2005). This suggested that the risk of progression from beryllium sensitization, to at least sub-clinical disease, is determined more by beryllium retained in the lung than by further exposure. Nonetheless the change in the nature and severity of disease with the progressive reduction in exposure in and outside the workplace suggests the potential benefit from avoiding further exposure in those found to have evidence of disease.

Identification of a case of CBD also has potential benefits for others employed in the same place of work. The diagnosed case should be considered a 'sentinel' event, which indicates the need for investigation of the workplace and workforce to identify any further cases, to minimize exposure to beryllium and reduce the risk of disease.

CONCLUSION

The increasing use of beryllium worldwide suggests the need for further studies to determine how frequently a diagnosis of sarcoidosis is in fact chronic beryllium disease, for enquiry to be made of patients with sarcoidosis of possible exposure to beryllium in their work, past and present, and for BeLPT to be undertaken in patients with sarcoidosis with a history of occupational beryllium exposure.

REFERENCES

Cullen MR, Kominsky JR, Rossman MD *et al.* (1987). Chronic beryllium disease in a precious metal refinery. *Am Rev Respir Dis* **135**: 201–8.

Cummings KC, Stefaniak AB, Virji MA, Kreiss K (2009). A reconsideration of acute beryllium disease. *Environ Health Perspect* **117**: 1250–6.

Curtis GH (1959). The diagnosis of beryllium disease with special reference to the patch test. *Arch Ind Hlth* **19**: 150–3.

De Nardi JM, Van Orstrandt HS, Carmody MG (1949). Acute dermatitis and pneumonitis in beryllium workers. *Ohio State Med J* 45: 567–5.

Editorial (1951). *Lancet* i: **1357**–8.

Eisenbud M, Lisson J (1983). Epidemiological aspects of beryllium-induced non-malignant lung disease: a 30-year update. *J Occup Med* 25: 196–202.

Eisenbud M, Wanta RC, Dustan C et al. (1949). Non-occupational berylliosis. *J Industr Hyg Toxicol* 31: 281–94.

Fireman E, Hainsky E, Noiderfer M et al. (2003). Misdiagnosis of sarcoidosis in patients with chronic beryllium disease. *Sarcoid Vasc Diff Lung Dis* 20: 144–8.

Hamilton A, Hardy HL (1974). *Beryllium in Industrial Toxicology*, 3rd edn. Publishing Sciences Group, p. 51.

Hardy HL, Tabershaw IR (1946). Delayed chemical pneumonitis in workers exposed to beryllium compounds. *J Ind Hyg Toxicol* 28: 197–211.

Hardy HL, Rabe EW, Lorch S (1967). United States Beryllium Case Registry, 1952–1966. *J Occup Med* 9: 271–6.

Hasan FM, Kazemi H (1974). Chronic beryllium disease: a continuing epidemiologic hazard. *Chest* 65: 289–93.

Jackson AJ (1950). In: Vorwald AJ (ed.). *Beryllium Alloys in Pneumoconiosis*. Hoeber, New York.

Kreiss K, Mroz MM, Zhen B et al. (1993a). Epidemiology of beryllium sensitization and disease in nuclear workers. *Am Rev Respir Dis* 148: 985–91.

Kreiss K, Wasserman S, Mroz MM, Newman LS (1993b). Beryllium disease screening in the ceramics industry. *J Occup Med* 35: 267–74.

Kreiss K, Mroz MM, Zhen B et al. (1997). Risks of beryllium disease related to work processes at a metal alloy and oxide production plant. *Occup Environ Med* 54: 605–12.

Lieben J, Metzner F (1959). Epidemiological findings associated with beryllium extraction. *Am Indust Hyg Assoc J* 20: 494–9.

Maier LA, Martyny JW, Liang J, Rossman MD (2008). Recent chronic beryllium disease in residents surrounding a beryllium facility. *Am J Respir Crit Care Med* 177: 1012–17.

Mroz MM, Kreiss K, Lezotte D et al. (1991). Re-examination of the blood lymphocyte transformation test in the diagnosis of chronic beryllium disease. *J Allergy Clin Immunol* 88: 54–60.

Muller-Quernheim J, Gaede KI, Fireman E, Zissel G (2006). Diagnoses of chronic beryllium disease within cohorts of sarcoidosis patients. *Eur Respir J* 27: 1190–5.

Newman LS (1995). Beryllium disease and sarcoidosis: clinical and laboratory links. *Sarcoidosis* 12: 7–19.

Newman LS, Kreiss K, King TE et al. (1989). Pathologic and immunologic alterations in early stages of beryllium disease. *Am Rev Respir Dis* 139: 479–86.

Newman LS, Mroz MM, Maier LA et al. (2001). Efficacy of serial medical surveillance for chronic beryllium disease in a beryllium machining plant. *J Occup Environ Med* 43: 231–7.

Newman LS, Mroz MM, Balkissoon R, Maier LA (2005). Beryllium sensitization progresses to chronic beryllium disease. *Am J Respir Crit Care Med* 171: 54–60.

Pott GB, Palmer BE, Sullivan AK et al. (2005). Frequency of beryllium-specific Th1-type cytokine expressing CD4 + T-cells in patients with beryllium-induced disease. *J Allergy Clin Immunol* 115: 1036–42.

Richeldi L, Kreiss K, Mroz MM et al. (1997). Interaction of genetic and exposure factors in the prevalence of berylliosis. *Am J Indust Med* 32: 337–40.

Richeldi L, Sorrentino R, Saltini C (1993). HLA DPB1 glutamate 69: a genetic marker of beryllium disease. *Science* 262: 242–4.

Rom WN, Lockey JE, Bang KM et al. (1983). Reversible beryllium sensitisation in a prospective study of beryllium workers. *Arch Env Hlth* 38: 302–7.

Rossman MD, Kern JA, Elias A et al. (1988). Proliferative response of bronchoalveolar lymphocytes to beryllium. *Ann Intern Med* 108: 687–93.

Snyder JE, Demchuk KE, McCanlies EC et al. (2008). Impact of negativity charged patches on the surface of MHC class II antigen-presenting proteins on risk of chronic beryllium disease. *J R Soc Interface* 5: 749–58.

Sprince NL, Kanarek DJ, Weber AL et al. (1989). Reversible respiratory disease in beryllium workers. *Am Rev Respir Dis* 117: 1011–17.

Sterner JH, Eisenbud M (1951). Epidemiology of beryllium intoxication. *Arch Ind Hyg Occup Med* 4: 123–51.

Tepper LB, Hardy HL, Chamberlain RI (1961). *Toxicity of Beryllium Compounds*. Elsevier, Amsterdam.

36

Human immunodeficiency virus infection

HELEN L BOOTH AND ROBERT F MILLER

EPIDEMIOLOGY OF HIV INFECTION AND THE USE OF ANTIRETROVIRAL THERAPY

In 2008, 33.4 million people worldwide were living with HIV: 31.3 million adults and 2.1 million children under 15 years of age (Table 36.1). Worldwide, two-thirds of people living with HIV infection are in Sub-Saharan Africa, which has a prevalence rate of 52 per 1000 population and accounts for 68 percent of new infections. In 2008 in the UK, an estimated 83000 people (1.3 per 1000 population; 1.8/1000 men, 0.9/1000 women) were living with HIV infection, although over a quarter were unaware of their HIV status (Health Protection Centre for Infections: www.hpa.org.uk/hiv).

In Sub-Saharan Africa the major route of transmission is by heterosexual sexual activity. In high-income countries, HIV is concentrated in particular risk groups: men who have sex with men, immigrants and injecting drug users. In the UK the two major risk groups affected are those who acquired their infection heterosexually (58 percent), the majority of whom are black Africans (67 percent) and female (63 percent), and men who have had sex with men (38 percent), the majority of whom are white (87 percent). The disproportionate impact of HIV among black African-Americans is also described; despite them making up only 12 percent of the population this group accounts for

46 percent of HIV prevalence (Hall *et al.* 2008a) and lifetime rates of seroconversion are 6.5 times and 19 times higher for men and women, respectively, compared to sex-matched white individuals (Hall *et al.* 2008b).

The number of people living with HIV worldwide continues to increase as a result of high rates of new infection and increased life expectancy resulting from advances in, and provision of, combination antiretroviral therapy (CART). Antiretroviral drugs have been widely available in high-income countries for over a decade. In 2008 in the UK, 75 percent of those with diagnosed HIV infection received antiretroviral therapy. This has had a huge impact on HIV mortality. The rate of excess mortality among HIV-positive patients compared with the HIV-negative population in 12 high-income countries has declined by 85 percent since the introduction of CART (Bhaskaran *et al.* 2008). Reduced HIV mortality is also being reported in resource-limited counties where access to CART has improved (Jahn *et al.* 2008). Between 2003 and 2008, overall access to CART has increased 10-fold in low- to middle-income countries; in Sub-Saharan Africa treatment coverage has increased from 2 to 44 percent of patients. Use of CART is increasing not only because of rising numbers of patients living with HIV and the increased availability of CART, but also because of recommendations that they

Table 36.1 Summary of incidence and prevalence of HIV and AIDS (2008).

	Worldwide	Sub–Saharan Africa	North America and western and central Europe	UK
Number of people living with HIV	33.4 million	22.4 million	2.3 million	83000
Number of new HIV infections	2.7 million	1.9 million	75000	7298
Number of children newly infected	430000	390000	<500	110
Number of AIDS-related deaths	2 million	1.4 million	38000	525

should be introduced earlier in the course of HIV disease, before the CD4 cell count falls below 350 cells/μL.

EPIDEMIOLOGY OF SARCOIDOSIS AND OF HIV INFECTION

The incidence of sarcoidosis varies widely around the world. However, this variability probably reflects genetic differences and environmental exposures as well as the diagnostic tools available between populations. Compared to HIV infection the incidence of sarcoidosis is relatively lower and the highest rate has been reported in Northern Europe, at 40 per 100 000 population (Pietinalho et al. 1995). However, there are some similarities in the populations at risk of developing sarcoidosis and acquiring HIV infection in that they are both diseases of young adults, and incidence rates are increased among black Africans compared to white individuals.

The prevalence of previously diagnosed sarcoidosis in patients with newly diagnosed HIV infection appears to be very low as only a handful of cases have been described in the literature, despite being two reasonably common diseases that occur in a similar at-risk population (Table 36.2). Trevenoli and associates reviewed the literature until 2003 and identified only 14 cases of co-existent sarcoidosis in HIV patients not receiving CART; in 13 the diagnosis of sarcoidosis preceded their HIV diagnosis (Trevenoli et al. 2003). This rarity may in part be due to under-reporting of sarcoidosis in patients with new HIV diagnoses. The need to record a sarcoidosis history, which may be distant, in newly diagnosed HIV patients is highlighted by the increasing recognition of a sarcoidosis-like 'immune reconstitution inflammatory' syndrome (IRIS) after starting CART (Lenner et al. 2001. Alternatively, the reduced incidence of prior sarcoidosis in the population with HIV could reflect the severity and likely duration of immunosuppression at the time of HIV diagnosis which might affect the clinical expression of sarcoidosis. In the UK, one-third of patients have CD4 cell counts below 200 cells/μL at their HIV diagnosis. Earlier diagnosis of HIV infection with screening programs may be expected to increase the number of patients with both diseases if this was the case. More speculatively, having sarcoidosis may be 'protective' against acquiring HIV either through its direct effect on the immune system or underlying genetic factors. The human leukocyte antigen (HLA) molecules are important in antigen presentation, and both HLA-DRB1 and HLA-DQB1 alleles have been associated with susceptibility to sarcoidosis (Voorter et al. 2007) and with different clinical phenotypes (Sato et al. 2002). No HLA haplotype has been associated with acquiring HIV infection (Just 1995), but HLA B35 has been associated with HIV progression to AIDS (Gao et al. 2001), and HLA A2, B27, B51 and B57 have been associated with slower disease progression (Hendel et al. 1999).

The occurrence of new diagnoses of sarcoidosis in patients with known HIV infection and who are not receiving CART is rare, and patients usually have CD4 counts above 200 cells/μL and/or have asymptomatic HIV infection. Morris and co-workers identified only seven known HIV-positive patients who had developed symptomatic sarcoidosis between 1994

and 2002 in an urban academic HIV referral center, but only two were not receiving CART (Morris et al. 2003). Haramati and co-workers retrospectively identified 10 patients at four hospitals during an 8-year period between 1989 and 1997. Six of these patients had established HIV infection and were not receiving CART. Two patients in this series and four others had synchronous diagnoses of both HIV and sarcoidosis (Haramati et al. 2001). In the case report by Gowda and associates, a chest radiograph performed as part of the routine work-up of a patient with newly diagnosed HIV infection and a CD4 lymphocyte count of 570 cells/μL showed stage II sarcoidosis confirmed on transbronchial biopsy (Gowda et al. 1990). Interestingly, chest radiographs from 2 years previously were reviewed and showed similar changes. This case highlights the difficulty in establishing which diagnosis predated the other.

It is increasingly being recognized that a sarcoidosis-like reaction may occur when some HIV-positive patients start CART (French et al. 2000). Sarcoidosis-like IRIS has not been associated with a specific CART regimen but is a consequence of generic CART. It has been reported that between one-quarter and one-third of patients started on CART experience an IRIS to some degree (Murdoch et al. 2007), and it is likely to depend on the prevalence of infections and genetic factors in a given population (Lawn et al. 2005). The incidence of sarcoidosis-like IRIS is uncommon but is likely to rise as the use of CART increases. Of the 65 case reports of sarcoidosis in HIV-infected patients reviewed, 40 (61 percent) were receiving CART at the time of the sarcoidosis diagnosis (see Table 36.2). Additionally, five cases of HIV-infected patients who had a flare-up of their known sarcoidosis when CART was started have been described. In the author's center over the last 10 years, which currently cares for 3500 HIV-infected patients, three cases have had sarcoidosis diagnosed as part of an IRIS; two are described in more detail later.

The overall picture of the incidence of HIV and sarcoidosis is described in a survey of twelve pneumology departments in Paris over a 4-year period to 2000. Only five of the departments reported cases of sarcoidosis among HIV-infected patients. These departments described 11 cases, of whom 8 were receiving CART. The incidence of HIV-associated sarcoidosis was estimated to be 3.2–7.24 per 1000 sarcoidosis-patient-years (Foulon et al. 2004). Among the 65 cases reviewed with dual diagnoses of sarcoidosis and HIV (Table 36.2), 23 (35 percent) were female – a lower proportion than for sarcoidosis in the general population – and 37 (57 percent) were white. These are similar to the gender and ethnicity rates of HIV infection in the UK.

Ages are as expected in these diseases, with adults ranging from 22 to 64 years. One child with perinatally acquired HIV has been reported with sarcoidosis developing at 13 years (Viani 2002).

IMMUNOLOGY OF HIV INFECTION AND IRIS

Since the first description of the acquired immunodeficiency syndrome in 1981, our understanding of the immunopathology of HIV infection and its consequences has increased substantially.

The virus enters the host CD4+ T-lymphocytes and/or monocytes via interaction of the virus gp120 receptor and the CD4 cell-surface and chemokine receptors on the host cells. Once inside the cell cytoplasm, HIV RNA is reverse transcribed into complementary DNA and is then transported to the nucleus where it integrates into the host cell genome. The resulting effect on the immune system is diverse and depends on both viral factors as well as the host immune response to the HIV infection.

The two major types of the virus are HIV-1 and HIV-2. The latter is mainly identified in people from West Africa. The two types are defined by different genetic sequences of the envelope and structural proteins. Although epidemiological studies are difficult it may be that different subtypes of HIV differ in their transmissibility and virulence, but no data exist on the subtype found in patients with sarcoidosis. Some HIV-infected patients remain asymptomatic and with normal CD4 lymphocyte count for long periods (so-called non-progressors), suggesting that an immune response that contains HIV infection can be mounted – and this appears to consist of a continued low-level viremia, Th1 cytokine production, HIV-specific CD4+T-lymphocyte proliferation, and CD8+ T-lymphocyte cytotoxic activity (Rosenberg et al. 1997). The humoral immune response does not appear to have a major role in containing HIV infection (Poignard et al. 1999).

The hallmark of progression of HIV infection is the reduction in peripheral blood CD4 T-lymphocyte numbers, and this is used both as surrogate marker of progressive immune deficiency and as an indicator for starting co-trimoxazole, as prophylaxis of Pneumocystis jirovecii pneumonia (PCP), and starting CART. Although HIV preferentially infects memory CD4+T-lymphocytes (CD45RO+), the largest impact is on naive T-lymphocyte numbers (CD45RA+ CD62L+).

The immunopathogenesis of sarcoidosis is also complex. However, as with HIV, sarcoidosis is also associated with a reduction in circulating CD4 lymphocytes – but this is thought to be secondary to a recruitment of these cells to affected organs such as the lungs (Hunninghake and Crystal 1981). Their role is important in triggering and promoting the Th1 immune response by the release of interferon-γ and interleukin-2 cytokines which are pivotal in attracting and activating mononuclear cells and the formation of granulomas which characterize sarcoidosis. It may be expected, therefore, that the incidence of sarcoidosis would be reduced in patients with HIV and the reports of their occurrence together have been described as an 'immune paradox' (Almeida et al. 2006). However, given the rarity of their co-existence – and that, when they do, it is usually in patients with CD4 counts above 200 cells/μL, and that the clinical features of sarcoidosis improve or stabilize as CD4 lymphocyte numbers drop with advancing HIV infection, and that the sarcoidosis-like IRIS corresponds with increasing CD4 counts – underscores the importance of the CD4 lymphocyte in the immunopathogenesis of sarcoidosis. In all the series reviewed here the median CD4 lymphocyte count was 254 cells/μL with a wide range (25–916). Excluding the series

with the lowest CD4 count, in the remaining 50 patients with CD4 counts recorded, the median was 166 cells/μL. However, there must be other immunological pathways for granuloma formation as they can form in HIV patients with low CD4 counts in association with infections such as tuberculosis and P. jirovecii pneumonia (Kadakia et al. 1993).

In the retrospective review by Morris et al. (2003), the seven patients identified with dual HIV and sarcoidosis had significantly higher CD4 lymphocyte counts (median 383 cell/μL) when compared to 16 HIV-positive patients with other diseases causing granulomatous inflammation (median 143 cell/μL). Interestingly, Amin and colleagues describe two patients who were both able to mount a granulomatous reaction to the Kveim reagent but had very different CD4 counts and HIV stage (Amin et al. 1992). The first patient had had sarcoidosis diagnosed 4 months before presenting with P. jirovecii pneumonia and a new HIV diagnosis. At this time the patient's CD4 count was 200 cells/μL and there was no evidence of active sarcoidosis other than a positive Kveim test. By contrast, the second patient had a positive Kveim test performed at the time of active skin sarcoidosis and was simultaneously diagnosed with asymptomatic HIV infection and a CD4 count of 900 cells/μL.

Among healthy, adult, non-smoking controls, the CD4/CD8 lymphocyte ratio is approximately 1.6 in both blood and bronchoalveolar lavage (BAL) fluid. In sarcoidosis the peripheral blood ratio is usually less than 1, but the reverse is found in BAL fluid where CD4/CD8 ratios up to 10 are described and the proportion of lymphocytes is also increased from normal (≤10 percent) to an average of 30 percent. These BAL abnormalities are often used to support a diagnosis of sarcoidosis and to exclude other granulomatous conditions such as hypersensitivity pneumonitis. In HIV-infected patients there is also a BAL lymphocytosis, but this is due to an increase in CD8 lymphocytes which by contrast with sarcoidosis results in low CD4/CD8 ratios and reflects the changes seen in peripheral blood. In the small number of HIV patients not receiving CART with sarcoidosis, the picture appears to be mixed, with BAL lymphocytosis reported in all cases but low CD4/CD8 ratios in nearly all patients. That there is an absolute increase in lymphocytes in the lungs of HIV patients with sarcoidosis suggests the possibility that co-existent sarcoidosis might affect the natural history of HIV infection by further reducing circulating CD4 counts, which may not only affect monitoring of disease progression but also increase the risk of opportunistic infection. Indeed there are case reports of HIV-negative sarcoidosis patients with diseases often associated with immunosuppression, in particular HIV infection, such as Kaposi's sarcoma (Corda et al. 1996) and P. jirovecii pneumonia. These reports are rare and may simply be coincidental or related to treatment of the sarcoidosis with corticosteroids or other immunosuppressive agents. However, from case reports and series this would not appear to happen. The low BAL CD4/CD8 ratio found in the majority of sarcoidosis/HIV patients not on CART might be more characteristic of HIV infection rather than sarcoidosis but does not appear to predict prognosis or response to treatment (Whitlock et al. 1990; Newman et al. 1992; Foulon et al., 2004). By contrast, BAL findings in HIV-infected

Table 36.2 Clinical characteristics of case reports/series of sarcoidosis in HIV patients.

Reference	No. of cases	Age (years)	Gender	Ethnicity	HIV risk factor	Sarcoidosis diagnosis relative to HIV diagnosis	Duration CART (months)	Sarcoidosis organ involvement	Treatment	Outcome
Ailani et al.	1	36	M	Black	MSM	IRIS	84	Intrathoracic Spinal	Steroids	Improved
Almeida et al.	1	41	F	Black	1 Het	Simultaneous Symptoms with CART	NA (48)	Intrathoracic Skin Hypercalcemia	Steroids	Improved
Amin et al.	2	37	F	White	Het	Pre 4 months	NA	Intrathoracic Muscle	Steroids	Died of AIDS
		36	F	NR	NR	Simultaneous	NA	Intrathoracic Skin (EN) Lymph nodes	No	Improved
Blanche et al	1	36	M	White	PostTx	IRIS (plus IL-2)	36	Intrathoracic Liver Salivary gland	IL–2 stopped	Improved
Coots et al.	1	29	M	Black	NR	Simultaneous	NA	Intrathoracic	None	Stable
Ferrand et al.	1	58	M	White	MSM	IRIS	12	Skin Salivary glands Hypercalcemia Kidney	Steroids	Improved
Foulon et al.	11	Median 37 Range 30–48	8 M 3 F	8 White 3 Black	6 Het 2 IVDU 3 MSM	3 post (1 flare on CART) 8 IRIS	Median 36 Range 3–43	11 Intrathoracic 3 Skin 3 Spleen 2 Liver 1 Muscle 3 Salivary glands	5 No 3 Steroids 1 Doxycycline 1 Hydroxychloroquine	4 Improved 1 Stable 5 Improved
Gomez et al.	1	53	M	White	NR	IRIS	14	Skin (EN)	Steroids	Improved
Gowda et al.	1	29	M	NR	MSM	Simultaneous	NA	Intrathoracic	No	Stable
Granieri et al.	1	42	M	Black	MSM	Simultaneous	NA	Intrathoracic Muscle Bone cysts	Steroids	Improved

Study	n	Age	Sex	Race	Risk factor	Timing	CXR stage	Organ involvement	Treatment	Outcome
Haramati et al.	10	Median 32.5 Range 26–66	3 M 7 F	NR	5 Het 5 IVDU 2 NR	2 Simultaneous 6 Post (1 flare with CART) 2 IRIS	NR	8 Intrathoracic 1 Liver + Spleen 1 Salivary gland	NR	NR
Hill et al.	1	50	F	Black	NR	IRIS	NR	Intrathoracic	NR	NR
Lassalle et al.	14	Median 30 Range 22–55	10 M 4F	14 White	2 Het 6 IVDU 6 MSM	14 IRIS	Median 5 Range 3–11	7+ Intrathoracic 2 Skin 6 Lymph nodes	NR	NR
Lee et al.	1	38	M	Black	NR	IRIS	NR	Uveitis	Steroids	NR
Lenner et al.	2	50	F	Black	Het	Pre 15 years Symptoms with CART	23	Intrathoracic	Steroids + Hydroxychloroquine	Improved
		64	M	Black	NR	Pre approx 40 years Symptoms with CART	NR	Intrathoracic	Steroids	Improved
Morris et al.	7	Median 40.5 Range 26–52	5 M 2 F	4 White 3 Black	NR	2 Post 5 IRIS	NA NR	7 Intrathoracic 3 Skin (1EN)	NR	NR
Naccache et al.	2	45	M	White	MSM	IRIS	15	Intrathoracic Salivary gland	No	Stable
Newman et al.	1	34	F	White	NR	IRIS (plus IL–2)	3	Intrathoracic	IL–2 stopped	Improved
		35	M	Hispanic	IVDU	Post	NA	Intrathoracic	Steroids	Improved
Okosun et al.	1	35	M	White	NR	IRIS	2	Pancytopenia Liver + Spleen Kidney Hypercalcemia	Steroids	Improved
Papadaki et al.	1	47	M	White	NR	NR	NR	Conjunctivitis	Topical steroids	Improved
Trevenzoli et al.	1	44	M	White	IVDU	IRIS	20	Intrathoracic Skin	Steroids	Improved
Viani	1	13	M	Black	Perinatal	IRIS	≈2	Salivary gland Uveitis Hypercalcemia Liver + spleen Kidney	Inhaled steroids	Improved
Whitlock et al.	1	37	M	White	NR	Pre 10 years	NA	Intrathoracic	None	Stable
Wittram et al.	1	45	F	NR	NR	IRIS	16	Intrathoracic	Steroids	Improved

BAL, bronchoalveolar lavage; CART, combined antiretroviral therapy; Cx LN, cervical lymph node; CXR stage, Scadding chest radiograph stage; EN, erythema nodosum; IRIS, immune reconstitution inflammatory syndrome; LN, lymph node; Med LN, mediastinal lymph node; MSM, men who have sex with men; ND, not detected; NR, not recorded; PostTx, post transfusional; SACE, serum angiotensin-converting enzyme; TBB, transbronchial biopsy.

patients on CART with sarcoidosis are similar to those found in sarcoidosis in the general population, with significantly higher proportion of lymphocytes at a mean of 39 ± 19 percent and high CD4/CD8 ratios 3.5 ± 2.5 compared with controls, but ratios up to 16 have been reported (Ailani et al. 2009).

Sarcoidosis and HIV infection share immunological similarities other than peripheral CD4 lymphopenia. They include polyclonal hypergammaglobulinemia and cutaneous anergy to recall antigens such as tuberculin PPD. In one review of cases, 17 tuberculin tests had been performed and all were reported as non-reactive. In one case the patient had had a positive Mantoux result at the time of the HIV diagnosis but had then become anergic at the time of the sarcoidosis diagnosis (Naccache et al. 2009).

As detailed above, CART has been shown to reduce HIV-related morbidity and mortality and its success is monitored clinically in individuals by reductions in viral load and increasing CD4 T-lymphocyte numbers (Moore and Chaisson 1999). Despite laboratory measured markers showing response to CART, some patients experience a clinical deterioration when they start treatment and this has been termed IRIS (Shelbourne et al. 2002). A proportion of these cases are due to recovery of antigen-specific immune responses resulting in an over-exuberant inflammatory reaction to organisms not recognized (dormant) or partially treated (overt) prior to starting CART. The onset of this form of IRIS, regardless of infectious pathogen, is within a few weeks of starting CART. Non-infectious antigens, including host-derived antigens, may be the precipitant for the autoimmune and sarcoidosis-like reactions seen as part of the IRIS spectrum as no microbiological cause has been identified (Lassalle et al. 2006). The quantitative and qualitative restoration of the immune response induced by CART may also be important in the pathogenesis of sarcoidosis-like IRIS. In the cases reviewed it occurred a median 11 months (range 3–84) after starting CART when CD4 counts had recovered and there was a marked reduction in HIV viral load, suggesting that some defect or delay in immune restoration rather than an infectious cause accounted for its development. Studies describing baseline CD4 lymphocyte counts and HIV viral load and their rate of change for the risk of developing IRIS in response to CART give conflicting results. HIV viral loads at the time of sarcoidosis / IRIS range from undetectable to 31 000 copies per milliliter, suggesting perhaps that the virological response to CART is less important than the immune restoration. A significant increase in peripheral CD4 lymphocyte counts has been described at time of diagnosis of sarcoidosis. Among the 65 patients reviewed, the median CD4 count at diagnosis of sarcoidosis / IRIS was 346 cells/μL (range 211–916). It has been postulated that this timeline for developing sarcoidosis-like IRIS corresponds with the recovery of naive CD4 lymphocytes at between 3 and 6 months – as opposed to memory CD4 lymphocytes which recover early, at 3–6 weeks, after starting CART. That it is the quality and/or quantity of the immune restoration which may be important in sarcoidosis-like IRIS is further supported by the observation that use of adjunctive immunomodulators such as IL-2 and interferon-α therapy for HIV disease and simultaneous

chronic hepatitis C infection, respectively, may be an additional risk for developing a sarcoidosis-like IRIS (Naccache et al. 1999; Blanche et al. 2000), by shortening the interval between CART introduction and clinical presentation with sarcoidosis. Certainly IL-2 has been shown to have a role in active pulmonary sarcoidosis (Hunninghake et al. 1983), and interferon-α-induced sarcoidosis has been described in the HIV-negative general population. Reports of patients with a remote history of sarcoidosis relapsing after starting CART, which is unusual in the natural history of sarcoidosis, suggests some form of immunological memory or a loss of immunological tolerance. Furthermore, although rates of opportunistic infection are markedly reduced after initiation of CART, there is no similar reduction in incidence of other infections and lymphoma, suggesting that the T-cell repertoire is not completely restored (Connors et al. 1997; Noursadeghi et al. 2006). These observations may be important in furthering an understanding of how the immune system recovers in response to CART and may provide important insights into the immunopathogenesis of sarcoidosis.

CLINICAL PRESENTATION IN HIV-POSITIVE INDIVIDUALS

See Table 36.3 for a summary of cases reviewed in this chapter.

It is clear that sarcoidosis and HIV infection may co-exist but not whether they are independent diagnoses or are associated with each other. Furthermore the presence of one disease may potentially affect the natural history and clinical phenotype of the other.

A diagnosis of sarcoidosis is established by the demonstration of non-caseating granulomas in a compatible clinical context with other diseases excluded. This should embrace HIV, given the similar epidemiology of these two conditions and the wider differential diagnosis of clinical symptoms and signs in the context of an HIV diagnosis. This recommendation is supported by updated UK national guidelines, which advocate offering an HIV test to any adult accessing hospital care. The diagnosis of HIV infection is currently made using a combined antigen and antibody test, using a peripheral blood sample.

Securing a diagnosis of sarcoidosis is often difficult but may be even harder in the context of HIV infection as there is a wider differential diagnosis for the patient's symptoms and signs. For example, musculoskeletal complications may arise from HIV itself, secondary to HIV-related problems such as infection, directly from drug toxicity either from CART (zidovidune-induced myopathy), or from statins used to counteract CART-induced hyperlipidemia, or as IRIS. Two cases of sarcoid myopathy presenting with proximal muscle weakness have been reported in HIV-positive patients with advanced HIV infection (Amin et al. 1992) and/or low CD4 counts (Granieri et al. 1995). However, HIV-associated polymyositis is a more likely cause of muscular complications occurring in 2–7 percent of HIV-positive patients.

Among HIV-infected individuals with sarcoidosis, involvement of the lungs and/or mediastinal lymph nodes is almost universal. In the cases reviewed, only 2 of 65 did not have symptomatic or radiological evidence of intrathoracic involvement. One had isolated ocular sarcoidosis (Papadaki *et al.* 2006), the second had systemic extrapulmonary sarcoidosis affecting parotid, skin, eyes and kidney and hypercalcemia (Ferrand *et al.* 2007).

In general, although the differential diagnosis is wider, clinical presentation and symptoms of sarcoidosis in HIV-positive patients are similar and are as diverse as among the HIV-uninfected general population. As in HIV-negative patients, sarcoidosis may be asymptomatic and be identified on routine chest radiology screening (Coots and Lazarus 1989; Newman *et al.* 1992). Organ involvement by sarcoidosis among HIV-infected patients appears to be similar whether or not they are receiving CART. After pulmonary/mediastinal lymph nodes, sites affected in order are skin, extrathoracic lymph nodes, salivary glands, muscle, spleen, eyes, liver and kidney. Sarcoidosis skin lesions reported include erythema nodosum, subcutaneous nodules and a hypopigmented annular macular rash. Hypercalcemia in the context of IRIS has been described in three patients with sarcoidosis, but clinically must be differentiated from infectious causes of IRIS such as tuberculosis and cryptococcosis which can cause similar biochemical abnormalities. Renal failure secondary to granulomatous kidney involvement is rare but appears to be over-represented among HIV-infected patients.

CASE REPORT 1

A 58-year-old homosexual white male with a 21-year history of HIV infection started CART 12 months prior to presentation with fatigue, weight loss, painless subcutaneous nodules on the arms, back and thighs, and red, itchy eyes. He then developed arthralgia and bilateral parotid swelling. His blood results were as follows: CD4 count 500 cells/µL and HIV viral load undetectable; impaired renal function with a creatinine 372 µmol/L, urea 20.9 mmol/L, creatinine clearance 22 mL/min (normal range 71–151), serum calcium 3.34 mmol/L (normal 2.2–2.6), urinary calcium excretion 10.7 mmol/24-h (normal 2.5–8.0), and SACE 110 U/L (normal 16–59). Chest radiography and thoracic CT imaging were normal. Parotid gland fine-needle aspiration of a skin nodule and kidney all showed epitheliod non-caseating granulomas. Mycobacterial cultures of all samples and a tuberculin skin test were negative. Symptoms, signs and calcium levels normalized and renal function improved after starting oral steroids which were reduced over the next 12 months. CART was continued and the patient remained well 5 years later.

Comment: This case illustrates that multiple biopsies from different sites are often taken to confirm the diagnosis, as the differential diagnosis is wide in HIV-positive patients. This case was unusual in that there was no pulmonary involvement, and granulomas in the renal parenchyma are a rare finding in sarcoidosis.

CASE REPORT 2

A 47-year-old white male presented with recent onset of a cough; he was a non-smoker. He had known HIV infection for 14 years and had been taking CART for 10 years. Current CD4 lymphocyte count was 310 cells/µL and viral load was undetectable. Investigations included a chest radiograph and CT scan which showed mediastinal and hilar lymphadenopathy, an elevated SACE and a negative Mantoux tuberculin test. Pulmonary function testing showed FEV_1 71 percent of predicted, FVC 80 percent of predicted, TLco 95 percent of predicted and Kco 128 percent of predicted. Endoscopic ultrasound revealed hypoechoic subcarinal lymph nodes. Biopsy and aspirate of these nodes showed discrete granulomas without necrosis; mycobacterial culture was negative. BAL showed a predominantly lymphocytic infiltrate and was also negative for mycobacterial culture. A presumptive diagnosis of sarcoidosis was made. Repeat CT scanning was performed 4 years later which showed further increase in the lymph node size. Although he remained well and the CD4 lymphocyte count was 300 cells/µL and viral load was undetectable, a repeat bronchoscopy was performed. Transbronchial biopsies showed ill-formed granulomas. In BAL fluid there was a 52 percent lymphocytosis; mycobacterial culture was negative. SACE was 76 and pulmonary function testing was unchanged. A diagnosis of chronic sarcoidosis was made. The patient remained off treatment for this but continued on CART.

Comment: This case shows that sarcoidosis-like IRIS can persist for years without causing any clinically significant pathology or adverse effect on the natural history of HIV infection.

DIAGNOSIS AND MANAGEMENT IN HIV-POSITIVE PATIENTS

IMAGING

The tests used to diagnose sarcoidosis in HIV-infected patients are the same as those used for the HIV-negative general population. Chest radiological findings are similar in both groups. In the retrospective series by Haramati *et al.* (2001), all 10 patients had chest radiograph abnormalities, the most common (70 percent) being mediastinal or hilar lymphadenopathy. Although this was a small series, 90 percent had parenchymal abnormalities on plain chest radiology and by contrast with the general population there was less upper-lobe predominance. CT findings also appear to be very similar with nodules ranging from 0.5 to 1 cm distributed along the bronchovascular bundles, subpleurally and interlobular septae being the most common abnormality. If atypical CT findings are present (e.g. cavitation), this should provoke a search to exclude alternative or co-existing pathology, such as an opportunistic infection.

Pulmonary fibrosis has not been described in HIV-infected sarcoidosis patients radiologically. However, given

Table 36.3 Investigations undertaken in case reports/series of sarcoidosis in HIV patients.

Reference	At sarcoidosis diagnosis CD4 (cells/µL)	Viral load (copies/mL)	CXR stage	Biopsy site	SACE (N 8–52 U/l)	Mantoux	BAL lymphocyte (%)	BAL CD4/CD8	Lung function pattern
Ailani et al.	231	ND	I	TBB	NR	NR	NR	16	NR
Almeida et al.	435	NR	III	TBB	56	NR	72	1.4	Restrictive
Amin et al.	200 900	NR	1 III 1 I	1 TBB 2 Kveim 1 Skin	119 Normal	NR	NR	NR	2 Normal
Blanche et al.	183	ND	III	Lung Liver Salivary gland	105	NR	52	0.65	NR
Coots et al.	666	NR	I	Med LN Lung	NR	Negative	NR	NR	NR
Ferrand et al.	500	ND	0	Parotid Kidney	110	Negative	NR	NR	NR
Foulon et al.	Median 418 ± 234 Range 166–771	<20–31 000	2 I 4 II 5 III	9 Lung 2 Skin 3 Med LN	Increased in 5	10 Negative 1 NR	37	Post 0.65, 2 IRIS 3.5	3 Restrictive 1 Obstructive 7 Normal
Gomez et al.	235	ND	I	TBB	NR	Negative	NR	NR	NR
Gowda et al.	570	NR	II	TBB	57	NR	NR	NR	Normal
Granieri et al.	110	NR	II	TBB Med LN	80	Negative	NR	NR	NR

Haramati et al.	Mean 213 Range 25–390	NR	1 I, 6 II, 3 III	8 TBB, 1 Lung, 1 Med LN	Increased in 5 of 6	NR	NR	NR	NR
Hill et al.	>700	ND	I	Cx LN	NR	NR	NR	NR	NR
Lassalle et al.	Median 273.5 Range 208–333	NR	NR	2 Skin, 7 Med LN, 5 Cx LN	NR	NR	NR	NR	NR
Lee et al.	NR	NR	NR	NR	NR	NR	NR	NR	NR
Lenner et al.	253	<40	III	TBB		NR	NR	NR	Restrictive
	371	ND	III	TBB		NR	NR	NR	Restrictive
Morris et al.	Median 383 Range 210–916	NR	3 I, 1 II, 3 III	2 Lung, 3 Skin, 2 LN	NR	NR	NR	NR	NR
Naccache et al.	219	<500	III	TBB	>100	Negative	45	7.7	NR
	318	<500	III	TBB	>100	Negative	46	5	Restrictive
Newman et al.	310	NR	II	TBB	NR	NR	70	0.09	Restrictive
Okosun et al	103	NR	NR	1 Bone marrow, 1 Liver	139	NR	NR	NR	NR
Papadaki et al.	NR	NR	NR	Conjunctival	NR	Negative	NR	NR	NR
Trevenzoli et al.	510	3500	II	Skin	200	Negative	9	1.2	NR
Viani	441	nd	II	Liver, Kidney, Duodenum	NR	NR	Lymphocytic	2.3	Restrictive
Whitlock et al.	NR	NR	NR	Med LN (pre)	NR	Negative	28	0.34	Normal
Wittram et al.	550	<50	III	Lung	NR	NR	NR	NR	Restrictive

BAL, bronchoalveolar lavage; CART, combined antiretroviral therapy; Cx LN, cervical lymph node; CXR stage, Scadding chest radiograph stage; EN, erythema nodosum; IRIS, immune reconstitution inflammatory syndrome; LN, lymph node; Med LN, mediastinal lymph node; MSM, men who have sex with men NA, not applicable; ND, not detected; NR, not recorded; PostTx, post transfusional; SACE, serum angiotensin–converting enzyme; TBB, transbronchial biopsy.

that this appearance usually results from chronic disease it could reflect lead-time bias in that patients are identified early and duration of follow-up has been limited. In one case report an open lung biopsy revealed pulmonary fibrosis (Wittram et al. 2001). Gallium-67 scanning has been used to assess extrathoracic and pulmonary involvement in HIV-infected patients with sarcoidosis; however, ^{18}F-fluorodeoxy-glucose positron emission tomography (18FDG PET) has not been described, despite its role in diagnosis of other HIV-associated infectious and malignant processes.

HISTOLOGY

The differential diagnosis of sarcoidosis is much larger in the context of HIV infection, so histological confirmation of well-formed non-caseating granulomas is required to make the diagnosis – although these may be less well formed as immunodeficiency progresses (Morris et al. 2003). Even in an HIV-positive patient on CART who presented with a clinical pattern of Löfgren's syndrome, in which a diagnosis of sarcoidosis without biopsy might be reasonably made, Gomez and colleagues confirmed granulomas on a trans-bronchial biopsy even though there was no parenchymal disease on CT scanning (Gomez et al. 2000). In the case reports reviewed, lung biopsies were the site most commonly positive for granulomas where the route of sampling was specified, which were as follows: 18 transbronchial biopsies, one CT-guided core needle lung biopsy of a lung nodule, and two open lung biopsies. The second most common positive biopsy site was mediastinal lymph nodes. Endobronchial ultrasound is an increasingly available and relatively non-invasive method, compared to mediastinoscopy, of sampling mediastinal lymph nodes and has a high yield for sarcoidosis and can be combined with other bronchoscopic sampling techniques (see Chapter 11). Bronchoalveolar lavage is often performed and can provide supportive evidence with a lymphocytosis and high CD4/CD8 lymphocyte ratio, although, as discussed above, the reverse is the usual pattern in patients not receiving CART. Other sites that have been successfully biopsied include skin, cervical lymph node, parotid, liver, bone marrow and conjunctiva.

Even if granulomas are confirmed, rigorous exclusion of other causes needs to be undertaken, particularly infectious causes of granulomatous disease such as *Cryptococcus neoformans*, *Histoplasma capsulatum*, *P. jirovecii*, mycobacterial infection including *Mycobacterium avium* complex, and *M. tuberculosis*, and protozoal infection including *Toxoplasma gondii*. In a retrospective review of 474 cases with a final pathological diagnosis of 'granulomas' reported between 1994 and 2002, Morris et al. (2003) identified 150 with no obvious pathological cause, of whom 24 were found to be HIV-infected. Detailed review of these 24 cases revealed a cause for the granulomas in 16: *M. avium* complex (4), *M. tuberculosis* (3), *Mycobacterium fortuitum* (1), *Mycobacterium leprae* (1), chronic *Staphylococcus aureus* lymphadenitis (1), hypersensitivity pneumonitis (1), lymphoma (2), and non-sarcoidal granulomatous dermatitis (3). One case was excluded, which left seven HIV-infected patients with a diagnosis of sarcoidosis. That mycobacterial

disease is well represented in this differential diagnosis perhaps underlines the usefulness of Mantoux testing. All HIV-infected patients with sarcoidosis who have had tuberculin tests performed have been found to be anergic. Conversely, Hill and associates report a case of sarcoidosis in an HIV-infected patient whose lymph node biopsy was initially incorrectly reported as showing budding yeast forms; on subsequent review these were found to be Hamazaki–Wesenberg bodies (Hill et al. 2003). The most common condition in which these are found is sarcoidosis, present in up to 68 percent of cases, but they can be found in normal lymph nodes. These bodies are differentiated from fungi as they are present within the sinusoids and not the granulomas, vary in size, and are not associated with an inflammatory response.

OTHER TESTS

The SACE in patients with dual diagnosis is significantly elevated in about 50 percent of cases, showing similar inconsistencies to those observed among the HIV-negative general population with sarcoidosis.

TREATMENT AND PROGNOSIS

Treatment

Treatment for HIV-infected patients with sarcoidosis follows the same principles as for treatment in the general population. Of note there are significant drug interactions between protease inhibitor drugs and corticosteroids, ciclosporin and mycophenolate; additionally there are interactions between mycophenolate and the nucleoside analogs abacavir and zidovudione and non-nucleoside drugs. When using immune-modifying agents to treat sarcoidosis in an HIV-infected patient who is receiving CART, advice should be sought from a specialist pharmacist and clinician who has expertise in the use of CART. Useful information on drug interactions may be obtained from www.hiv_druginteractions.org/.

Prognosis

The prognosis of sarcoidosis in HIV-infected patients is similarly to good that observed in HIV-negative patients. In the 11 cases reviewed by Foulon et al. (2004), three spontaneously resolved completely, two improved and one remained stable without treatment. The remainder were successfully treated with corticosteroids (3), doxycycline for skin lesions (1), and hydroxychloroquine for constitutional symptoms (1). Two cases that relapsed have been reported, one at a dose of prednisolone 10 mg/day and the other after non-adherence with corticosteroid treatment. No complications during long-term corticosteroid treatment, such as reactivation of herpes zoster or tuberculosis, have been reported.

In no cases reported, even in sarcoidosis-like IRIS, has CART had to be stopped. In two patients in whom therapy with subcutaneous interleukin-2 might have been implicated in the pathogenesis of sarcoidosis, cessation of this treatment resulted in remission or stability of the sarcoidosis without need for corticosteroid therapy. In general in patients with both diagnoses, the HIV infection is asymptomatic and stable.

CONCLUSION

The populations at risk of developing sarcoidosis and acquiring HIV are similar. Although uncommon, the two conditions can occur together and this highlights the importance of offering HIV testing to patients with a diagnosis of sarcoidosis. The clinical presentation, investigation, treatment and prognosis in HIV-positive patients appears to be similar to HIV-negative patients, although kidney involvement may be more common. Understanding the immunological response to CART and the development of sarcoidosis-like IRIS provides a unique opportunity to explore the immunopathogenesis of sarcoidosis.

REFERENCES

Ailani J, Graber J, Fagan I et al. (2009). Neurosarcoidosis in a patient with AIDS. AIDS Reader, 17 November.

Almeida FA, Sager JS, Eiger G (2006). Coexistent sarcodiosis and HIV infection: an immunological paradox. J Infect 52: 195–201.

Amin DN, Sperber K, Brown LK et al. (1992). Positive Kveim test in patients with coexisting sarcoidosis and human immunodeficiency virus infection. Chest 101: 1454–6.

Bhaskaran K, Hamouda O, Sannes M et al. (2008). Changes in the risk of death after HIV seroconversion compared with mortality in the general population. J Am Med Assoc 300: 51–9.

Blanche P, Gombert B, Rollot F et al. (2000). Sarcoidosis in a patient with acquired immunodeficiency syndrome treated with interleukin-2. Clin Infect Dis 31: 1493–4.

Connors M, Kovacs JA, Krevat S et al. (1997). HIV induces changes in CD4+T-cell phenotype and depletions within the CD4+ T-cell repertoire that are not immediately restored by antiviral or immune-based therapies. Nat Med 3: 533–40.

Coots L, Lazarus AA (1989). Sarcoidosis diagnosed in a patient with known HIV infection. Chest 96: 201–2.

Corda L, Benerecetti D, Ungari M et al. (1996). Kaposi's disease and sarcoidosis. Eur Respir J 9: 383–5.

Ferrand RA, Cartledge JD, Connolly J et al. (2007). Immune reconstitution sarcoidosis presenting with hypercalcaemia and renal failure in HIV infection. Int J STD AIDS 18: 138–9.

Foulon G, Wislez W, Naccache J-M et al. (2004). Sarcoidosis in HIV-infected patients in the era of highly active antiretroviral therapy. Clin Infect Dis 38: 418–25.

French MA, Lenzo N, John M et al. (2000). Immune restoration disease after the treatment of immunodeficient HIV infected patients with highly active antiretroviral therapy. HIV Med 1(2): 107–15.

Gao X, Nelson GW, Karacki P et al. (2001). Effect of a single amino acid change in MHC class 1 molecules in the rate of progression to AIDS. New Engl J Med 344: 1688–75.

Gomez V, Smith PR, Burack J et al. (2000). Sarcoidosis after antiretroviral therapy in a patient with acquired immunodeficiency syndrome. Clin Infect Dis 31: 1278–80.

Gowda KS, Mayers I, Shafran SD (1990). Concomitant sarcoidosis and HIV infection. Can Med Assoc J 142: 136–7.

Granieri J, Wisniewski JJ, Graham RC et al. (1995). Sarcoid myopathy in a patient with human immunodeficiency virus infection. Southern Med J 88: 591–5.

Hall HI, Song R, Rhodes P et al. (2008a). Estimation of HIV incidence in the United States. J Am Med Assoc 300: 520–9.

Hall HI, An Q, Hutchinson AB, Sansom S (2008b). Estimating the lifetime risk of a diagnosis of the HIV infection in 33 states, 2004–2005. J Acquir Immun Def Synd 49: 294–7.

Haramati LB, Lee G, Singh A et al. (2001). Newly diagnosed pulmonary sarcoidosis in HIV-infected patients. Radiology 218: 242–6.

Hendel H, Caillat-Zucman S, Lebuanec H et al. (1999). New class 1 and class II HLA alleles strongly associate with opposite patterns of progression to AIDS. J Immunol 162: 6942–6.

Hill KA, Till M, Laskin WB (2003). Pulmonary symptoms and lymphadenopathy in a human-immunodeficiency virus-infected woman. Arch Pathol Lab Med 127: 111.

Hunninghake GW, Crystal RG (1981). Pulmonary sarcoidosis: a disorder mediated by excess helper T-lymphcoyte activity at sites of disease activity. New Engl J Med 305: 429–34.

Hunninghake GW, Bedell GN, Zavala DC et al. (1983). Role of interleukin-2 release by lung cells in active pulmonary sarcoidosis. Am Rev Respir Dis 128: 634–8.

Jahn A, Floyd S, Crampin AC et al. (2008). Population-level effect of HIV on adult mortality and early evidence of reversal after introduction of antiretroviral therapy in Malawi. Lancet 371: 1603–11.

Just JJ (1995). Genetic predisposition to HIV-1 infection and acquired immunodeficiency virus syndrome: a review of the literature examining associations with HLA. Hum Immunol 44: 159–66.

Kadakia J, Kiyabu M, Sharma OP et al. (1993). Granulomatous response to Pneumocystis carinii in patients infected with HIV. Sarcoidosis 104: 352–61.

Lassalle S, Selve E, Hofman V et al. (2006). Sarcoid-like lesions associated with the immune restoration inflammatory syndrome in AIDS: absence of polymerase chain reaction detection of Mycobacterium tuberculosis in granulomas isolated by laser capture microdissection. Virchows Arch 449: 689–96.

Lawn SD, Bekker LG, Miller RF (2005). Immune reconstitution disease associated with mycobacterial infections in HIV-infected individuals receiving antiretrovirals. Lancet Infect Dis 5: 361–73.

Lee AK, Chronister CL (1999). Sarcodiosis-related anterior uveitis in a patients with human immunodeficiency virus. J Am Optom Assoc 70: 384–90.

Lenner R, Bregman Z, Teirstein AS et al. (2001). Recurrent pulmonary sarcodiosis in HIV-infected patients receiving highly active antiretroviral therapy. Chest 119: 978–81.

Moore RD, Chaisson RE (1999). Natural history of HIV infections in the era of combination antiretroviral therapy. AIDS 13: 1933–42.

Morris DG, Jasmer RM, Huang L et al. (2003). Sarcoidosis following HIV infection: evidence for CD4+ lymphocyte dependence. Chest 124: 929–35.

Murdoch DM, Venter WDF, van Rie A et al. (2007). Immune reconstitution inflammatory syndrome (IRIS): review of common infectious manifestations and treatment options. AIDS Res Ther 4: 9.

Naccache J-M, Antoine M, Wislez M et al. (1999). Sarcoid-like pulmonary disorder in human immunodeficiency virus-infected patients receiving antiretroviral therapy. Am J Respir Crit Care Med 159: 2009–13.

Newman TG, Minkowitz S, Hanna A et al. (1992). Coexistent sarcoidosis and HIV infection: a comparison of bronchoalveolar and peripheral blood lymphocytes. Chest 102: 1899–901.

Noursadeghi M, Katz DR, Miller RF (2006). HIV-1 infection of mononuclear phagocytic cells: the case for bacterial innate immune deficiency in AIDS. *Lancet Infect Dis* 6: 794–804.

Okosun J, Martin F, Murphy M *et al.* (2008). Sarcoid-like immune restoration inflammatory syndrome (IRIS) presenting with hypercalcaemia and renal failure in HIV infection. *HIV Med* 9(Suppl. 1): 31.

Papadaki TG, Kafkala C, Zacharopoulos IP *et al.* (2006). Conjunctival non-caseating granulomas in a human immunodeficiency virus positive patient attributed to sarcoidosis. *Ocul Immunol Inflamm* 14: 309–11.

Pietinalho A, Hirago Y, Hosoda Y *et al.* (1995). The frequency of sarcoidosis in Finland and Hokkaido, Japan: a comparative epidemiology study. *Sarcoidosis* 12: 61–7.

Poignard P, Sabbe R, Pichio GR *et al.* (1999). Neutralizing antibodies have limited effects on the control of established HIV-1 infection *in vivo*. *Immunity* 10: 431–8.

Rosenberg ES, Billingsley JM, Caliendo AM *et al.* (1997). Vigorous HIV-1 specific CD4+ T-cell responses associated with control of viraemia. *Science* 278: 1447–50.

Sato H, Grutters JC, Pantelides P *et al.* (2002). HLA-DQB1*0201 a marker for good prognosis in British and Dutch patients with sarcoidosis. *Am J Respir Cell Mol Biol* 27: 406–12.

Shelbourne SA, Hamill RJ, Rodriguez-Barradas MC *et al.* (2002). Immune reconstitution inflammatory syndrome during highly active antiretroviral therapy. *Medicine (Baltimore)* 81: 213–27.

Trevenzoli M, Cattelan AM, Marino F *et al.* (2003). Sarcoidosis and HIV infection: a case report and a review of the literature. *Postgrad Med J* 79: 535–8.

Viani RM (2002). Sarcoidosis and interstitial nephritis in a child with acquired immunodeficiency syndrome: implications of immune reconstitution syndrome with indinavir-based regimen. *Paedtr Infect Dis J* 21: 435–8.

Voorter CE, Amicosante M, Berretta F *et al.* (2007). HLA class II amino acid epitopes as susceptibility markers of sarcoidosis. *Tissue Antigens* 70: 18–27.

Whitlock WL, Lowery WS, Dietrich RA (1990). Bronchoalveolar lavage in sarcoidosis and HIV infection. *Chest* 98: 517.

Wittram C, Fogg J, Farber H (2001). Immune restoration syndrome manifested by pulmonary sarcoidosis. *Am J Roentgen* 177: 1427.

Neoplasia, chemotherapy and rare local lesions

STEPHEN SPIRO AND DONALD MITCHELL

INTRODUCTION

The clinical course of sarcoidosis is often prolonged and may be preceded by a varying period in which granulomatous changes are present in various organs without causing symptoms. It is also certain that some individuals go through the entire course of sarcoidosis to spontaneous resolution without symptoms, or with only trivial ones, although granulomas, if sought, would be found in involved organs. Thus it is to be expected that a proportion of patients will show evidence of some other disease during the course of known sarcoidosis; and that also during the investigation of patients found to be suffering from some other disease, evidence of previously unsuspected sarcoidosis will be found occasionally.

The associations of particular interest are, therefore, those that may cause diagnostic difficulty because one disease masks the other; and those in which there is some possibility of a pathogenic relationship through a common immunological, genetic or other factor between sarcoidosis and the other disease, or through some feature of sarcoidosis that predisposes to the other disease. It is important to determine whether these associations occur more frequently than one would expect as if by chance. Because of uncertainty of the total incidence of sarcoidosis, including undiagnosed and asymptomatic cases, estimates of the expected frequency of associations with other diseases are subject to considerable error.

Another source of uncertainty arises from the occurrence of local granulomatous reactions in adjacent tissues and (in particular) lymph nodes to malignant disease. Because of such reactions, convincing evidence of more generalized granulomatosis is required before the additional diagnosis of sarcoidosis is accepted in patients with diseases of these types.

MALIGNANT TUMORS

There is no consistent evidence that the frequency of malignant tumors in general, or of any particular tumor with the possible exception of lymphoma (see below), differs from the general expectation in patients with sarcoidosis. There appears no basis to the suggestion that the immunological peculiarities of sarcoidosis may predispose to tumors. Although there is an abnormality of T-cell function in sarcoidosis which results in diminished ability to express delayed hypersensitivity, this does not impair immune defenses.

A Danish central registry of cases collected between 1962 and 1971 was maintained, and was correlated with the Danish Cancer Registry (Brincker and Wilbeck 1974). Among 2561 registered patients with sarcoid, 65 were also recorded in the cancer register. In 17 of these, the diagnosis of malignant disease preceded that of sarcoidosis. Thus among 2544 patients with sarcoidosis and no previous history of malignant disease, 48 were subsequently registered with malignant disease. This number significantly exceeded the number expected, namely 33.8. The excess was attributed principally to malignant lymphoma of which six cases, 11 times the expected number, were reported; and partly to lung cancer of which nine cases, three times the expected number, were found. Rômer (1978) reviewed these 48 cases through individual case records, and found that the diagnosis of sarcoidosis had not been established in ten, and of cancer in three. Removal of these cases brought the levels of cancers to that expected, while the level of lymphoma remained six times that expected, although there were only three cases. As would be expected if sarcoidosis and cancer occurred together by chance, ages of onset of sarcoidosis in those later found to develop cancer showed a distribution peaking past middle age, 94 percent being over

37

40 years old when sarcoidosis was diagnosed, as compared with the peak in young adult life seen in unselected series of patients with sarcoidosis.

It is probably because the occasional concurrence of a common cancer with sarcoidosis is not unexpected, that many case reports of this concurrence have been reported.

Adrenal pheochromocytoma has been described in a patient with bilateral lymphadenopathy biopsy-proven to be sarcoidosis, and the case of a 20-year-old girl with sarcoidosis associated with fibrolamellar carcinoma of the liver (Pila Pérez et al. 2007; Kim et al. 2009) are almost certainly coincidental. The increased incidence of lung cancer in patients with pulmonary fibrosis is well known and sarcoidosis has also been implicated (Bouros et al. 2002; Sharma and Lamb 2003). In testicular seminomas, relapse in the mediastinum is rare, but there are reports of testicular cancers and sarcoid and/or sarcoid-like processes in the mediastinum, emphasizing the importance of making a histological diagnosis of any mediastinal lymphadenopathy following treatment of testicular tumors (Jegannathen et al. 2009).

The presence of autoimmune disease can be associated with an increased risk of sarcoidosis. In a population-based case–control study in Scandinavia, 32 separate autoimmune and related conditions were identified in individuals with Hodgkin's lymphoma, compared to matched controls (Landgren et al. 2006). They found a significantly increased risk of Hodgkin's associated with personal histories of rheumatoid arthritis, systemic lupus erythematosus, sarcoidosis and a family history of sarcoidosis and of ulcerative colitis. A similar pooled analysis of more than 29 000 participants in Sweden from 12 case–control studies confirmed an association with non-Hodgkin's lymphoma and Sjögren's syndrome, SLE and with hemolytic anemia, but not for sarcoidosis (Ekstrom et al. 2008).

It has also been hypothesized that certain chemotherapeutic agents are associated with an increased risk of sarcoidosis (Merchant et al. 1994; Hurst and Mauro 2005). However, in studies looking at the association of malignancy, treatment and the development of sarcoidosis, there is no clear association between the use of any particular chemotherapeutic agent and sarcoidosis; in fact, many patients who later developed sarcoidosis after treatment for malignancy did not receive any chemotherapy (Hunt et al. 2009).

LYMPHOMA

Brincker (1972), in a survey of 1500 cases of various types of malignant lymphoma, found five in whom the diagnosis of sarcoidosis was made on acceptable grounds, in three before and in two after the lymphoma was diagnosed. Those in whom the sarcoidosis appeared first do not seem especially remarkable; in two chronic lymphatic leukemia was diagnosed 14 and 27 years after erythema nodosum and lymphadenopathy attributed to sarcoidosis, and in the other, Hodgkin's disease developed in a patient with chronic pulmonary sarcoidosis which had been diagnosed 8 years earlier. Of the two in whom lymphoma appeared first, both

had Hodgkin's disease, successfully treated; in one, cutaneous sarcoidosis with radiographic evidence of sarcoid changes in a metatarsal bone appeared 5 years later, and in the other erythema nodosum and bilateral hilar lymphadenopathy (BHL) 17 years later. In both, sarcoid-like granulomas had been seen in the lymph nodes which had provided the initial diagnosis of Hodgkin's disease, or part of a widespread sarcoid granulomatosis that later became clinically apparent.

As mentioned above, Brincker and Wilbek (1974) reported a high incidence of malignant lymphomas in their survey of 2544 patients with sarcoidosis, which, even after review by Rômer (1978) had removed dubious diagnoses, was six times that expected for the general population; the number of cases, however, was only three. Among about 500 cases of sarcoidosis followed by varying periods by Scadding (1972), three developed malignant lymphomas – 1, 9 and 11 years after the initial diagnosis of sarcoidosis which was following a chronic course.

A more recent report from Sweden was a retrospective cohort study testing the hypothesis that there was an increased risk of lymphoma and of lung cancer, as well as cancers of other organs affected by sarcoidosis (Askling et al. 1999). They studied 474 patients diagnosed to have sarcoidosis from an incidence study, and 8541 sarcoidosis patients gathered from the Swedish Inpatient Register over a 30-year period (1964–94). They assessed the relative risks for cancers using the standardized incidence ratio (SIR). The 474 incidence patients were consecutively diagnosed cases at Uppsala University Hospital between 1966 and 1980. Cases were identified either from symptoms or because of regular health screening which included a chest X-ray, and represent all detected cases of pulmonary sarcoidosis in patients older than 15 years in a defined catchment area. The inpatient cohort was all patients in the country admitted to hospital for investigations and treatment in whom a discharge diagnosis of sarcoidosis was reached. All those where the diagnosis seemed uncertain, and all those in whom sarcoidosis was a contributory factor and not the main diagnosis, were excluded, leaving 8541 subjects for follow-up. End of follow-up was date of death, date of diagnosis of cancer, or the end of 1995. In the Uppsala Hospital cohort there were 50 cases of cancer corresponding to an SIR of 1.2 (95 percent confidence interval 0.9–1.6). The risks were higher in men than women (1.5 to 1.1) and similar whether older or younger than 60 years at diagnosis. Five cases of lung cancer occurred, and although the numbers are small, there was a significantly increased risk during the years 5–9 of follow-up (SIR 5.7; CI 1.2–17), but no increase thereafter. Also, five cases of malignant melanoma occurred (SIR 3.3), all after more than 10 years of follow-up. There were three cases of non-melanomatous skin cancers and four of liver cancer (SIR 3.9; CI 1.1–9.9). Two cases of breast cancer occurred against 7.6 expected. There were no cases of Hodgkin's disease but two cases of non-Hodgkin's lymphoma and one case of chronic lymphocytic leukemia.

In the inpatient study, 653 cancers occurred, an SIR of 1.3 (95 percent CI 1.2–1.4). The risk was higher among men than women. The risk for lung cancer was doubled during the first 10 years of follow-up, but decreased to a significant deficit thereafter, perhaps related to the low smoking history of the cohort.

Both melanoma and non-melanomatous skin cancers occurred with greater frequency, and the risk was increased in both genders. There was also an increased risk for stomach cancers, cancers of the small intestine (4 carcinoids), and a small increase in risk of colorectal cancers. Breast, uterine, ovarian, prostatic and testicular cancers occurred at the expected rates, while bladder cancer occurred at less than the expected rate.

For lymphomas, the excess of Hodgkin's disease was confined to the first decade following entry to the cohort, and the risk for non-Hodgkin's (29 cases) followed the same pattern.

This large and interesting study makes the point that the increased incidence of some cancers after sarcoidosis is similar to the rates found after other inflammatory conditions or chronic diseases such as diabetes, inflammatory bowel diseases and rheumatoid arthritis. In lung cancer, misdiagnosis could be an explanation for the early increase in risk, but with its poor prognosis this will not explain the increased risk seen for years 5–9 of follow-up. The same argument should apply to the cases of lymphoma. The reason why both melanomatous and non-melanomatous skin cancers are increased after sarcoidosis is not clear as only non-melanomatous lesions are associated with immunosuppressive therapies. However, skin sarcoid is associated with scarring and this may be the common stimulant. In general, there remains no clear theory why sarcoidosis predisposes to some cancers, albeit in relatively small numbers.

The literature contains many isolated case studies of lymphoma or other hematological malignancy in the presence of previous, established, sarcoidosis. A series of five such cases reported in 1996 followed each patient with a previously apparently secure histological diagnosis of sarcoidosis (Karakantza et al. 1996). The malignancies developed within 18 months and 28 years of the diagnosis of sarcoidosis. The cases comprised non-Hodgkin's lymphoma, Hodgkin's disease, plasmacytoma, large granular lymphocytic lymphoma, and a mantle cell lymphoma. In the first case, when the original histology of the mediastinal lymph node biopsy in which sarcoidosis was diagnosed was reviewed, the diagnosis was revised to non-Hodgkin's lymphoma, and the patient probably never had sarcoidosis. This illustrates the problem of clear histological diagnoses, which is an ever-present factor. Thus four of these five patients represent the 'sarcoidosis–lymphoma' syndrome (Brincker 1986). The three main features are:

- the lymphoid malignancy occurs after a preceding history of sarcoid;
- the median age of onset of sarcoidosis is 10 years above that of unselected patients with the disease;
- Hodgkin's disease occurs more frequently than other types of lymphoma.

The authors of these reports speculate on several pathogenic mechanisms that may predispose to malignancy. Possibly there is sufficient disturbance of the immune system by the initial sarcoidosis to allow malignancy to develop. In sarcoidosis, there is a well-documented increase in CD4+ T-cells and a reduction in CD8+ T-cells within the affected tissues. The CD4+ cells express activation markers and respond vigorously to mitogenic and antigenic stimulation, and spontaneously release interleukin-2 and interferon-α.

The low number of CD8+ T-cells has been interpreted as indicating dysfunction in the immunoregulatory pathways leading to the formation of granulomas. Cytokines released by activated lymphocytes react and stimulate macrophages. Thus in an environment where there is defective regulation by suppressor T-cells, a clone may escape, resulting in the development of a lymphoid malignancy. In this context, this is more likely to happen on the background of chronic rather than acute sarcoidosis. In addition, steroid treatment, a common phenomenon in chronic sarcoidosis, may be another predisposing immunosuppressive factor that can act synergistically with those described above to enhance the malignant process (Karakantza et al. 1996).

An alternative hypothesis suggested by Reich (1985) and quoted by Karakantza is that sarcoid is a generalized cell-mediated immune response to tumor antigens. This may explain in part why true sarcoidosis and reactive, sarcoid-like granuloma formation is associated with the same type of lymphoma, for example Hodgkin's disease. It may also explain why cases of lymphoma arise shortly after the diagnosis of sarcoid, although of course this is not always the case.

LOCAL 'SARCOID' REACTIONS

Localized groups of epitheloid tubercles of sarcoid-type may be observed in a variety of tissues as a response both to foreign bodies and to the infiltrating processes of malignant disease.

Sarcoid-type tubercles may be found in lymph nodes draining malignant tumors (Nickerson 1937; Gorton and Linell 1957), or a bronchial adenoma (Anderson 1942; Symmers 1951) and also within ovarian tumors (Schattenburg and Harris 1946). These localized granulomas may be a stromal reaction to a lipoid produced by a tumor and may depend on the response pattern of the subject.

Similar granulomas have been found in association with Hodgkin's disease and other lymphomas (Nickerson 1937; Kadin et al. 1970; Brincker 1972) in both lymph nodes and other tissues affected by the lymphoma, as well as not so affected tissues. Kadin and associates performed multiple biopsies at staging laparotomy in 185 patients with Hodgkin's disease, and found granulomatous reactions in 31 of them; of these, eight were in tissues affected by Hodgkin's disease and 23 in not so affected areas. Among these 23, granulomas were found in the liver in 17, spleen in 17, and in lymph nodes in 5 (Kadin et al. 1970). In no case was there clinical evidence of sarcoidosis, but there was no long-term follow-up report. Brincker surveyed 1500 cases of malignant lymphoma and found epithelioid granulomas in 19. Of these, five showed evidence of generalized sarcoidosis. In the remaining 14, there was no clinical evidence of sarcoidosis during follow-up periods of up to 7 years. Granulomas were found in tissues affected by lymphoma in 11, and in unaffected tissues in 7, both showing granulomas in 4. In ten of the 14, the lymphoma was classified as Hodgkin's disease (Brincker 1972).

The histology of local sarcoid reactions may be indistinguishable from that of generalized sarcoidosis, and may be so extensive within an affected lymph node or may be even more widely disseminated so as to be misleading. Diagnosis depends on search for evidence of granulomas at other sites and for a possible cause for a local reaction.

Local sarcoid reactions have been described in association with a plethora of tumor types, including lymphomas, breast cancer, primary lung cancer, renal cell, ovarian and stomach cancers. They are defined by their limited distribution. Much less commonly, multi-organ granulomas consistent with systemic sarcoidosis develop simultaneously or shortly following the development of cancer, or following chemotherapy. The most established associations are with testicular cancer and lymphoma. In these situations, sarcoidosis usually presents with mediastinal or hilar lymphadenopathy, or occasionally with pulmonary interstitial infiltrates or nodules. Both the primary malignancy and the associated granulomatous nodules from sarcoidosis may demonstrate ^{18}F-fluorodeoxyglucose (FDG) uptake on PET scanning. In these cases, the diagnosis of sarcoidosis is usually established by mediastinal biopsy, or open lung biopsy because of the concern of recurrent malignancy.

A review of mediastinoscopies in 565 patients collected over a 5-year period in Seattle, where all were investigated for mediastinal adenopathy, found that there were 41 biopsy-proven cases of sarcoidosis, of which 21 were diagnosed after a diagnosis of cancer. Although, historically, sarcoidosis has been associated with Hodgkin's disease and testicular cancer (Brincker 1986; Merchant et al. 1994; Parra et al. 2004), in this study there were 10 cases of breast cancer and only 2 with Hodgkin's disease (Hunt et al. 2009). The patients with sarcoidosis were predominantly female and only a third were smokers. The average time between a diagnosis of cancer and then sarcoid was 3 years. The patients with sarcoidosis alone were younger than those who had cancer. Most of the patients also had a PET/CT with positive nodal uptake in the range of SUV 4–15, similar to uptake in malignancy.

CONCLUSION

In lymphoma, particularly Hodgkin's lymphoma, there does appear to be an association of greater risk in the presence of sarcoidosis. This is less clear-cut for non-Hodgkin's disease. Solid cancers are common and the association with previous sarcoidosis is likely to be fortuitous. There is no evidence that cancer chemotherapy predisposes to sarcoidosis. However, there is a strong suggestion that sarcoidosis may be more common in patients with established autoimmune diseases. The immunological link between sarcoidosis and malignancy, if any, is far from clear.

REFERENCES

Anderson WM (1942). Bronchial adenoma with metastases to the liver. J Thorac Surg 12: 351–60.

Askling J, Grunewald J, Eklund A et al. (1999). Increased risk for cancer following sarcoidosis. Am J Respir Crit Care Med 160: 1668–72.

Bouros D, Hatzakis K, Lambrakis H, Zeibecoglou K (2002). Association of malignancy with diseases causing interstitial pulmonary changes. Chest 121: 1278–89.

Brincker H (1972). Sarcoid reactions and sarcoidosis in Hodgkin's disease and other malignant lymphomata. Br J Cancer 26: 120–8.

Brincker H (1986). The sarcoidosis–lymphoma syndrome. Br J Cancer 54: 467–73.

Brincker H, Wilbeck E (1974). The incidence of malignant tumors in patients with respiratory sarcoidosis. Br J Cancer 29: 247–51.

Ekstrom SK, Vajdic CM, Falster M et al. (2008). Autoimmune disorders and risk of non-Hodgkin lymphoma subtypes: a pooled analysis within the InterLymph Consortium. Blood 111: 4029–38.

Gorton G, Linell AG (1957). Malignant tumors and sarcoid reactions in regional lymph nodes. Acta Radiol 47: 381–92.

Hunt BM, Vallieres E, Buduhan G et al. (2009). Sarcoidosis as a benign cause of lymphadenopathy in cancer patients. Am J Surg 197: 629–32.

Hurst EA, Mauro T (2005). Sarcoidosis associated with PEGylated interferon alpha and ribavarin treatment for chronic hepatitis C: a case report and review of the literature. Arch Dermatol 141: 865–8.

Jegannathen A, Taylor MB, Jones M, Logue JP (2009). Testicular seminoma with mediastinal lymphadenopathy: a diagnostic pitfall. Br J Radiol 82: e85–6.

Kadin ME, Donaldson SS, Dorfman RF (1970). Isolated granulomas in Hodgkin's disease. New Engl J Med 283: 859–61.

Karakantza M, Matutes E, MacLennon K et al. (1996). Association between sarcoidosis and lymphoma revisited. J Clin Path 49: 208–12.

Kim KA, Kim SW, Park G et al. (2009). Simultaneous adrenal pheochromocytoma and sarcoidosis. South Med J 102: 537–41.

Landgren O, Engels EA, Pfeiffer RM et al. (2006). Autoimmunity and suspceptibility to Hodgkin lymphoma: a population-based case–control study in Scandanavia. J Natl Cancer Inst 98: 1321–30.

Merchant TE, Filippa DA, Yahalom J (1994). Sarcoidosis following chemotherapy for Hodgkin's disease. Leuk Lymphoma 13: 339–47.

Nickerson DA (1937). Boeck's sarcoid: report of 6 cases in which autopsies were made. Arch Pathol 24: 19–29.

Parra ER, Canzian M, Saber AM et al. (2004). Pulmonary and mediastinal 'sarcoidosis' following surgical resection of cancer. Pathol Res Pract 200: 701–5.

Pila Pérez PR, Pelaez R, Rosales TP et al. (2007). Sarcoidosis and fibrolamellar carcinoma of the liver. Ann Med Interna 24: 431–4.

Reich J (1985). Acute myeloblastic leukaemia and sarcoidosis. Cancer 55: 366–9.

Rômer FK (1978). Sarcoidosis and cancer: a critical view. In: Jones Williams W, Davies BH (eds). Proceedings of the 8th International Conference on Sarcoidosis and Other Granulomatous Diseases. Alpha Omega, Cardiff, pp. 567–71.

Scadding JG (1972). Skin infiltrations in 500 cases of sarcoidosis. Praxis 61: 133–6.

Schattenberg HJ, Harris WH (1946). Malignant granulosa-cell tumor with pseudo-tubercles. Am J Pathol 22: 539–49.

Sharma OP, Lamb C (2003). Cancer in interstitial pulmonary fibrosis and sarcoidosis. Curr Opin Pulm Med 9: 398–401.

Symmers WStC (1951). Localized tuberculoid granulomas associated with carcinoma: their relationship to sarcoidosis. Am J Pathol 27: 493–521.

Antibody deficiency

PETER KELLEHER AND ROBERT WILSON

INTRODUCTION

Primary immunodeficiency disorders (PIDs) comprise many diseases caused by genetic defects affecting the immune system. Over the last 25 years, 214 diseases have been identified with more than 120 genetic defects identified to date (Notarangelo et al. 2007). The incidence of PIDs is low, but their prevalence can range from 1 in 500 to 1 in 500 000 in the general population depending on clinical awareness and medical resources available in different countries. Multi-organ granulomatous disease of unknown etiology can occur in a number of PID including common variable immune deficiency (CVID), severe combined immunodeficiency, ataxia telangiectasia, Wiskott Aldrich syndrome and unclassified combined immunodeficiency. All these conditions are characterized by functional defects in the humoral and cell mediated immune systems. It remains a matter of debate as to whether granulomatous disease associated with PID represents an immune response to an as yet unidentified pathogen, the occurrence of sarcoidosis in an immune deficient patient, or in the case of CVID a unique disease. CVID is the most common symptomatic PID affecting adults, so this chapter will largely concentrate on granulomatous disease in CVID.

EPIDEMIOLOGY

Common variable immune deficiency is the most common clinically relevant PID. The European Society for Immunodeficiencies (ESID) internet-based database on distribution of PID shows that 20.7 percent of patients have CVID (Gathmann et al. 2009). The incidence of CVID is believed to be 1 in 75 000 live births with an estimated prevalence in Europe and North America between 1 per 25 000 and 1 per 200 000 individuals (Park et al. 2008). In the UK it is likely that one in four consultant physicians and one in fifteen general practitioners will see a patient with CVID during their working life. Males and females are equally affected. Age at presentation has a bimodal distribution: patients can present in early childhood or in the second or third decade of adult life. A large US cohort of 248 patients with CVID showed that the mean age of onset of symptoms was 23 years for males and 28 years for females (Cunningham-Rundles and Bodian 1999). As in other studies there was a significant delay in diagnosis of CVID from onset of symptoms, with a mean age at diagnosis of 29 and 33 years for males and females, respectively.

Almost all epidemiological data on CVID are derived from Caucasian populations of European origin. Although this may reflect ascertainment bias, as a result of differences in access to medical care, it is likely that the prevalence of CVID will be influenced by ethnic background. In the New York cohort of 248 CVID patients there were only 4 black Americans and 11 Hispanics, the remaining patients being Caucasians of European origin (Cunningham-Ruddles and Bodian 1999). IgA deficiency shares similar genetic susceptibility factors; in some cases it can evolve over time into CVID and is more common in first-degree relatives of patients with CVID than in the general population. There is significant variability in the prevalence of IgA deficiency in different ethnic groups, ranging from about 165 per 100 000 in Caucasians to 5.5 per 100 000 in the Japanese population (Hammarstrom *et al.* 2000).

THE GENETICS OF CVID

Monogenic defects in CVID have been found in 10–20 percent of patients (Park *et al.* 2008). The first genetic defect described in CVID was in the gene for the inducible co-stimulator (ICOS) molecule which encodes a protein on T-cells that promotes germinal center B-cell maturation and differentiation (Grimbacher *et al.* 2003). Patients with ICOS deficiency have low B-cells, few or absent memory B-cells, and impaired T-cell-dependent class switch. Clinical features include recurrent bacterial infections, autoimmune neutropenia, intestinal lymphoid hyperplasia, splenomegaly, and neoplasia (Salzer *et al.* 2004).

ICOS mutations are uncommon in CVID and the numbers of patients described to date are too small to allow any conclusions to be made regarding any association with granulomatous disease. The most common mutation identified in CVID is in a gene called TNFRSF13B which encodes the transmembrane activator and calcium-modulating interactor (TACI) (Bacchelli *et al.* 2007). The TACI protein is a member of the TNF receptor superfamily and is involved in the regulation of memory B-cell survival. Patients with TACI mutation have reduced memory B-cells, impaired T-cell-independent class switch recombination, and B-cell lymphoproliferation. The clinical phenotype includes recurrent bacterial infection, autoimmune disease and splenomegaly, but there have been no reports of granulomatous disease. Two other mutations in genes encoding CD19 and the B-cell activation factor of the TNF family receptor (BAFF-R) have been described in CVID, but they account for less than 1 percent of all cases and granulomatous disease has not been noted in individuals with these disorders (Bacchelli *et al.* 2007). Although a small proportion of patients with CVID have a single gene defect, it is likely that there is a large group of patients who have a polygenic disorder resulting from genetic susceptibility factors and environmental triggers.

IMMUNOLOGY

Protective humoral immune responses involve close cooperation between antigen-presenting cells (APCs) and antigen-specific T- and B-cells within germinal centers of secondary lymphoid tissue. Studies of the immune system in patients with CVID show multiple phenotypic and functional abnormalities involving B-cells, T-cells, natural killer cells, macrophages, monocytes and dendritic cells. This, in part, reflects the enormous complexity of the immune system and the fact that CVID is a heterogeneous condition with varying phenotypes.

The cause of granulomas in CVID is not known. The role of recurrent or persistent infection has been investigated with no great success to date. A number of immunological findings – including alteration in function of cells of the innate immune system (reduced dendritic cell numbers and function and macrophage activation), abnormal T-cell counts/function, and impairment in B-cell maturation – have been associated with the presence of granulomas in CVID. Some of the disturbances in the immune system that have been described are likely to play a significant role in the development of tissue granulomas.

Infections

Granulomas are known to develop in response to microbial or insoluble agents and some infections (EBV, congenital CMV, rubella) that can give rise to antibody deficiency (Conley *et al.* 1999). As the lungs are commonly involved in CVID, clinical investigators have searched for environmental agents that could trigger this condition. Most granulomas in CVID patients are non-caseating, but there have reports of caseating granulomas, raising the possibility that some cases of this condition may be caused by a microbial agent. A case of CVID with granulomatous and lymphoproliferative disease following acute *Toxoplasma gondii* infection has been described in a 12-year-old girl (Mrusek *et al.* 2004). In 2005, a study from Denver showed the presence of human herpes virus 8 (HHV-8) in pulmonary and bone marrow samples of some CVID with granulomatous lymphocytic interstitial lung disease (Wheat *et al.* 2005). The results of this study were not confirmed by other investigators and in most patients with CVID no microorganism has yet been identified.

The issue of the role, if any, of infections in the pathogenesis of CVID remains to be clarified, although in time the use of more sophisticated means to identify microbes may provide more information on this matter.

Abnormalities of the innate immune system in CVID

In recent years a number of research groups have shown there are defects in antigen-presenting cells and function in CVID. Dendritic cells (DCs) are antigen-presenting cells derived from bone marrow. There are two main dendritic cell subsets:

- myeloid dendritic cells which secrete the cytokine IL-12, promote Th1 CD4 cytokine responses (IL-2 and IFN-α) and facilitate the provision of CD4 T-cell help to B-cells in the germinal center of lymph nodes to produce class-switched immunoglobulin;
- plasmacytoid dendritic cells which traffic directly from blood to the lymph nodes, secrete the cytokine IFN-α which can act directly on B-cells and in conjunction with other circulating cytokines and Toll-like receptor ligands induce class-switched immunoglobulin synthesis in the absence of T-cell help.

Dendritic cells and other antigen-presenting cells such as monocytes/macrophages express proteins known as Toll-like receptors (TLRs). These receptors bind to invariant microbial structures expressed by bacteria, viruses and fungi and initiate a complex set of immune responses, including T- and B-cell activation and the elimination of pathogens by neutrophils and monocytes/macrophages.

Several groups have shown that myeloid and plasmacytoid DC counts are reduced in patients with CVID and are associated with granulomatous disease (Viallard *et al.* 2005; Yong *et al.* 2008). One factor that may increase the likelihood of granulomatous disease in CVID patients is a defect in TLR9 signaling as TLR9 knockout mice have increased granuloma formation after challenge with mycobacterial antigens (Ito *et al.* 2007). A recent study has shown that activation of plasmacytoid DC and B-cells in CVID patients by the TLR9 agonist CpG DNA is impaired in CVID and, if confirmed, this may potentially be important in the future management of this condition (Cunningham-Rundles *et al.* 2006). IL-12 is a cytokine believed to be important in the development of granulomatous inflammation. Data on the role of IL-12 in CVID are conflicting, but increased intracellular IL-12 expression by monocytes has been described in patients with CVID (Cambronero *et al.* 2000). However, other studies have identified a defect in IL-12 secretion by DC in CVID patients (Bayry *et al.* 2004; Cunningham-Rundles and Radigan 2005). Some of the discrepancies may be explained by the fact that regulation of IL-12 may vary in different cell types, the failure to discriminate between IL-12 and IL-23, and the difference in patient populations studied and experimental techniques used. The relationship between alteration in IL-12 secretion and disease complications has not yet been formally assessed.

As TNF-α plays a key role in formation and maintenance of granulomas in animal models and human disease, this cytokine has attracted a lot of attention in CVID. The absence of TNF or TNF receptors in experimental models is associated with defective granuloma formation due to inefficient dendritic cell function and lack of T-cell infiltration (Roach *et al.* 2002). It is clear that patients with the granulomatous complication of CVID have a distinct immunological profile characterized by macrophage activation. A small study of CVID patients found that granulomas were associated with reduced CD4 T-cell counts and splenomegaly. Increased serum neopterin (a marker of macrophage activation), elevated concentration of TNF-α and both forms of the soluble TNF-α (p50 and p75) receptors were seen in this CVID patient subset (Aukrust *et al.* 1996). A UK multicenter study showed that CVID patients with granulomatous disease were more likely to have an unusual TNF-α allele (TNF + 488A), compared to other patients without this complication, although TNF-α protein concentration was not determined (Mullighan *et al.* 1997).

T–cell dysfunction in CVID

Defects in the phenotype and function of T-cells in patients with CVID have been recognized over the last 40 years. The presence of granulomas is strongly associated with reduced CD4 T-cell counts, depletion of naive CD4 T-cells (CD4 + CD45RA + CD62L +), increased CD8 + CD57 + percentage, and reduced T-cell proliferative responses (Mechanic *et al.* 1997; Mullighan *et al.* 1997; Cunningham-Rundles and Bodian 1999).

Other features of T-cell dysfunction in CVID include increased expression of markers of cellular apoptosis, restriction of the T-cell receptor repertoire, defects in early T-cell receptor-protein tyrosine phosphorylation (failure to recruit ZAP-70 to the TCR complex, secondary to reduced *Vav1* expression, reduced lipid raft formation), and impairment of TNF receptor p75 activation (Paccani *et al.* 2005; Aspalter *et al.* 2007; Giovanetti *et al.* 2007).

A limited number of patients have been studied to date and the relationship between observed functional T-cell defects and granulomatous disease needs further confirmation. Alteration in T-cell-derived cytokines including IL-2, IL-4, IL-7, IL-10 and IFN-α have been noted in CVID patients. Increased expression of IFN-α has been detected in CVID with low numbers of naive CD4 T-cells: an immune defect associated with the presence of granulomatous disease (Aspalter *et al.* 2007).

B-CELL DEFECTS IN CVID

One of the hallmarks of CVID is failure of terminal B-cell maturation resulting in decreased synthesis of IgG and IgA antibodies. The interaction between T- and B-cells in lymph node germinal centers gives rise to class-switch recombination which generates IgG, IgA and IgE antibodies and somatic hypermutation, resulting in development of high-affinity antibodies.

There has been considerable progress in the use of cell surface proteins to identify antigen experienced memory B-cells. CD27 is a well-accepted biomarker which can distinguish between circulating blood naive (CD19 + CD27−) and memory (CD19 + CD27 +) B-cells. The expression of immunoglobulin isotypes can be used to characterize subsets of memory B-cells into class-switched memory B-cells (CD19 + CD27 + IgM−IgD−) which respond to T-cell-dependent protein antigens and marginal zone-like or IgM memory cells (CD19 + CD27 + IgM + IgD) that are involved in the generation of T-cell independent carbohydrate immune responses. In healthy adults almost all circulating B-cells express high levels of the complement receptor 2 protein (CD21) which is one of the subunits of the B-cell receptor complex. Activated B-cells have reduced expression of CD21, increased levels of inflammatory chemokines and preferentially home to sites of tissue inflammation. Increased numbers of CD21low B-cells have been identified in patients with autoimmune diseases such as systemic lupus erythematosus (SLE) and rheumatoid arthritis, as well as in CVID patients (Kim and Berek 2000; Warnatz *et al.* 2002; Wehr *et al.* 2004).

Numerous studies have shown that the composition of distinct peripheral blood B-cell subsets in patients with CVID is markedly different from that seen in healthy adults. The most consistent findings observed have been a marked reduction in class-switched (CD19 + IgM−IgD−CD27 +) memory B-cells (80 percent of CVID patients) and an expansion of CD21low B-cells (Warnatz *et al.* 2002; Piqueras *et al.* 2003; Sanchez-Ramon *et al.* 2008; Wehr *et al.* 2008). A number of studies of patients with CVID have shown an association between a reduction in class-switched memory B-cells and the presence of granulomatous disease (Warnatz *et al.* 2002; Piqueras *et al.* 2003; Sanchez-Ramon *et al.* 2008; Wehr *et al.* 2008). It is possible that impaired B-cell maturation may be a contributory factor to the development of granulomatous disease in CVID. One study has also found that increased CD21low B-cells were more commonly observed in granulomatous CVID compared with patients who had other CVID disease complications (Warnatz *et al.* 2002). In CVID patients with increased numbers of circulating CD21low B-cells, there was preferential accumulation of CD21low B-cells in bronchoalveolar space compared with lymph nodes or spleen, which indicates that this B-cell subset may also play an important role in the development of pulmonary inflammatory responses (Rakhmanov *et al.* 2009).

CLINICAL PRESENTATIONS

CVID is a disorder characterized by low serum antibody levels, poor antibody responses and recurrent bacterial infections. CVID patients have a high incidence of autoimmune disease, lymphoid proliferation and malignancy. Some patients develop granulomatous inflammation with non-caseating granulomas in the lungs, spleen, skin, lymph nodes, eyes and other parts of the body (Bronsky and Dunn 1965; Fasano *et al.* 1996; Mechanic *et al.* 1997; Martinez-Garcia *et al.* 2001; Artac *et al.* 2009). In general these cases do less well. There may be a subgroup of patients who are characterized by histological appearances of lymphocytic interstitial pneumonia, lymphoid hyperplasia or follicular bronchiolitis in association with granulomatous inflammation who have a worse prognosis (Bates *et al.* 2004). There is a spectrum of disease ranging from isolated granulomatous inflammation in a single organ, to widespread granulomatous inflammation at several sites that may be difficult to distinguish from the usual clinical syndrome of sarcoidosis. There are, however, a number of clinical, laboratory and radiological features of granulomatous CVID that may be helpful in distinguishing this condition from sarcoidosis (Table 38.1).

The majority of patients presenting for the first time with granulomatous CVID involving the lung give a history of recurrent infections due to CVID, rather than, or in addition to, symptoms characteristic of sarcoidosis such as breathlessness. Infections caused by encapsulated bacteria, such as *Streptococcus pneumoniae*, non-typeable *Haemophilus influenzae* and *Moraxella catarrhalis*, occur in the upper and/or lower respiratory tracts.

Pneumonia is the most common presenting feature of CVID (Webster 2005). Recurrent bacterial pneumonia should always lead to consideration of an underlying immunodeficiency. Bronchitis with purulent sputum production occurs much more frequently, and because the illness is less serious it is unlikely to be investigated until the symptoms have recurred over a prolonged period. The damage caused by repeated infections leads to the development of bronchiectasis, and at this time the symptoms of cough productive of purulent sputum may have become chronic. Symptoms of rhinosinusitis include nasal blockage, purulent anterior and posterior nasal discharge, and facial pain. Other prominent infectious complications in CVID include otitis media, giardia, salmonella and campylobacter enteritis and cutaneous herpes zoster (Cunningham-Rundles and Bodian 1999; Oksenhendler *et al.* 2008). When a patient with known CVID subsequently develops granulomatous inflammation in the lung, the onset may be insidious, with worsening cough that is usually dry, and increased breathlessness leading to reduced exercise tolerance (Webster 2005). Granulomatous disease in CVID can be found in association with autoimmunity, in particular immune thrombocytopenic purpura, (ITP) or autoimmune hemolytic anemia (AIHA) (Ardeniz and Cunningham-Rundles 2009).

The estimated prevalence of granulomatous inflammation in CVID has varied in different series (8–22 percent) and is influenced by geographic region and physician willingness to perform relevant tissue biopsy. The largest single-center cohort of granulomatous disease in CVID has recently been reported by Ardeniz and Cunningham-Rundles (2009). The authors described clinical and laboratory characteristics of

Table 38.1   Comparison of clinical, radiological and laboratory features in sarcoidosis and CVID (Arnold *et al.* 2008).

	Sarcoidosis	CVID granulomatous disease
Recurrent infections	No	Yes
Dyspnea	Yes	Yes
Autoimmune disease	Not usually present	Common
Serum immunoglobulins	Polyclonal increase in IgG and IgA	Low IgG and IgA and/or IgM
Primary antibody response failure	No specific studies	Low antibody post test immunization
Raised ACE levels	Common	Uncommon
IL-12/23 expression by APC	Increased	Decreased
T-cell dysfunction	Common	Common
B-cell differentiation	No specific studies	Failure of B-cell maturation
Pulmonary function test	Restrictive and reduced gas transfer	Restrictive and reduced gas transfer
Splenomegaly on ultrasound	15%	Very common
Chest radiology	Bilateral hilar lymphadenopathy: fibrosis	Bronchiectasis, fibrosis
Treatment	Steroids/none	IgG/steroids/antibiotics

ACE, angiotensin-converting enzyme; APC, antigen-presenting cell; CVID, common variable immune deficiency.

37 patients with granulomatous CVID (defined on biopsy) in a patient cohort of 455. The median age at diagnosis was 26 years (range 2–59) and almost 40 percent (14 patients) had granulomas 1–18 years before diagnosis of CVID. As noted previously, the lungs were the most common site of granulomatous disease, but 20 percent of patients had no evidence of symptomatic or radiological lung disease. Auto-immune disease, in particular idiopathic thrombocytopenic purpura (ITP), was commonly found in patients with granulomatous CVID. Over a 25-year follow-up there was no significant difference in mortality in patients with granulomatous CVID compared with other CVID patient subgroups, and patients with lung granulomas had a similar mortality to those with granulomas in other tissues.

In a separate study, 18 patients were selected from a CVID clinic on the basis of lung function abnormalities and/or histologically proven granulomatous disease (Park *et al.* 2005). Thirteen patients had diffuse reticulation, which varied from fine to coarse with features of fibrosis. Nodules were found in eight patients, usually associated with reticulation. This study suggests that granulomatous inflammation in CVID is prone to cause fibrosis. Bronchiectasis was found as the only abnormality in three patients and in association with reticulation/nodules in another three. Therefore, in 33 percent of patients bronchiectasis had developed at the time of assessment. This is a lower frequency of bronchiectasis than is found in a general CVID population, a fact that has been noted in another study (Torrigan *et al.* 2008). One possible explanation is that granulomatous CVID is a more symptomatic condition that presents earlier, before serious or repeated infections cause bronchiectasis.

INVESTIGATIONS

The chest radiograph in multi-organ granulomatous CVID (Fig. 38.1) may suggest a diagnosis of sarcoidosis, but in

addition there may be changes caused by infection such as pneumonia or bronchiectasis. In these circumstances, particularly if there is a positive history of infection, it is important for the clinician to include serum immunoglobulins together with specific antibodies to pneumococcus (polysaccharide antigen) and tetanus (protein antigen) in the investigations of sarcoidosis.

CVID is a diagnosis of exclusion and is defined by reduction in IgG and IgA and/or IgM with evidence of impaired vaccine responses to polysaccharide and/or protein antigens (Conley *et al.* 1999; Notarangelo *et al.* 2007). A reduction in IgG levels may be secondary to steroid therapy, but vaccine responses are not affected by corticosteroids. Other causes of decreased immunoglobulins (Box 38.1) should be excluded in patients with suspected CVID. A fall in serum IgG level in patients on replacement immunoglobulin is a useful clue to an inflammatory (granulomatous) process somewhere in the body, probably caused by increased catabolism of IgG by activated macrophages. The level of C-reactive protein is an unreliable measure of granulomatous inflammation, and serum angiotensin-converting enzyme (SACE) is often normal (Webster 2005).

The majority of CVID patients suffer from recurrent bronchitis/pneumonia and ultimately develop bronchiectasis (Webster 2005). There are currently no predictive features that will identify patients at higher risk of developing lung disease, but patients diagnosed late are more at risk. High-resolution CT scanning of patients with granulomatous inflammation will show features of sarcoidosis such as reticulonodular shadowing, fibrosis, hilar and mediastinal

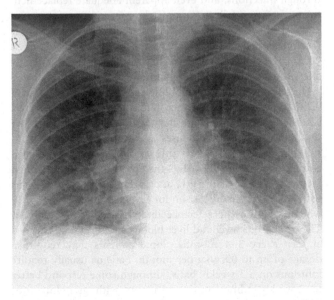

Figure 38.1   Chest radiograph of a patient with granulomatous common variable immunodeficiency. Note the bilateral hilar and paratracheal lymphadenopathy together with mid- and lower-zone nodular opacification and patches of consolidation.

Box 38.1 Differential diagnosis of common variable immune deficiency (CVID)

B cell lymphoproliferative disorders
- Multiple myeloma
- Chronic lymphatic leukemia
- Non-Hodgkin's lymphoma

Protein-losing diseases
- Nephrotic syndrome
- Celiac disease
- Intestinal lymphangiectasia

Infection
- Epstein–Barr virus
- Cytomegalovirus
- Rubella

Drugs
- Corticosteroids
- Sulphasalazine
- Phenytoin
- Carbamazepine

Good's syndrome
- Thymoma, hypogammaglobulinemia

Primary immunodeficiency
- X-linked agammaglobinemia
- CD40 ligand deficiency
- X-linked lymphoproliferative syndrome

lymphadenopathy; in addition there may be bronchiectasis, 'tree-in-bud' exudative bronchiolitis and patches of consolidation (Fig. 38.2). Fibrosis due to sarcoidosis may cause traction bronchiectasis, but in cases associated with antibody deficiency the bronchiectasis and associated changes are seen in areas distant from areas of scarring (Park *et al.* 2005). Idiopathic bronchiectasis and sarcoidosis are not rare conditions and they may co-exist, so not all patients with these features will have a unifying diagnosis of CVID.

Lung function tests should be performed annually in CVID and are used as a non-invasive method of assessing patient stability. Patients who develop bronchiectasis due to CVID have abnormal lung function tests. In moderate bronchiectasis there is mild-to-moderate airflow obstruction, which is usually not responsive to inhaled bronchodilators; there is gas trapping and signs of abnormal small airways function (MEF50) that are more impaired than FEV_1. Gas transfer corrected for alveolar gas distribution, which may be impaired by mucus plugging, is usually well preserved in all but severe cases. However, in the presence of co-existent granulomatous inflammation the gas transfer is often markedly impaired and this is usually associated with a restrictive defect.

In a recent study of long-term follow-up of a cohort of bronchiectasis patients with various etiologies, impaired gas transfer and airflow obstruction in the presence of lung restriction were important independent predictors of mortality (Loebinger *et al.* 2009). Although there are no prospective studies of granulomatous lung disease in CVID, these results would suggest that the prognosis is worse than CVID without this complication.

Granulomatous inflammation in CVID most commonly affects the lung, liver and spleen. Abnormal liver function tests and abnormalities such as low platelets in the blood count may be present. Other features of sarcoidosis are less commonly seen. Histological confirmation may be required, particularly in the absence of typical radiological features in the lung or in cases of severe granulomatous inflammation in the liver. The histology of granulomas in CVID is similar to that observed in sarcoidosis.

MANAGEMENT

Treatment of CVID is by immunoglobulin replacement. Antibiotics are used to treat infections and, particularly in cases with frequent infections that have caused bronchiectasis, they may be used as prophylaxis. Prednisolone and other immunosuppressive therapy may be required to control the granulomatous inflammation.

IMMUNOGLOBULIN

The decision to begin immunoglobulin replacement is made after considering the patient's infection history, the level of serum immunoglobulins (particularly Ig G) and the degree of structural and functional lung impairment (Webster 2005). Immunoglobulin is prepared from pooled donor plasma after screening for viral diseases. It can be administered intravenously or subcutaneously and either route has similar efficacy (Chapel *et al.* 2000). There are several different commercial preparations available and all donors are carefully screened. However, there are risks of transmissible disease as with any blood product, both real (hepatitis C) and theoretical (variant CJD).

Replacement therapy increases life expectancy and reduces frequency and severity of infections, antibiotic use and hospital admissions. Patients remain susceptible to breakthrough infections, and even apparent adequate replacement treatment may fail to completely prevent progression of established disease complications such as bronchiectasis (Kainulainen *et al.* 1999; Pettit *et al.* 2002; Herriot and Sewell 2008). There is no evidence that immunoglobulin therapy alters the natural history of granulomatous disease.

Intravenous immunoglobulin is given as an initial dose of 0.2–0.4 g/kg per month, either in hospital as a day case or via a home IV program. Thereafter the dosage is determined by the patient's clinical responses and trough IgG level, measured just before the next infusion of immunoglobulin is administered. The aim of IgG therapy is to achieve a trough IgG level greater than 5 g/L, and in Europe most physicians with an interest in CVID aim for trough IgG levels 7–8 g/L – which is within the reference interval for healthy controls. The trough IgG level and liver blood tests should be checked at least every 3–4 months. Some patients may require a dosage of up to 0.8 g/kg per month. Patients usually require infusions on a 3-weekly basis, although some respond better to 2-weekly administration. Patients with granulomatous CVID tend to require the higher dosage.

Adverse reactions become apparent within the first hour of the infusion and are usually mild (e.g. temperature, shivering, headache). They are more common if the patient

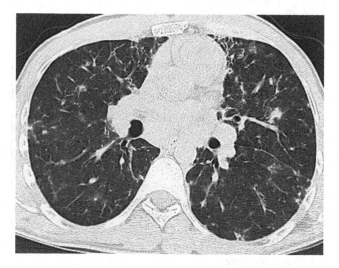

Figure 38.2   High-resolution CT scan through the mid-zones of a patient with granulomatous common variable immunodeficiency. The section shows mildly bronchiectatic airways anteriorly (there was more overt bronchiectasis in the lower lobes). Bilateral hilar and subcarinal lymphadenopathy is present. There are multiple nodules ranging in size from 3 mm to 9 mm, as well as a reticular pattern with associated distortion of lung parenchyma.

has an intercurrent infection, and it may then be best to delay the infusion for a few days while antibiotics are administered. Moderate allergic reactions can be controlled by prior administration of intravenous hydrocortisone and an anti-histamine. More severe reactions and anaphylaxis are rare (Webster 2005; Herriot and Sewell 2008).

Subcutaneous immunoglobulin is used when there is poor venous access, for those intolerant of IV immunoglobulin, and when patients prefer this mode of delivery. Patients with eczema or those on anticoagulant therapy are excluded. The monthly dosage is the same, but it is administered every 7–10 days. The patient is trained to have the infusions at home but must also have a trained infusion partner, both to assist in the administration, and to be present if there is an adverse reaction.

PREDNISOLONE

If the patient's condition allows, several months of immunoglobulin therapy, and antibiotic treatment of any intercurrent infection, should be given before deciding that additional prednisolone treatment is required. This decision is usually based on clinical symptoms and the degree of impairment of lung function. The usual approach is taken of gaining maximal response with a high dosage of prednisolone, 30–60 mg daily, for one month before gradually reducing the dose, while monitoring response. Many patients relapse if the maintenance dosage is reduced below 10 mg/day (Webster 2005), but the lowest dosage that maintains maximal improvement should be established.

The role of other immunosuppressants is uncertain, but hydroxychloroquine may be a useful steroid sparing agent (Moller 2005).

ANTIBIOTICS

Acute respiratory tract infections are treated with appropriate antibiotics guided by sputum cultures and antibiotic sensitivities when available. Acute severe infection is a medical emergency requiring admission to hospital for intravenous antibiotics and consideration of additional immunoglobulin. Chronic infections stimulate a neutrophilic inflammatory response which may cause further damage to the lung. Infection can also stimulate granulomatous inflammation. For this reason patients with chronic infection should be considered for continuous antibiotic treatment to suppress the level of infection, and in this way reduce inflammation (Loebinger and Wilson 2007). This is particularly common with Gram-negative pathogens such as Pseudomonas aeruginosa that are more likely to establish chronic infection.

If continuous antibiotic treatment for P. aeruginosa is given by the oral route, gastrointestinal side-effects and emergence of bacterial antibiotic resistance are common. Antibiotic delivery by inhalation (e.g. tobramycin or colomycin) is an alternative. The advantage of the inhaled route is that high concentrations of the antibiotic can be achieved in the airway, reducing the risk of emergence of resistance, without the same effect on the gut bacterial flora that occurs with oral treatment. Unfortunately some patients cannot tolerate the inhaled antibiotic because of coughing and bronchospasm even when the antibiotics are given with bronchodilators. For this reason a trial of inhaled antibiotic under medical supervision should always be performed with spirometry before and after the drug.

Intravenous antibiotics can also be given on a regular planned basis to suppress the bacterial infection in the lung. This may require admission to hospital, although some hospitals have a nurse-led home IV service; or patients can be trained to administer the treatment themselves, provided the first dose has been supervised. Long-term antibiotic treatment with macrolide antibiotics, particularly azithromycin, has been used successfully in bronchiectasis, including patients with chronic Pseudomonas infection, and may have the added advantage of an anti-inflammatory action (Crosbie and Woodhead 2009).

The natural pulmonary history of CVID may be the development of progressive bronchiectasis, respiratory failure and pulmonary hypertension. Management in this circumstance is very difficult and the experience of lung transplantation in this setting is limited. In a UK study of pulmonary complications of CVID, a single patient had lung transplantation because of bronchiectasis and respiratory failure. The explanted lung showed granulomatous disease and obliterative bronchiolitis. The patient died of respiratory failure 30 months post-transplant, and the transplanted lung also had granulomatous disease, demonstrating that granulomatous disease in CVID is a systemic disorder that is likely to recur following transplant (Thickett et al. 2002). This suggests that lung transplantation to treat respiratory failure caused by severe lung scarring from granulomatous CVID may not give longlasting benefit.

MONITORING RESPONSE TO TREATMENT

Patient symptoms, chest X-ray and lung function tests will inform decisions about response to treatment. However, there is concern that bronchiectasis can develop and progress silently in patients with immunoglobulin deficiency (Kainulainen et al. 1999). For this reason an interval CT scan should be performed, but there is no consensus about how often this should be. Clinical judgment has to be made in each case based on frequency of infections and improvement in other parameters balanced against concerns about radiation exposure.

Deterioration in lung function may be secondary to infection, when airway abnormalities may predominate, or interstitial lung disease when gas transfer is more likely to be the parameter affected (Martinez-Garcia et al. 2001). Serum ACE is elevated in a proportion of patients, and if this is the case the level can be monitored. Sputum bacteriology and C-reactive protein will give additional information indicating an infective etiology, and in patients with bronchiectasis sputum cultures should be performed regularly to guide future antibiotic treatment and screen for acquisition of difficult species such as Pseudomonas. When Pseudomonas is first isolated, eradication can be attempted before chronic infection is established (Loebinger and Wilson 2007).

CONCLUSION

Granulomatous disease is a well-recognized complication of CVID. Granulomas may precede the onset of immune deficiency and in this setting it can be very difficult to distinguish this condition from sarcoidosis. A history of recurrent infection and/or the onset of autoimmune disease (ITP, AIHA) should prompt reconsideration of the diagnosis of sarcoidosis. Recognition of CVID is important as its management differs from sarcoidosis.

REFERENCES

Ardeniz O, Cunningham-Rundles C (2009). Granulomatous disease in common variable immunodeficiency. *Clin Immunol* **133**: 198–207.

Arnold DF, Wiggins J, Cunningham-Rundles C et al. (2008). Granulomatous disease: distinguishing primary antibody deficiency from sarcoidosis. *Clin Immunol* **128**: 18–22.

Artac H, Bozkurt B, Talim B, Reisli I (2009). Sarcoid-like granulomas in common variable immunodeficiency. *Rheumatology Int* **10**: 1007.

Aspalter RM, Eibl M, Wolf HM (2007). Defective T cell activation caused by impairment of the TNF receptor 2 costimulatory pathway in common variable immunodeficiency. *J Allergy Clin Immunol* **120**: 1193–200.

Aukrust P, Lien AK, Kristofferson F et al. (1996). Persistent activation of the tumor necrosis factor system in a subgroup of patients with common variable immunodeficiency: possible immunologic and clinical consequences. *Blood* **87**: 674–81.

Bacchelli C, Buckridege S, Thrasher AJ, Gaspar HB (2007). Translational mini-review series on immunodeficiency: molecular defects in common variable immunodeficiency. *Clin Exp Immunol* **149**: 401–9.

Bates CA, Ellison MC, Lynch DA et al. (2004). Granulomatous lymphocytic lung disease shortens survival in common variable immunodeficiency. *J Allergy Clin Immunol* **114**: 415–21.

Bayry L, Lacroix-Desmazes, Kazatchkine MD et al. (2004). Common variable immunodeficiency associated with defective functions of dendritic cells. *Blood* **101**: 2441–3.

Bronsky D, Dunn YOL (1965). Sarcoidosis with hypogammaglobulinaemia. *Am J Med Sci* **250**: 11.

Cambronero R, Sewell WA, North ME et al. (2000). Upregulation of IL-12 in monocytes: a fundamental defect in common variable immunodeficiency. *J Immunol* **164**: 488–94.

Chapel HM, Spickett GP, Erison D et al. (2000). Comparison of the efficacy and safety of intravenous versus subcutaneous immunoglobulin therapy. *J Clin Immunol* **20**: 94–100.

Conley ME, Notarangelo LD, Etzioni A (1999). Diagnostic criteria for primary immunodeficiencies. *Clin Immunol* **93**: 190–7.

Crosbie PAJ, Woodhead MA (2009). Long-term macrolide therapy in chronic inflammatory airway diseases. *Eur Respir J* **33**: 171–81.

Cunningham-Rundles C, Bodian C (1999). Common variable immunodeficiency: clinical and immunological features in of 248 patients. *Clin Immunol* **92**: 34–48.

Cunningham-Rundles C, Radigan L (2005). Deficient IL-12 and dendritic cell function in common variable immune deficiency. *Clin Immunol* **115**: 147–53.

Cunningham-Rundles C, Radigan L, Knight AK et al. (2006). TLR9 activation is defective in common variable immune deficiency. *J Immunol* **176**: 1978–87.

Fasano MB, Sullivan KE, Sarpong SB et al. (1996). Sarcoidosis and common variable immunodeficiency. *Medicine* **75**: 251–61.

Gathmann B, Grimbacher B, Beaute J et al. (2009). The European internet-based patient and research database for primary immunodeficiencies: results 2006–2008 (Need ESID database). *Clin Exp Immunol* **157**(Suppl. 1): 3–11.

Giovanetti A, Pierdominici M, Mazetta F et al. (2007). Unravelling the complexity of T-cell abnormailities in common variable immunodeficiency. *J Immunol* **178**: 3932–43.

Grimbacher B, Hutloff A, Schleiser M et al. (2003). Homozygous loss of ICOS is associated with adult-onset common variable immunodeficiency. *Nat Immunol* **4**: 261–8.

Hammarstrom L, Vorechovsky I, Webster D (2000). Selective IgA deficiency and common variable immunodeficiency. *Clin Exp Immunol* **120**: 225–31.

Herriot R, Sewell WAC (2008). Antibody deficiency. *J Clin Pathol* **61**: 994–1000.

Ito T, Schaller M, Hogaboam CM (2007). TLR activation is a key event for the maintenance of a mycobacterial antigen-elicited pulmonary granulomatous response. *Eur J Immunol* **37**: 2847–55.

Kainulainen L, Varpula M, Liippo K et al. (1999). Pulmonary abnormalities in patients with primary hypogammaglobulinemia. *J Allergy Clin Immunol* **104**: 1031–6.

Kim HJ, Berek C (2000). B-cells in rheumatoid arthritis. *Arthritis Res* **2**: 126–31.

Loebinger MR, Wells AU., Hansell DM (2009). Mortality in bronchiectasis: a long-term study of the factors influencing survival. *Eur Respir J* **34**: 843–9.

Loebinger MR, Wilson R (2007). Pharmacotherapy for bronchiectasis. *Expert Opin Pharmacother* **8**: 3183–93.

Martinez-Garcia MA, De Rojas MD, Nauffal Manzur MD et al. (2001). Respiratory disorders in common variable immunodeficiency. *Respir Med* **95**: 191–5.

Mechanic LJ, Dikman S, Cunningham-Rundles C (1997). Granulomatous disease in common variable immunodeficiency. *Ann Intern Med* **127**: 613–17.

Moller DR (2005). Rare manifestations of sarcoidosis. In: Drent M, Costabel U (eds). *Sarcoidosis*. European Respiratory Monograph 32, pp. 233–50.

Mrusek S, Marx A, Kummerle-Descher J et al. (2004). Development of granulomatous common variable immunodeficiency subsequent to infection with *Toxoplasma gondii*. *Clin Exp Immunol* **137**: 578–83.

Mullighan CG, Fanning HM, Chapel HM, Welch KI (1997). TNF and lymphotoxin-alpha polymorphisms associated with common variable immunodeficiency: role in the pathogenesis of granulomatous diseases. *J Immunol* **159**: 6236–41.

North ME, Webster AD, Farrant J et al. (1998). Primary defect in CD8 + lymphocytes in the antibody deficiency disease (common variable immunodeficiency): abnormalities in intracellular production of interferon-gamma in CD28 + ('cytotoxic') and CD28- ('suppressor') CD8 + subsets. *Clin Exp Immunol* **111**: 70–5.

Notarangelo LD, Fischer A, Geha RS et al. (2007). Primary immunodeficiency diseases: 2009 update from the International Union of Immunological Societies Primary Immunodeficiency Classification Committee. *J Allergy Clin Immunol* **120**: 776–94.

Oksenhendler E, Gerard L, Fieschi C et al. (2008). Infections in 252 patients with common variable immunodeficiency. *Clin Infect Dis* **46**: 1547–54.

Paccani SR, Boncristiano M, Patrussi L et al. (2005). Defective Vav expression and impaired F-actin reorganization in a subset of patients with common variable immunodeficiency characterized by T-cell defects. *Blood* **106**: 626–34.

Park JES, Beal I, Dilworth JP et al. (2005). The HRCT appearances of granulomatous pulmonary disease in common variable immunodeficiency. *Eur J Radiol* **54**: 359–64.

Park MA, Li JT, Hagan JB *et al.* (2008). Common variable immunodeficiency: a new look at an old disease. *Lancet* **372**: 489–502.

Pettit SJ, Bourne H, Spickett GP (2002). Survey of infection in patients receiving antibody replacement treatment of immune deficiency. *J Clin Pathol* **55**: 577–80.

Piqueras B, Lavenu-Bombled C, Galicier L *et al.* (2003). Common variable immunodeficiency patient classification based upon on impaired B-cell memory differentiation correlates with clinical aspects. *J Clin Immunol* **23**: 385–400.

Rakhmanov M, Keller B, Gutenberger S *et al.* (2009). Circulating CD21low B-cells in common variable immunodeficiency resemble tissue homing, innate-like B cells. *Proc Natl Acad Sci USA* **106**: 13451–6.

Roach DR, Bean AG, Demangel C *et al.* (2002). TNF regulates chemokine induction essential for cell recruitment, granuloma formation, and clearance of mycobacterial infection. *J Immunol* **168**: 4620–7.

Salzer U, Maul-Pavick , Cunningham Rundles C *et al.* (2004). ICOS deficiency in patients with common variable immunodeficiency. *Clin Immunol* **113**: 324–40.

Sanchez-Ramon A, Radigan L, Yu JE *et al.* (2008). Memory B cells in common variable: clinical associations and sex differences. *Clin Immunol* **128**: 314–21.

Thickett KM, Kumararatne DS, Banerjee AK *et al.* (2002). Common variable immunodeficiency: respiratory manifestations, pulmonary function and high-resolution CT findings. *Q J Med* **95**: 655–62.

Torrigan DA, LaRosa DF, Levinson AI *et al.* (2008). Granulomatous-lymphocytic interstitial lung disease associated with common variable immunodeficiency: CT findings. *J Thorac Imaging* **23**: 162–9.

Viallard JF, Camou F, Andre M *et al.* (2005). Altered dendritic cell distribution in patients with common variable immunodeficiency. *Arthritis Res Ther* **7**: R1052–5.

Warnatz K, Denz A, Drager R *et al.* (2002). Severe deficiency of switched memory B cells (CD27+IgM-IgD-) in subgroups of patients with common variable immunodeficiency: a new approach to classify a heterogeneous disease. *Blood* **99**: 1544–51.

Webster ADB (2005). Humoral immunodeficiency and the lung. In: Verleden GM *et al.* (eds). *Pulmonary Manifestations of Systemic Diseases.* European Respiratory Monogragh 34, pp. 220–33.

Wehr C, Eibel H, Masilamani M *et al.* (2004). A new CD21low B-cell population in the peripheral blood of patients with SLE. *Clin Immunol* **113**: 161–71.

Wehr C, Kivoja T, Schmitt C *et al.* (2008). The EUROclass trial; defining subgroups in common variable immunodeficiency. *Blood* **111**: 77–85.

Wheat WH, Cool CD, Morimoto Y *et al.* (2005). Possible role of human herpesvirus 8 in the lymphoproliferative disorders in common variable immunodeficiency. *J Exp Med* **202**: 479–84.

Yong PF, Workman S, Wahid F *et al.* (2008). Selective deficits in blood dendritic cell subsets in common variable and X-linked agammaglobulinaemia but not specific polysaccharide deficiency. *Clin Immunol* **127**: 34–42.

Concomitant diseases
1. Infections with agents causing granulomatous inflammation

ELSPETH POTTON AND JEREMY S BROWN

INTRODUCTION

The clinical manifestations of sarcoidosis vary from asymptomatic disease to inflammation within a single organ or multiple organs, often causing relatively non-specific symptoms and signs. A diagnosis of sarcoidosis may therefore need to be considered in a range of clinical scenarios, many of which have infectious disease as their differential diagnosis. Infectious diseases also commonly cause granulomas so may have a histological resemblance to sarcoid. Sarcoidosis can also co-exist with infectious diseases, and cases of concomitant infection and sarcoid have led to the suggestion that in some cases sarcoidosis has been *caused* by infection.

This chapter reviews the relationship between sarcoidosis and infectious diseases, discussing cases of the latter that may be confused with sarcoid. As treatment of sarcoidosis often requires immunosuppressive therapy, misdiagnosis of an infectious disease as sarcoid could have severe consequences. In addition, deterioration in the clinical condition of a patient with sarcoid who is being treated with immunosuppressive therapy may not be due to worsening sarcoid but could be caused by a superadded opportunistic infection with a clinical presentation that overlaps.

The risk and presentation of infection with different microorganisms is heavily dependent on epidemiological and clinical factors such as country of habitation, country of origin, age, ethnic background, vaccination history, occupation, past medical history and current drug therapy – factors that can also affect the likelihood of sarcoidosis (Pietinalho *et al.* 1995; Baughman *et al.* 2001; Thomas and Hunninghake 2003). As a consequence, epidemiological factors will often help define the potential infectious differential diagnosis in patients presenting with sarcoid or in whom granulomas have been identified in a tissue biopsy.

PULMONARY DISEASE

The two most common diseases that cause granulomatous disease within the thoracic cavity are sarcoidosis and tuberculosis (TB), and differentiating between these is a common clinical conundrum. Other infectious diseases that may be confused with sarcoid include non-tuberculous mycobacterial (NTM) infections, actinomycosis, aspergillosis, and infections caused by *Nocardia* or endemic fungi such as *Histoplasma* or *Cryptococcus*.

In general, chronic pulmonary sarcoidosis causes little systemic upset and is not rapidly progressive, so clinically is unlikely to be confused with most infections. In contrast, acute pulmonary involvement with sarcoid by definition is associated with new radiological changes and can be associated with occasionally marked systemic upset, and infectious disease has to be considered. To avoid missing an infectious cause, it is vital that histological samples containing granulomas be examined using specific stains for microbiological causes, including the following:

- stains for acid-fast bacilli to identify *Mycobacterium* and *Nocardia*;
- methanamine silver, periodic acid-Schiff silver or Grocott staining for fungal pathogens;
- Gram staining for bacterial pathogens such as *Actinomyces*.

Specific features of granulomas may also indicate a particular cause, with caseation suggesting TB as the most obvious example. Features and diagnostic tests that may help differentiate lung disease due to sarcoidosis from infectious diseases that are sometimes associated with granulomas are summarized in Tables 39.1A and 39.1B.

Tuberculosis probably should always be considered when granulomas are identified in pulmonary samples, especially in patients who have an ethnic or clinical background associated with a high incidence of tuberculosis. Fortunately, with the exception of enlarged mediastinal nodes, in general there is little overlap in the clinical picture associated with the classical presentations of sarcoidosis and TB. Occasionally the rare necrotizing forms of sarcoid can be mistaken for an infectious disease, and the radiological appearance of micronodular sarcoid confused with miliary tuberculosis or endemic fungal infection. Both tuberculosis and sarcoid often manifest in other organ systems simultaneously with the lung. Hence, the clinical assessment of the patient with suspected granulomatous lung disease should always incorporate a thorough assessment of other systems. Targeted investigations for common extrapulmonary manifestations – close inspection of the skin for areas of lupus pernio, serum calcium levels, serum transaminase levels to identify subclinical liver disease, imaging for abdominal lymphadenopathy or terminal ileal/mesenteric pathology etc. – may allow a firm diagnosis to be made without invasive investigations of the lung. Specific clinical presentations when infectious disease needs to be considered in the differential diagnosis of sarcoidosis are discussed below.

Mediastinal lymphadenopathy

Enlarged mediastinal lymph nodes occur in the majority of patients with sarcoidosis and are the primary manifestation of tuberculosis in 9 percent of adult cases (Health Protection Agency 2009). When presented with a patient with mediastinal lymphadenopathy, the various factors that can help differentiate between TB and sarcoidosis as the likely cause are discussed below and summarized in Table 39.2.

EPIDEMIOLOGY

Sarcoid is uncommon in children, making tuberculosis the more likely cause of enlarged mediastinal nodes in children, but the age range affected in adults is similar for both diseases. However, the incidence of TB varies enormously, with certain predictable epidemiological factors allowing at-risk subjects to usually be readily identified. Tuberculosis needs to be considered in the differential diagnosis mainly for:

- patients born in high-risk countries (especially if recent immigrants, that is within 2 or 3 years) (Health Protection Agency 2009);
- the elderly, who may have been infected with TB when the incidence in the country of residence was much higher;
- selected high-risk groups such as the homeless, prison populations and people who use intravenous drugs (Story et al. 2007).

The pre-existing risk of tuberculosis is compounded by disease or treatment that impairs T-cell immunity, such as corticosteroids, anti-TNF-α treatment, or malignancy. Certain ethnic groups such as subjects from the Indian subcontinent are also

more likely to have extrapulmonary tuberculosis, including mediastinal lymphadenopathy. Although in areas with a high incidence there is some 'spillover' of infection from high-risk populations into low-risk individuals, in general outside of these risk groups TB is a much less likely diagnosis. Hence knowing the place of birth, whether the person has lived in high-risk countries, has had close contacts with someone with TB, social circumstances, medical history and present treatment will readily identify patients at risk of tuberculosis. Unfortunately, some of these risk factors overlap with those for sarcoid. For example, the incidence of TB and sarcoidosis are both raised in patients of African origin, with an annual incidence of sarcoid in black Americans of 35.5 per 100000, and possibly a similar incidence for black Africans (Rybicki et al. 1997).

In practice, although epidemiological factors cannot exclude the possibility of TB or sarcoidosis in a particular patient, they do allow the recognition of most cases of mediastinal lymphadenopathy in whom tuberculosis has to be considered.

CLINICAL FEATURES

Local symptoms attributable to the enlarged nodes do not differentiate between sarcoidosis and tuberculosis, but marked constitutional symptoms such as night sweats and weight loss occur in only some 12 percent of cases of sarcoidosis and are more suggestive of TB. Mediastinal lymphadenopathy does not usually lead to detectable clinical signs, but clinical examination may identify other sites of disease that can differentiate between sarcoidosis and TB. For example, the presence of lupus pernio or widespread low-volume symmetrical adenopathy and hepatosplenomegaly would suggest sarcoidosis rather than TB. Erythema nodosum (EN) is associated with both diseases, with a prevalence of 8.3 percent in sarcoidosis (Baughman et al. 2001), and is common in primary but not secondary tuberculosis (Mert et al. 2004). At bronchoscopy, sarcoid can cause a cobblestone appearance of the endobronchial tree (Chapman and Mehta 2003), but this appearance may also be seen in TB (Lee et al. 1992).

RADIOLOGY

In many cases of mediastinal adenopathy, the associated radiological features of lung involvement on the plain chest X-ray or on CT scanning usually distinguish between sarcoid and tuberculosis. Tuberculosis causes asymmetric areas of cavitation, 'tree-in-bud' infiltrations, pleural effusions, macronodules and/or patches of consolidation, whereas micronodular infiltration (especially along fissures and the pleura) is more suggestive of sarcoid (Traill et al. 1997). However, military TB also causes symmetrical micronodular infiltration throughout the lungs, and there are rarer radiological presentations of sarcoid that can mimic the changes seen in TB, such as necrotizing sarcoid (see below). In patients without lung parenchymal involvement, radiological features of the enlarged nodes are not able to conclusively differentiate mediastinal adenopathy due to sarcoid from TB, but the following features often provide important pointers to the diagnosis.

Table 39.1A Comparative clinical features of sarcoid and granulomatous infections.

	Sarcoidosis	Tuberculosis	Non-tuberculous mycobacteria	Actinomycosis	Nocardia
Epidemiology	African American and African populations Scandinavia	TB endemic regions, e.g. Sub-Saharan Africa, Asia Homeless, prison populations, drug abuse	Variable	Rare Sporadic	Rare Sporadic
Increased susceptibility	HLA association Family history (5- fold risk)	Defects in cell-mediated immunity, HIV	Chronic respiratory diseases HIV infection (CD4 count <50)	Bad dentition Recent oral or head and neck surgery	Defects in cell-mediated immunity
Serum ACE Blood tests	SACE elevated 87%	SACE elevated 4% Role of IGRA tests unclear	SACE elevated in 13%	–	–
Mantoux test	Negative 90%	Positive 65–94%	May be positive due to previous TB exposure or BCG vaccination	May be positive due to previous TB exposure or BCG vaccination	May be positive due to previous TB exposure or BCG vaccination
Radiological presentations	Symmetrical hilar and mediastinal lymphadenopathy Diffuse or micronodular interstitial infiltrates Upper-lobe fibrosis Rarely diffuse alveolitis or cavitating masses	Assymetrical hilar and mediastinal lymphadenopathy, necrosis common Upper-lobe infiltrates with cavitation, tree-in-bud, nodular infiltrates	Assymetrical hilar and mediastinal lymphadenopathy, necrosis common Upper-lobe infiltrates with cavitation Multifocal bronchiectasis, tree-in-bud, small nodules/ cavitatory lesions	Focal consolidation, pleural or chest wall involvement, or cavitation Hilar lymphadenopathy 33%	Macronodules that can cavitate, diffuse pulmonary infiltrates Occasional associated hilar lymphadenopathy
Histology/microscopy	Defined non-necrotizing granulomas	Caseating granulomas 'Acid-fast' positive bacilli	Necrotizing granulomas 'Acid-fast' positive bacilli	Ill-defined granulomas without giant cells Filamentous branching bacilli 'Sulfur' granules 25%	Occasional necrotizing granulomas 'Acid-fast' branching beaded filamentous bacilli
Culture	Culture negative	Positive for *M. tuberculosis*	Culture positive for non-tuberculous mycobacteria	Prolonged anaerobic culture necessary	Culture of variable sensitivity

HLA, human leukocyte antigen; IGRA, interferon-gamma release assay; SACE, serum angiotensin-converting enzyme

Table 39.1B   Comparative clinical features of sarcoid and granulomatous infections.

	Cryptococcus	Aspergillosis	Coccidiodomycosis (endemic mycosis)	Blastomycosis (endemic mycosis)	Histoplasmosis (endemic mycosis)
Epidemiology	Rare Sporadic	Rare Sporadic	Travel to endemic areas, e.g. southern USA, Central and South America	Travel to endemic areas, e.g. North and South America	Travel to endemic areas, e.g. Mississippi and Ohio river valleys Exposure to bird or bat guano
Increased susceptibility	Defects in cell-mediated immunity	Neutropenia Corticosteroids Chronic lung disease	Defects in cell-mediated immunity	Defects in cell-mediated immunity	Defects in cell-mediated immunity COPD
Serum ACE and blood tests	Serum cryptococcal antigen positive in disseminated disease, limited utility in lung disease	Cell-wall antigen tests *Aspergillus* specific IgG and IgE	SACE elevated 7% Serum precipitin test positive 90%	Serum serological tests of limited value	SACE elevated 14% Serum serology usually positive
Mantoux test	May be positive due to previous TB exposure or BCG vaccination	May be positive due to previous TB exposure or BCG vaccination	May be positive due to previous TB exposure or BCG vaccination	May be positive due to previous TB exposure or BCG vaccination	May be positive due to previous TB exposure or BCG vaccination
Radiological presentations	Macronodules, segmental consolidation, reticulonodular infiltrates Rarely hilar lymphadenopathy	Macronodules, pulmonary infiltrates, halo or crescent signs Bronchial wall thickening, tree-in-bud Hilar lymphadenopathy rare	Pulmonary nodules, alveolar infiltrates or consolidation, cavitation Hilar or paratracheal lymphadenopathy common	Alveolar infiltrates or consolidation, cavitation Commonly hilar or paratracheal lymphadenopathy	Pulmonary nodules, alveolar infiltrates or consolidation, cavitation Hilar or paratracheal lymphadenopathy common Chronic progressive cavitation (if pre-existing COPD)
Histology/microscopy	Can form non-caseating granulomas Cryptococci visible with methanamine silver or periodic–acid Schiff staining	Occasional necrotizing granulomas Dichotomous branching septate hyphae	Caseating granulomas Methanimine silver or periodic–acid Schiff often positive for spherules	Non-caseating granulomas Methanimine silver or periodic–acid Schiff stains usually show organisms	Necrotizing and non-necrotizing granulomas Methanamine silver or periodic–acid Schiff stains positive for yeast forms
Culture	Often culture positive	Culture positive 50%	Often culture positive	Often culture positive	Culture negative in acute disease

COPD, chronic obstructive pulmonary disease; SACE, serum angiotensin–converting enzyme

Table 39.2   Clinical and radiological features of mediastinal lymphadenopathy caused by sarcoid or tuberculosis.

	Sarcoidosis	Tuberculosis
Symptoms and signs	Constitutional symptoms 12% cases EN 8.3% (39% with Löfgren's syndrome)	Constitutional symptoms usual, fever 66% EN incidence unclear
Site of enlarged nodes	Hilar, mediastinal, paratracheal	Paratracheal, mediastinal Bilateral hilar nodes uncommon
Node size and symmetry	Symmetrical in size and distribution	Usually asymmetrical distribution and variable in size
Node morphology	No necrosis Clearly defined	Central necrosis common Can adhere to mediastinal structures and form fistulas
Histology, microscopy and culture	Caseation in minority Negative for acid-fast bacilli and on culture	Caseating 76% Acid-fast bacilli positive 8% Culture positive 30+%

- *Site.* Sarcoid causes enlargement of hilar, tracheal and central mediastinal nodes (Sider and Horton 1990), whereas TB most commonly causes tracheal node enlargement with hilar involvement being less common.
- *Size and symmetry.* Sarcoid usually causes a symmetrical enlargement of hilar and mediastinal nodes, whereas TB usually causes asymmetrical enlargement (Andreu *et al.* 2004) with often massive enlargement of one or two mediastinal nodes.
- *Morphology.* Sarcoid causes smooth enlargement of mediastinal nodes with well-defined margins, and significant nodal coalescence or adhesion to other mediastinal structures suggests an infective cause. Low attenuation within nodes, associated with peripheral rim enhancement and obliteration of the perinodal fat on CT scanning, is suggestive of central necrosis, a sign that is associated with active TB but is rare in sarcoidosis (Moon *et al.* 1997). Calcification has been observed in 53 percent and 46 percent of cases of sarcoid and tuberculosis patients, respectively, but classically in sarcoid has an 'eggshell' pattern whereas in tuberculosis calcification tends to be localized central foci and suggests inactive disease (Gawne-Cain and Hansell 1996).

HISTOLOGICAL AND MICROBIOLOGICAL FEATURES

A confirmed diagnosis of sarcoid in most cases will require biopsy to identify granulomas. Enlarged mediastinal nodes can be biopsied surgically (via mediastonoscopy or mediastinotomy), or sometimes by CT-guided biopsies for nodes in the anterior mediastinum. In addition they can be aspirated via the bronchial tree or esophagus using endobronchial ultrasound (EBUS) or endoscopic ultrasound with a diagnostic yield of up to 92 percent (Wong *et al.* 2007; Tournoy *et al.* 2009). The sarcoid granuloma classically is well formed, compact, with no central necrosis, whereas tuberculous granulomas tend to caseate. However, caseation has sometimes been reported in sarcoidosis and 24 percent of tuberculous granulomas are non-caseating (Cutler *et al.* 1994). In practice, in patients at high risk of TB the presence of caseation strongly suggests this is the diagnosis, but lack of caseation does not exclude TB.

Although almost 100 percent specific, staining nodal biopsies for acid-fast bacilli is insensitive and is positive in fewer than 10 percent of cases of tuberculosis (Cutler *et al.* 1994). Lymph node culture for *M. tuberculosis* is positive in around 30 percent of cases of TB but takes up to 6 weeks (Gulati *et al.* 2000). PCR amplification of mycobacterial DNA from nodal material is possible; but given that latent tuberculosis may be present within mediastinal nodes, and that mycobacterial DNA can be amplified from sarcoid tissues, a positive PCR may not be that helpful. Even if the radiology suggests there is no obvious lung parenchymal involvement, transbronchial or endobrochial biopsies will identify pulmonary granulomas in 40–90 percent of sarcoid cases (Koonitz *et al.* 1976; Gilman and Wang 1980), but are rarer in TB except in miliary disease.

As well as the enlarged node, other samples such as sputum and bronchoalveolar lavage (BAL) fluid should be cultured if mycobacterial disease is suspected, as a significant proportion will be culture-positive for *M. tuberculosis* even in the absence of clinically obvious disease within the lung.

PURIFIED PROTEIN DERIVATIVES AND INTERFERON–GAMMA RELEASE ASSAYS

Immunological tests may provide some help in differentiating sarcoidosis from tuberculosis. Intradermal injection of purified protein derivatives (PPDs) of *M. tuberculosis* provokes a type-4 hypersensitivity reaction manifested as an area of dermal induration in subjects previously sensitized to mycobacterial peptides, such as individuals with past, active or latent tuberculous infection, previous BCG vaccination, or exposure to atypical mycobacteria. PPD tests are positive in approximately 80 percent of cases of active TB, but a negative result does not exclude TB. In contrast, over 90 percent of patients with sarcoidosis have anergy to tuberculous antigens and a negative skin reaction to PPDs, so a positive skin reaction to PPDs should prompt a thorough investigation for tuberculosis (Smith-Rohrberg and Sharma 2006). Immunosuppression due to diseases such as HIV or lymphoma, or secondary to immunosuppression, can also cause negative reactions to PPD.

Interferon-γ release assays (IGRAs) identify circulating lymphocytes that recognize antigens specific to *M. tuberculosis* and are therefore more specific for previous exposure to tuberculosis than PPDs. These assays have an established role in identifying patients with latent TB, but have not been fully validated for diagnosing active TB, or distinguishing tuberculosis from sarcoidosis as yet. Given the high incidence of anergy to PPD in subjects with sarcoidosis, IGRAs might also be expected to be negative.

BLOOD TESTS

Blood tests are not particularly helpful in differentiating tuberculosis from sarcoidosis. Markedly raised levels of inflammatory markers such as C-reactive protein and the erythrocyte sedimentation rate (ESR) are unusual in cases of sarcoidosis, and more common in patients with TB but less when infection is restricted to nodal disease. Conversely the serum angiotensin-converting enzyme (ACE) is raised in only 50–85 percent of cases of sarcoid (Studdy et al. 1983), and can also be high in 4 percent of cases of TB (Studdy et al. 1983) or other granulomatous diseases. Raised calcium would suggest sarcoid but is present in only 2.3 percent of cases (Baughman et al. 2001). Abnormal liver function tests suggestive of sarcoid infiltration are found in 11.5 percent of cases of sarcoidosis (Baughman et al. 2001), but again also occur with tuberculosis.

CYTOLOGY AND LYMPHOCYTE RATIOS

A BAL lymphocytosis of greater than 50 percent is unlikely with tuberculosis and suggests sarcoid is the diagnosis, but occurs in only a minority of patients (Greco et al. 2005). A BAL CD4/CD8 lymphocyte ratio greater than 3.5 may indicate sarcoidosis, but is also found in 29 percent of patients with culture-proven tuberculosis (Greco et al. 2005). Overall, BAL cytology and lymphocyte subset ratios are not often helpful in differentiating sarcoid and tuberculosis.

OTHER INFECTIOUS DISEASES THAT CAN CAUSE ISOLATED MEDIASTINAL LYMPHADENOPATHY

Although many infectious diseases can cause mediastinal lymphadenopathy, this is usually in combination with patterns of pulmonary parenchymal diseases that clearly suggest sarcoidosis is not the diagnosis. However, infection with the endemic fungus Histoplasma capsulatum (histoplasmosis) can present with hilar and mediastinal lymphadenopathy and should be considered in at-risk populations in the differential diagnosis (Kauffman 2007). Previous H. capsulatum infection can cause asymptomatic non-progressive calcified hilar nodes that can be mistaken for sarcoid, but does not represent active disease so does not usually require investigation. Acute pulmonary histoplasmosis can closely mimic acute sarcoid, presenting with bilateral hilar lymphadenopathy, arthralgia and EN (Thornberry et al. 1982). Recognition depends on a high index of suspicion, which depends on knowing the geography of exposure to H. capsulatum (mainly the Ohio and Mississippi river valleys in the USA, rare in Europe, but also not uncommon in parts of Africa and Asia), and serological testing. In addition, histoplasmosis can cause asymmetric enlarged coalesced mediastinal nodes, often with local effects such as superior vena cava obstruction, but this presentation is usually clinically distinct to sarcoid.

Diagnosis of histoplamosis requires sending samples for specific fungal stains, which should identify fungi within affected nodal tissue. Culture of H. capsulatum takes up to 6 weeks and is usually negative in acute histoplasmosis. Serological tests for Histoplasma become positive by 6 weeks after infection but are often positive in people from endemic regions, so are mainly useful at suggesting histoplasmosis should be included in the differential diagnosis. An antigen test exists, but there are few data on its utility in acute histoplasmosis in non-HIV patients.

Other endemic fungal infections such as blastomycosis or coccidiomycosis can also cause mediastinal lymphadenopathy, usually with some lung parenchymal involvement, and so on occasions might be confused with sarcoidosis (Sheflin et al. 1990). Isolated lymphadenopathy is a relative common presentation for infections caused by NTM, especially in HIV-positive individuals, but the nodes affected are usually extrathoracic and mycobacteria are readily identified by microscopy or culture of nodal tissue. Other infections that can cause significant mediastinal adenopathy such as nocardiosis and actinomycosis will usually have dominant pulmonary parenchymal involvement so are less readily confused with sarcoidosis.

SUMMARY

Although there is considerable overlap in the clinical features of isolated mediastinal lymphadenopathy caused by sarcoid or tuberculosis, the diagnosis is frequently suggested by epidemiological factors, radiological features, and the presence or absence of caseation in granulomas found in biopsies. Bilateral symmetrically enlarged nodes including hilar nodes in an individual at low risk of TB is likely to be sarcoid, especially if the patient has EN and is only mildly systemically unwell, whereas asymmetric nodal disease with central necrosis on CT in a high-risk patient would make tuberculosis more likely. Microscopy and culture are able to unequivocally confirm the presence of mycobacterial infection, but unfortunately these tests have a significant false-negative rate and culture takes up to 6 weeks, and even histology is not diagnostic. The sensitivity and specificity of newer tests such as PCR or IGRAs are unlikely to be adequate to make a certain diagnosis. In the future, analysis of nodal lymphocytes using modified IGRAs or other immunological tests may provide an effective test for differentiating sarcoid and tuberculous lymphadenopathy. In some cases of mediastinal lymphadenopathy it will not be possible to be sure whether infection or sarcoid is the cause, and a balanced clinical judgment whether a trial of anti-tuberculous or anti-fungal therapy is warranted may be required.

Pulmonary nodules and cavitation

Although unusual, sarcoidosis can present with CT evidence of parenchymal macronodules (Traill et al. 1997), the differential diagnosis of which includes infections with Aspergillus species, endemic fungi, *Cryptococcus*, brucella, and parasites (e.g. paragonimiasis) if the patient lives in or has visited the appropriate geographical areas. The rare necrotizing sarcoid granulomatosis causes dry cavitating pulmonary lesions often with significant systemic symptoms, a presentation that can readily be confused with several infections including tuberculosis, NTM, semi-invasive forms of aspergillosis, *Nocardia*, actinomycosis, and endemic fungal infections.

Appropriate serological tests will help identify infectious causes, and prolonged culture of sputum, bronchial washings and biopsy samples for fungi, mycobacteria and unusual bacterial pathogens are necessary. Biopsies of the affected areas can be diagnostic of sarcoid as long as specific stains for microorganisms are performed.

Although granulomas may be present with many of these infections they are usually poorly defined and fragmentary compared to sarcoid granulomas, and specific stains should identify infective elements.

Micronodular infiltrations

The radiological appearances of diffuse micronodular infiltration through both lungs due to sarcoid is similar to that of miliary tuberculosis and some cases of acute histoplasmosis or other endemic fungal infections (Kauffman 2007). Sarcoid micronodules characteristically form along fissures (Traill *et al.* 1997) and the pleura and tend to spare the lower lobes, whereas miliary infection is more uniform in its distribution (Andreu *et al.* 2004). Patients with miliary infection should be significantly unwell whereas micronodular sarcoid can be surprisingly asymptomatic. Transbronchial biopsies will identify granulomas in a high proportion of both sarcoid and miliary TB; in sarcoid they tend to be confined to the interstitium, following the bronchovascular bundles and interlobular septae, and do not involve the airspaces, whereas in TB the granulomas tend to be rounded and bronchiolar involvement is common (Andreu *et al.* 2004).

Pleural disease

Pleural involvement is rare in sarcoidosis and the identification of pleural granulomas strongly suggests tuberculosis. Pleural sarcoid may need to be considered in patients with known sarcoid or who are at low risk of TB.

Apical fibrosis

Longstanding sarcoid may cause apical fibrosis, which can also be a consequence of previous tuberculosis and chronic indolent *Aspergillus* infection and endemic mycoses. Apical fibrosis due to sarcoid may cause dyspnea but is often asymptomatic, and is static or only slowly progressive, symmetrical in distribution and the patient may have a clear history of a diagnosis of sarcoid many years earlier. Significant systemic symptoms, asymmetrical or more rapidly progressive disease should prompt investigations for an alternative

diagnosis with bronchoscopy, BAL, and serological tests for fungi.

Diffuse alveolitis

Acute sarcoidosis may present with a diffuse widespread ground-glass pattern suggestive of an alveolitis (Traill *et al.* 1997), and marked dyspnea with a dry cough. This clinical presentation is similar to those seen during infection with *Pneumocystis jirovecii* or cytomegalovirus, but these infections are rare unless the patient is immunosuppressed or HIV-positive. However, bronchoscopy for BAL and transbronchial biopsies will usually be necessary to exclude an infectious cause of this presentation.

NEUROLOGICAL DISEASE

Neurosarcoid occurs in up to 15 percent of patients with sarcoid, and can affect any part of the neurological system with a wide range of presentations including cranial nerve palsies, aseptic meningitis, hydrocephalus, cerebral lesions (including pituitary syndromes), seizures, psychiatric syndromes, spinal syndromes and peripheral neuropathies (Zajicek *et al.* 1999; Hoitsma *et al.* 2004). A prior diagnosis of sarcoidosis suggests new neurological symptoms are likely to be caused by sarcoid, but an opportunistic infection needs to be considered if the patient is receiving immunosuppressive therapy. Most infectious diseases affecting the nervous system will cause an unremitting deterioration in the patient's clinical status, contrasting with the often more variable and chronic presentation of neurosarcoid. However, some clinical presentations of neurosarcoid can be confused with infectious disease, and published criteria for the diagnosis of neurosarcoidosis (Hoitsma *et al.* 2004) state a definite diagnosis depends on exclusion of all other causes. Again the epidemiological background of the patient is important and this often suggests whether there is a risk for specific infectious diseases. Systemic features of sarcoid or infectious disease should be sought, including the use of ACE levels, reaction to PPD and IGRA tests as described earlier, and evidence of systemic sarcoidosis should prompt biopsies of non-neurological anatomical sites to provide histological evidence of the diagnosis. In the absence of alternative extracranial disease that can be biopsied, then brain biopsies with specific staining and culture for mycobacterial and fungal organisms may be necessary to differentiate sarcoid from infective causes of neurological disease.

Aseptic meningitis

Aseptic meningitis affects 7–18 percent of patients with neurosarcoid (Ginsberg and Kidd, 2008), sometimes associated with focal masses usually affecting the basal aspects of the brain. Infectious diseases that may also present with 'culture-negative' meningitis include tuberculosis, *Cryptococcus neoformans*, disseminated histoplasmosis, Lyme disease and neurosyphilis. In addition, malignant disease (e.g.

neurolymphomas and leptomeningeal metastases) should be considered. Features of sarcoid and infectious causes of meningitis are summarized in Table 39.3.

Presentation of all these diseases tends to be insidious, but headache and fever are much more common in meningitis due to tuberculosis (≥90 percent) or fungi (56 percent for *C. neoformans*) than neurosarcoid (24 percent of cases) (Hoitsma *et al.* 2004; Garg 2010). The neuroradiological changes associated with sarcoid meningitis (thickening and enhancement of the basal leptomeninges) are generally indistinguishable from those of tuberculous or fungal meningitis (Smith *et al.* 2004; Terushkin *et al.* 2010).

The typical cerebrospinal fluid (CSF) examination of a patient with meningitis caused by sarcoid, tuberculosis or fungi is similar, with a mild pleocytosis, high protein content and slightly low glucose concentration. Increases in the concentration of CSF ACE, oligoclonal bands and CD4/CD8 lymphocyte ratios have been reported with neurosarcoid but are not sensitive or specific enough to exclude infection. CSF is only positive for acid-fast bacilli in 5–30 percent, culture positive in 45–90 percent (Garg 2010), and PCR positive in 56 percent of cases of tuberculosis meningitis (Pai *et al.* 2003). All patients presenting with an aseptic meningitis should have an HIV test, the main risk factor for cryptococcal meningitis. CSF and blood cryptococcal antigen is positive in around 90 percent of patients with cryptococcal meningitis, and microscopy of CSF using Indian ink staining will identify cryptococci in 50–95 percent of cases. Interestingly, there

Table 39.3 Features that distinguish meningitis caused by neurosarcoid or infectious diseases.

Clinical feature/test	Neurosarcoid	Tuberculous meningitis	Cryptococcal meningitis	Disseminated histoplasmosis	Lyme disease	Syphilis
At-risk populations	African American and other African origin populations Scandinavia	TB endemic regions, e.g. Sub-Saharan Africa, Asia Homeless, prison populations, drug abuse Defects in cell-mediated immunity	Defects in cell-mediated immunity, HIV	Travel to endemic areas, e.g. Mississippi and Ohio river valleys Exposure to bird or bat guano Defects in cell-mediated immunity	Exposure to deer-borne ticks, e.g. eastern USA, northern Europe	Homosexuality History of sexually transmitted infections
Clinical features	Insidious Fever 19%, meningism 12%, headache 24% Cranial nerve palsies common	Insidious Fever 91%, meningism 79%, headache 96% Cranial nerve palsies 25%	Insidious Fever 56%, meningism 24%, headache 73% Cranial nerve palsies unusual	Insidious Fever, meningism, headache Cranial nerve palsies common	Symptoms weeks after skin lesions Cranial nerve palsies (especially 7th nerve)	Often asymptomatic and very chronic
CSF findings	Lymphocytosis Normal or slightly low CSF glucose Raised CSF protein Raised CSF ACE Oligoclonal bands matched with serum	Lymphocytosis Decreased CSF glucose Very raised CSF protein AFB positive 5–30% Culture positive 4–90%	Lymphocytosis Decreased glucose Very raised CSF protein India ink stain positive 50–95% Cryptococcal antigen positive 90% Culture often positive	Lymphocytosis or mononuclear cells Decreased glucose Very raised CSF protein Yeast forms within macrophages on silver staining Culture usually negative	Lymphocytosis Normal glucose Raised CSF protein CSF IgM for *B. burgdoferi* often positive Culture negative	Lymphocytosis Normal glucose Raised CSF protein Oligoclonal bands Treponemal serology positive Culture negative
Other specific tests	Evidence of other organ involvement SACE	Evidence of lung disease Hyponatremia common Skin test with PPD/IGRA	HIV test Serum cryptococcal antigen	Evidence of other organ involvement Serum serology	Serum *B. burgdoferi* serology	Serum treponemal serology

AFB, acid-fast bacilli; CSF, cerebrospinal fluid; IGRA, interferon-gamma release assay; PPD, purified protein derivative; SACE, serum angiotensin-converting enzyme have been reports of concomitant sarcoidosis and crypto-coccal meningitis (Ross and Katz 2002). In meningitis due to disseminated histoplasmosis, CSF culture is usually negative, although yeast forms may be seen within mononuclear cells. Although meningitis caused by neurosyphilis is usually very chronic or asymptomatic, it can present more acutely on occasions and should be considered in the differential diagnosis. CSF glucose is usually normal, and treponemal serology will be positive.

Lyme disease, caused by infection with the spirochete *Borrelia burgdorferi* acquired from tick bites, can cause meningitis associated with cranial nerve (especially facial nerve) palsies. Affected patients should have a history of exposure to *B. burdoferi* infected ticks, which are limited to specific geographical areas (e.g. eastern USA). The initial skin lesions may have occurred a number of weeks earlier, and CSF glucose will be normal. Serology for *B. burgdorferi* will usually but not always be positive, with detection of serum or CSF IgM to *B. burgdorferi* confirming the diagnosis.

Other neurological presentations

Although both sarcoidosis and Lyme disease can cause bilateral seventh nerve palsies, in practice the presence of enlarged parotids makes a diagnosis of sarcoid obvious. Cranial nerve palsies are also a complication of basal meningitis-like tuberculosis, the differentiation of which from sarcoid is discussed above. Granulomas due to neurosarcoid can form small or large intracranial space-occupying lesions. They can occupy extradural, subdural and parenchymous locations. Hence infectious diseases that also cause intracranial focal lesions may need to be considered in the differential diagnosis, including TB, viral and fungal infections. However, sarcoid does not cause ring-enhancing lesions, making infectious diseases unlikely in most circum-stances. Rarely, sarcoid can cause a large-fiber peripheral neuropathy, and nerve biopsy may show epineural and perineural granulomas. Nerve granulomas also occur in leprosy, caused by *Mycobacterium leprae*, but leprosy is very rare outside endemic areas such as Asia. *M. leprae* bacilli can be seen in nerve biopsies and the diagnosis confirmed with Fite staining.

LIVER DISEASE

In patients with sarcoidosis, hepatomegaly and/or raised serum transanimases or alkaline phosphatase is not uncom-mon, and liver biopsies often contain granulomas, but liver involvement is usually asymptomatic. In a patient known to have sarcoid, hepatic granulomas can generally be assumed to be caused by sarcoid. However, if there is no established diagnosis of sarcoid there is a wide range of causes of hepatic granulomas that need to be considered, including several infectious diseases.

As well as identification of extrahepatic clinical features, there are specific histological features that differentiate between sarcoid and other causes of hepatic granulomas

(summarized in Table 39.4). Sarcoid hepatic granulomas are typically non-caseating, round and well demarcated, and occur within the portal or periportal tract. The granulomas characteristically heal by fibrosis, occasionally causing portal hypertension. Typical features were found in 81 percent of cases in one study, with the remaining cases showing atypical features such as necrosis and/or no associated fibrosis (Drebber *et al.* 2008). Features suggesting particular infec-tious diseases are discussed below.

Tuberculosis, NTM and leprosy

Hepatic granulomas are common in disseminated tubercu-losis, but are AFB (acid-fast bacillus) or culture-positive in only 54 percent of cases (Amarapurkar *et al.* 2008). Caseation is found in 78 percent of cases. Disseminated BCG infection (developing after BCG vaccination or BCG immunotherapy for bladder cancer) can also cause hepatic granulomas and should be considered in the right clinical context. Dissemi-nated NTM occurs predominately in HIV-positive patients with low CD4 counts and cause poorly formed hepatic granulomas containing large numbers of AFBs within histiocytes or Kupffer cells, so is unlikely to be confused with hepatic sarcoid. The clinical manifestations of leprosy are distinctive and unlikely to be confused with sarcoidosis, especially as hepatic granulomas are more prevalent in lepromatous leprosy which is characterized by extensive skin lesions, clinically palpable peripheral nerves, and less well formed granulomas containing numerous bacilli.

Brucellosis

Brucellosis is a zoonosis caused by *Brucella* species, usually contracted from swine, goats or cattle and therefore pre-dominantly seen in farmers, butchers and vets. Patients present with intermittent fevers and myalgia, and often have hepatosplenomegaly. Hepatic granulomas due to brucellosis have few features and can cause diagnostic confusion with sarcoid as there is usually no obvious localized site of extrahepatic infection. *Brucella* are most often isolated from blood or bone marrow.

Other infectious disease

A range of other infectious diseases may occasionally need to be considered in the differential diagnosis of hepatic granulomas. These include Q fever (*Coxiella burnetii*), cat scratch disease (*Bartonella henselae*), listeriosis (*Listeria monocytogenes*), *Yersinia* infections, toxoplasmosis (*Toxoplasma gondii*), and infection with cytomegalovirus (CMV) or Epstein–Barr virus (EBV). Hepatic granulomas associated with these infections are usually ill-defined and often associated with specific unusual features, such as a fibrin ring in Q fever or histiocytic granulomas with CMV and EBV. Fungal infections can also cause hepatic granulomas. Endemic fungal infections (e.g. disseminated histoplasmosis) are most likely to be confused with sarcoidosis, as hepatic infections due to *Aspergillus* or

Table 39.4 Features of liver granulomas associated with sarcoid or infectious diseases.

	Sarcoid	Tuberculosis	NTM	Leprosy	Brucellosis	Viruses (e.g. CMV, EBV, HSV)	Fungal infections (e.g. Histoplasma, Aspergillus, Candida)	Schistosomiasis
Histological features of granulomas	Non-caseating 99%, round, well demarcated Frequently in the periportal tract	Caseating 78%, tend to coalesce Common in cases of disseminated disease	Can be caseating	Commoner in lepromatous leprosy	No distinguishing features	CMV commonly associated with fibrin ring granulomas	Often poorly formed, can be necrotizing	Eosinophils common
Other histological features	Occasionally portal hypertension and granulomatous destruction of portal veins	Positive for acid-fast bacilli in 54%	AFBs readily identified inside histiocytes or Kupffer cells	M. leprae commonly identified on acid-fast and Fite staining Rarely culture-positive	Rarely culture-positive		Silver stains may identify fungal elements	Fragments of schistosomal eggs may be visible
Important general features	See Table 39.1A/Table 39.1B	See Table 39.1A/Table 39.1B	See Table 39.1A/Table 39.1B	Geographic exposure SACE raised in 34%	Exposure to farm animals Blood and bone marrow culture Serum agglutinin titer	Viral PCR quantification of CMV and EBV Serological tests	Immunosuppressed (Candida, Aspergillus) Geographic exposure (endemic mycoses) See Table 39.1A/Table 39.1B	Geographic exposure Schistosomal eggs in feces or on rectal biopsy

AFB, acid-fast bacilli; CMV, cytomegalovirus; EBV, Epstein–Barr virus; HSV, herpes simplex virus; NTM, non-tuberculous mycobacterium; PCR, polymerase chain reaction; SACE, serum angiotensin-converting enzyme

Candida liver are generally restricted to severely immunocompromised patients. In patients with the correct environmental exposure, parasitic infections such as schistosomiasis should be considered, but can be distinguished from sarcoid by a predominance of eosinophils and evidence of egg fragments associated with the granulomas.

OTHER ORGANS

Cutaneous disease

Acute sarcoid is a common cause of EN, but EN is also associated with infectious diseases including tuberculosis, streptococcal and *Salmonella* infections, leprosy, cat scratch disease, EBV and CMV. The clinical picture and the results of some simple investigations (e.g. serology, throat swab culture, antistreptolysin O (ASO) titers, chest X-ray) will identify the cause in the majority of cases. Lupus pernio is clinically distinctive and is unlikely to be confused with other conditions, but tuberculosis, leprosy, NTMs (e.g. Buruli ulcer caused by *Mycobacterium marinum*), cutaneous leishmaniasis, endemic fungal infections (e.g. paracoccidioidomycosis) cause slowly progressive, potentially destructive granulomatous skin infiltrations and may need to be considered in the differential diagnosis of sarcoid.

Nodal disease

Disseminated lymphadenopathy due to sarcoid can cause palpable inguinal, cervical (mainly in the posterior triangle) and axillary lymph nodes. Extrathoracic nodal sarcoid can be confused with a variety of infectious diseases that also cause granulomatous lymphadenopathy, including tuberculosis, NTMs, cat scratch fever, brucellosis and endemic fungal infections. In sarcoidosis the enlarged nodes are usually discrete, mobile, non-tender, and although asymmetric they tend not to be massively enlarged. Large nodal masses that are fixed to other tissues, fluctuant or forming sinuses suggest an infective cause. EBV, CMV and toxoplasmosis may present with non-specific symptoms and widespread lymphadenopathy and could clinically be mistaken for sarcoidosis, but the nodal involvement tends to be symmetrical and small volume and these infections are readily identified by viral PCR or serological tests.

Other organ involvement

As sarcoid can cause granulomatous infiltrations of almost any organ, a differential diagnosis of sarcoid or a granulomatous infection such as tuberculosis, endemic fungi, leishmania or brucellosis may have to be considered on occasions in a wide variety of clinical situations associated with biopsy evidence of granulomas, including granulomatous infiltration of the genitourinary tract or bone marrow.

CONCLUSION

Differentiating sarcoidosis from granulomatous infectious diseases can be a diagnostic conundrum, but untreated infection can be fatal, and mistaken use of immunosuppression could exacerbate an underlying infection. Although tuberculosis is the most important infectious disease that needs to be considered, a variety of other infections – including endemic fungi, NTM, brucellosis and parasitic infections – can also form part of the differential diagnosis for some presentations of sarcoid. Epidemiological features often define which infectious diseases could be present, thereby allowing targeted investigations for an appropriate differential diagnosis. To identify or exclude infectious disease, histological specimens containing granulomas will need microscopy and culture for fungal and bacterial pathogens. Concomitant disease with infectious agents should be considered if there is a clinical deterioration in a patient with sarcoid despite treatment.

REFERENCES

Amarapurkar DN, Patel ND, Amarapurkar AD (2008). Hepatobiliary tuberculosis in western India. *Indian J Pathol Microbiol* 51: 175–81.

Andreu J, Caceres J, Pallisa E, Martinez-Rodriguez M (2004). Radiological manifestations of pulmonary tuberculosis. *Eur J Radiol* 51: 139–49.

Baughman RP, Teirstein AS, Judson MA et al. (2001). Clinical characteristics of patients in a case control study of sarcoidosis. *Am J Respir Crit Care Med* 164: 1885–9.

Brett GZ (1965). Epidemiological trends in tuberculosis and sarcoidosis in a district of London between 1958 and 1963. *Tubercle* 46: 413–16.

Chapman JT, Mehta AC (2003). Bronchoscopy in sarcoidosis: diagnostic and therapeutic interventions. *Curr Opin Pulm Med* 9: 402–7.

Cutler RR, Baithun SI, Doran HM, Wilson P (1994). Association between the histological diagnosis of tuberculosis and microbiological findings. *Tuber Lung Dis* 75: 75–9.

Drebber U, Kasper HU, Ratering J et al. (2008). Hepatic granulomas: histological and molecular pathological approach to differential diagnosis – a study of 442 cases. *Liver Int* 28: 828–34.

Garg RK (2010). Tuberculous meningitis. *Acta Neurol Scand* 122: 75–90.

Gawne-Cain ML, Hansell DM (1996). The pattern and distribution of calcified mediastinal lymph nodes in sarcoidosis and tuberculosis: a CT study. *Clin Radiol* 51: 263–7.

Ghossein RA, Ross DG, Salomon RN, Rabson AR (1994). A search for mycobacterial DNA in sarcoidosis using the polymerase chain reaction. *Am J Clin Pathol* 101: 733–7.

Gilman MJ, Wang KP (1980). Transbronchial lung biopsy in sarcoidosis: an approach to determine the optimal number of biopsies. *Am Rev Respir Dis* 122: 721–4.

Ginsberg L, Kidd D (2008). Chronic and recurrent meningitis. *Pract Neurol* 8: 348–61.

Greco S, Marruchella A, Massari M, Saltini C (2005). Predictive value of BAL cellular analysis in differentiating pulmonary tuberculosis and sarcoidosis. *Eur Respir J* 26: 360–1; author reply 362.

Gulati M, Venkataramu NK, Gupta S et al. (2000). Ultrasound guided fine needle aspiration biopsy in mediastinal tuberculosis. *Int J Tuberc Lung Dis* 4: 1164–8.

Health Protection Agency (2009). *Tuberculosis in the UK.* Annual report on tuberculosis surveillance in the UK, available at www.hpa.org.uk/web/hpawebfile/hpaweb_c/1259152022594.

Hoitsma E, Faber CG, Drent M, SHARMA OP (2004). Neurosarcoidosis: a clinical dilemma. *Lancet Neurol* 3: 397–407.

Kauffman CA (2007). Histoplasmosis: a clinical and laboratory update. *Clin Microbiol Rev* 20: 115–32.

Koonitz CH, Joyner LR, Nelson RA (1976). Transbronchial lung biopsy via the fiberoptic bronchoscope in sarcoidosis. *Ann Intern Med* 85: 64–6.

Lee JH, Park SS, Lee DH *et al.* (1992). Endobronchial tuberculosis: clinical and bronchoscopic features in 121 cases. *Chest* 102: 990–4.

Mert A, Ozaras R, Tabak F, Ozturk R (2004). Primary tuberculosis cases presenting with erythema nodosum. *J Dermatol* 31: 66–8.

Moon WK, Im JG, Yeon KM, Han MC (1997). Tuberculosis of the central airways: CT findings of active and fibrotic disease. *Am J Roentgen* 169: 649–53.

Pai M, Flores LL, Pai N *et al.* (2003). Diagnostic accuracy of nucleic acid amplification tests for tuberculous meningitis: a systematic review and meta-analysis. *Lancet Infect Dis* 3: 633–43.

Pietinalho A, Hiraga Y, Hosoda Y *et al.* (1995). The frequency of sarcoidosis in Finland and Hokkaido, Japan: a comparative epidemiological study. *Sarcoidosis* 12: 61–7.

Ross JJ, Katz JD (2002). Cryptococcal meningitis and sarcoidosis. *Scand J Infect Dis* 34: 937–9.

Rybicki BA, Major M, Popovich J *et al.* (1997). Racial differences in sarcoidosis incidence: a 5-year study in a health maintenance organization. *Am J Epidemiol* 145: 234–41.

Sheflin JR, Campbell JA, Thompson GP (1990). Pulmanary blastomycosis: Findings on chest radiographs in 63 patients. *AJR Am J Roentgenol* 154(6): 1177–80.

Sider L, Horton ES (1990). Hilar and mediastinal adenopathy in sarcoidosis as detected by computed tomography. *J Thorac Imaging* 5: 77–80.

Smith-Rohrberg D, Sharma SK (2006). Tuberculin skin test among pulmonary sarcoidosis patients with and without tuberculosis: its utility for the screening of the two conditions in tuberculosis-endemic regions. *Sarcoid Vasc Diff Lung Dis* 23: 130–4.

Smith JK, Matheus MG, Castillo M (2004). Imaging manifestations of neurosarcoidosis. *Am J Roentgen* 182: 289–95.

Story A, Murad S, Roberts W *et al.* (2007). Tuberculosis in London: the importance of homelessness, problem drug use and prison. *Thorax* 62: 667–71.

Studdy PR, Lapworth R, Bird R (1983). Angiotensin-converting enzyme and its clinical significance: a review. *J Clin Pathol* 36: 938–47.

Terushkin V, Stern BJ, Judson MA *et al.* (2010). Neurosarcoidosis: presentations and management. *Neurologist* 16: 2–15.

Thomas KW, Hunninghake GW (2003). Sarcoidosis. *J Am Med Assoc* 289: 3300–3.

Thombemy DK, Wheat LT, Brand KD, Rosenthal J (1982). Histoplasmosis presenting with joint pain and hilar adenopathy: pseudosarcoidosis. *Arthirtis Rheum* 25(12): 396–402.

Tournoy KG, Rintoul RC, Van Meerbeeck JP *et al.* (2009). EBUS-TBNA for the diagnosis of central parenchymal lung lesions not visible at routine bronchoscopy. *Lung Cancer* 63: 45–9.

Traill ZC, Maskell GF, Gleeson FV (1997). High-resolution CT findings of pulmonary sarcoidosis. *Am J Roentgen* 168: 1557–60.

Wong M, Yasufuku K, Nakajima T *et al.* (2007). Endobronchial ultrasound: new insight for the diagnosis of sarcoidosis. *Eur Respir J* 29: 1182–6.

Zajicek JP, Scolding NJ, Foster O *et al.* (1999). Central nervous system sarcoidosis: Diagnosis and Management. *QJM* 92(2): 103–17.

39

2. Miscellaneous diseases

SIDDHARTHA PARKER AND DAVID CAVE

INTRODUCTION

Sarcoidosis is an enigmatic systemic condition with a worldwide distribution. The etiology remains unknown and treatment remains empirical. The histological hallmark of the 'sarcoid granuloma' has led to the concept that a number of diseases with a granulomatous component to their histopathology may have a common or linked pathogenesis. Other conditions that may co-exist may share a common genetic milieu and/or similar immune-pathogenetic pathways. Different disorders demonstrating non-caseating granulomas as part of their pathology has led to many reports consisting of either small case series or case reports purporting a linkage between them and sarcoidosis. This concept has been challenged by a recent large-scale epidemiological study that provides a reassessment of sarcoid-associated diseases. This chapter reviews the old and new associations. However, until the etiologies of sarcoid are elucidated, the validity of even this approach will remain observational. It does minimize the risk of unwarranted associations being investigated.

The fundamental immunology of sarcoidosis is mediated primarily by CD4+ T-helper cells and cells derived from mononuclear phagocytes that allow for the direct association with a number of other systemic and immunologically mediated diseases. This autoimmune pathophysiology, which includes auto-antibodies, immune complexes and altered lymphocyte function, suggests a common predisposition among those with symptoms consistent with multiple disorders. In some cases, sarcoidosis may itself mimic the presentation of associated disorders, but the clinical challenge is to identify those circumstances when the diagnosis of sarcoidosis may be made independently, perhaps with a change in the management, outcomes and prognosis. The presence of non-caseating granulomas in the gastrointestinal (GI) tract may be seen in Crohn's disease. This histological connection has led to a variety of hypotheses; this issue will be discussed below.

LITERATURE SEARCH

A comprehensive literature search returns a wide variety of evidence suggesting associations between sarcoidosis and various other diseases, the great majority of which are immune-mediated chronic inflammatory diseases. The preponderance of this evidence is observational and supported only by case reports.

The most convincing basis for association is provided by a large-scale epidemiological study (Rajoriya et al. 2009). This retrospective study of more than 600 000 people in the Oxford Record Linkage Study (ORLS) database was analyzed for the presence of patients with the diagnosis of sarcoidosis both before and/or after diagnosis with a wide variety of immune-mediated or chronic inflammatory diseases. The data covered more than a 30-year period in the northern region of the United Kingdom with a median follow-up of 19.5 years. The authors identified over 1510 patients with sarcoidosis and found significant associations in patients with:

- ulcerative colitis – observed number 12, expected 5.6 (adjusted rate ratio 2.14, 95% confidence interval 1.11–3.74);
- celiac disease – observed number 5, expected 1.6 (ARR 3.13, CI 1.01–7.29);
- systemic lupus erythematosus (SLE) – observed 5, expected 0.6 (ARA 8.33, CI 2.71–19.4);
- thyrotoxicosis – observed 16, expected 6.5 (ARA 2.46, CI 1.41.–4.00);
- myxoedema – observed 13, expected 6.0 (ARA 1.51, CI 1.15.–3.71);

- autoimmune chronic hepatitis – observed number 4, expected 0.6 (ARR 6.67, CI 1.82–17.1);
- multiple sclerosis – observed number 13, expected 4.4 (ARA 3.25, CI 1.7–5.6).

A weaker association was found with found with type 2 diabetes. Perhaps surprisingly, no significant associations were found with Crohn's disease (observed number 7, expected 4.6; ARR 1.52, CI 0.61–3.14), primary biliary cirrhosis, Sjögren's disease or scleroderma, among others. The study was limited by the size of the regional population, but it does provide the best epidemiological evidence to date of associations between sarcoidosis and immune-mediated diseases.

Box 39b.1 lists diseases associated with sarcoidosis and those previously suspected but not confirmed to be associated with sarcoidosis based on this epidemiological study.

An even larger study, using the Multigenerational Register in Sweden, found a familial link of both Crohn's disease and ulcerative colitis with sarcoidosis. This linkage, along with

---

Box 39.1 Disorders with and without association with sarcoidosis

Disorders associated with sarcoidosis
- Chronic active hepatitis
- Celiac disease
- Multiple sclerosis
- Myxedema
- Systemic lupus erythematosus
- Thyrotoxicosis
- Ulcerative colitis

Disorders not associated with sarcoidosis
- Crohn's disease
- Pernicious anemia
- Psoriasis
- Rheumatoid arthritis

---

that of other autoimmune disorders, suggested a genetic basis for the observations (Hemminki *et al.* 2010).

RHEUMATOLOGICAL ASSOCIATIONS

Sarcoidosis may present with connective tissue or musculoskeletal symptoms depending on the systems involved. However, positive rheumatoid factor and antinuclear antibodies, common in rheumatologic disease, may also be found in sarcoidosis. Similar clinical and pathological outcomes suggest related immune-pathogenic mechanisms, as are commonly seen among patients with connective tissue disorders. There is well-documented support of a close relationship between systemic lupus erythematosus and rheumatoid arthritis and a similar association between SLE and systemic sclerosis (scleroderma).

A comprehensive literature review returns numerous reports of concomitant sarcoidosis and rheumatologic and connective tissue disease. Several case reports note the presentation of sarcoidosis concomitant with a number of

separate rheumatologic disorders including Sjögren's syndrome (SjS), SLE, systemic sclerosis (SyS), rheumatoid arthritis (RA), gout, psoriasis, and various vasculitides. Many of these manifestations may be the direct result of sarcoidosis, which may mimic other disease patterns owing to broad systemic effects. Similarly, identifying true associations is complicated by the incidental and simultaneous co-existence of two different diseases. However, there is some evidence, primarily from case reports and limited reviews over the last 50 years, that sarcoidosis may co-exist with rheumatic disease more frequently than chance alone would suggest.

The epidemiological study by Rajoriya and associates in 2009 found a significant association with SLE in 1510 sarcoidosis patients, with an odds ratio of 8.3. Although limited in size and scope, the study did report investigating for associations with a broad range of immune-mediated and rheumatologic diseases including ankylosing spondylitis, dermatomyositis, psoriasis, rheumatoid arthritis, scleroderma, and Sjögren's syndrome. Interestingly, only SLE was found to have an increased association.

Systemic lupus erythematosus

SLE is an autoimmune disorder characterized by the production of antinuclear antibodies and commonly affecting multiple organ systems. There is a strong genetic component and well documented associations with other autoimmune and rheumatologic disease (Sharma 2002). Until recently, the rare co-existence of sarcoid and SLE which may have similar presentations was believed to be primarily related to similar autoimmune disease mechanisms.

However, the sometimes similar presentations of SLE and sarcoidosis also creates the possibility of misdiagnosis and mimicry. Both SLE and sarcoidosis may present with hyperglobulinemia, positive ANA, and decreased lymphoid responsiveness. There are multiple case reports of misdiagnosis including a patient who initially met the diagnostic criteria for SLE and improved with steroid therapy. After subsequent deterioration in her liver function, she was diagnosed with sarcoidosis when liver biopsy revealed non-caseating granuloma (Collins and Bourke 1996). Similarly, in 1964, Telium described two young women diagnosed with SLE who presented with rash, joint pain, anemia, leukopenia, pleurisy and peripheral lymphadenopathy. At autopsy, both were found to have non-caseating granulomas in the lungs, lymph nodes and blood vessels consistent with sarcoidosis.

Sarcoidosis and SLE have similar genetic predispositions. In addition to an increased incidence in Afro-Caribbean and African-American populations there is limited evidence suggesting up to 32 percent of patients with sarcoidosis will have positive ANA screening (Begum *et al.* 2002), suggesting that an association could be due in part to similar genetic predisposition. There are rare but well-documented cases of SLE and sarcoidosis in the same patient (Migita *et al.* 2005), including 19 cases in the English literature from 1979 to 2007 (Nakayama *et al.* 2007). One hospital review identified 300 SLE patients over 22 years at a single UK institution, with three associated case reports of sarcoidosis, consistent with a previous review of a variety of autoimmune diseases (including SLE, SyS and RA) and which also found co-existent sarcoidosis in approximately 6 of 569 subjects (Begum *et al.* 2002). More recently, the previously mentioned retrospective epidemiological study found supportive evidence of a significant association (odds ratio of 8.3) between sarcoidosis and SLE (Rajoriya *et al.* 2009).

The increasing epidemiological evidence of an association between sarcoidosis and SLE, combined with case reports of co-existing disease and similar clinical presentation, suggests that the co-existence may be under-reported and supports evidence of association. However, every effort should be made to narrow the diagnosis to a single disease, whether sarcoidosis or SLE, with continued monitoring as necessary for new or refractory symptoms that might suggest concomitant disease.

Systemic sclerosis

Systemic sclerosis (SSc), commonly known as scleroderma, is a systemic disorder characterized by microvascular inflammation with the deposition of collagen in skin and internal organs (primarily the gastrointestinal tract, lung, heart, and kidney). Sarcoidosis is typically diagnosed years after the onset of SSc and the symptoms are usually more severe and refractory to treatment (Cox *et al.* 1995; De Bandt *et al.* 1997).

There is limited case evidence of co-existing disease, the majority of which is reported in two case reviews. One describes the presentation and subsequent death of a 48-year-old woman initially seen for Raynaud's phenomenon, sclerodactyly, skin changes, and pulmonary fibrosis at age 29. Although initial chest X-ray showed bilateral hilar lymphadenopathy and nodular shadows, she was not diagnosed with sarcoidosis until 4 years later when lymph node biopsy showed non-caseating granuloma (Ishioka *et al.* 1999). Another case of a 3-year-old girl diagnosed with sarcoidosis on the basis of histology, hypercalcemia, and elevated angiotensin-converting enzyme (ACE) was reported (Ho *et al.* 2009). Although she had skin findings consistent with SSc, the authors point out that the symptoms were adequately explained by sarcoidosis alone.

Although SSc was included in the survey along with a number of immune-mediated and chronic inflammatory diseases, no association with sarcoidosis was found in Rajoriya's recent epidemiological review of sarcoidosis patients over a 30-year period (Rajoriya *et al.* 2009). Case reports support mimicry and/or overlap with difficulty attributing flares and worsening symptoms to SSc versus sarcoidosis. The current criteria for diagnosis of SSc are broad, and may be mimicked by atypical sarcoidosis.

Rheumatoid arthritis

Sarcoidosis often involves musculoskeletal findings including both acute and chronic arthritis in addition to tendonitis, myopathy and bone changes which may be more commonly seen with today's advanced imaging techniques. Even so, there is limited evidence of any direct association with rheumatoid arthritis (RA). Rare cases of concomitant RA and sarcoidosis have been reported (Ishioka *et al.* 1999). In addition, rheumatoid factor was present in 20–40 percent of patients with sarcoidosis, but of 94 patients with confirmed sarcoidosis only one case of RA was found (Sharma 2002). The epidemiological study by Rajoriya and associates (2009) found no evidence of an association, with an adjusted rate ratio of 0.89, identifying fewer cases of RA in the sarcoidosis population than would be expected based on the control population.

There is currently limited case-report evidence of rheumatoid arthritis in patients with sarcoidosis. Given the incidence of sarcoidosis and RA at the population level, co-existence would be expected by chance alone.

As discussed in Chapter 42, anti-tumor necrosis factor alpha (anti-TNF-α), in particular infliximab, a common therapeutic intervention for RA, is increasingly being used to treat refractory sarcoidosis (Farah and Shay 2007). Interestingly, there are case reports of patients on anti-TNF-α therapy with etanercept (also used for treatment of RA, psoriatic arthritis but not effective for treating sarcoidosis and inflammatory bowel disease), who have subsequently developed sarcoidosis. For example, sarcoidosis was diagnosed in two rheumatoid factor-positive females within 1 year of starting etanercept for RA. The sarcoidosis symptoms improved with cessation of the etanercept in both patients (Verschueren *et al.* 2007). While both infliximab and etanercept have the same general end-effect, TNF-α blockade, the mechanisms of action are different. It is unclear whether the underlying autoimmune process or systemic inflammation acts as a catalyst for sarcoidosis or the medication itself plays a role, but what is apparent is that infliximab may be useful in treating refractory sarcoid, while etanercept is permissive for its development.

Gout

While the association of gout with sarcoidosis has long been suggested and there are many case reports, the common occurrence of gout combined with a relatively common presentation of sarcoidosis suggests that association may be by chance. After identifying three cases of concomitant sarcoidosis, psoriasis and gout, Kaplan and Klatskin reviewed 73 cases of histologically confirmed sarcoidosis and 100 randomly selected cases of gout; none of the 73 sarcoidosis patients exhibited psoriasis and similarly there was no histologic confirmation of sarcoidosis in the 100 gout subjects (Kaplan and Klatskin 1960).

While case reports of gout and sarcoidosis have been made, the incidence of gout alone is likely adequate to explain the occasional co-existence. This was further confirmed inferentially by the fact that there was no association reported in the epidemiological study of Rajoriya *et al.* (2009).

Psoriasis

Cutaneous sarcoidosis has been documented with scaling plaques that resemble psoriasis, although this clinical presentation is rare and primarily reported in individuals with darker skin (Marchell and Judson 2007). One case report noted the diagnosis of sarcoidosis in a patient with existing psoriasis, suggesting sarcoidosis was the result of a Koebner reaction in psoriasis rather than cutaneous sarcoidosis (Burgoyne and Wood 1972). The same report also discusses the co-existence of psoriasis and sarcoidosis reported in rare case reports as early as 1925 and evaluated in retrospective reviews dating back to 1960.

As already noted, one report of three cases of concomitant sarcoidosis, psoriasis and gout reviewed 73 cases of histologically confirmed sarcoidosis and 100 random selected cases of psoriasis (Kaplan and Klatskin 1960). None of the 73 patients with sarcoidosis exhibited psoriasis, and there was no histologic confirmation of sarcoidosis in the 100 psoriatic subjects. A total of five case reports described concomitant sarcoidosis and psoriasis but included no evidence of both diseases in the same lesion. A subsequent retrospective study in 1966 by Zimmer and Demis reviewed 647 subjects with psoriasis, gout or sarcoidosis and did not identify any unequivocal cases with sarcoidosis.

Rajoriya and associates included psoriasis in their epidemiological study in 2009, but found no association with sarcoidosis. There are limited but well-documented case reports of concomitant sarcoidosis and psoriasis as well as rare cutaneous sarcoidosis with psoriaform-like lesions.

The evidence supports the co-existence of sarcoidosis and psoriasis but no increased association.

Vasculitis

Systemic vasculitis, although uncommon, is a well-documented complication of sarcoidosis and may affect small, medium and/or large vessels. The clinical presentation varies based on the organ systems involved, but sarcoid vasculitis appears to affect small and medium-sized pulmonary vessels most commonly (refer to Chapter 5 for additional details). Active disease may present with cutaneous lesions, neuropathy, pulmonary hypertension, systemic vasculitis, and more rarely aortitis (Torralba and Quismorio 2009). Extrapulmonary manifestations include cutaneous vascular sarcoidosis and granulomatous vasculitis in addition to reports of aortitis, which may be confused with Takayasu's arteritis (Fernandes et al. 2000).

Takayasu's arteritis

Takayasu's arteritis (TA) is an idiopathic large-vessel vasculitis that typically affects the aorta and associated major branches. The disease disproportionately affects women in their reproductive years (Kerr et al. 1994) and is difficult to differentiate from aortitis, a rare feature of sarcoidosis. The rare reports of pulmonary arterial involvement in TA can further complicate the diagnosis, and this has led to misdiagnosis (Karadag et al. 2008). At least five cases of Takayasu's arteritis have been reported years after initial diagnosis with sarcoidosis (Weiler et al. 2000). The rare incidence of both TA and aortitis in sarcoidosis suggests either a common pathogenic association or – perhaps more likely – misdiagnosis, as aortitis in patients with sarcoidosis may exclude TA.

Polyarteritis nodosa

Polyarteritis nodosa (PAN) is a systemic vasculitis, sometimes called systemic necrotizing vasculitis. It most commonly demonstrates cutaneous involvement. PAN was recently reviewed along with a number of immune-mediated and chronic inflammatory diseases, finding no association with sarcoidosis over a 30-year period (Rajoriya et al. 2009).

Overall, the evidence supports the diagnosis of vasculitis as part of the broad systemic affects of sarcoidosis. Fernandes and associates summarized numerous case reports of vasculitis in sarcoidosis throughout the literature, in addition to reporting six new cases, concluding that sarcoid vasculitis can mimic hypersensitivity vasculitis, polyarteritis nodosa, Takayasu's arteritis or microscopic polyangiitis (Fernandes et al. 2000).

The current literature suggests that vasculitis is either a component of sarcoidosis or mimicry resulting in misdiagnosis.

ENDOCRINE DISORDERS

The association between sarcoidosis and autoimmune thyroid disease has been reported in multiple case series and cohort studies. One study found females with sarcoidosis to be at increased risk of clinical hypothyroidism and Graves' disease (Antonelli et al. 2006), and a retrospective review of 78 patients with sarcoidosis found evidence of endocrine autoimmunity in 20 percent (Papadopoulos et al. 1996). Most recently, the systematic review by Rajoriya and associates in 2009 found a statistically significant but modest association.

There has been little research to address the underlying cause of autoimmune thyroid disease in patients with sarcoidosis. Again, given the broad systemic effects of sarcoidosis and the known involvement of endocrine glands, we may simply be observing the clinical presentation of systemic extrapulmonary sarcoidosis. Additional clinical study is necessary, and closely following thyroid function, especially in women, is recommended for patients with sarcoidosis.

Autoimmune chronic hepatitis and primary biliary cirrhosis

There are multiple case reports of concomitant autoimmune hepatitis and various inflammatory or autoimmune processes. Rajoriya and associates describe a significant association between sarcoidosis and autoimmune chronic hepatitis (Rajoriya et al. 2009). The literature is also notable for a limited number of cases describing interferon-induced sarcoidosis in patients treated for chronic hepatitis C (Adla *et al.* 2008). It remains unclear whether the trigger for sarcoidosis is the hepatitis C or the medication itself.

Additional epidemiological studies would be necessary to establish a direct relationship and further rule out mimicry. However, there does appear to be mounting evidence of sarcoidosis developing in association with an autoimmune response that may be influenced not only by associated disease patterns but with the treatment of those diseases (refer to above-referenced cases of sarcoidosis after treatment with anti-TNF-α therapy for rheumatoid arthritis).

Multiple sclerosis

There is no published evidence to support the co-existence of sarcoidosis and multiple sclerosis, as suggested by the significant epidemiological association described by Rajoriya *et al.* (2009). Given the broad systemic effects of sarcoidosis, including neurosarcoidosis, there is certainly a potential for mimicry and misdiagnosis of multiple sclerosis.

MISCELLANEOUS PULMONARY DISORDERS

Sarcoidosis is a multi-organ systemic disease although characterized by pulmonary involvement in the majority of patients. Both bronchiectasis and pulmonary hypertension are broad pathologic processes that may be found in patients with a variety of diseases.

Bronchiectasis is characterized by abnormal and irreversible dilation of the bronchi. There are reports of bronchiectasis in patients with normal chest X-ray, and wide associations with a variety of systemic rheumatological and autoimmune diseases including many covered in this chapter, such as Sjögren's syndrome, rheumatoid arthritis, ankylosing spondylitis and SLE (Cohen and Sahn 1999). Even so, any association between bronchiectasis and sarcoidosis can best be explained by the pulmonary pathophysiology.

COMMON VARIABLE IMMUNE DEFICIENCY SYNDROME

Chapter 38 covers sarcoid and antibody deficiency syndromes.

INTESTINAL DISORDERS

There is good evidence that sarcoid can involve the gastro-intestinal (GI) tract as part of its multisystem propensity (Ebert *et al.* 2008). This may be clinically detectable in up to 1 percent of patients with sarcoidosis, but inapparent granulomas are probably much more common. The most common organ to be involved is the stomach and this may be associated with peptic ulceration (Fireman *et al.* 1997; Liang *et al.* 2010) or luminal narrowing from granulomatous infiltration (Friedman *et al.* 2007). Clinically, epigastric pain of a varying nature is the most frequent symptom.

Diagnosis is usually by endoscopic biopsy and the finding of non-caseating granulomas. Granulomas do occur with other GI disorders such as Crohn's disease, tuberculosis, fungal infections and Whipple's disease. Unless the sarcoidosis is systemic, the diagnosis of sarcoid in the GI tract may be difficult.

The remainder of the GI tract can be involved and cases of sarcoid involving the esophagus, appendix (Cullinane *et al.* 1997), colon, rectum (Hilzenrat *et al.* 1995) and pancreas (Limaye *et al.* 1997) have been described.

Crohn's disease

Since the 1940s, Crohn's disease has attracted a number of investigators because of the propensity of the disease to form sarcoid-like granulomas. This common histological feature has stimulated a significant number of case reports (Fries *et al.* 1995; Brunner *et al.* 2006) and small case series that have suggested a commonality between the two disorders. A familial element to this was noted in three reports (Willoughby *et al.* 1971; Gronhagen-Riska *et al.* 1983; Bambery *et al.* 1991).

The approach of implying a greater or lesser degree of commonality based on case reports and small series is vulnerable to serious bias, as has been demonstrated by the much more powerful tool of a large-scale epidemiological study (Rajoriya *et al.* 2009). The epidemiological data from this study provided no support for an association of Crohn's disease and sarcoidosis; the odds ratio for the association was 1.52 with a confidence interval of 0.16–3.14. Rather unexpectedly it did yield a relationship with ulcerative colitis.

Reconciliation between these different strategies may be explained by genome-wide association analysis. A 100k genome-wide association study with 83 360 single-nucleotide polymorphisms (SNPs) was performed on 382 Crohn's disease patients, 398 sarcoid patients and 394 controls. The 24 most strongly associated SNPs were then re-analyzed in another population of Crohn's disease and sarcoid patients. The most significant single nucleotide polymorphism, rs1398024, was found on chromosome 10p12.2 ($p = 4.24 \times 10^{-6}$; Franke *et al.* 2008). This suggested a common susceptibility locus on 10p12.2, implying that both diseases have a common susceptibility gene. This then could explain the rather rare co-existence of both diseases, one occurring before, concurrently or subsequent to the other without implying a common etiology.

Taking these observations further, the analysis of families with Crohn's disease and sarcoidosis, using standardized risk ratios determined from the multigenerational register in Sweden, showed a just significant familial connection between the two disorders (Hemminki *et al.* 2010).

It is helpful to add to this discussion earlier work that hypothesized that both sarcoid and Crohn's disease may have an infectious basis. The fact that this fell into abeyance does not preclude that possibility, if one considers the parallel of hepatitis C. This viral disease proved very difficult to identify as such, and demonstrated a very low spousal transmission rate, despite large numbers of circulating viral particles. Similarly the prion disease, Creutzfeld–Jacob disease, has more infectious particles per gram of brain tissue than any other disease, yet its prevalence is so low as to never have been considered an infectious disease until the work of Gajdusek and Prusiner (Gajdusek et al. 1967; Prusiner et al. 1982).

Based on the successful transmission of leprosy to mouse foot-pads, which suggested that the local environment of the foot-pad provided a microenvironment for difficult-to-grow mycobacteria (Palmer et al. 1965), several investigators explored the possibility that there may be an infectious origin for sarcoidosis. The transmission of sarcoid granulomas to mouse foot-pads was reported, but there was very limited success in passaging tissue to a second generation of mice (Mitchell and Rees 1969; Mitchell et al. 1976). Characterization of the putative agent suggested that it would pass a 0.2 μm filter and was destroyed by autoclaving, irradiation storage at −200°C for more than a week and by radiation. This would be consistent with a small infectious particle; but the difficulty in reproducing the findings, and the very long incubation time (6–9 months) for the evolution of granulomatous change, has largely led to the abandonment of this line of research. Passage of the granulomatous changes to a second generation of mice was reported along with successful induction of Kveim positivity (Mitchell et al. 1976).

Based on histological similarities of ulcerative colitis and Crohn's disease, attempts were made to perform similar transmission experiments with Crohn's disease and ulcerative colitis tissues (Cave et al. 1973,1976). Reproduction has been limited and the very long duration of these studies has been a problem. Thus, to date Koch's postulates have not been fulfilled and the infectious hypothesis has fallen from favor. Limited first-generation passage was achieved in mice, based on histological changes. However, in the absence of good markers for any of these diseases, it is very difficult to fully evaluate the significance of histology alone as a marker for transmission, as evidence of an infectious origin for these diseases. Das and colleagues further explored the infectious hypothesis using nude mice (Das et al. 1980,1983). They showed an increased incidence of lymphoma in these mice and that an antibody in Crohn's sera recognized an antigen in the murine lymphomas (Das et al. 1986). Again, this work has not been extended.

Ulcerative colitis

Ulcerative colitis, a chronic inflammatory condition of the colon, is not associated with granuloma formation, but it is generally regarded as being at the other end of a spectrum of non-specific inflammatory bowel disorders including Crohn's disease and has rarely been reported to be associated with sarcoid (Barr et al. 1986). These authors considered the relationship to be based on an immunologically induced pathogenic mechanism because of the frequency of HLA B8 associated with some of the additional manifestations of sarcoid and ulcerative colitis, including erythema nodosum and iritis. Up until 2001 there had been only 18 patients with the association of ulcerative colitis and sarcoidosis. Nilubol and co-workers reported an additional case with ulcerative

colitis presenting in a background of quiescent sarcoidosis (Nilubol et al. 2001). Surprisingly, ulcerative colitis was shown to have an epidemiological association based on the observations of Rajoriya et al. (2009). This observation was also noted by Hemminki and co-workers in their analysis of the multigeneration registry in Sweden, suggesting that there was genetic sharing (Hemminki et al. 2010).

Celiac disease

Celiac disease an immunogenetic disorder, characterized by villous atrophy of the proximal small intestine. It occurs in response to an allergy to gluten and has been associated with sarcoidosis at the case-report level (Ludvigsson et al. 2007) and epidemiologically (Rajoriya et al. 2009). Again this suggests a prerequisite of a common genetic background and an appropriate immunological stimulus that is permissive for development of the disease.

CONCLUSION

It is clear that a variety of disorders that are associated with sarcoidosis appear on the basis of a common genetic milieu. The presence of a granulomatous response, as is the case with Crohn's disease, based on recent epidemiological studies, does not imply a common etiology but simply histological overlap.

REFERENCES

Adla M, Downey KK, Ahmad J (2008). Hepatic sarcoidosis associated with pegylated interferon alfa therapy for chronic hepatitis C: case report and review of literature. Dig Dis Sci 53: 2810–12.

Antonelli A, Fazzi P, Fallahi P et al. (2006). Prevalence of hypothyroidism and Graves' disease in sarcoidosis. Chest 130: 526–32.

Bambery P, Kaur U, Bhusnurmath SR, Dilawari JB (1991). Familial idiopathic granulomatosis: sarcoidosis and Crohn's disease in two Indian families. Thorax 46: 919–21.

Barr GD, Shale DJ, Jewell DP (1986). Ulcerative colitis and sarcoidosis. Postgrad Med J 62: 341–5.

Begum S, Li C, Wedderburn LR et al. (2002). Concurrence of sarcoidosis and systemic lupus erythematosus in three patients. Clin Exp Rheumatol 20: 549–52.

Brunner J, Sergi C, Muller T et al. (2006). Juvenile sarcoidosis presenting as Crohn's disease. Eur J Pediatr 165: 398–401.

Burgoyne JS, Wood MG (1972). Psoriasiform sarcoidosis. Arch Dermatol 106: 896–8.

Cave DR, Mitchell DN, Kane SP, Brooke BN (1973). Further animal evidence of a transmissible agent in Crohn's disease. Lancet ii: 1120–2.

Cave DR, Mitchell DN, Brooke BN (1976). Evidence of an agent transmissible from ulcerative colitis tissue. Lancet 1: 1311–15.

Cohen M, Sahn SA (1999). Bronchiectasis in systemic diseases. Chest 116: 1063–74.

Collins DA, Bourke BE (1996). Systemic lupus erythematosus: an occasional misdiagnosis. Ann Rheum Dis 55: 421–2.

Cox D, Conant E, Earle L et al. (1995). Sarcoidosis in systemic sclerosis: report of seven cases. J Rheumatol 22: 881–5.

Cullinane DC, Schultz SC, Zellos L, Holt RW (1997). Sarcoidosis manifesting as acute appendicitis: report of a case. Dis Colon Rectum 40: 109–11.

Das KM, Valenzuela I, Morecki R (1980). Crohn disease lymph node homogenates produce murine lymphoma in athymic mice. Proc Natl Acad Sci USA 77: 588–92.

Das KM, Valenzuela I, Williams SE (1983). Studies of the etiology of Crohn's disease using athymic nude mice. Gastroenterology 84: 364–74.

Das KM, Simon MR, Valenzuela I et al. (1986). Serum antibodies from patients with Crohn's disease and from their household members react with murine lymphomas induced by Crohn's disease tissue filtrates. J Lab Clin Med 107: 95–100.

De Bandt M, Perrot S, Masson C, Meyer O (1997). Systemic sclerosis and sarcoidosis, a report of five cases. Br J Rheumatol 36: 117–19.

Ebert EC, Kierson M, Hagspiel KD (2008). Gastrointestinal and hepatic manifestations of sarcoidosis. Am J Gastroenterol 103: 3184–92.

Farah RE, Shay MD (2007). Pulmonary sarcoidosis associated with etanercept therapy. Pharmacotherapy 27: 1446–8.

Fernandes SRM, Singsen BH, Hoffman GS (2000). Sarcoidosis and systemic vasculitis. Semin Arthritis Rheum 30: 33–46.

Fireman Z, Sternberg A, Yarchovsky Y et al. (1997). Multiple antral ulcers in gastric sarcoid. J Clin Gastroenterol 24: 97–9.

Franke A, Fischer A, Nothnagel M et al. (2008). Genome-wide association analysis in sarcoidosis and Crohn's disease unravels a common susceptibility locus on 10p12.2. Gastroenterology 135: 1207–15.

Friedman M, Ali MA, Borum ML (2007). Gastric sarcoidosis: a case report and review of the literature. South Med J 100: 301–3.

Fries W, Grassi SA, Leone L et al. (1995). Association between inflammatory bowel disease and sarcoidosis: report of two cases and review of the literature. Scand J Gastroenterol 30: 1221–3.

Gajdusek C, Gibbs CJ, Alpers M (1967). Slow-acting virus implicated in kuru. J Am Med Assoc 199: 34.

Gronhagen-Riska C, Fyhrquist F, Hortling L, Koskimies S (1983). Familial occurrence of sarcoidosis and Crohn's disease. Lancet i: 1287–8.

Hemminki K, Li X, Sundquist K, Sundquist J (2010). Familial association of inflammatory bowel diseases with other autoimmune and related diseases. Am J Gastroenterol 105: 139–47.

Hilzenrat N, Spanier A, Lamoureux E et al. (1995). Colonic obstruction secondary to sarcoidosis: nonsurgical diagnosis and management. Gastroenterology 108: 1556–9.

Ho AC, Hasson N, Singh-Grewal D (2009). Sarcoidosis or scleroderma? An unusual case of sarcoidosis in a 3-year-old Caucasian girl. Rheumatology (Oxford) 48: 1172–3.

Ishioka S, Yamanishi Y, Hiyama K et al. (1999). Sarcoidosis associated with connective tissue diseases: report of three cases. Intern Med 38: 984–7.

Kaplan H, Klatskin G (1960). Sarcoidosis, psoriasis, and gout: syndrome or coincidence? Yale J Biol Med 32: 335–52.

Karadag B, Kilic H, Duman D et al. (2008). Takayasu disease with prominent pulmonary artery involvement: confusion with pulmonary disease leading to delayed diagnosis. Mod Rheumatol 18: 507–10.

Kerr GS, Hallahan CW, Giordano J et al. (1994). Takayasu arteritis. Ann Intern Med 120: 919–29.

Liang DB, Price JC, Ahmed H et al. (2010). Gastric sarcoidosis: case report and literature review. J Natl Med Assoc 102: 348–51.

Limaye AP, Paauw D, Raghu G et al. (1997). Sarcoidosis associated with recurrent pancreatitis. South Med J 90: 431–3.

Ludvigsson JF, Wahlstrom J, Grunewald J et al. (2007). Coeliac disease and risk of sarcoidosis. Sarcoid Vasc Diff Lung Dis 24: 121–6.

Marchell RM, Judson MA (2007). Chronic cutaneous lesions of sarcoidosis. Clin Dermatol 25: 295–302.

Migita K, Udono M, Kinoshita A et al. (2005). Lupus erythematosus and sarcoidosis. Clin Rheumatol 24: 312–13.

Mitchell DN, Rees RJ (1969). A transmissible agent from sarcoid tissue. Lancet ii: 81–4.

Mitchell DN, Rees RJ, Goswami KK (1976). Transmissible agents from human sarcoid and Crohn's disease tissues. Lancet ii: 761–5.

Nakayama S, Mukae H, Morisaki T et al. (2007). Sarcoidosis accompanied by systemic lupus erythematosus and autoimmune hepatitis. Intern Med 46: 1657–61.

Nilubol N, Taub PJ, Venturero M et al. (2001). Ulcerative colitis and sarcoidosis. Mt Sinai J Med 68: 400–2.

Palmer E, Rees RJ, Weddell AG (1965). Site of multiplication of human leprosy bacilli inoculated into the foot-pads of mice. Nature 206: 521–2.

Papadopoulos KI, Hornblad Y, Liljebladh H, Hallengren B (1996). High frequency of endocrine autoimmunity in patients with sarcoidosis. Eur J Endocrinol 134: 331–6.

Prusiner SB, Gajdusek C, Alpers MP (1982). Kuru with incubation periods exceeding two decades. Ann Neurol 12: 1–9.

Rajoriya N, Wotton CJ, Yeates DG et al. (2009). Immune-mediated and chronic inflammatory disease in people with sarcoidosis: disease associations in a large UK database. Postgrad Med J 85: 223–7.

Sharma OP (2002). Sarcoidosis and other autoimmune disorders. Curr Opin Pulm Med 8: 452–6.

Telium G (1964). Miliary epithelioid cell granulomas in lupus erythematosus disseminatus. Acta Pathol Microbiol Scand 22: 39–43.

Torralba KD, Quismorio FP (2009). Sarcoidosis and the rheumatologist. Curr Opin Rheumatol 21: 62–70.

Verschueren K, Van Essche E, Verschueren P et al. (2007). Development of sarcoidosis in etanercept-treated rheumatoid arthritis patients. Clin Rheumatol 26: 1969–71.

Weiler V, Redtenbacher S, Bancher C et al. (2000). Concurrence of sarcoidosis and aortitis: case report and review of the literature. Ann Rheum Dis 59: 850–3.

Willoughby JM, Mitchell DN, Wilson JD (1971). Sarcoidosis and Crohn disease in siblings. Am Rev Respir Dis 104: 249–54.

Zimmer JG, Demis J (1966). Associations between gout psoriasis and sarcoid. Ann Int Med 64: 786–96.

PART VIII

CHILDHOOD SARCOID

40

Pulmonary and extrapulmonary involvement in childhood

ANDREW BUSH

INTRODUCTION

Sarcoidosis is rarely diagnosed in childhood, but the manifestations are so disparate that the possibility of the diagnosis should at least be considered in many common and rare clinical scenarios. Most studies of the pathophysiology and treatment are in adults, and these are discussed elsewhere in this volume. This chapter will focus only on specifically pediatric aspects of pathophysiology, epidemiology in children, the clinical manifestations over the span of childhood, prognosis, and such data as exist on the treatment of children.

PATHOPHYSIOLOGY

Sarcoidosis is a chronic, multisystem, granulomatous disease in childhood, as in adults. No particular differences have been reported in the microscopic and immuno-pathology across the age range, probably largely because it is such a rare disease in children that few if any such comparative studies have been done.

The main justification for a separate pathophysiology section in a pediatric chapter is because there are important differences in the way that adults and children respond to a given stimulus. This is likely a necessary future focus for understanding sarcoid in children, in particular if it turns out to be an infectious disease. The differences are most starkly shown in childhood interstitial lung disease (chILD). Surfactant protein-C deficiency is an autosomal dominant, gain-of-function mutation responsible for family kindreds of ILD (Mulugeta et al. 2005). In adult-onset disease, the histology is usual interstitial pneumonia (UIP); but, in the same family, childhood-onset disease causes a cellular non-specific interstitial pneumonia (NSIP), or occasionally desquamative interstitial pneumonia (DIP) (Thomas et al. 2002; Beers and Mulugeta 2005). Furthermore, in the related autosomal recessive ABCA3 deficiency, histological patterns of chILD are very variable between children, and change over time in the same child (Doan et al. 2008).

The reasons for these differences are not clear, but there are many possibilities. During early life, there is rapid growth of the airways to a degree never seen again, and particularly of the alveolar–capillary membrane (Hislop et al. 1986). The exact nature of the growth factors which drive the increase in size and maturation of the lung are not fully understood, but are likely unique to this early time period. The immune system normally shows a change from the pregnancy-associated Th2 to a neonatal Th1 bias, and the infant has to switch from reliance on maternal humoral immunity during pregnancy to the development of immune responses and immune memory functions (Holt and Jones 2000). The developing airway and immune system have to interact with environmental pollutants, which may act as immune adjuvants, and are often exposed to acid and alkaline aspirated gastric fluids. Novel proteins and infective agents are encountered for the first time. Allergen exposure in this crucial time window may have long-term effects, and the lesson of occupational asthma is that it is at the time of early exposure that sensitization is most likely to occur, if it is to happen. Finally, the response to infection may be very different. Varicella and Severe acute respiratory syndrome (SARS), for example, are usually relatively trivial illnesses in children, but can be very severe and even fatal in adults (Wong et al. 2003). Any or all of the above may account for the characteristic and different sarcoid presentation triad (rash, uveitis, arthritis) which is only seen in pre-school children (see later).

So, in summary, there is no reason to suppose the immunology and pathophysiology of sarcoid is the same at all ages, and thus disease manifestations might differ greatly as the child ages. However, this has unfortunately not been explored, not least because of the rarity of the condition in children and the lack of a newborn or young adult animal model.

EPIDEMIOLOGY

Perhaps the most comprehensive population-based dataset comes from the Denmark registry (Hoffman et al. 2004; Milman and Hoffman 2008; Milman et al. 2009). Over a 15-year period, 5536 patients were reported to the national registry, in whom only 81 were age <15 years. Of these, 33 were incorrectly diagnosed, meaning that childhood sarcoidosis accounts for less than 1 percent of the total, or 0.29 cases per 100 000 (child) person-years. The peak age of presentation was adolescence. There were only three children under age 5 years, two of whom were monozygotic twins. There was no significant gender difference in children. Other sources suggest that there are probably the same racial patterns in children as in adults (Kendig and Niitu 1980; Pattishall and Kendig 1996; Milman et al. 1998), although this is controversial, because in the USA the high Afro-Caribbean predominance reported in children elsewhere is not seen (Newman et al. 1997; Lindsley and Petty 2000). There has been no change in prevalence over the last 30 years in Denmark (Milman et al. 1998).

A combined Danish and Finnish twin study (Sverrild et al. 2008), which included children, has established a genetic basis for the disease: 210 of 61 662 pairs had at least one proband with sarcoid, 160 dizygotic (DZ) and 50 monozygotic (MZ). Although the affected numbers are small, in particular of monozygotic twins, there was an 80-fold risk in the proband of MZ twins as against a 7-fold risk for DZ. The numbers precluded looking for an age effect, but one might predict that if genetic factors were most important, then the effect would be strongest for early-onset sarcoidosis, if environmental, the converse. Phenotypic differences between MZ and DZ twins could not be determined. An Irish study, also including children, showed that nearly 10 percent of affected patients (most of whom presented as adults) had an affected sibling (Brennan et al. 1984). Again, whether there was an age-related difference in the prevalence of an affected sibling was not determined.

CLINICAL MANIFESTATIONS BY AGE AND ORGAN

General

Childhood sarcoidosis is a spectrum, but with a characteristic pre-school presentation. The pre-school form is characterized by the triad of uveitis, arthritis and skin lesions (Rosenberg et al. 1983; Clark 1987; Hetherington, 1987) which closely mimics juvenile chronic arthritis. The pre-school form may be difficult to diagnose (Falcini et al. 1999), especially if the earliest feature is a relatively non-specific skin rash (Rasmussen 1981; Falcini et al. 1999). Granulomatous tendon sheath synovitis and effusion are typical, and important clues to the diagnosis. The childhood and adolescent form by contrast is characterized by lung, ocular and lymph node disease, often with systemic symptoms such as malaise, cough, dyspnea and a non-specific exanthema (Gibson and Winklemann 1986; Faye-Petersen 1991; Singal et al. 2005). Also seen in this age group are various forms of cutaneous and systemic vasculitis. Late adolescent sarcoid is similar to the adult disease.

The Danish Registry study showed that all but one of 48 children had systemic symptoms such as weight loss, fever and abdominal discomfort (Hoffman et al. 2004). Other common features at presentation were respiratory symptoms (65 percent), lymphadenopathy (40 percent), ocular disease (29 percent), neurological problems (25 percent) and joint involvement (10 percent, similar to adults in this series – Milman and Selroos 1990a). Eye features are more common in children than in adults, and this is confirmed by other series which report prevalences of between 24 and 58 percent (Kendig 1974; Hetherington 1982; Pattishall et al. 1986). Arthritis has been reported as more common in other series (45–58 percent; Hetherington 1982; Milman et al. 1998; Pattishall and Kendig 1996). Erythema nodosum was the only manifestation of sarcoid vasculitis in the Danish series (Hoffman et al. 2004; Milman and Hoffman 2008). Hepatosplenomegaly at presentation was rare in this series, but only very few had an abdominal ultrasound performed; others report a prevalence of 43 percent at some stage of the disease (Pattishall et al. 1986). On chest X-ray, only 10 percent had a normal film, 71 percent had bilateral hilar lymphadenopathy (stage I), 8.3 percent also had parenchymal involvement (stage II), 8.3 percent had only parenchymal involvement (stage III), and none had evidence of irreversible fibrosis (stage IV). High-resolution CT data were not reported. Spirometry and other pulmonary function tests were reported too infrequently for any comment to be made. Serum angiotensin-converting enzyme (ACE) was elevated in 11 of 20 patients in whom levels were reported. Forty percent had a raised erythrocyte sedimentation rate (ESR). High or low white cell count, and raised immunoglobulins were frequent. Very importantly, hypercalcemia was present in 30 percent. Histological confirmation of the disease was not possible in only 13 of 48 children. Lymph node biopsy was the most common histological diagnostic modality.

Another source of data, which does not have the total population denominator as reliably as the Danish work, is an international registry. Between 1991 and 1996, 53 patients from 14 countries were recorded (Lindsley and Petty 2000). All the patients had definite histological evidence of sarcoidosis: non-caseating granulomas of the skin (31), synovium (15), liver (10), lymph node (8), lung (5), muscle (4), conjunctiva (3) or kidney (1). All but nine patients developed polyarthritis; 38 of 44 had persistent arthritis. Of those with persistent polyarthritis, arthritis occurred at presentation in 16 of 38 patients and inflammation of the uveal tract occurred in 44 with involvement of both anterior and posterior segments in 21. One patient had become blind. Other ocular complications included chorioretinitis, glaucoma and phthisis bulbi. Laboratory abnormalities included mild anemia and elevated ESR (39/45). Angiotensin-converting enzyme levels were elevated in 14 out of 37 patients.

Organ systems

The remainder of this section comprises descriptions of the manifestations of childhood sarcoidosis by organ system.

RESPIRATION

Pulmonary disease is rare in very young children. In older children, symptoms are often mild, such as dry hacking cough or breathlessness, or there may be none (Hetherington 1982) – prevalences probably reflecting the difficulty in diagnosis. Skin manifestations can be divided into specific and non-specific; examples of the latter being erythema nodosum, which has numerous other causes, and non-specific exanthems. Specific manifestations include firm, red or yellow–brown papules with a predilection for the nares, nasolabial folds and eyelids; lupus pernio; keloid-like lesions and scar sarcoidosis (Singhal et al. 2005); generalised erythematous macules and papules; acquired icthyosis; erythroderma; hypopigmented macules, which are particularly obvious in Afro-Caribbean children; papules; plaques or nodules; ulcers; scarring alopecia; a psoriasis-like dermatitis; and granulomatous cheilitis (Yanardag et al. 2003; Singhal et al. 2005; Kwon et al. 2007).

Histology is typically of classic sarcoid granulomas, but many other appearances have been reported (Rosen et al. 1977; Kauh et al. 1978; Herzlinger et al. 1979; Batres et al. 1982; Kuramoto et al. 1988; Alexis 1994; Goldberg et al. 1994; Magro et al. 1996; Okamoto 1999; Callen 2001; Crowson et al. 2003; Shirodaria et al. 2003; Ball et al. 2004).

However, atypical and overlap forms of cutaneous sarcoidosis are described. One child with ocular and cutaneous sarcoid had a rash resembling granuloma annulare, which on histology had overlap features of sarcoidosis, granuloma annulare and palisading neutrophilic and granulomatous dermatitis (Kwon et al. 2007). There was a dramatic response to ocular and systemic prednisolone.

EYES

The typical ocular manifestations of sarcoid in children are anterior uveitis, granulomatous corneal precipitates, and nodules – either or both of Koeppe (nodules seen at the inner margin of the iris in patients with granulomatous anterior uveitis, consisting of epithelioid cells and giant cells surrounded by lymphocytes) and Busacca (inflammatory, granulomatous nodules located away from the pupillary margin of the iris). Posterior chamber involvement is typical but not inevitable, and if present, this feature distinguishes sarcoid eye disease from that of juvenile chronic arthritis. Multifocal choroiditis, choroidal granuloma, vasculitis and perivascular sheathing are typical. Corneal opacities have

rarely been described in pre-school sarcoidosis (de Boer et al. 2009). Unilateral proptosis due to orbital sarcoidosis has been described (Khan et al. 1986).

RHEUMATOLOGY

Synovial sheath involvement is a characteristic presentation of sarcoid in the pre-school years, and biopsy reveals typical sarcoid granulomas (Morris et al. 1996). Sarcoid arthritis is typically large joint, persistent and non-destructive (Thomas et al. 1983). There may be large, boggy tendon sheath effusions. Typically movement is little affected and radiographs are normal. Lytic bone lesions are rarely seen in children, and when present are often seen in conjunction with skin lesions (Neville et al. 1977). This combination may cause confusion with juvenile-onset histiocytosis X.

NEUROSARCOIDOSIS

This was reported in five of the Danish children (Hoffman et al. 2004), two with peripheral neuropathy and three with central manifestations, including obstructive hydrocephalus. The biggest review in childhood reported 29 cases up to 2003, and a further case (Baumann and Robertson 2003) was added; these were compared to adult-presenting neurosarcoid. The new case presented with a non-specific encephalopathy, and, as is common in the literature, sarcoid was only considered as a diagnostic possibility late on. Reviewing the literature, children were more likely to have seizures, less likely to have cranial nerve palsies (and these were said to be seen only after puberty), and perhaps more likely to have a space-occupying lesion. Hypothalamic dysfunction is not uncommon, with growth failure, failure of sexual maturation and diabetes insipidus being common features. Space-occupying masses may be asymptomatic. In those who have been followed through adolescence, progression to a more adult pattern is reported, with fewer seizures and more cranial neuropathy. If cerebrospinal fluid is examined, mild lymphocytocis and elevation of proteins with oligoclonal bands, and reduced sugar is seen (Nowak and Widenka 2001). This is not specific to sarcoidosis. Brain MRI typically shows some or all of periventricular high-signal lesions on T2-weighted images, meningeal involvement and a space-occupying mass, and is the preferred neuro-imaging modality in children.

There are a number of case reports highlighting the protean manifestations of neurosarcoidosis. A case with a Guillain–Barré like presentation, diagnosed by endobronchial ultrasound-guided fine-needle lymph node aspiration, was recently reported (Wurzel et al. 2009). Sarcoid was first suspected when mediastinal lymphadenopathy was demonetrated on MRI scanning looking for cord compression! A child with combined uveitis and hearing loss due to neurosarcoidosis was reported; the differential diagnosis included neurosyphilis, tuberculosis, Cogan's syndrome (interstitial keratitis, hearing loss and vasculitis in children and young adults), Vogt–Koyanagi–Harada syndrome (a granulomatous systemic disease involving various melanocyte-containing organs characterized by bilateral panuveitis associated with cutaneous, neurologic and auditory abnormalities), and Behçet's disease.

OTHER ORGAN SYSTEMS

The true prevalence of renal sarcoidosis in children is not known. Four of the Danish series had renal disease (Hoffman et al. 2004), three secondary to hypercalcemia and one to nephrocalcinosis. Glomerulonephritis and renovascular complications of sarcoid have been described (Gross et al. 1986; Dimitriades et al. 1999). Granulomatous renal disease has been described in children (Turner et al. 1977; Martini et al. 1980; Morris et al. 1996) as has interstitial nephritis, usually as part of multisystem involvement (Coutant et al. 1999), but rarely isolated (Thumfart et al. 2004). In one case, hypertension and growth failure were features (Morris et al. 1996). The cause for the latter is unclear, but it was thought not to be related to steroid treatment. Granulomatous renal sarcoid may manifest as a pseudotumoral involvement, with echogenic masses on ultrasound. The differential diagnosis includes angiomyolipoma, focal pyelonephritis and nephrogenic adenofibromas (Comerci et al. 1996). On CT, low-density lesions with mottled contrast enhancement may be seen (Herman et al. 1997); in some cases the lesions are invisible unless intravenous contrast is given (Hughes and Wilder 1988; Bottone et al. 1993; Gazaigne et al. 1995).

Although mild derangement of liver function tests is not uncommon, sarcoid hepatitis is rare in children (Pattishall et al. 1986). A granulomatous myopathy may be the presenting feature of sarcoidosis (Rossi et al. 2001)). Intrascrotal sarcoidosis has been described (Marty and Kwong 2009). Confusingly, there is a reported association between testicular cancer and sarcoid and also granulomatous reactions (Paparel et al. 2007). Testicular cancer may precede the diagnosis of sarcoid. Cardiac sarcoidosis is important in adults, but primary recent literature in children is scant, and it must be assumed to be a very rare complication of a rare disease. Indeed, there are no cases reported in recent big autopsy series (Sharma et al. 1993; Syed and Myers, 2004). Ventricular arrhythmia due to cardiac sarcoid has been described in a child (Serwer et al. 1978). Recommendations for screening are based on adult studies (Hunninghake et al. 1999), but there is no evidence that these are applicable to children. Involvement of the stomach, pancreas and tonsils by sarcoid granulomas has been reported (Baculard et al. 2001).

DIFFERENTIAL DIAGNOSIS

Depending on the presentation, sarcoid may enter the differential diagnosis of most pediatric respiratory diseases, especially including tuberculosis. In this section, rather than exhaustively list every possible condition that might mimic sarcoidosis, particular issues described in the literature as being important differentials will be highlighted. It should be noted that misdiagnosis is common, being nearly 50 percent in the Danish Registry (Hoffman et al. 2004). A general point is that the lack of a true diagnostic 'gold standard' for pediatric sarcoidosis means that there are a number of reports of sarcoid-like features in association with other poorly characterized syndromes, and it is unclear whether in fact these are true cases of sarcoid, or an overlap syndrome, or a granulomatous reaction to an unrelated problem. However, it may be that the study of rare genetic or acquired conditions that are characterized by granulomatous disease may shed light on the pathophysiology of sarcoid (for examples, see below).

Necrotizing sarcoidosis is rare in children (Heinrich et al. 2003), and there is debate as to whether it is an overlap syndrome with Wegener's or Churg–Strauss. It is very rare in children (Tauber et al. 1999). Some consider it a specific form of sarcoisosis, with a relatively good outlook. Spontaneous resolution is usual, although occasionally steroids may be needed (Currie et al. 2007). Diagnosis is by finding necrotizing granulomas and vasculitis on a granulomatous background. It may rarely be extrapulmonary; central nervous system and ocular involvement has been reported in children (Beach et al. 1980; Sigh et al. 1981; Lazzarini et al. 2008). There are no specific laboratory features in children. An interesting family kindred in which sarcoid and necrotizing sarcoidosis occurred in different family members reinforces the likelihood that they are protean manifestation of the same disease (Lazzarini et al. 2008).

The skin lesions of juvenile rheumatoid arthritis, macular or maculopapular exanthematous erruptions may be confused clinically with those of sarcoidosis. The histology is different, consisting of mild dermal edema and a mild perivascular mixed infiltrate (Kwon et al. 2007). Rheumatoid-like nodules are characterized histologically by deep dermal palisading granulomas surrounding areas of fibrinoid necrosis, sometimes with areas suggestive of palisading neutrophilic dermatitis. Juvenile arthritis is obviously a multisystem disease, and the eye and joint manifestations can add further confusion. Posterior uveitis is said not to be a feature of ocular juvenile rheumatoid.

Blau's syndrome is a familial, early-onset granulomatous disease that may affect the skin, eyes and joints. There is no pulmonary or lymph node involvement. ACE levels may be elevated, and distinction from sarcoidosis may be difficult. The cardinal genetic feature is mutations in the Caspase-Recruitment Domain-Containing Protein 15 (CARD15) gene. Interestingly, CARD15 mutations have been found in some children with early-onset sarcoidosis (Kanazawa et al. 2005; Rose et al. 2005), which leads one to speculate whether they are truly separate diseases or share common etiological or pathophysiological pathways (see below).

Melkersson–Rosenthal syndrome (MRS) is a rare disease characterized by localized swelling (usually of the lips) which on biopsy is due to non-caseating epithelioid granuloma, which may be confused with sarcoid (Scerri et al. 1996). Treatment is with clofazimine unless there is complete spontaneous remission (Sussman et al. 1992). Anderson–Fabry disease (alpha galactosidase A deficiency (α-GAL A, encoded by GLA) causing multisystem globotriaosylceramide accumulation) may mimic both conditions (Young et al. 1978). Sarcoid granulomatous reactions to neuroblastoma (Hojo et al. 2000) and hepatoblastoma (Schmidt et al. 1985) have rarely been described; the prognostic significance is not known.

Granulomatous disease may be the first presentation of an immunodeficiency (Skinner and Masters, 1970; Siegfried et al. 1991; Levine et al. 1994). Hyper-IgM syndrome is a rare condition, either X-linked, autosomal recessive or acquired, characterized by reduced or absent IgG, IgA and IgE levels, but normal or raised IgM. The X-linked form results from mutations in the CD40 ligand gene. Presentation with granulomatous skin disease, without the more characteristic autoimmune disease or oral ulcers, was recently described in a 5-year-old boy (Gallerani et al. 2004).

Many primary skin conditions may enter the differential diagnosis of juvenile sarcoidosis. Granuloma annulare may mimic sarcoid, as well as complicate both sarcoid and Blau's syndrome. It is a benign, self-limiting condition, and specifically ocular complications are rare. Childhood granulomatous periorificial dermatitis is usually but not invariably found in Afro-Caribbean children, and is characterized by a papular monomorphic eruption around the nose, mouth and eyes. Although usually it is transient, and the histology, a mixed inflammatory infiltrate, is usually easily distinguished from sarcoid, overlap granulomatous forms have been described (Ball et al. 2004).

Koeppe and Busacca nodules are not specific to sarcoid, and can be seen in a number of conditions that may cause diagnostic confusion, including TB, leprosy, Lyme disease, brucellosis, syphilis and Vogt–Koyanagi–Harada syndrome (Moorthy et al. 1995).

Finally, the co-existence of sarcoid and cystic fibrosis has been reported in five children (Cooper et al. 1987; Soden et al. 1989; Rettinger et al. 1989; Burton et al. 2005). Whether this represents a true association, coincidence, undiagnosed atypical mycobacterial disease (common in CF) or an atypical granulomatous reaction to inflammation is not known. In one case there was a prompt beneficial response to steroids (Burton et al. 2005), so the possibility of an association should be borne in mind in atypical CF.

INVESTIGATIONS

Investigations may be pursued in four clinical contexts:

- making the diagnosis of a condition which mimics sarcoid, in order to exclude the condition, such as TB or immunodeficiency;
- establishing the diagnosis of sarcoidosis in a child with an undiagnosed illness;
- seeking evidence of sarcoidosis elsewhere, when the child has presented with localized disease, usually ocular, which may be compatible with a diagnosis of sarcoidosis (also in this category is the investigation of a child diagnosed with sarcoidosis in whom other disease manifestations are to be excluded);
- monitoring the child with known sarcoidosis

The range of diagnostic testing for mimics of sarcoidosis is outside the scope of this chapter. In passing, it should be noted that it is worth at least considering 'could this be sarcoidosis?' in many clinical scenarios, despite the rarity of

the condition. Likewise 'could there be co-existent sarcoid?' is also always worth at least a thought.

In terms of establishing a diagnosis of sarcoidosis, in most cases pediatricians will want to pursue a tissue diagnosis, because of the rarity of the disease. ACE levels may be elevated, but this is generally held to be an insufficiently sensitive or specific test on which to commit a child to potentially toxic therapy; most other laboratory tests are even less sensitive and specific. Tuberculin anergy is a diagnostic clue, but is not specific. If the child has a brisk tuberculin reaction, however, sarcoid is unlikely. Biopsy is easy with skin or peripheral lymph node involvement but, in the author's view, mediastinoscopy and biopsy are justified if there is intrathoracic lymphadenopathy and no peripheral targets. A child presenting with lung nodules or an interstitial lung disease will probably undergo lung biopsy, preferably using video-assisted thoracoscopic surgery (VATS). A blind liver biopsy may confirm the diagnosis, because asymptomatic hepatic granulomatous involvement is common. Other tissues that may be biopsied include synovium and conjunctiva, and very exceptionally, endomyocardial biopsy may be considered. Granulomas are of course not specific to sarcoid, and the differential diagnosis includes the whole spectrum of childhood granulomatous disease. A careful examination may reveal unsuspected skin or scar lesions, and the finding of granulomas on biopsy, in the setting of a multi-organ disease, may be enough to establish the diagnosis (Singal et al. 2005).

In the child with a known or suspected diagnosis of sarcoid, further testing should be considered. There are no evidence-based guidelines to help the pediatrician. The usual clinical scenario in my practice is the child with apparently isolated uveitis referred from the ophthalmology department. A full clinical history and examination, with particular attention to skin, joints and the respiratory system, is performed. All patients should have blood tests, which as well as basic hematology and biochemistry should include serum calcium, ESR and immunoglobulins. A 24-hour urine calcium should be performed, because hypercalcuria even without hypercalcemia may affect renal function. A baseline abdominal ultrasound is performed. My practice is also to obtain a chest X-ray, and full lung function testing (spirometry, lung volumes, carbon monoxide transfer) and an exercise test with earlobe saturation monitoring. If these are normal, I do not routinely perform a CT scan of the chest because of radiation, and the extreme unlikelihood of finding an abnormality that will result in a change in treatment. However, if non-invasive testing is normal, I would at least consider performing a CT and also a bronchoscopy; BAL reveals a lymphocytic picture with an increased CD4/CD8 ratio (Milman and Selroos 1990b; Chadelat et al. 1993; Tessier et al. 1996) but this is not specific to sarcoidosis. A neutrophilic lavage may be associated with a worse prognosis. Bronchoscopy is also indicated if there is any evidence of large airway compression. I would take the opportunity to perform a mucosal biopsy, because it is so safe, even though the yield in children is not known. Transbronchial biopsy is not performed, because it is too risky and too unlikely to be positive in my view. If lung tissue is needed, VATS biopsy is performed. As to whether a brain MRI is indicated in an otherwise asymptomatic child with anterior uveitis, there are no data; although silent space-occupying lesions in sarcoid have been described, I suspect most would not routinely perform this test. Given the rarity of cardiac sarcoid, I doubt that many perform a routine echocardiogram, although perhaps it should be done, given that it is a non-invasive test, and our lack of knowledge may reflect a lack of ascertainment. Any child with suspected sarcoid must be seen by an ophthalmologist, because inadequate treatment can lead to blindness (Lindsley and Petty 2000).

In terms of monitoring the child with known sarcoidosis, I know of no biomarkers of disease activity. Ocular monitoring is as for any case of uveitis, pulmonary sarcoid with lung function tests and intermittent, often limited HRCT. I do not routinely perform blood or urine tests in an asymptomatic child with apparently quiescent sarcoid. Since BAL lymphocytosis does not correlate with disease activity, surveillance bronchoscopy is not indicated (Chadelat et al. 1993). However, there is an urgent need for evidence on which to base recommendations.

TREATMENT

Given the likelihood of spontaneous remission in many forms of childhood sarcoidosis, and the likelihood of side-effects from treatment, it is first important to consider whether any therapy is necessary. There are no randomized controlled trials of treatment in pediatric sarcoid; evidence is at the level of case series or even case reports. Based on these and adult series, if treatment is given, oral corticosteroids are first line for systemic sarcoidosis. There are no evidence-based regimens for children; I would start with 1 mg/kg prednisolone, tapering slowly over time as the disease permits, on an individual basis. Typically, 18 months of treatment may be needed for pulmonary sarcoid (Fauroux and Clement 2005). Inhaled corticosteroids have been proposed to maintain remission, but the evidence of efficacy is poor (Kiper et al. 2001). If the disease is severe, or there is life-threatening organ involvement, I would consider pulsed methylprednisolone. In particular, neurosarcoidosis usually responds to prednisolone (Baumann and Robertson 2003). There is very little experience in childhood sarcoidosis with steroid sparing agents; low-dose methotrexate has been used successfully (Gedalia et al. 1997), including for the treatment of sarcoid iritis (Shetty et al. 1999). Hydroxychloroquine has also been used (Hilton et al. 1997). Mycophenylate has also been reported to be successful in a 12-year-old with ocular sarcoidosis, who was subsequently able to come off therapy. This child was included in a larger adult series (Bhat et al. 2009).

The basic treatment for anterior uveitis is corticosteroids, but these have considerable morbidity. There is no evidence for a sarcoid-specific treatment regimen for pediatric ocular sarcoid. Antimetabolites, alkylating agents and T-cell inhibitors have all been deployed (Mochizuki et al. 1993). In one series, 23 children with refractory uveitis, including one with sarcoidosis, were treated with biological modifying agents. Eligibility was failure or intolerance of standard therapy. Other

diagnoses included juvenile idiopathic arthritis, keratouveitis, Adamantiades–Behçets disease, and idiopathic. Ocular involvement was bilateral. Treatment with inliximab ($n=13$), adalimumab, both TNF-α blockers ($n=5$) or daclizumab, which binds to CD25, part of the IL-2 receptor expressed on activated T-cells ($n=5$), led to improvement in inflammation and visual acuity, with the best results in the infliximab group (Gallagher et al. 2007). The 12-year-old sarcoid patient responded to daclizumab, but prednisolone could not be discontinued. The medications were well tolerated. There are other small series in which a variety of cytotoxic and cytokine specific therapies have been used (Rosenbaum 1994; Mochizuki et al. 1996; Kilmartin et al. 1998; Walton et al. 1998; Goldstein et al. 2002; Baltatzis et al. 2003). Successful treatment with infliximab has also been reported in sarcoid interstitial nephritis (Thumfart et al. 2004). There is anecdotal evidence of successful anti-TNF strategies, combined with low-dose methotrexate, in non-ocular sarcoid (Antoniou 2010).

Treatment of other manifestations of sarcoid are based on adult regimens, and are discussed elsewhere in this volume. There are no child-specific, evidence-based regimens.

The use of these potentially toxic agents is not without risks. Death from acute leukemia has been described (Milman and Hoffman 2008). Rarely, the disease may flare during etanercept treatment (Hashkes and Shajrawi 2003). Furthermore, sarcoidosis has been reported to develop in a 9-year-old boy immunosuppressed with tacrolimus and mycophenylate after cardiac transplantation for complex congenital heart disease at 3 months of age; there was a good response to prednisolone (Bartram et al. 2006).

PROGNOSIS

Generally, the prognosis for adult survivors of childhood sarcoidosis is good. Most recover within 6 years of the onset of the disease (Milman and Hoffman 2008). In the Danish series, 46 adults were diagnosed with sarcoid aged <15 years between 1979 and 1994 (Milman and Hoffman 2008; Milman et al. 2009). Thirty-seven had a follow-up examination, of whom 30 had recovered completely. Two had permanent organ damage (loss of vision and lung fibrosis, respectively); five had ongoing disease activity, and three were dead (neurosarcoidosis and leukemia, the latter probably due to cytotoxic treatment). Erythema nodosum, scar sarcoidosis and peripheral lymphadenopathy were all good prognostic features, whereas iridocyclitis, hypercalcemia and neurosarcoidosis patients did less well. Height, weight and laboratory tests were largely normal. Thirty-one of 39 in whom chest X-rays were available had normal imaging, and 30 of 33 had normal lung function.

Quality of life was assessed in 34 patients. They scored normally in the SF-36. Of the nine who did not complete the questionnaire, one had neurosarcoid with pituitary insufficiency, and one was said to have asthma. The quality of life for those followed from childhood was much better than patients with adult-onset, active sarcoidosis (Cox et al. 2003, 2004). However, whether this reflects different disease severity or different responses to the same severity is not clear. Prognosis may be much less good for early childhood sarcoidosis, with a progressive, multisystem picture and a high mortality rate (Fink and Cimaz 1997).

Although the prognosis is generally good, given the small size of even the best series, my practice would be to follow up all children with sarcoid, to detect relapse and new manifestations of the disease.

CONCLUSION

Pediatric sarcoidosis is a true orphan disease. If we are to make progress, an international registry is urgently needed, and protocols for investigation and follow-up devised to ensure uniform data collection. These can then be used to understand prognosis and monitoring and carry out proper randomized controlled trials of treatment, thus putting the management of pediatric sarcoid on a firm footing. This collaborative approach would also hopefully lead to pathophysiological studies in children. In particular, the curious triadic presentation in pre-schoolers is unexplained, and may throw light on the underlying cause of the disease. However, above all, we need to go from case series to cohorts if we are to make progress.

REFERENCES

Alexis JB (1994). Sarcoidosis presenting as cutaneous hypopigmentation with repeatedly negative skin biopsies. *Int J Dermatol* **33**: 44–5.

Antoniou SA (2010). Targeting the TNF-alpha pathway in sarcoidosis. *Expert Opin Ther Targets* **14**: 21–9.

Baculard A, Blanc N, Boule M et al. (2001). Pulmonary sarcoidosis in children: a follow-up study. *Eur Respir J* **17**: 628–35.

Ball NJ, Kho GT, Martinka M (2004). The histological spectrum of cutaneous sarcoidosis: a study of 28 cases. *J Cutan Pathol* **31**: 160–8.

Bartram U, Thul J, Bauer J et al. (2006). Systemic sarcoidosis after cardiac transplantation in a 9-year-old child. *J Heart Lung Transplant* **25**: 1263–7.

Baltatzis S, Tufail F, Yu EN et al. (2003). Mycophenylate mofetil as an immunomodulatory agent in the treatment of chronic ocular inflammatory disorders. *Ophthalmology* **110**: 1061–5.

Batres E, Klima M, Tschen J (1982). Transepithelial elimination in cutaneous sarcoidosis. *J Cutan Pathol* **9**: 50–4.

Baumann RJ, Robertson WC (2003). Neurosarcoid presents differently in children than in adults. *Pediatrics* **112**: e480–6.

Beach RC, Corrin B, Scopes JW, Graham E (1980). Necrotizing sarcoid granulomatosis with neurologic lesions in a child. *J Pediatr* **97**: 950–3.

Beers MF, Mulugeta S (2005). Surfactant protein C biosynthesis and its emerging role in conformational lung disease. *Ann Rev Physiol* **67**: 663–96.

Bhat P, Cervantes-Castaneda RA, Doctor PP et al. (2009). Mycophenylate mofetil therapy for sarcoidosis-associated uveitis. *Ocul Immunol Inflamm* **17**: 185–90.

Bottone AC, Labarbera M, Asadourian A et al. (1993). Renal sarcoidosis coexisting with hypernephroma. *Urology* **41**: 157–9.

Brennan NJ, Crean P, Long JP, Fitzgerald MX (1984). High prevalence of familial sarcoidosis in an Irish population. *Thorax* **39**: 14–18.

Burton CM, Pressler T, Milman N (2005). Pulmonary sarcoidosis in a child with cystic fibrosis. *Pediatr Pulmonol* **39**: 473–7.

Callen JP (2001). The presence of foreign bodies does not exclude the diagnosis of sarcoidosis. *Arch Dermatol* **137**: 485–6.

Chadelat KC, Baculard MD, Grimfeld A et al. (1993). Pulmonary sarcoidosis in children: serial evaluation of bronchoalveolar lavage cells during corticosteroid treatment. *Pediatr Pulmonol* **16**: 41–7.

Clark SK (1987). Sarcoidosis in children. *Pediatr Dermatol* **4**: 291–9.

Comerci SCD, Levin TL, Ruzal Shapiro C et al. (1996). Benign adenomatous kidney neoplasms in children with polycythemia: imaging findings. *Radiology* **198**: 265–8.

Cooper T, Day A, Weller P, Geddes DM (1987). Case report: sarcoidosis in two patients with cystic fibrosis. A chance association? *Thorax* **42**: 818–20.

Cox CE, Donohue JF, Brown CD et al. (2003). The Sarcoidosis Health Questionnaire: a new measure of health-related quality of life. *Am J Respir Crit Care Med* **168**: 323–9.

Cox CE, Donohue JF, Brown CD et al. (2004). Health-related quality of life of persons with sarcoidosis. *Chest* **125**: 997–1004.

Crowson AN, Mihm MC, Magro CM (2003). Cutaneous vasculitis: a review. *J Cutan Pathol* **30**: 161–73.

Coutant R, Leroy B, Niaudet P et al. (1999). Renal granulomatous sarcoid in childhood: a report of 11 cases and a review of the literature. *Eur J Paediatr* **13**: 154–9.

Currie GP, Kerr KM, Legge JS (2007). Relapsing necrotising sarcoid granulomatosis in a young patient. *Eur Respir J* **29**: 816.

Dimitriades C, Shetty AK, Vehaskari M et al. (1999). Membranous nephropathy associated with childhood sarcoidosis. *Pediatr Nephrol* **13**: 444–7.

de Boer JH, Sijssens KM, Smeekens AE, Rothova A (2009). Keratitis and arthritis in children with sarcoidosis. *Br J Ophthalmol* **93**: 835.

Doan ML, Guillerman RP, Dishop MK et al. (2008). Clinical, radiological and pathological features of ABCA3 mutations in children. *Thorax* **6**: 366–73.

Falcini F, Battini ML, Ceruso M, Cimez R (1999). A 4-year-old with a rash. *Lancet* **354**: 40.

Fauroux B, Clement A (2005). Pediatric sarcoidosis. *Pediatr Resp Rev* **6**: 128–33.

Faye-Petersen O, Frenkel SR, Schulman PE et al. (1991). Giant cell vasculitis with extravascular granulomas in an adolescent. *Paediatr Pathol* **11**: 281–95.

Fink CW, Cimaz R (1997). Early onset sarcoidosis is not a benign disease. *J Rheumatol* **24**: 174–7.

Gallagher M, Qumories K, Cervantes-Castenada RA et al. (2007). Biological response modifier therapy for refractory childhood uveitis. *Br J Ophthalmol* **91**(10): 1341–3.

Gallerani I, Innocenti DD, Coronella G et al. (2004). Cutaneous sarcoid-like granulomas in a patient with X-linked hyper-IgM syndrome. *Pediatr Dermatol* **21**: 39–43.

Gazaigne J, Mozziconacci JG, Mornet M, Provendier B (1995). Epididymal and renal sarcoidosis. *Br J Urol* **75**: 413–14.

Gedalia A, Molina JF, Ellis GSJ et al. (1997). Low-dose methotrexate therapy for childhood sarcoidosis. *J Pediatr* **130**: 25–9.

Gibson LE, Winkelmann RK (1986). Chronic granulomatous vasculitis: its relationship to systemic disease. *J Am Acad Dermatol* **14**: 492–501.

Goldberg LJ, Goldberg N, Abrahams I et al. (1994). Giant cell lichenoid dermatitis: a possible manifestation of sarcoidosis. *J Cutan Pathol* **21**: 47–51.

Goldstein DA, Fontanilla FA, Kaul S et al. (2002). Long-term follow-up of patients treated with short-term high dose chlorambucil for sight-threatening ocular inflammation. *Ophthalmology* **109**: 370–3.

Gross KR, Malleson PN, Culham G et al. (1986). Vasculopathy with renal artery stenosis in a child with sarcoidosis. *J Pediatr* **108**: 724–6.

Hashkes PJ, Shajrawi I (2003). Sarcoid-related uveitis occurring during etanercept therapy. *Clin Exp Rheumatol* **21**: 645–6.

Heinrich D, Gordjani N, Trusen A et al. (2003). Necrotizing sarcoid granulomatosis: a rarity in childhood. *Pediatr Pulmonol* **35**: 407–11.

Herman TE, Shackelford GD, McAlister WH (1997). Pseudotumoral sarcoid granulomatous nephritis in a child: case presentation with sonographic and CT findings. *Pediatr Radiol* **27**: 752–4.

Herzlinger DC, Marland AM, Barr RJ (1979). Verrucous ulcerative skin lesions in sarcoidosis: an unusual clinical presentation. *Cutis* **23**: 569–72.

Hetherington S (1982). Sarcoidosis in young children. *Am J Dis Child* **136**: 13–15.

Hetherington SV (1987). Sarcoidosis in children. *Pediatr Dermatol* **4**: 291–9.

Hilton JM, Cooper DM, Henry RL (1997). Hydroxychloroquine therapy of diffuse pulmonary sarcoidosis in two Australian male children. *Respirology* **2**: 71–4.

Hislop AA, Wigglesworth JS, Desai R (1986). Alveolar development in the human fetus and infant. *Early Hum Dev* **13**: 1–11.

Hoffman AL, Milman N, Byg K-E (2004). Childhood sarcoidosis in Denmark 1979–1994: incidence, clinical features and laboratory results at presentation in 48 children. *Acta Pediatr* **93**: 30–36.

Hojo H, Suzuki S, Kikuta A et al. (2000). Sarcoid reaction in primary neuroblastoma: case report. *Pediatr Devel Pathol* **3**: 584–9.

Holt PG, Jones CA (2000). The development of the immune system during pregnancy and early life. *Allergy* **55**: 688–97.

Hughes JJ, Wilder WW (1988). Computed tomography of renal sarcoidosis. *J Comput Assist Tomogr* **12**: 1057–8.

Hunninghake GW, Costabel U, Ando M et al. (1999). Statement on sarcoidosis. *Am J Respir Crit Care Med* **160**: 736–55.

Kanazawa N, Okafuji I, Kambe N et al. (2005). Early-onset sarcoidosis and CARD15 mutations with constitutive nuclear factor-κB activation: common genetic etiology with Blau syndrome. *Blood* **105**: 1195–7.

Kauh YC, Goody HE, Luscombe HA (1978). Ichthyosiform sarcoidosis. *Arch Dermatol* **114**: 100–1.

Kendig EL (1974). The clinical picture of sarcoidosis in children. *Pediatrics* **54**: 289–92.

Kendig E, Niitu Y (1980). Sarcoidosis in Japanese and American children. *Chest* **51**: 4–6.

Khan JA, Hoover DL, Giangiacomo J, Singsen BH (1986). Orbital and childhood sarcoidosis. *J Pediatr Ophthalmol Strabismus* **23**: 190–4.

Kilmartin DJ, Forrester JV, Dick AD (1998). Cyclosporin therapy in refractory non-infectious childhood uveitis. *Br J Ophthalmol* **82**: 737–42.

Kiper N, Anadol D, Ozcelik U, Goomen A (2001). Inhaled corticosteroids for maintenance treatment in childhood pulmonary sarcoidosis. *Acta Paediatr* **90**: 953–6.

Kuramoto Y, Shindo Y, Tagami H (1988). Subcutaneous sarcoidosis with extensive caseation necrosis. *J Cutan Pathol* **15**: 188–90.

Kwon EJ, Hivnor CM, Yan AC et al. (2007). Interstitial granulomatous lesions as part of the spectrum of presenting cutaneous signs in pediatric sarcoidosis. *Pediatr Dermatol* **24**: 517–24.

Lazzarini LCO, Teixera MdeFdoA, Rodrigues RS, Valiante PMN (2008). Necrotizing sarcoid granulomatosis in a family of patients with sarcoidosis reinforces the association between both entities. *Respiration* **76**: 356–60

Levine TS, Price AB, Boyle S, Webster ADB (1994). Cutaneous sarcoid-like granulomas in primary immunodeficiency disorders. *Br J Dermatol* **130**: 118–20.

Lindsley CB, Petty RE (2000). Overview and report on international registry of sarcoid arthritis in childhood. *Curr Rheumatol Rep* **2**: 343–8.

Magro CM, Crowson AN, Regauer S (1996). Granuloma annulare and necrobiosis lipoidica tissue reactions as a manifestation of systemic disease. *Hum Pathol* **27**: 50–6.

Martini A, Serena Scotta M, Magrini U (1980). Granulomatous sarcoidosis of the kidneys with renal insufficiency in a 12 year old girl. *Nephrologie* **1**: 117–19.

Marty CL, Kwong PC (2009). Intrascrotal sarcoidosis in a pediatric patient. *Cutis* **83**: 133–7.

Milman N, Hoffman AL (2008). Childhood sarcoidosis: long-term follow up. *Eur Respir J* **31**: 592–8.

Milman N, Hoffman AL, Byg KE (1998). Sarcoidosis in children: epidemiology in Danes, clinical features, diagnosis and prognosis. *Acta Paediatr* **87**: 871–8.

Milman N, Selroos O (1990a). Pulmonary sarcoidosis in the Nordic countries 1950–1982: epidemiology and clinical picture. *Sarcoidosis* **7**: 50–7.

Milman N, Selroos O (1990b). Pulmonary sarcoidosis in the Nordic countries 1950–1982. II: Course and prognosis. *Sarcoidosis* **7**: 113–18.

Milman N, Svendsen CB, Hoffman AL (2009). Health-related quality of life in adult survivors of childhood sarcoidosis. *Respir Med* **103**: 913–18.

Mochizuki M, Masuda K, Sakane T et al. (1993). A clinical trial of FK506 in refractory uveitis. *Am J Ophthalmol* **115**: 763–9.

Morris KP, Coulthard MG, Smith PJ, Craft AW (1996). Renovascular and growth effects of childhood sarcoid. *Arch Dis Child* **75**: 74–5.

Moorthy RS, Inomata H, Rao NA (1995). Vigt–Koyanagi–Harada syndrome. *Surv Ophthalmol* **39**: 265–92.

Mulugeta S, Nguyen V, Russo SJ et al. (2005). A surfactant protein C precursor protein BRICHOS domain mutation causes endoplasmic reticulum stress, proteasome dysfunction, and caspase 3 activation. *Am J Respir Cell Mol Biol* **32**: 521–30.

Neville E, Carstairs LS, James DG (1977). Sarcoidosis of bone. *Q J Med* **46**: 215–27.

Newman LS, Rose CS, Maher LA (1997). Sarcoidosis. *New Engl J Med* **336**: 1224–34.

Nowak DA, Widenka DC (2001). Neurosarcoidosis: a review of its intracranial manifestations. *J Neurol* **248**: 363–72.

Okamoto H (1999). Epidermal changes in cutaneous lesions of sarcoidosis. *Am J Dermatopathol* **21**: 229–33.

Paparel P, Devonec M, Perrin P (2007). Association between sarcoidosis and testicular carcinoma: a diagnostic pitfall. *Sarcoid Vasc Diff Lung Dis* **24**: 95–101.

Pattishall EN, Kendig EL (1996). Sarcoidosis in children. *Pediatr Pulmonol* **22**: 195–203.

Pattishall EN, Strope GL, Spinola SM, Denny FD (1986). Childhood sarcoidosis. *J Pediatr* **108**: 169–77.

Rasmussen JE (1981). Sarcoidosis in young children. *J Am Acad Dermatol* **5**: 566–70.

Rettinger S, Trulock E, Mackay B, Auerbach HS (1989). Case report: sarcoidosis in an adult with cystic fibrosis. *Thorax* **44**: 829–30.

Rose CD, Doyle TM, McIlvain-Simpson G et al. (2005). Blau syndrome mutation of CARD15/NOD2 in sporadic early-onset granulomatous arthritis. *J Rheumatol* **32**: 373–5.

Rosen Y, Moon S, Huang CT et al. (1977). Granulomatous pulmonary angiitis in sarcoidosis. *Arch Pathol Lab Med* **101**: 170–4.

Rosenbaum JT (1994). Treatment of severe refractor uveitis with intravenous cyclophosphamide. *J Rheumatol* 21: 123–5.

Rosenberg AM, Yee EH, MacKenzie JW (1983). Arthritis in childhood sarcoidosis. *J Rheumatol* 10: 987–90.

Rossi GA, Battistini E, Celle ME *et al.* (2001). Long-lasting myopathy as a major clinical feature of sarcoidosis in a child: case report with a 7-year follow-up. *Sarcoid Vasc Diff Lung Dis* 18: 196–200.

Scerri L, Cook LJ, Jenkins EA, Thomas AL (1996). Familial juvenile systemic granulomatosis (Blau's syndrome). *Clin Exp Dermatol* 21: 445–8.

Schmidt D, Harms D, Lang W (1985). Primary malignat hepatic tumours in childhood. *Virchows Arch A Pathol Anat* 407: 387–405.

Serwer GA, Edwards SB, Benson DW *et al.* (1978). Ventricular tachyarrhythmia due to cardiac sarcoidosis in a child. *Pediatrics* 62: 322–5.

Sharma O, Maheshwari A, Thaker K (1993). Myocardial sarcoid. *Chest* 103: 253–8.

Shetty AK, Zganjar BE, Ellis GS *et al.* (1999). Low-dose methotrexate in the treatment of severe juvenile rheumatoid arthritis and sarcoid iritis. *J Pediatr Ophthalmol Strabismus* 36: 125–8.

Shirodaria CC, Nicholson AG, Hansell DM *et al.* (2003). Lesson of the month: necrotising sarcoid granulomatosis with skin involvement. *Histopathology* 43: 91–3.

Siegried EC, Prose NS, Friedman NJ, Paller AS (1991). Cutaneous granulomas in children with combined immunodeficiency. *J Am Acad Dermatol* 25: 761–6.

Sigh N, Cole S, Krause PJ *et al.* (1981). Necrotizing sarcoid granulomatosis with extrapulmonary involvement. *Am Rev Respir Dis* 124: 189.

Singal A, Thami GP, Goraya JS (2005). Scar sarcoidosis in childhood: case report and review of the literature. *Clin Exp Dermatol* 30: 244–6.

Skinner MD, Masters R (1970). Primary acquired agammaglobulinemia with granulomas of the skin and internal organs. *Arch Dermatol* 102: 109–10.

Soden M, Tempany E, Bresnihan B (1989). Case report: sarcoid arthropathy in cystic fibrosis. *Br J Rheumatol* 28: 341–3.

Sussman GL, Yang WH, Steinberg S (1992). Melkersson–Rosenthal syndrome: clinical, pathologic, and therapeutic considerations. *Ann Allergy* 69: 187–94.

Sverrild A, Backer V, Kyvik KO *et al.* (2008). Heredity in sarcoidosis: a registry-based twin study. *Thorax* 63: 894–6.

Syed J, Myers R (2004). Sarcoid heart disease. *Can J Cardiol* 20: 89–93.

Tauber E, Wojnarowski C, Horcher E *et al.* (1999). Necrotizing sarcoid granulomatosis in a 14-year-old female. *Eur Respir J* 13: 703–5.

Tessier V, Chadelat K, Baculard A *et al.* (1996). BAL in children: a controlled study of differential cytology and cytokine expression profiles by alveolar cells in pediatric sarcoidosis. *Chest* 109: 1430–8.

Thomas AQ, Lane K, Phillips J *et al.* (2002). Heterozygosity for surfactant protein C gene mutation associated with usual interstitial pneumonitis and cellular nonspecific interstitial pneumonitis in one kindred. *Am J Respir Crit Care Med* 165: 1322–8.

Thomas AL, Thomas CL, Dodge JA, Jessop JD (1983). A case of sarcoid arthritis in a child. *Ann Rheum Dis* 42: 343–6.

Thumfart J, Muller D, Rudolph B *et al.* (2004). Isolated sarcoid granulomatous interstitial nephritis responding to infliximab therapy. *Am J Kidney Dis* 45: 411–14.

Turner MC, Shin ML, Ruley EJ (1977). Renal failure as a presenting sign of diffuse sarcoidosis in an adolescent girl. *Am J Dis Child* 131: 997–1000.

Yanardag H, Pamuk ON, Karayel T (2003). Cutaneous involvement in sarcoidosis: analysis of the features in 170 patients. *Respir Med* 97: 978–82.

Walton RC, Nussenbltt RB, Whitcip SM (1998). Cyclosporine therapy for severe sight-threatening uveitis in children and adolescents. *Ophthalmology* 105: 2028–34.

Wong GW, Li AM, Ng PC, Fok TF (2003). Severe acute respiratory syndrome in children. *Pediatr Pulmonol* 36: 261–6.

Wurzel DW, Steinfort DP, Massie J *et al.* (2009). Paralysis and a perihilar protuberance: an unusual presentation of sarcoidosis in a child. *Pediatr Pulmonol* 44: 410–14.

Young WG, Sauk JJ, Pihlstrom B, Fish AJ (1978). Histopathology and electron and immunofluorescence microscopy of gingivitis granulomatosa associated with glossitis and cheilitis in a case of Anderson–Fabry disease. *Oral Surg Oral Med Oral Pathol* 46: 540–54.

PART **IX**

DIAGNOSIS AND TREATMENT

41

Diagnosis of sarcoidosis

DONALD N MITCHELL, SUVEER SINGH, STEPHEN SPIRO AND ATHOL WELLS

INTRODUCTION

The diagnosis and, where appropriate, the differential diagnosis of sarcoidosis involving individual organs and tissues are detailed in other chapters. This chapter relates to the more general aspects of the diagnosis of sarcoidosis to be considered by clinicians.

The diagnosis should be based on a summary of all available data and is more secure if histological confirmation of compatible granulomatous changes has been obtained from one or more sites. However, there are some clinical presentations so characteristic of sarcoidosis, which in most cases proceed to spontaneous resolution, that the best interests of the patient justify an expectant policy without recourse to biopsy. Conversely, there are patients in whom diagnostic uncertainty will persist, even after compatible tissue biopsy has been obtained. Additionally, supportive immunological and biochemical findings or evidence of asymptomatic involvement of organs frequently affected may increase the probability of sarcoidosis, without being conclusive.

PRESUMPTIVE DIAGNOSIS OF SARCOIDOSIS WITHOUT BIOPSY

Erythema nodosum (EN)

The histology of EN is in general similar whatever the cause of the erythema. Löfgren and Wahlgren studied the histology of 64 cases divided into groups associated with tuberculous streptococcal infection with confirmed or suspected sarcoidosis and of uncertain association (Löfgren and Wahlgren 1949). Similar changes were found in all groups, affecting the deep dermis and subcutaneous tissue. The epidermis showed no changes. Occasionally, EN appears in a patient in whom bilateral hilar lymphadenopathy has already been detected radiographically: a few cases have been reported in which the chest radiograph was normal when the EN appeared, and radiographic or other evidence of sarcoidosis was found later (Macpherson 1970). Accordingly, biopsy of EN should be avoided since histopathology shows no granuloma but nonspecific inflammation and vasculitis.

However, the proportion of patients with sarcoidosis in which EN occurs varies widely between studies: 74 percent of 170 patients (James 1961), 8 percent of 179 patients (Löfgren 1946) and 29 percent of 401 patients (Mikhail et al. 1978). In the BTTA study, there was a considerable difference between geographical regions in the proportion of men with sarcoidosis who had EN (British Thoracic and Tuberculosis Association 1969). This ranged from 11 percent in Cornwall to 29 percent in East Anglia; the proportions among women varied less, ranging between 30 and 38 percent.

Most patients with EN associated with sarcoidosis have some joint pain, and in about half of them it is the most prominent symptom. The larger joints, ankles and knees are most frequently affected. In some, especially men, painful ankle swelling is more prominent than EN. This clinical picture merges into features at presentation in a few patients, consisting of febrile arthropathy, without EN, and has the same place in the national history of sarcoidosis as does EN. It is noteworthy that, in the USA and Japan, EN is a much less frequent manifestation of sarcoidosis (James 1976), although EN is frequent among Puerto Ricans with sarcoidosis in New York (Siltzbach 1958).

Löfgren's syndrome

This syndrome is characterized by the radiological appearance of bilateral hilar lymphadenopathy associated with EN, ankle arthritis and/or arthropathy, and constitutional symptoms such as fever, sweating and loss of weight. Löfgren's syndrome has a remission rate of 70–80 percent, whereas patients with lupus pernio or fibrocystic pulmonary sarcoidosis rarely undergo remission (Joint Statement 1999). Sipathi Demirkok and colleagues examined the seasonality of sarcoidosis in symptomatic recently diagnosed patients with Löfgren's syndrome which was diagnosed in 87 of 492 patients (18 percent) with sarcoidosis (Sipathi Demirkok et al. 2006). Among these 87 patients, the distribution of cumulative monthly presentations peaked in May and was lowest in January and November.

Is histological support always required?

The classical clinical presentation of Löfgren's syndrome usually justifies an expectant policy of management without recourse to tissue biopsy. It has been argued, in a comprehensive review of sarcoidosis, that a diagnosis without biopsy as permissible only in patients who present with Löfgren's syndrome (Iannuzi et al. 2007). However, among sarcoidosis patients presenting to us in the UK, we have felt justified in adopting a somewhat more liberal view. In patients presenting with other recognizable syndromes, including those associated with bilateral hilar lymphadenopathy, the confidence with which a diagnosis of sarcoidosis may be acceptable without biopsy, especially with the advent of high-resolution CT (HRCT), will depend on the experience of the observer. A detailed history and clinical examination with special reference to evidence of extrathoracic involvement, in particular peripheral lymphadenopathy, conjunctival follicles, or nodular infiltrates over the nasal septum or inferior turbinates, may be helpful in clinical confirmation of a diagnosis of sarcoidosis, without recourse to a tissue biopsy or to an appropriate form of bronchopulmonary biopsy. Access to any previous radiograph which may depict features in keeping with a diagnosis of sarcoidosis is obviously of cardinal importance. Obviously, where further radiological resolution may be helpful, HRCT may assist in radiological clarification (Wells 1998).

A further crucial consideration is the view of the informed patient in cases in which there is no histological confirmation but the diagnosis is highly probable on clinical grounds. Dogmatic statements that diagnosis is not 'permissible' without biopsy, except in Löfgren's syndrome (Iannuzi et al. 2007), are very redolent of the last century and disempower the patient. In the modern era, it is generally accepted that when medical decisions are a very close call, the final decision should be determined by the wishes of the patient. When sarcoidosis is suspected, with a diagnostic probability of 90–95 percent but no histological confirmation, many patients have strong views on whether they wish to undergo bronchoscopy or other semi-invasive procedures, or would prefer an empirical diagnosis. In the latter scenario, it is essential that the patient be made aware of alternative diagnostic possibilities and the need for meticulous monitoring with a view to further diagnostic tests if atypical features emerge. However, the authors believe strongly that patient involvement in marginal decisions regarding invasive diagnostic tests is as important as in treatment decisions.

Other general considerations

In a minority of patients presenting with Heerfordt's syndrome, as characterized by a protracted course, low fever, localization in the parotid gland and in the uveal tract and the frequent appearance of complicating paresis of the cerebrospinal nerves, especially the facial, a diagnosis of sarcoidosis, as designated by Heerfordt, may also be acceptable without recourse to biopsy tissue (Heerfordt 1909).

All patients in whom a provisional or definitive diagnosis of sarcoidosis is proposed (with or without the intention of proceeding to biopsy) should complete tuberculin and interferon-γ release assay tests with clarification of chest radiograph appearances (HRCT) where appropriate. Where biopsy tissue is obtained, special stains for acid-fast bacilli and fungi as well as cultures for such organisms are essential.

It is relevant that recent data have strongly endorsed the view that the predisposition to sarcoidosis is genetically determined and that genetics also appears to account for the variability of clinical phenotype and behavior (Spagnolo and du Bois 2007), with the association between Löfgren's syndrome and the extended HLA D.R BIx0301/DQ BIx0201 haplotype probably the most extensively reproduced. These authors add, however, that our understanding of the biological evidence of variations in the genome is still incomplete and that the reported associations need to be verified in populations of different ethnicities (see Chapter 7). It is not yet clear whether genetic associations will add usefully to non-histological diagnosis.

Bronchoalveolar lavage

Although non-specific, BAL may be helpful in differentiating sarcoidosis from other disorders. In active sarcoidosis, BAL fluid characteristically shows a predominance of lymphocytes with a normal or elevated total cell count. In rare instances, the percentage of eosinophils may be significantly elevated and very rarely a peripheral eosinophilia may be evident. Plasma cell and foamy alveolar macrophage counts are usually normal.

Drent and colleagues reported the development of a computer program for BAL data using logistic regression, which clearly showed that a BAL CD4 + CD8 + ratio of > 3.5 has a sensitivity of 52–59 percent and a specificity of 94–96 percent and is, therefore, highly supportive of a probable diagnosis of sarcoidosis (Drent et al. 2001). In another study, transbronchial biopsy of lung had a specificity of 89 percent for the differentiation between sarcoidosis and other diffuse lung diseases and was no better than the CD4/CD8 ratio for this differentiation (Winterbauer et al. 1973), with similar findings reported by Costabel (Costabel et al. 1992). Higher numbers of neutrophils in BAL fluid have been observed in groups of patients in whom sarcoidosis deteriorated during follow-up, although this finding was not always present in individual patients (Drent et al. 1999; Ziegenhagen et al. 2003).

A reduction in vascular endothelial growth factor (VEGF) in BAL from patients with radiographic evidence of pulmonary infiltration only or pulmonary fibrosis suggests that impaired angiogenesis is associated with parenchymal fibrotic lesions (Fireman *et al.* 2009; see Chapter 12).

Compatible clinical features

AGE RANGE

Sarcoidosis may occur at any age including the very young. Of the recorded cases below the age of 15 years, most have been in older children (see Chapter 40). A higher proportion of young children than of adults present with unusual features such as chronic polyarthritis, basal granulomatous meningitis, hepatomegaly and jaundice, purpura, myositis and fever. Conversely, EN and hilar lymphadenopathy are infrequent in children. However, in countries where children have been included in mass radiographic surveys, both have been seen; thus, Mandi (1964) found that of 14 children below the age of 15 years, 10 had asymptomatic bilateral hilar lymphadenopathy (BHL). Thus, in very young children, sarcoidosis is rare and tends to present in unusual forms. In late childhood, the frequency of sarcoidosis increases and assumes clinical features and a prognosis very similar to that in adults. Among adults, the incidence is highest in both sexes at some point between 20 and 40 years. There is a small increase of incidence in women past middle age, which accounts for most of the slightly higher excess incidence in women (see Chapter 3).

ORGAN INVOLVEMENT

Baughman and colleagues reviewed the multisystem organ involvement that may be present among patients presenting with a diagnosis of sarcoidosis: intrathoracic manifestations tend to predominate (Baughman *et al.* 2001) (Figs 41.1 to 41.9). These, together with the investigation, diagnosis, management and prognosis of sarcoidosis involving extrapulmonary organs and tissues, are the subjects of other chapters in this book.

SOURCES OF BIOPSY MATERIAL

Lymph nodes

Palpable lymph nodes are a very fruitful source for biopsy confirmation of a diagnosis of sarcoidosis and should be sought in all suspected cases. Subcutaneous nodules, which are more prevalent in the early acute stages, are also a favorable source of tissue for biopsy. Mediastinoscopy, in which lymph nodes are removed from the anterior part of the superior mediastinum through a skin incision over the suprasternal notch, was introduced by Carlens in 1959. In 1964, he reported confirmation of the diagnosis of sarcoidosis in 118 (96 percent) of 123 cases in whom sarcoidosis was suspected. Mikhail and colleagues reported that, of 227 patients in whom a diagnosis of sarcoidosis was thought likely and who were investigated by mediastinoscopy, 187 (82 percent) yielded lymph nodes showing sarcoid type granulomas: the proportion was lower (55 percent) in those with lung infiltration, but without evident hilar node enlargement (Mikhail *et al.* 1979).

Although largely replaced by more recent techniques, mediastinoscopy continues to be a helpful method of obtaining biopsy of lymph node tissue from patients in whom clinical or radiographic features have led to a suspicion of tuberculosis or malignancy. It is of paramount importance that lymph node tissue be set aside for auromine and Ziehl–Neelson staining and for culture on Lowenstein medium for mycobacteria. Where malignancy is suspected, tissue should also be set aside for immunopathological examination. The interpretation of granulomatous changes in lymph nodes is complicated both by the occurrence of non-caseating changes without discernible mycobacteria in nodes remote from a focus of caseating mycobacterial tuberculosis, and by the phenomenon of sarcoid reactions in nodes draining areas thath are the site of malignant disease, and in association with Hodgkin's and other lymphomas.

Liver

Liver biopsy has been widely used in the past in the diagnosis of sarcoidosis, as granulomas are found in a needle biopsy of liver in some 70 percent of patients with active sarcoidosis with or without clinical or other evidence of liver dysfunction. Its value is limited by the large number of possible causes of granulomas in the liver, between most of which histology does not discriminate (see Chapter 24).

Skin

In all patients suspected of sarcoidosis, a search for abnormalities of the skin which the patient may not have noticed or mentioned should be made, including old scars (Figs 41.7 to 41.9). A simple punch biopsy of any such abnormalities submitted to histology has a high likelihood of yielding a positive result if the diagnosis of sarcoidosis is correct (see Chapter 30).

Bronchi

Biopsy of the bronchial mucosa may show granulomas in a varying but high proportion of patients with BHL and radiologically clear lungs. Similar findings result among patients with evident lung changes. Biopsies from thickened or otherwise abnormal mucosa and from normal-looking mucosa alike frequently show specific changes (see Chapters 12 and 43).

Conjunctiva

Careful inspection of the conjuctiva may show suspicious abnormalities, especially accompanying uveitis. If so, a biopsy can be performed easily and safely by an expert and may well show granulomas in a patient with sarcoidosis. Biopsy of a normal-looking mucosa is unlikely to be productive (see Chapter 31).

Nasal mucosa

Inspection of the mucosa over the nasal septum and over the inferior turbinates may show abnormalities. If so, biopsy by an expert may yield granulomas in a patient with sarcoidosis. Biopsy of the normal mucosa in such circumstances is unlikely to be productive and may give rise to significant bleeding (see Chapter 21).

Skeletal muscle

Random biopsy of skeletal muscle in patients with early active sarcoidosis, especially with fever, arthropathy or EN, shows granulomas in a significant proportion of cases. Later in the disease, biopsy of muscle is unlikely to show granulomas except in those rare cases with clinical evidence suggesting muscle involvement (see Chapter 32).

Spleen

Selroos performed percutaneous fine-needle biopsy of the spleen, after confirming a normal platelet count in 77 patients with verified sarcoidosis (Selroos 1976). The procedure was performed without local anesthesia. The aspirated material, spread on slides, air-dried and stained, showed recognizable granulomas in 41 (53 percent). Five of six with enlarged spleens, 47 percent with BHL as the only clinical sign of disease, and 67 percent of those with detected extrathoracic disease showed granulomas. This experience cannot be extrapolated to obscure cases (see Chapter 26).

Lung

Fiberoptic bronchoscopy with mucosal biopsy, transbronchial lung biopsy, transbronchial needle aspiration using ultrasound guidance, and bronchoalveolar lavage are now the procedures of choice (Hunninghake et al. 1999). The yield of transbronchial lung biopsy (TLB) for sarcoidosis patients with hilar adenopathy alone is approximately 50 percent. In the past, the alternative approach was mediastinoscopy (the results of which are summarized earlier) which, overall, was associated with significant cost and morbidity (Reich et al. 1998). Transbronchial needle aspiration (TBNA) is an emerging bronchoscopic diagnostic sampling modality for sarcoidosis. It is known to be safe, easy to pick up and, provided larger needles (e.g. 19 gauge) are used and material is reviewed by an experienced cytologist, the yield is encouraging. This may be performed with other sampling modalities to maximize yield (Bilaceroglu et al. 1999; Trisoloni et al. 2003,2008). Of a total of 137 patients, among whom sarcoidosis was diagnosed in 115, endoscopic ultrasound following negative flexible bronchoscopy avoided a surgical procedure in 47 of 80 patients (Tournoy et al. 2010).

Recently, the diagnostic yield from endobronchial needle aspiration has approached 90 percent when ultrasound guidance was used (Garwood et al. 2007). Thus, many cases of BHL that were assumed to be due to sarcoidosis because of the risks of mediastinoscopy can now be diagnosed with lower risk, at lower cost, and as an outpatient procedure (Judson 2008). Exceptionally, recourse to open lung biopsy may be needed (see Chapters 11 and 43).

OTHER TESTS CONTRIBUTING TO THE DIAGNOSIS OF SARCOIDOSIS

A number of tests, immunological, biochemical and radiological, may contribute to the diagnosis of sarcoidosis, either generally or in particular contexts, without being specific.

Pulmonary function tests

Although sarcoidosis is traditionally viewed as a restrictive lung disease, patterns of ventilatory impairment include airflow obstruction, lung restriction and, commonly, a mixed pattern, usually in association with a reduction in the diffusing capacity of carbon monoxide – more so in patients with stage III and IV radiographic appearances. In apparently idiopathic fibrotic lung disease, the presence of a marked obstructive defect increases the likelihood of a diagnosis of sarcoidosis. It is more usual for lung function to be normal at presentation, with exercise desaturation indicative of more advanced disease (Dunn et al. 1988). Endobronchial sarcoidosis may lead to airflow obstruction (Karetsky and McDonough 1996). Overall, only 20 percent of patients with stage 1 disease show abnormalities, compared to 40–70 percent in other stages of sarcoidosis (Lynch et al. 1977).

Tuberculin test and other delayed skin reactions

The serum generally depressed reactivity to agents causing type IV reactions observed in patients with sarcoidosis is of limited diagnostic value. The significance of non-reactivity to 'recall' antigens (those of infective agents to which the subject has been exposed previously) depends on the proportion of reactors to be expected in the general population. When most adults reacted to tuberculin, a negative tuberculin test gave general support to the diagnosis of sarcoidosis, although a positive test was (and is) entirely compatible with it; in communities where the general level of tuberculin sensitivity is now low, the significance of non-reactivity to tuberculin has been reduced to making the diagnosis of caseating tuberculosis very unlikely. Similarly, the significance of skin reactivity to histoplasmin and coccidiodin varies with the local prevalence of the relevant infections.

High proportions of adults are reactive to Candida, Trichophyton and mumps antigens, and failure to respond, especially to more than one of these, supports a diagnosis of sarcoidosis. This support may be useful in a doubtful case, but is not conclusive enough to justify the routine use of these tests (see Chapter 17).

Serum angiotensin-converting enzyme and lysozyme levels

Levels of certain enzymes, notably angiotensin-1-converting enzyme (ACE) and lysozyme, have been found to be elevated significantly in the serum of patients with active sarcoidosis, and to be related to the extent and activity of the disease. ACE and lysozyme have been demonstrated in macrophages, epithelioid cells and giant cells in the sarcoid granuloma. The following discussion concerns the diagnostic value of estimation of these enzymes.

Elevated serum lysozyme levels have been found in patients with sarcoidosis (Pascual et al. 1973; Selroos and Klockars 1997). Those with both BHL and lung infiltration and those with both extra- and intrathoracic changes showed higher levels than those with BHL only. There are similar elevations in pulmonary tuberculosis, levels being related to the activity of the disease, though correlating poorly with the presence of tubercle bacilli in the sputum (Khan *et al.* 1973). The diagnostic value of serum lysozyme levels in sarcoidosis is thus limited principally to discrimination from non-granulomatous disease.

Using a modification of the spectrophotometric assay described by Cushman and Cheung in 1971, Lieberman found that levels of ACE in the serum of many patients with active sarcoidosis were raised, and fell on resolution of therapeutic suppression of activity with prednisone. Even high levels found in Gaucher's disease, but raised levels were infrequent in diseases likely to be confused with sarcoidosis (Lieberman 1975). These observations were extended in 391 patients with sarcoidosis, of whom 58 percent had levels more than 2 standard deviations above the mean of values in a control group; excluding 91 who were being treated with corticosteroids of whose disease was thought to be inactive, 76 percent had raised levels (Lieberman *et al.* 1979). Values tended to be higher in black than in white patients, and in children than in adults. Among patients started on treatment, mean values fell to less than half pre-treatment levels. Elevated levels were found in 5 percent of a group of patients with miscellaneous other pulmonary diseases. In a number of other studies, serum ACE levels have been elevated in about half of patients with untreated sarcoidosis (Fanberg *et al.* 1976; Silverstein *et al.* 1976; Studdy *et al.* 1978; Turton *et al.* 1979; Grönhagen-Riska *et al.* 1979).

General parallelism has been reported between serum ACE levels and the clinical course, including the response to corticosteroids (De Remee and Rohrbach 1980). In another study, both ACE and lysozyme levels fell rapidly towards normal in five sarcoidosis patients after treatment with corticosteroids, with falls of 28 and 24 percent in ACE and lysozyme levels, and in nine patients receiving corticosteroids for other diseases (Turton *et al.* 1979).

In Gaucher's disease, serum ACE levels even higher than those found in some cases of sarcoidosis are usual (Lieberman 1975). This disease is unlikely to be confused with sarcoidosis; but moderately raised levels have been reported in some patients with pulmonary tuberculosis, leprosy, extrinsic allergic alveolitis (hypersensitivity pneumonitis), primary biliary cirrhosis and pneumoconiosis, all of which is some circumstances might be confused with sarcoidosis. In tuberculosis, Silverstein and Friedland reported that 6.5 percent of patients with active and 10.5 percent of those with inactive disease had raised levels, though generally levels were lower than in sarcoidosis (Silverstein and Friedland 1979). Studdy and colleagues found raised levels in 9 percent of those with active tuberculosis (Studdy *et al.* 1978). In some other reports, lower proportions of patients with tuberculosis showed raised levels; but without information about the extent and character of the disease, especially whether it was in an actively granulomatous stage, it is difficult to interpret these findings. Similar considerations apply to the varied reports in leprosy and in chronic beryllium disease, in both of which some have shown a moderate proportion of patients

with raised levels and other levels similar to those in control groups. In one report, serum ACE levels in 22 patients with chronic beryllium disease were similar to those in 84 controls: while those with beryllium disease were mostly longstanding cases, with the duration of symptoms ranging from 5 to 36 years, the duration of illness for the sarcoidosis patients was not stated (Sprince *et al.* 1978).

In Finland, raised ACE levels were found in a significant minority of patients with asbestosis or silicosis (Grönhagen-Riska *et al.* 1979). Of patients with primary biliary cirrhosis, 12 of 57 in London and seven of 14 in Rochester, Minnesota, had elevated levels.

Thus, it is evident that serum ACE levels are of little use in discriminating between sarcoidosis and other diseases in which levels may be raised. However, a high level would favor sarcoidosis in the discrimination of sarcoidosis from diseases in which ACE levels are rarely or never raised; these include Hodgkin's disease, primary lung cancer, chronic lung disease with persistent airflow limitation, and asthma (Studdy and James 1983). Another complicating factor is that levels may be raised in diabetes mellitus: in a cited oral communication, 18 percent of 265 diabetic patients in California were said to have raised levels (Studdy and James 1983).

The value of serum ACE estimations in diagnosis is thus limited and its value as a diagnostic test has diminished (Baughman 2004). In patients whose serum ACE is significantly raised on diagnosis, ACE values (in the absence of steroid therapy) are useful in monitoring the course of sarcoidosis: revised normal ranges corrected for the ACE genotype may be used to improve interpretation. As a diagnostic tool, the measurement of serum ACE levels lacks both sensitivity and specificity (Kruit *et al.* 2007) (see Chapter 17).

Hypercalcuria

Hypercalcuria among patients with sarcoidosis is approximately three times more common than hypercalcemia. It is probably more common in males than females and in London (UK), in Caucasian than in West Indian patients. The urinary excretion rate of calcium is based on the filtered load of calcium when corrected for urinary calcium excretion; the tabular maximum reabsorptive rate for calcium is not increased in sarcoidosis (Broulik *et al.* 1990). These findings suggest that calcitriol has no direct effect on renal calcium handling and that hypercalcuria is due to the flow of calcium from gut and bone (see Chapters 17 and 28).

Enzyme-linked immunospot ('ELISpot') assay

This new assay was developed by Ajit Lalvani (Lalvani *et al.* 2001a,b; Lalvani 2003). The assay detects interferon-γ molecules in the immediate vicinity of the T-cell from which they were secreted, while still at a high concentration. Thus, each spot represents the footprint of an antigen-specific T-cell that secretes interferon-γ (spot-forming cell) (see Chapter 15).

Examinations for mycobacteria and other organisms causing granulomatous inflammation

In patients with pulmonary infiltrations, routine examination for mycobacteria and other organisms by microscopy and culture of sputum (when present) and bronchial secretions (when available) is mandatory. All biopsy material should be similarly examined. Where the differential diagnosis rests between sarcoidosis and caseating tuberculosis, the finding of tubercle bacilli will, of course, support the latter diagnosis, especially if bacilli are repeatedly present. The problem presented by the patient with a syndrome characteristic of sarcoidosis, in association with observation of acid-fast bacilli, or culture of tubercle bacilli on one or a few occasions, is discussed in Chapter 4.

Imaging

In a study of prognosis, Scadding (1961) divided patients into four descriptive groups, according to the radiographic findings at the beginning of the observation period (Fig. 41.1), as follows:

- group 1 – BHL with radiographically clear lungs;
- group 2 – apparently non-fibrotic lung changes with concurrent or previously observed BHL;
- group 3 – apparently non-fibrotic lung changes without BHL either currently or previously observed;
- group 4 – lung changes interpreted as fibrotic.

Grouping of radiographs in this fashion became widely adopted, usually with the groups renamed stages, and with group 2 including only cases with concurrent BHL and lung changes and group 3 consisting of those with lung changes without concurrent BHL, whether or not BHL had been observed previously; often with the addition of a 'stage 0' to designate cases in which the chest radiograph is normal.

The use of the term 'stage' to refer to descriptive groups is unfortunate, since it unjustifiably implies that a numbering 0–4 corresponds to a temporal sequence. Although the sequence of BHL, the appearance of lung infiltration, and the subsidence of BHL with persistence of lung disease occurs in many cases, there are also many important exceptions. Lung infiltration without BHL may be the earliest detected change, occasionally in patients who have had a normal chest radiograph so recently that preceding BHL is unlikely. Rarely, BHL with radiographically clear lungs persists indefinitely and may be accompanied by progressive granulomatous changes in other organs. Likewise, plain radiographic appearances designated 'stage IV' may include, in addition to reticular opacities, appearances suggestive of cavitation, areas of consolidation, calcification or cyst formation (Hours et al. 2008). The advent of high-resolution CT may change perceptions of the relative frequency of these patterns. Nonetheless, the plain radiographic designations of stages II–V provide a convenient 'hat-peg' of reference for descriptive purposes.

Pleural involvement

Pleural involvement, which is not reviewed in other chapters, is covered in greater detail here.

It is probable that some granulomas are present in or immediately under the visceral pleura in most cases of pulmonary sarcoidosis, but symptoms due to pleural involvement are infrequent. Willen and colleagues reviewed lung biopsies from 11 patients with pulmonary sarcoidosis who showed no radiographic evidence of pleural changes and found pleural granulomas in 4 individuals (Willen et al. 1974). Similarly, in lung biopsies from two patients presenting with radiographic abnormalities in the lungs, but with no radiographic evidence of pleural involvement, there was histological evidence of granulomatous changes in pleura as well as lung (Beekman et al. 1976).

Effusions not attributable to some other cause and presumed, or in some cases confirmed by biopsy, to be related to sarcoidosis have been reported in approximately 3–4 percent of most large series of patients with sarcoidosis. Among 150 patients in Los Angeles, of whom 80 percent were black, 6 (all black) had pleural effusion at some time (Sharma and Gordenson 1975). The effusions were small in all cases, and bilateral in two. Open biopsy showed granulomas in the visceral pleura, as well as in lung in one patient; in the others, needle biopsy of the pleura showed only non-specific changes. In all cases, the effusions cleared spontaneously in three and after corticosteroid treatment in three. Two presented with pleural effusions, the others developing at intervals of 4 months to 6 years from the original diagnosis of sarcoidosis. This series was later extended to 250 cases, of whom 12 had effusions at some time (Sharma 1978).

Small pleural effusions accompanying active intrathoracic sarcoidosis, resolving spontaneously or in response to

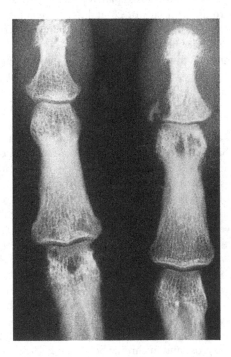

Figure 41.1   Macroradiograph of bone cysts in fingers.

corticosteroid treatment, and showing no evidence of other cause, can be accepted as a manifestation of sarcoidosis, without biopsy confirmation of the presence of granulomas in the pleura. Needle biopsy cannot be relied on, since in the presence of an effusion it produces only a small sample of parietal pleura. A number of reported cases have occurred at an early stage of the disease, with BHL with or without lung changes, often without local symptoms, although sometimes with pain, pleuritic in type, and limited in duration.

In a few cases, large pleural effusions have been a prominent feature. Mikhail and colleagues reported the case of a 37-year-old black man who presented with a large right pleural effusion, and no radiographic evidence of hilar node enlargement. Pleural biopsy showed thickening with

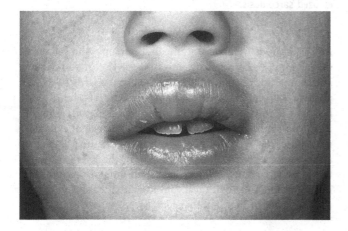

Figure 41.2   Orofacial granulomatosis. Courtesy of Dr John Warner.

non-caseating granulomas. In spite of a negative tuberculin test and failure to demonstrate acid-fast bacilli, antimyco-bacterial treatment was started, together with a short period of corticosteroid treatment (Mikhail *et al.* 1976). The pleural effusion disappeared, but on cessation of corticosteroid therapy it recurred and later a widespread pulmonary infiltration appeared. Mediastinal lymph node biopsy now showed non-caseating granulomas and a Kveim test gave a granulomatous response. Antimycobacterial treatment was stopped and reinstitution of corticosteroid was followed by clearing of the effusion, and diminution of the infiltration.

Pleural thickening in the later stages of pulmonary sarcoidosis cannot be attributed with certainty to sarcoidosis without histological confirmation. Nevertheless, pleural thickening, for which no other cause was evident, was seen in 8 of 227 patients with sarcoidosis; all 8 had chronic and extensive pulmonary sarcoidosis (Willen *et al.* 1974). Biopsies in five of these cases showed fibrotic pleura with interspaced granulomas.

Most of the published reports giving data on the characteristics of effusions have described them as exudates with specific gravities ranging from 4.0 to 6.0 gD; the cells have been predominantly up to 100 percent lymphocytes. Exceptionally, in the series of Willen and colleagues cited above, in six of the eight patients with active sarcoidosis and transient pleural effusions, with biopsies showing parietal granulomas, the effusions had the characteristic of transu-dates with specific gravities between 1.011 and 1.016, and protein contents between 1.3 and 2.3 gD; no cells were found in five and a few lymphocytes in three (Willen *et al.* 1974).

Two reported cases illustrate difficulties that may arise in deciding whether a pleural effusion is to classified as

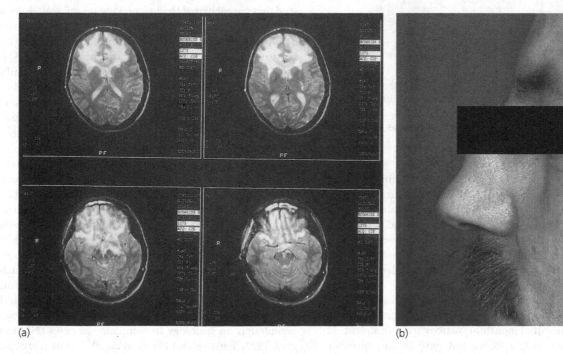

(a)   (b)

Figure 41.3   Nasal involvement with granulomatosis transgressing cribriform plate.

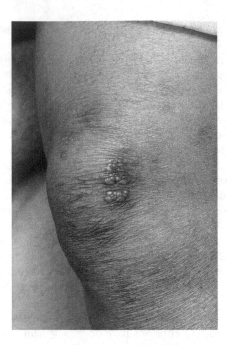

Figure 41.4   Infiltration of skin over knee at site of childhood injury.

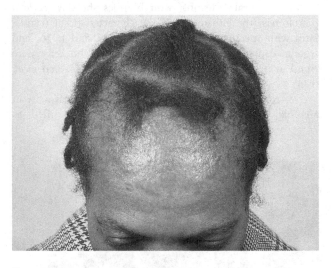

Figure 41.5   Alopecia in West Indian sarcoidosis patient.

associated with sarcoidosis or as due to mycobacterial tuberculosis (Mikhail *et al.* 1970). These occurred in Irish twin brothers aged 21 years shown by blood-group studies to be probably monozygotic, who came to England at the same time, and lived in the same household. One presented with a pleural effusion, biopsy showing epithelioid and giant cell granulomas with some caseation in the pleura; and a tuberculin test with 10 IU was positive – though no mycobacteria could be found on culture of the fluid. The effusion cleared under antimycobacterial treatment for 18 months, with an initial month of corticosteroid treatment. At the end of treatment, a Kveim test gave an unequivocally granulomatous response. The other twin, examined as a contact of his brother, was found to have symptomless BHL.

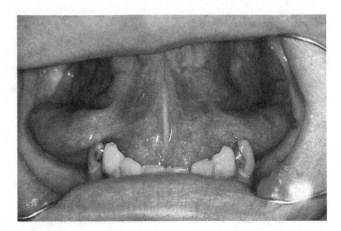

Figure 41.6   Enlarged sublingual glands attributable to generalized sarcoidosis.

A lymph node removed at mediastinoscopy showed confluent granulomas with hyalinization, a Kveim test gave a granulomatous response, and a tuberculin test with 10 IU was positive. On the evidence of the tuberculin tests, both twins had had a mycobacterial infection and both gave granulomatous responses to Kveim tests. On the balance of evidence, most observers would probably categorize the first as having a tuberculous pleural effusion in spite of the Kveim test and the second as showing the typical syndrome of sarcoid BHL in spite of the tuberculin test. But in neither case would it be unreasonable to hold another view (see Chapter 8).

CT scanning

Computerized tomography is better than chest X-ray for studying parenchymal lesions, picking up micronodules and peribronchovascular thickening, and mediastinal lymphadenopathy. It also allows differential diagnosis and more sensitive monitoring of changes in disease severity (Hantous-Zannad *et al.* 2003) (Fig. 41.3). Typical findings include hilar and mediastinal lymphadenopathy, beaded or irregular thickening of the bronchovascular bundles with nodules, ground-glass opacification, parenchymal masses of consolidation, cysts, traction, bronchiectasis and fibrosis with distortion of the lung architecture (Wells 1998).

In patients with advanced pulmonary fibrosis due to sarcoidosis, HRCT imaging is often an important component of the diagnosis, adding usefully to clinical features and chest radiographic findings. In this group of patients, histologic confirmation of the diagnosis is often elusive, with lung biopsy sometimes impracticable in severe disease. Within this difficult patient group, ancillary HRCT features such as non-smoking-related bullae, hilar retraction cephalad, tracheal deviation and 'tenting' of the diaphragm are strongly suggestive of sarcoidosis. Ground-glass attenuation is less diagnostically specific, correlating with peribronchovasular granulomas on histology in some sarcoid cases (Nishimura *et al.* 1993; Teirstein and Norgenthan 2009), but representing fine fibrosis in others. Some of the HRCT features and extent of disease correlate with respiratory functional impairment at

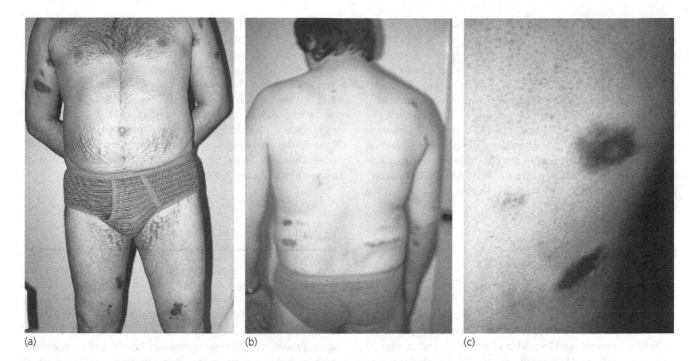

(a)   (b)   (c)

Figure 41.7   Ulcerative granulomatous lesions in patient with sarcoidosis.

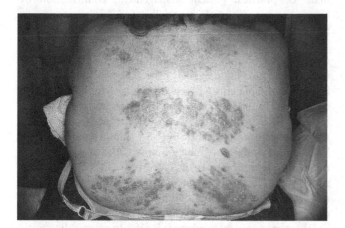

Figure 41.8   Granulomatous lesions over skin of back and forearms, mimicry of psoarisis.

rest and after maximal exercise (Drent *et al.* 2003). Nevertheless, its role in assessing disease activity remains controversial (Hantous-Zannard *et al.* 2003).

Indeed, some experts suggest that CT scanning is indicated only in about one-third of cases presenting to specialist centers – for atypical clinical or radiological appearances, high clinical suspicion with a clear radiograph, presumed complex lung disease (i.e. bronchiectasis, mycetomas, fibrotic complications) or intercurrent infection/malignant concerns (see Chapter 8).

PET scanning

Positive emission tomography using ^{18}F-fluorodeoxyglucose (18F-FDG) identifies two-thirds of patients with known stage

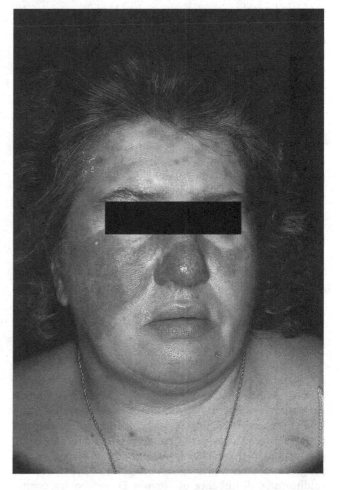

Figure 41.9   Lupus pernio in patient with sarcoidosis. Granulomatous lesions over skin of face, mimicry of psoarisis.

II or III disease. It is poor in picking up activity in stages 0, I and IV, and does not differentiate sarcoidosis from malignancy, as 18F-FDG PET may be positive in both processes. It may play some role in identifying sites of occult granulomas and steroid-reversible disease in stage II and III disease (Teirstein et al. 2007; Teirstein and Norgenthan 2009). However, in a small study (24 sarcoid, 17 lung cancer), the combination of 18F-FDG and 18F-FMT (L-[3-[18F]-methyl-tyrosine) PET scanning allowed differentiation between sarcoidosis and malignancy; sarcoid lesions were positive on 18F-FDG PET, but negative on 18F-FMT PET (both are positive in patients with cancer) (Kaira et al. 2007; see Chapter 9).

Gallium-67 scanning

Scanning after intravenous injection of gallium-67 citrate was introduced for detection of the spread of malignant disease (Edwards and Hayes 1969). Gallium is taken up, not only by malignant tumors, but also by inflammatory processes, including tuberculosis (Lavender et al. 1971) and at sites of active sarcoidosis (McKusick et al. 1973). Heshiki and colleagues found that radiographically normal lungs showed no abnormal uptake, and uptake in the lungs and hila correlated poorly with clinical activity (Heshiki et al. 1974). The diagnostic value of gallium scanning in sarcoidosis is therefore limited; whether or not it allows an accurate assessment of the degree of alveolitic inflammation is also unclear (Beaumont et al. 1982). With the advent of other current investigative procedures, its use in the diagnosis of sarcoidosis has become restricted.

Other radionuclide tracers have been investigated. Technetium-labeled depreotide binds to somatostatin receptors. In a pilot study of 22 patients with sarcoidosis, 18 patients (81 percent) had positive scans, and 4 patients had negative total body scans with normal plain chest radiographs (Shorr et al. 2004; see Chapter 14).

Serum proteins

Serum protein changes are of no diagnostic value in sarcoidosis, though they may reflect the activity of the disease (see Chapter 17).

Serum calcium

Although symptoms caused by abnormal calcium metabolism occasionally lead to the diagnosis of sarcoidosis, routine estimation of the serum calcium level rarely gives diagnostic help in patients who present with other manifestations. In patients with sarcoidosis, the inappropriate endogenous overproduction of the metabolic calcitriol by activated macrophages and granulomas is responsible for hypercalcemia. Additionally, disturbance of vitamin D metabolism contributes to a state of disordered homeostasis (see Chapters 17 and 28).

Radiography of the hands and feet

Changes in the bones of the hands and feet rarely occur without active and generally extensive sarcoidosis (see Fig. 41.1). For this reason, radiography of hands and feet in the search for changes characteristic of sarcoidosis in patients in whom the diagnosis is in doubt is only rarely productive. Even if compatible changes are found, the histological confirmation which is desirable in such cases is preferably sought from a more easily accessible site (see Chapter 32).

CONCLUSION

The diagnosis of sarcoidosis is a statement of belief or knowledge that non-caseating epithelioid cell granulomas, or their hyalinized remnants, are present in a number of affected organs or tissues. This concept is justified in the presence of a combination of clinical, radiological (including HRCT where appropriate) and laboratory findings known to be associated with such changes, supported by a compatible clinical course. However, some clinical presentations are so characteristic that, for practical patient management, confirmation by biopsy is not essential, especially if a benign course is probable.

In doubtful cases, BAL and biopsy are required and, in those with symptoms calling for treatment with corticosteroids, support for the diagnosis from biopsy of suitable tissue is desirable. In patients with enlarged hilar lymph nodes, with or without pulmonary changes, further investigation will include BAL with tissue biopsy, selected from TBNA, endoscopic ultrasound (EUS/EBUS), transbronchial biopsy, VATS or, very rarely, open lung biopsy. Other tests, including tuberculin and ELISpot and measurement of ACE, may support the diagnosis of sarcoidosis in patients with active and extensive disease but are unlikely to be helpful in obscure cases.

There are some cases where it is safer to reserve diagnostic judgment, even though there are granulomatous changes in a single organ or tissue biopsy. Such findings do not establish, though they may suggest, the diagnosis of sarcoidosis. In patients presenting discordant elements in the clinical syndrome, multiple biopsies may be required before the diagnosis can be accepted.

Finally, the need for confirmation by biopsy varies inversely with the confidence with which the clinical syndrome is recognized. This of necessity depends to a large extent on the experience of the clinician.

REFERENCES

Baughman RP (2004). Pulmonary sarcoidosis. Clin Chest Med 25: 521–30.

Baughman RP, Teirstein AS, Judson MA et al. (2001). Clinical characteristics of patients in case control study of sarcoidosis. Am J Respir Crit Care Med 164: 1885–9.

Beaumont D, Herry JY, Sapene M et al. (1982). Gallium-67 in the evaluation of sarcoidosis: correlations with serum angiotensin-converting enzyme and bronchoalveolar lavage. Thorax 37: 11–18.

Beekman JF, Zimmet SM, Chun BK et al. (1976). Spectrum of pleural involvement in sarcoidosis. Arch Intern Med 136: 323–30.

Bilaceroglu S, Perim K, Günel O et al. (1999). Combining transbronchial aspiration with endobronchial and transbronchial biopsy in sarcoidosis. Monaldi Arch Chest Dis 54: 217–23.

British Thoracic and Tuberculosis Association (1969). Geographic variations in the incidence of sarcoidosis in Great Britain; a comparative study of four areas. Tubercle 50: 211–32.

Broulik P, Votava V, Pacovsky V (1990). The tubular maximum for calcium reabsorption in patients with chronic active thoracic sarcoidosis. Eur Respir J 3: 447–9.

Carlens E (1959). Mediastinoscopy: a method for inspection and tissue biopsy in the superior mediastinum. Dis Chest 36: 343–52.

Carlens E (1964). Biopsies in connection with bronchoscopy and mediastinoscopy in sarcoidosis: a comparison. Acta Med Scand 425: s237–8.

Costabel U, Zaiss AW, Juraman T (1992). Sensitivity and specificity of BAL findings in sarcoidosis. Sarcoidosis 9(Suppl. 1): 211–14.

Cushman DW, Cheung HS (1971). Spectrophotometric assay and properties of angiotensin-converting enzyme of rabbit lung. Biochem Pharmacol 20: 1637–48.

De Remee RA, Rohrbach MS (1980). Serum angiotensin-converting enzyme activity in evaluating the clinical course of sarcoidosis. Ann Intern Med 92: 361–5.

Drent M, Jacobs JA, De Vries J et al. (1999). Does the cellular bronchoalveolar lavage fluid profile reflect the severity of sarcoidosis? Eur Respir J 13: 1338–44.

Drent M, Jacobs JA, Cobben NA et al. (2001). Computer program supporting the diagnostic accuracy of cellular BALF analysis: a new release. Respir Med 95: 781–6.

Drent M, De Vries J, Lenters M et al. (2003). Sarcoidosis: assessment of disease severity using HRCT. Eur Radiol 13: 2462–71.

Dunn TL, Watters LC, Hendrix C et al. (1988). Gas exchange at a given degree of volume restriction is different in sarcoidosis and idiopathic pulmonary fibrosis. Am J Med 85: 221–4.

Edwards CL, Hayes RL (1969). Tumor scanning with 67Ga citrate. J Nucl Med 10: 103–5.

Fanberg B, Schoenberger MD, Bachus B, Snider GL (1976). Elevated serum angiotensin converting enzyme in sarcoidosis. Am Rev Respir Dis 114: 525–8.

Fireman E, Gilburd D, Marmor S (2009). Angiogenic cytokines in induced sputum of patients with sarcoidosis. Respirology 14: 117–23.

Garwood S, Judson MA, Silvestri G et al. (2007). Endobronchial ultrasound for the diagnosis of pulmonary sarcoidosis. Chest 132: 1298–304.

Grönhagen-Riska C, Kurppa K, Fyhrquist F, Selroos O (1978). Angiotensin-converting enzyme and lysozyme in silicosis and asbestosis. Scand J Respir Dis 59: 228–31.

Hantous-Zannad S, Charrada L, Zidi A et al. (2003). Value of CT scanning in the investigation of thoracic sarcoidosis. Rev Mal Respir 20: 207–13.

Heerfoodt CT (1909). Ubereine 'febris' uveo-parotidia silbefromica. Graefes Arch Opthalmol 70: 254–73.

Heshiki A, Schutz SL, McKussick KA et al. (1974). Gallium-67 citrate scanning in patients with pulmonary sarcoidosis. Am J Roentgen Radium Ther Nucl Med 122: 744–9.

Hours S, Nunes H, Kambouchner M et al. (2008). Pulmonary cavitory sarcoidosis: clinical-radiologic characteristics and natural history of a rare form of sarcoidosis. Medicine (Baltimore) 87: 142–51.

Hunninghake GW, Costabel U, Ando M et al. (1999). American Thoracic Society/European Thoracic Society/World Association of Sarcoidosis and other Granulomatous Disorders. Statement on sarcoidosis. Sarcoid Vasc Diff Lung Dis 16: 149–73.

Iannuzzi MC, Rybicki BA, Teirstein AS (2007). Sarcoidosis. New Engl J Med 357: 2153–65.

James DG (1961). Erythema nodosum. Br Med J 1: 853–7.

James DG (1976). A world-wide review of sarcoidosis. Am NY Acad Med 278: 321–34.

Joint Statement (1999). American Thoracic Society (ATS), European Respiratory Society (ERS) and World Association of Sarcoidosis and Other Granulomatous Disorders (WASOG). Joint statement. Am J Respir Crit Care Med 160: 736–55.

Judson MA (2008). The diagnosis of sarcoidosis. Clin Chest Med 29: 415–27.

Kaira K, Oriuchi N, Otami Y et al. (2007). Diagnostic usefulness of fluorine-18-alpha-methyltyrosine positron emission tomography in combination with 18F-fluorodeoxyglucose in sarcoidosis patients. Chest 131: 1019–27.

Karetzky M, McDonough M (1996). Exercise and resting pulmonary function in sarcoidosis. Sarcoid Vasc Diff Lung Dis 13: 43–9.

Khan K, Perillie PE, Finch SC (1973). Serum lysozyme in pulmonary tuberculosis. Am J Med Sci 265: 297–302.

Kruit A, Grutters JC, Gerritsen WB et al. (2007). ACE I/D-corrected Z-scores to identify normal and elevated ACE activity in sarcoidosis. Respir Med 101: 510–15.

Lalvani A (2003). Spotting latent infection: the path to better tuberculosis control [editorial]. Thorax 58: 916–18.

Lalvani A, Pathan A, Durkan H et al. (2001a). Enhanced contact tracing and spatial tracking of Mycobacterium tuberculosis infection by enumeration of antigen specific T cells. Lancet 357: 2017–21.

Lalvani A, Pathan A, McShane H et al. (2001b). Rapid detection of Mycobacterium tuberculosis infection by enumeration of antigen-specific T cells. Am J Respir Crit Care Med 163: 824–8.

Lavender JP, Lowe J, Barker JR et al. (1971). Gallium-67 citrate scanning in neoplastic and inflammatory lesions. Br J Radiol 44: 361–6.

Lieberman J (1975). Elevation of serum angiotensin-converting enzyme (ACE) level in sarcoidosis. Am J Med 59: 365–72.

Lieberman J, Nosal A, Schlessner A, Sastre-Foken A (1979). Serum angiotensin-converting enzyme for diagnosis and therapeutic evaluation of sarcoidosis. Am Rev Respir Dis 120: 329–35.

Löfgren S (1946). Erythema nodosum; studies on aetiology and pathogenesis of 185 adult cases. Acta Med Scand 124(Suppl. 174): 1–197.

Löfgren S, Wahlgren F (1949). On the histopathology of erythema nodosum. Acta Derm Venereol 29: 1–13.

Lynch JP, Kazerooni EA, Gay SE (1997). Pulmonary sarcoidosis. Clin Chest Med 18: 755–85.

Macpherson P (1970). A survey of erythema nodosum in a rural community between 1954 and 1968. Tubercle 51: 324–7.

Mandi L (1964). Thoracic sarcoidosis in childhood. Acta Tuberc Pneumol Scand 45: 256–70.

McKusick KA, Soin JS, Ghiladi A, Wagner HN (1973). Gallium-67 accumulation in pulmonary sarcoidosis. J Am Med Assoc 223: 688.

Mikhail JR, Mitchell DN, Druby RA (1970). Identical twins, one presenting with tuberculosis, the other with sarcoidosis. Am Rev Respir Dis 102: 636–40.

Mikhail JR, Lovel D, McGhee KI (1976). Sarcoidosis presenting with a pleural effusion. Tubercle 57: 123–5.

Mikhail JR, Mitchell DN, Sutherland I, McNicol MW (1978). Sarcoidosis presenting in a district general hospital. In: Jones Williams W,

Davies BH (eds). *Proceedings of the 8th International Conference on Sarcoidosis*. Alpha Omega, Cardiff, pp. 532–42.

Mikhail JR, Shepherd M, Mitchell DN (1979). Mediastinal lymph node biopsy in sarcoidosis. *Endoscopy* 11: 5–8.

Nishimura K, Itoh H, Kitaichi M *et al.* (1993). Pulmonary sarcoidosis: correlation of CT and histopathologic findings. *Radiology* 189: 105–9.

Pascual RS, Gee JB, Finch SC (1973). Usefulness of serum lysozyme measurement in diagnosis and evaluation of sarcoidosis. *New Eng J Med* 289: 1074–6.

Reich JM, Brouns MC, O'Connor EA, Edwards MJ (1998). Mediastinoscopy in patients with presumptive stage 1 sarcoidosis: a risk/benefit cost/benefit analysis. *Chest* 113: 147–53.

Scadding JG (1961). Prognosis of intrathoracic sarcoidosis in England. *Br Med J* 2: 1165–72.

Selroos C (1976). Fine needle aspiration biopsy of spleen in diagnosis of sarcoidosis. *Ann NY Acad Sci* 278: 511–20.

Selroos O, Klockars M (1977). Serum lysozyme in sarcoidosis: evaluation of its usefulness in determination of disease activity. *Scand J Respir Dis* 58: 110–16.

Sharma OP (1978). Unusual manifestations of pulmonary sarcoidosis. In: Jones Williams W, Davies BH (eds). *Proceedings of the 8th International Conference on Sarcoidosis*. Alpha Omega, Cardiff, pp. 278–85.

Sharma OP, Gordonson J (1975). Pleural effusion in sarcoidosis; a report of six cases. *Thorax* 30: 95–101.

Shorr AF, Helman DL, Lettieri CJ *et al.* (2004). Depreotide scanning in sarcoidosis: a pilot study. *Chest* 126: 1337–43.

Silverstein E, Friedland J (1979). Serum angiotensin-converting enzyme in sarcoidosis and other diseases. *Lancet* i: 382–3.

Silverstein E, Friedland J, Lyons H, Gourin A (1976). Elevation of angiotensin converting enzyme in granulomatous lymph nodes and serum in sarcoidosis: clinical and possible pathogenic significance. *Ann NY Acad Sci* 278: 498–513.

Sipathi Demirkok S, Basaranoglu M, Dervis E *et al.* (2006). Analysis of 81 patients with Löfgren's syndrome and the pattern of seasonality of subacute sarcoidosis. *Respirology* 11: 456–61.

Siltzbach LE (1958). Clinical conference on sarcoidosis. *J Mt Sinai Hosp* 25: 548.

Spagnolo P, de Bois RM (2007). Genetics of sarcoidosis. *Clin Dermatol* 25: 242–9.

Sprince NL, Kazensi H, Fanberg BL (1978). Serum angiotensin 1 converting enzyme in chronic beryllium disease. In: Jones Williams W, Davies BH (eds). *Proceedings of the 8th International Conference on Sarcoidosis*. Alpha Omega, Cardiff, pp. 287–9.

Studdy PR, James DG (1983). The specificity and sensitivity of serum antiotensin converting enzyme in sarcoidosis and other diseases: experience in twelve centres in six different countries. In: Cretien J, Marsac J, Saltiel JC (eds). *Proceedings of the 9th International Conference on Sarcoidosis*. Permagon Press, Oxford, pp. 332–44.

Studdy PR, Bird R, James FD, Sherlock S (1978). Serum angiotensin-converting enzyme (SACE) in sarcoidosis and other granulomatous disorders. *Lancet* ii: 1331–4.

Teirstein AS, Norgenthan AS (2009). End-stage pulmonary fibrosis in sarcoidosis. *Mt Sinai J Med* 76(1): 30–6.

Teirstein AS, Machac J, Almeida O *et al.* (2007). Results of 188 whole-body fluorodeoxyglucose positron emission tomography scans in 137 patients. *Chest* 132: 1949–53.

Tournoy KG, Bolly A, Aerts JG *et al.* (2010). The value of endoscopic ultrasound after bronchoscopy to diagnose thoracic sarcoidosis. *Eur Respir J* 35: 1329–35.

Trisolini R, Lazzari Agli L, Cancellieri A *et al.* (2003). The value of flexible transbronchial needle aspiration in the diagnosis of stage 1 sarcoidosis. *Chest* 124: 2126–30.

Trisolini R, Tinelli C, Cancellieri A *et al.* (2008). Transbronchial needle aspiration in sarcoidosis: yield and predictors of a positive aspirate. *J Thorac Cardiovas Surg* 135: 837–42.

Turton CW, Grundy E, Firth G *et al.* (1979). Value of measuring serum angiotensin 1 converting enzyme and serum lysozyme in the management of sarcoidosis. *Thorax* 34: 57–62.

Wells A (1998). High resolution comuted tomography in sarcoidosis. *Sarcoid Vasc Diff Lung Dis* 15: 140–6.

Willen SB, Rabinowitz JG, Ulreich S, Lyons HA (1974). Pleural involvement in sarcoidosis. *Am J Med* 57: 200–9.

Winterbauer RH, Belie N, Moores KD (1973). Clinical interpretation of bilateral hilar lymphadenopathy. *Ann Intern Med* 78: 65–71.

Ziegenhagen MW, Rothe ME, Sehlaak M, Muller-Quernheim J (2003). Bronchoalveolar and serological parameters reflecting the severity of sarcoidosis. *Eur Respir J* 21: 407–13.

42

Treatment of sarcoidosis

ATHOL WELLS, SUVEER SINGH, STEPHEN SPIRO AND DONALD MITCHELL

INTRODUCTION

The treatment of sarcoidosis is governed by a number of considerations drawn from clinical experience of the highly variable natural history of the disease. The absence of an identifiable inciting agent, historical observations of effects of various treatments on the clinical course, and similar observations from clinical studies over a number of years, have shaped current recommendations. Current management strategies in individual patients include observation without treatment and a variety of steroid, immunomodulatory and cytotoxic regimens. The wide variety of regimens following initial treatment reflects the highly variable disease, ranging from spontaneous regression of disease activity to ongoing chronic inflammation which, in some but not all cases, precedes and leads to severe fibrosis. The lack of a proven etiological agent has led to a number of pathogenetic hypotheses which, in turn, have given rise to a variety of empirical treatments.

Some agents have been tried in sarcoidosis because of their benefits in other chronic disease processes, although this approach has sometimes been highly speculative, with little true clinical or pathophysiological overlap between the sarcoidosis and other diseases from which therapeutic interventions have been extrapolated. Historical treatments based on microbial etiological hypotheses consisted of agents used to treat leprosy in the 1930s (Lomholt 1934) and tuberculin or antituberculous drugs (Gougerot and Burnier 1935; Irgang 1939). Other therapies have included gold (Bureau *et al.* 1933), vitamin D, radiotherapy (based on a possible analogy with mediastinal lymphoma), potassium, para-aminobenzoic acid (based on early favorable results reported in scleroderma), arsenic, and vitamin C.

THE RATIONALE AND BROAD GOALS OF TREATMENT

The treatment of sarcoidosis is aimed at suppressing the inflammatory response, and reducing the burden of granulomas, based in part on the assumption that there is progression from granulomatous inflammation to chronic fibrotic disease. In the modern era, anti-inflammatory agents are the cornerstone of active therapy. Corticosteroids are generally regarded as first-line treatment, with immunosuppressive agents such as methotrexate and azathioprine introduced in refractory disease. However, no single broad management approach applies to all cases, owing to the highly heterogeneous nature of the disease. Specifically, treatment should not be introduced merely because a diagnosis of sarcoidosis has been made. Furthermore, guideline statements specifying standardized recommendations for all treated patients should be viewed with suspicion. More than in most chronic diseases, the decision to treat sarcoidosis and the choice of therapeutic agent must be tailored to the clinical presentation and observed disease course.

In many patients with self-limiting disease, treatment is not required. This can be readily understood if the primary goals of therapy are considered. The long list of indications for active intervention, specified in many texts, can be subdivided into two broad *reasons to treat*:

- danger from disease;
- unacceptable loss of quality of life.

This essential distinction profoundly influences both the selection of treatment and the way in which decisions are negotiated between the physician and the patient.

However, in a great many cases, the disease poses no immediate danger, either to life or to major organs, and the loss of quality of life resulting from active disease does not, in itself, justify intervention. *In this setting, the correct management approach is therapeutic inaction, coupled with meticulous observation.* The difficulty with this approach is the need to suspend judgment at presentation in many instances and to tailor treatment decisions to the observed evolution of disease.

It should be stressed, however, that treatment decisions made rapidly, based on a perceived need to treat overt disease for its own sake, are often repented at leisure. In particular, if distinctions are not drawn between dangerous disease and disease that should be suppressed solely for symptomatic reasons, treatment goals are difficult to define. Failure to deconstruct the indication(s) for intervention leads to major confusion as to the choice of agent, the indications for second-line therapy, and the timing of the modulation of treatment during follow-up. Lack of clarity as to the broad goals of treatment inevitably communicates itself to the patient, often leading, in turn, to lack of compliance and an early decision to withdraw from follow-up.

Up to one-third of sarcoidosis patients are asymptomatic in most series and do not require treatment unless major organ involvement is detected on investigation (Hunninghake et al. 1994; Rizzato et al. 1998; Nagai et al. 1999). The series with the highest reported use of systemic therapy at presentation (in 67 percent of patients) included mainly African-American subjects, who have an increased tendency to more aggressive disease (Gottlieb et al. 1997). In essence, treatment should be instituted only when it is is clearly required.

This principle can be extrapolated usefully to cases in which an acute presentation, associated with bilateral hilar lymphadenopathy, can reasonably be expected to regress spontaneously in the short term. It is often possible to relieve symptoms resulting from short-term inflammation, such as arthralgia, fever and erythema nodosum, with non-steroidal anti-inflammatory drugs. By this means, the side-effects associated with corticosteroid therapy can be avoided. Even when corticosteroids are required in this setting, because of unacceptable morbidity from active disease, early reductions (over a few months) and, often, withdrawal of treatment are possible in many cases. In classic acute sarcoidosis, active granulomatous inflammation is usually readily suppressed by corticosteroids, although the dose required varies from individual to individual, as does the duration of the active stage of disease. The recrudescence of symptoms as treatment is withdrawn provides an easy means of ascertaining whether longer term treatment is required.

Prognostic evaluation at presentation provides a useful guide as to the likely need for longer term therapy. Among major organ involvements, pulmonary disease is the most frequent indication for prolonged treatment. Neville and colleagues identified the frequency of resolution of chest radiograph changes after 2 years in patients with a wide variety of clinical features (Neville et al. 1983). Factors that portended an increased chance of resolution were (in descending order): erythema nodosum, stage I chest radiographic abnormalities, and ocular involvement. Erythema nodosum (EN) and stage I radiographic findings were associated with complete regression of disease in over 80 and 70 percent of cases, respectively. By contrast, pulmonary disease regressed less frequently with the presence of eye involvement (regression rate of 50 percent) or cardiac involvement (30 percent). The presence of renal calculi denotes a high likelihood of chronic disease (Rizzato and Colombo 1996).

However, it must be stressed that prognostic evaluation at presentation provides only an approximate guide to long-term treatment needs. In important subgroups of patients with 'benign' presentations, major organ involvement may be overt at presentation or may develop during follow-up (Mana et al. 1999). In patients with a less favorable course, granulomatous inflammation may evolve into a more fibrotic, less treatment-responsive course, as seen most often with pulmonary and cutaneous disease. Pulmonary involvement is the most prevalent scenario in which sarcoidosis follows an unfavorable course, leading to progressive functional impairment and, sometimes, to life-threatening disease. Thus, there is no substitute for careful staging of disease at presentation, to identify major organ involvement, followed by a detailed discussion of the loss of quality of life due to active disease.

The deconstruction of the goals of treatment is captured by the following questions which provide a rationale for management.

1. Is there evidence of dangerous organ involvement? If so, there is a need for immediate treatment.
2. If there is no organ-threatening or life-threatening disease, is the patient symptomatic?
3. If so, are symptoms sufficiently severe to require treatment?
4. Can symptoms due to granulomatous inflammation be controlled by non-steroidal anti-inflammatory agents?
5. If corticosteroid therapy seems to be needed to suppress symptoms, does morbidity from active disease exceed the likely morbidity from treatment side-effects?
6. If so, does the patient agree that current symptoms justify a trial of treatment?
7. If not, and it is considered that immediate treatment is not warranted, or the patient declines immediate symptomatic treatment, is it apparent at follow-up that there is progression towards a chronic disease state?

The distinction between dangerous disease and active symptomatic disease, without significant involvement of major organs, lies at the heart of accurate management. It should be recognized that occasionally the distinction is difficult. For example, cutaneous involvement usually falls into the latter category but major skin involvement, likely to lead to disfigurement and the psychological consequences of that, should be viewed as 'dangerous' disease requiring aggressive intervention, irrespective of the level of short-term morbidity. Plainly, a subset of patients lie somewhere between these poles and the same is broadly true of other patterns of organ involvement. However, in most patients, clear distinctions are possible and serve to inform both management and the nature of the discussion between doctor and patient.

CLINICALLY SIGNIFICANT PULMONARY DISEASE: WHEN TREATMENT SHOULD BE INSTITUTED

It has been estimated that sarcoidosis reduces life expectancy in approximately 5 percent of cases. The most frequent causes of death (in descending order) are pulmonary, cardiac, neurological and hepatic disease (Baughman *et al.* 1997; Ferriby *et al.* 2001; Reich 2002), with fatal renal involvement or hypercalcemia less prevalent. In pulmonary disease, indicators of an increasing likelihood of death from respiratory failure include a low vital capacity (of less than 1 liter) (Baughman *et al.* 1997) and the presence of pulmonary hypertension (Judson 1998; Arcosy *et al.* 2001; Shorr *et al.* 2003). In an important additional group of patients, there is danger of disability without, necessarily, a risk to life, as in less advanced pulmonary disease, retinal involvement (with a risk of blindness), some types of neurological involvement, disfiguring cutaneous involvement and major musculoskeletal involvement. In these settings, the need for aggressive therapy is usually evident to the patient; and when this is not obvious, the physician can usually make this case without difficulty. In striking contrast to treatment decisions made solely for reasons of quality of life (discussed later), the rationale for therapy is based on accumulated medical experience as to the likelihood of a poor outcome. Although always important, the wish of a patient to avoid treatment if possible must be overcome by a strong statement of the likely consequences of non-intervention.

The discussion that follows relates predominantly to pulmonary disease. For other forms of life-threatening and organ-threatening disease, the reader is referred to chapters dealing with specific patterns of organ involvement.

From the outset, it must be stressed that the recommendations that follow for pulmonary disease are based more on anecdotal medical experience, accumulated in sarcoidosis clinics around the world, than on formal controlled treatment trials. There are several reasons for this deficiency. By and large, studies of corticosteroid therapy (discussed later) have contained a wide spectrum of disease severity, ranging from relatively mild parenchymal involvement to end-stage disease. In treatment studies, it has not been possible to distinguish between predominantly inflammatory disease, in which regression of disease is a logical treatment goal, and fibrotic disease, in which disease regression is an unrealistic aim with current treatments, but stabilization of disease and the prevention of progression may be achievable. With the advent of high-resolution computed tomography (HRCT), the striking variation in morphological abnormalities in pulmonary sarcoidosis has been highlighted: the major distinction between widespread nodular disease, representing intense granulomatous inflammation, and predominantly reticular disease, representing irreversible fibrotic disease, is not always well captured. However, no definitive study of treatment has been based on HRCT appearances and, for the most part, distinctions have been drawn from radiographic staging. In a minority of cases with clear-cut stage IV radiographic appearances, disease is overtly predominantly fibrotic but no formal comparison has been made, confined to these cases, to establish whether treatment prevents disease progression. In stage II and, especially, in stage III disease, the relative proportion of inflammatory and fibrotic disease is highly heterogeneous. Until a clear distinction has been drawn in treatment studies between these disease subsets, with a clear separation in the goals of treatment between achieving disease regression and achieving disease stabilization, recommendations on treatment will continue to be tailored to individual patients, rather than applied inflexibly by protocol.

The definition of the primary end-points in treatment studies in pulmonary sarcoidosis is a further difficult problem. It is generally accepted, in interstitial lung disease, that pulmonary function tests better reflect the intensity of the underlying histopathological process than chest radiography or symptoms (Keogh and Crystal 1980). However, the morphological heterogeneity of sarcoidosis is mirrored by a striking variation in the pattern of pulmonary function impairment. Distinct patient subgroups exist with patterns of airflow obstruction, lung restriction, mixed ventilatory defects and disproportionate reduction in gas transfer (which may represent either diffuse – rather than airway-centered – disease or pulmonary vascular involvement). Broad statements of the average changes in individual pulmonary function indices, designated as primary end-points, fail to address this issue. In essence, uncritical statements of mean changes in pulmonary function indices in treatment studies can be regarded as 'meaningless mean' statements, when it comes to treatment decisions in individual patients.

It is sometimes argued that, although treatment of sarcoidosis may result in short-term gains, it has not been established that the natural history of sarcoidosis is improved in the longer term. However, while this conclusion may be correct with reference to relatively short-term treatment trials, it does not address the possibility that gains during treatment may be preserved by longer term low-dose maintenance therapy. Once again, the distinction between suppression of active inflammatory disease and the prevention of progression of fibrotic disease is a crucial confounder. Moreover, as discussed later, a suspicion exists that many patients included in treatment trials did not necessarily require treatment on a case-by-case basis, whether because of a high likelihood of spontaneous regression of disease in a significant subset, or because disease was fibrotic but not progressive. In these subgroups, treatment would not be expected to influence the natural course of disease but their inclusion in treatment studies necessarily obscures important treatment benefits in a minority of cases.

One highly influential treatment study was performed by the British Thoracic Society (Gibson *et al.* 1996). In this evaluation of asymptomatic pulmonary sarcoidosis (with definite parenchymal involvement), continuous corticosteroid therapy in pulmonary sarcoidosis was compared to an empirical approach, in which intermittent courses of corticosteroids were introduced during follow-up if the disease course appeared to warrant intervention (in 19 percent of cases). At the end of the study period of 18 months, outcome differences favoring continuous treatment were seen in some end-points, including breathlessness, vital capacity and carbon monoxide diffusing capacity (DLco) pulmonary function. In another placebo-controlled study, evaluating a regimen of 3 months of corticosteroids, followed by 15 months of inhaled corticosteroid therapy, active treatment was associated with significantly higher DLco levels and a favorable radiographic course at the end of the treatment period in patients with stage II radiographic abnormalities (but not in patients with stage 1 disease). Moreover, a higher frequency of deterioration requiring oral corticosteroid therapy was seen in the placebo group during 5 years of follow-up.

The average treatment effect on pulmonary function variables was small in both studies, although statistically significant; but for the reasons discussed above, it is likely that these mean statements represented important treatment benefits in a subgroup of patients, diluted by a non-benefit in patients with spontaneous disease remission or stable fibrotic disease.

The view that treatment studies do not properly capture treatment benefits is widely accepted in the international community and accounts for the existence of recommended approaches in selecting patients for treatment and in treatment regimens, in the absence of a definitive evidence base for these statements. The challenge to the clinician, in the absence of such an evidence base, lies in identifying the subset of patients in whom treatment benefits are likely to be major. Indications for treatment, stated in a great many texts, can be summarized as follows:

- worsening pulmonary symptoms, including breathlessness, cough, chest pain and hemoptysis;
- severe pulmonary function impairment or deterioration in pulmonary function indices (Box 42.1);
- evidence of significant progression on chest radiography, such as the development of cavities or honeycombing, major worsening of interstitial opacities, or evidence of pulmonary hypertension.

However, it should be stressed that none of the above indications can be applied in all cases in a formulaic fashion. Cough and chest pain are highly non-specific and, when due to sarcoidosis, are not necessarily associated with clinically significant interstitial lung disease. Hemoptysis is infrequent in sarcoidosis, in the absence of co-existent infection. Increasing exertional dyspnea is the most reliable pulmonary

symptomatic indication for treatment. However, pulmonary hypertension is present in approximately half of sarcoidosis patients with chronic exercise intolerance (Baughman et al. 2006b), with important therapeutic implications (see Chapter 20); and in other cases, exertional dyspnea is not due to cardiopulmonary limitation. Similarly, although treatment is warranted when pulmonary function impairment is severe, no exact validated severity threshold exists that can be used in isolation as a basis for treatment decisions. The significance of serial pulmonary function and chest radiographic trends is difficult to interpret when functional impairment is mild. Thus, decisions on treatment require the integration of the indications listed above in an assessment of the overall clinical significance of disease. In many cases, judgment on the need for treatment must be suspended in the short-term, with re-evaluation of disease at 3- to 6-monthly intervals (Box 42.2).

A common difficulty is the presence of persistent, moderately extensive parenchymal infiltrates in an asymptomatic patient with mild pulmonary function impairment. In the absence of evident disease progression, there are currently no data that guide the clinician on whether treatment is warranted. Some clinicians argue that disease that is stable but persistent for 12 months merits treatment, in the hope of switching off 'disease activity' and preventing evolution to chronic non-responsive fibrotic disease. Others advocate continued observation in view of the likelihood of adverse effects and lack of evidence of long-term benefits from treatment. As the cases for and against intervention are finely balanced in this scenario, it is appropriate to discuss the uncertainties with the patient, as strong patient preferences should influence the decision in marginal situations.

Box 42.2 Deferment of therapy on pulmonary grounds

Immediate therapy on pulmonary grounds is not indicated in the following groups:

- asymptomatic patients with stage I radiographic abnormalities (bilateral hilar lymphadenopathy alone);
- patients with stage II radiographic abnormalities and mildly abnormal lung function which does not progress at 6–12 months (50% of patients will have radiographic resolution at 3 years);
- patients with stage III radiographic abnormalities and mildly abnormal lung function not progressing at 6 months (one-third of patients will have disease resolution at 5 years, although a majority may still require treatment at some stage during follow-up).

Box 42.1 Pulmonary function deterioration

Pulmonary function deterioration is assessed by serial evaluation at 3- to 6-monthly intervals, with significant decline defined as a reduction in forced vital capacity of over 10% or a reduction in DLco of over 15% from baseline values – see Chapter 10.

TREATMENT ON SYMPTOMATIC GROUNDS

The indications for treatment on quality-of-life grounds, in the absence of major organ involvement, are difficult to quantify and must be adapted to the individual patient. Disabling fatigue, arthralgia, severe night sweats and other symptoms may be unrelenting, with devastating consequences in daily life, despite the absence of a dangerous complication. Persistent lower-grade symptoms, although not severe enough to require treatment in the short term, are also an important cause of disability. It should be emphasized that treatment is needed for unacceptable loss of quality of life as often as for major organ involvement.

However, the whole treatment approach differs radically from that used in dangerous sarcoidosis. No single laboratory parameter quantifies the overall impact of the disease on quality of life, so treatment decisions are highly subjective. The level of morbidity associated with fatigue, for example, is known only to the patient. Thus, it is necessary for the patient and physician, in partnership, to weigh the morbidity of disease (defined by the patient) against the likely morbidity of treatment (defined by the physician), with a frank appraisal of the anticipated side-effects of corticosteroid and immunosuppressive agents. It is essential that the patient be empowered with regard to treatment decisions made for quality-of-life reasons. Ideally, the final decision on whether to start treatment should be made by the patient, guided by the physician, in contrast to treatment decisions taken in relation to major organ involvement.

Similarly, a flexible approach is required, with input from the patient, as to the choice, dose and duration of treatment. As discussed below, high-dose corticosteroid therapy is usual as initial treatment for major organ involvement. By contrast, based on patient choice, low-dose treatment is often warranted (e.g. prednisolone 15 mg daily) with a comparison of symptoms with and without treatment, and adjustment of the dose accordingly. The essential conundrum, in the selection of therapy for impaired quality of life, is whether treatment results in a net symptomatic benefit or increases morbidity as a result of treatment side-effects. An understanding of this dilemma provides a rational basis for patients to accept or decline treatment and to adjust corticosteroid dosages to find the best balance of disease morbidity and treatment side-effects.

The problem of fatigue poses particular management difficulties. Fatigue is highly prevalent in active sarcoidosis and is often disabling. However, it is often dismissed, by family members and medical practitioners alike, as a psychological phenomenon, especially when not associated with objective evidence of ongoing disease activity. There is sometimes no option but to determine whether fatigue is abolished by the institution of treatment and it is often useful to begin with an intermediate corticosteroid dose (e.g. prednisolone 25 mg daily for 4 weeks), rather than low-dose therapy, in order to establish definitively whether treatment is helpful. In the longer term, the primary goal is to identify, by gradual dose reduction, the minimum dose that meets the needs of the patient. This aim is helped greatly if a marker of disease activity (such as the serum ACE level or inflammatory indices) can be identified. Chronic depression, an alternative common cause of fatigue in sarcoidosis, is an important confounding factor and should be suspected and discussed with the patient before the institution of therapy, and especially when fatigue is not helped by treatment.

SECOND-LINE THERAPIES: INDICATIONS AND CHOICE OF AGENT

Alternative treatments to corticosteroid therapy, discussed below, may be required as steroid sparing agents or because an additional treatment effect is required. Second-line agents may be categorized as immunosuppressive, cytotoxic antimalarial and other drugs. Specific agents include methotrexate, azathioprine, cyclophosphamide, mycophenolate mofetil, chloroquine and its analog hydroxychloroquine, ciclosporin, pentoxifylline, and monoclonal antibodies against tumor necrosis factor, such as infliximab.

The decision to introduce a second-line agent is often far from straightforward, as the side-effects from immunosuppressive agents are usually greater than seen with long-term low-dose corticosteroid treatment (e.g. prednisolone 10 mg daily). In life-threatening disease and when there is severe organ involvement, it is often obvious that a second-line treatment will be required and the early introduction of azathioprine or methotrexate is warranted. However, the decision is more often marginal and it is appropriate to delay the introduction of other agents until the minimum dose of corticosteroid meeting the needs of the patient has been established. As a general rule of thumb, the introduction of a steroid sparing agent is likely to increase morbidity with no therapeutic gain if disease is well controlled in the longer term by a dose of prednisolone of 10 mg daily or lower, although it should be stressed that evidence of an increased predilection to corticosteroid side-effects in individual patients should be taken into account. By contrast, if higher long-term corticosteroid doses are required to control unacceptable disease morbidity, or to prevent disease relapse in major organs, the introduction of a second-line agent is amply justified.

The choice of agent is critically dependent on the corticosteroid dose required to control disease. If it is considered that a relatively minor steroid sparing effect is required (e.g. to allow a reduction in prednisolone dosage from 15 to 10 mg daily), hydroxychloroquine is usually well tolerated and has the major advantages of safety and the lack of need for blood-test monitoring. On average, the treatment effect of hydroxychloroquine equates to a prednisolone dose of 5–7.5 mg daily, but in occasional patients the effect is considerably greater and may hold the key to long-term management.

When a greater treatment effect is required, the initial choice generally lies between methotrexate and azathioprine. No controlled comparison exists between these agents; but the overall clinical consensus, based on accumulated worldwide experience, is that methotrexate is, on average, more efficacious. However, when a second-line agent is introduced, it is essential to stress to the patient that side-effects are unpredictable and will sometimes dictate an early change to an alternative agent.

CORTICOSTEROID THERAPY

Owing to their ability to suppress the inflammatory response, glucocorticoids remain the mainstay of treatment for sarcoidosis. Their current role is justified both by symptom relief and by their control of disability as a result of systemic involvement (Sharma 1993; du Bois 1994). Following the earliest reported success of cortisone for sarcoidosis (Siltzbach 1952), there were a number of further uncontrolled studies confirming the efficacy of corticosteroids in partially or completely suppressing the extrathoracic manifestations of disease (James *et al.* 1967; Young *et al.* 1970; Hapke and Meek 1971; Israel *et al.* 1973; Mikami *et al.* 1974; Selroos and Sellergen 1979; Eule *et al.* 1980; Yamamoto *et al.* 1983), reducing the size of enlarged lymph nodes, and diminishing or clearing radiographic infiltrates in the majority of cases.

These early reports were followed by a number of controlled studies of corticosteroid therapy in pulmonary sarcoidosis in which short-term benefits were not sustained after the cessation of treatment. Regimens compared with randomly selected or matched control groups – with observation for the same time periods – included:

- prednisolone 15 mg/day for 6 months (Hapke and Meek 1971);
- high-dose prednisolone (starting at 60 mg/day) for at least 6 months (Young *et al.* 1970);
- prednisolone 15 mg/day for 3 months (Israel *et al.* 1973);
- prednisolone 30 mg/day initially, with subsequent dosage reduction for 6 months (Mikami *et al.* 1974);
- methylprednisolone (24–32 mg/day for 2 weeks, with subsequent dosage reduction) for 7 months (Selroos and Sellergen 1979);
- prednisolone 40 mg/day initially, with reduction to 10–15 mg/day for either 6 or 12 months (Eule *et al.* 1980).

In all these studies, with variable entry criteria, radiographic and/or pulmonary function variables improved during the period of treatment, but these differences were not sustained 1 to 15 years later. There were similar findings in the only longer term study (which included a large subgroup with stage I disease), in which treatment consisted of prednisolone 60 mg on alternate days initially, gradually reducing to 5 mg on alternate days over 18 months (Yamamoto *et al.* 1983).

These findings have caused some physicians to adopt a nihilistic approach to the treatment of pulmonary sarcoidosis in general, without due consideration of the benefits of therapy in an important subgroup of cases (Paramothayan and Jones 2002; Paramothayan *et al.* 2005). Treatment was not selectively studied in patients meeting criteria for the institution of treatment discussed earlier. Symptomatic patients tended to receive treatment and were largely excluded. In large patient subgroups, therapy would not now be instituted (bilateral hilar lymphadenopathy without pulmonary infiltration on chest radiography, inactive burnt-out disease, mild or transient pulmonary disease with stage II or III chest radiographic appearances). In such patients, no lasting 'treatment benefit' was ever likely at long-term follow-up. Moreover, in those patients in whom treatment would now be widely used, the duration of treatment was inappropriately brief.

Taken together, these studies do, at least, show conclusively that a worthwhile long-term treatment benefit in appropriate cases will not generally be achieved if treatment is withdrawn completely after 6–12 months, as the active stage of disease usually persists for much longer in severe disease, although usually burning out eventually. Moreover, the accumulated evidence effectively rebuts a policy of routine treatment in all patients with pulmonary sarcoidosis. However, the broad conclusion often drawn – that corticosteroid therapy does not alter the natural course of disease in the long term – is essentially flawed. The alternative view, drawn from widespread clinical experience, and supported by subsequent studies (as discussed earlier), is that longer term treatment is required in selected patients with dosage reduction tailored in individual cases to evidence of relapse. The underlying goal of longer term intervention is to protect the lungs from progressive fibrotic damage as long as disease remains active, while identifying the minimum dose that meets this aim, with the use of second-line therapy if the side-effects of steroid monotherapy are unacceptable or if the required maintenance corticosteroid dose is high. This principle also applies to patients with progressive predominantly fibrotic disease.

Inhaled glucocorticoids have been suggested for the treatment of pulmonary sarcoidosis (Arcosy *et al.* 2001). The use of inhaled budesonide was more efficacious than placebo in maintenance treatment in two studies (Zych *et al.* 1993; Alberts *et al.* 1995), but had no effect on outcomes in open (du Bois *et al.* 1999) and blinded (Milnam *et al.* 1994) placebo-controlled randomized studies. Overall, there are no adequate data supporting the efficacy of inhaled therapy in unselected patients (Paramothayan and Jones 2002; Paramothayan *et al.* 2005). However, some clinicians argue for this approach when there is prominent cough, evidence of bronchial hyper-reactivity, early pulmonary disease associated with mild symptoms, and as an alternative to oral prednisolone in those requiring long-term low-dose prednisolone (5–10 mg). Commonly used inhaled steroids have included budesonide (800–1600 µg twice daily), triamcinolone, and fluticasone.

Glucocorticoids alter the action of B- and T-lymphocytes, which play important roles in pathogenesis of sarcoidosis. Glucocorticoids bind to their receptors within the cytoplasm causing heat shock proteins to dissociate. Reconfiguration leads to the steroid receptor complex entering the nucleus, binding to responsive elements on the gene, resulting in modulation of gene transcription (du Bois 1994). Inactivation of nuclear factor kappa B (NFκB) prevents synthesis of tumor necrosis factor alpha (TNF-α), granulocyte stimulating factor (GMSCF), and interferon-1 and -6. All these effects are thought to be important in the attenuation of the inflammatory process of sarcoidosis.

Since the optimal dose of glucocorticoids is not known, the principles guiding the choice of dose require balance of (a) the likelihood of response with risk of adverse effects (Sharma 1993; du Bois 1994; Paramothayan and Jones 2002), and (b) the minimum necessary dose for optimal benefit in those with steroid responsiveness (Judson 1999). Six phases of corticosteroid therapy have been suggested:

- the initial dose;
- tapering regimen to maintenance;
- the maintenance dose;
- tapering-off regimen;
- the observation period;
- the relapse dosing regimen.

One such recommended regimen is:

- For the first 4–6 weeks, give a daily dose of between 0.5 and 1 mg/kg ideal bodyweight (approximately 13–16 mg/day).
- On re-evaluation, identified improvement or stability should enable tapering by 5–10 mg decrements every 4–8 weeks, down to 0.25–0.5 mg/kg (usually 15–30 mg/day).
- If stability or improvement continues, a maintenance dose of 10–15 mg/day, for 6–9 months, is usual, with a tapering regimen thereafter, so enabling a treatment period of approximately 12 months.

The maintenance period requires a longer duration in patients sustaining symptomatic relapses such as cough, breathlessness and chest pain, usually managed by shorter course of higher doses (10–20 mg above the maintenance dose for up to 4 weeks) and a return to an adequate maintenance dose.

Alternate-day corticosteroid therapy treatment has been suggested. One such regimen is: a starting dose of 40 mg per alternate day for 3 months, followed by dose-tapering by 10 mg per alternate day every 3 months, and continued for at least one year to achieve remission, followed by withdrawal thereafter. Another approach is alternate-day therapy following initial daily therapy with prednisolone. The rationale behind alternate-day therapy is the belief that it may reduce side-effects, as seen with daily therapy above 10 mg/day for over a year (Baughman et al. 2003a). However, no controlled comparisons exist to justify this approach, as opposed to more traditional regimens (Deremee 1995).

High-dose oral corticosteroid therapy (80–100 mg/day) or pulsed intravenous methylprednisolone (e.g. 750 mg weekly for up to 8 weeks with prednisolone 20 mg daily on intervening days) is recommended in those with cardiac, neurological, retinal/optic nerve or severe upper airways disease, followed by dosage reduction and maintenance therapy when disease activity is controlled. These organ-specific regimens are discussed further elsewhere (see Chapters 19, 21 and 27).

There is no controlled evidence to suggest that long-term corticosteroid therapy is detrimental to the natural course of disease, although this concern has been expressed (Izumi 1994). In a non-randomized study of 37 patients, a higher relapse rate was observed when remission has been induced by corticosteroids than in patients with spontaneous remission (24 vs 20 percent; Gottlieb et al. 1997), leading to speculation that rebound exacerbations might occur on withdrawal of treatment. However, this observation is likely to reflect the fact that patients receiving treatment have, on average, greater disease activity.

OTHER SPECIFIC PHARMACOLOGICAL TREATMENTS

Deflazacort

It has been claimed that deflazacort has fewer adverse effects, especially on bone mineral content, than prednisolone, based on a prospective comparison of deflazacort and prednisolone in patients with histologically confirmed sarcoidosis needing long-term corticosteroid therapy (Rizzato et al. 1997). Overall, 69 patients completed one year, 59 two years, 46 three years and 24 four years of treatment. Six atraumatic fractures occurred in the prednisolone-treated group but only one in those receiving deflazacort. Two patients among those receiving deflazacort and eight among those receiving prednisolone required corrective measures for bone loss or bone pain. Deflazacort and prednsiolone were similar in efficacy.

Methotrexate

The antifolate metabolite, methotrexate, has both immuno-suppressant and anti- inflammatory properties and is widely used in the management of chronic inflammatory or autoimmune disorders such as rheumatoid arthritis, cirrhosis and severe resistant asthma.

Methotrexate was first reported as a treatment of sarcoidosis in 1968 (Lacher 1968) and was initially used as a very short-term treatment, often for less than 6 months, because of concerns about hepatotoxicity. Although no large studies have established that methotrexate is superior to other immunosuppressive therapies, a large amount of accumulated experience in individual cases and in small case series has established its efficacy in patients with pulmonary and extrapulmonary disease (Fenton et al. 1985; Lower and Baughman 1990,1995; Suda et al. 1994; Henderson et al. 1994). Methotrexate has been beneficial in cutaneous lesions (Baughman and Lower 2007; Webster et al. 1991), pulmonary disease (Baughman and Lower 1999), arthritis (Gedalia et al. 1997), ophthalmic manifestations (Dev et al. 1999; Bradley et al. 2002), and neurosarcoidosis (Agbogu et al. 1995; Lower et al. 1997). Methotrexate also has a role as a steroid sparing agent in acute sarcoidosis, as demonstrated in a double-blind randomized studies (Baughman et al. 2000). Overall, methotrexate has been beneficial in half to two-thirds of patients, even in refractory disease (Lower and Baughman 1990; Baughman et al. 2000) and is now widely viewed as the second-line agent of first choice.

Methotrexate is usually administered orally at weekly intervals, although occasionally it is given intramuscularly. In most regimens, an initial dose of 7.5 mg weekly is increased by 2.5 mg every 2–4 weeks, usually to 15 mg per week. However, in refractory disease, doses as high as 20 mg or 25 mg per week may be required and treatment for 6 months may be needed, in order to demonstrate a benefit, as with other immunosuppressive agents. For this reason, an initial treatment period of 4–6 months is usually appropriate, before efficacy is evaluated (Baughman and Lower 1997b).

Methotrexate has both acute and chronic adverse effects. Acute toxicities, which include gastrointestinal (GI) side-effects and mucositis, tend to be dose-related, often respond to dose reduction, and are minimized by the use of folic acid, at 5 mg once a week or 1 mg daily (Morgan et al. 1994), recommended in patients receiving a methotrexate dose of over 10 mg per week.

Methotrexate is cleared by the kidneys and is contra-indicated in patients with significant renal impairment. An early drug-induced hepatitis may occur and blood dyscrasia is a very rare side-effect. Liver function tests and a full blood count should be monitored weekly as the dose of methotrexate is gradually increased, with monthly monitoring, once the long-term dose has been instituted (Baughman et al. 2003b).

The major chronic toxicities of methotrexate occur in the lungs and the liver. Methotrexate-induced interstitial lung disease was first reported in patients with rheumatoid lung and appears to be much more prevalent in that context than in sarcoidosis or psoriasis. As in rheumatoid arthritis, methotrexate lung is sometimes indistinguishable from pulmonary disease progression due to the underlying disease. Pulmonary toxicity from methotrexate may occur at any dose, although seen more often in association with higher cumulative doses (White et al. 1989; Zisman et al. 2001). In idiosyncratic toxicity, developing within days of starting treatment, cough and dyspnea are often associated with systemic symptoms, including generalized malaise, fever and arthralgia. A peripheral eosinophilia, present in approximately 50 percent of cases, is a useful pointer to methotrexate toxicity. Other occasional features include hilar lymphadenopathy, pleural effusions and poorly formed granulomas on lung biopsy (White et al. 1989; Zisman et al. 2001). However, methotrexate toxicity may also develop insidiously, with symptoms confined to non-productive cough or exertional dyspnea. Pulmonary side-effects are often wholly reversible on withdrawal of methotrexate (White et al. 1989). However, severe pulmonary toxicity should be treated with high-dose corticosteroid therapy and may result in residual pulmonary fibrotic abnormalities.

Hepatotoxicity usually takes the form of a reversible hepatitis, often associated with systemic symptoms. However, hepatotoxicity may also be clinically silent, necessitating regular liver function tests. Some groups advocate liver biopsies when the total dose exceeds 1 g or after 18 months of regular therapy, even in the absence of signs of hepatic injury (Baughman et al. 2003a), but other groups confine monitoring to regular blood tests, with the performance of a liver biopsy or discontinuation of methotrexate if there is a persistent elevation of transaminases (Vicunic 2002). Baughman and colleagues identified methotrexate-associated changes at biopsy in 14 of 68 patients, with sarcoid-related abnormalities present in 47 cases: 10 percent of patients eventually developed hepatotoxicity if treated for more than 2 years (Baughman et al. 2003b), although irreversible liver damage was not seen.

In practice, the distinction between methotrexate hepatotoxicity and hepatic sarcoidosis seldom causes major difficulty if liver function tests are normal when methotrexate is introduced, as liver function test abnormalities due to methotrexate usually normalize with cessation of therapy. However, the use of methotrexate in patients with pre-existing hepatic sarcoidosis is problematic, as liver toxicity from methotrexate is more difficult to detect.

Azathioprine

Azathioprine, a purine analog, is converted to 6-mercaptopurine, which acts by arresting RNA and DNA synthesis. Thiopurine S-methyl transferase (TMTP) enzymatically deactivates 6-mercaptopurine, with azathioprine-related toxicity occurring in patients with genetic polymorphisms of TMTP: some groups measure TMTP levels before starting treatment. Azathioprine is often used to treat the fibrotic idiopathic interstitial pneumonias and other interstitial lung diseases (Demedts et al. 2005), perhaps explaining its widespread use in sarcoidosis.

As with other immunosuppressive agents, the evidence-based literature supporting the use of azathioprine in sarcoidosis is very limited. In a number of small series, limited success has been reported in the short-term control of disease (Pachecho et al. 1985; Agbogu et al. 1995; Muller-Quernheim et al. 1999), with response rates of less than 20 percent in two reports (Lewis et al. 1999; Mosam and Morar 2004). However, these observations are likely to reflect the selective use of azathioprine in longer standing disease which is often fibrotic and irreversible. The prevention of progression may be a more realistic goal in this context, with azathioprine essentially acting as a steroid sparing agent: in one series, disease remission or stabilization was achieved with azathioprine use in 19 of 35 patients (Baughman and Lower 1997a).

Azathioprine is usually given 2–2.5 mg/kg (up to 200 mg/day), as a single morning dose. It is initiated incrementally, usually starting at 50 mg/day for 2–4 weeks, increasing by 25–50 mg every 2–4 weeks until the required dose is reached.

The most frequent short-term side-effects are systemic symptoms (malaise, lethargy, fever), gastrointestinal (most commonly nausea, vomiting and a drug-induced hepatitis) and hematological suppression. During the initiation of therapy, a full blood count and liver function tests should be performed at weekly intervals as early hepatotoxicity is occasionally encountered and there are rare reports of profound neutropenia, due to homozygous TMPT deficiency. Hepatotoxicity and marrow suppression may also occur with longer term use, but neutropenia due to TMPT deficiency will occur only shortly after the introduction of azathioprine; therefore, blood tests can be monitored at 6-weekly intervals once the target dose is achieved. Azathioprine may have teratogenic effects and so must be used with caution in woman of child-bearing age. In a small subset of patients, recurrent infection is a major problem.

In general, although side-effects are very seldom dangerous, azathioprine is often poorly tolerated with approximately 20–25 percent of patients unable to remain on the drug in some series.

Azathioprine has probably been the most widely used second-line agent after methotrexate. Although no direct comparison has been made, accumulated experience suggests that methotrexate has a better benefit/toxicity ratio in the majority of patients. However, the lesser hepatotoxicity of azathioprine is sometimes a major advantage. Most practitioners reserve azathioprine for patients unable to tolerate methotrexate and, especially, when there is active hepatic sarcoidosis (Kennedy *et al.* 2006) or long-term usage of methotrexate has caused concerns about liver toxicity.

Cyclophosphamide

Cyclophosphamide is relatively infrequently used as a steroid sparing agent but has been successful in patients with neurological disease and in other 'rescue' situations (Demeter 1988; Lower *et al.* 1997; Doty *et al.* 2003). Cyclophosphamide is an alkalizing agent that is metabolized by the hepatic system into aldophosphamide, oxidized to the active metabolite carboxyphoshphamide. Some aldophosphamide is converted to phoshoramide mustard and acrolein, which are toxic to the bladder epithelium. Cyclophosphamide is lymphocytotoxic and, possibly, anti-inflammatory at the doses used. In contrast to other autoimmune diseases such as Wegener's granulomatosis and systemic lupus erythematosus, where episodic intravenous doses are given to reduce the overall toxicity, it is generally given as an oral single daily dose of 25–50 mg in sarcoidosis, increasing over weeks to maintain a white cell count between 4000 and 7000/mm^2. A total daily dose of 150 mg/day is usually the maximum used. It is recommended that there should be adequate oral fluid hydration, with monthly monitoring of urine for red cells. Patients should be informed of the risk of hemorrhagic cystitis, bladder cancer and teratogenicity.

Intravenous pulsed therapy in refractory disease may require single doses of 500–1000 mg for over 30 to 60 minutes every 2–4 weeks. Treatment is recommended for at least 3–6 months to assess a response. In addition the usual recommendations are adequate oral fluid hydration and monthly monitoring of urine for red cells.

Leflunomide

Leflunomide was developed as an analog of methotrexate with significantly less toxicity and, especially, with little or no lung toxicity. Leflunomide was efficacious in 25 of 32 sarcoidosis patients (78 percent) in one report (Baughman and Lower 2004), including 12 of 15 patients treated with both methotrexate and leflunomide. Leflunomide was well tolerated with only 3 of 32 patients (9 percent) discontinuing treatment because of GI toxicity. Leflunomide and methotrexate are similarly efficacious in rheumatoid arthritis (Emery *et al.* 2000) and, as their mechanisms of action differ, there is a biochemical basis for the use of both drugs in a combined regimen in refractory disease (Kremer 1999) – although that approach has yet to be evaluated formally in sarcoidosis.

Ciclosporin

Ciclosporin A may be used in the treatment of sarcoidosis at a dose of 5–7 mg/kg for several months along with conventional doses of oral prednisolone in a tapered regimen (York *et al.* 1990). Unfortunately, an elevation of the mean serum creatinine concentration is often noted after 3–6 months of treatment, and there is a considerable risk of infection among patients receiving this drug. Its use in sarcoidosis has been largely confined to small series of patients with optic neuropathy (Bielory and Frohman 1991) and chronic sarcoidosis (York *et al.* 1990). In a study from the National Institutes of Health, ciclosporin suppressed the spontaneous release of interleukin-2 and monocyte chemotactic factor by T-cells from patients with active sarcoidosis *in vitro*, but did not reduce the percentage of activated T-cells or improve pulmonary function tests in treated patients (Martinet *et al.* 1988), suggesting that this agent was unlikely to be generally effective. Similarly, in a comparison between prednisolone therapy and prednisolone in combination with ciclosporin, combination therapy conferred no additional short- or long-term therapeutic benefit (over prednisolone alone) and was associated with significantly more side-effects (Wyser 1997). Thus, although ciclosporin has been used successfully in a patient with severe pulmonary sarcoidosis unresponsive to corticosteroid therapy (O'Callaghan *et al.* 1991), there is no current basis for its routine use.

Chlorambucil

Chlorambucil, an alkylating agent, has been used as a steroid sparing agent in sarcoidosis. However, although short-term responses were observed in 8 of 10 treated patients with progressive pulmonary or systemic disease, longer term follow-up in that series did not demonstrate a curative effect and one patient with severe neurosarcoidosis died from the disease (Kataria 1980). As chlorambucil is associated with an increased risk of myeloproliferative malignancies, there is no current basis for its routine use.

Chloroquine and hydroxychloroquine

These drugs were used historically in the treatment of malaria. They have been used in sarcoidosis for many years as steroid sparing agents and have had particular utility in the treatment of cutaneous disease (Zic *et al.* 1991). In an early report of the use of chloroquine in cutaneous sarcoidosis, a daily dose of 500 mg for 6 months produced greater beneficial changes in cutaneous disease than in pulmonary sarcoidosis (Morse *et al.* 1961) – an observation that was supported by subsequent accumulated experience (Stilzbach and Tierslein 1964; British Tuberculosis Association 1967; Johns *et al.* 1983; Baltzan *et al.* 1999).

In 43 patients treated with 500 mg daily for between 4 and 17 months, hilar lymphadenopathy regressed in 11 of 14 cases (with 6 relapses), pulmonary infiltration improved in 20 of 29 cases (with 5 relapses), and cutaneous sarcoidosis improved in 14 of 14 cases (with 5 relapses) (Stilzbach and Tierstein 1964). The British Tuberculosis Association conducted a controlled study in pulmonary sarcoidosis, in which subjects were randomly allocated to chloroquine 600 mg/day for 8 weeks and 400 mg/day for a further 8 weeks. Improvements in dyspnea, ventilatory function and radiological appearances were apparent at 6 months in the treated group, but were not sustained, when compared with the control group, 8 months after the end of the treatment period (British Tuberculosis Association 1967). In a randomized trial, 23 patients with pulmonary sarcoidosis completed 6 months of chloroquine therapy followed by randomization to maintenance treatment with chloroquine or observation. The group receiving maintenance therapy demonstrated statistically significant benefits improvement in FEV_1 levels and the prevalence of relapse at 20 months of follow-up (Baltzan et al. 1999).

These data suggest that, as with corticosteroid therapy, chloroquine and hydroxychloroquine have short-term therapeutic benefits that are lost with the early cessation of treatment. Thus, these agents should be introduced with a view to longer term treatment. Fortunately, both agents are often effective when used at relatively low doses for cutaneous sarcoidosis (i.e. hydroxychloroquine 200 mg/day; Jones and Callen 1990), with avoidance of gastrointestinal side-effects in most cases. Hydroxychloroquine tends to be preferred as it has fewer GI side-effects than chloroquine. The observation of reversible corneal changes and irreversible retinopathy stimulated initial recommendations that there should be regular ophthalmic review before and during treatment. Subsequently, the Royal College of Ophthalmologists in the UK endorsed increases in the dosage of hydroxychloroquine to 400 mg daily but recommended that the integrity of the visual fields should be monitored at regular intervals, as a safeguard against the development of retinal toxicity. However, retinal toxicity is extraordinarily rare with the use of low-dose therapy (Sharma 1996).

Melatonin

Melatonin was reported to be efficacious in two patients with chronic sarcoidosis that was unresponsive to long-term corticosteroid therapy (Cagnoni et al. 1995). After treatment with melatonin 20 mg/day, tapering to 10 mg/day over 6 months to a year, resolution of symptoms, pulmonary disease and skin lesions was noted. In one case, resurgence of disease responded to treatment for a further 3 months, with no side-effects observed. Subsequently, open therapy with melatonin was instituted in 18 patients with chronic sarcoidosis that was refractory to other treatments, and improvements were noted in pulmonary and systemic markers of active disease (Pignone et al. 2006). These findings must be interpreted with caution in the absence of a control group, given the regression of disease activity with time in many cases. However, melatonin is an extremely safe treatment and this justifies its occasional empirical usage in refractory disease, pending further controlled evaluation.

Ketoconazole

The antifungal drug ketoconazole, a known inhibitor of cytochrome P450 steroid oxidase, lowers circulating calcitriol and serum calcium levels (Adams et al. 1990; Ejaz et al. 1994). Sarcoidosis patients receiving ketoconazole should avoid

sunlight, curtail major dietary sources of vitamin D and calcium, and ensure a high intake of fluids. The occasional use of this drug in the authors' sarcoidosis clinic has been helpful in controlling hypercalcemia that was otherwise severe and refractory to other treatments (see Chapter 28). A dose of 100 mg daily is often efficacious, but there is a risk of profound hypocalcemia with higher doses (e.g. 200 mg/day). Thus, meticulous clinical and laboratory monitoring are required.

Tetracycline analogs

Minocycline and doxycycline have both been helpful in the treatment of cutaneous sarcoidosis (Bachelez et al. 2001). Their mode of action is not understood. It is relevant that tetracyclines are bactericidal for Propionibacterium acnes, which has been the subject of considerable interest as a possibly etiological agent in sarcoidosis (Eishi et al. 2002; see also Chapter 30).

IMMUNOMODULATORY AGENTS

Pentoxifylline

As a suppressor of cytokine release by alveolar macrophages, pentoxyfylline may be more effective against tumor necrosis factor (TNF) than other drugs known to suppress TNF release, such as thalidomide (Marques et al. 1999; Tong et al. 2003). Uncontrolled data suggest some efficacy in the treatment of patients with active sarcoidosis (Zabel et al. 1987; Baughman and Iannuzzi 2003). However, further controlled data are required before this agent can be integrated into the routine treatment of chronic active sarcoidosis.

Thalidomide

Thalidomide has been efficacious in cutaneous sarcoidosis (Carlesimo et al. 1995; Baughman et al. 2002b; Oliver et al. 2002; Nguyen et al. 2004), and has been used to treat other manifestations of chronic disease, including lupus pernio (Lee and Koblenzer 1998). In one study, cutaneous sarcoidosis responded in all 14 patients to 200 mg daily, with 12 of 14 responding to 100 mg daily, without significant adverse effects (Baughman et al. 2002b). However, thalidomide appears to be relatively ineffective in non-cutaneous disease in most patients, perhaps because most toxicities (hypersomnolence, rashes, constipation) are dose-dependent and occur at the doses required for control of systemic disease. Furthermore, a sensory peripheral neuropathy is frequently experienced at doses required to suppress active cutaneous disease. Thalidomide is absolutely contraindicated in pregnancy as teratogenicity can occur at any dose.

Thalidomide is known to suppress TNF release by alveolar macrophages (Tavares et al. 1997; Ye et al. 2006). However, no changes in TNF levels were seen in skin biopsies before and after treatment, in a study in which skin lesions improved (Oliver *et al.* 2002). Thus, it appears that other pathogenetic pathways are modulated by treatment, in keeping with the observation of drug effects on a number of cytokines involved in sarcoidosis inflammation (Oliver *et al.* 2002; Ye *et al.* 2006).

Anti-TNF therapy

Anti-TNF therapy has recently been explored as a third-line treatment in refractory sarcoidosis. Early studies established that treatment effects are much more likely with infliximab than with etanercept, which offered no benefit in a placebo-controlled study of the treatment of chronic ocular sarcoidosis (Baughman *et al.* 2002a) and was ineffective in most patients with pulmonary sarcoidosis in another clinical trial (Utz *et al.* 2003). The efficacy of infliximab may result from its action as an antibody, whereas etanercept is a TNF receptor antagonist: infliximab may produce cellular apoptosis (Van den Brande 2003) whereas etanercept may act as a partial antagonist, with binding on cell surfaces leading to the release of TNF.

The benefits of inflixiamb were first reported in small numbers of sarcoidosis patients with cutaneous, pulmonary, ocular and neurological disease (Yee and Pochapin 2001; Baughman and Lower 2001; Petersen *et al.* 2002; Roberts *et al.* 2003). It has become clearer with increasing experience that the likelihood of a response to infliximab is unpredictable in both pulmonary and extrapulmonary disease. In the only moderately large placebo-controlled evaluation of infliximab in pulmonary sarcoidosis, a statistically significant treatment benefit was seen on the forced vital capacity but the amplitude of the effect was low – a 4 percent effect in favor of active therapy (Baughman *et al.* 2006a).

Although the clinical significance of this treatment effect has been questioned, it can also be argued that the biases inherent in the selection of patients for placebo-controlled studies must inevitably reduce treatment effects. Enrolment in placebo-controlled studies, as opposed to open therapy, tends to be reserved for patients with less severe and less progressive disease, especially when the therapy on trial is also available as open therapy for patients with more aggressive disease, as in the infliximab study of Baughman and colleagues (2006a). If a therapy acts, at least in part, to prevent disease progression, it is less likely to be demonstrably beneficial in the subset of patients with non-progressive disease, and the amplitude of any treatment effect must necessarily be low. Moreover, in a population of patients with milder disease, more striking responses in a minority of outlying patients will be diluted to a low average treatment effect, which can be seen as a 'meaningless mean value'.

Based on these considerations and the striking effects reported in some patients, infliximab therapy cannot currently be recommended as routine treatment in sarcoidosis, but should be reserved as a speculative therapy, which might or might not radically improve the outcome in individual patients with aggressive disease when routine therapies are ineffective. Exactly the same conclusions apply to extrapulmonary disease. Judson and colleagues evaluated the likelihood of regression of extrapulmonary involvement, in patients enrolled in the placebo-controlled trial of infliximab therapy in pulmonary sarcoidosis (Judson *et al.* 2008). As with pulmonary disease, a statistically significant treatment effect in favor of infliximab was observed; but once again, the clinical significance of the effect was difficult to interpret. The evaluation of an extrapulmonary treatment effect was a post-hoc analysis, with the ad-hoc construction of a multisystem end-point in which dangerous end-organ involvement and minor extrapulmonary manifestations were grouped together indiscriminately.

A critical view of current evidence for the early use of infliximab therapy is important, both because of its uncertain efficacy in individual patients, and because of the potential seriousness of adverse effects. The increase in active tuberculosis and other infections with infliximab is now well established (Keane *et al.* 2001; Kroesen *et al.* 2003). Furthermore, allergic reactions have been reported with infliximab and with other anti-TNF therapies, with infliximab reported to cause severe anaphylaxis. The duration of a beneficial effect from infliximab remains uncertain, as follow-up remains short. It appears that beneficial effects, if any, are generally evident within 6 months of the initiation of therapy, allowing an early decision to be made on the rationale for longer term treatment.

However, given all these uncertainties, it would seem that a well-defined role for anti-TNF therapy is still some way from definition. This does create difficulties for clinicians that are greater than with any other sarcoidosis treatment. Funding for expensive therapies is often impossible to obtain in the absence of a definitive evidence base, but barriers to funding do effectively disenfranchise patients with unusually aggressive disease, in whom an intervention may be life-saving. The current evidence does at least allow clinicians to argue strongly for infliximab in dangerous refractory sarcoidosis but further studies are urgently required.

NON-PHARMACOLOGICAL THERAPIES

Radiotherapy

Radiotherapy has been administered empirically for various general manifestations of sarcoidosis (Florangi 1910; Jackson 1925) but there is no current evidence that it has any beneficial effect (Donlan 1938), other than in neurosarcoidosis.

There are several reports of the treatment of refractory neurosarcoidosis with cranial irradiation (Rubenstein *et al.* 1988; Menninger *et al.* 2003; Bruns *et al.* 2004). Although evidence-based recommendations cannot be provided, radiation therapy may be considered as a treatment of last resort in patients suffering from life-threatening neurosarcoidosis refractory to medical therapy.

Organ transplantation

Transplantation of either a single lung, both lungs or heart and lungs for end-stage sarcoidosis is now an accepted form of treatment. Transplantation assessment should not be delayed until disease is end-stage and the patient is physically too debilitated to undergo the procedure. The 5-year survival rates in sarcoidosis patients undergoing transplantation are broadly comparable to those seen in other pulmonary disorders. Transplantation is discussed in detail in Chapter 44.

REFERENCES

Adams JS, Sharma OP, Diz MM, Endres DB (1990). Ketoconazole decreases the serum 1,25-dihydroxyvitamin D and calcium concentration in sarcoid-associated hypercalcaemia. *J Clin Endocrin Metab* 70: 1090–5.

Agbogu BN, Stern BJ, Sewell C, Yang G (1995). Therapeutic considerations in patients with refractory neurosarcoidosis. *Arch ·Neurol* 52: 875–9.

Alberts C, van der Mark TW, Jansen HM; Dutch Study Group on Pulmonary Sarcoidosis (1995). Inhaled budesonide in pulmonary sarcoidosis: a double-blind, placebo-controlled study. *Eur Respir J* 8: 682.

Arcosy SM, Christie JD, Pochettino A *et al.* (2001). Characteristics and outcomes of patients with sarcoidosis listed for lung transplantation. *Chest* 120: 873–80.

Bachelez H, Senet P, Cadranel J *et al.* (2001). The use of tetracyclines for the treatment of sarcoidosis. *Arch Dermatol* 137: 69–73.

Baltzan M, Mehta S, Kirkham TH, Cosio MG (1999). Randomized trial of prolonged chloroquine therapy in advanced pulmonary sarcoidosis. *Am J Respir Crit Care Med* 160: 192–7.

Baughman RP, Iannuzzi M (2003). Tumour necrosis factor in sarcoidosis and its potential for targeted therapy. *BioDrugs* 17: 425–31.

Baughman RP, Lower EE (1997a). Steroid-sparing alternative treatments for sarcoidosis. *Clin Chest Med* 18: 853–64.

Baughman RP, Lower EE (1997b). Alternatives to corticosteroids in the treatment of sarcoidosis. *Sarcoid Vasc Diff Lung Dis* 14: 121–30.

Baughman RP, Lower EE (1999). A clinical approach to the use of methotrexate for sarcoidosis. *Thorax* 54: 742–6.

Baughman RP, Lower EE (2001). Infliximab for refractory sarcoidosis. *Sarcoid Vasc Diff Lung Dis* 18: 70–4.

Baughman RP, Lower EE (2004). Leflunomide for chronic sarcoidosis. *Sarcoid Vasc Diff Lung Dis* 21: 43–8.

Baughman RP, Lower EE (2007). Evidence-based therapy for cutaneous sarcoidosis. *Clin Dermatol* 25: 334–40.

Baughman RP, Winget DB, Bowen EH, Lower EE (1997). Predicting respiratory failure in sarcoidosis patients. *Sarcoidosis Vasc Diffuse Lung Dis* 14: 154–8.

Baughman RP, Winget DB, Lower EE (2000). Methotrexate is steroid sparing in acute sarcoidosis: results of a double blind, randomized trial. *Sarcoid Vasc Diff Lung Dis* 17: 60–6.

Baughman RP, Bradley DA, Raymond LA *et al.* (2002a). Double-blind randomized trial of a tumor necrosis factor recpetor antagonist (etanercept) for treatment of chronic ocular sarcoidosis. *Am J Respir Crit Care Med* 165: A495.

Baughman RP, Judson MA, Teirstein AS *et al.* (2002b). Thalidomide for chronic sarcoidosis. *Chest* 122: 227–32.

Baughman RP, Lower EE, du Bois RM (2003a). Sarcoidosis. *Lancet* 36̇1: 1111–18.

Baughman RP, Koehler A, Bejarano PA *et al.* (2003b). Role of liver function tests in detecting methotrexate-induced liver damage in sarcoidosis. *Arch Intern Med* 163: 615–20.

Baughman RP, Drent M, Kavuru M *et al.* (2006a). Infliximab therapy in patients with chronic sarcoidosis and pulmonary involvement. *Am J Respir Crit Care Med* 174: 795–802.

Baughman RP, Engel PJ, Meyer CA *et al.* (2006b). Pulmonary hypertension in sarcoidosis. *Sarcoid Vasc Diff Lung Dis* 23: 108–16.

Bielory L, Frohman LP (1991). Low-dose cyclosporine therapy of granulomatous optic neuropathy and orbitopathy. *Ophthalmology* 98: 1732–6.

Bradley DA, Baughman RP, Raymond L, Kaufman AH (2002). Ocular manifestations of sarcoidosis. *Semin Respir Crit Care Med* 23: 543–8.

British Tuberculosis Association (1967). Chloroquine in the treatment of sarcoidosis: a report. *Tubercle* 48: 257–72.

Bruns F, Pruemer B, Haverkamp U, Fischedick AR (2004). Neurosarcoidosis: an unusual indication for radiotherapy. *Br J Radiol* 77: 777–9.

Bureau Y, Picard R, Barrire H (1933). Ichthyosis acquire et maladee de Hodgkin. *Arch Dermatol Syphilol* 27: 231–4.

Cagnoni ML, Lombardi A, Cerinic MC *et al.* (1995). Melatonin for treatment of chronic refractory sarcoidosis. *Lancet* 346: 1229–30.

Carlesimo M, Giustini S, Rossi A *et al.* (1995). Treatment of cutaneous and pulmonary sarcoidosis with thalidomide. *J Am Acad Derrmatol* 32: 866–9.

Demedts M, Behr J, Buhl R *et al.* (2005). High-dose acetylcysteine in idiopathic pulmonary fibrosis. *New Engl J Med* 353: 2229–42.

Demeter SL (1988). Myocardial sarcoidosis unresponsive to steroids: treatment with cyclophosphamide. *Chest* 94: 202–3.

Deremee RA (1995). Sarcoidosis. *Mayo Clin Proc* 70: 177–81.

Dev S, Macallum RM, Jaffe GJ (1999). Methotrexate for sarcoid-associated panuveitis. *Ophthalmology* 106: 111–18.

Donlan CP (1938). X-ray therapy of Boeck's sarcoid. *Radiology* 51: 237–40.

Doty JD, Mazur JE, Judson MA (2003). Treatment of corticosteroid-resistant neurosarcoidosis with a short-course cyclophosphamide regimen. *Chest* 124: 2023–6.

du Bois RM (1994). Corticosteroids in sarcoidosis: friend or foe? *Eur Respir J* 7: 1203–9.

du Bois RM, Greenhalgh PM, Southcott AM *et al.* (1999). Randomized trial of inhaled fluticasone propionate in chronic stable pulmonary sarcoidosis: a pilot study. *Eur Respir J* 13: 1345–50.

Eishi Y, Suga M, Ishige I *et al.* (2002). Quantitative analysis of mycobacterial and propionibacterial DNA in lymph nodes of Japanese and European patients with sarcoidosis. *J Clin Microbiol* 40: 198–204.

Ejaz AA, Zabaneh RI, Tiwari P *et al.* (1994). Ketoconazole in the treatment of recurrent nephrolithiasis associated with sarcoidosis. *Nephrol Dial Transplant* 9: 1492–4.

Emery P, Breedveld FC, Lemmel EM *et al.* (2000). A comparison of the efficacy and safety of leflunomide and methotrexate for the treatment of rheumatoid arthritis. *Rheumatology* (Oxford) 39: 655–65.

Eule H, Roth I, Weide W (1980). Clinical and functional results of a controlled clinical trial of the value of prednisolone therapy in sarcoidosis. In: Jones Williams W, Davies BH (eds). *Proceedings of the International Conference on Sarcoidosis*. Cardiff, Alpha Omega, pp. 624–31.

Fenton DA, Shaw M, Black MM (1985). Invasive nasal sarcoidosis treated with methotrexate. *Clin Exp Dermatol* 10: 279–83.

Ferriby D, de Seze J, Stojkovic T *et al.* (2001). Long-term follow-up of neurosarcoidosis. *Neurology* 57: 927–9.

Florangi A (1910). Uber einmen Fall von Lupus pernio und seine Reaktion auf Rotgenbestrahlung. *Dermatol* 17: 558–64.

Gedalia A, Molina JF, Ellis GS et al. (1997). Low-dose methotrexate therapy for childhood sarcoidosis. J Pediatr 130: 25–9.

Gibson GJ, Prescott RJ, Muers MF et al. (1996). British Thoracic Society sarcoidosis study: effects of long-term corticosteroid therapy. Thorax 51: 238–47.

Gougerot and Burnier 1935. Traitement local par les sels d'or d'un lupus erythemateux delaface: résultat esthétique éloigné excellent. Bull Soc Franc Dermat 42: 906.

Gottlieb JE, Israel HL, Steiner RM et al. (1997). Outcome in sarcoidosis: the relationship of relapse to corticosteroid therapy. Chest 111: 623–31.

Hapke EJ, Meek JC (1971). Steroid treatment in pulmonary sarcoidosis. In: Levinsky L, Macholda F (eds). Proceedings of the 5th International Conference on Sarcoidosis. Universita Karlova, Prague, pp. 621–5.

Henderson CA, Ilchyshyn A, Curry AR (1994). Laryngeal and cutaneous sarcoidosis treated with methotrexate. J R Soc Med 87: 632–3.

Hunninghake GW, Gilbert S, Pueringer R et al. (1994). Outcome of the treatment for Sarcoidosis. Am J Respir Crit Care Med 149: 893–8.

Irgang S (1939). Sarcoid of Boeck: report of a case of generalized cutaneous distribution and pulmonary involvement with clinical cure with tuberculin. Arch Derm Syphilol 40: 35–44.

Izumi T (1994). Are corticosteroids harmful to sarcoidosis? Sarcoidosis 11(Suppl. 1): 119.

Israel HF, Fouts DW, Beggs RA (1973). A controlled trial of prednisone treatment of sarcoidosis. Am Rev Respir Dis 107: 609–14.

Jackson BH (1925). Use of X-ray in uveoparotitis. Ann Opthalmol 8: 361.

James DG, Carstairs LS, Trowell J, Sharma OP (1967). Treatment of sarcoidosis: report of a therapeutic trial. Lancet ii: 526–8.

Johns CJ, Zachary JB, Macgregor MI et al. (1983). The longitudinal study of chronic sarcoidosis. Trans Am Clin Climatol Assoc 94: 173–81.

Jones E, Callen JP (1990). Hydroxychloroquine is effective therapy for the control of cutaneous sarcoid granulomas. J Am Acad Dermatol 23: 487–9.

Judson MA (1998). Lung transplantation for pulmonary sarcoidosis. Eur Respir J 11: 738–44.

Judson MA (1999). An approach to the treatment of pulmonary sarcoidosis with corticosteroids. Chest 115: 1158–65.

Judson MA, Baughman RP, Costabel U et al. (2008). Efficacy of infliximab in extrapulmonary sarcoidosis: results from a randomised trial. Eur Respir J 31: 1189–96.

Kataria Y (1980). Chlorambucil in sarcoidosis. Chest 78: 36–43.

Keane J, Gershon S, Wise RP et al. (2001). Tuberculosis associated with infliximab, a tumor necrosis factor-alpha neutralizing agent. New Engl J Med 345: 1098–104.

Keogh BA, Crystal RG (1980). Pulmonary function testing in interstitial pulmonary disease. What does it tell us? Chest 78: 856–64.

Kennedy PT, Zakaria N, Modawi SB et al. (2006). Natural history of hepatic sarcoidosis and its response to treatment. Eur J Gastroenterol Hepatol 18: 721–6.

Kremer JM (1999). Methotrexate and leflunomide: biochemical basis for combination therapy in the treatment of rheumatoid arthritis. Semin Arthritis Rheum 29: 14–26.

Kroesen S, Widmer AF, Tyndall A et al. (2003). Serious bacterial infection in patients with rheumatoid arthritis under anti-TNF-alpha therapy. Rheumatology (Oxford) 42: 617–21.

Lacher MJ (1968). Spontaneous remission or response to methotrexate in sarcoidosis. Ann Intern Med 69: 1247–8.

Lee JB, Koblenzer PS (1998). Disfiguring cutaneous manifestation of sarcoidosis treated with thalidomide: a case report. J Am Acad Dermatol 39: 835–8.

Lewis SJ, Ainslie GM, Bateman ED (1999). Efficacy of azathioprine as second-line treatment in pulmonary sarcoidosis. Sarcoid Vasc Diff Lung Dis 16: 87–92.

Lomholt S (1934). Douze cas de sarcoides de Boeck traites a l'antileprol. Bull Soc Franc Dermatol Syph 41: 1354.

Lower EE, Baughman RP (1990). The use of low dose methotrexate in refractory sarcoidosis. Am J Med Sci 299: 153–7.

Lower EE, Baughman RP (1995). Prolonged use of methotrexate for sarcoidosis. Arch Intern Med 155: 846–51.

Lower EE, Broderick JP, Brott TG, Baughman RP (1997). Diagnosis and management of neurologic sarcoidosis. Arch Intern Med 157: 1864–8.

Mana J, Gomez VC, Montero A et al. (1999). Löfgren's syndrome revisited: a study of 186 patients. Am J Med 107: 240–55.

Marques LJ, Zheng L, Poulakis N et al. (1999). Pentoxifylline inhibits TNF-alpha production from human alveolar macrophages. Am J Respir Crit Care Med 159: 508–11.

Martinet Y, Pinkston P, Saltini C et al. (1988). Evaluation of the in-vitro and in-vivo effects of cyclosporine on the lung T-lymphocyte alveolitis of active pulmonary sarcoidosis. Am Rev Respir Dis 138: 1242–8.

Menninger MD, Amdur RJ, Marcus RB (2003). Role of radiotherapy in the treatment of neurosarcoidosis. Am J Clin Oncol 26: E115–18.

Mikami R, Hitagi Y, Iwai K et al. (1974). A double-blind controlled trial on the ffect of corticosteroid therapy in sarcoidosis. In: Iwai K, Hosoda Y (eds). Proceedings of the International Conference on Sarcoidosis. University of Tokyo Press, Tokyo, pp. 533–8.

Milnam N, Graudal N, Grode G et al. (1994). No effect of high dose inhaled steroids in pulmonary sarcoidosis: a double-blind placebo-controlled study. J Intern Med 236: 285–90.

Morgan SL, Baggot JE, Vaughn WH et al. (1994). Supplementation with folic acid during methotrexate therapy for rheumatoid arthritis. Ann Intern Med 121: 833–41.

Morse Si, Cohn ZA, Hirsch JG, Schaeder RW (1961). The treatment of sarcoidosis with chloroquine. Am J Med 30: 779–84.

Mosam A, Morar N (2004). Recalcitrant cutaneous sarcoidosis: an evidence-based approach. J Dermatolog Treat 15: 353–9.

Muller-Quernheim J, Kienast K, Held M et al. (1999). Treatment of chronic sarcoidosis with an azathioprine/prednisolone regimen. Eur Respir J 14: 1117–22.

Nagai S, Shigematsu M, Hamada K et al. (1999). Clinical courses and prognoses of pulmonary sarcoidosis. Curr Opin Pulm Med 5: 293–8.

Neville E, Walker AN, James DG (1983). Prognostic factors predicting the outcome of sarcoidosis; an analysis of 818 patients. Q J Med 208: 525–33.

Nguyen YT, Dupuy A, Cordoliani F et al. (2004). Treatment of cutaneous sarcoidosis with thalidomide. J Am Acad Dermatol 50: 235–41.

O'Callaghan CA, Wells AU, Lalvani A et al. (1991). Effective use of cyclosporin in sarcoidosis: a treatment strategy based on computed tomography scanning. Eur Respir J 7: 2255–6.

Oliver SJ, Kikuchi T, Krueger J et al. (2002). Thalidomide induces granuloma differentiation in sarcoid skin lesions associated with disease improvement. Clin Immunol 102: 225–36.

Pachecho Y, Marechal C, Marechal F et al. (1985). Azathioprine treatment of chronic pulmonary sarcoidosis. Sarcoidosis 2: 107–13.

Paramothayan S, Jones PW (2002). Corticosteroid therapy in pulmonary sarcoidosis: a systematic review. J Am Med Assoc 287: 1301–7.

Paramothayan NS, Lasserson TJ, Jones PW (2005). Corticosteroids for pulmonary sarcoidosis. Cochrane Database Systemaic Review, CD001114.14,15.

Petersen JA, Zochodne DW, Bell RB et al. (2002). Refractory neurosarcoidosis responding to infliximab. Neurology 59: 1660–1.

Pignone AM, Ross AD, Fiori G et al. (2006). Melatonin is a safe and effective treatment for chronic pulmonary and extrapulmonary sarcoidosis. J Pineal Res 41: 95–100.

Reich JM (2002). Mortality of intrathoracic sarcoidosis in referral vs population-based settings: influence of stage, ethnicity, and corticosteroid therapy. Chest 121: 32–9.

Rizzato G, Colombo P (1996). Nephrolithiasis as a presenting feature of chronic sarcoidosis: a prospective study. Sarcoidosis 13: 167–72.

Rizzato G, Riboldi A, Imbimbo B et al. (1997). The long-term efficacy and safety of two different corticosteroids in chronic sarcoidosis. Respir Med 91: 449–60.

Rizzato G, Montemurro L, Colombo P (1998). The late follow up of chronic sarcoid patients previously treated with corticosteroids. Sarcoidosis 15: 52–8.

Roberts SD, Wilkes DS, Burgett RA et al. (2003). Refractory sarcoidosis responding to infliximab. Chest 124: 2028–31.

Rubenstein I, Gray TA, Moldofsky H, Hoffstein V (1988). Neurosarcoidosis associated with hypersomnolence treated with corticosteroids and brain irradiation. Chest 94: 205–6.

Selroos O, Sellergen T-L (1979). Corticosteroid therapy of pulmonary sarcoidosis: a prospective evaluation of alternate day and daily dosage in stage II disease. Scand J Respir Dis 60: 215–21.

Sharma OP (1993). Pulmonary sarcoidosis and corticosteroids. Am Rev Respir Dis 147: 1598–600.

Sharma OP (1996). Vitamin D, calcium and sarcoidosis. Chest 109: 535–9.

Shorr AF, Davies DB, Nathan SD (2003). Predicting mortality in patients with sarcoidosis awaiting lung transplantation. Chest 124: 922–8.

Siltzbach LE (1952). Effects of cortisone in sarcoidosis: a study of thirteen patients. Am J Med 2: 139–60.

Stilzbach LE, Tierstein AS (1964). Chloroquine therapy in 43 patients with intrathoracic and cutaneous sarcoidosis. Acta Med Scand 425: 302–6s.

Suda T, Sato A, Toyoshima M et al. (1994). Weekly low-dose methotrexate therapy for sarcoidosis. Intern Med 33: 437–40.

Tavares JL, Wangoo A, Dilworth P et al. (1997). Thalidomide reduces tumour necrosis factor-alpha production by human alveolar macrophages. Respir Med 91: 31–9.

Tong Z, Dai H, Chen B, Abdoh Z et al. (2003). Inhibition of cytokine release from alveolar macrophages in pulmonary sarcoidosis: comparison with dexamethasone. Chest 124: 1526–32.

Utz JP, Limper AH, Kalra S et al. (2003). Etanercept for the treatment of stage II and stage III progressive pulmonary sarcoidosis. Chest 124: 177–85.

Van den Brande JM, Braat H, van den Brink GR et al. (2003). Infliximab but not etanercept induces apoptosis in lamina propria T-lymphocytes from patients with Crohn's disease. Gastroenterology 124: 1774–85.

Vucinic VM (2002). What is the future of methotrexate in sarcoidosis? A study and review. Curr Opin Pulm Med 8: 470–6.

Webster GF, Razsi LK, Sanchez M, Shupack JL (1991). Weekly low-dose methotrexate therapy for cutaneous sarcoidosis. J Am Acad Dermatol 24: 451–4.

White DA, Rankin JA, Stover DE et al. (1989). Methotrexate pneumonitis bronchoalveolar lavage findings suggest an immunologic disorder. Am Rev Respir Dis 139: 18–21.

Wyser CP, van Schalkwyk E, Alheit B et al. (1997). Treatment of progressive pulmonary sarcoidosis with cyclosporin A. Am J Respir Crit Care Med 156: 1371–6.

Yamamoto M, Saito N, Tachibana T, et al. (1983). Effects of an 18-month corticosteroid therapy on stage I and stage II sarcoidosis patients (a control trial). In:Proceedings of the 9th International Conference on Sarcoidosis. Pergamon Press, Oxford. pp. 470–4.

Ye Q, Chen B, Tong Z et al. (2006). Thalidomide reduces IL-18, IL-8 and TNF-alpha release from alveolar macrophages in interstitial lung disease. Eur Respir J 28: 824–31.

Yee AMF, Pochapin MB (2001). Treatment of complicated sarcoidosis with infliximab anti-tumour necrosis-alpha therapy. Ann Intern Med 135: 27–31.

York EL, Kovithathongs T, Man SF et al. (1990). Cyclosporin and chronic sarcoidosis. Chest 98: 1026–9.

Young RL, Harkelroad LE, Lorden RE et al. (1970). Pulmonary sarcoidosis: a prospective evaluation of glucocorticoid therapy. Ann Intern Med 73: 207–12.

Zabel P, Eritzian P, Dalhoff K, Schlaak M (1987). Pentoxifylline in treatment for sarcoidosis. Am J Respir Crit Care Med 155: 1665–9.

Zic JA, Horowitz DH, Arzubiaga C, King LE (1991). Treatment of cutaneous sarcoidosis with chloroquine: review of the literature. Arch Dermatol 127: 1034–40.

Zisman DA, McCune WJ, Tino G, Lynch JP (2001). Drug-induced pneumonitis: the role of methotrexate. Sarcoid Vasc Diff Lung Dis 18: 243–52.

Zych D, Pawlicka L, Zielinski J (1993). Inhaled budesonide vs prednisone in the maintenance treatment of pulmonary sarcoidosis. Sarcoidosis 10: 56–61.

PART X

SURGICAL INVESTIGATION, MANAGEMENT AND FUTURE RESEARCH

43

Surgical investigation and management

ERIC LIM

INTRODUCTION

In general, the role of surgery in the management of sarcoidosis is confined to obtaining confirmatory tissue diagnosis. Surgery may be required to manage complications such as pericarditis or laryngeal sarcoidosis, but this is not usually specific to the disease.

The diagnostic methods obtain either lymph node or lung tissue using minimally invasive techniques.

BRONCHOSCOPY AND MEDIASTINAL LYMPH NODE AND LUNG BIOPSIES

With a move towards less-invasive techniques, flexible bronchoscopy and transbronchial needle biopsy of lymph nodes are increasingly being evaluated for clinical use in the diagnosis of suspected sarcoidosis. Patients may be admitted for a day-case procedure under local anesthetic. Needle aspiration of the lymph nodes at bronchoscopy can be undertaken either blind or using ultrasound guidance. A recent randomized trial reported a higher yield when ultrasound-guided needle aspiration was performed (Tremblay et al. 2009).

Flexible bronchoscopy can be used to obtain transbronchial lung biopsies. The sensitivity for transbronchial lymph node aspiration has been reported as 66 percent and that for transbronchial lung biopsy as 63 percent, but with a joint sensitivity of 94 percent for stage I and II sarcoidosis (Trisolini et al. 2004).

MEDIASTINOSCOPY AND LYMPH NODE BIOPSIES

The standard method for confirmatory diagnosis of sarcoidosis is to obtain mediastinal lymph node tissue by mediastinoscopy. A 2–3 cm cervical incision (above the suprasternal notch) is performed under anesthesia and dissection undertaken to the pretracheal fascia to facilitate the passage of a mediastinoscope. The lymph nodes are identified (Fig. 43.1), dissected and biopsied; multiple biopsies are undertaken. The specimens are usually sent fresh to the pathologist. In general, mediastinoscopy and lymph node biopsy is a safe procedure with a complication rate of 2 percent, which includes major bleeding, injury to the trachea or esophagus and recurrent laryngeal nerve palsy (Luke et al. 1986).

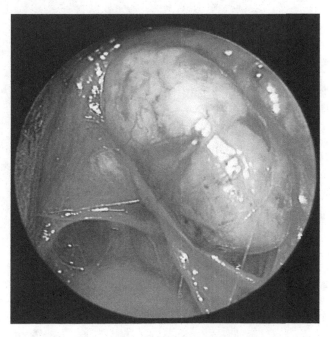

Figure 43.1   Mediastinoscopy view of an enlarged lymph node due to sarcoidosis.

SURGICAL LUNG BIOPSIES

Surgical lung biopsy is less commonly performed as a primary method for the diagnosis of sarcoidosis. It is

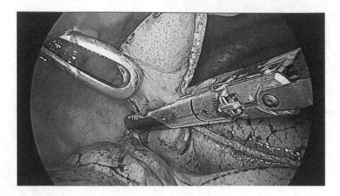

Figure 43.2   Video-assisted lung biopsy.

usually undertaken in the absence of mediastinal lymphadenopathy or for the diagnosis of a diffuse pulmonary parenchymal disorder with sarcoidosis as an incidental diagnosis.

Surgical biopsy can be undertaken using a video-assisted technique (Fig. 43.2) with an instrument that simultaneously cuts and seals the edges of the lung tissue with rows of buttressing staples.

In the presence of dense adhesions, or if the lung disease is so severe that the patient cannot tolerate single lung ventilation, then surgical lung biopsy can be undertaken via a thoracotomy.

REFERENCES

Luke WP, Pearson FG, Todd TR *et al.* (1986). Prospective evaluation of mediastinoscopy for assessment of carcinoma of the lung. *J Thorac Cardiovasc Surg.* **91**: 53–6.

Tremblay A, Stather DR, Maceachern P *et al.* (2009). A randomized controlled trial of standard vs endobronchial ultrasonography-guided transbronchial needle aspiration in patients with suspected sarcoidosis. *Chest* **136**: 340–6.

Trisolini R, Lazzari Agli L, Cancellieri A *et al.* (2004). Transbronchial needle aspiration improves the diagnostic yield of bronchoscopy in sarcoidosis. *Sarcoid Vasc Diff Lung Dis* **21**: 147–51.

44

Lung transplantation

LAURA TANNER, MATTHEW LANE AND PAUL A CORRIS

INTRODUCTION

Lung transplantation is established as a successful treatment option for those with end-stage lung disease that is unresponsive to maximal medical therapy and where no effective medical therapy exists. Over 2000 lung transplants are performed each year worldwide (Christie *et al.* 2009). In carefully selected patients, transplantation confers both quality-of-life and survival benefits, with many recipients now surviving more than 10 years.

REFERRAL FOR TRANSPLANT ASSESSMENT

There is a window of opportunity for transplantation where the potential benefits outweigh the risks of the operation. Each individual must be assessed and the possibility of all outcomes weighed. Early referral is key to ensuring that there is enough time for unhurried assessment, patient education, and management of any outstanding areas of concern before active listing. It is advised that the patient be referred for assessment when his or her predicted survival at 2 years is less than 50 percent.

Waiting time is variable and depends on numerous factors such as:

- recipient characteristics, including size and blood group;
- type of transplant;
- availability of a donor;
- the local arrangement for donor allocation.

Patients tend to wait longer for a transplantation if female, small, or excessively tall, or if they have a blood group other than AB.

GENERAL CONSIDERATIONS FOR LUNG TRANSPLANTATION

The overall aim of lung transplantation is to confer a survival benefit. Despite huge advances in the field, the procedure carries a significant perioperative mortality rate, and the numerous factors that may influence the outcome must be weighed carefully in each patient. The factors considered below are in no way an exhaustive list but rather an overview of some of the more frequently occurring and important considerations.

Major contraindications

The list of contraindications is standard for all lung transplant recipients and requires little further elaboration (Box 44.1).

> **Box 44.1 Contraindications to lung transplantation**
>
> - Malignancy in the last 5 years (excluding squamous and basal cell carcinomas of the skin)
> - Untreatable advanced dysfunction of another major organ system
> - Significant chest wall or spinal deformity
> - Documented non-adherence
> - Untreatable psychiatric or psychological condition associated with inability to cooperate with follow-up
> - Absence of reliable consistent social support
> - Current substance addiction or use
> - Active extrapulmonary infections and sepsis

Relative contraindications

Age

While there is no absolute upper age limit, those over 60 years have a poorer overall post-transplant survival. It is very rare for patients over 65 years to be accepted in the UK.

Nutritional status

Transplant candidate should be within 15 kg of their ideal bodyweight. The perioperative period is a highly catabolic state and patients invariably lose weight during this time. Those with a body mass index (BMI) less than 17 kg/m^2 are most at risk of severe nutritional deficiency and subsequent poor wound healing and infection. Conversely those with a BMI greater than 30 kg/m^2 are less likely to achieve early mobilization and rehabilitation.

Osteoporosis

Systemic corticosteroids are widely used in many end-stage lung diseases, including sarcoidosis. This, together with the debility and decreased mobility associated with advanced lung disease, leads to a high risk of osteoporosis. The ability to undertake early mobilization is hindered by symptomatic osteoporosis, and a loss in bone mineral density of 16 percent has been described after lung transplantation.

Presence of other major organ dysfunction

In view of the potential for calcineurin inhibitor toxicity, preserved renal function is important. A creatinine clearance of 50 mL/min is taken as the lower limit of acceptability. Patients with significant coronary artery disease may undergo percutaneous intervention prior to transplantation or, rarely, coronary artery bypass grafting during the procedure itself.

All other medical co-morbidity, including diabetes mellitus, systemic hypertension and gastroesophageal reflux disease, should be well controlled prior to transplantation.

Psychological factors

Transplantation listing, and the postoperative period, is a hugely stressful time for patients and their families. The patient's ability to cope with the psychological demands must be given serious consideration prior to listing. Of particular concern would be known previous non-compliance with treatment or failure to attend follow-up. In addition to this, patients must have an adequate social support network. Psychiatric illness that is not amenable to treatment, and substance abuse within the last 6 months, is almost universally considered as a contraindication to transplantation.

SPECIAL CONSIDERATIONS IN SARCOIDOSIS

Extrapulmonary organ involvement

Sarcoidosis is a multisystem disease, so extrapulmonary involvement needs to be evaluated. Evidence of uncontrolled progressive extrapulmonary disease can represent an absolute contraindication. Sarcoid cardiomyopathy with a decreased LV ejection fraction is a contraindication to isolated lung transplantation; heart–lung transplantation may be considered. Hepatic involvement is common and not an absolute contraindication provided the synthetic function of the liver is preserved. Neurological involvement, particularly meningeal, would usually represent an absolute contraindication. It must be emphasized that these are generalities and each patient should be discussed on a case-by-case basis by specialists.

Infection

A high proportion of patients with stage IV sarcoidosis have co-existent traction bronchiectasis. Bacterial colonization and aspergilloma(s) are more prevalent in this group. This is of importance, not only in considering the available antibiotic options in the peri- and postoperative periods, but in deciding which operation will be most appropriate.

The decision to perform either single- or double-lung transplantation in patients with sarcoidosis is often based on the presence or absence of infection. Single-lung replacement is not an option for those with bacterial or fungal colonization. The presence of a subpleural aspergilloma is a relative contraindication to lung transplantation.

LUNG TRANSPLANTATION IN SARCOIDOSIS

General points

Since 1990, over 600 lung transplants for sarcoidosis have been performed and reported worldwide (Christie et al. 2009). Transplantation is now an accepted therapy for end-stage sarcoidosis and this is reflected in the updated ISHLT guidelines.

Sarcoidosis currently represents 2.6 percent of all indications for adult lung replacements: 2.1 percent single-lung transplantation (SLT), 2.9 percent bilateral lung transplantation (BLT) (Christie et al. 2009). Outcomes in this group are comparable to many of the other major indications, including idiopathic pulmonary fibrosis (IPF), chronic obstructive pulmonary disease (COPD) and idiopathic pulmonary arterial hypertension (IPAH).

Kaplan–Meier survival rates in patients with sarcoidosis indicate survival of 72 percent at 1 year, 52 percent at 5 years, and 37.4 percent at 10 years (Christie et al. 2009). A clear quality-of-life benefit has been demonstrated with over 90 percent of surviving recipients having no functional limitations of activity at the end of the first year (Christie et al. 2009).

Predictors of survival in patients with sarcoidosis awaiting lung transplantation

Mortality in those with sarcoidosis awaiting transplantation is of the order of 29 percent (Shorr et al. 2002) to 53 percent (Arcasoy et al. 2001). Although sarcoidosis is a multisystem disease, 75 percent of mortality is due to advanced lung disease (Huang et al. 1981).

Attempts to improve outcomes in patients with sarcoidosis awaiting transplantation have focused on identifying those most at risk. While mortality prediction models for these patients have only demonstrated moderate predictive value, several poor prognostic factors have been identified (Shorr et al. 2003):

- severity of hypoxemia;
- pulmonary hypertension;
- elevated right atrial pressure.

Supplementary oxygen requirements and the mean pulmonary artery pressure are two major variables identified as differentiating survivors and non-survivors on the transplant registry.

Spirometric values have been noted to be worse in patients with sarcoidosis at assessment for transplantation compared to patients with IPF (FEV$_1$ 36.0 percent and FVC 42.6 percent predicted vs FEV$_1$ 46.0 percent and FVC 45.0 percent, respectively). Mean pulmonary artery pressure is also noted to be significantly higher in the sarcoidosis group (34.4 mmHg vs 25.6 mmHg, respectively) (Shorr et al. 2002). Studies support the referral of patients with FEV$_1$ < 40 percent and FVC < 50 percent predicted (Shorr et al. 2002).

Finally, an elevated right atrial pressure above 15 mmHg emerges as an ominous sign, with a high short-term mortality rate, and serves to emphasize the importance of thorough cardiac work-up and hemodynamic surveillance in those with advanced sarcoidosis (Arcasoy et al. 2001).

Pulmonary hypertension

Pulmonary hypertension (PH) deserves further mention, given its prognostic significance for those on the transplant registry. Pulmonary hypertension (defined as a resting mean pulmonary artery pressure > 25 mmHg) is common in advanced sarcoidosis, with a prevalence of over 70 percent in those awaiting transplantation (Shorr et al. 2005).

Supplemental oxygen requirements have been shown to be an independent predictor of PH in this group. When used as a screening test for detecting PH, the need for supplementary oxygen has a sensitivity of over 90 percent (Shorr et al. 2005).

One study discussed 22 patients with sarcoidosis-associated pulmonary hypertension. Seven patients had PH in the absence of pulmonary fibrosis, raising the possibility of a sarcoidosis-specific vasculopathy (Nunes et al. 2006).

Mycetoma

Mycetoma is a major contraindication in many transplant centers. Patients with fungal contamination of fibrobullous cavities also have increased risk of mortality and morbidity post-transplantation compared to other transplants (Judson 1998; Hadjiliadis et al. 2002; Shah 2007). Tissue colonized with *Aspergillus* or a mycetoma needs to be fully removed as there is a high chance of invasive fungal disease with associated high mortality in the context of immunosuppression if infected tissue is left behind. Patients with pleural disease or mycetoma adjacent to the pleura with pleural reaction are at increased risk of seeding at the time of transplantation and are estimated to be at higher risk of fungal empyema (Arcasoy et al. 2001; Shah 2007). Bilateral lung transplantation remains the treatment of choice in patients with mycetomas.

Although studies have shown reduced survival post-transplantation, with careful patient selection and aggressive antifungal treatment pre- and postoperatively, these patients can be successfully transplanted (Hadjiliadis et al. 2002).

Suggested disease–specific criteria for referral

A high mortality rate seen in patients with sarcoidosis awaiting lung transplantation may be related to late referral for transplant consideration. Early referral is strongly encouraged in those with functional limitation despite maximal medical therapy. See Box 44.2 for a useful guide as to when referral to the transplant center is appropriate.

It should also be emphasized that the approach should be individualized, taking into account the patient's wishes, his or her overall quality of life, and the referring physician's impression of the patient's prospects. Early referral allows time for the appropriate pre-transplantation work-up and patient education and can lead to improved outcomes regardless of whether the patient ultimately receives a transplant or not.

Box 44.2 Guide to referral to the transplant center

Impairment of exercise tolerance (NYHA functional class III or IV) in those with stage IV sarcoidosis and any of the following:

- vital capacity deteriorating and reaching less than 50% predicted
- hypoxemia at rest
- pulmonary hypertension

Donor–recipient matching

Recipients are matched to donor organs using:

- ABO blood grouping;
- predicted total lung capacity (TLC), using donor height, sex and age to make the prediction;

Relevant human leukocyte antigens (HLAs) are avoided in patients with preformed anti-HLA antibodies.

The majority of donor lungs are from patients declared brainstem dead with no major lung infection or disease. When a provisional offer of a donor lung is made to the transplant center, it must meet certain criteria to be suitable. If these initial criteria are met, potential recipients will be contacted to come to the hospital. Graft suitability is based on function (gas exchange and compliance) and appearance (macroscopic, bronchoscopic and radiographic) (Box 44.3).

The shortfall in donor lungs has led to the additional use of lungs retrieved from non-heart-beating donors who have irreversible circulatory failure, donation after circulatory determination of death (DCD).

In the UK and Europe, donor lungs are offered to each transplant center from a defined zone and allocated to a recipient by the center based on matching and clinical need. In the USA, all transplant-listed patients are allocated a formal 'lung allocation score' (LAS) which assesses both risk of dying on the waiting list and the chance of surviving transplant surgery.

Box 44.3 Standard ('ideal') lung donor criteria (Van Raemdonck et al. 2009)

- Age < 55 years
- Clear serial chest X-ray
- Normal gas exchange: $Pao_2 > 300\,mmHg$ on $Fio_2 = 1.0$, PEEP = 5 cmH$_2$O
- Absence of chest trauma
- No evidence of aspiration or sepsis
- Absence of purulent secretions at bronchoscopy
- Absence of organisms on sputum Gram stain
- No history of primary pulmonary disease or active pulmonary infection
- Tobacco history less than 20 pack-years
- ABO compatibility
- No prior cardiopulmonary surgery
- Appropriate size match with prospective recipient

OUTCOMES AFTER LUNG TRANSPLANTATION

Medium- and long-term survival rates for sarcoidosis patients are comparable to patients undergoing lung replacement for other diseases (Fig. 44.1; Walker et al. 1998; Nunley et al. 1999; Boehler 2001; Milman et al. 2005a; Willie et al. 2008).

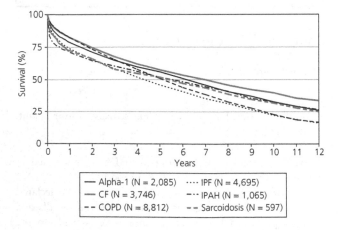

Figure 44.1   Results of lung transplantation for sarcoidosis in comparison with other indications (adapted from the registry of the International Society for Heart and Lung Transplant).

Both recipient race and donor race significantly have affected short-term survival, with higher perioperative mortality (almost 50 percent) in African-American recipients than in Causcasians (Shorr et al. 2004). Recurrence of sarcoidosis in the transplanted lung appears to be more frequent in African-American patients (Nunley et al. 1999).

CHOICE OF TRANSPLANT OPERATION

Choice of transplant is decided on an individual basis, taking into account factors that may affect the outcome.

Single-lung transplantation

In this operation the native lung with the poorest function on the basis of a quantitative perfusion scan is transplanted. The advantage of SLT is that it is the shortest operation and can be performed with or without the need for cardiopulmonary bypass, depending on hemodynamic stability during surgery.

Many patients with end-stage pulmonary sarcoidosis have elevated right heart pressures and right ventricular dysfunction at the time of transplantation which may lead to high preoperative mortality. SLT is still a viable option if the patient has PH as right heart pressures normalize after transplantation (Bjortuft et al. 1996). However, while afterload is immediately reduced, right ventricular dysfunction does not immediately improve and hemodynamic instability may be problematic in the period immediately after transplant with patients requiring prolonged duration of inotropes (National PH Centres 2008). Patients with pulmonary hypertension pre-transplant are at increased risk of early lung injury but this may not result in prolonged ventilator dependence or intensive-treatment stay (Shah 2007).

Single-lung transplants enable more transplants to be performed and may be considered a more judicious use of scarce resources. SLT is associated with lower absolute pulmonary function and FEV$_1$ values, but this has not been shown in studies to equate to reduced function or exercise performance (Judson 1998).

Bilateral lung transplantation

In this operation (BLT) both the native lungs are removed and transplanted sequentially (one after the other) resulting in two separate anastomoses at each main bronchus. Previous analysis of results indicated a small survival advantage for BLT over SLT (Meyer et al. 2000; Studer et al. 2004), but more recent data from the ISHLT registry have shown no difference in short-term survival at 1 and 3 years.

Bronchiectasis and mycetoma are common findings in end-stage fibrocystic sarcoidosis. In patients with poor clearance from bronchiectatic lungs colonized with bacteria, BLT should be performed to prevent overwhelming infection in the context of immunosuppression (Shah 2007).

Heart–lung transplantation

This operation (HLT) is now performed very rarely owing to the scarcity of adequate organ blocks and the improvement in outcomes of the other transplant options. The vast majority of patients with pulmonary sarcoidosis are suitable for SLT or BLT.

ROUTINE MANAGEMENT AFTER TRANSPLANTATION

Transplantation requires an enormous, continuous commitment from the patient and lifelong adherence to immunosuppressive medication. Subjects must attend clinic regularly and undergo lung function and blood tests to monitor drug levels, renal function, glucose and lipids. All allografts are subject to lifelong threat from alloimmune rejection.

Following lung transplantation most patients will receive triple immunosuppressive therapy:

- calcineurin inhibitor (ciclosporin or tacrolimus);
- cell-cycle inhibitor (azathioprine or mycophenolate mofetil);
- corticosteroids (prednisolone).

A small proportion of patients receive the mTOR inhibitors sirolimus or everolimus, and currently these are sometimes introduced to replace calcineurin inhibitors in patients with worsening renal function. There is an ongoing multicenter trial comparing everolimus with mycophenolate in combination with ciclosporin and prednisolone.

COMPLICATIONS AFTER TRANSPLANTATION

Primary graft dysfunction

Primary graft dysfunction is a form of acute lung injury, similar to acute respiratory distress syndrome (ARDS), with alveolar damage and increased vascular permeability leading to interstitial edema and reduction in pulmonary blood flow. Primary graft dysfunction accounts for 30.5 percent of deaths in the first 30 days post-transplantation (Studer et al. 2004). The lungs become poorly compliant and require increased positive end-expiratory pressure (PEEP) to enable adequate ventilation. Prolonged mechanical ventilation at high pressures inevitably leads to risk of increasing the lung injury, and ventilator strategies similar to those used for ventilating patients with ARDS are adopted. Patients may require consideration of support via extracorporeal membrane oxygenators and the use of inhaled nitric oxide.

Early airway complications

Early airway complications, such as dehiscence and necrosis and bronchial stensosis, are due to ischemia of the donor bronchus. Anastomotic healing has improved with reduced complications owing to improved surgical techniques and perioperative management, including shorter recipient bronchus and non-telescoping anastomosis (Wilson et al. 1996).

Dehiscence has a high mortality and usually occurs early within the first few weeks (Santacruz and Mehta 2009). Confirmation of the diagnosis is made at bronchoscopy and usually requires surgical repair (Mughal et al. 2005).

Strictures can be an early or late complication but are commonly seen 2–9 months after transplantation (Santzcruz and Mehta 2009). The incidence has been reported to be as low as 1.6 percent (Wilson et al. 1996). Stenosis occurs where there has been an area of ischemia. It causes a monophonic wheeze and reduction in lung function with a characteristic change on flow volume loop showing a biphasic pattern indicative of a two-compartment emptying pattern (Santacruz and Mehta 2009). Diagnosis is via flexible bronchoscopy. Potential treatments include dilatation, balloon bronchoplasty, laser and stent insertion.

Infection

Infection is omnipresent post-transplantation and can be viral, bacterial or fungal. An additional difficulty in managing the post-transplant patient is that localizing signs and symptoms and markers of severity present in an immunocompetent patient are often lacking in the context of immunosuppressive therapy.

Infections are the most common cause of morbidity and mortality at any time point following lung transplantation. Bacterial infections are one of the major causes of mortality in the early postoperative period (Lyu and Zamora 2009). The incidence of infection is higher in lung transplant recipients than following transplantation of any other solid organ (Kotloff and Ahya 2004). This is due to a combination of higher levels of immunosuppression and direct exposure of the lung allograft to the external environment. Other predisposing conditions include denervation with impaired mucocilliary clearance, reduced cough, and ischemic injury to the bronchial mucosa.

BACTERIAL INFECTIONS

Bacterial infections are most common in the first month. The prevalence then falls, only to rise later as a complication of chronic allograft dysfunction. The incidence of bacterial infection in the first postoperative month has been reported as 16 percent (Kotloff and Ahya 2004). In the early postoperative period, the most common pathogens to cause infection are those colonizing the donor/recipient and those known to populate the local intensive-care unit (Lau and Patterson 2003). Recipients undergo bronchoalveolar lavage (BAL) at the time of implantation so that potential pathogens are identified early. The risk of early postoperative infections is reduced by initiating early prophylactic antibiotics at the time of transplantation based on the preoperative organisms of the recipient, which are then modified when the results of the lavage are obtained.

Although opportunistic infection must always be considered in the immunosuppressed transplant patient, typical respiratory pathogens are more likely to cause infection beyond 6 months. *Pseudomonas* infection is particularly troublesome in the context of chronic allograft dysfunction, due to bronchiolitis obliterans syndrome (BOS; Lau and Patterson 2003).

Treatment of community-acquired lower respiratory tract infections or pneumonias should avoid the use of macrolide antibiotics without a reduction in calcineurin inhibitor dosage and close monitoring of levels since there is a danger of precipitating acute renal failure.

VIRAL INFECTIONS

Cytomegalovirus (CMV) is the most common viral pathogen isolated in the postoperative period (Kotloff and Ahya 2004). CMV infection can occur passively via transmission from the donor lung allograft or be reactivated recipient virus in a CMV-positive recipient. The incidence of disease has been significantly reduced by the introduction of prophylactic valganciclovir and polymerase chain reaction (PCR) surveillance, but CMV infection remains problematic post-transplantation. CMV IgG-negative recipient and CMV IgG-positive donor combinations (CMV mismatch) are at highest risk of developing severe, invasive disease (Lau and Patterson 2003). CMV disease has long-term implications as it has been associated with the development of bronchiolitis obliterans syndrome (Kotloff and Ahya 2004).

All lung transplant patients receive acyclovir prophylaxis for the first 3 months to protect against herpes simplex infection.

Respiratory viral infections can occur at any time post-transplantation, and in common with the general population occur seasonally. They can range from causing a mild coryzal illness to severe fulminant infection and are often complicated by secondary bacterial infections. Seasonal flu vaccination is recommended for all lung transplant recipients.

FUNGAL INFECTIONS

Candida and *Aspergillus* account for the majority of fungal infections. Colonization is frequent, but the prevalence will vary considerably between centers and depend on local environment and changes in environment. Infection with *Aspergillus* may be environmental or associated with pre-transplant colonization which is not uncommon in sarcoidosis. Any disturbance of surrounding soil associated with new buildings, for example, will lead to an increase in environmental *Aspergillus* spores. Colonization rates for *Aspergillus* alone are 29–46 percent (Kotloff and Ahya 2004). *Aspergillus* is often asymptomatic and detected on surveillance bronchosopy and lavage. True invasive *Aspergillus* infection is seen in approximately 5 percent of lung transplant recipients, with only 3 percent of those colonized progressing to invasive disease. However,

Aspergillus colonization has been linked to airway complications such as bronchial stenosis (Kotloff and Ahya 2004).

Voricanazole is the current treatment of choice. Care must be taken to reduce calcineurin inhibitor doses and monitor levels, because azole antifungals interact, resulting in an increase in calcineurin inhibitor levels which can rapidly become toxic and lead to acute renal failure.

Mortality from *Pneumocystis jiroveci* used to be significant, but with the introduction of lifelong prophylaxis in the form of co-trimoxazole the incidence of infection has decreased. Alternative prophylaxis includes trimethoprim-dapsone, fansidar or azithromycin.

Acute cellular rejection

Acute allograft rejection is common, with most patients experiencing more than one episode in the first year (Lau and Patterson 2003). Mortality relating to acute rejection is relatively low, accounting for 4.9 percent of early deaths (Studer *et al.* 2004). Acute rejection produces a perivascular infiltrate of mononuclear cells including lymphocytes into the allograft; these can be identified on lung biopsies obtained via transbronchial biopsy (TBB) during fiberoptic bronchoscopy. Many transplant centers perform regular bronchoscopy and TTB in addition to spirometry in the first year, to enable early diagnosis and treatment of asymptomatic rejection, with the aim of preserving graft function and protecting against later chronic allograft rejection.

Acute rejection can be asymptomatic or present with low-grade fever, lethargy and dyspnea associated with lung infiltrates, a pleural effusion and a drop in pulmonary function. Classification is according to histological criteria found on transbronchial biopsy and ranges from none (A0) to severe (A4).

The incidence of acute rejection in sarcoidosis patients is still debated as studies have produced conflicting results. Initially these patients appeared to have higher rates of severe acute rejection and early graft failure (Johnson *et al.* 1993; Shorr *et al.* 2004), but further studies have shown similar incidences of both acute and chronic rejection and no difference in mortality (Judson 1998; Nunley *et al.* 1999; Boehler 2001; Morgenthau *et al.* 2008).

Rejection grade A2 or above is usually treated with intravenous methylprednisolone (10 mg/kg) followed by a tapering dose of augmented oral prednisolone (initially 1 mg/kg). Recurrent episodes of rejection and lymphocytic bronchiolitis are risk factors for chronic allograft rejection and dysfunction, with acute rejection being the single most important risk factor for the development of bronchiolitis obliterans syndrome (Scott *et al.* 2005; Table 44.1). After the first episode of rejection, immunosuppression may be increased and ciclosporin substituted by tacrolimus.

Other treatment options for steroid-resistant rejection include T-cell ablation with anti-thymocyte globulin or similar medications. Total lymphoid irradiation (TLI) has been shown to be effective at controlling the frequency of rejection when drug-based immunosuppression has failed in patients with recurrent acute rejection (Fisher *et al.* 2005).

Table 44.1 Pathological grading of lung rejection (Martini *et al.* 2009).

Category	Grade	Meaning	Appearance
A = acute rejection	0	None	Normal lung parenchyma
	1	Minimal	Inconspicuous small mononuclear, perivascular infiltrates
	2	Mild	More frequent, more obvious, perivascular infiltrates; eosinophils may be present
	3	Moderate	Dense perivascular infiltrates, extension into interstitial space; can involve endotheliasis, eosinophils and neutrophils
	4	Severe	Diffuse perivascular, interstitial and airspace infiltrates with lung injury; neutrophils may be present
B = airway inflammation (lymphocytic bronchiolitis)	0	None	No evidence of bronchiolar inflammation
	1R	Low-grade	Infrequent, scattered or single layer mononuclear cells in bronchiolar submucosa
	2R	High-grade	Larger infiltrates of larger and activated lymphocytes in bronchiolar submucosa; can involve eosinophils and plasmatid cells
	X	Ungradeable	No bronchiolar tissue available

Chronic allograft dysfunction (BOS)

The greatest obstacle to improving long-term survival remains chronic allograft dysfunction, or bronchiolitis obliterans syndrome. This affects up to 50–60 percent of patients surviving more than 5 years and is ultimately responsible for more than 30 percent of all deaths 3 years after the procedure (Boehler and Estenne 2003).

The histological lesion of chronic rejection is obliterative bronchiolitis (OB), which is an increase in fibrous tissue between the muscularis mucosa and the epithelium of

membranous and proximal respiratory bronchioles, often in the form of fibrous plaques, eventually leading to occlusion of the bronchiole by fibrous tissue (Scott *et al.* 2005). The mechanism is thought to be due to repeated injury and inflammation causing airway epithelial damage and loss, resulting in an exaggerated healing response and fibro-proliferation (Boehler and Estenne 2003; Scott *et al.* 2005).

Obliterative bronchiolitis can be patchy in distribution and is not invariably seen on TBB, despite a typical functional decline. Positive histology (grade C1) is not therefore required to make a diagnosis of BOS. Bronchiolitis obliterans syndrome is characterized by progressive airflow obstruction and is a clinical diagnosis, defined by a persistent, irreversible drop in pulmonary function (FEV_1, FVC, FEF_{25-75}) and supported by histological or radiological findings on high-resolution CT – such as bronchial dilatation, 'tree-in-bud' appearance and mosaicism with air-trapping. BOS is a diagnosis of exclusion and can be made only when other causes of drop in FEV_1 (i.e. acute rejection, infection and bronchial anastomotic stricture) have been excluded.

The timing of onset is highly variable, ranging from months to years, with a median time from transplantation of 16–20 months (Fietta and Meloni 2008). The consequences of BOS are increased morbidity and mortality: a 5-year survival after onset of BOS of 30–40 percent; and 55 percent of those affected die as a direct consequence (Scott *et al.* 2005). It also results in significantly reduced health-related quality of life, with more than 80 percent being functionally limited 2 years after diagnosis.

The importance of detecting early, subclinical BOS before irreversible fibro-proliferative disease becomes established has been recognized, so a new stage of BOS, 0-p, has been added (Table 44.2).

Table 44.2 Severity criteria for bronchiolitis obliterans syndrome (BOS).

Stage	Spirometry
BOS 0	FEV_1 >90% baseline, FEF_{25-75} >75% baseline
BOS 0-p	FEV_1 81–90% baseline or FEF_{25-75} ≤ 75% baseline
BOS 1	FEV_1 66–80% baseline
BOS 2	FEV_1 51–65% baseline
BOS 3	FEV_1 ≤ 50% baseline

In established disease, patients experience repeated symptomatic infection followed by persistent colonization with organisms such as *Pseudomonas* and *Aspergillus*. It is unclear whether *Pseudomonas* infection is a risk factor for development of BOS or simply a representation of damaged airways that are prone to colonization. Studies have shown that patients with BOS have small, distal airway obstruction and central bronchial dilatation, and they are often colonized with *Pseudomonas* and *Aspergillus* (Belperio *et al.* 2009). It has been shown that the development of pseudomonal colonization can predate any functional change by many months, providing evidence as to *Pseudomonas* colonization being causal.

Table 44.3 Risk factors for development of bronchiolitis obliterans syndrome (BOS).

	Alloimmune	Non-alloimmune
Recurrent acute rejection (A2 or above)	Primary graft dysfunction	Ischemic–reperfusion injury
Lymphocytic bronchiolitis on BAL	Viral infections	CMV pneumonitis Community respiratory virus
HLA mismatching Anti-HLA antibodies	Bacterial infection Gastric reflux Airway ischemia Medication non-compliance Older donor age, prolonged graft ischemic time	Pseudomonas

BAL, bronchoalveolar lavage; CMV, cytomegalovirus; HLA, human leukocyte antigen

The rate of progression of disease is variable. An acute onset occurring earlier after surgery is associated with a worse prognosis (Boehler and Estenne 2003).

There are many risk factors, both hypothesized and proven, for developing BOS. These risk factors can be categorized into alloimmune and non-alloimmune types (Belperio et al. 2009; Table 44.3).

ALLOIMMUNE RISK FACTORS

These include number and severity of episodes of acute rejection, lymphocytic bronchiolitis and HLA mismatching (Husain et al. 1999; Schulman et al. 2001).

Acute rejection is the most significant risk factor for development of chronic rejection (Scott et al. 2005). In multivariate analysis, three or more episodes of A2 grade or above acute rejection were highly associated with the development of BOS (Bando et al. 1995). Late episodes of acute rejection are also associated with subsequent development of BOS (Husain et al. 1999). Recent studies suggest any grade of acute rejection will increase the risk of developing BOS compared with a patient who has never had histological evidence of rejection.

Lymphocytic bronchitis/bronchiolitis has been shown to be a risk factor for BOS independent of the presence of acute perivascular rejection (Husain et al. 1999).

NON-ALLOIMMUNE RISK FACTORS

CMV pneumonitis is a recognized risk factor for BOS (Husain et al. 1999; Schulman et al. 2001; Scott et al. 2005). The increased use of prophylactic antiviral agents for CMV mismatches has reduced the incidence of CMV pneumonitis.

Other viral and bacterial infections have been implicated, as well as gastroesophageal reflux, medication non-compliance leading to low immunosuppression levels, and airway ischemia and injury (Bando et al. 1995).

Community respiratory viruses (respiratory syncytial virus, parainfluenza, influenza A), bacterial and fungal infections and chlamydial infections have all been implicated in the development of BOS (Scott et al. 2005; Khalifah et al. 2004). Evidence suggests that the number of respiratory infections is important in the development of BOS and that early, aggressive treatment of infection can slow the rate of progression to BOS.

GASTROESOPHAGEAL REFLUX

About two-thirds of patients suffer gastroesophageal reflux after lung transplantation. It appears to be due to a combination of medication-induced gastroparesis and damage to the vagal nerve during surgery causing delayed gastric emptying and altered lower esophageal sphincter function (Boehler and Estenne 2003; Verleden et al. 2005). Denervation of the lungs abolishes the cough reflex and the likelihood of silent aspiration is increased. This continuous micro-aspiration of gastric contents and bile acids may promote chronic inflammation, airway damage and bacterial infection/colonization, all of which could predispose to BOS (Boehler and Estenne 2003).

Gastroesophageal reflux has also been demonstrated to be a reversible cause of allograft dysfunction. Fundoplication may improve pulmonary function and in such patients improves survival (Davis et al. 2003; Verleden et al. 2005).

Patients with sarcoidosis have been shown in studies to have similar rates of BOS and long-term outcomes to those patients transplanted for other diseases (Willie et al. 2008). Potential risk factors should be modified where possible in all patients, but there are emerging treatments for BOS after diagnosis.

TREATMENT

Azithromycin is already used in the treatment of asthma, bronchiectasis, pan-bronchiolitis and cystic fibrosis because of its anti-inflammatory and immunomodulatory effects (Fietta and Meloni 2008). Studies to date have been on small numbers but have given promising results. Responders showed significant improvement in lung function, and a large proportion of 'non-responders' showed an arrest of decline in FEV_1 (Scott et al. 2005; Yates et al. 2005; Fietta and Meloni 2008). Response appears to be better in patients with higher levels of neutrophils and IL-8 on BAL and those who started treatment earlier post-transplantation (Verleden et al. 2006). Randomized controlled trials to substantiate this effect are ongoing.

Other potential treatments include cytolytic therapy, photophoresis, total lymphoid irradiation, cyclophosphamide and methotrexate (Fietta and Meloni 2008). TLI has been shown to significantly slow the rate of decline of FEV_1, with some patients gaining lung function (Fisher et al. 2005).

Post-transplant lymphoproliferative disorder (PTLD)

INCIDENCE AND CLASSIFICATION

Malignancy is increased after solid-organ transplantation. This is probably related to immunosuppressive therapy with

Table 44.4   WHO classification of post-transplant lymphoproliferative disorder (PTLD).

Category	Subtype
Early lesions	Reactive plasmacytic hyperplasia
Polymorphic	Polyclonal or monoclonal
Monomorphic	Diffuse large B-cell lymphomas
	Burkitt's/Burkitt's-like lymphoma
	Plasma-cell myeloma
T cell lymphomas	Peripheral T-cell lymphoma
Others	Myeloma
	Hodgkin's disease-like
	Plasmacytoma-like

subsequent co-infection with oncogenic viruses such as Epstein–Barr (Zafar *et al.* 2008). After skin cancers, PTLD is the most common malignancy following transplantation. Lung transplantation has the highest reported incidence of PTLD (4–10 percent) owing to the higher degree of immunosuppression needed to prevent rejection (Hopwood and Crawford 2000; LaCasce 2006). PTLD is categorized according to the WHO classification (Table 44.4).

An increase in the incidence of PTLD has been linked to the introduction of more effective immunosuppressive agents such as ciclosporin A and T-cell ablative therapy (Hopwood and Crawford 2000; Studer *et al.* 2004). The incidence of PTLD is highest in the first year, especially in lung recipients (Zafar *et al.* 2008; Lyu and Zamora 2009).

The majority of cases of PTLD are associated with Epstein–Barr virus (EBV) which is normally suppressed by a functioning immune system. In the context of immunosuppression, there is abnormal lymphoid proliferation of EBV-infected B-cells which are allowed to replicate unchecked, leading to the development of PTLD. Diagnosis can be difficult: a high index of suspicion is needed for diagnosis owing to the varied clinical and histological presentation. Symptoms can be constitutional including malaise, sweats and weight loss or due to the site and extent of disease. Any organ can be affected, including extranodal sites such as the gastrointestinal tract, central nervous system, skin and allograft. The most common extranodal sites involved are the allograft (69–89 percent) and the GI tract (20–34 percent) (Lyu and Zamora 2009). Excisional biopsies should be obtained wherever possible for histology and determination of EBV status.

TREATMENT

Initial treatment of PTLD is reduced immunosuppression – up to a half respond to this reduction alone (LaCasce 2006). No clear benefit has been shown for antiviral therapy.

More than 90 percent of PTLD after solid-organ transplant are CD20-positive, defining a role for anti-CD20 antibodies which have been associated with complete remission (Kotloff and Ahya 2004; Oertel *et al.* 2005). Rituximab is preferred to chemotherapy because it is less toxic and better tolerated. Response rates with rituximab are around 60 percent, which is similar to chemotherapy with CHOP (cyclophosphamide, hydroxydaunorubicin, oncovin, prednisolone) (Zafar *et al.* 2008). Chemotherapy is reserved for patients with aggressive or CNS disease or those failing treatment with reduced immunosuppression or rituximab.

Combination chemotherapy has been shown to have better outcomes than using a single agent. CHOP alone or with rituximab (CHOP-R) are the most frequently used regimens (LaCasce 2006; Zafar *et al.* 2008). CNS disease is treated with radiotherapy.

Other important complications

METABOLISM

Many metabolic complications can occur after transplantation. Initially the most important is hypomagnesemia, often requiring both intravenous and oral supplementation. It can present as visual disturbance with flashing lights, tremor and lethargy. Hypomagnesemia in combination with hypertension and high ciclosporin levels can precipitate seizures. Other common electrolyte disturbances include hypo- or hyperkalemia, hypocalcemia and hypophosphatemia. Hyponatremia is also commonly encountered and can be due to the syndrome of inappropriate antidiuretic hormone hypersecretion (SIADH) or a salt-wasting picture associated with immunosuppressive medication.

Diabetes mellitus and dyslipidemia occur commonly following lung transplantation and are caused or worsened by immunosuppression, including calcineurin inhibition, particularly by tacrolimus. The reported incidence is about 24 percent at 1 year and 33 percent at 5 years (Lyu and Zamora 2009).

OSTEOPOROSIS

Osteoporosis is an important cause of morbidity and has the potential to compromise a good outcome owing to poor mobility and pain secondary to fractures despite adequate graft function. Studies have shown that patients lose approximately 5 percent of bone mineral density (BMD) within the first transplant year, with an osteoporosis prevalence of 78 percent and fracture rate of 18 percent (Spira *et al.* 2000). Therefore, pre-existing osteopenia or osteoporosis should be treated adequately with bisphosphonates and calcium supplementation before the procedure.

CALCINEURIN INHIBITOR NEPHROTOXICITY

Calcineurin inhibitors are nephrotoxic and lead to hypertension. Ninety-three percent of transplantation patients exhibit a decrease in renal function at 6 months (Kotloff and Ahya 2004; Lyu and Zamora 2009). A doubling of serum creatinine was demonstrated in 34 percent at 1 year, 43 percent at 2 years, and 53 percent at 5 years; and 4.6 percent eventually required hemodialysis for established renal failure (Kotloff and Ahya 2004). The use of tacrolimus in the first 6 months may be associated with reduced renal dysfunction (Lyu and Zamora 2009; Ishani et al. 2002).

The presence of hypertension has been linked to more severe renal dysfunction requiring aggressive blood pressure control with ACE inhibitors or angiotensin-receptor blockers (Kotloff and Ahya 2004). Factors worsening chronic renal failure include hypertension, hyperlipidemia and diabetes mellitus (Lyu and Zamora 2009) which should be aggressively treated.

RECURRENT SARCOIDOSIS IN THE ALLOGRAFT

Sarcoidosis is the most common disease reported to recur following lung transplantation (Johnson et al. 1993; Judson 1998; Walker et al. 1998; Nunley et al. 1999; Studer et al. 2004; Ma et al. 2007). Surveillance bronchoscopy and TBB have shown that sarcoidosis and granulomas frequently recur in the allograft. In Caucasian patients the recurrence rate is approximately 50 percent (Milman et al. 2005b). Generally, this is asymptomatic with no corresponding radiographic evidence or clinical symptoms (Milman et al. 2005a).

Recurrence occurs in 30–50 percent of patients (Boehler et al. 2001; Milman et al. 2005b; Ionescu et al. 2005). In some studies it is as high as 60 percent if centers perform an extensive surveillance program. The mean time to diagnosis is 224 days post-transplantation (Morgenthau et al. 2008).

If any deterioration is present in the form of symptoms or radiographic changes, these respond favorably to increased corticosteroids (Nunley et al. 1999; Boehler 2001; Milman et al. 2005a; Morgenthau et al. 2008).

Immunofluoresence and hybridization techniques have established that recurrent sarcoid granulomas are recipient in origin (Ionescu et al. 2005; Morgenthau et al. 2008; Milman et al. 2005b). The milder course of recurrent sarcoidosis may be due in part to the immunosuppressive medication and does not appear to affect graft function (Ionescu et al. 2005).

Recurrence appears to be of little clinical relevance. It produces few or no symptoms and no deterioration in lung function. It has not been shown to affect survival or increase rates of BOS (Judson 1998; Walker et al. 1998; Nunley et al. 1999; Ionescu et al. 2005; Milman et al. 2005b; Ma et al. 2007; Shah 2007).

CONCLUSION

Lung transplantation is a well-established therapy for patients with advanced life-threatening pulmonary sarcoidosis. Despite the prevalence of potential complications it has been demonstrated to improve both quality of life and survival in such patients. Overall survival has improved over the years, so that at least 40 percent of current recipients will survive for more than 10 years, and the majority will be able to enjoy all activities of daily living.

REFERENCES

Arcasoy SM, Christie JD, Pochettino A et al. (2001). Characteristics and outcomes of patients with sarcoidois listed for lung transplantation. Chest 120: 873–80.

Bando K, Paradis IL, Similo S et al. (1995). Obliterative bronchiolitis after lung and heart-lung transplantation: an analysis of risk factors and management. J Thorac Cardiovasc Surg 110: 4–13.

Belperio JA, Weigt SS, Fishbein MC, Lynch JP (2009). Chronic lung allograft rejection: mechanisms and therapy. Proc Am Thorac Soc 6: 108–21.

Bjortuft O, Simonsen S, Geiran OR et al. (1996). Pulmonary haemodynamics after single-lung transplantation for end stage pulmonary parenchymal disease. Eur Respir J 9: 2007–11.

Boehler A (2001). Lung transplantation for cystic lung diseases: lymphangioleiomyomatosis, histiocytosis X, and sarcoidosis. Sem Respir Crit Care Med 22: 509–16.

Boehler A, Estenne M (2003). Post-transplant bronchiolitis obliterans. Eur Respir J 22: 1007–18.

Christie JD, Edwards LB, Aurora P et al. (2009). Twenty-sixth official adult lung and heart–lung transplantation report. J Heart Lung Transplant 28: 1031–49.

Davis RD, Lau CL, Eubanks S et al. (2003). Improved lung allograft function after funcoplication in patients with gastroesophageal reflux disease undergoing lung transplantation. J Thorac Cardiovasc Surg 125: 533–42.

Fietta AM, Meloni F (2008). Lung transplantation: the role of azithromycin in the management of patients with bronchiolitis obliterans syndrome. Curr Med Chem 15: 716–23.

Fisher AJ, Rutherford RM, Bozzino J et al. (2005). The safety and efficacy of total lymphoid irradiation in progressive bronchiolitis obliterans syndrome after lung transplantation. Am J Transplant 5: 537–43.

Hadjiliadis D, Sporn TA, Perfect JR et al. (2002). Outcome of lung transplantation in patients with mycetomas. Chest 121: 128–34.

Hopwood P, Crawford DH (2000). The role of EBV in post-transplant malignancies: a review. J Clin Pathol. 53: 248–54.

Huang CT, Heurich AE, Sutton AC, Lyons HA (1981). Mortality in sarcoidosis: a changing pattern in the cause of death. Eur J Respir Dis 62: 231–8.

Husain AN, Siddiqui MT, Holmes EW et al. (1999). Analysis of risk factors for the development of bronchiolitis obliterans syndrome. Am J Respir Crit Care Med 159: 829–33.

Ionescu DN, Hunt JL, Lomago D, Yousem SA (2005). Recurrent sarcoidosis in lung transplant allografts: granulomas are of recipient origin. Diagn Mol Pathol 14: 140–5.

Ishani A, Erturk S, Hertz MI et al. (2002). Predictors of renal function following lung or heart–lung transplantation. Kidney Int 61: 2228–34.

Johnson BA, Duncan SR, Ohori NP et al. (1993). Recurrence of sarcoidosis in pulmonary allograft recipients. Am Rev Respir Dis 148: 1373–7.

Judson MA (1998). Lung transplantation for pulmonary sarcoidosis. Eur Respir J 11: 738–44.

Khalifah AP, Hachem RR, Chakinala MM et al. (2004). Respiratory viral infections are a distinct risk for bronchiolitis obliterans syndrome and death. Am J Respir Crit Care Med 170: 181–7.

Kotloff RM, Ahya VN (2004). Medical complications of lung transplantation. Eur Respir J 23: 334–42.

LaCasce AS (2006). Post-transplant lymphoproliferative disorders. Oncologist 11: 674–80.

Lau CL, Patterson GA (2003). Current status of lung transplantation. *Eur Respir J Suppl* **47**: 57–64s.

Lyu DM, Zamora MR (2009). Medical complications of lung transplantation. *Proc Am Thorac Soc* **6**: 101–7.

Ma Y, Gal A, Koss MN (2007). The pathology of pulmonary sarcoidosis: update. *Semin Diagn Pathol* **24**: 150–61.

Martinu T, Chen DF, Palmer SM (2009). Acute rejection and humeral sensitization in lung transplant recipients. *Proc Am Thorac Soc* **6**: 54–65.

Meyer DM, Bennett LE, Novick RJ, Hesenpud JD (2000). Effect of donor age and ischaemic time in intermediate survival and morbidity after lung trasplantation. *Chest* **118**: 1255–62.

Milman N, Burton C, Andersen CB et al. (2005a). Lung transplantation for end-stage pulmonary sarcoidosis: outcome in a series of seven consecutive patients. *Sarcoid Vasc Diff Lung Dis* **22**: 222–8.

Milman N, Andersen CB, Burton CM, Iversen M (2005b). Recurrent sarcoid granulomas in a transplanted lung derive from recipient immune cells. *Eur Respir J* **26**: 549–52.

Morgenthau AS, Michael C, Lannuzzi M (2008). Lung transplantation in sarcoidosis. *Minerva Pneumol* **47**: 63–72.

Mughal MM, Gildea TR, Murthy S et al. (2005). Short-term deployment of self-expanding metallic stents facilitates healing of bronchial dehiscence. *Am J Respir Crit Care Med* **172**: 768–71.

National PH Centres of the UK and Ireland (2008). Consensus statement on the management of pulmonary hypertension in clinical practice in the UK and Ireland. *Thorax* **63**(Suppl. II): ii1–41.

Nunes H, Humbert M, Capron F et al. (2006). Pulmonary hypertension associated with sarcoidosis: mechanisms, haemodynamics and prognosis. *Thorax* **61**: 68–74.

Nunley DR, Hattler B, Keenan RJ et al. (1999). Lung transplantation for end-stage pulmonary sarcoidosis. *Sarcoid Vasc Diff Lung Dis* **16**: 93–100.

Oertel SHK, Verschuuren E, Reinke P et al. (2005). Effect of anti-CD 20 antibody rituximab in patients with post-transplant lymphoproliferaive disorder (PTLD). *Am J Transplant* **5**: 2901–6.

Santacruz JF, Mehta AC (2009). Airway complications and management after lung transplantation: ischemia, dehiscence and stensois. *Proc Am Thorac Soc* **6**: 79–93.

Schulman LL, Weinberg AD, McGregor CC et al. (2001). Influence of donor and recipient HLA locus mismatching on development of obliterative bronchiolitis after lung transplantation. *Am J Respir Crit Care Med* **163**: 437–42.

Scott AIR, Sharples LD, Stewart S (2005). Bronchiolitis obliterans syndrome: risk factors and therapeutic strategies. *Drugs* **65**: 761–71.

Shah L (2007). Lung transplantation in sarcoidosis. *Semin Respir Crit Care Med* **28**: 134–40.

Shorr AF, Davies DB, Nathan SD (2002). Outcomes for patients with sarcoidosis awaiting lung transplantation. *Chest* **122**: 233–8.

Shorr AF, Davies DB, Nathan SD (2003). Predicting mortality in patients with sarcoidosis awaiting lung transplantation. *Chest* **124**: 922–8.

Shorr AF, Helman DL, Davies DB, Nathan SD (2004). Sarcoidosis, race, and short-term outcomes following lung transplantation. *Chest* **125**: 990–6.

Shorr AF, Helman DL, Davies DB, Nathan SD (2005). Pulmonary hypertension in advanced sarcoidosis: epidemiology and clinical characteristics. *Eur Respir J* **25**: 783–8.

Spira A, Gutierrez C, Chaparro C et al. (2000). Osteoporosis and lung transplantation: a prospective study. *Chest* **117**: 476–81.

Studer SM, Levy RD, McNeil K, Orens JB (2004). Lung transplant outcomes: a review of survival, graft function, physiology, health-related quality of life and cost-effectiveness. *Eur Respir J* **24**: 674–85.

Van Raemdonck D, Neyrinck A, Verleden GM et al. (2009). Lung donor selection and management. *Proc Am Thorac Soc* **6**: 28–38.

Verleden GM, Dupont LJ, Van Raemdonck DE (2005). Is it bronchiolitis obliterans syndrome or is it chronic rejection: a reappraisal? *Eur Respir J* **25**: 221–4.

Verleden GM, Vanaudenaerde BM, Dupont LJ, Raemdonck DE (2006). Azithromycin reduces airway neutrophilia and interleukin-8 in patients with bronchiolitis obliterans syndrome. *Am J Respir Crit Care Med* **174**: 566–70.

Walker S, Mikhail G, Banner N et al. (1998). Medium term results of lung transplantation for end stage pulmonary sarcoidosis. *Thorax* **53**: 281–4.

Willie KM, Gaggar A, Hajari AS et al. (2008). Bronchiolitis obliterans syndrome and survival following lung transplantation for patients with sarcoidosis. *Sarcoid Vasc Diff Lung Dis* **25**: 117–24.

Wilson IC, Hasan A, Healey M et al. (1996). Healing of the bronchus in pulmonary transplantation. *Eur J Cardio-thorac Surg* **10**: 521–6.

Yates B, Murphy DM, Forrest IA et al. (2005). Azithromycin reverses airflow obstruction in established bronchiolitis obliterans syndrome. *Am J Respir Crit Care Med* **172**: 772–5.

Zafar SY, Howell DN, Gockerman JP (2008). Malignancy after solid organ transplantation: an overview. *Oncologist* **13**: 769–78.

45

Physiotherapy

PENNY AGENT AND HELEN PARROTT

INTRODUCTION

Physiotherapy aims to optimize functional ability, health and wellbeing, through a holistic problem-oriented approach to maximize quality of life. There is little evidence to support or refute physiotherapeutic intervention for individuals with sarcoidosis. However, in clinical practice a problem-based approach indicates the areas where physiotherapy can be of benefit in symptom management. The characteristic symptoms of interstitial lung disease (ILD) such as sarcoidosis where physiotherapy may be appropriate are:

- dyspnea – progressive, often resulting in altered breathing patterns and anxiety;
- cough – dry, irritable and possibly productive;
- deconditioning and associated peripheral muscle dysfunction – resulting in loss of exercise tolerance and functional capability.

DYSPNEA

Dyspnea has been defined by Comroe (1965) as:

the persistent and unpleasant sensation of shortness of breath that includes the perception of difficult breathing as well as the reaction to the sensation.

In individuals with sarcoidosis, dyspnea may be due to a number of causes, but in all cases it is progressive and impacts on functional capability and quality of life. Primary causes of dyspnea include hypoxemia, peripheral muscle dysfunction and deconditioning, and increased work of breathing (due to greater effort required during inspiration to maintain adequate ventilation) (Pryor and Prasad 2008a).

In addition to the pathophysiological reasons, anxiety and disordered breathing may heighten the individual's perception of dyspnea.

Physiotherapy treatment strategies to alleviate or desensitize symptoms of dyspnea can range from simple positioning advice to controlled breathing exercises and relaxation. These strategies are best taught in the early stages of disease as they can prove to be valuable coping mechanisms.

POSITIONING ADVICE

Commonly in individuals with respiratory disease, lying supine is poorly tolerated and can exacerbate dyspnea owing to the mechanical disadvantage of the diaphragm in this position, and it is not recommended. Diaphragmatic excursion is optimized in the upright position. In particular, positions such as forward-lean sitting with supported arms or high-side lying are considered favorable for use at rest. Forward-lean positions increase transdiaphragmatic pressure, improve thoraco-abdominal movements and reduce activity of the scalenes and sternomastoid muscles (Pryor and Prasad 2008b). If this position is combined with relaxed upper-limb support, this allows the pectoral muscles to contribute significantly to rib-cage elevation (Gosselink 2004). On exertion, these positions may be used during a pause in mobilization, but positions such as supported standing (e.g. leaning back or laterally against a wall) or perched sitting may be more convenient. Positioning combined with breathing control and relaxation techniques are used in an attempt to decrease the work of breathing and eliminate unnecessary muscular activity (O'Neill and McCarthy 1983; Gosselink 2004).

BREATHING CONTROL

Breathing control consists of relaxed normal tidal breathing using the lower chest, encouraging relaxation of the upper chest and shoulders (Pryor and Prasad 2008b). Breathing control is usually used in conjunction with the positioning advice above and is best taught in a position of comfort. It should not be forced at all and expiration should be passive. Breathing control is useful at the onset of dyspnea as it alleviates the sensation of breathlessness and conserves energy expenditure. It may be used during exertion to maintain control of breathing and to quicken recovery.

BREATHING PATTERN RETRAINING

Hyperventilation (over-breathing) can be a co-existing complication of chronic lung disease and can occur at any stage of disease severity. Disordered breathing patterns can emerge following episodes of acute exacerbation, but these patterns may become habitual despite resolution of the exacerbation. With habitual disordered breathing patterns a great number of symptoms may arise in addition to dyspnea. These may include chest pain and tightness, peripheral paresthesia, dizziness, air hunger, diminished concentration and feelings of a lack of oxygen. Disordered breathing patterns in interstitial lung disease can present with excessive movement of the upper chest with rapid, shallow breaths, poor coordination of breathing and speech, mouth breathing with overuse of accessory muscles of respiration, and excessive sighing, yawning and a persistent dry cough. However, many of these symptoms listed are characteristic of sarcoidosis and therefore a referral to and assessment by a specialist trained physiotherapist is required in individuals where disordered breathing pattern is suspected.

Breathing pattern retraining utilizes the key principles of breathing control in order to optimize respiratory function and encourage a change in pattern using relaxation. This takes place over a series of weeks or months and typically involves daily practice of the exercises and techniques such as nose breathing, breathing control at rest and during exertion and with speech and eating. Although breathing pattern retraining can be labor-intensive for both the individual and therapist, it can be a useful adjunct to pharmacological therapies in the reduction of anxiety and enable individuals to cope with their symptoms (Chaitow et al. 2002).

OXYGEN THERAPY

There is no evidence that oxygen therapy influences quality of life or long-term survival in patients with ILD (Crockett et al. 2001). It may provide subjective relief of dyspnea. There is a lack of controlled studies of long-term, short-burst and ambulatory oxygen therapy in sarcoidosis and other ILDs, and readers are referred to published recommendations (O'Driscoll et al. 2008).

Physiotherapists may be involved in the optimization of oxygen delivery for patients with sarcoidosis, ensuring fixed-flow devices are used with sufficient flow rates to overcome peak inspiratory flow demands so that air hunger is not experienced, and adequate oxygen saturation is achieved. High-flow oxygen systems may be required that can provide an accurate FiO_2, but appropriate humidification also needs

to be considered owing to the uncomfortable drying nature of these delivery systems.

COUGH

Typically in sarcoidosis, an irritable dry cough predominates that may be improved with advice on breathing control. However, if there is a co-existent respiratory disease such as chronic obstructive pulmonary disease (COPD), the individual may experience a productive cough with excess secretions that are difficult to clear. In these situations, airway clearance techniques may be of benefit and assessed on an individual basis. Despite a paucity of evidence in the use of these techniques in sarcoidosis or other interstitial lung diseases, clinical experience supports the use of various techniques such as active cycle of breathing techniques (ACBT), autogenic drainage (AD) and positive expiratory pressure (PEP). Further details of airway clearance techniques can be found in physiotherapy texts (Pryor and Prasad 2008b).

DECONDITIONING AND PERIPHERAL MUSCLE DYSFUNCTION

It is established that peripheral muscle weakness is predictive of exercise intolerance in interstitial lung disease (Nishiyama et al. 2005; Spruit et al. 2005), but the physiological basis of exercise limitation differs substantially from that seen in COPD (Holland et al. 2008).

In sarcoidosis and other ILDs, the mechanisms of reduced exercise capacity and deconditioning are multifactorial. Fatigue and general weakness in patients with sarcoidosis may result in exercise intolerance (Drent et al. 1999; Sharma 1999). In interstitial lung disease, circulatory impairment results from pulmonary capillary destruction and vasoconstriction, leading to pulmonary hypertension and cardiac dysfunction, and is closely associated with exercise performance (Hansen and Wasserman 1996; Harris-Eze et al. 1996). Impaired gas exchange, as a result of capillary bed destruction, leading to ventilation/perfusion mismatch and limitations in oxygen diffusion (Agusti et al. 1988), characterizes exercise-induced hypoxemia (Chetta et al. 2001; Lama et al. 2003). Peripheral muscle dysfunction as a result of physical deconditioning has a significant role in limiting exercise capacity (Holland and Hill 2009), coupled with potential drug-induced myopathies from chronic corticosteroid and immunosuppressive therapy. However, despite reporting the presence of skeletal muscle weakness in patients with sarcoidosis who complain of fatigue, one study reports no difference in muscle strength between patients taking or not taking steroids (Spruit et al. 2005).

The combination of dyspnea with activity leads patients into a vicious cycle of inactivity, worsening exercise capacity and increasing symptoms (Holland and Hill 2009). Nevertheless, this should not deter clinicians from providing exercise training to patients with ILD as evidence demonstrates that, while maximum exercise capacity is constrained by the pathophysiology of the disease, submaximal exercise capacity is amenable to training, and exercise training in ILD is safe and results in short-term improvements in functional exercise capacity, dyspnea and quality of life for up to 6 months (Holland *et al.* 2008). Exercise training programs are usually provided as comprehensive pulmonary rehabilitation programs.

PULMONARY REHABILITATION

Pulmonary rehabilitation 'is an evidence-based, multi-disciplinary, and comprehensive intervention for patients with chronic respiratory diseases who are symptomatic and often have decreased daily life activities' (Ries *et al.* 2007). Although pulmonary rehabilitation is delivered in a group setting, it focuses on individualized treatment aimed to reduce symptoms, optimize functional status, increase participation and reduce healthcare costs through stabilizing or reversing systemic manifestations of the disease. Pulmonary rehabilitation is optimal if it combines individual patient assessment, a group-based education and exercise training program and psychosocial support.

While there is a wealth of published evidence supporting the use of pulmonary rehabilitation in COPD (Ries *et al.* 2007), this is not the case for sarcoidosis or other restrictive lung diseases. In spite of this, in the few studies evaluating pulmonary rehabilitation for restrictive lung disease, results for non-COPD patients are as good (Foster and Thomas 1990; Ando *et al.* 2003; Ferreira *et al.* 2006), or better (Congleton *et al.* 1997; Dix *et al.* 2002) than for COPD. Generally, patients with restrictive lung disease should be referred for pulmonary rehabilitation as early as possible in the disease process (Wells and Hirani 2008; Bott *et al.* 2009) in order to provide opportunities to educate and train patients in adapting to complex treatment interventions such as immunosuppressive and oxygen therapy.

BEST SUPPORTIVE CARE

In diseases such as sarcoidosis, which are progressive and have uncomfortable symptoms impacting on functional ability and quality of life, 'best supportive care' should be considered by the whole multidisciplinary team. This care, which is proactive and incorporates all aspects of palliative care, is defined by the World Health Organization as:

> an approach that improves the quality of life of patients and their families facing the problem associated with life-threatening illness, through the prevention and relief of suffering by means of early identification and impeccable assessment of pain and other problems, physical, psychosocial and spiritual.

Physiotherapy is aimed at symptom alleviation and, through its strategies such as dyspnea management, exercise training and pulmonary rehabilitation, it provides important components of best supportive care.

CONCLUSION

With a focus on maximizing quality of life, physiotherapists are valuable members of the multidisciplinary team and can be introduced when required to help address patient-specific problems such as progressive breathlessness, reduced functional capacity, anxiety or pain. Despite a lack of evidence for physiotherapeutic interventions, individuals with sarcoidosis can benefit from physiotherapy assessment and treatment at many stages of disease severity.

Respiratory physiotherapists are skilled in the holistic, problem-oriented management of chronic respiratory disease. Many strategies that are well supported for other chronic diseases – such as pulmonary rehabilitation, airway clearance techniques and breathing pattern retraining – can be used when appropriate. The advice and education can be a useful adjunct to pharmacological and medical therapies in enabling individuals to cope with progressive and debilitating symptoms.

REFERENCES

Agusti AG, Roca J, Rodriguez-Roisin R *et al.* (1988). Different patterns of gas exchange response to exercise in asbestosis and idiopathic pulmonary fibrosis. *Eur Respir J* 1: 510–16.

Ando M, Mori A, Esaki H *et al.* (2003). The effect of pulmonary rehabilitation in patients with post-tuberculosis lung disorder. *Chest* 123: 1988–95.

Bott J, Blumenthal S, Buxton M *et al.* (2009). Guidelines for the physiotherapy management of the adult, medical spontaneously breathing patient. *Thorax* 64(Suppl. 1): 1–51.

Chaitow C, Bradley D, Gilbert C (2002). *Multidisciplinary Approaches to Breathing Pattern Disorders.* Churchill Livingstone, Oxford, pp. 56–9.

Chetta A, Aielo M, Foresi A *et al.* (2001). Relationship between outcome measures of six-minute walk test and baseline lung function in patients with interstitial lung disease. *Sarcoid Vasc Diff Lung Dis* 18: 170–5.

Comroe JH (1965). Some theories of the mechanisms of dyspnoea. In: Howell JB, Campbell EJM (eds). *Breathlessness.* Blackwell Scientific, Oxford, pp. 1–7.

Congleton J, Bott J, Hindell A *et al.* (1997). Comparison of outcome of pulmonary rehabilitation in obstructive lung disease, interstitial lung disease and chest wall disease. *Thorax* 52: A11.

Crockett AJ, Cranston JM, Antic N (2001). Domiciliary oxygen for interstitial lung disease. Cochrane Database Systematic Review, CD002883.

Dix K, Daly C, Garrod R *et al.* (2002). Pulmonary rehabilitation in restrictive lung disease. *Thorax* 57: iii48–94.

Drent M, Wirnsberger RM, de Vries J *et al.* (1999). Association of fatigue with an acute phase response in sarcoidosis. *Eur Respir J* 13: 718–22.

Ferreira G, Feuerman M, Spiegler P (2006). Results of an 8-week, outpatient pulmonary rehabilitation program on patients with and without chronic obstructive pulmonary disease. *J Cardiopulm Rehab* 26: 54–60.

Foster S, Thomas HM (1990). Pulmonary rehabilitation in lung disease other than chronic obstructive pulmonary disease. *Am Rev Respir Dis* 141: 601–4.

Gosselink R (2004). Breathing techniques in patients with chronic obstructive pulmonary disease. *Chron Respir Dis* 1: 163–7.

Hansen JE, Wasserman K (1996). Pathophysiology of activity limitation in patients with interstitial lung disease. *Chest* **109**: 1566–76.

Harris-Eze AO, Sridhar G, Clemems RE *et al.* (1996). Role of hypoxemia and pulmonary mechanics in exercise limitation in interstitial lung disease. *Am J Respir Crit Care Med* **154**: 994–1001.

Holland A, Hill C (2009). Physical training for interstitial lung disease. *Cochrane Database of Systematic Reviews* **4**: CD006322.

Holland AE, Hill CJ, Conron M *et al.* (2008). Short-term improvement in exercise capacity and symptoms following exercise training in interstitial lung disease. *Thorax* **63**: 549–54.

Lama VN, Flaherty KR, Toews GB *et al.* (2003). Prognostic value of desaturation during a 6-minute walk test in idiopathic interstitial pneumonia. *Am J Respir Crit Care Med* **168**: 1084–90.

Nishiyama O, Taniguchi H, Kondoh Y (2005). Quadriceps weakness is related to exercise capacity in idiopathic pulmonary fibrosis. *Chest* **127**: 2028–33.

O'Driscoll BR, Howard LS, Davison AG (2008). BTS guideline for emergency oxygen use in adult patients. *Thorax* **63**: vi1–68.

O'Neill S, McCarthy DS (1983). Postural relief of dyspnoea in severe chronic airflow limitation: relationship to respiratory muscle strength. *Thorax* **38**: 595–600.

Pryor JA, Prasad SA (eds). (2008a). *Physiotherapy for Respiratory and Cardiac Problems: Adults and Paediatrics*, 4th edn. Churchill Livingstone, Oxford, p. 228.

Pryor JA, Prasad SA (eds). (2008b). *Physiotherapy for Respiratory and Cardiac Problems: Adults and Paediatrics*, 4th edn. Churchill Livingstone, Oxford, pp. 155–9.

Ries AL, Bauldoff GS, Carlin BW *et al.* (2007). Pulmonary rehabilitation: joint ACCP/AACVPR evidence-based clinical practice guidelines. *Chest* **131**(Suppl. 5): 4–42.

Sharma OP (1999). Fatigue and sarcoidosis. *Eur Respir J* **13**: 713–14.

Spruit MA, Thomeer MJ, Gosselink R *et al.* (2005). Skeletal muscle weakness in patients with sarcoidosis and its relationship with exercise intolerance and reduced health status. *Thorax* **60**: 32–8.

Wells AU, Hirani N on behalf of the BTS Interstitial Lung Disease Guideline Group (2008). Interstitial lung disease guideline. *Thorax* **63**(Suppl. 5): v1–58.

46

Rehabilitation, long-term oxygen therapy and quality of life

MICHAEL I POLKEY AND LUCY PIGRAM

REHABILITATION

Rehabilitation as a therapy in lung disease

The most common lung disease in adults is chronic obstructive pulmonary disease (COPD; Jemal et al. 2005), and for this condition it is clearly established that pulmonary rehabilitation is effective in improving patient function – judged by performance on an exercise test, quality of life, and indeed in terms of unplanned hospital attendance (Griffiths et al. 2000; Troosters et al. 2000). The mechanism of improvement is unknown and, interestingly, is not confined to those with either good or poor pre-rehabilitation exercise performance (Singh et al. 2008). There is consensus, however, that the improvement is not achieved by alteration in lung function. It is most likely that improvements in peripheral muscle function are a key element of a successful rehabilitation program. Peripheral muscle weakness is common in COPD (Seymour et al. 2010), so this is a plausible hypothesis.

Components of a rehabilitation program

A typical rehabilitation program in COPD will comprise some 16 to 18 visits (typically 3 times a week for 6 weeks or twice weekly for 8 weeks) and will be supervised in hospital or an appropriate community facility. In different healthcare systems more extreme variations may be observed (Sewell et al. 2006; Pitta et al. 2008), and historically there have been fewer rehabilitation programs in the USA. Aside from the exercise component (see below), the program will be multidisciplinary and contain disease education and drug optimization, nutritional and psychological input. An important aspect of the rehabilitation program is its social component so that patients meet other people with similar conditions. Very frequently patients keep in touch after the program or may meet to do their own maintenance exercise.

The exercise program will include resistance exercise for the legs (e.g. weight lifts or pushes) combined with endurance exercise which may be in the form of cycling or walking. There is some evidence that a more intense program delivers greater benefit than a less intense program (Casaburi et al. 1991). Further details have been provided by Nici and associates (Nici et al. 2006).

Rehabilitation in sarcoidosis

As discussed in Chapter 32, peripheral muscle involvement in sarcoidosis is frequent, but there are no studies in which the frequency and extent of muscle weakness have been systematically evaluated, nor have there been any reported studies of pulmonary rehabilitation in the condition. A Cochrane review found only two studies in pulmonary fibrosis considered more generally (Holland and Hill 2008), and there has been one subsequent uncontrolled study published in the French language (Rammaert et al. 2009). Quadriceps weakness has been described in pulmonary fibrosis (Nishiyama et al. 2005).

Nishiyama and co-workers randomized 30 patients with idiopathic pulmonary fibrosis (IPF) to receive a 10-week program of pulmonary rehabilitation. Consistent with the COPD experience, there was no change in lung function but there was a mean improvement, compared with placebo, in the 6-minute walking distance of 46.3 m (95 percent confidence interval 8.3–84.4; $p < 0.05$; Nishiyama *et al.* 2008). Holland and co-workers randomized 57 patients to receive an 8-week program of rehabilitation or to a control group who received telephone support only (Holland *et al.* 2008). Four of the participants had granulomatous lung disease including sarcoid. A significant improvement in 6-minute walking distance (mean 35 m) was observed at 9 weeks, but this was entirely lost after 6 months.

The combined data are summarized in Fig. 46.1. Overall, as one might expect, PR is associated with a short-term improvement in exercise performance in lung fibrosis, which might reasonably also be expected in sarcoid. Studies are urgently warranted to confirm this. Because in general the progression of sarcoid is less aggressive than IPF, the benefits might be longer lasting, particularly if a maintenance program were also used subsequently – although this has not so far proved effective in COPD (Spencer *et al.* 2010).

Care should, of course, be taken to ensure patient safety. In sarcoidosis patients, evaluation of cardiac function and the integrity of the cardiac conduction system should be assured before beginning strenuous exercise.

LONG-TERM OXYGEN THERAPY

The case for domiciliary oxygen therapy in chronic obstructive pulmonary disease was conclusively shown by two studies. This therapy reduced mortality (NOTT 1980; Medical Research Council 1981). Based on these studies (and in the absence of specific studies in sarcoidosis), long-term oxygen

therapy is recommended in sarcoid patients when the resting Pao_2 is $\leq 7.3\,\text{kPa}$ on two occasions separated by a minimum of 3 weeks in the absence of a remediable cause, and is then prescribed for 16 hours a day. Policies with regard to ambulatory oxygen vary, but in the authors' institution the indications would be confined to patients with a demonstrable increase in performance on a field walking test (e.g. incremental shuttle walking distance) in association with oxygen desaturation when walking without supplemental oxygen.

Oxygen is commonly available in two supply types in the UK: compressed gas cylinders and concentrator. Concentrators are clearly the most appropriate source for home use. They work on the principle that free air is approximately 79 percent nitrogen and 21 percent oxygen. The concentrator works by removing the nitrogen from air by a molecular sieve, leaving the oxygen available. This sieving is achieved by compressing air and passing it through a 'zeolite tower' filled with aluminum silicate. Nitrogen is *adsorbed* onto these granules (a reversible reaction and not a chemical reaction). The resulting gas that flows out from the tower contains about 93 percent oxygen. As the zeolite tower becomes saturated with nitrogen (typically within a few seconds), the system switches to a second zeolite tower to maintain a constant flow of oxygen. At this point, the first tower is vented to atmosphere, and the adsorbed nitrogen is expelled. Thus all that is required are two towers that regularly switch from one to the other to keep up a steady flow of oxygen.

Compressed gas is available in a variety of sizes of cylinder for the patient to carry, but the limiting factors with this are (a) the ability of the patient to carry the cylinder, and (b) the flow rate required by the patient. For example, a standard E cylinder will last about 5 hours at a flow rate of 2 L/min.

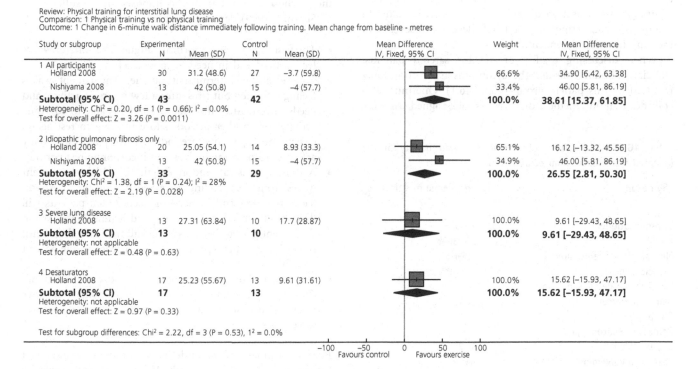

Figure 46.1   Meta-analysis of outcome judged by a 6-minute walk test immediately after a program of pulmonary rehabilitation. Reproduced with permission from Holland and Hill (2008).

A conserver device has recently become standard issue on ambulatory cylinders; this confines the patient's supply of oxygen to the inspiratory phase rather than a continuous flow, thus extending the usage.

Oxygen concentrators used not to be portable, but battery-powered devices weighing as little as 3 kg are now available and patients may choose to wheel or carry these. There are no data to support their use in sarcoidosis. Interestingly, even in patients with COPD, the data to support the postulate that oxygen significantly improves walking distance are controversial (Keilty et al. 1994; Roberts et al. 1996). The available data do suggest, however, that liquid oxygen is equally effective as a portable oxygen concentrator (Nasilowski et al. 2008).

QUALITY OF LIFE

As sarcoidosis is often a long-term disease, physicians aim to reduce its impact on the individual patient's quality of life (QoL) mainly through the intermittent use of corticosteroids.

Assessments

When reviewing a patient's quality of life it is important to take a detailed history of the symptoms that actually affect the person, as diagnostic tests used to detect physical decline do not always give the medical team a meaningful analysis of how the disease is affecting the patient. Typically, lung function tests (LFTs) may not decline but the patient will report feeling more breathless on exertion or not being able to complete tasks without stopping (Drent et al. 1999). Very commonly the sensation of fatigue is not directly related to angiotensin-converting enzyme (ACE) level or to severity of the lung function derangement.

When discussing quality of life for sarcoid patients, clinicians should consider the symptoms most commonly reported by this patient group (Table 46.1). One must also consider that any medical diagnostic tool designed will only

Table 46.1   Symptoms of sarcoid affecting quality of life (adapted from Aladesanmi et al. 2004).

Symptom	Prevalence in sufferers
Chronic fatigue	30%
Cough	20–30%
Neurological / depression	10%
Muscle aches	25–40%
Respiratory: decreased lung function	20–30%
Skin involvement	30%
Sleep apnea	30%
Palpable hepatomegaly	20%
Eye involvement	9–25%
Cardiac involvement	5%
Weight loss	30%
Fever	30%

give the examiner a score of ability and not a score of perceived ability – which sometimes do not coincide.

This mismatch impacts on the patient's quality of mental health and life in general. An example is the patient stating that he is able to walk only 100 m on the flat, whereas on a 6-minute walking test he is able to achieve 250 m without stopping. Victorson and associates give an interesting explanation for this phenomenon by arguing that the granulomatous inflammation process in sarcoid releases cytokines which may be responsible for the symptoms commonly complained of, such as fatigue, pain, weight loss and fever (Victorson et al. 2008). Even so, such a biological explanation cannot explain the straightforward disparity illustrated in the example above, suggesting that factors related to the *perceived* exertion in completing a 100 m task may color the patient's recollection. It should also be appreciated that both doctors and patients are poor at estimating distances in real life (Sharrack and Hughes 1997), so a complaint of an 'inability to walk 100 m' may be a more general assessment by the patient of their health.

Fatigue

Quality-of-life research in sarcoidosis has mainly concentrated on fatigue, as this symptom is known to have a negative effect on QoL scores.

Michielsen and associates demonstrated in their research comparing healthy controls with sarcoid sufferers that fatigue was the most frequently mentioned symptom and negatively affected the sarcoid group's QoL scores (Michielsen et al. 2006). This could be explained by the greater dependency in activities of daily living (ADLs) resulting from fatigue, and the psychosocial limitations this imposes on the sufferer.

Sharma (1999) describes four types of fatigue.

- The first type is early-morning fatigue. The sufferer wakes feeling tired and in need of more sleep.
- The second is intermittent fatigue. The patient wakes feeling refreshed but tires after a few hours of activity and needs to rest. After this rest he or she is able to continue activity for another period before needing to rest again. Often these patients are advised to plan their daily activities to pace themselves and incorporate rest periods.
- A third type is 'afternoon fatigue' in which the patient wakes from sleep feeling refreshed but by the afternoon feels exhausted and in need of sleep. Often patients will describe this tiredness as heavy and aching limbs. When the patient goes to bed he or she will then stay there until the morning. This type of fatigue clearly leaves the patient socially isolated.
- The fourth type is post-activity 'sarcoid chronic fatigue'. This occurs typically in 5 percent of patients who have otherwise diagnostically recovered from a period of active sarcoidosis.

Beyond treatment of the underlying condition, treatment of fatigue in sarcoidosis is difficult. There is probably a role for rehabilitation, but an innovative study reported that an amphetamine, dexmethylphenidate hydrochloride, improved fatigue scores though not walking distance (Lower *et al.* 2008). In our view, amphetamines are unlikely to be widely used in the UK for this purpose; but newer, and perhaps safer, vigilance-enhancing drugs such as modafanil may merit investigation as an adjunctive treatment for fatigue in sarcoidosis patients.

Gender comparisons

Sarcoidosis is believed to be marginally more common in women than men, although this has been shown to vary according to ethnicity.

When QoL scores were taken in a study by Drent and co-workers, it was found that female patients showed more emotional problems and encountered more sleep problems than males. The study also demonstrated that female suffers had more perceived problems with body care and movement (Drent *et al.* 1999). This and other studies found that both men and women reported being affected by the same issues, but men considered these to be less problematic to their quality of life. All participants, regardless of gender, were shown to be affected – physically by their fatigue, emotionally by the disease limiting their social interactions and hobbies, and psychologically by the impact on their inability to perform well at work and sleep disturbances.

A limitation of gender research performed to date is that the null hypothesis, of course, is that sarcoidosis behaves differently in male and female patients, thus accounting for the difference in complaints of symptoms between genders.

Pain

A number of patients will report pain as a symptom affecting their quality of life. Sarcoidosis patients frequently suffer from arthralgia (Michielsen *et al.* 2007). Less commonly reported, but still important to quality of life, are headaches, muscle aches and chest pain. Pain is important to consider as it will affect the patient's functioning and level of fatigue.

The SHQ

As result of studies mentioned earlier, a sarcoid health questionnaire (SHQ) has been devised (Cox *et al.* 2003). This is a short tool consisting of 29 questions covering three areas:

- daily functioning;
- physical functioning;
- emotional functioning.

A limitation of this tool is that fatigue argued earlier to be the single most important symptom related to QoL in sarcoid is represented in only one question. Rigorous research is warranted to confirm whether this tool is completely representative of the patient's quality of life.

CONCLUSION

Quality of life for sarcoidosis patients is dependent on symptom control. Owing to the nature of the disease – with its active and remission stages – quality of life can be variable. Psychological support for these patients should never be underestimated.

With the introduction of the SHQ, respiratory physicians have one tool by which to assess their patients' quality of life. With serial completion of the SHQ, physicians can obtain data to test a correlation between active phases and remission phases, and have a guide to individualized treatment strategies. However, research in the future needs to investigate the SHQ to check its reliability, and needs to continue to test novel pharmacological and non-pharmacological interventions.

REFERENCES

Aladesanmi OA (2004). Sarcoidosis: an update for the primary care physician. *Med Gen Med* 6: 7.

Casaburi R, Patessio A, Ioli F *et al.* (1991). Reductions in exercise lactic acidosis and ventilation as a result of exercise training in patients with obstructive lung disease. *Am Rev Respir Dis* 143: 9–18.

Cox CE, Donohue JF, Brown CD *et al.* (2003). The Sarcoidosis Health Questionnaire: a new measure of health-related quality of life. *Am J Respir Crit Care Med* 168: 323–9.

Drent M, Wirnsberger RM, de Vries J *et al.* (1999). Association of fatigue with an acute phase response in sarcoidosis. *Eur Respir J* 13: 718–22.

Griffiths TL, Burr ML, Campbell IA *et al.* (2000). Results at 1 year of outpatient multidisciplinary pulmonary rehabilitation: a randomised controlled trial. *Lancet* 355: 362–8.

Holland A, Hill C (2008). Physical training for interstitial lung disease. *Cochrane Database Systematic Review*, CD006322.

Holland AE, Hill CJ, Conron M *et al.* (2008). Short-term improvement in exercise capacity and symptoms following exercise training in interstitial lung disease. *Thorax* 63: 549–54.

Jemal A, Ward E, Hao Y *et al.* (2005). Trends in the leading causes of death in the United States, 1970–2002. *J Am Med Assoc* 294: 1255–9.

Keilty SE, Ponte J, Fleming TA *et al.* (1994). Effect of inspiratory pressure support on exercise tolerance and breathlessness in patients with severe stable chronic obstructive pulmonary disease. *Thorax* 49: 990–4.

Lower EE, Harman S, Baughman RP (2008). Double-blind, randomized trial of dexmethylphenidate hydrochloride for the treatment of sarcoidosis-associated fatigue. *Chest* 133: 1189–95.

Medical Research Council Working Party (1981). Long-term domicilliary oxygen therapy in chronic hypoxic cor pulmonale complicating chronic bronchitis and emphysema, *Lancet* i: 681–6.

Michielsen HJ, Drent M, Peros-Golubicic T *et al.* (2006). Fatigue is associated with quality of life in sarcoidosis patients. *Chest* 130: 989–94.

Michielsen HJ, Peros-Golubicic T, Drent M *et al.* (2007). Relationship between symptoms and quality of life in a sarcoidosis population. *Respiration* 74: 401–5.

Nasilowski J, Przybylowski T, Zielinski J *et al.* (2008). Comparing supplementary oxygen benefits from a portable oxygen concentrator and a liquid oxygen portable device during a walk test in

COPD patients on long-term oxygen therapy. *Respir Med* 102: 1021–5.

Nici L, Donner C, Wouters E *et al.* (2006). American Thoracic Society/European Respiratory Society statement on pulmonary rehabilitation. *Am J Respir Crit Care Med* 173: 1390–413.

Nishiyama O, Kondoh Y, Kimura T *et al.* (2008). Effects of pulmonary rehabilitation in patients with idiopathic pulmonary fibrosis. *Respirology* 13: 394–9.

Nishiyama O, Taniguchi H, Kondoh Y *et al.* (2005). Quadriceps weakness is related to exercise capacity in idiopathic pulmonary fibrosis. *Chest* 127: 2028–33.

NOTT (1980). Nocturnal Oxygen Therapy Trial Group: Continuous or nocturnal oxygen therapy in hypoxemic chronic obstructive lung disease. *Ann Intern Med* 93: 391–8.

Pitta F, Troosters T, Probst VS *et al.* (2008). Are patients with COPD more active after pulmonary rehabilitation? *Chest* 134: 273–80.

Rammaert B, Leroy S, Cavestri B *et al.* (2009). Home-based pulmonary rehabilitation in idiopathic pulmonary fibrosis. *Rev Mal Respir* 26: 275–82.

Roberts CM, Bell J, Wedzicha JA (1996). Comparison of the efficacy of a demand oxygen delivery system with continuous low flow oxygen in subjects with stable COPD and severe oxygen desaturation on walking. *Thorax* 51: 831–4.

Sewell L, Singh SJ, Williams JE *et al.* (2006). How long should outpatient pulmonary rehabilitation be? A randomised controlled trial of 4 weeks versus 7 weeks. *Thorax* 61: 767–71.

Seymour JM, Spruit MA, Hopkinson NS *et al.* (2010). The prevalence of quadriceps weakness in COPD and the relationship with disease severity. *Eur Respir J* 36: 81–8.

Sharma OP (1999). Fatigue and sarcoidosis. *Eur Respir J* 13: 713–14.

Sharrack B, Hughes RA (1997). Reliability of distance estimation by doctors and patients: cross sectional study. *Br Med J* 315: 1652–4.

Singh SJ, Jones PW, Evans R *et al.* (2008). Minimum clinically important improvement for the incremental shuttle walking test. *Thorax* 63: 775–7.

Spencer LM, Alison JA, McKeough ZJ (2010). Maintaining benefits following pulmonary rehabilitation: a randomised controlled trial. *Eur Respir J* 35: 571–7.

Troosters T, Gosselink R, Decramer M (2000). Short- and long-term effects of outpatient rehabilitation in patients with chronic obstructive pulmonary disease: a randomized trial. *Am J Med* 109: 207–12.

Victorson DE, Cella D, Judson MA (2008). Quality of life evaluation in sarcoidosis: current status and future directions. *Curr Opin Pulm Med* 14: 470–7.

47

Immunization and vaccination

BERNIE GRANEEK

INTRODUCTION

The immunological responses related to immunization are closely linked to those contributing to the pathology of sarcoidosis. Following vaccination the cellular responses to antigen presentation via MHC class I molecules depend on intact CD8+ cytotoxic T-lymphocytes. In addition, antigen presentation via MHC class II molecules stimulates CD4+ T-helper-1 lymphocytes, involved with cytotoxic and delayed hypersensitivity responses as well as granuloma formation, and CD4+ T-helper-2 lymphocytes, which support the humoral response involving B-lymphocytes, leading to antibody production. The amplification of regulatory T-cells in sarcoidosis, which control the proliferation of CD4+ and CD8+ lymphocytes, is unable to completely inhibit the secretion of factors involved with granuloma formation, but the associated T regulatory/memory disequilibrium is a possible mechanism for anergy in sarcoidosis, most commonly recognized as the absence of a response to the tuberculin skin test (Miyara et al. 2006). Given the shared immunological pathways, the impact of the disease on the ability of the host to react to foreign antigens, and the persisting questions regarding the contribution of infection to the etiology of the disease, it is worth exploring the relationship between immunization/vaccination and sarcoidosis.

DOES VACCINATION CONTRIBUTE TO DISEASE?

Following its first use in humans in 1921, the Bacillus Calmette-Guérin (BCG) vaccination did not become widespread until 1945. The universal vaccination program for adolescents in the UK was introduced in 1953; the possible therapeutic effect of immunization in sarcoidosis was considered at this time. During the 1950s there were isolated case reports of sarcoidosis occurring in BCG-vaccinated individuals. But the large Medical Research Council trial of BCG, which followed over 54000 participants for more than 10 years post-vaccination, showed no difference in the incidence of sarcoidosis between the vaccinated and non-vaccinated groups (Sutherland et al. 1965). It was concluded that BCG vaccination neither protected against nor promoted the disease.

Since then there have been several more case reports of sarcoidosis developing after BCG vaccination. These included cutaneous lesions subsequently diagnosed as juvenile sarcoidosis in a 2-year-old boy, which developed 5 months after the vaccination, and pulmonary lesions in an 11-year-old boy with associated lymphopenia. A T-helper cell alveolitis, thought to be sarcoidosis, has also been reported in a patient receiving BCG immunotherapy for a bladder tumor. It has been suggested that mycobacterial heat-shock proteins in both *Mycobacterium tuberculosis* and BCG could be involved in the development of autoimmunity favoring granuloma formation and sarcoidosis in genetically susceptible individuals. Alternatively, it is possible that in certain individuals exposure to mycobacteria, such as *M. bovis* in the BCG vaccination, provokes a strong granulomatous response, associated with effective elimination of the bacteria, continuing analogous to a hypersensitivity response.

Several studies have explored the association of sarcoidosis with hepatitis C, suggesting that sarcoidosis occurs more frequently in those receiving immunotherapy with interferon-α, with or without ribavirin, than those who are treatment-naive (Goldberg et al. 2006). It is believed that interferon-α increases CD4+ Th1 lymphocyte production of interferon-γ and interleukin-2, thereby increasing MHC class II expression, provoking further activation of CD4+ lymphocytes in excess of that which can be controlled by regulatory T-cells, resulting in granuloma formation. Concomitant treatment with ribavirin could enhance this effect by inhibiting Th2 production while preserving Th1 responses. Specific allergen immunotherapy has also been suggested as a factor promoting disease in one case series.

DOES ANERGY AFFECT THE RESPONSE TO VACCINATIONS?

Anergy in sarcoidosis is well recognized, and is most commonly associated with the apparent absence of sensitivity to tuberculoprotein. A negative tuberculin skin test has been shown to have a high sensitivity for the diagnosis of sarcoidosis in a population with a high prevalence of tuberculin sensitivity. Also the tuberculin skin test has a high specificity, but low sensitivity for identifying co-morbid tuberculosis in sarcoidosis patients in tuberculosis endemic regions.

Absence of immunity to other infectious diseases has also been reported in other cases of sarcoidosis. An 8-year-old girl with necrotizing sarcoid granulomatosis was shown to have a lack of specific antibodies to diphtheria toxoid despite previous vaccination. In a study of the response to hepatitis B (HBV) vaccination in 16 longstanding sarcoidosis patients with no evidence of a primary humoral immune deficiency, there was a complete absence of antibody response to a standard vaccination course compared with an 85.7 percent response rate among 35 age- and sex-matched controls (Mert *et al.* 2000). The humoral response to hepatitis B virus is a T-helper-1 mediated process. It has been suggested that T-cell and macrophage-dependent induction of B-cell immunoglobulin production might be defective in sarcoidosis, which might account for the lack of response to hepatitis B vaccination compared with other viruses that stimulate B-cell immunoglobulin production through an alternative pathway, such as Epstein–Barr virus, herpes simplex, rubella, measles and parainfluenza viruses. In this study almost half the original cohort of sarcoidosis patients were found to have natural immunity to hepatitis B, but it was not known if they had been exposed to the virus before or after development of sarcoidosis. Therefore, whether this absence of response to vaccination is related to a difference in the nature of antigen stimulation between the natural virus and the recombinant HBV vaccine has yet to be determined. While vaccine-unresponsive healthy subjects are seen, this seems to be an invariable finding in sarcoidosis.

The recognized alternative pathways for immunoglobulin production following exposure to different microorganisms, and the absence of seroconversion following recombinant hepatitis B vaccination, raise questions about the efficacy of other vaccination/immunization programs in sarcoidosis patients: whether, given an understanding of the immunological processes involved, their efficacy could be predicted, or whether the use of live vaccines could be problematic. In the UK, the recommendations of the Joint Committee on Vaccination and Immunisation (www.dh.gov.uk/ab/JCVI/) are that there is a risk of disseminated infection and associated serious complications from live vaccination in

those receiving high doses of corticosteroids systemically for more than a week, or lower doses over the longer term or in combination with other cytotoxic agents, or those with evidence of impaired cell-mediated immunity. This might include more complicated longstanding cases of sarcoidosis, depending on their treatment protocol.

There is a lack of data on the efficacy of other vaccinations in sarcoidosis patients. However, as the cellular interactions associated with the granulomatous process in sarcoidosis become better understood, the theoretical basis for hypotheses regarding the immunological mechanisms and outcome of vaccinations might also become apparent. CD1d-restricted natural killer T (NKT) cells recognize glycolipid antigens found in a wide range of pathogens, including *M. tuberculosis*, presented by CD1 antigen-presenting molecules. Activated NKT cells produce numerous cytokines, which influence the immune response; animal studies confirm their importance in protection against infection. The CD1d-restricted T-cells are also believed to have an immunoregulatory role in CD4+ T-helper-1 lymphocyte immune responses; they have been shown to be either absent or significantly deficient in sarcoidosis patients, which might contribute to granuloma formation as a disproportionate unregulated response (Ho *et al.* 2005), and might also hypothetically influence the response to vaccination with antigens that CD1 antigen-presenting molecules would recognize.

In-vitro studies have demonstrated significantly reduced proliferation of T-lymphocytes in sarcoidosis patients in response to several recall antigens. The reduced cellular and humoral immune response to recall antigen has also been demonstrated in normal subjects who failed to respond to hepatitis A vaccination. There was a direct correlation between antibody response, antigen-specific cytokine levels and the expression of the hepatitis A cellular receptor 1 (HAVcr-1) on CD4+ lymphocytes, associated with immunomodulatory properties (Garner-Spitzer *et al.* 2009). These data suggest that impaired lymphocyte function might have a negative impact on the effective immunological response to vaccination.

While the efficacy of vaccinations in sarcoidosis is for the most part unknown, this should not prevent vaccination programs for certain infections, such as pneumococcal pneumonia or influenza, as they would be recommended for those with chronic respiratory conditions or those with immunodeficiency due to disease or treatment. Deficient antibody production following polyvalent pneumococcal polysaccharide vaccination has been identified in HIV-positive patients. In one study the lack of antibody response was associated with low total CD4+ cell counts; in another study there was no correlation between CD4+ cell count and level of antibody response. These results conflict with another study examining the antibody response to influenza, tetanus and pneumococcal vaccines in HIV patients compared with healthy controls. Normal antipneumococcal antibody responses were demonstrated in the HIV patients, but vaccination with tetravalent influenza vaccine and tetanus toxoid provoked significantly reduced antibody responses, which were correlated with the CD4+ cell count. It was suggested that the difference in humoral response was related to whether it was T-lymphocyte dependent (influenza and tetanus) or independent (pneumococcal). Other studies of influenza vaccination in HIV patients have shown generally poorer humoral responses compared with healthy control subjects, but this was thought to be related to the types of antigen used and not the CD4+ cell count. Antibody responses to pneumococcal vaccination have been shown to be satisfactory in kidney transplant patients, as have responses to influenza vaccination. However, there are conflicting results between studies of influenza vaccine efficacy in patients with end-stage renal failure; patients on hemodialysis have a lower antibody response than patients on peritoneal dialysis, possibly due to reduced production of interleukin-2 and interferon-γ in the former group, with resultant reduction in CD4+ cell proliferation. Overall response rates following influenza vaccination in patients with malignant disease are satisfactory; some studies show better results when vaccination is given more than a month after chemotherapy is discontinued, whereas other studies show no difference in the immune response between patients undergoing chemotherapy and healthy controls (Brydak and Machala 2000).

In a study comparing intradermal and intramuscular influenza vaccination in groups of healthy control subjects and immunocompromised patients, which included subjects receiving treatment with antitumor necrosis factor, HIV-positive subjects and stem-cell transplantation patients, there was no difference in humoral response associated with the route of vaccine administration, but significantly better responses in healthy control subjects than immunocompromised patients (Gelinck et al. 2009).

CAN VACCINATION TREAT SARCOIDOSIS?

There is strong support for the view that T-cell receptor AV2S3+ CD4+ lymphocytes, found in increased numbers in bronchoalveolar lavage fluid of HLA-DRB1*0301 and HLA-DRB3*0101 patients with sarcoidosis, preferentially recognize and proliferate in response to a sarcoidosis-specific antigen (Grunewald and Eklund 2007). The specificity of these cells in sarcoidosis has yet to be established, but *M. tuberculosis* extracts have been shown to preferentially stimulate peripheral blood AV2S3+ CD4+ T cells of healthy HLA-DRB1*0301-positive subjects. Whether the identification of a specific antigen facilitates the development of targeted immunotherapy remains to be seen. To date there are only a few studies exploring immunization or the use of immunoglobulin in the treatment of active disease.

Past claims have been made for positive outcomes in patients treated with old tuberculin, blood from highly tuberculin-sensitive donors, and BCG vaccination. However, no appropriately controlled studies were undertaken, and, given the duration of treatment, the probability of natural

resolution could not be excluded. This work has not been repeated.

A number of case reports have described the successful treatment of severe thrombocytopenia in sarcoidosis with human immunoglobulin. Platelet-associated IgG antibodies were present, and the patients had failed to respond to high-dose corticosteroids prior to the introduction of immunoglobulin treatment, used in isolation in one patient, and in combination with vincristine in a second (Larner et al. 1990). It has been suggested that the immunoglobulin competes with IgG-coated platelets for clearing at the reticuloendothelial system.

Intravenous human immunoglobulin has also been used in the treatment of vasculitic peripheral neuropathy associated with a number of diseases, including one case of sarcoidosis. While there was improvement or complete resolution in 80 percent of the study group this did not include the patient with sarcoidosis.

The many unanswered questions regarding the immunopathogenesis of sarcoidosis, the immunological paradoxes, and the limited understanding of their impact on vaccination responses, suggest that perhaps this is an area where further investigation could assist our knowledge of this intriguing disease.

REFERENCES

Brydak LB, Machala M (2000). Humoral immune response to influenza vaccination in patients from high risk groups. *Drugs* 60: 35–53.

Garner-Spitzer E, Kundi M, Rendi-Wagner P et al. (2009). Correlation between humoral and cellular immune responses and the expression of the hepatitis A receptor HAVcr-1 on T-cells after hepatitis A revaccination in high- and low-responder vaccinees. *Vaccine* 27: 197–204.

Gelinck LB, van den Bemt BJ, Marijt WA et al. (2009). Intradermal influenza vaccination in immunocompromised patients is immunogenic and feasible. *Vaccine* 27: 2469–74.

Goldberg HJ, Fiedler D, Webb A et al. (2006). Sarcoidosis after treatment with interferon-α: a case series and review of the literature. *Respir Med* 100: 2063–8.

Grunewald J, Eklund A (2007). Role of CD4+ T-cells in sarcoidosis. *Proc Am Thorac Soc* 4: 461–4.

Ho LP, Urban BC, Thickett DR et al. (2005). Deficiency of a subset of T-cells with immunoregulatory properties in sarcoidosis. *Lancet* 365: 1062–72.

Larner AJ, Dollery CT, Cox TM et al. (1990). Life-threatening thrombocytopenia in sarcoidosis: response to vincristine, human immunoglobulin, and corticosteroids. *Br Med J* 300: 317–19.

Mert A, Bilir M, Ozara R et al. (2000). Results of hepatitis B vaccination in sarcoidosis. *Respiration* 67: 543–5.

Miyara M, Amoura Z, Parizot C et al. (2006). The immune paradox of sarcoidosis and regulatory T-cells. *J Exper Med* 203: 359–70.

Sutherland I, Mitchell DN, D'Arcy Hart P (1965). Incidence of intrathoracic sarcoidosis among young adults participating in a trial of tuberculosis vaccines. *Br Med J* 2: 497–503.

48

Future research into etiology, diagnosis, investigations and management

DONALD MITCHELL, ATHOL WELLS AND STEPHEN SPIRO

INTRODUCTION

Although a great many research questions remain unanswered, the key issues for several decades have been the lack of a robust etiologic model in sarcoidosis and lack of a validated investigation and management algorithm for pulmonary sarcoidosis, which remains the most prevalent form of major organ involvement. Better understanding of the etiology would cast light on many other aspects of pathogenesis. Similarly, more accurate staging of pulmonary disease and the development of more effective treatments would have immediate relevance to the investigation and management of other less prevalent patterns of major organ involvement.

ETIOLOGY

A better understanding of the etiology of sarcoidosis is likely to depend on the continued use of proteonomic methodology in order to identify unique proteins, in sarcoid tissue and Kveim reagent, which may be acting as antigens in sarcoidosis. In this regard, the development and validation of an in-vitro 'Kveim' reaction may prove to be fruitful (see Chapter 16). Given a high level of selectivity and specificity for sarcoidosis, the identification of the antigen or antigens that selectively incite granulomatous responses may greatly facilitate understanding of the etiology and pathogenesis of the disease. It has long been apparent that some carefully validated suspensions may induce granulomatous responses in some patients with conditions other than sarcoidosis, thus displaying a 'relative selectivity' among other granulomatous and non-granulomatous disorders. It can be hoped that

in-vitro testing will disclose further information regarding the possibility that the Kveim reaction detects a discrete form of reactivity, rather than a specific infective agent. This hypothesis is entirely compatible with current data, including the reactivity of sarcoidosis patients all over the world to a suspension from a single source and the indirect evidence for a number of different inciting infective agents.

A similar model of pathogenesis has provided key insights in celiac disease, which was found to have a higher prevalence among patients with sarcoidosis in studies performed by Rutherford and colleagues (2004), who accordingly advised routine screening of their sarcoidosis population for this disorder. However, although Papadopoulos and co-workers had shown gastric autoimmunity and gluten-associated immune reactivity in some 40 percent of patients with sarcoidosis, the frequency of pernicious anemia or of celiac disease was not found to be greater than in a control population (Papadopoulos et al. 1996). The immune characteristics of celiac disease may also be linked to an increased risk of sarcoidosis (Ludvigsson et al. 2007). It is relevant to note that Dr Janet Marks working with Dr Alex Watson and Dr Sam Shuster discovered in 1966 the celiac syndrome of dermatitis herpetiformis for which she was accorded the Parkes–Webber and Archibald Gray medals.

The advent of an internationally validated in-vitro Kveim test will enable large numbers of patients to be tested, thus enhancing further epidemiological studies. The suggestion that stratification of data by clinical phenotypes may discover genetic associations that analysis of disease susceptibility alone would fail to detect was mooted by Spagnolo and associates in a report of environmental triggers and susceptibility factors in idiopathic granulomatous diseases (Spagnolo et al. 2008). An in-vitro Kveim test study of sarcoidosis patients and apparently healthy matched controls with an evaluation of findings against conventional clinical criteria may provide crucial pathogenetic insights.

In-vitro Kveim investigations may also include patients presenting with orofacial granulomatosis (Melkesson–Rosenthal syndrome; Grave *et al.* 2009). It may also be of interest to include patients presenting with idiopathic pulmonary fibrosis and non-specific interstitial pneumonia as there is occasional evidence of an 'overlap' between these disorders and sarcoidosis in some patients (Maher *et al.* 2009). The overall findings of the above investigations may complement those of the ACCESS Research Group (Rybicki *et al.* 2001). Furthermore, since a high proportion of human cancer tumors contain elevated levels of the tolomerase enzyme (Cooper 2009), it may be informative to explore the measurement of this enzyme in lymph node tissues removed from sarcoidosis patients for diagnostic purposes.

The results of in-vivo Kveim tests among patients with active sarcoidosis have shown, across the world, granulomatous responses in only some 62 percent of those tested. The large proportion of non-granulomatous responses has been attributed to the form of presentation of sarcoidosis and/or the duration of disease, but the importance of the genetic determination of the granulomatous response remains uncertain. Thus, it would be of interest to examine in-vitro Kveim testing among patients with active sarcoidosis in genetic subgroups, irrespective of the form or presentation of disease.

DIAGNOSIS

With the advent of high-resolution computerized tomography (HRCT) and the undoubted diagnostic utility it provides in many difficult cases, a reappraisal of the diagnostic algorithm for pulmonary sarcoidosis is long overdue. The inflexible statement that a histological diagnosis is mandatory, except in a small minority of patients with absolutely typical clinical features, is no longer acceptable. In the modern era, patient views should be sought when the diagnosis is highly probable and a decision needs to be made on more invasive investigation. Patients will often choose to decline a biopsy, deciding instead to remain under observation with a view to further investigation if the subsequent course of disease suggests diagnostic concerns. When these views are strongly held, the clinician must expect to support the views of the patient but also has a responsibility to indicate when this approach is imprudent. However, the exact diagnostic accuracy of non-invasive approaches has not been properly evaluated in the HRCT era.

In this context, there is an urgent need to apply studies in which specific combinations of clinical, bronchoalveolar lavage (BAL) and HRCT appearances are examined against histological findings, and to extend these studies to the long-term evaluation of the accuracy of non-invasive diagnostic algorithms, both in terms of their accuracy and their 'safety' in the avoidance of adverse outcomes due to misdiagnosis.

In this regard, the prevailing difficulty is the failure to integrate clinical, BAL, HRCT and other non-invasive data in current diagnostic studies. In part, this problem reflects the fact that centers differ radically in their use of these tests, with HRCT viewed as a pivotal test by some, but distrusted in other units, in which there is a continuation of the historical emphasis on bronchoscopic diagnostic techniques. The hostility towards the diagnostic use of HRCT, articulated by some experts, probably largely reflects the contrasting uses made of HRCT and bronchoscopic techniques in current diagnostic algorithms. As is usually the case in clinical practice, views tend to be held more strongly when not informed by robust clinical data. For example, it remains unclear whether bronchoscopic evaluation is always diagnostically useful when HRCT appearances are typical, and whether a diagnostic surgical lung biopsy is really warranted when the pre-biopsy likelihood of a diagnosis of sarcoidosis exceeds 90 percent. Without these studies, the value added by more advanced bronchoscopic sampling techniques is difficult to quantify.

INVESTIGATIONS TO STAGE AND MONITOR SARCOIDOSIS

Given that no uniform treatment protocol can be applied to all patients with sarcoidosis, and that observation without treatment is often appropriate, the identification of disease at higher risk of progression is central to accurate management. It should be stressed that this problem is equally important in pulmonary and extrapulmonary disease but is most easily studied in pulmonary disease, the most prevalent form of major organ involvement.

The need to stage activity in sarcoidosis has been highlighted for several decades, but use of the term 'disease activity' has hindered a logical appraisal of the problem. In pulmonary sarcoidosis, the most dangerous form of the disease consists of ongoing progression from inflammation to fibrosis, leading to disability and death in some cases; parallel pathways are evident also in cardiac sarcoidosis and other major systemic forms of disease. This pattern of disease evolution contrasts sharply with a larger patient subset in which there is prominent inflammation, with little or no progression to fibrotic disease and eventual regression of disease activity. It appears intuitively unlikely that these sharply contrasting patterns of disease can usefully be unified in pathogenetic models and studies of 'disease activity'. Pathogenetic considerations aside, the latter subset of patients tend to be identified by a short trial of oral prednisolone, which often serves to demonstrate the reversibility of disease and the absence of major residual fibrotic change. By contrast, a short-term trial of treatment will not identify the form of disease activity that results in ongoing progressive fibrosis. In many cases of longer duration, there has already been considerable progression to fibrotic disease and ongoing inflammation is more difficult to detect using current tests.

This crucial distinction has not been addressed in studies of 'disease activity', in which indices of inflammation and specific mediators have been sought across the whole spectrum of sarcoidosis. The primary need is not for the identification of inflammation or 'activity' per se, but for a biomarker that is linked to future progression from inflammatory to fibrotic disease. Ideally, such a biomarker might be used to refine the selection of treatments used to prevent disease progression in the longer term, with efficacious agents shown to reduce biomarker levels in the shorter term. However, even if this utopian goal is not met, the more accurate identification of progressive fibrotic disease would have incalculable benefits in both routine management and the selection of patients for treatment trials. Preliminary work using positron emission tomography (PET) in fibrotic pulmonary disease appears promising, but the ideal biomarker needs to be more immediately available and readily repeatable than is the case with complex imaging techniques. One possible approach is to use HRCT appearances to identify unequivocally irreversible disease and to explore biomarkers selectively in that patient subset, before examining their utility more widely in sarcoidosis in general. However, that approach does require confrontation of the inexplicable hostility towards HRCT evaluation that has been evident in statements made by some authorities in recent years.

A further consideration, highlighted in recent treatment studies in interstitial lung disease (both in sarcoidosis and in non-granulomatous fibrosing disease), has been the lack of a single validated end-point for pulmonary disease progression. In sarcoidosis, it is widely accepted that chest radiographic and spirometric monitoring are the cornerstone of routine monitoring, but there has been a paucity of studies to validate this view. The lack of studies evaluating the quantification of change on chest radiography and its clinical utility is particularly surprising, although this deficiency is now beginning to be addressed. In reality, monitoring of this sort probably meets the needs of the majority of patients, but not all cases. In particular, pulmonary hypertension (PH) develops in an important patient subset. Despite a low prevalence in unselected sarcoidosis patients, PH is confirmed during right heart study in up to 50 percent of sarcoidosis patients with chronic exercise intolerance. The earlier detection of this complication would require the monitoring of non-invasive markers of pulmonary vascular disease. However, no consensus exists on the importance of gas transfer monitoring in established pulmonary disease and further clinical research in this area is needed.

The identification of best end-points in the evaluation of disease progression in extrapulmonary disease is equally important. The principles discussed above can be applied equally to all major forms of organ involvement, as discussed in a number of other chapters. The lack of a validated tool to monitor extrapulmonary sarcoidiosis was highlighted in a recent study of infliximab therapy in extrapulmonary disease: this required the ad-hoc construction of a non-validated staging system (Judson *et al.* 2003). In cardiac sarcoidosis, for example, it is increasingly clear that MRI scanning is a very sensitive tool in the identification of active inflammation. However, neither the use of MRI scanning to identify patients at higher risk of progression to cardiac fibrosis nor the best use of MRI to monitor cardiac disease have been explored definitively. It can be argued that the more urgent research need is not the identification of more sensitive means of detecting inflammation but, rather, the focused evaluation of current techniques in the correct patient subsets, in prognostic evaluation and monitoring.

TREATMENTS

The three key issues that need to be addressed in future research studies apply equally to pulmonary and extrapulmonary disease.

First, there is an ongoing need for more effective therapies to suppress dangerous inflammation in major organs, in the minority of patients who do not respond to conventional treatment. New agents that show promise include anti-TNF therapies, with most data relating to the use of infliximab, and there is ongoing interest in rituximab, based on encouraging results in other difficult inflammatory diseases. New immunosuppressive agents such as mycophenolate mofetil, that have provided added benefits in other inflammatory diseases, need to be tested in sarcoidosis. However, equally important is the examination of combinations of current agents, including combinations of immunomodulatory therapies. Hydroxychloroquine has been empirically combined with more potent immunosuppressive drugs for several decades and the anecdotally reported benefits need to be evaluated more formally. Anecdotal reports of increased efficacy when methotrexate is combined with low-dose azathioprine should also be taken further.

The second key goal in future research is to develop a more flexible treatment algorithm that can be better adapted to the heterogeneous nature of sarcoidosis, in both pulmonary and extrapulmonary disease. The era of treating all patients with sarcoidosis has now passed. However, most clinicians continue to use a single 'approved' treatment protocol in all patients needing treatment, starting with high-dose corticosteroid therapy and weaning to intermediate-dose maintenance therapy, with or without a second-line agent. This approach tends to meet the needs of the minority of patients with dangerous disease. However, a larger patient subgroup have need of treatment because there is an unacceptable loss of quality of life, without significant involvement of major organs. In many cases, low-dose treatment suffices and higher dose therapy merely results in a net loss of quality of life due to drug side-effects. Flexible treatment approaches, in which the patient titrates the level of therapy against changes in quality of life, need to be validated in clinical studies. This problem was highlighted in a recent study of infliximab in extrapulmonary disease, in which serious organ involvement (e.g. cardiac disease) was amalgamated with clinically insignificant disease such as lymphadenopathy. This non-discriminatory approach, although perhaps necessary in explorations of novel treatment effects, is unhelpful in routine practice.

Finally, there is an ongoing need to confront the two-dimensional nihilistic conclusion that there is no evidence that treatment influences the natural history of fibrotic sarcoidosis – an approach that has sometimes been used to justify non-intervention as disease progresses to end-stage fibrosis. It is perfectly obvious that, in some patients, failure to treat is associated with inexorable progression which is halted by therapy. In many cases it is eventually possible to withdraw therapy without relapse, with a higher level of organ function than would otherwise have been the case. It can certainly be argued that, in these cases, there is no evidence that treatment has shortened the duration of active disease. However, it is equally clear that, in these patients, treatment protects against ongoing damage during a high-risk period (whether or not that period is shortened by therapy); and in that sense, the 'natural consequences' of disease have indeed been radically altered for the better. The skill lies in choosing the right patients in whom to institute this approach.

CONCLUSION

Nihilism must be confronted and, to that end, longer term studies of the use of therapy to prevent ongoing damage to major organs need to be constructed. Unless this happens, some physicians will continue to cite a group of studies in which sarcoidosis was not 'cured' by 6–12 months of therapy – the basis of the view that therapy offers little in the longer term. To understand the intellectual poverty of this view, one need only consider how it would be received by rheumatologists in the treatment of systemic lupus erythematosus. However, a skeptical approach that is long held can, in the end, only be influenced by robust data. To design longer term treatment studies in the right patient

subgroups with the correct end-points represents a major challenge, but it is a challenge that needs to be overcome.

REFERENCES

Cooper J (2009). Elevated levels of telomerase enzyme in human cancer tumors. *Br Med J* 339: b4120.

Grave B, McCullough M, Wiesenfeld D (2009). Orofacial granulomatosis: a 20-year review. *Oral Dis* 1: 46–51.

Judson MA, Braughman RP, Thompson BW, Teirstein AS *et al.* (2003). Two-year prognosis in sarcoidosis: The ACCESS experience. *Sarcoid Vase Diff Lung Dis* 20(3): 204–11.

Ludvigsson JF, Wahlstrom J, Grunewald J *et al.* (2007). Coeliac disease and risk of sarcoidosis. *Sarcoid Vasc Diff Lung Dis* 24: 121–6.

Maher TM, Wells AU (2009). Lost in translation: From animal models of pulmonary fibrosis to human disease. *Respirology* 14(7): 915–6.

Papadopoulos KI, Hornblad Y, Liljebladh H, Hallengrem B (2006). High frequency of endocrine autoimmunity in patients with sarcoidosis. *Eur J Endocrin* 134: 331–6.

Rutherford RM, Brutsche MH, Kearns M *et al.* (2004). HLA-DR2 predicts susceptibility and disease chronicity in Irish sarcoidosis patients. *Sarcoid Vase Diff Lung Dis* 3: 191–8.

Rybicki BA, Iannuzi MC, Frederick MM *et al.* (2001). Familial aggregation of sarcoidosis: a case–control etiological study of sarcoidosis (ACCESS). *Am J Respir Crit Care Med* 164: 2085–91.

Spagnolo P, Richeldi L, du Bois RM (2008). Environmental triggers and susceptibility factors in idiopathic granulomatous diseases. *Semin Respir Crit Care Med* 6: 610–19.

Index

Printed in the United States
by Baker & Taylor Publisher Services